Hands-On Ablation:
The Experts' Approach

Hands-On Ablation:
The Experts' Approach

EDITORS

Amin Al-Ahmad MD, FACC, FHRS
Stanford University, Stanford, California

David J. Callans MD
University of Pennsylvania, Philadelphia, Pennsylvania

Henry H. Hsia MD, FACC, FHRS
Stanford University, Stanford, California

Andrea Natale MD, FACC, FHRS, FESC
Texas Cardiac Arrhythmia Institute at St. David's Medical Center, Austin, Texas

Oscar Oseroff MD, FHRS
Bazterrica Clinic, Buenos Aires, Argentina

Paul J. Wang MD, FACC, FHRS
Stanford University, Stanford, California

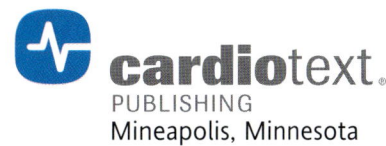

cardiotext
PUBLISHING
Mineapolis, Minnesota

© 2013 Amin Al-Ahmad, David J. Callans, Henry H. Hsia, Andrea Natale, Oscar Oseroff, Paul J. Wang

Cardiotext Publishing, LLC
3405 W. 44th Street
Minneapolis, Minnesota 55410
USA

www.cardiotextpublishing.com

Any updates to this book may be found at: www.cardiotextpublishing.com/titles/detail/9781935395249

Comments, inquiries, and requests for bulk sales can be directed to the publisher at: info@cardiotextpublishing.com.

All rights reserved. No part of this book may be reproduced in any form or by any means without the prior permission of the publisher.

All trademarks, service marks, and trade names used herein are the property of their respective owners and are used only to identify the products or services of those owners.

This book is intended for educational purposes and to further general scientific and medical knowledge, research, and understanding of the conditions and associated treatments discussed herein. This book is not intended to serve as and should not be relied upon as recommending or promoting any specific diagnosis or method of treatment for a particular condition or a particular patient. It is the reader's responsibility to determine the proper steps for diagnosis and the proper course of treatment for any condition or patient, including suitable and appropriate tests, medications, or medical devices to be used for or in conjunction with any diagnosis or treatment.

Due to ongoing research, discoveries, modifications to medicines, equipment and devices, and changes in government regulations, the information contained in this book may not reflect the latest standards, developments, guidelines, regulations, products, or devices in the field. Readers are responsible for keeping up to date with the latest developments and are urged to review the latest instructions and warnings for any medicine, equipment, or medical device. Readers should consult with a specialist or contact the vendor of any medicine or medical device where appropriate.

Except for the publisher's website associated with this work, the publisher is not affiliated with and does not sponsor or endorse any websites, organizations, or other sources of information referred to herein.

The publisher and the authors specifically disclaim any damage, liability, or loss incurred, directly or indirectly, from the use or application of any of the contents of this book.

Unless otherwise stated, all figures and tables in this book are used courtesy of the authors.

Library of Congress Control Number: 2012949102

ISBN: 978-1-935395-24-9

Printed in the United States of America

CONTENTS

Contributors．．．xi

Foreword．．．xix

Preface．．．xxi

Abbreviations．．xxiii

SECTION I: Ablation of Supraventricular Tachycardia．．．．．．．．．．．．．．．．．．．．．．1

Chapter 1: How to Rapidly Diagnose Supraventricular Tachycardia (SVT)
in the Electrophysiology Lab．．3
Luis F. Couchonnal, Bradley P. Knight

Chapter 2: How to Ablate Typical and Reverse Atrial Flutter．．．11
John C. Evans, Donald D. Hoang, Mintu P. Turakhia

Chapter 3: How to Ablate Atrial Flutter Postsurgery．．．23
George F. Van Hare

Chapter 4: The Ablation of Atrial Tachycardia．．33
Patrick M. Heck, Peter M. Kistler, Andrew W. Teh, Jonathan M. Kalman

Chapter 5: How to Ablate Atrial Tachycardias in Patients with Congenital Heart Disease．．．．．．．．．．．．．39
John K. Triedman

Chapter 6: How to Perform Radiofrequency and Cryoablation Ablation
for AV Nodal Reentrant Tachycardia．．．51
Paul J. Wang, Zhongwei Cheng

Chapter 7: Ablation of Left-Lateral Accessory Pathways．．59
Abram Mozes, Mark S. Link, Ann C. Garlitski, Jonathan Weinstock, Munther Homoud, N. A. Mark Estes III

Chapter 8: Catheter Ablation of Accessory Pathways．．．64
Hiroshi Nakagawa, Warren M. Jackman

Chapter 9: Right-Sided Accessory Pathways 72
Anne M. Dubin

Chapter 10: How to Diagnose, Map, and Ablate AVRT Due to Atriofascicular Conduction Fibers 81
Melvin M. Scheinman, David S. Kwon

Chapter 11: How to Ablate Accessory Pathways in Patients with Ebstein's Syndrome 85
Christina Y. Miyake

SECTION II: Ablation of Atrial Fibrillation 95

Chapter 12: How to Perform a Transseptal Puncture... 97
Gregory E. Supple, David J. Callans

Chapter 13: How to Utilize ICE for Optimal Safety and Efficacy with AF Ablation................. 107
Mathew D. Hutchinson

Chapter 14: How to Perform Pulmonary Vein Antrum Isolation for
Atrial Fibrillation 120
Marco V. Perez, Amin Al-Ahmad, Andrea Natale

Chapter 15: How to Perform Circumferential Ablation for Atrial Fibrillation 129
Carlo Pappone, Vincenzo Santinelli

Chapter 16: How to Perform Ablation of Atrial Fibrillation by Targeting Complex
Fractionated Atrial Electrograms 139
Koonlawee Nademanee, Montawatt Amnueypol

Chapter 17: How to Ablate Long-Standing Persistent Atrial Fibrillation
Using a Stepwise Approach (The Bordeaux Approach).............................. 147
Daniel Scherr, Michala Pedersen, Ashok J. Shah, Sébastien Knecht, Pierre Jaïs

Chapter 18: How to Ablate Long-Standing Persistent Atrial Fibrillation
Using a Stepwise Approach (The Natale Approach)................................. 159
Luigi Di Biase, Pasquale Santangeli, Andrea Natale

Chapter 19: How to Use Balloon Cryoablation for Ablation of Atrial Fibrillation 167
Pipin Kojodjojo, D. Wyn Davies

Chapter 20: How to Perform Pulmonary Vein Isolation Using Laser Catheter Ablation 175
Edward P. Gerstenfeld

Chapter 21: The Combined Surgical/Endocardial Ablation Procedure for Atrial Fibrillation........... 182
Rodney P. Horton, Luigi Di Biase, Andrew T. Hume, James R. Edgerton,
Javier E. Sánchez, Andrea Natale

Chapter 22: How to Perform a Hybrid Surgical Epicardial and Catheter Endocardial Ablation
for Atrial Fibrillation 189
Srijoy Mahapatra, Gorav Ailawadi

Chapter 23: How to Ablate the Vein of Marshall... 202
Seongwook Han, Peng-Sheng Chen, Chun Hwang

Chapter 24: Diagnosis and Ablation of Atrial Tachycardias Arising in the Context of
Atrial Fibrillation Ablation... 210
Amir S. Jadidi, Ashok J. Shah, Mélèze Hocini, Michel Haïssaguerre, Pierre Jaïs

Chapter 25: How to Perform 3-Dimensional Entrainment Mapping to Treat Post–AF
Ablation Atrial Tachycardia/AFL... 220
Philipp Sommer, Christopher Piorkowski, Gerhard Hindricks

Chapter 26: Catheter Ablation of Autonomic Ganglionated Plexi in Patients with
Atrial Fibrillation 227
Hiroshi Nakagawa, Benjamin J. Scherlag, Warren M. Jackman

Chapter 27: How to Use Electroanatomic Mapping to Rapidly Diagnose and Treat
Post–AF Ablation Atrial Tachycardia and Flutter 234
Aman Chugh

Chapter 28: How to Utilize Frequency Analysis to Aid in Atrial Fibrillation Ablation................. 248
Yenn-Jiang Lin, Li-Wei Lo, Shih-Ann Chen

Chapter 29: Utilization of the Hansen Robotic Catheter Navigation System:
The Austin Approach... 259
G. Joseph Gallinghouse, Luigi Di Biase, Andrea Natale

Chapter 30: How to Perform Atrial Fibrillation Ablation Using Remote Magnetic Navigation 267
J. David Burkhardt, Matthew Dare, Luigi Di Biase, Pasquale Santangeli, Andrea Natale

Chapter 31: How to Perform Accurate Image Registration with
Electroanatomic Mapping Systems 275
Francesco Perna, Moussa Mansour

Section III: Ablation of Ventricular Tachycardia........................ 281

Chapter 32: How to Localize Ventricular Tachycardia Using a 12-Lead ECG 283
Hicham El Masry, John M. Miller

Chapter 33: How to Diagnose and Ablate Ventricular Tachycardia from
the Outflow Tract and Aortic Cusps... 292
Takumi Yamada, G. Neal Kay

Chapter 34: How to Diagnose and Ablate
Fascicular Ventricular Tachycardia 302
Frederick T. Han, Nitish Badhwar

Chapter 35: How to Map and Ablate Hemodynamically Tolerated Ventricular Tachycardias............ 313
Kojiro Tanimoto, Henry H. Hsia

Chapter 36: How to Map and Ablate Unstable Ventricular Tachycardia:
The University of Pennsylvania Approach 331
Wendy S. Tzou, Francis E. Marchlinski

Chapter 37: How to Map and Ablate Unstable Ventricular Tachycardia:
The Brigham Approach 341
Usha B. Tedrow, William G. Stevenson

Chapter 38: How to Map and Ablate Ventricular Tachycardia Using Delayed Potential
in Sinus Rhythm.. 350
Eduardo Castellanos, Jesús Almendral, Carlos De Diego

Chapter 39: How to Utilize Electroanatomical Mapping to Identify Critical Channels for
Ventricular Tachycardia Ablation 360
Henry H. Hsia, Kojiro Tanimoto

Chapter 40: How to Use Noncontact Mapping for Catheter Ablation of Ventricular Tachycardia 373
Jason T. Jacobson

Chapter 41: How to Use ICE to Aid in Catheter Ablation of Ventricular Tachycardia 385
Marc W. Deyell, Mathew D. Hutchinson, David J. Callans

Chapter 42: How to Perform an Epicardial Access 399
Mauricio I. Scanavacca, Sissy Lara Melo, Carina A. Hardy, Cristiano Pisani, Eduardo Sosa

Chapter 43: Transcoronary Ethanol Ablation for Ventricular Tachycardia. 407
Karin K. M. Chia, Paul C. Zei

Chapter 44: How to Perform Epicardial Ablation in Postcardiac Surgery Patients 414
Sheldon M. Singh, James O. Coffey, Andre d'Avila

Chapter 45: How to Perform Endocardial/Epicardial Ventricular Tachycardia Ablation. 419
J. David Burkhardt, Luigi Di Biase, Matthew Dare, Pasquale Santangeli, Andrea Natale

Chapter 46: How to Ablate Ventricular Fibrillation Arising from the Structurally Normal Heart 428
Shinsuke Miyazaki, Ashok J. Shah, Michel Haïssaguerre, Mélèze Hocini

Chapter 47: How to Ablate Ventricular Tachycardia in Patients with Congenital Heart Disease 435
Katja Zeppenfeld

Chapter 48: Catheter Ablation of Ventricular Tachycardia in Sarcoidosis /
Hypertrophic Cardiomyopathy. 450
Kyoko Soejima, Akiko Ueda, Masaomi Chinushi

Chapter 49: How to Ablate Ventricular Tachycardia in Patients with
Arrhythmogenic Right Ventricular Cardiomyopathy/Dysplasia. 462
Fermin C. Garcia, Victor Bazan

Chapter 50: How to Perform Hybrid VT Ablation in the Operating Room 471
Paolo Della Bella, Giuseppe Maccabelli, Francesco Alamanni

Index. 487

To Rola, Maya, Dana, and Mohammad, for the constant love and support.

—Amin Al-Ahmad

This book is dedicated to my lovely wife Linda, who loves me despite all the time I invest in projects such as this, and to all students and teachers of cardiac electrophysiology.

—Dave Callans

To my family, for their continuous support and guidance; to my parents, for their encouragement and illumination.

—Henry H. Hsia

To my lovely wife Marina and our beautiful daughters Veronica and Eleonora.

—Andrea Natale

To my loving wife Solange, my sons Pablo and Martin, my parents, and my brother, for their endless understanding and support.

—Oscar Oseroff

To my lovely wife Gloria, my wonderful daughters Margaret and Katie, and the memory of my parents, Samuel and Lillian.

—Paul Wang

CONTRIBUTORS

Editors

Amin Al-Ahmad, MD, FACC, FHRS
Assistant Professor, Department of Medicine, Stanford University School of Medicine; Associate Director of the Cardiac Arrhythmia Service and Director of the Cardiac Electrophysiology Laboratory, Stanford University, Stanford, California

David J. Callans, MD
Professor of Medicine, University of Pennsylvania School of Medicine, Department of Medicine, Division of Cardiovascular Medicine, Philadelphia, Pennsylvania

Henry H. Hsia, MD, FACC, FHRS
Associate Professor of Medicine, Stanford University School of Medicine; Cardiac Electrophysiology and Arrhythmia Service, Stanford University, Stanford, California

Andrea Natale, MD, FACC, FHRS, FESC
Executive Medical Director, Texas Cardiac Arrhythmia Institute, St. David's Medical Center, Austin, Texas; Consulting Professor, Division of Cardiology, Stanford University, Palo Alto, California; Clinical Professor of Medicine, Case Western Reserve University, Cleveland, Ohio; Director, Interventional Electrophysiology, Scripps Clinic, San Diego, California; Senior Clinical Director, EP Services, California Pacific Medical Center, San Francisco, California

Oscar Oseroff, MD, FHRS
Chief of Pacing and Electrophysiology, Electrophysiology Department, Bazterrica Clinic, Buenos Aires, Argentina

Paul J. Wang, MD, FACC, FHRS
Professor, Department of Medicine, Stanford University School of Medicine; Director of the Cardiac Arrhythmia Service, Stanford University, Stanford, California

Contributors

Gorav Ailawadi, MD
Associate Professor, TCV Surgery, University of Virginia; Biomedical Engineering, University of Virginia, Charlottesville, Virginia

Francesco Alamanni, MD
Department of Cardiac Surgery, University of Milan, Centro Cardiologico, Monzino, Italy

Jesús Almendral, MD, PhD, FESC
Unidad de Electrofisiología Cardíaca y Arritmología Clínica, Grupo Hospital de Madrid, Universidad CEU-San Pablo, Madrid, Spain

Montawatt Amnueypol, MD
Pacific Rim Research Institute at White Memorial Hospital, Los Angeles, California; Bangkok Medical Center, Bangkok, Thailand

Nitish Badhwar, MBBS, FACC, FHRS
Director, Cardiac Electrophysiology Training Program; Associate Chief, Cardiac Electrophysiology, Medicine/Cardiology, University of California, San Francisco, California

Victor Bazan, MD, PhD
Attending Physician, Electrophysiology Unit, Cardiology Department, Hospital del Mar, Barcelona, UAB, Barcelona, Spain

J. David Burkhardt, MD, FACC, FHRS
Director of Research, Texas Cardiac Arrhythmia Institute, Austin, Texas; Director of Complex Arrhythmia Ablation, Scripps Clinic, La Jolla, California

Eduardo Castellanos, MD, PhD
Unidad de Electrofisiología Cardíaca y Arritmología Clínica, Grupo Hospital de Madrid, Universidad CEU-San Pablo, Madrid, Spain

Peng-Sheng Chen, MD, FHRS
Medtronic Zipes Chair in Cardiology; Director, Krannert Institute of Cardiology; Chief, Division of Cardiology, Department of Medicine, Indiana University School of Medicine, Indianapolis, Indiana

Shih-Ann Chen, MD, FHRS
Professor, Institute of Clinical Medicine, and Cardiovascular Research Center, National Yang-Ming University, Taipei, Taiwan; Division of Cardiology, Department of Medicine, Taipei Veterans General Hospital, Taipei, Taiwan

Zhongwei Cheng, MD
Cardiologist, Department of Cardiology, Peking Union Medical College Hospital, Peking Union Medical College and Chinese Academy of Medical Sciences, Beijing, China

Karin K. M. Chia, MBBS, FRACP
Staff Specialist Cardiac Electrophysiologist, Senior Lecturer, Royal Brisbane and Women's Hospital, The University of Queensland, Herston, Queensland, Australia

Masaomi Chinushi, MD, PhD
Associate Professor, School of Health Science, Niigata University School of Medicine, Niigata, Japan

Aman Chugh, MD, FACC
Associate Professor of Medicine, Section of Electrophysiology, Division of Cardiology, University of Michigan Medical School/University of Michigan Hospital, Ann Arbor, Michigan

James O. Coffey, MD
Assistant Professor of Medicine, Department of Cardiac Electrophysiology, Miller School of Medicine, University of Miami, Miami, Florida

Luis F. Couchonnal, MD
Electrophysiologist, Alegent Creighton Health Omaha, Nebraska

Andre d'Avila, MD, PhD
Associate Professor of Medicine; Co-Director Cardiac Arrhythmia Service, Helmsley Cardiac Arrhythmia Service, Mount Sinai School of Medicine, New York, New York

Matthew Dare, CEPS
Research, Technology, and Education Coordinator, Texas Cardiac Arrhythmia Institute, St. David's Medical Center, Austin, Texas

D. Wyn Davies, MD, FRCP, FHRS
Consultant Cardiologist, Department of Cardiology, St. Mary's Hospital, Imperial College Healthcare NHS Trust, London, United Kingdom

Carlos De Diego, MD
Unidad de Electrofisiología Cardíaca y Arritmología Clínica, Grupo Hospital de Madrid, Universidad CEU-San Pablo, Madrid, Spain

Paolo Della Bella, MD, FESC
Arrhythmia Unit and Electrophysiology Laboratories, Department of Cardiology and Cardiothoracic Surgery, San Raffaele Hospital, Milan, Italy

Marc W. Deyell, MD, MSc
Electrophysiology Fellow, Department of Medicine, Division of Cardiovascular Diseases, University of Pennsylvania School of Medicine, Philadelphia, Pennsylvania

Luigi Di Biase, MD, PhD, FHRS
Cardiologist, Electrophysiologist, Senior Researcher, Texas Cardiac Arrhythmia Institute at St. David's Medical Center, Austin, Texas; Adjunct Associate Professor, Department of Biomedical Engineering, University of Texas at Austin, Austin, Texas; Clinical Assistant Professor, Department of Cardiology, University of Foggia, Foggia, Italy

Anne M. Dubin, MD
Associate Professor of Pediatrics; Director, Pediatric Arrhythmia Center, Department of Pediatrics, Lucile Packard Children's Hospital, Stanford University, Palo Alto, California

James R. Edgerton, MD, FACS, FACC, FHRS
Co-Director, Arrhythmia Center of Innovation; Director of Research, Education, and Training, The Heart Hospital, Plano, Texas

Hicham El Masry, MD
Director of Cardiac Electrophysiology, Marion General Hospital, Marion, Indiana

N. A. Mark Estes III, MD, FACC, FHRS, FAHA, FESC
Professor of Medicine, Tufts University School of Medicine, New England Cardiac Arrhythmia Center, Tufts Medical Center, Boston, Massachusetts

John C. Evans, MD
Clinical Cardiac Electrophysiologist, Renown Institute for Heart and Vascular Health, Reno, Nevada

G. Joseph Gallinghouse, MD
Cardiac Electrophysiologist, Texas Cardiac Arrhythmia Institute, St. David's Medical Center, Austin, Texas

Fermin C. Garcia, MD
Cardiac Electrophysiologist, Hospital of the University of Pennsylvania, University of Pennsylvania, Perelman School of Medicine, Philadelphia, Pennsylvania

Ann C. Garlitski, MD, FACC, FHRS
Assistant Professor of Medicine, Tufts University School of Medicine, New England Cardiac Arrhythmia Center, Tufts Medical Center, Boston, Massachusetts

Edward P. Gerstenfeld, MD, FACC, FHRS
Associate Professor of Medicine; Chief, Cardiac Electrophysiology, Section of Cardiac Electrophysiology, Department of Medicine, University of California, San Francisco, California

Michel Haïssaguerre, MD
Hôpital Cardiologique du Haut-Lévêque and the Université Victor Segalen Bordeaux II, Bordeaux, France

Frederick T. Han, MD
Medicine/Cardiology, University of California, San Francisco, California

Seongwook Han, MD, PhD, FHRS
Central Utah Clinic—Cardiology, Provo, Utah

Carina A. Hardy, MD
Medical Staff of Cardiac Arrhythmia Unit, Instituto do Coração (InCor), Faculdade de Medicina da Universidade de São Paulo (Heart Institute, University of São Paulo Medical School), São Paulo, Brazil

Patrick M. Heck, BM, BCh, DM
Consultant Cardiologist, Department of Cardiology, Papworth Hospital, Cambridge, United Kingdom

Gerhard Hindricks, MD, PhD
Head of Department, Department of Electrophysiology, Heart Center, University of Leipzig, Leipzig, Germany

Donald D. Hoang, BA
Research Associate, Department of Cardiology, Cardiac Electrophysiology Section, Veterans Affairs Palo Alto Health Care System, Palo Alto, California

Mélèze Hocini, MD
Hôpital Cardiologique du Haut-Lévêque and the Université Victor Segalen Bordeaux II, Bordeaux, France

Munther Homoud, MD, FACC, FHRS
Director, CCEP Fellowship Program; Associate Professor of Medicine, New England Cardiac Arrhythmia Center, Tufts University School of Medicine, Tufts Medical Center, Boston, Massachusetts

Rodney P. Horton, MD
Texas Cardiac Arrhythmia Institute, Adjunct Professor, Department of Biomedical Engineering, Cockrell School of Engineering, University of Texas, Austin; Adjunct Assistant Professor, Division of Cardiology, Department of Medicine, University of Texas Health Sciences Center, San Antonio, Texas

Andrew T. Hume, MD
Director of Surgical Arrhythmias, St. David's Medical Center, Austin, Texas

Mathew D. Hutchinson, MD, FACC, FHRS
Assistant Professor of Medicine, Cardiovascular Division, Department of Medicine, University of Pennsylvania, Perelman School of Medicine Philadelphia, Pennsylvania

Chun Hwang, MD, FACC, FHRS
Director of Electrophysiology, Utah Valley Regional Medical Center, Central Utah Clinic—Cardiology, Provo, Utah

Warren M. Jackman, MD, FACC, FHRS
Professor of Medicine; George Lynn Cross Research Professor, University of Oklahoma Health Sciences Center, Oklahoma City, Oklahoma

Jason T. Jacobson, MD, FACC
Assistant Professor; Director, Cardiac Electrophysiology, Columbia University Division of Cardiology at Mount Sinai Medical Center, Miami Beach, Florida

Amir S. Jadidi, MD
Department of Cardiac Arrhythmias, Hôpital Cardiologique du Haut-Lévêque, CHU de Bordeaux, Pessac-Bordeaux, France; Department of Cardiac Arrhythmias, University Heart Centre Freiburg—Bad Krozingen, Bad Krozingen, Germany

Pierre Jaïs, MD
Arrhythmia Department, Hôpital Haut-Lévêque, University of Bordeaux, Bordeaux, France

Jonathan M. Kalman, MBBS, PhD
Professor, Department of Cardiology, Royal Melbourne Hospital, Melbourne, Australia

G. Neal Kay, MD, FACC, FAHA
Professor of Medicine, Division of Cardiovascular Disease, University of Alabama at Birmingham, Birmingham, Alabama

Peter M. Kistler, MBBS, PhD
Associate Professor, Department of Cardiology, Alfred Hospital and Baker IDI, Melbourne, Australia

Sébastien Knecht, MD, PhD
Professor, Electrophysiology, CHU Brugmann, Brussels, Belgium

Bradley P. Knight, MD, FACC, FHRS
Medical Director, Center for Heart Rhythm Disorders, Bluhm Cardiovascular Institute, Northwestern Memorial Hospital; Cooley Professor of Medicine, Northwestern University, Feinberg School of Medicine, Chicago, Illinois

Pipin Kojodjojo, MRCP, PhD
Clinical Senior Lecturer in Cardiac Electrophysiology, Department of Cardiology, St. Mary's Hospital, Imperial College Healthcare NHS Trust, London, United Kingdom

David S. Kwon, MD, PhD
Associate Director Clinical Research, Cardiovascular Therapeutic Area, Gilead Sciences, Foster City, California

Yenn-Jiang Lin, MD, PhD
Assistant Professor, School of Medicine, National Yang-Ming University, Taipei, Taiwan; Division of Cardiology, Department of Medicine, Taipei Veterans General Hospital, Taipei, Taiwan

Mark S. Link, MD, FACC, FHRS
Professor of Medicine, Tufts University School of Medicine, New England Cardiac Arrhythmia Center, Tufts Medical Center, Boston, Massachusetts

Li-Wei Lo, MD
Assistant Professor, School of Medicine, National Yang-Ming University, Taipei, Taiwan; Division of Cardiology, Department of Medicine, Taipei Veterans General Hospital, Taipei, Taiwan

Giuseppe Maccabelli, MD
Arrhythmia Unit and Electrophysiology Laboratories, Department of Cardiology and Cardiothoracic Surgery, San Raffaele Hospital, Milan, Italy

Srijoy Mahapatra, MD, FHRS
Medical Director and Vice President of Clinical and Therapy Development, AF Division, St. Jude Medical, St. Paul, Minnesota

Moussa Mansour, MD
Director, Cardiac Electrophysiology Laboratory, Massachusetts General Hospital, Harvard Medical School, Boston, Massachusetts

Francis E. Marchlinski, MD, FACC
Director, Cardiac Electrophysiology, Department of Medicine, Division of Cardiovascular Medicine, Hospital of the University of Pennsylvania, Philadelphia, Pennsylvania

Sissy Lara Melo, MD, PhD
Assistant Professor, Arrhythmia Unit, Instituto do Coração (InCor), Faculdade de Medicina da Universidade de São Paulo (Heart Institute, University of São Paulo Medical School), Sao Paulo, Brazil

John M. Miller, MD
Director of Cardiac Electrophysiology, Indiana University Health; Director, Electrophysiology Training Program, Indiana University School of Medicine, Indianapolis, Indiana

Christina Y. Miyake, MD
Instructor of Pediatrics, Department of Pediatrics, Division of Pediatric Cardiology, Lucile Packard Children's Hospital, Stanford University, Palo Alto, California

Shinsuke Miyazaki, MD
Hôpital Cardiologique du Haut-Lévêque and the Université Victor Segalen Bordeaux II, Bordeaux, France

Abram Mozes, MD
Clinical Fellow in Cardiac Electrophysiology, New England Cardiac Arrhythmia Center, Tufts Medical Center, Boston, Massachusetts

Koonlawee Nademanee, MD, FACC, FAHA, FHRS
Pacific Rim Research Institute at White Memorial Hospital, Los Angeles, California; Bangkok Medical Center, Bangkok, Thailand

Hiroshi Nakagawa, MD, PhD
Professor of Medicine; Director, Clinical Catheter Ablation Program; Director, Translational Electrophysiology, Heart Rhythm Institute, University of Oklahoma Health Sciences Center, Oklahoma City, Oklahoma

Carlo Pappone, MD, PhD, FACC
Department of Arrhythmology, Maria Cecilia
Hospital, Cotignola, Ravenna, Italy

Michala Pedersen, MD, DPhil
Hôpital-Haut-Lévêque, Service Rhythmologie;
Hôpital-Haut-Lévêque & Université Victor
Segalen, Bordeaux II, Bordeaux-Pessac, France

Marco V. Perez, MD
Clinical Instructor, Cardiac Arrhythmia Service,
Division of Cardiovascular Medicine, Stanford
University, Stanford, California

Francesco Perna, MD, PhD
Cardiology Department, Agostino Gemelli
Hospital, Catholic University of the Sacred Heart,
Rome, Italy

Christopher Piorkowski, MD
EP Consultant, Department of Electrophysiology,
Heart Center, University of Leipzig, Leipzig,
Germany

Cristiano Pisani, MD
Assistant Professor, Arrhythmia Unit, Instituto do
Coração (InCor), Faculdade de Medicina da
Universidade de São Paulo (Heart Institute,
University of São Paulo Medical School), São Paulo,
Brazil

Javier E. Sánchez, MD
Cardiac Electrophysiologist, Texas Cardiac
Arrhythmia Institute, St. David's Medical Center,
Austin, Texas

Pasquale Santangeli, MD
Texas Cardiac Arrhythmia Institute, St. David's
Medical Center, Austin, Texas

Vincenzo Santinelli, MD
Department of Arrhythmology, Maria Cecilia
Hospital Cotignola, Ravenna, Italy

Mauricio I. Scanavacca, MD, PhD
Director of Cardiac Arrhythmia Unit, Instituto do
Coração (InCor), Faculdade de Medicina da
Universidade de São Paulo (Heart Institute,
University of São Paulo Medical School), São Paulo,
Brazil

Melvin M. Scheinman, MD
Professor of Medicine; Walter H. Shorenstein
Endowed Chair of Cardiology, Cardiac
Electrophysiology, University of California,
San Francisco, California

Benjamin J. Scherlag, PhD, FHRS
Professor of Medicine, Division of Cardiology,
Heart Rhythm Institute, University of Oklahoma
Health Sciences Center, Oklahoma City, Oklahoma

Daniel Scherr, MD, PD
Assistant Professor of Medicine, Division of
Cardiology, Department of Medicine, Medical
University of Graz, Graz, Austria

Ashok J. Shah, MD
Hôpital Cardiologique du Haut-Lévêque and the
Université Victor Segalen Bordeaux II, Bordeaux,
France

Sheldon M. Singh, MD, FRCPC, FACC
Assistant Professor of Medicine, Schulich Heart
Program, Sunnybrook Health Sciences Center,
Faculty of Medicine, University of Toronto, Toronto,
Ontario, Canada

Kyoko Soejima, MD
Associate Professor, Cardiovascular Division, Kyorin
University School of Medicine, Tokyo, Japan

Philipp Sommer, MD
EP Consultant, Department of Electrophysiology,
Heart Center, University of Leipzig, Leipzig,
Germany

Eduardo Sosa, MD, PhD
Clinic Arrhythmia and Pacemaker Unit, Instituto do
Coração (InCor), Heart Institute, University of São
Paulo Medical School, São Paulo, Brazil

William G. Stevenson, MD
Professor of Medicine, Harvard Medical School,
Cardiovascular Division, Department of Medicine,
Brigham and Women's Hospital, Boston,
Massachusetts

Gregory E. Supple, MD
Assistant Professor of Medicine, University of Pennsylvania School of Medicine, Department of Medicine, Division of Cardiovascular Medicine, Philadelphia, Pennsylvania

Kojiro Tanimoto, MD
Instructor, Cardiology Division, Keio University School of Medicine, Tokyo, Japan

Usha B. Tedrow, MD, MSc
Assistant Professor of Medicine, Harvard Medical School; Director, Clinical Cardiac Electrophysiology Program, Cardiovascular Division, Department of Medicine, Brigham and Women's Hospital, Boston, Massachusetts

Andrew W. Teh, MBBS, PhD
Physician, Department of Cardiology, Royal Melbourne Hospital, Melbourne, Australia

John K. Triedman, MD, FACC, FHRS
Professor of Pediatrics, Harvard Medical School, Arrhythmia Service, Department of Cardiology, Boston Children's Hospital, Boston, Massachusetts

Mintu P. Turakhia, MD, MAS
Acting Assistant Professor of Medicine; Director of Cardiac Electrophysiology, Veterans Affairs Palo Alto Healthcare System, Stanford University School of Medicine, Stanford, California

Wendy S. Tzou, MD, FHRS
Assistant Professor of Medicine, Cardiology Division, Electrophysiology Section, University of Colorado Anschutz Medical Campus, Aurora, Colorado

Akiko Ueda, MD
Doctor, Department of Cardiology, Tokyo Metropolitan Hiroo Hospital, Tokyo, Japan

George F. Van Hare, MD
Director, Pediatric Cardiology; Louis Larrick Ward Professor of Pediatrics; Co-Director, St. Louis Children's and Washington University Heart Center, Washington University School of Medicine, St. Louis, Missouri

Jonathan Weinstock, MD, FACC, FHRS
Assistant Professor of Medicine, Tufts University School of Medicine, New England Cardiac Arrhythmia Center, Tufts Medical Center, Boston, Massachusetts

Takumi Yamada, MD, PhD
Assistant Professor of Medicine, Division of Cardiovascular Disease, University of Alabama at Birmingham, Birmingham, Alabama

Paul C. Zei, MD, PhD, FHRS
Clinical Associate Professor, Cardiac Electrophysiology; Chief, Cardiovascular Clinics; Director, Electrocardiology, Stanford University, Stanford, California

Katja Zeppenfeld, MD, PhD, FESC
Professor of Cardiology, Electrophysiology, Department of Cardiology, Leiden University Medical Centre, Leiden, The Netherlands

FOREWORD

How Not to Get "Lost in Translation"

Cardiac electrophysiology started when intracardiac signals were first recorded using catheters in the late 1950s. It has matured over the last half-century into an internationally recognized cardiovascular subspecialty. We can now diagnose most cardiac arrhythmias, though at times we may not be able to define the exact arrhythmia mechanism in a given patient. In concert with advances in our diagnostic abilities, advances in arrhythmia surgery paved the way to curative procedures. It was a natural extension to deliver energy through catheters after a definitive diagnosis was reached, and thus we entered the catheter ablation era in the 1980s.

We have a vast body of literature that defines how a particular arrhythmia is diagnosed and how it should be ablated. Electrophysiologic diagnosis depends on observation of intracardiac electrograms and response to certain electrical perturbations, at times using pharmacological agents. This has been an international endeavor and continues to evolve. These advances need to be translated into safe, effective, and efficient approaches for diagnosis and treatment in the electrophysiology laboratory. For example, newer electrophysiologic maneuvers have been described for differentiating various paraseptal arrhythmias: the use of parahisian pacing, observations about VA relationships after entrainment, and the use of PPI-TCL intervals and VA linking. Differentiating arrhythmia mechanisms is the first step toward developing safe, effective, and efficient treatment strategies. This is illustrated by the evolution of our approach to LBBB-inferior axis VT. Initially, these were thought to arise in the RVOT. As knowledge and experience have evolved, we have come to realize that these VTs can arise from either the left or the right outflow regions, aorto-mitral continuity, aortic cusps, aorta, pulmonary artery, or the epicardial surface. Being able to ascertain the likely site of origin of these VTs preoperatively helps in discussions with patients about procedural risks, procedure planning, and outcomes.

The editors of *Hands-On Ablation: The Experts' Approach* are to be congratulated for a comprehensive table of contents that covers arrhythmias amenable to curative ablation. The book is divided into three sections—supraventricular tachycardias, atrial fibrillation, and ventricular tachycardias—and each chapter translates the existing literature into practical steps of how to confirm the diagnosis in the electrophysiology laboratory and how to ablate it.

The book will be invaluable to fellows training in cardiac electrophysiology and to experienced electrophysiologists to remind them of the additional diagnostic maneuvers that may be needed to differentiate diagnostic challenges. It will be a valuable reference in every electrophysiology laboratory when difficult diagnostic dilemmas arise. A how-to approach will help the clinician avoid getting "lost in translation" between the existing literature and clinically useful approaches for effective diagnosis and ablation.

The book is written in a user-friendly manner using a how-to approach to make the information clinically relevant. It is beautifully and amply illustrated, following the adage "A picture is worth a thousand words." The authors are thought leaders in the field of electrophysiology, and they possess a command of their respective fields, thereby providing an expert's approach to each problem.

In summary, this book translates the existing electrophysiologic literature into useful approaches for clinical decision making. It's meant for hands-on electrophysiologists who deal with real-life clinical problems in the EP lab, as it provides an expert's approach on how to deal with common clinical scenarios and will keep the clinician from getting "lost in translation."

—Ranjan K. Thakur, MD, MPH, FHRS
Professor of Medicine
Michigan State University
Editor, *Cardiac Electrophysiology Clinics*

PREFACE

The field of catheter ablation continues to advance with innovations in technology and a deeper understanding of the pathophysiology of arrhythmias. The practitioner must keep up with these advances in order to deliver the most state-of-the-art care for his or her patients. Journal publications offer a first look into new ideas and innovations, but often lack the practical details that help translate something new into practice.

The aim of this book is to give the reader an inside look at leading electrophysiology labs in the world with chapters that focus on the more practical aspects of ablation procedures. This book is unique in attempting to answer the question of "how to" perform procedures including supraventricular tachycardia ablation, atrial fibrillation ablation, and ventricular tachycardia ablation. Each chapter highlights the practical knowledge of the expert authors with a specific procedure. In addition, each chapter has multiple images and/or videos that aid in illustrating concepts.

Our goal is to provide the reader with practical knowledge and tips that previously could only be obtained by directly observing experts in action.

We hope that practicing electrophysiologists, electrophysiology trainees, and allied professionals and industry professionals will find this text to be a useful resource and educational tool.

—Amin Al-Ahmad
David J. Callans
Henry H. Hsia
Andrea Natale
Oscar Oseroff
Paul J. Wang

ABBREVIATIONS

A-A-V	atrial-atrial-ventricular	EGM	electrogram
ACT	activated clotting time	E-IDC	electrograms with isolated delayed components
AF	atrial fibrillation		
AFCL	atrial fibrillation cycle length	EP	electrophysiology
AFL	atrial flutter	ERP	effective refractory period
AIVV	anterior interventricular vein	EUS	electrical unexcitable scar
AMC	aorto-mitral continuity	GCV	great cardiac vein
AP	accessory pathway	HA	His-atrial
APC	atrial premature contraction	HB	His bundle
ARVC/D	arrhythmogenic right ventricular cardiomyopathy/dysplasia	HB-RB	His bundle-right bundle branch
		HPS	His-Purkinje system
ASC	aortic sinus cusp	HRA	high right atrium
ASD	atrial septal defect	HRP	His-refractory PVCs
AT	atrial tachycardia	IABP	intra-aortic balloon pump
ATP	antitachycardia pacing	IART	intra-atrial reentrant tachycardia
AV	atrial-ventricular or atrioventricular	IAS	interatrial septum
AVN	atrioventricular node	ICD	implantable cardioverter-defibrillator
AVNRT	atrioventricular nodal reentry	ICE	intracardiac echocardiography
AVRT	atrioventricular reciprocating tachycardia	ICM	ischemic cardiomyopathy
BBB	bundle branch block	ICU	intensive care unit
BBRVT	bundle branch reentrant ventricular tachycardia	IDCM	idiopathic dilated cardiomyopathy
		INR	international normalized ratio
bpm	beats per minute	IPV	inferior pulmonary vein
CAD	coronary artery disease	IVC	inferior vena cava
CFAE	complex fractionated atrial electrograms	IVS	interventricular septum
CL	cycle length	IVT	inferior ventricular tachycardia
CS	coronary sinus	JET	junctional ectopic tachycardia
CT	computed tomography	LA	left atrium/atrial
CTI	cavotricuspid isthmus	LAA	left atrial appendage
ECG	electrocardiogram	LAD	left anterior descending coronary artery

LAO	left anterior oblique	**PSVT**	paroxysmal supraventricular tachycardia
LBBB	left bundle branch block	**PTT**	partial thromboplastin time
LBRS	left bundle branch block-right superior	**PV**	pulmonary vein
LCC	left coronary cusp	**PVAD**	peripheral left ventricular assist devices
LCx	left circumflex coronary artery	**PVAI**	pulmonary vein antrum isolation
LFA	left femoral artery	**PVC**	premature ventricular contraction
LFV	left femoral vein	**PVI**	pulmonary vein isolation
LI-MI	left inferior pulmonary vein to mitral isthmus	**RA**	right atrium/atrial
		RAA	right atrial appendage
LIPV	left inferior pulmonary vein	**RAAS**	retrograde atrial activation sequence
LOM	ligament of Marshall	**RAMP**	right atrial multipurpose
LPA	left pulmonary artery	**RAO**	right anterior oblique
LPF	left posterior fascicle	**RBLI**	right bundle branch block-left inferior
LPV	left pulmonary vein	**RBRS**	right bundle branch block-right superior
LSPV	left superior pulmonary vein	**RCA**	right coronary artery
LV	left ventricle/ventricular	**RCC**	right coronary cusp
LVEF	left ventricular ejection fraction	**RF**	radiofrequency
LVO	left ventricular outflow region	**RFA**	right femoral artery
MAC	monitored anesthesia care	**RFV**	right femoral vein
MAT	multifocal atrial tachycardia	**RIPV**	right inferior pulmonary vein
MB	Marshall bundle	**RPA**	right pulmonary artery
MCV	middle cardiac vein	**RPV**	right pulmonary vein
MDI	maximum deflection index	**RSPV**	right superior pulmonary vein
MDP	mid-diastolic potential	**RV**	right ventricle/ventricular
MDT	maximum deflection time	**RVA**	right ventricular apex
MI	myocardial infarction	**RVOT**	right ventricular outflow tract
MRI	magnetic resonance imaging	**SA**	stimulus to atrial interval
MRT	macro reentrant tachycardia	**SA-VA**	stimulus to atrial interval minus the VA interval
NCC	noncoronary cusp		
NF	nodofascicular	**SH**	stimulus to His
NICM	nonischemic cardiomyopathy	**ST**	sinus tachycardia
NIPS	noninvasive programmed stimulation	**SVC**	superior vena cava
NPV	negative predictive value	**SVT**	supraventricular tachycardia
NV	nodoventricular	**TCEA**	transcoronary ethanol ablation
ORT	orthodromic reentrant tachycardia	**TCL**	tachycardia cycle length
PAC	premature atrial contractions	**TEE**	transesophageal echocardiogram/echocardiography
PFO	patent foramen ovale		
PJRT	permanent junctional reciprocating tachycardia	**TIA**	transient ischemic attack
		TTE	transthoracic echocardiogram/echocardiography
PNV	peak negative voltage		
PPI	postpacing interval	**VA**	ventriculo-atrial
PPI-TCL	postpacing interval minus the tachycardia cycle length	**VOM**	vein of Marshall
		VT	ventricular tachycardia
PPV	positive predictive value	**WPW**	Wolfe-Parkinson-White syndrome

SECTION I

ABLATION OF SUPRAVENTRICULAR TACHYCARDIA

CHAPTER 1

How to Rapidly Diagnose Supraventricular Tachycardia (SVT) in the Electrophysiology Lab

Luis F. Couchonnal, MD; Bradley P. Knight, MD

Introduction

The differential diagnosis of SVT includes a variety of conditions, including ST, AVNRT, AVRT, AT, JET, AFL, AF, and MAT (**Figure 1.1**). The term *paroxysmal* supraventricular tachycardia (PSVT) is used to refer to regular SVTs that have a sudden onset and termination, namely AVNRT, AVRT, and AT.[1] AVNRT accounts for 60% of PSVTs, and AVRT and AT account for 30% and 10%, respectively (**Figure 1.2**). This chapter will focus on the diagnosis of AVNRT, AVRT, and AT in the EP laboratory. The discussion of AVRT will be focused on ORT, which exhibits retrograde activation via the AP, and anterograde conduction via the AV node, resulting in a narrow QRS complex tachycardia in the absence of aberration. The diagnosis of the PSVT mechanism is dependent on evaluation of 3 key elements: (1) baseline findings prior to tachycardia initiation; (2) tachycardia characteristics; and (3) tachycardia response to atrial and ventricular pacing maneuvers.

Preprocedure Planning

Before performing an EP study on a patient with PSVT, a detailed history and physical should be performed. The patient's age at onset of PSVT may give insight into the underlying mechanism. Greater than 70% of patients with AVRT present before the age of 20 years (median age 23 ± 14 years). In contrast, 60% of patients with AVNRT present after the age of 20 years (median age 32 ± 18 years).[2] Atrial tachycardia is also influenced by age, accounting for 23% of PSVTs over the age of 70 years. The mechanism of SVT is also influenced by gender. In a study of 1700 patients presenting with PSVT, the majority of patients with AVRT were men (54%), while the majority of

Causes of Supraventricular Tachycardia

1. Sinus tachycardia
2. AV nodal reentry (AVNRT) } PSVT
3. AV reciprocating tachycardia (AVRT) } PSVT
4. Atrial tachycardia (AT) } PSVT
5. Junctional ectopic tachycardia (JET)
6. Atrial flutter (AFl)
7. Atrial fibrillation (AF)
8. Multifocal AT (MAT)

Figure 1.1 Causes of SVT. The different mechanisms of SVT are listed. The term *PSVT* is reserved for tachycardias caused by AVNRT, AVRT, and AT.

Hands-On Ablation: The Experts' Approach © 2013 Amin Al-Ahmad, David J. Callans, Henry H. Hsia, Andrea Natale, Oscar Oseroff, Paul J. Wang, eds.
Cardiotext Publishing, ISBN: 978-1-935395-24-9.

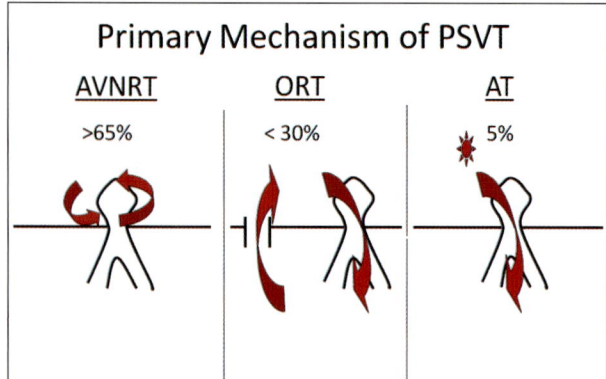

Figure 1.2 Primary mechanism of PSVT. AVNRT is a reentrant tachycardia that uses the AV nodal and perinodal tissues to sustain the tachycardia. In typical AVNRT, antegrade conduction proceeds via the slow pathway and retrograde conduction proceeds via the fast pathway, resulting in a septal VA time of < 70 ms. In atypical AVNRT, antegrade conduction proceeds via the fast pathway and retrograde conduction proceeds via the slow pathway, resulting in a septal VA time of > 70 ms. In AVRT, antegrade conduction is via the AV node and retrograde conduction is via the AP, with a septal VA time > 70 ms. Septal pathways may exhibit a concentric retrograde atrial activation sequence, while lateral pathways exhibit varying degrees of eccentric atrial activation. The mechanism of AT can be focal in nature or due to reentry within the atria. Unlike AVNRT and AVRT, AT is independent of AV nodal conduction to maintain the arrhythmia. The VA time of atrial tachycardia is variable.

patients presenting with AVNRT and AT were women (70% and 62%, respectively).[3]

The baseline ECG should be assessed for evidence of manifest preexcitation. The ECG during PSVT with 1:1 AV conduction should be evaluated for the P-wave morphology and the R-P interval. A short R-P tachycardia (defined as an R-P interval < 50% of the R-R interval) with evidence of superiorly directed P waves suggests a diagnosis of typical (slow-fast) AVNRT, AVRT, or AT. A short R-P tachycardia with an abnormal P-wave morphology suggests a diagnosis of AT. A long R-P tachycardia (defined as an R-P interval > 50% of the R-R interval) with superiorly directed P waves suggests a diagnosis of atypical (fast-slow) AVNRT, or AVRT with a slowly conducting AP. A long R-P tachycardia with abnormal P-wave morphology suggests an AT. When no P waves are discernable, the terminal portion of the QRS complex should be evaluated in lead V1 to assess for a pseudo R′ related to retrograde atrial activation. When the P wave is hidden within the QRS complex or is just visible in the terminal portion of the QRS, the rhythm is very likely AVNRT. However, the observer should base the diagnosis using the ECG with caution. Studies looking at ECG criteria to differentiate between AVNRT, AVRT, and AT incorrectly classified the tachycardia 20% of the time.[4]

Vascular Access and Catheter Placement

Informed consent and labs (complete blood count, coagulation studies, and chemistries) are obtained in the cardiac surveillance unit on or before the day of the procedure. The majority of patients undergoing an EP procedure for PSVT receive intravenous sedation administered by the EP nursing staff under the direction of the attending physician. Most EP procedures for PSVT can be performed using access via a single femoral vein. Standard sheaths for an EP procedure for PSVT include 3 sheaths from the right femoral vein. After the patient is prepped and draped, access to the right femoral vein is performed. When the suspicion is high that the PSVT mechanism is AVNRT, a long guiding sheath can be placed initially, and an ablation catheter can be used for the diagnostic portion of the study. A standard 4-mm electrode-tip deflectable ablation catheter is typically used. A soft-tip quadripolar catheter is positioned at the RV apex. A steerable quadripolar catheter is positioned in the HRA. The ablation catheter or the HRA catheter can later be moved to the CS to assess for eccentric or concentric atrial activation. After catheters are positioned, the patient receives an intravenous bolus of heparin (3000 U) followed by an additional 1000 U every hour to prevent thrombus formation. A multipolar catheter can be placed in the CS at the beginning of the procedure if there is evidence of preexcitation suggestive of a left-sided pathway. An advanced 3-dimensional mapping system is not needed for most PSVT cases, but can be used for challenging cases.

Baseline Observations in the EP Lab

Before initiation of SVT in the EP lab, several baseline observations should be made to determine the baseline substrate and to look for clues that might support a specific mechanism of tachycardia.[5] For example, evidence of ventricular preexcitation during sinus rhythm has a positive predictive value (PPV) of 86% and negative predictive value (NPV) of 78% that the patient will have AVRT. Preexcitation may be manifest on the 12-lead ECG and is defined as an HV interval of less than 35 ms. Dual AV node physiology, defined as an increase of ≥ 50 ms in the A2H2 interval with atrial extrastimuli A1A2 interval decremented in 10- to 20-ms steps, has a PPV for AVNRT of 86%. Although evidence of preexcitation or dual AV node physiology both carry a relatively high PPV, 10% of patients with ventricular preexcitation will have inducible AVNRT, and approximately 15% of patients with evidence of dual AV node physiology will have either AVRT or AT. Lack of baseline VA conduction at a ventricular pacing CL of ≥ 600 ms makes the diagnosis of AVRT highly unlikely. However, 5% of patients without evidence of VA conduction at baseline will have inducible AVRT, as retrograde conduction of the AP may be dependent on catecholamine stimulation.[6] Furthermore, evidence of decremental VA conduction with ventricular extrastimuli makes the presence of an AP unlikely. However, a small percentage of pathways do exhibit decremental conduction. Evidence of intra-atrial conduction delay or atrial scar, as determined by low voltage or fractionated atrial electrograms, may suggest atrial tachycardia as the culprit mechanism. Rarely do we administer adenosine in the baseline state to look for evidence of extranodal conduction while performing atrial or ventricular pacing. However, absence of VA block after administration of adenosine is not diagnostic for the presence of an AP because retrograde fast pathway conduction is not blocked in 38% of patients with typical AVNRT.[7]

Parahisian Pacing

Parahisian pacing can be utilized at baseline to determine the presence or absence of retrograde conduction over a septal AP.[8] To perform this maneuver, the pacing catheter is positioned at the basal RV septum. The distal pacing electrodes should record both His and ventricular electrograms. To avoid inadvertent atrial capture, atrial electrograms should be minimized at the distal pacing electrode. Pacing should initially be performed at higher outputs (5–10 mA) to ensure HB-RB capture and decremented until loss of HB-RB capture.

Parahisian pacing results in both antegrade and retrograde conduction via the HPS. The antegrade wavefront conducts via the HPS, resulting in a relatively narrow QRS morphology. In the absence of an AP, the retrograde wavefront conducts over the His bundle, with a SH interval of 0 ms, followed by atrial activation, with a SA interval equal to the HA interval. As the pacing output is decreased, loss of HB-RB capture results in widening of the QRS as a result of antegrade conduction occurring directly over slowly conducting ventricular myocardium. Retrograde His bundle capture is delayed as conduction first occurs over ventricular myocardium, followed by retrograde activation of the right bundle, with resultant activation of the His bundle. This delayed His activation results in prolongation of the SA interval, which is a sum of the SH and HA interval. This is typical of a nodal response to parahisian pacing (**Figure 1.3A**). In the setting of a septal AP, the SA interval remains constant, with loss of HB-RB capture as atrial activation depends only on the retrograde conduction properties of the AP connecting the ventricular myocardium to the atrium (**Figure 1.3B**).

In order to properly interpret the results of parahisian pacing, the retrograde atrial activation sequence (RAAS) must be closely observed.[9] When there is evidence of loss of HB-RB capture with the same SA interval and no change in the RAAS, conduction is via only an AP. However, if there is a change in the RAAS after loss of HB-RB capture, conduction is likely occurring either via multiple APs, simultaneous conduction up the fast and

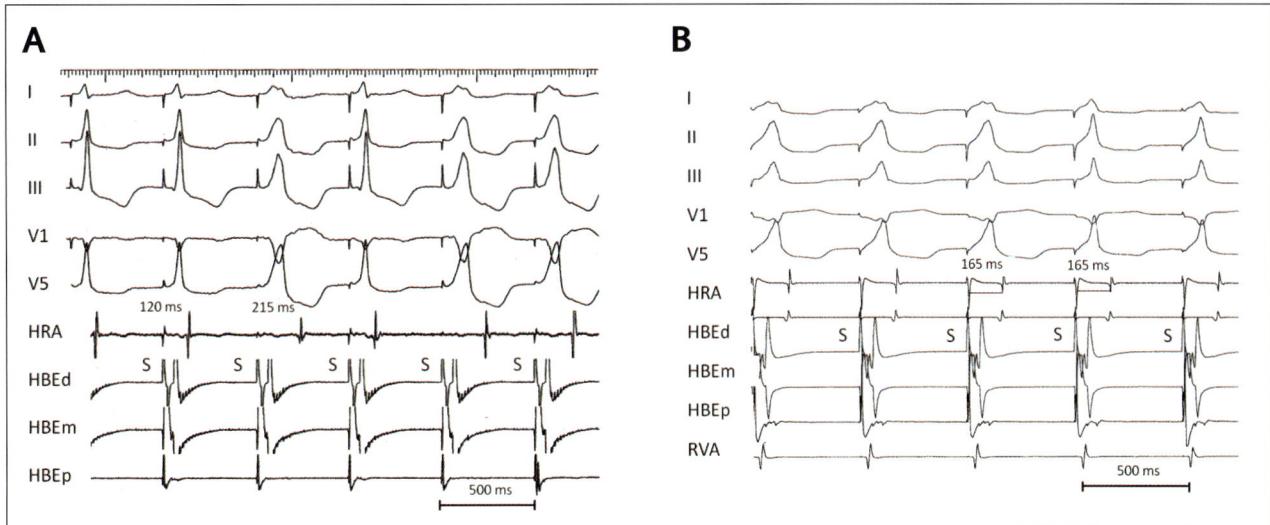

Figure 1.3 A. Nodal response to parahisian pacing. In this example, the pacing output in decreased while pacing at the His position. The third beat shows widening of the QRS complex, consistent with loss of His capture. With loss of His capture, there is a corresponding increase in the stimulus to HRA interval, consistent with a nodal response to parahisian pacing. **B.** Extranodal response to parahisian pacing. In the example above, pacing is performed from a quadripolar catheter positioned at the His position. As the pacing output is held constant, intermittent capture of the His bundle results in a narrow complex QRS (last 2 beats), The stimulus to HRA interval is 165 ms with and without His capture, consistent with an extranodal response to parahisian pacing. This finding demonstrates the presence of a septal AP.

slow AV nodal pathways, or concomitant conduction up the AV node and an AP. To differentiate between these, the HA interval should be evaluated. If the HA interval remains fixed, then conduction is dependent on retrograde AV nodal conduction with concomitant AP conduction. However, if there is evidence of HA interval shortening, which implies HA dissociation, then conduction is related to 1 of 2 pathways, concomitant fast and slow AV nodal conduction, or concomitant AV node and pathway conduction. The sensitivity of the extranodal response to parahisian pacing for detecting the presence of an AP is 46%. This likely reflects the fact that an extranodal response is less likely to be elicited for pathways farther from the AV node (ie, lateral pathways). The specificity of this finding is 96%.

Differential RV Pacing

Another maneuver utilized to determine the presence of a septal AP is to perform differential RV pacing.[10] Ventricular pacing is performed at both apical and basal RV sites at the same pacing cycle length (CL) and the interval from the RV pacing stimulus to the HRA is measured. In the absence of an AP, the VA interval is longer when pacing basally compared to pacing apically, because conduction from the base must proceed over the septal myocardium before entering the HPS at the RV apex. However, in the presence of an AP, the VA interval is shorter when pacing basally compared to apically, as retrograde atrial activation is dependent on conduction via the basally located AP. The VA index can be calculated, which is the difference in the VA intervals apically compared to basally (VAapical – VAbasal). A VA index of > 10 ms had a sensitivity, specificity, and PPV of 100% for detecting the presence of a posteroseptal AP.

Tachycardia Characteristics

After initiation of SVT, there are several observations that can be made to determine the tachycardia mechanism. The TCL gives insight into the mechanism of the tachycardia, although there is significant overlap. In general, AVNRT tends to be slower than AVRT. Slow tachycardias (CL > 500 ms) tend to be AVNRT, with a PPV of 83%. The first measurement made at the initiation of the tachycardia is the septal VA interval, measured from the beginning of the surface QRS to the earliest septal atrial electrogram. A septal VA time of less than 70 ms excludes AP-mediated tachycardias and makes typical AVNRT highly likely. Less than 1% of ATs will exhibit a VA time less than 70 ms.

When tachycardia is initiated, spontaneous oscillations ("wobble") in the TCL should be noted. If changes in the A-A interval precede changes in the H-H interval (the As are driving the Vs), the mostly likely mechanism is AT. However, if changes in the H-H interval precede changes in the A-A intervals, the most likely mechanism is AVNRT or ORT.

If the septal VA time is greater than 70 ms, the CS catheter can be used to determine whether the RAAS during tachycardia is concentric or eccentric. During typical AVNRT, the RAAS is concentric, as the area of earliest atrial activation is near the fast pathway that inserts near the His at the apex of the triangle of Koch. With atypical AVNRT, the earliest atrial activation is near the CS ostium. With the exception of paraseptal AVRT and AT, AVRT and AT will demonstrate varying degrees of eccentric atrial activation, depending on the pathway or foci locations relative to the AV node. Evidence of eccentric activation excludes most all forms of AVNRT as the tachycardia mechanism. However, a small number of patients with AVNRT have evidence of eccentric atrial activation and can only be successfully ablated from within the CS or along the mitral annulus, related to leftward extension of the slow pathway.

Zones of transition, including tachycardia initiation, aberration, and spontaneous termination, give insight into the tachycardia mechanism. When tachycardia induction is reproducibly dependent on a prolongation of the AH interval with atrial pacing, the most likely diagnosis is AVNRT, with a PPV of 91%. This prolongation is related to block in the fast pathway and "jumping" to the slow pathway, usually with a change in the AH interval of at least 50 ms with an atrial extrastimulus. Initiation of AVRT may also demonstrate some AV delay, but delay can also occur anywhere within the circuit, including intramyocardial conduction delay. As AT is independent of the AV node, AV nodal delay is not required for tachycardia induction.

The development of LBBB is more commonly seen with ORT, with a PPV of 92%. There are several reasons for this phenomenon. The faster rate of ORT likely favors the development of aberrant conduction. The occurrence of LBBB aberration also promotes the development of ORT by allowing the AP time to recover to allow for retrograde conduction to occur. Furthermore, as induction of AVNRT is dependent on the development of AV nodal delay, resulting in a longer H1-H2 interval, the development of aberration is unlikely. In contrast, a critical AH delay is not required for initiation of ORT. Therefore, the short AH interval during tachycardia initiation encroaches on the refractoriness of the HPS, resulting in aberration. An increase in the VA time by greater than 20 ms with bundle branch block (BBB) is diagnostic of ORT using an AP that is ipsilateral to the side of block, with a PPV of 100%. This increase in the VA time is related to relatively slower intramyocardial conduction caused by the BBB. This increase in the VA time may result in a corresponding increase in the TCL. However, the increased VA time may

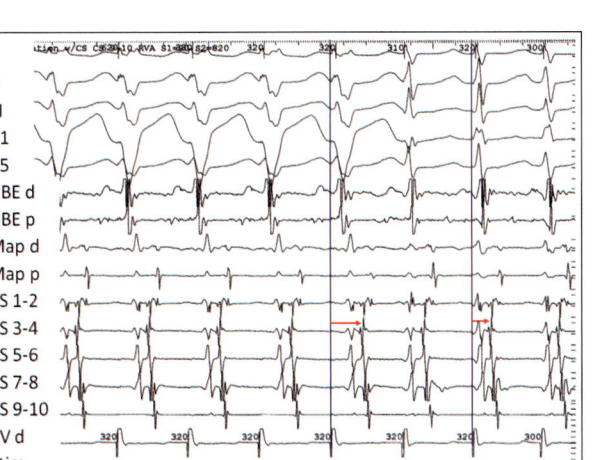

Figure 1.4 Example of an increase in the VA interval with LBBB during ORT in a patient with left free-wall AP. The VA time during tachycardia with concomitant left bundle aberrancy is longer than with a narrow complex QRS. This proves that the tachycardia mechanism is AVRT with an AP that is ipsilateral to the site of bundle branch block.

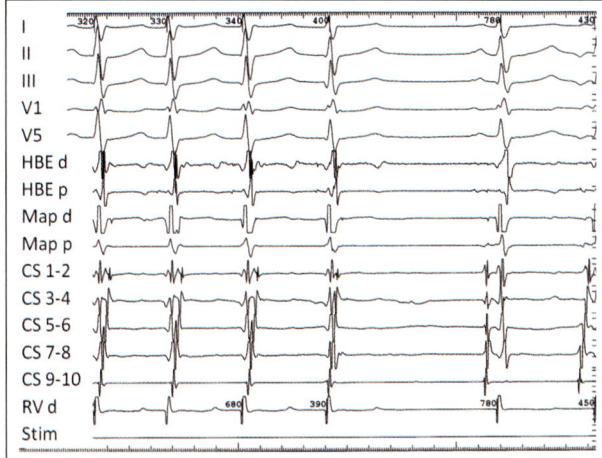

Figure 1.5 Example of spontaneous termination with AV block. The spontaneous termination of tachycardia with an atrial electrogram is consistent with an AV nodal-dependent tachycardia mechanism (either AVNRT or AVRT). In this example, the last electrogram noted is an atrial beat as block occurs in the AV node, preventing ventricular depolarization. The simultaneous atrial and ventricular activation excludes AVRT. Therefore, the tachycardia must be typical AVNRT.

also result in a compensatory decrease in the AH interval, resulting in no apparent change in the TCL (**Figure 1.4**).

Evidence of AV block during SVT excludes ORT, as the ventricle is obligate for continuation of the reentrant circuit. AV block can be seen in both AT and AVNRT, with block occurring infranodally in the latter.

A spontaneous termination of tachycardia should be inspected carefully for clues as to the tachycardia mechanism. Typically, spontaneous termination of AVNRT and ORT is caused by antegrade block in the AV node. As a result, AVNRT and ORT usually terminate with a P wave not followed by a QRS (**Figure 1.5**). Conversely, when AT with 1:1 conduction terminates, the last atrial beat typically conducts to the ventricle. The simultaneous termination of the AT with AV block would be an exceedingly rare phenomenon. Therefore, a tachycardia that terminates spontaneously with a P wave excludes AT. However, a tachycardia that terminates with QRS does not differentiate between AVNRT, AVRT, or AT.

Pacing Maneuvers During Tachycardia

Ventricular Pacing Maneuvers

After evaluation of the baseline findings and the tachycardia characteristics, pacing maneuvers are performed to further define the tachycardia mechanism. The first pacing maneuver performed is entrainment from the ventricle. To perform entrainment, the ventricle is paced at a CL 10 to 40 ms less than the TCL, with the goal of accelerating the atrium to the pacing CL. With cessation of ventricular pacing, the tachycardia should return to its original CL. After ensuring acceleration of the atrial CL, the RAAS of the tachycardia is compared to the entrained activation. If the paced atrial activation sequence differs from the tachycardia, either a bystander pathway or an atrial tachycardia is suspected. If the atrial activation sequence is the same, the electrogram sequence after the last paced ventricular complex is evaluated to determine whether the conduction sequence can be described as atrial-ventricular (A-V) or atrial-atrial-ventricular (A-A-V). An A-V response is consistent with either AVNRT or AVRT, as the last entrained atrial beat travels via the retrograde limb of the circuit (ie, AV nodal pathway or AP) and then antegrade down the AV node (**Figure 1.6A**). However, an A-A-V response is consistent with atrial tachycardia because during entrainment, retrograde conduction occurs via the AV node, and the last entrained atrial beat finds the AV node refractory (**Figure 1.6B**).

The calculation of the postpacing interval minus the TCL (PPI-TCL) after entrainment can also be utilized to differentiate atypical AVNRT from a septal AP. A value > 115 ms suggests atypical AVNRT, while a value < 115 ms is suggestive of a septal AP (**Figure 1.7**).[11] As the ventricle is an obligate component of the AVRT circuit, entrainment from the ventricle results in a shorter PPI compared to the PPI during AVNRT, where the entire circuit is near the AV node. This explains why septal pathways have a PPI-TCL shorter than that of atypical AVNRT. The SA interval minus the VA interval during tachycardia (SA-VA) can also be utilized to differentiate atypical AVNRT from a septal AP. A SA-VA time < 85 ms suggests a septal

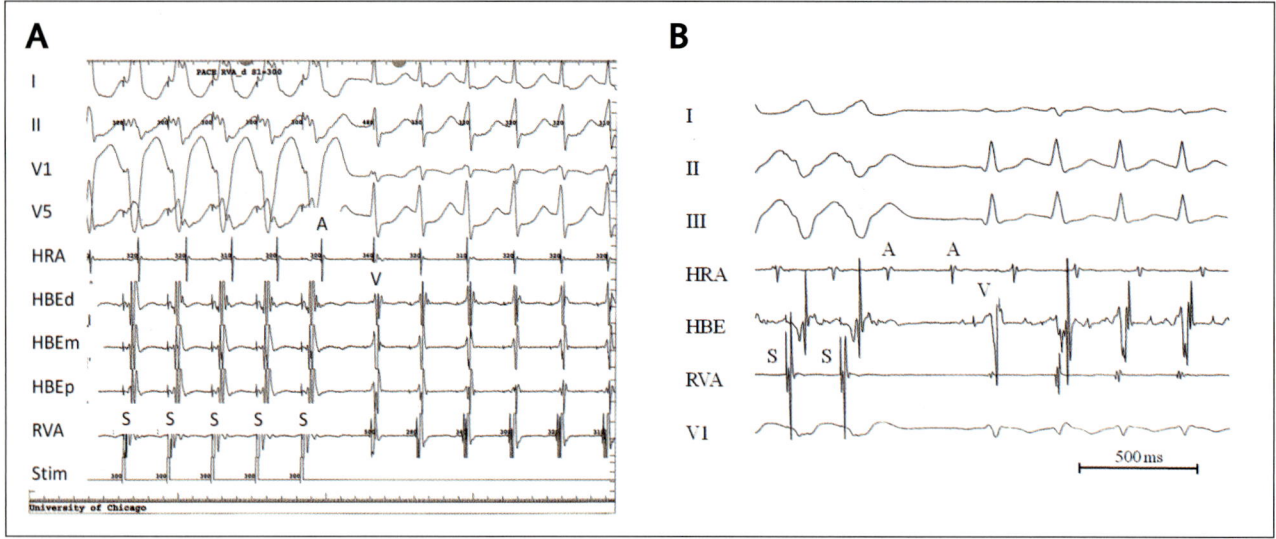

Figure 1.6 A. V-A-V response during AVNRT. During SVT, entrainment is performed from the ventricle. After ensuring that entrainment has occurred, by measuring that the A-A interval is the same as the S-S interval, the return beat is examined. After cessation of pacing, there is evidence of a V-A-V response. With a VA time < 70 ms and a VAV response, the diagnosis of typical (slow-fast) AVNRT is made. **B.** V-A-A-V response during AT. After entrainment from the ventricle is performed, the return beat demonstrates a V-A-A-V response, consistent with AT.

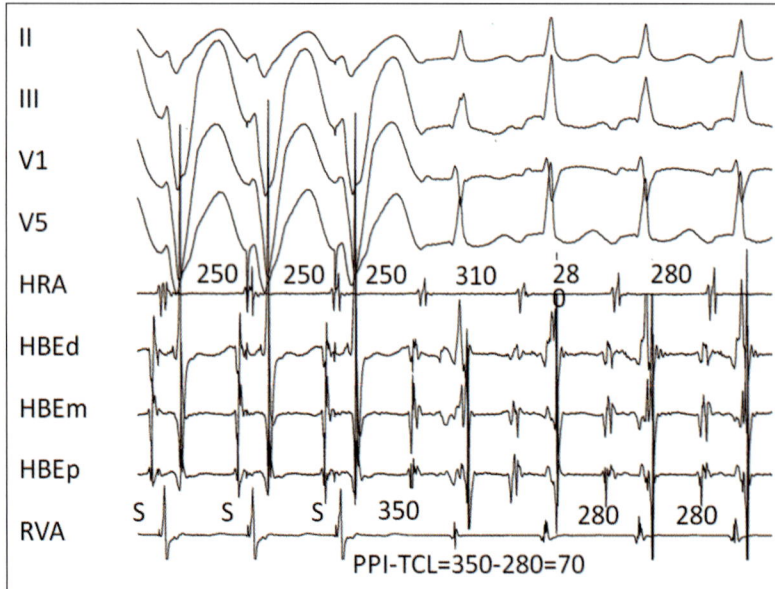

Figure 1.7 Example of long R-P tachycardia with a PPI < 115, consistent with ORT. After ventricular entrainment, the PPI is 350 ms. The PPI-TCL is 70 ms, consistent with ORT using a septal AP.

pathway, while a value > 85 ms suggests atypical AVNRT. The SA-VA time calculation has the benefit of only measuring the differences of VA conduction, whereas the PPI-TCL also takes into account anterograde AV conduction, where decremental properties can falsely prolong the PPI, resulting in an incorrect diagnosis.

If attempts at entrainment result in termination of the tachycardia with no evidence of conduction to the atrium, AT can be excluded as the cause of the tachycardia, as termination could only have occurred by making refractory either an AV nodal pathway or accessory (**Figure 1.8**). Another pacing maneuver employed is pacing the RV at a CL of 200 to 250 ms for 3 to 6 beats to determine if the ventricle can be dissociated from the atrium. If tachycardia persists despite full capture and dissociation of the ventricle, then ORT can be excluded.

His Refractory PVCs

To distinguish between atypical AVNRT and a septal AP, His-refractory PVCs (HRP) can be utilized. During tachycardia, premature ventricular stimuli delivered during His bundle refractoriness can help determine the presence of an AP. In order to deliver an HRP, the PVC should be delivered at the onset of the QRS complex or 30 to 50 ms pre-His. If an HRP results in advancement of atrial

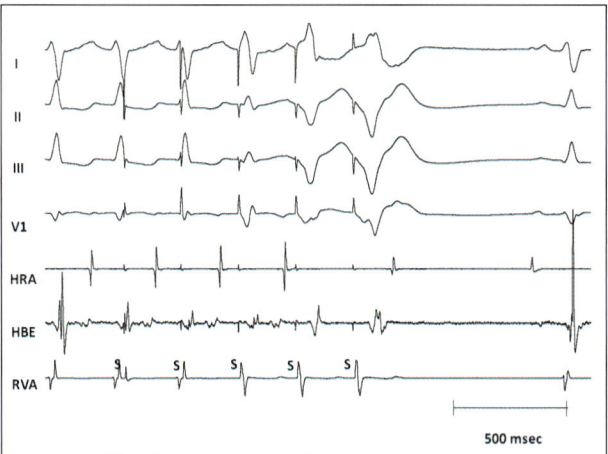

Figure 1.8 In the figure above, the ventricle is paced with evidence of ventricular fusion and full capture of the ventricle on the 4th and 5th beat. The 4th paced beat from the ventricle results in termination of the tachycardia without activation of the atrium, ruling out AT as the mechanism.

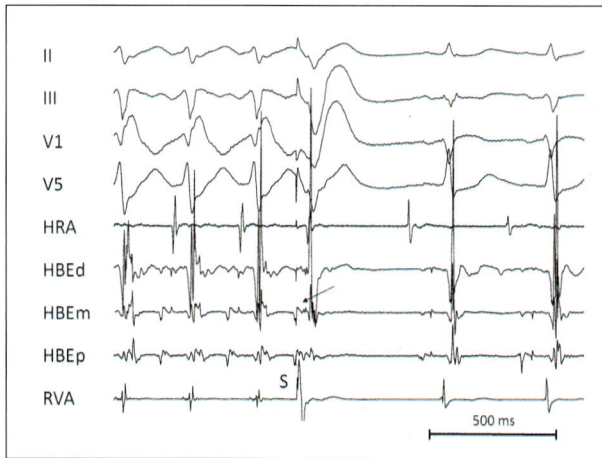

Figure 1.9 A ventricular extrastimuli delivered while the His is refractory. The tachycardia terminates without preexciting the atrium, consistent with AVRT.

activation, an AP is present but does not necessarily prove participation in the tachycardia. If an HRP advances the atrial activation with a change in the activation sequence, the pathway does not participate in the tachycardia. However, an HRP that terminates the tachycardia without preexciting the atrium is diagnostic for an AP that is participating in the tachycardia (**Figure 1.9**).

Atrial Pacing Maneuvers

If a diagnosis is not made after performing ventricular pacing maneuvers, atrial pacing maneuvers are employed. The first atrial pacing maneuver performed is atrial entrainment at 10 to 40 ms shorter than the TCL. The VA interval of the return beat is observed. A fixed VA interval ("VA linking") indicates that the tachycardia is dependent on VA conduction, ruling out AT (**Figure 1.10**). The next pacing maneuver employed is atrial entrainment at the longest CL that results in AV block. The AH interval preceding termination of the tachycardia is observed. If the AH interval at tachycardia termination is longer than the AH interval during tachycardia, this suggests the tachycardia is dependent on AV node conduction, ruling out AT.

Conclusions

Prior to performing ablation, the electrophysiologist must incorporate baseline findings, tachycardia characteristics, and pacing maneuvers in order to properly elucidate the tachycardia mechanism. The combination of 2 tachycardia characteristics, the septal VA time and the retrograde atrial activation, and the utilization of entrainment to determine the return response (eg, A-V vs. A-A-V) provides a diagnosis in 65% of cases. In addition, these maneuvers can also exclude one mechanism in 27% of cases. **Figure 1.11** depicts an algorithm for the rapid diagnosis of PSVT.

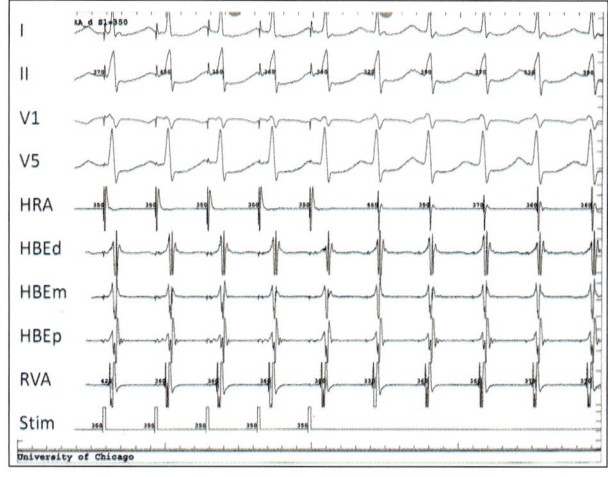

Figure 1.10 VA linking during AVNRT. Atrial entrainment is performed and the first return beat is examined. If the return beat consistently demonstrates the same VA interval as during tachycardia (VA linking), the tachycardia is dependent on AV nodal conduction and the tachycardia mechanism is either AVNRT or AVRT. AT is ruled out, as the tachycardia mechanism is independent of AV nodal conduction.

References

1. Blomstrom-Lundqvist C, Scheinman MM, et al. ACC/AHA/ESC guidelines for the management of patients with supraventricular arrhythmias—executive summary: A report of the American College of Cardiology/American Heart Association Task Force on Practice Guidelines and the European Society of Cardiology Committee for Practice

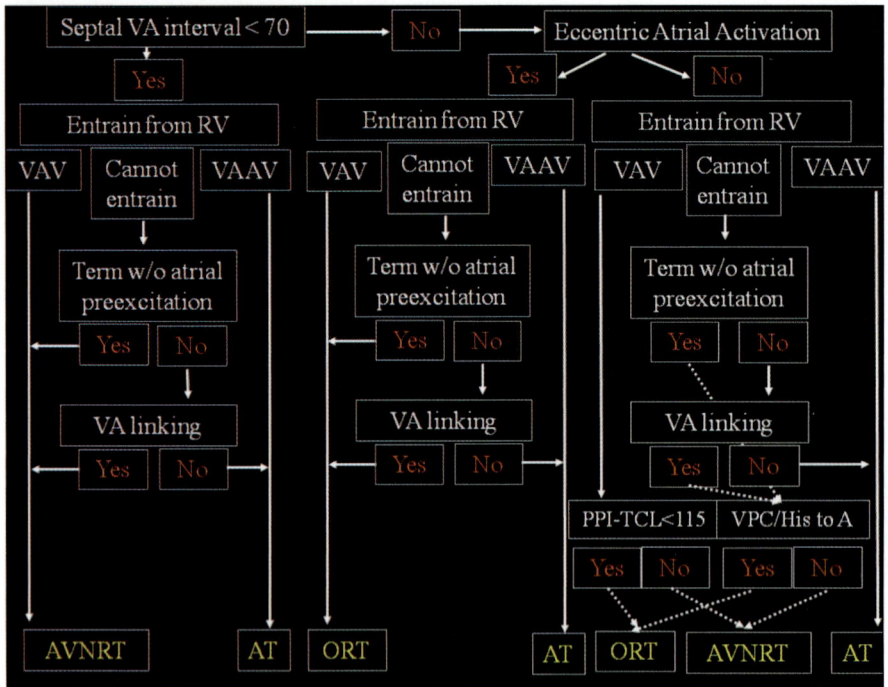

Figure 1.11 Algorithm employed for the rapid diagnosis of PSVT in the EP lab. If the VA time is < 70 ms, entrainment is performed from the RV to differentiate between AVNRT and AT. If the VA time is > 70 ms, retrograde atrial activation sequence is analyzed. If there is eccentric atrial activation, RV entrainment is performed to differentiate between an AVRT and AT. If the VA time is > 70 ms and there is concentric atrial activation, entrainment is performed to differentiate AT from AVNRT and AVRT. If a V-A-V response is present, the observer must differentiate between a septal AP and atypical (fast-slow) AVNRT. If the PPI-TCL is < 115 ms, the tachycardia mechanism is a septal AP. If the PPI-TCL is > 115 ms, the tachycardia mechanism is atypical AVNRT. When ventricular entrainment results in tachycardia termination, entrainment from the atrium can be performed to look for VA linking to differentiate AT from AVNRT and AVRT.

Guidelines (Writing Committee to Develop Guidelines for the Management of Patients With Supraventricular Arrhythmias). *Circulation*. 2003;108(15): 1871–1909.
2. Goyal R, Zivin A, Souza J, et al. Comparison of the ages of tachycardia onset in patients with atrioventricular nodal reentrant tachycardia and AP-mediated tachycardia. *Am Heart J*. 1996;132(4):765–767.
3. Porter MJ, Morton JB, Denman R, et al. Influence of age and gender on the mechanism of supraventricular tachycardia. *Heart Rhythm*. 2004;1(4):393–396.
4. Kalbfleisch SJ, el Atassi R, Calkins H, Langberg JJ, Morady F. Differentiation of paroxysmal narrow QRS complex tachycardias using the 12-lead electrocardiogram. *J Am Coll Cardiol*. 1993;21(1):85–89.
5. Knight BP, Ebinger M, Oral H, et al. Diagnostic value of tachycardia features and pacing maneuvers during paroxysmal supraventricular tachycardia. *J Am Coll Cardiol*. 2000; 36(2):574–582.
6. Yamamoto T, Yeh SJ, Lin FC, Wu DL. Effects of isoproterenol on AP conduction in intermittent or concealed Wolff-Parkinson-White syndrome. *Am J Cardiol*. 1990; 65(22):1438–1442.
7. Souza JJ, Zivin A, Flemming M, et al. Differential effect of adenosine on anterograde and retrograde fast pathway conduction in patients with atrioventricular nodal reentrant tachycardia. *J Cardiovasc Electrophysiol*. 1998;9(8):820–824.
8. Hirao K, Otomo K, Wang X, et al. Parahisian pacing. A new method for differentiating retrograde conduction over an accessory AV pathway from conduction over the AV node. *Circulation*. 1996;94(5):1027–1035.
9. Nakagawa H, Jackman WM. Parahisian pacing: useful clinical technique to differentiate retrograde conduction between accessory atrioventricular pathways and atrioventricular nodal pathways. *Heart Rhythm*. 2005;2(6):667–672.
10. Martinez-Alday JD, Almendral J, et al. Identification of concealed posteroseptal Kent pathways by comparison of ventriculoatrial intervals from apical and posterobasal right ventricular sites. *Circulation*. 1994;89(3):1060–1067.
11. Michaud GF, Tada H, Chough S, et al. Differentiation of atypical atrioventricular node re-entrant tachycardia from orthodromic reciprocating tachycardia using a septal AP by the response to ventricular pacing. *J Am Coll Cardiol*. 2001; 38(4):1163–1167.

CHAPTER 2

How to Ablate Typical and Reverse Atrial Flutter

John C. Evans, MD; Donald D. Hoang, BA; Mintu P. Turakhia, MD, MAS

Introduction

Typical AFL is a right atrial macroreentrant arrhythmia dependent upon conduction across the CTI. AFL is common and relatively refractory to medical therapies for rate and rhythm control. AFL may be an isolated arrhythmia or occur in conjunction with AF. Even when AFL presents in the absence of AF or structural heart disease, it may have serious adverse effects, including stroke and systemic embolism, extreme tachycardia, myocardial ischemia, pulmonary venous congestion, tachycardia-induced cardiomyopathy, and heart failure. Because catheter ablation of typical flutter is generally straightforward, success rates are high and complication rates are quite low. Ablation can also be performed without advanced EP laboratory equipment such as electroanatomic mapping, intracardiac ultrasound, or non-contact mapping catheters, although these tools can be useful in complex cases or when the diagnosis is difficult to establish. For these reasons, catheter ablation of typical AFL is one of the most common procedures performed in invasive cardiac EP.

AFL Terminology

Since its discovery in 1920 by Sir Thomas Lewis,[1] numerous terms have been used to describe AFL. Specifically, these terms have been used to characterize the flutter circuits based on direction of conduction around the tricuspid annulus (*counterclockwise* or *clockwise*), whether it is right- or left-sided, whether its conduction is dependent upon the CTI (*isthmus-dependent* and *non-isthmus dependent*), or a combination of these factors (*typical*, *reverse typical*, *atypical*, *type 1*, *type 2*).[2] In 2001, a consensus document recommended standardized terminology for AFL.[3] CTI-dependent, RA macro-reentrant tachycardia in the counterclockwise direction of propagation around the tricuspid annulus is defined as "typical" AFL. "Reverse typical flutter" is defined as using the same anatomic circuit but propagating in the clockwise direction. For this article, we refer to both typical and reverse forms collectively as AFL.

Anatomy and Physiology

The CTI is bounded anteriorly by the tricuspid annulus and posteriorly by the inferior vena cava Eustachian ridge (**Figure 2.1**). These structures provide anatomical or functional barriers of conduction, which allow for depolarization through a protected zone of slow conduction and propagation of the arrhythmia. Slow conduction is predominantly in the CTI, where conduction may be 30 to 50% of the AFL tachycardia CL.[4] In typical AFL, depolarization of atrial myocardium proceeds from the lateral portions of the isthmus to the medial portions, with continuation up the septal atrium and around the roof. With both the crista terminalis and Eustachian ridge serving as anatomic or functional barriers to conduction, the depolarization

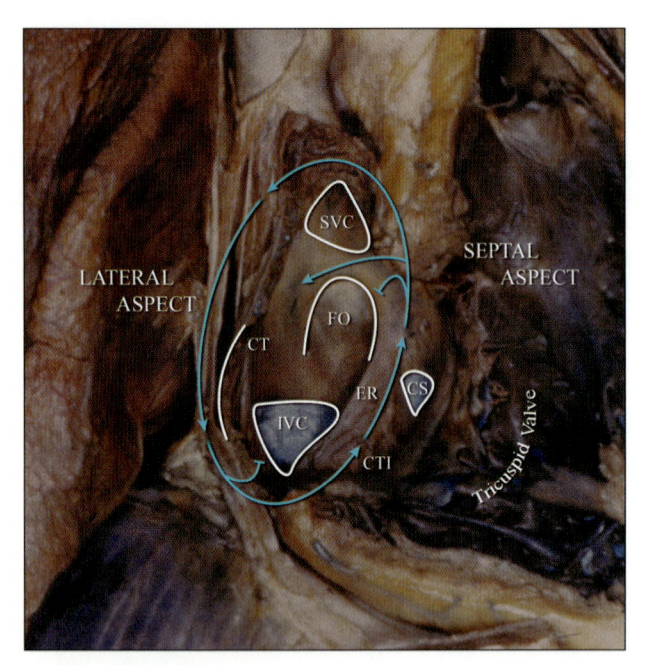

Figure 2.1 Anatomic Figure of circuit. Depolarization proceeds from the lateral portions of the isthmus to the medial portions, up the septal atrium, around the roof, and then anterior to the crista terminalis to reenter the isthmus. (Photograph reprinted with permission from the Stanford Medical History Center.)

wavefront coming around the roof is then funneled anterior to the crista terminalis to reenter the isthmus. Therefore, disruption of conduction across the CTI eliminates the slow conduction that provides an adequate wavelength for reentry relative to atrial conduction velocities[5] and represents the preferred ablation strategy. Sustained bidirectional block across the CTI is the goal and endpoint of the procedure.

ECG Diagnosis

As seen in **Figure 2.2**, typical AFL is classically recognized on the surface 12-lead ECG by regular negative flutter waves in the inferior limb leads (II, III, AVF) and positive flutter waves in V_1.[2,6,7] The atrial rate is typically greater than 240 bpm in the absence of antiarrhythmic drugs. The rate can be slowed in the presence of antiarrhythmic drugs, including both class I and class III antiarrhythmic drugs. QRS widening due to rate-related fascicular block, BBB, or class Ic drug effect may also be observed. Clockwise, or reverse typical flutter (**Figure 2.3**) (using the same anatomic circuit but traveling clockwise around the CTI), is typically described as having positive flutter waves in the inferior leads with a similar CL,[6] but the pattern is much less specific than that of counterclockwise typical flutter.

The classical appearance of 12-lead ECG of typical flutter is specific but not sensitive for a counterclockwise CTI-dependent circuit. The morphology of the flutter waves may markedly different in the setting of a structurally abnormal atrium, as in the case of congenital heart disease or previous cardiac surgery. In these situations, flutter waves may have markedly reduced amplitude in the limb leads, reflecting slow isthmus or interatrial conduction, usually from severe left atrial scar or recurrence after prior isthmus ablation.

Indications for Ablation

The 2003 American Heart Association, American College of Cardiology, and European Society of Cardiology *Guidelines for the Management of Patients with Supraventricular Arrhythmias* address management of primary AFL. These joint guidelines recommend catheter

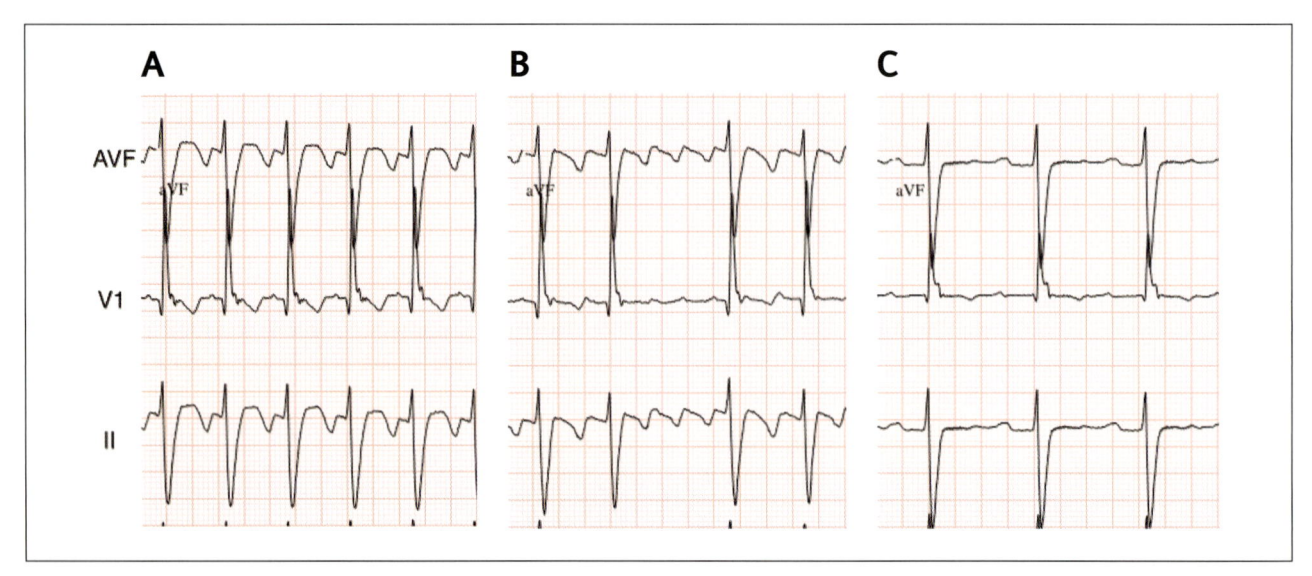

Figure 2.2 Electrocardiogram of a patient with AFL. **A.** Leads AVF, V_1, and II in a patient with a regular narrow complex tachycardia with right BBB and left anterior fascicular block. A small P wave is seen before the QRS, making the tracing appear suspicious for a long RP SVT. **B.** ECG after administration of adenosine. The ventricular rate is slowed and flutter waves are easily discerned. The flutter waves are (+) in V_1 and (−) and II, III (not shown), and AVF, which is consistent with typical counterclockwise CTI dependent flutter. **C.** demonstrated sinus rhythm with persistent bivascular block in sinus rhythm. The P-wave axis has changed and is consistent with sinus rhythm.

ablation for typical flutter that is recurrent or poorly tolerated (class I indication; Level of Evidence: B). The guidelines also assert that it is reasonable to perform catheter ablation for the first episode of well-tolerated typical flutter (class IIa indication; Level of Evidence: B). Catheter ablation is also recommended for AFL appearing after use of class Ic agents or amiodarone for the treatment of AF (class I; Level of Evidence: B).[8]

Following the publication of these guidelines, a randomized controlled clinical trial has compared catheter ablation to amiodarone treatment as a first-line therapy after only one symptomatic episode of AFL.[9] This study showed that, compared to amiodarone therapy, ablation had better long-term success, unchanged risk of subsequent AF, and fewer antiarrhythmic drug side effects. Cardioversion, with or without antiarrhythmic therapy, may still be attempted as the first-line therapy, but this strategy is usually reserved for acute management, as cardioversion alone would not alter the electrophysiologic substrate to prevent recurrence. Antiarrhythmic drug therapy is generally ineffective in preventing or terminating AFL, and the recurrence after cardioversion is extremely high (70–90%).[10]

Adjunctive ablation for typical AFL is generally recommended in patients undergoing ablation for AF who have documented typical AFL as a clinical arrhythmia.[11] Empiric ablation for inducible AFL (without clinical documentation) and prophylactic isthmus ablation in patients with AF is controversial.[12] However, ablation of the CTI in patients treated with class Ic antiarrhythmic agents for AF who organize into AFL is reasonable, particularly since slowed isthmus conduction from class Ic agents may paradoxically result in 1:1 ventricular conduction, particularly in situations of high sympathetic tone.[11]

Preprocedure Planning

Anticoagulation

AFL is believed to confer a stroke risk similar to AF. Therefore, risk stratification and therapy for stroke prevention should parallel management of AF.[6,11] Termination of AFL from catheter ablation should be viewed no differently than cardioversion. Therefore, for patients presenting for the procedure in AFL, a preprocedure TEE should be performed prior to ablation to exclude left atrial thrombus. Alternatively, for patients taking warfarin, documentation of therapeutic anticoagulation for 4 weeks prior and up to the procedure is reasonable to avoid TEE. We prefer to document 4 weekly therapeutic prothrombin time or INR measurements as proof of therapeutic anticoagulation. Dabigatran etexilate is an approved direct thrombin inhibitor that may safely be used prior to cardioversion.[13]

Low-molecular-weight heparin at 0.75 to 1.0 mg/kg every 12 hours may be used for periprocedural anticoagulation bridging with warfarin. Direct thrombin inhibitors

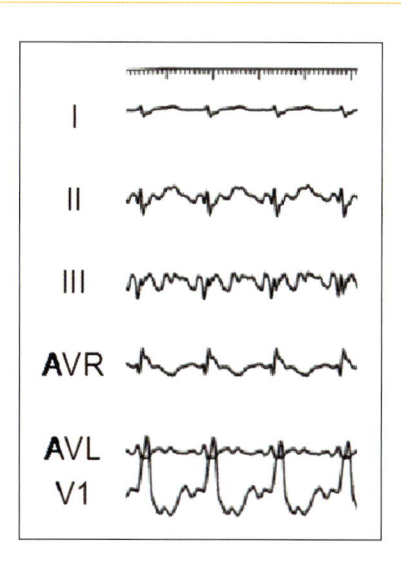

Figure 2.3
Clockwise flutter. The positive flutter wave noted in inferior leads is best seen immediately preceding the QRS complex in lead II.

such as dabigatran may be cost-effective alternatives to warfarin that could eliminate the requirement for bridging with injectable heparin.[14] Several experienced centers and operators have demonstrated the safety and efficacy of performing catheter ablation during therapeutic INRs and without warfarin discontinuation.[15,16] For patients presenting in normal sinus rhythm in whom the ECG diagnosis is classic, diagnostic, and specific for AFL, ablation of the CTI may be performed in sinus rhythm without induction or termination or flutter, potentially obviating the need for TEE. Still, we recommend induction of the clinical arrhythmia unless there are extenuating circumstances.

Procedure

Patient Preparation

We perform CTI ablation on patients in the postabsorptive state, after a fast of at least 6 hours. Due to the short procedure duration, a urinary catheter is typically not required. The majority of our patients undergo CTI ablation with the aid of conscious sedation with fentanyl and midazolam rather than general anesthesia. We emphasize the use of fentanyl because it will aid in pain control when ablating near the IVC, which can be exquisitely painful for many patients.

Vascular Access and Catheter Configuration

It is important to note that there are no systematic comparisons of procedural efficacy between different catheter configurations; thus, catheter configurations vary greatly among operators. There are several catheters that can have a role in CTI ablation. The most important consideration is to ensure that there are sufficient electrodes about the CTI to test for bidirectional block.

For diagnostic catheters, there must be electrodes at various points around the circuit. We favor a comprehensive approach where RA activation can be assessed to determine the full path of the AFL circuit (**Figure 2.4**). A duodecapolar catheter with electrodes extending from the HRA catheter to the inferior RA lateral to the CTI allows for mapping of activation anterior to the crista and may be helpful in identifying flutter variants that break through the crista. A His-bundle catheter can be helpful for both the identification of the septum and as a marker of the His-bundle electrogram for added safety. A CS catheter provides useful information on both left atrial activation, which may change during RF ablation or mimic AFL in coarsely organized fibrillation, and direction of propagation across the atrial septum when compared to a more superiorly located His catheter. Extending electrodes to the left side via the CS also ensures that the left atrium is not an obligatory part of the circuit. Inserting the duodecapolar catheter across the isthmus and into the CS can obviate the need for separate RA and CS catheters, but it can interfere with the ablation catheter as it lies in the isthmus. If this approach is used, careful attention must be used to ensure that the ablation catheter is below any catheter straddling the isthmus for optimum contact and ablation. Finally, a right ventricular catheter is generally not necessary, but it may be useful to preempt pauses or asystole upon termination of AFL in patients with severe sinus node dysfunction. In cases where a preemptive right ventricular catheter has not been placed, pacing from the distal electrodes of the His bundle catheter can be used for backup ventricular pacing.

Vascular access, including the number of catheters, is tailored to each patient's case and depends on catheter configuration and patient preferences. We limit the femoral veins to 3 catheters and the internal jugular to a single access. When a 4-catheter setup is required, using ablator, RA, CS, and His, we defer to patient preference when deciding between placing the CS from the neck with 3 catheters in the groin or dividing up 2 catheters in each groin (**Figure 2.5**). However, the risk of groin complications is most likely reduced when femoral access is obtained from only one side, especially when patients are anticoagulated after the procedure. Unilateral femoral access also better facilitates same-day discharges for elective procedures. To minimize the risk of catheter-associated venous thrombosis, we recommend low-volume infusion of heparinized saline in all vascular access ports. Alternatively, a small intravenous heparin bolus of 30 to 50 U/kg may be given after venous sheaths are in place.

Fluoroscopic Orientation of Catheters

Figure 2.5 demonstrates typical catheter positions for the ablation of the CTI. Fluoroscopy should demonstrate the CS proximal electrode at the CS ostium. More distally placed CS catheters may make it more difficult to ascertain bidirectional isthmus block with differential pacing or to recognize slow residual isthmus conduction. In the LAO view, the proximal CS catheter should be positioned nearly

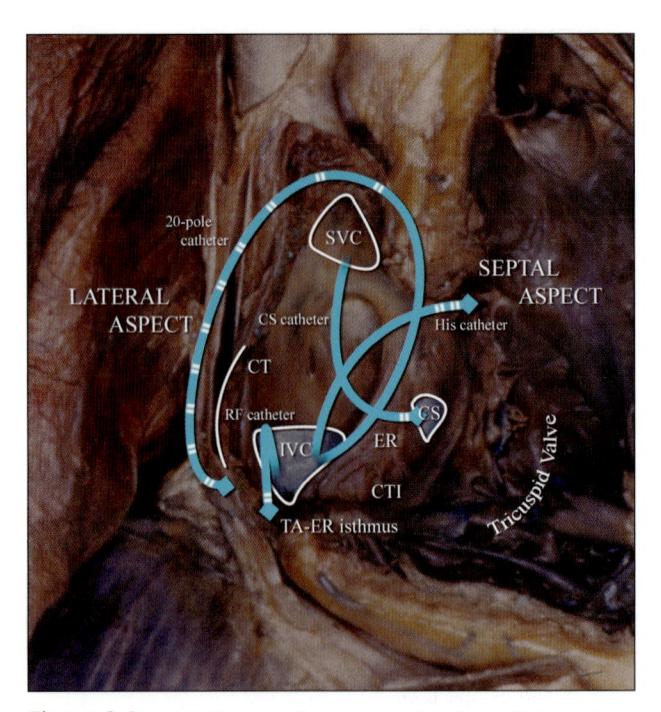

Figure 2.4 LAO diagram of our comprehensive catheter setup. This comprehensive setup allows real-time mapping of the full path of the flutter circuit and can be useful in identifying variants of typical flutter, or secondary atrial arrhythmias after termination of flutter, macroreentrant arrhythmias in which the CTI is not a critical component of the circuit. The duodecapolar or tricuspid annular (TA) catheter has electrodes extending from the HRA medial and anterior to the SVC down to the lateral RA, just anterior to the lower crista terminalis and lateral to the CTI. The His bundle catheter identifies regions of the compact AV node, His bundle, and septum medial to the isthmus. The CS catheter, inserted from a superior approach, provides useful information on left atrial activation, which may change during RF ablation or mimic AFL in coarsely organized fibrillation. This catheter also allows real-time information on the direction of propagation across the atrial septum when compared to a more superiorly located His catheter. Extending electrodes to the left side via the CS also ensures that the left atrium is not an obligatory part of the circuit. The RF catheter is shown at the 6 o'clock position, which is where we recommend making the CTI ablation line. (Photograph reprinted with permission from the Stanford Medical History Center.)

as leftward as the His catheter. The importance of having the crista terminalis catheter placed anteriorly cannot be understated, as the activation patterns can be deceiving with variable block across the crista terminalis. If the catheter is placed too anteriorly, as can happen with some duodecapolar catheters with an anterior bias to facilitate placement, the distal electrodes may extend across the tricuspid annulus and into the right ventricle, which can be identified by electrograms or fluoroscopically. The RAO projection best demonstrates the position of this catheter. In cases with significant RA enlargement or significant tricuspid regurgitation, extra large curves of duodecapolar catheters may improve stability. In cases with a small RA, a standard- or large-curve duodecapolar can often be placed across the CTI and into the proximal CS.

Chapter 2: Ablation of AFL • 15

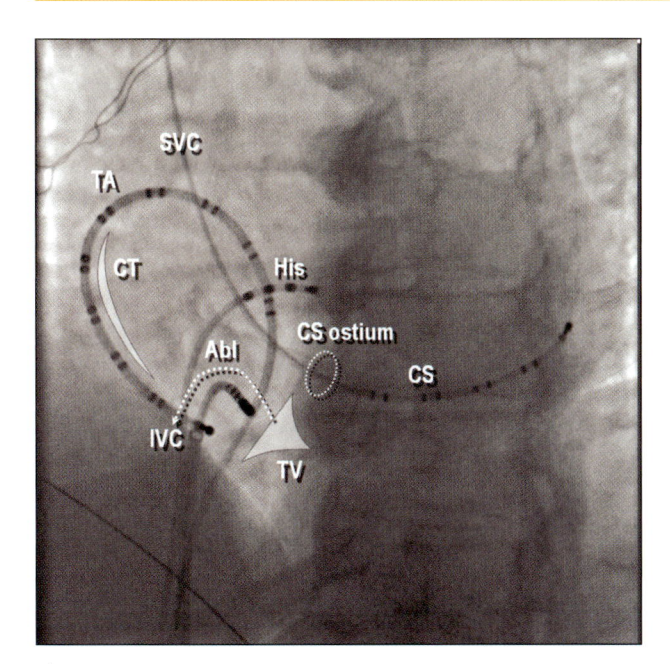

Figure 2.5 Fluoroscopic image of catheters. Partial left anterior oblique fluoroscopic projection of our catheter configuration for typical flutter. The CS catheter (CS) is placed from the right internal jugular vein with the proximal electrodes placed just inside the CS ostium. The CS catheter will help to exclude left-sided tachycardia or left atrial dissociation. The bundle of His catheter (His), right atrial catheter (TA) and ablation catheter (Abl) are all placed from the right femoral vein via 3 separate access sheaths. This approach avoids bilateral groin access, increasing procedural safety and facilitating same-day discharges in uncomplicated cases. The TA catheter is placed to span the septal and lateral walls and positioned just anterior to the crista terminalis (CT). In counterclockwise flutter, TA activation occurs from proximal to distal. The Abl catheter is positioned in the CTI. The dotted line indicates the approximate path of the catheter for placement of the ablation line extending from the tricuspid valve (TV) annulus to the inferior vena cava (IVC). Note the generous distance from the Abl catheter, which is in the medial isthmus, to the His bundle.

Use of Electroanatomic Mapping

For CTI ablation, electroanatomic mapping is not necessary as long as catheters are positioned to ensure appropriate assessment of RA activation and isthmus conduction. Electroanatomic mapping is more useful and recommended in situations where ECG patterns are atypical or when AFL variants such as upper or lower loop reentry may be suspected. Mapping may also be useful in atrial arrhythmias after CTI ablation, as the differential diagnosis is quite broad. Patients with prior RA surgical incisions may harbor complex circuits involving slow conduction across an incision or using an incision as an anatomic barrier of macroreentry.

For straightforward typical flutter, electroanatomic mapping can be used to create an activation map, but it is most useful for in marking catheter potentials, His potentials, and ablation lesions. The position of the His bundle can be noted on an electroanatomical map (**Figure 2.6**), obviating the added safety provided by having a His catheter. The position of the ablation catheter can also be noted to allow the ablation catheter to return to the same location if the operator needs to maneuver around other catheters, such as a duodecapolar catheter, extending across the isthmus and into the CS. This is especially useful in labs that have only monoplace fluoroscopy, where the mapping system can be used to complement a single LAO or RAO view. Marking ablation lesions can also be useful in identifying gaps in the ablation line or in ensuring that a line is continuous, which can be challenging in cases with tortuous or difficult CTI anatomy. In prospective studies, the use of mapping systems has been shown to reduce fluoroscopy times.[17] The mapping system can be used to demonstrate a stable position of the catheter thus reducing and nearly eliminating fluoroscopy exposure.

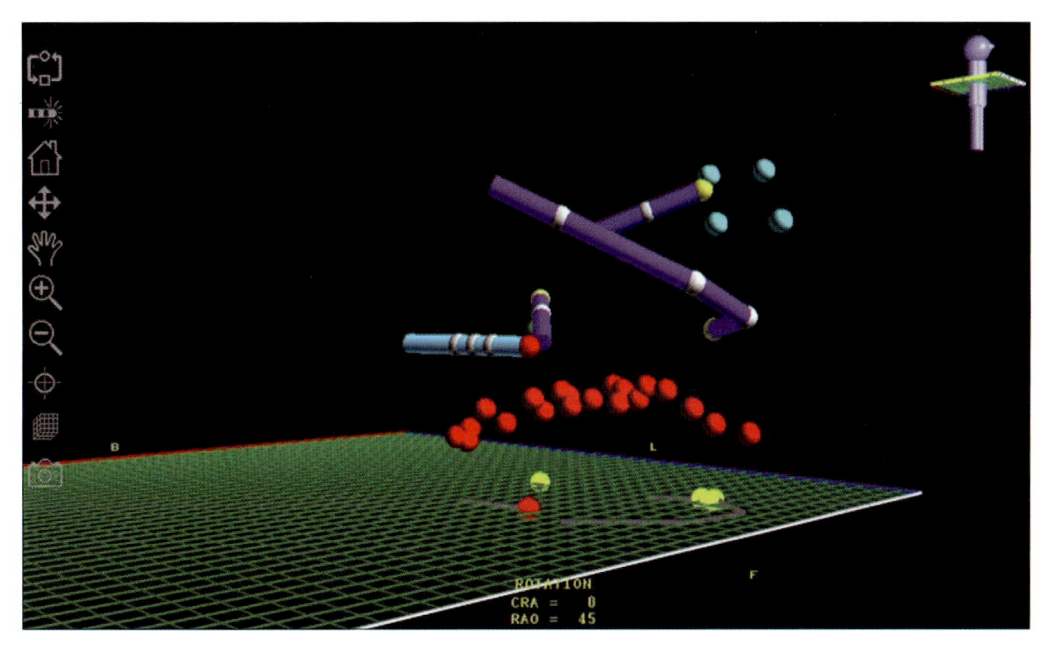

Figure 2.6 Electroanatomical map of ablation lines. The Figure demonstrates the ability of a mapping system to mark the location of catheters, His electrogram positions (blue dots), and ablation lesions (red dots). In this RAO view, the His cloud is seen superior and anterior to the ablation lesions, which span the CTI. Although modern mapping systems can be used to define atrial geometry and even merge radiographic and ultrasound images, these features are typically unnecessary for uncomplicated typical flutter procedures.

Diagnostic Electrophysiologic Study

Initiation of AFL When Presenting in Sinus Rhythm

In patients presenting in normal sinus rhythm, we first pace from the medial and lateral isthmus to confirm rapid transisthmus conduction in both medial-to-lateral (clockwise) and lateral-to-medial (counterclockwise). In those with previous ablation and discernable double potentials, an interval between them < 90 ms was always associated with intact conduction across the isthmus, and an interval ≥ 110 ms was always associated with local block.[18] Slow transisthmus conduction (> 140 ms) does not eliminate the possibility of AFL.[19] The initial transisthmus conduction time is nonetheless useful in patients without previous ablation, because lack of an increase in the transisthmus interval by ≥ 50% in both directions after ablation has an excellent NPV in determining complete bidirectional transisthmus block.[20]

In the cases with slow initial transisthmus conduction times or intermediate intervals between double potentials, we perform differential pacing (described below) to exclude slow transisthmus conduction, which can mimic block. Next, we perform programmed atrial stimulation with atrial overdrive pacing and single extrastimuli from the HRA to define the atrioventricular and atrial conduction properties, including atrioventricular and atrial nodal effective refractory periods. Usually, these maneuvers will not induce AFL.

We will then perform atrial burst pacing at CLs of 250 to 350 ms, or double or triple atrial extrastimuli near that atrial effective refractory period. Most often, these maneuvers will not induce AFL. If these maneuvers fail, then AFL can be induced in any number of ways that exploit the anisotropic conduction properties and functional block of the RA. For example, proximal CS burst pacing, double or triple atrial extrastimuli from the HRA or CS, or sensed extrastimuli from both locations can usually induce flutter. To avoid inadvertent induction of AFL, burst pacing should be performed for only brief periods (3 to 7 seconds); tight coupling intervals (< 160 ms) should be avoided. If AFL is still not induced, we will begin an infusion of isoproterenol, beginning at 1 mcg/min and titrated up by 1 mcg/min until the sinus rate has increased by 10 to 20% of baseline. Isoproterenol can induce other arrhythmias such as AF, which may or may not be clinically significant. Once flutter is induced, we continue as for patients that present in AFL outline below.

Induction and termination of AFL in the laboratory harbors a theoretical risk of left atrial appendage clot embolization, although clinical studies have never directly confirmed this. Therefore, our practice is to attempt to induce tachycardia in all situations except when the clinical, preprocedure ECG shows the highly specific ECG pattern for counterclockwise isthmus-dependent flutter.

AF precludes the determination of CTI block, so in patients who have a history of AF or present to the lab in AF, we will cardiovert with either 1 mg of ibutilide over 10 minutes or with direct current. If only AF rather than AFL is repeatedly induced, then the clinical confidence of the ECG pattern of tachycardia should inform the decision for empiric CTI ablation, AF ablation, or both.

Confirmation of CTI-Dependence in AFL

When the patient presents in AFL or after AFL is induced, we utilize our catheters in the RA, specifically the catheters along the crista terminalis, CTI, proximal CS and His to see that the majority of the CL is represented (**Figure 2.7**). Ideally, we will entrain the tachycardia from the CTI with pacing at a CL 10 to 20 ms shorter than tachycardia CL to ensure that there is concealed entrainment with intracardiac activation during pacing matching that during tachycardia and that the PPI is less than 20 ms greater than the tachycardia CL (**Figure 2.8**).

Confirmation of concealed entrainment must be performed carefully and meticulously. First, entrainment must be confirmed by ensuring that the tachycardia CL matches the paced CL. Next, the PPI or return cycle must be measured from the electrogram of the pacing electrode to the first intrinsic deflection of tachycardia. When pacing from within the flutter circuit, the PPI is generally within 10 ms

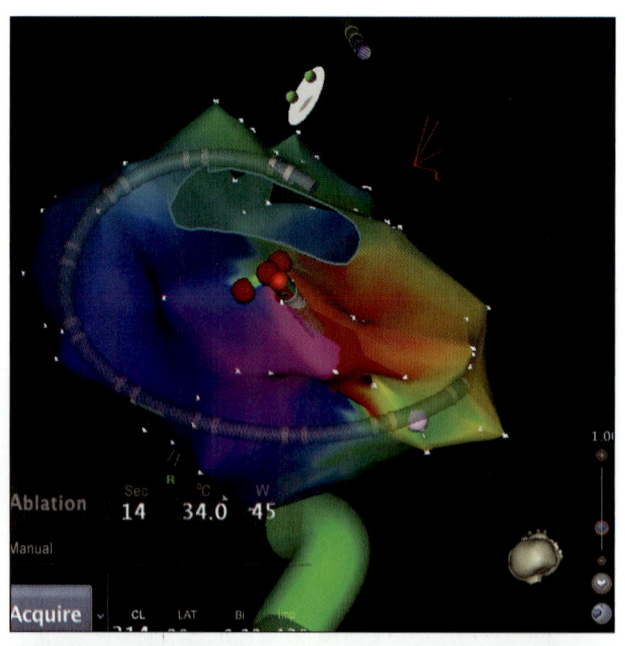

Figure 2.7 Activation of typical flutter is shown in this LAO caudal view of an electroanatomical activation map of the RA obtained during AFL. The duodecapolar catheter location is seen, as well as the ablation catheter with the initial ablation lesions (red) performed anteriorly at the tricuspid annulus. Reentry is inferred from electroanatomic maps based on 2 criteria: the timing from earlier to latest spans over 90% of the tachycardia CL; early and late activation meet, suggesting reentry. Early and late activation do not have to meet in the CTI but should meet over a critical part of the flutter circuit. Typically over 60% of the flutter CL is subtended by the CTI. These mapping features are consistent, but not diagnostic for reentry, for which entrainment mapping remains the gold standard.

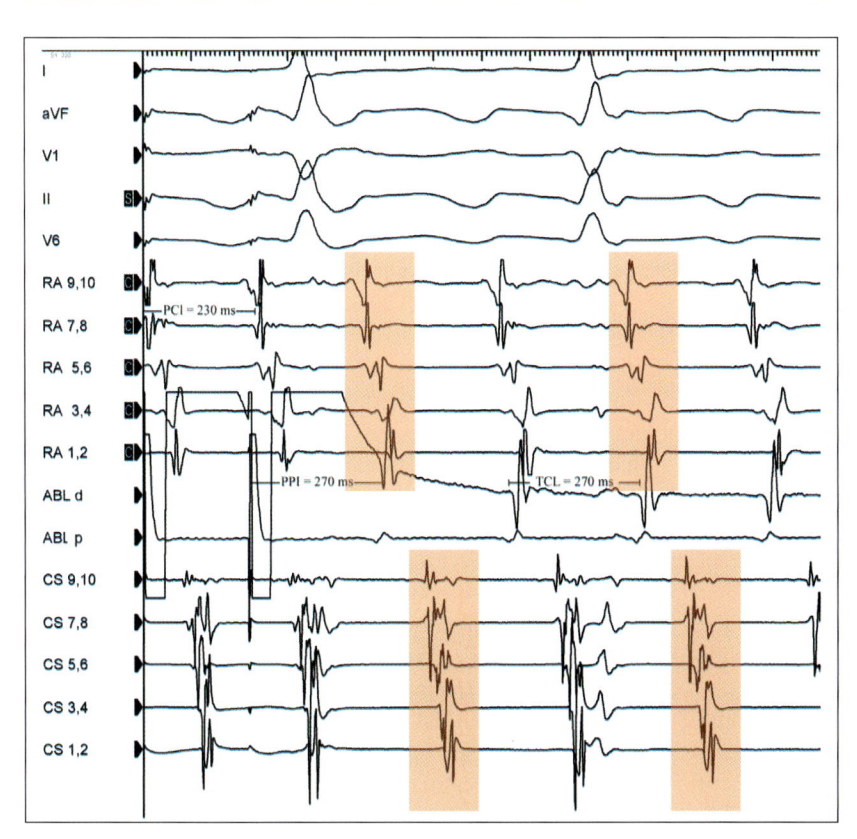

Figure 2.8 Entrainment with concealed fusion. While in tachycardia, the heart was paced from the ablation catheter located in the 6 o'clock position of the CTI. Prior to pacing, atrial activation extends from the high lateral RA wall (RA 9,10) and then to the proximal CS (CS 9,10) followed by late left atrial activation. This pattern is consistent but not diagnostic with the counterclockwise wavefront seen in typical, counterclockwise flutter. Burst pacing at a CL of 230 ms accelerates the tachycardia CL (TCL) from 270 ms to the pacing CL (PCL). Although the surface P-wave pattern is difficult to discern due to overlying T wave, concealed fusion is identified by the identical intracardiac activation (RA 10-1, CS 10-1) of the last paced beat and the tachycardia (highlighted in orange). With the cessation of pacing, the postpacing interval (PPI) or return CL, as measured from the pacing source (ablation catheter), is 270 ms, which is identical to the TCL. The finding of concealed entrainment is diagnostic that the pacing site in the CTI is in the circuit.

of the tachycardia CL, but this can prolong in many patients when the entrainment pacing is performed at CLs more than 10 ms shorter than the flutter CL due to decremental conduction. Finally, concealed entrainment is confirmed by ensuring constant fusion in which both the intracardiac activation and surface flutter waves during entrained pacing are identical to spontaneous activation in tachycardia.[21]

It is very important to note that the activation remains the same before and after entrainment pacing, as the rhythm can change with the maneuver, but when there are multiple arrhythmias, it is often helpful to ablate isthmus-dependent flutter in order to reproducibly map the other rhythms. The other risk of entraining flutter is that it also can induce AFL even when properly performed at only 10 ms shorter than tachycardia CL. In cases of flutter with slow conduction across the isthmus, decremental conduction may make it difficult to prove concealed entrainment based on return CLs and activation. For these cases, we recommend careful and meticulous pacing of only 5 ms below the tachycardia CL.

Ablation

Ablation Catheter Selection

Multiple types of ablation catheters and energy sources may be used for flutter ablation, ranging from traditional RF catheters and irrigated-tip RF catheters to cryoenergy catheters. Most of these catheters are available in a variety of electrode size, curvatures, and mapping system compatibility. The use of RF for energy delivery is the standard in performing CTI. An irrigated-tip catheter allows greater power delivery for larger lesions with the advantage of a smaller tip for finer mapping. Irrigated-tip catheters may have an advantage or better power delivery when contact is excessive due to isthmus ridges, for which convective cooling from circulatory blood flow may be inadequate for heat dissipation with nonirrigated catheters. In a randomized trial, the irrigated-tip catheter has been shown to be as safe as and more effective than conventional catheters in the ablation of the CTI.[22] For traditional RF catheters, we recommend avoiding 4-mm-electrode-size catheters and prefer using 8-mm or 10-mm electrode sizes. The advantage of larger-electrode catheters is more power delivery over a greater electrode area. The disadvantage is poor signal resolution, particularly with 10-mm electrodes. Sustained bidirectional block has also been demonstrated with cryoablation.[23] Proponents of cryoablation note that there is no pain with delivery of the lesions.

The curve of the catheter is selected based on several factors: (1) length of the isthmus (large curve if isthmus is long); (2) orientation of tricuspid annulus relative to IVC (avoid large curve if angle is acute). A bidirectional catheter with an asymmetric curve (standard and large curves) may afford the greatest flexibility. If a bidirectional catheter is not available or manufactured, then we recommend a large curve on our ablation catheter to access the isthmus. The deflectable catheter is passed into the ventricle and pulled back in the 6 o'clock position on the tricuspid annulus until there is a sharp atrial electrogram in the distal ablator. Moderate- or large-sized RA typically need sheaths to provide reach to the 6 o'clock position at the annulus (in the LAO view) because the catheter will otherwise have a tendency to back away from the isthmus to the posterior RA and posterior IVC. This may also occur in patients with normal-sized RA who have fairly distal and anterior tricuspid valves and right ventricular inflow tracts.

Once reaching the 6 o'clock position in the LAO view, we rehearse the creation of an ablation line by slowly pulling back the catheter to the IVC, noting any jumps in catheter position during the pullback. The contour of the isthmus is interrogated at the site of jumps. If there appears to be good contact with sharp electrograms throughout the pullback, we will again go to the 6 o'clock position on the annulus to begin ablation. In some patients, the catheter may have a tendency to go excessively medially or laterally. If there is difficulty with contact or stability during the pullback, a long sheath will be used because it can provide stability of location on the CTI as well as reach.

A sheath will generally provide greater stability and contact, even in patients with structurally normal hearts and unremarkable chamber dimensions. The choice of sheath depends on operator preference and the area of difficulty. An SR0 sheath can be used to orient the catheter anteriorly and is helpful in reaching the anterior portion of the isthmus if that is the site of difficulty. When a 180-degree bend on the catheter to reach the depths of the pouch and the anterior edge of a ridge is needed, a RAMP sheath can help provide stability throughout this maneuver. An SAFL sheath can be used to navigate both of these issues but can have a tendency to orient the catheter more septally (4 to 5 o'clock position in the LAO) than desired. In cases of complex isthmus anatomy, multiple sheaths may be required during ablation of different segments of the isthmus.

Ablation Technique

There are several approaches to isthmus ablation. Technique selection is best guided by operator experience and preference. The first approach is a "drag-and-burn" technique, in which the catheter is moved continuously to create a linear isthmus burn during a prolonged application of RF energy. Using an irrigated-tip catheter to make a linear line with point lesions, we begin with 30 W of energy and titrate to a maximum of 45 W, with a maximum temperature of 42°C and irrigation flow rate of 30 ml/second. The catheter is slowly moved in 2- to 4-mm increments once electrogram amplitude and slew rate are diminished on the distal electrode. We use the electrogram on the proximal electrode to guide the target site of where to move the distal electrode and will stop once the proximal electrode signal is seen on the distal electrode, being careful to avoid any gaps in the ablation line. With open irrigated catheters, impedance drops of 10 ohms usually confirm successful power delivery.

The second technique is a "spot burn" technique, where a series of consecutive point burns are used to create a linear isthmus line. This technique may be more useful in cases of complex isthmus anatomy where a simple "drag and burn" approach could lead to gaps in the ablation line around crests or ridges of the isthmus. With the 60-second lesion delivery, we will typically see an impedance drop of approximately 10 ohms with an open irrigated catheter that occurs in the first 20 to 30 seconds of ablation. The catheter is moved to target the proximal electrogram signal in much the same way as the "drag and burn" technique. Finally, some operators will perform electrogram-guided point ablation, only ablating the large and active points along the line until bidirectional block is achieved.[24]

When approaching the IVC-RA junction at the proximal isthmus, we may reduce the power delivery because this area is highly innervated with nerves and ablation may be quite painful. Prophylactic fentanyl administration, if safe, may reduce pain during RF application in this area.

When the initial pre-ablation drag is performed to assess for the need for a sheath, it is important to identify prominent ridges or pouches. The line should be moved accordingly. For prominent pouches, it may be easier to ablate more laterally, and for prominent pectinate musculature, a more medial approach may be easier.

For patients in normal sinus rhythm at the start of ablation, we will typically perform ablation while pacing from the proximal CS to be able to identify a change in activation around the CTI suggestive of block. For patients in AFL, we will ablate in the rhythm. Often, the TCL can be seen to prolong with each lesion. When the tachycardia breaks during ablation, we will typically mark this site and deliver an extra lesion very close to the lesion that broke the tachycardia. Termination of tachycardia does not imply bidirectional block. In fact, AFL may terminate in response to atrial or ventricular premature complexes associated with ablation or catheter manipulation. Therefore, when tachycardia terminates, it is useful to confirm termination in the isthmus (usually between the crista and CS electrodes), especially when preceded by flutter CL prolongation that is driven by isthmus conduction time prolongation. Once AFL terminates, we will pace from the CS to assess for block while completing the remainder of the isthmus line.

If atrial activation does not change with CS pacing or if AFL does not terminate, then we will continue the line to the IVC. When there does not appear to be block after the initial line, we interrogate the line, focusing on gaps in the electroanatomical map if available. We look for remaining atrial signal along the line and especially for fractionated signals. In areas of previous ablation, it is often possible to see double potentials along the line. These double potentials can be followed to narrowing between the potentials to find the site of residual conduction.

Procedural Endpoints for Ablation

Even when a patient is ablated in flutter and the rhythm terminates, the standard endpoint for ablation is bidirectional block across the CTI. There are several methods to determine if bidirectional block is present. All methods attempt to ascertain the direction of conduction to the opposite site of the isthmus (medial to lateral; lateral to medial). There are no systematic or head-to-head data reviewing the prognostic performance of each of these maneuvers. All maneuvers are fairly specific for confirmation of block. However, each of them has theoretical limitations in certain circumstances, thereby decreasing sensitivity for identification of residual isthmus conduction or leaks. Using several methods together can therefore increase sensitivity while maintaining high specificity.

In the simplest methods to confirm isthmus block, pacing is performed both medial and lateral to the line to note activation (**Figure 2.9**). With medial to lateral block, the activation should be high to low along the crista terminalis. The activation should always be toward the line of block once on the lateral isthmus if there is medial to lateral block. Likewise, with lateral pacing, there should be delay before activation of the medial isthmus and the CS. The atrial electrogram on the His bundle catheter should be activated prior to the proximal CS or medial isthmus. If there is breakthrough across the crista allowing activation in the mid crista prior to the HRA, then isthmus conduction may occur prior or on time with electrodes away from the line of block.

Differential Pacing

Differential pacing is a more sensitive method to exclude slow conduction or leaks across the isthmus and therefore confirm complete isthmus block. When block is present, the local activation gets shorter, moving away from the line when pacing on the opposite side of the line (**Figure 2.10**).[25] We typically wait for 30 minutes after the last RF lesion delivery to ensure that block has been maintained.

Troubleshooting

If the patient remains in atrial arrhythmia after completion of the CTI line, 2 possibilities must be considered: (1) ablation of tissue has been inadequate; and (2) CTI is not part of the circuit. To exclude these factors, the activation sequence should be carefully evaluated again to ensure

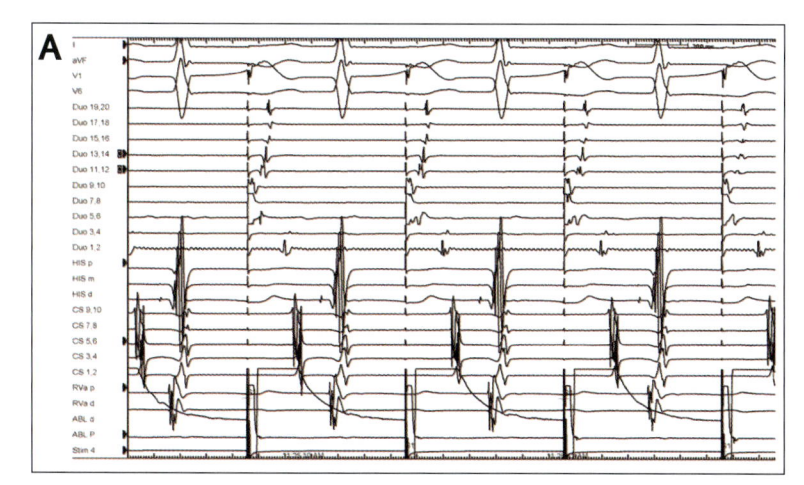

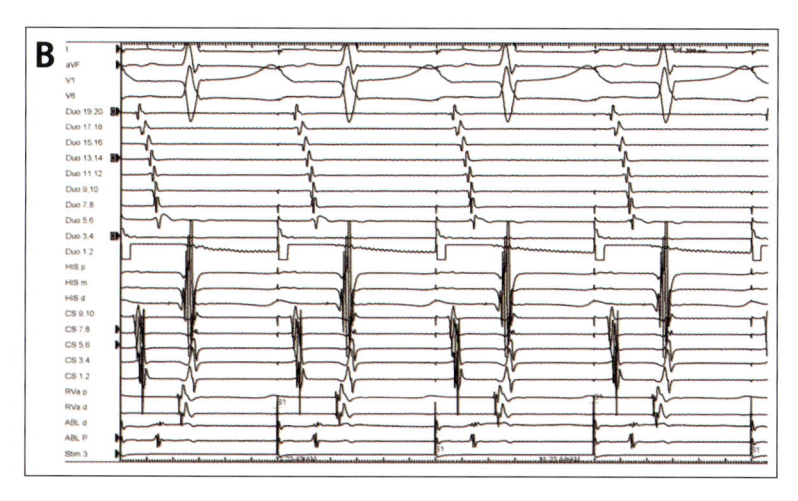

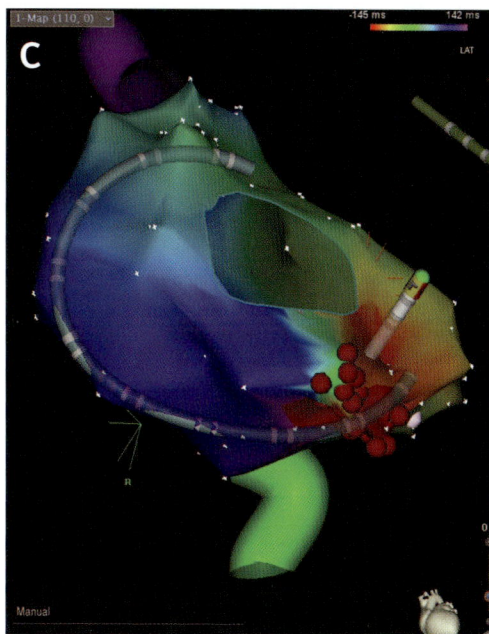

Figure 2.9 Bidirectional block. **A.** Lateral to medial block. Pacing from the ablation catheter lateral to the line demonstrates activation proceeding progression up the RA catheter sequentially from Duo 5,6 to Duo 19,20 and then the His catheter prior to reaching the CS electrodes. **B.** Medial to lateral block. Pacing in the distal duodecapolar catheter, medial to the ablation line, leads to activation proceeding along the crista from Duo 19,20 to Duo 5,6 at the line of block. **C.** Activation map confirming flutter. With medial pacing, the latest activation in the RA is just lateral to the line of block.

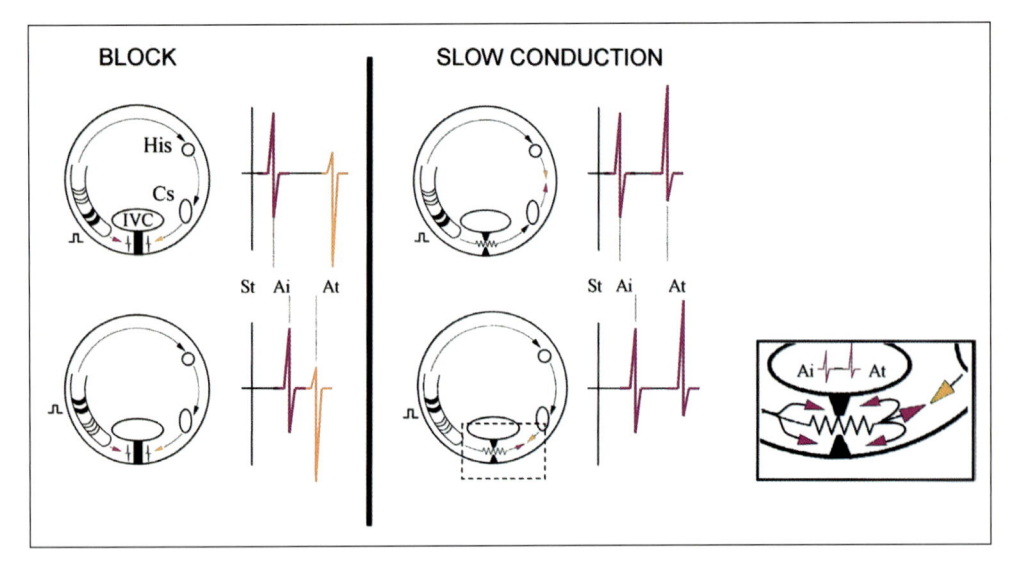

Figure 2.10 Differential pacing. Schematic representation of activation principles on which assessment is based. RA and selected key structures (IVC, His bundle, CS ostium [Cs]) are shown in a cartoon format. A quadripolar catheter is shown positioned as in Figure 2.1, and activation is pictured during distal bipole stimulation (top row) and proximal bipole stimulation (bottom row). Shown are activation patterns during complete isthmus block (left) and during persistent but slow isthmus conduction through a gap in ablation line (right). During complete isthmus block, double potentials separated by an isoelectric interval are recorded on ablation line as a result of 2 opposing fronts: a descending front (shown in pink) and another that detours around isthmus (in orange) give rise to double potentials Ai (initial potential) and At (terminal potential) (pink and orange, respectively). On changing to a proximal stimulation site, descending wavefront (in pink) has to travel a longer distance to reach line of block, whereas detouring wavefront (in orange) has a shorter distance to travel; as a result Ai (pink potential) is delayed and At (orange potential) is anticipated. During persistent isthmus conduction through a gap in ablation line, double potentials are recorded as a result of delayed activation of downstream isthmus by same pink front, and therefore both resulting potentials (Ai and At) are shown in pink (inset, far right). When stimulation is performed from a proximal site, activation pattern does not change, but descending wavefront (in pink) has a longer distance to travel to reach isthmus line; as a result, both pink potentials (Ai and At) are delayed. St indicates stimulus artifact. (Figure and legend reprinted with permission from: Shah D, et al. *Circulation*. 2000;102:1517.)

that there was no unnoticed change in activation sequence during ablation. Activation change may signify another circuit or reversal of the same typical flutter circuit. Often, with incomplete ablation of the CTI, the activation sequence will remain unchanged, but the CL of the tachycardia will prolong due to further slowing of conduction across the isthmus.

Next, entrainment should be repeated at both the medial and lateral CTI to ensure that both locations remain part of the circuit. If either medial or lateral isthmus has a long PPI, the circuit will need to be defined. When both have long PPIs, the activation will likely have changed, and the rhythm cannot be treated with CTI ablation. Attention can return to the isthmus for bidirectional block once the rhythm is terminated by either ablation or cardioversion. When one side of the isthmus remains in the circuit but the other is out, it may indicate intra-isthmus reentry or another circuit. With intra-isthmus reentry, consolidation of the flutter line on the side with PPI approximately equal to TCL may terminate the rhythm. If both medial and lateral isthmus remain in the circuit, attention must be focused on the adequacy of lesion delivery.

Inadequate ablation at the isthmus should lead the operator to evaluate lesion delivery. Troubleshooting should start with an evaluation of energy delivery. Problems with equipment or contact should have been noticed during the formation of the line with a lack of impedance changes and signal reduction at the sites of ablation. Attention should be paid to any potential gaps. These are much more likely to occur in ridges and gullies, which can be addressed with different catheter curves or sheaths.

When conduction continues across the isthmus, there are several approaches to successfully achieve block. If an electroanatomical mapping system has been used for the procedure, it can help to identify gaps in the line and can thus be used for a focused search when there does not appear to be block when the line is first completed. Even without electroanatomical mapping, the ablation line can be consolidated by adding a line of lesions either immediately medial or lateral to the line. If there are prominent muscular ridges due to the pectinates, we recommend going slightly medial to the original line, as the isthmus typically becomes smoother more medially. If a prominent pouch has been found, it is often less deep laterally, and therefore ablating slightly laterally to the original line may be useful. It can be helpful to change the rhythm to see the signals differently. In sinus rhythm, the CS pacing can be stopped to see an alternate activation. Likewise, flutter can be converted to sinus rhythm for sinus rhythm mapping if the gaps cannot be identified. Finally, these techniques can fail when there are small crevices on the isthmus that are not apparent with the catheter, and in these cases, with the electroanatomical mapping, a fine activation map can be constructed to identify the gaps. This approach is often much more time consuming than using the local signals, so it is reserved for when the line has been consolidated and there are no telling local signals.

When the patient is in sinus rhythm after completion of the line or terminating flutter with ablation, the main focus of troubleshooting is determining why bidirectional block across the isthmus has not been achieved. First and foremost, the appropriateness of catheter positions should be reconfirmed to make sure that the catheters are anterior to the crista terminalis for repeat testing for block. A catheter behind the crista can make it appear as though there is no block when one really is present. When the lack of bidirectional block is confirmed, it means that there is some gap along the line that can be approached the same as when patients remain in flutter.

Postprocedure Care

After a 30-minute waiting period of achieving bidirectional block, all catheters and sheaths are removed. Patients will typically lie flat for 4 to 6 hours after sheaths are pulled. For the patients who have had AFL or fibrillation in the preceding 48 hours, including those who were induced in the lab, we begin anticoagulation 6 to 8 hours after sheaths are pulled. We administer low-molecular-weight heparin (0.75 to 1.0 mg/kg twice a day) to maintain stroke prophylaxis and minimize bleeding complications until the warfarin is therapeutic. In patients without an indication for anticoagulation, we will typically administer one dose of 40 mg for venous thromboembolism prophylaxis. Patients are usually discharged on the same or next day. For patients who undergo the procedure with a therapeutic INR, low-molecular-weight heparin is not required. For patients presenting in sinus rhythm and at low risk of stroke, warfarin may be restarted without heparin bridging.

Follow-Up

Patients are typically seen 4 to 6 weeks after ablation. In patients without concomitant AF, anticoagulation can be stopped if it had been indicated for treatment of atrial flutter. In those with AF, we continue to use the CHADS2 score to guide anticoagulation for stroke risk. In patients who had a history of both AF and flutter, sinus rhythm may be easier to maintain with antiarrhythmic drugs, and rate control is typically much easier in AF than in AFL. Ambulatory ECG monitoring may be useful to evaluate for AF, even if patients are asymptomatic.

Repeat Ablation

Recurrence rates in the published literature vary from 80 to 100%.[2] However, if the diagnosis of typical flutter is correctly made, if entrainment mapping is performed to verify isthmus involvement, and if bidirectional block is carefully assessed with differential pacing after ablation, then the recurrence rate for CTI flutter is likely below 1%. Repeat ablation is performed with a focus on gaps, but we most often will perform another line to start the procedure.

Procedural Complications

Because the RA is a thin-walled structure, pericardial irritation manifesting as chest dullness can occur after the procedure. Pericarditis and effusions without hemodynamic compromise are sometimes noted following the procedure. Most asymptomatic effusions can be managed conservatively. Since many patients are anticoagulated following the procedure, the most common complications are vascular, including hematoma and arteriovenous fistulae. Less than 0.5% of patients suffer from a cerebrovascular accident. It is worth mentioning that the right coronary artery runs posterior to the CTI. If tissue heating during RF leads to heating or thermal injury of the vessel, then right coronary infarction may occur. This may be more common in situations where right coronary flow is already diminished (concomitant coronary stenosis or collateral grafts to right coronary artery). In these situations, the diminished flow may lead to decreased convective cooling of the ablation catheter tip, which paradoxically will lead to increased thermal injury and possibly vascular damage.

In patients with pacemakers and defibrillators, care must be taken to avoid dislodgement or damage to the leads. Pacing and sensing thresholds and fluoroscopic position should be checked before and after the start of the procedure.

Limitations of Ablation for Typical Flutter

For management of AFL, catheter ablation has many advantages over pharmacotherapy. As discussed earlier, recurrence rates are high with drug therapy, and the rate in AFL is often difficult to control. AFL ablation success rates are very high when performed carefully by experienced operators. However, the main limitation is that a large number of patients, approximately 30%, will develop other atrial arrhythmia within 2 years.

Conclusions

Radiofrequency catheter ablation has evolved to be a first-line treatment for typical flutter. CTI ablation is a safe, effective, and curative treatment for AFL that can be used as first-line therapy. The most effective approach for ablation is one in which atrial activation is carefully mapped with comprehensive catheter placement, isthmus conduction is confirmed, and bidirectional block is carefully assessed after ablation. Computerized electroanatomical mapping systems and irrigated ablation catheters are not essential but may be useful in difficult cases.

References

1. Lewis T, Feil HS, Stroud WD. Observations upon flutter and fibrillation. Part II: The nature of auricular flutter. *Heart*. 1920;7:191–245.
2. Sawhney NS, Anousheh R, Chen W-C, Feld GK. Diagnosis and management of typical atrial flutter. *Cardiol Clinics*. 2009;27(1):55–67.
3. Saoudi N, Cosio F, Waldo A, et al. Classification of atrial flutter and regular atrial tachycardia according to electrophysiologic mechanism and anatomic bases: a statement from a Joint Expert Group from the Working Group of Arrhythmias of the European Society of Cardiology and the North American Society of Pacing and Electrophysiology. *J Cardiovascular Electrophysiol*. 2001;12(7):852–866.
4. Kinder C, Kall J, Kopp D, Rubenstein D, Burke M, Wilber D. Conduction properties of the inferior vena cava-tricuspid annular isthmus in patients with typical atrial flutter. *J Cardiovascular Electrophysiol*. 1997;8(7):727–737.
5. Olgin JE, Kalman JM, Fitzpatrick AP, Lesh MD. Role of right atrial endocardial structures as barriers to conduction during human Type I atrial flutter: Activation and entrainment mapping guided by intracardiac echocardiography. *Circulation*. 1995;92(7):1839–1848.
6. Fuster V, Ryden LE, Cannom DS, et al. ACC/AHA/ESC 2006 guidelines for the management of patients with atrial fibrillation: A report of the American College of Cardiology/American Heart Association Task Force on Practice Guidelines and the European Society of Cardiology Committee for Practice Guidelines (Writing Committee to Revise the 2001 Guidelines for the Management of Patients with Atrial Fibrillation): developed in collaboration with the European Heart Rhythm Association and the Heart Rhythm Society. *Circulation*. 2006;114(7):e257–e354.
7. Poty H, Saoudi N, Nair M, Anselme F, Letac B. Radiofrequency catheter ablation of atrial flutter: Further insights into the various types of isthmus block: Application to ablation during sinus rhythm. *Circulation*. 1996;94(12):3204–3213.
8. Blomstrom-Lundqvist C, Scheinman MM, Aliot EM, et al. ACC/AHA/ESC guidelines for the management of patients with supraventricular arrhythmias—executive summary: A report of the American College of Cardiology/American Heart Association Task Force on Practice Guidelines and the European Society of Cardiology Committee for Practice Guidelines (Writing Committee to Develop Guidelines for the Management of Patients with Supraventricular Arrhythmias). *Circulation*. 2003;108(15):1871–1909.
9. Da Costa A, Thevenin J, Roche F, et al. Results from the Loire-Ardeche-Drome-Isere-Puy-de-Dome (LADIP) Trial on atrial flutter, a multicentric prospective randomized study comparing amiodarone and radiofrequency ablation after the first episode of symptomatic atrial flutter. *Circulation*. 2006;114(16):1676–1681.
10. Natale A, Newby KH, Pisanó E, et al. Prospective randomized comparison of antiarrhythmic therapy versus first-line radiofrequency ablation in patients with atrial flutter. *J Am Coll Cardiol*. 2000;35(7):1898–1904.
11. Camm AJ, Kirchhof P, Lip GYH, et al. Guidelines for the management of atrial fibrillation. *Eur Heart J*. 2010;31(19):2369–2429.
12. Calkins H, Brugada J, Packer DL, et al. HRS/EHRA/ECAS expert consensus statement on catheter and surgical ablation of atrial fibrillation: Recommendations for personnel, policy, procedures and follow-up. *Europace*. 2007;9(6):335–379.
13. Nagarakanti R, Ezekowitz MD, Oldgren J, et al. Dabigatran versus warfarin in patients with atrial fibrillation: An analysis of patients undergoing cardioversion. *Circulation*. 2011;123(2):131–136.
14. Freeman JV, Zhu RP, Owens DK, et al. Cost-effectiveness of dabigatran compared with warfarin for stroke prevention in atrial fibrillation. *Ann Intern Med*. 2011;154(1):1–11.
15. Wazni OM, Beheiry S, Fahmy T, et al. Atrial fibrillation ablation in patients with therapeutic international normalized ratio: Comparison of strategies of anticoagulation management in the periprocedural period. *Circulation*. 2007;116(22):2531–2534.
16. Hussein AA, Martin DO, Saliba W, et al. Radiofrequency ablation of atrial fibrillation under therapeutic international normalized ratio: A safe and efficacious periprocedural anticoagulation strategy. *Heart Rhythm*. 2009;6(10):1425–1429.
17. Kottkamp H, Hugl B, Krauss B, et al. Electromagnetic versus fluoroscopic mapping of the inferior isthmus for ablation of typical atrial flutter: A prospective randomized study. *Circulation*. 2000;102(17):2082–2086.
18. Tada H, Oral H, Sticherling C, et al. Double potentials along the ablation line as a guide to radiofrequency ablation of typical atrial flutter. *J Am Coll Cardiol*. 2001;38(3):750–755.
19. Zambito PE, Palma EC. DP+1: Another simple endpoint for atrial flutter ablation. *J Cardiovasc Electrophysiol*. 2008;19(1):10–13.
20. Oral H, Sticherling C, Tada H, et al. Role of transisthmus conduction intervals in predicting bidirectional block after ablation of typical atrial flutter. *J Cardiovasc Electrophysiol*. 2001;12(2):169–174.
21. Kalman JM, Olgin JE, Saxon LA, Fisher WG, Lee RJ, Lesh MD. Activation and entrainment mapping defines the tricuspid annulus as the anterior barrier in typical atrial flutter. *Circulation*. 1996;94(3):398–406.
22. Jaïs P, Shah DC, Haïssaguerre M, et al. Prospective randomized comparison of irrigated-tip versus conventional-tip catheters for ablation of common flutter. *Circulation*. 2000;101(7):772–776.
23. Kuniss M, Kurzidim K, Greiss H, et al. Acute success and persistence of bidirectional conduction block in the cavotricuspid isthmus one month post cryocatheter ablation of common atrial flutter. *Pacing Clin Electrophysiol*. 2006;29(2):146–152.
24. Redfearn DP, Skanes AC, Gula LJ, Krahn AD, Yee R, Klein GJ. Cavotricuspid isthmus conduction is dependent on underlying anatomic bundle architecture: Observations using a maximum voltage-guided ablation technique. *J Cardiovasc Electrophysiol*. 2006;17(8):832–838.
25. Chen J, Christian de Chillou, Basiouny T, et al. Cavotricuspid isthmus mapping to assess bidirectional block during common atrial flutter radiofrequency ablation. *Circulation*. 1999;100(25):2507–2513.

CHAPTER 3

How to Ablate Atrial Flutter Postsurgery

George F. Van Hare, MD

Introduction

This chapter will discuss current techniques for mapping and ablating AFL in patients who have previously undergone heart surgery. Catheter ablation, while often challenging, is an attractive option in patients who have undergone surgery for congenital heart disease. Experience has shown that such tachyarrhythmias are very unlikely to disappear spontaneously, and therefore, the need for antiarrhythmic therapy is likely to be lifelong, absent definitive therapy with ablation. There is an increased incidence of sinus node dysfunction in this patient population, and the addition of antiarrhythmic agents may cause a patient with sinus node disease to experience new or more serious symptoms. These symptoms may include syncope, mandating implantation of a permanent pacemaker in order to continue antiarrhythmic therapy. Similarly, this patient population often has coexisting ventricular dysfunction. Many of the most effective agents for the control of tachyarrhythmias have the potential to worsen ventricular dysfunction, especially beta blockers and sotalol.

The most common form of arrhythmia seen in the postoperative congenital heart disease patient population is AFL, also known as intra-atrial reentrant tachycardia (IART). To understand the techniques used in mapping of large macroreentrant circuits, several concepts need to be considered: the concept of barriers to impulse propagation, and the concept of sites that are "in the circuit" versus sites that are "outside the circuit." These concepts come originally from classic studies by Waldo, et al,[1] which were applied by various workers to the mapping and ablation of common AFL in adult patients[2-4] and subsequently extended for use in postoperative patients.[5-8]

Initial activation mapping studies of the typical form of AFL showed a "counterclockwise" reentrant activation in the RA,[9] with impulses spreading up the septum and down the RA freewall. From studies using concealed entrainment techniques, described below, as well as techniques for precise placement of ablative lesions, it is now well established that one critical element of the AFL reentrant circuit is the isthmus between the IVC and the tricuspid valve annulus.[10] This area of tissue is protected by these 2 barriers to impulse propagation, which prevent the reentrant wave from circling back and catching the "tail of refractoriness," and thereby being extinguished. The situation is more complex, however, than simply a small isthmus of tissue between 2 small barriers. In fact, as shown by Olgin et al and Kalman et al, it is not the IVC *per se* but actually the crista terminalis and its extension as the Eustachian valve ridge that acts as the barrier to impulse propagation.[2,4] The crista terminalis is formed at the junction between the sinus venosus portion and the true, heavily trabeculated portion of the RA; it runs along the posterolateral aspect of the RA, coursing inferiorly. As it reaches the region of the IVC, it is extended by the Eustachian valve ridge, which courses superiorly to the os of the CS, joining with the valve of the CS to form the tendon of Todaro. In patients with common AFL, the crista terminalis has been shown to act as a long line of intra-atrial block. This block seems to be anatomic and fixed rather than functionally determined in patients with clinical AFL. The tricuspid annulus constitutes the "anterior barrier" in typical flutter. Sites around the tricuspid annulus are activated sequentially and in a counterclockwise direction.

These 2 long barriers to impulse propagation form a "funnel" of conducting tissue in the RA. This funnel forces atrial activation to the narrow isthmus between the tricuspid annulus and the IVC, where, because of the short distance, the reentrant circuit is most amenable to successful ablation.

It is interesting that in the otherwise normal human heart, despite the fact that there are numerous potential barriers to impulse propagation (IVC, SVC, mouth of CS, tricuspid and mitral valve annuli, ostia of pulmonary veins, crista terminalis), the vast majority of atrial reentrant arrhythmias are due to common counterclockwise or clockwise AFL. This fact speaks to the importance of the crista terminalis and tricuspid annulus. One would expect these structures to also be important in IART, which is seen following congenital heart disease surgery. The effect of extensive atrial surgery is clearly complex and may involve several effects that make IART more likely. First, the creation of a long atriotomy with subsequent suture closure creates a long line of block of impulse propagation, which is superimposed on the existing RA anatomy described above. Second, such an atriotomy may modify the typical flutter circuit by making it longer, thereby lengthening the tachycardia cycle length and slowing the atrial tachycardia rate. Third, the placement of an atriotomy near the crista terminalis or the use of the crista terminalis for anchoring a suture line (as is done in the lateral Fontan modification) may cause the crista terminalis to begin to act as a line of conduction block.[11] Finally, extensive atrial surgery may cause slowing of conduction, making reentry more likely. At present, it is not known which of these possible mechanisms is most important. It is clear from clinical experience, however, that slow flutter involving the posterior flutter isthmus is very common in postoperative patients[12]; circuits that do not include the typical flutter zone and so are due to reentry involving incisional suture lines are also frequently seen.[13]

Preprocedure Planning

In preparation for mapping a patient with IART, it is important to carefully review the patient's cardiac anatomy, and, in particular, the exact surgical approach that was used. This will be facilitated by a review of the original operative report. The details of the exact placement of atriotomies, baffles, patches, and conduits will become important in the interpretation of the EP recordings and the results of mapping. If possible, the sites bounded by surgically created and anatomic obstacles to impulse propagation should be identified, and several possible candidate sites for ablation should be determined prior to the study. For example, for patients who have undergone simple surgery, such as repair of an atrial septal defect, such sites might be (a) the typical flutter isthmus, (b) between an atriotomy and the tricuspid annulus, or (c) between an atriotomy and the superior vena cava. The same sites are commonly found in patients with more complex surgery, such as repair of tetralogy of Fallot, because a long atriotomy is often employed in these repairs (**Figure 3.1**). The cardiologist must combine an intimate knowledge of the patient's congenital defect with knowledge of the details of the exact surgical procedure used previously to determine appropriate ablation sites.

Procedure

General Techniques for Mapping

In general, methods for mapping clinical atrial arrhythmias may be classified in 3 broad categories: single-site roving mapping, simultaneous multisite mapping, and "destructive" mapping. In practice, the typical atrial tachycardia ablation incorporates elements of all 3. Single-site mapping involves the use of a single, steerable catheter, which is maneuvered throughout the atrium during tachycardia. Electrograms from various sites are recorded, and the map is constructed from these nonsimultaneous measurements, ideally using a 3-dimensional mapping system to record timing of activation superimposed on the anatomy of the atrium. Unfortunately, with some patients, the tachycardia mechanism may change in the midst of a map, forcing the operator to stop to re-induce the original rhythm. For this reason, when confronted by a substrate with numerous tachycardia circuits, "substrate mapping" may be considered, in which a voltage map in sinus or paced rhythm is constructed, allowing for the identification of areas of scar, lines of block, suture lines, and other important anatomic details.[14]

Simultaneous multisite mapping involves various systems for introducing large numbers of electrodes into or onto the heart. These may include basket catheters or, more commonly, noncontact systems that compute virtual electrograms based on far-field intracavitary systems (eg, EnSite, St. Jude Medical). An advantage is the potential to obtain a map on one beat of tachycardia, yet still see the entire circuit. It is limited, however, by the basic inability to introduce electrodes in all parts of both atria in the catheterization laboratory. Also, in large chambers, resolution will not be adequate. Areas that are "in the circuit" may not easily be identified and separated from those that are "out of the circuit" without the ability to perturb the system— for example, by entrainment pacing.

"Destructive" mapping is defined as the direct interruption of an area of conducting myocardium, with subsequent

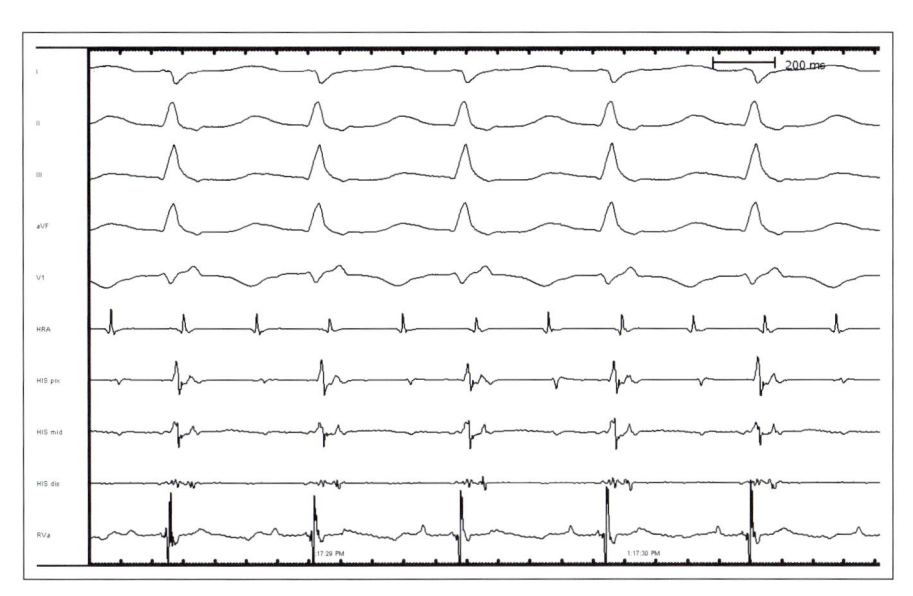

Figure 3.1 Intracardiac and surface ECG recordings in an 18-year-old patient who is s/p repair of tetralogy of Fallot. AFL at a cycle length of approximately 235 ms is evident, with 2:1 conduction. Flutter waves are not easily visible on the surface ECG leads, partly due to the 2:1 conduction and partly due to the preexisting right BBB, which is nearly always present following repair of tetralogy. Abbreviations: HRA: high RA. prx: proximal electrode pair. dis: distal electrode pair. mid: middle electrode pair. RVa: right ventricular apex.

observation to determine whether the target rhythm has been eradicated. This may be done by the delivery of RF or cryoablation lesions during tachycardia. Ideally, such lesions are directed by the use of detailed substrate maps to target these lesions. A successful RF lesion that terminates a tachyarrhythmia is perhaps the best evidence that the site chosen for ablation was critical for maintenance of the arrhythmia. In 1914, Mines[15] recognized the limitations of multisite mapping, saying in reference to AFL that "the test for a circulating excitation is to cut through the ring at one point thereby terminating the flutter." The advantage of this approach is that the lesion may very well be curative. The limitation, of course, is the potential for needless destruction of working myocardium that is not involved in the tachycardia, as well as the potential for lengthening the reentrant circuit, slowing the tachycardia, and making it more incessant.

Identification of Lines of Block

During the EP study, the goal is to identify an isthmus of tissue that is bounded by 2 long barriers. The identification, for example, of the tricuspid annulus, which often provides one important barrier in such patients, is not challenging, as one has fluoroscopic landmarks as well as local atrial electrogram characteristics. Specifically, on the tricuspid annulus, one normally records both atrial and ventricular electrograms, and these are approximately equivalent in size when the catheter is resting on the annulus. Other sites of conduction block are identified by the presence of double potentials, reflecting conduction up one side of the barrier and down the other side, with the bipolar electrogram recording both waves of atrial activation (**Figure 3.2**). Such double potentials are easily recorded in patients with common AFL along the crista terminalis and

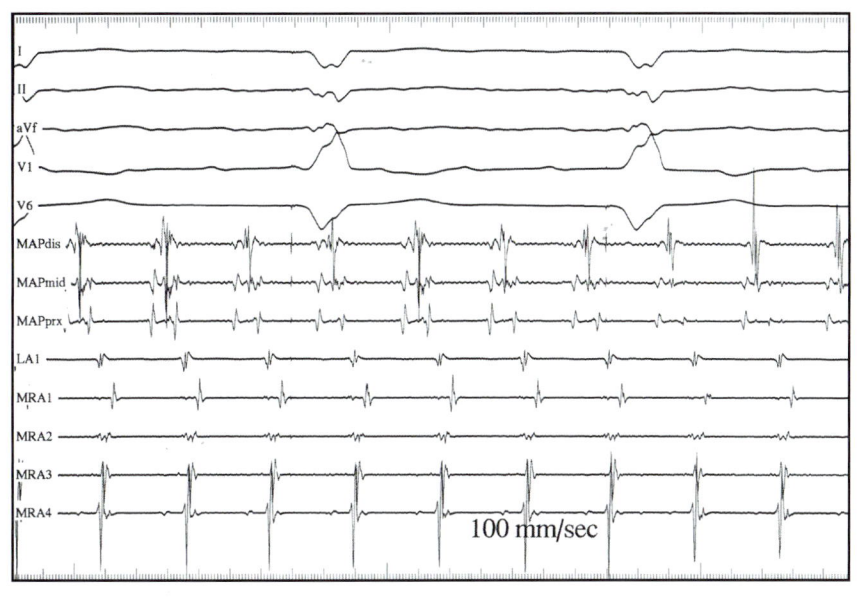

Figure 3.2 Intracardiac and surface ECG recordings during intra-atrial reentry tachycardia, in a patient with D-transposition, s/p Senning procedure, who also has a permanent dual-chamber transvenous pacing system. The recording demonstrates double potentials recorded from the anterior RA wall in the pulmonary venous atrium, most likely at the site of an atriotomy. Abbreviations: MAP: mapping/ablation catheter. MRA: mid-RA catheter, placed in the systemic venous atrium. dis: distal electrode pair. mid: middle electrode pair. prx: proximal electrode pair. (Reproduced with permission from Balaji S, Gillette PC, Case CL. *Cardiac Arrhythmias after Surgery for Congenital Heart Disease*. London: Arnold; 2001:309.)

the Eustachian valve ridge. In patients who have undergone atrial surgery, a long atriotomy is often identified along the anterior wall of the atrium and may be followed along the atrial wall for some distance. In patients after the Senning procedure for transposition, a long line of double potentials may be recorded along the edge of the baffle in the systemic venous atrium.[7]

It must be emphasized that the identification of a line of double potentials is not sufficient for the completion of the map, because such lines of double potentials are very common, and often are not associated in any way with the actual reentrant circuit. That is, both, either, or neither of the areas of atrial myocardium on either side of the line of block may be involved in the reentrant circuit. Areas that are uninvolved in the circuit are considered to be "bystander" areas. Confirmation that the line of block is critical for the tachycardia circuit must be obtained by assessment of the entrainment response from areas of viable tissue adjacent to these lines of block.

Assessment of the Entrainment Response

Current mapping techniques should include assessment of the entrainment response, partly for the confirmation of a reentrant mechanism and partly for identification of candidate sites for ablation. An understanding of these concepts is essential. Waldo described a number of criteria for transient entrainment,[1] and others have suggested additional criteria.[16] The demonstration of any one of these criteria establishes that the atrial tachycardia is a macroreentrant rhythm with an excitable gap. The most common of these criteria is the identification of constant fusion: pacing into tachycardia at a rate slightly faster than the AFL rate produces a P-wave morphology that is intermediate between the free-running tachycardia P-wave morphology and the morphology that would have been seen with simple pacing into sinus rhythm. Fusion is due to collision between the orthodromic wavefront and an antidromic wavefront emanating from the pacing site, thereby changing atrial activation sequence. The observation of constant fusion cannot be made in the case of a focal automatic tachycardia, in which fusion either would not be seen or would not be constant. In the situation of postoperative AFL, the distinction is important, as a focal tachycardia can occupy a potential reentrant circuit created by lines of block and masquerade as a reentrant rhythm. Electroanatomic mapping is unable to make the distinction. Therefore, it is always preferred to demonstrate one of the criteria for transient entrainment before proceeding with mapping and ablation.

"Concealed entrainment" has been defined as the inability to demonstrate the usual criteria for entrainment in an atrial rhythm that is otherwise known to be reentrant, despite demonstration of acceleration to the pacing rate and return to the tachycardia rate following pacing. One common cause for concealed entrainment is that of pacing from within a protected zone of slow conduction. There is no fusion, because the retrograde wave of activation collides with the antegrade wave in the protected zone, and the atrial activation sequence changes little. There is latency between the pacing stimulus and the onset of the P wave due to conduction within this protected zone. Furthermore, the degree of latency from the stimulus to the P-wave onset during entrainment pacing is similar to the latency, when not pacing, from the local electrogram at the pacing site to the onset of the P wave. Most importantly for the purposes of entrainment mapping, when one terminates pacing, the time necessary for return of the wave of activation to the pacing site, the postpacing interval (PPI), is the same as the tachycardia cycle length (TCL) (**Figures 3.3** and **3.4**). As pointed out by Stevenson with respect to ventricular tachycardia, the characteristic of PPI = TCL should be a reliable indication of whether a given site is within or outside of the reentry circuit.[17]

Unlike the situation of typical AFL, in which most atrial sites yield fast conduction (from which manifest entrainment may be demonstrated) and the protected slow zone is restricted to the tricuspid-IVC isthmus, in patients with complex atrial surgery, there may be multiple areas of slow conduction and conduction block, which may or may not be part of the reentrant circuit. For example, if one imagines a side branch of dead-end atrial myocardium in which conduction is slow, one can imagine that sites in this isolated patch of myocardium may activate so late that they appear "early" (ie, with local activation times of 30 or 40 ms in advance of the surface P wave). One should note that this situation is common in patients with the Senning or Mustard procedure for transposition in whom a large section of lateral systemic venous atrium often acts as a bystander branch (Figure 3.4).[7] If one paces from a site in this area, however, it is clear that the PPI will be much longer than the TCL, as the return time to this site will equal the total of (1) conduction time into the circuit, (2) conduction time around the entire circuit, and (3) conduction time back to the pacing site in the side branch.

One often may note in patients with complex atrial surgery that P waves are difficult to assess adequately, because they tend to have quite low voltage (Figure 3.1). Furthermore, they often lack sharp features, so that consistently judging the onset of the P wave in order to determine the latency and assess for fusion is difficult. This is particularly a problem with patients after the Senning or Mustard procedure, in which P waves are often nearly impossible to appreciate despite the presence of sinus rhythm. For these reasons, one should rely more heavily on determination of the PPI and its comparison to TCL than on any measurement or assessment in which P-wave morphology and timing are essential.

Technique of Mapping and Ablation

Anatomy and Surgical History

In practice, the standard ablation for postoperative AFL starts with an understanding of the congenital cardiac

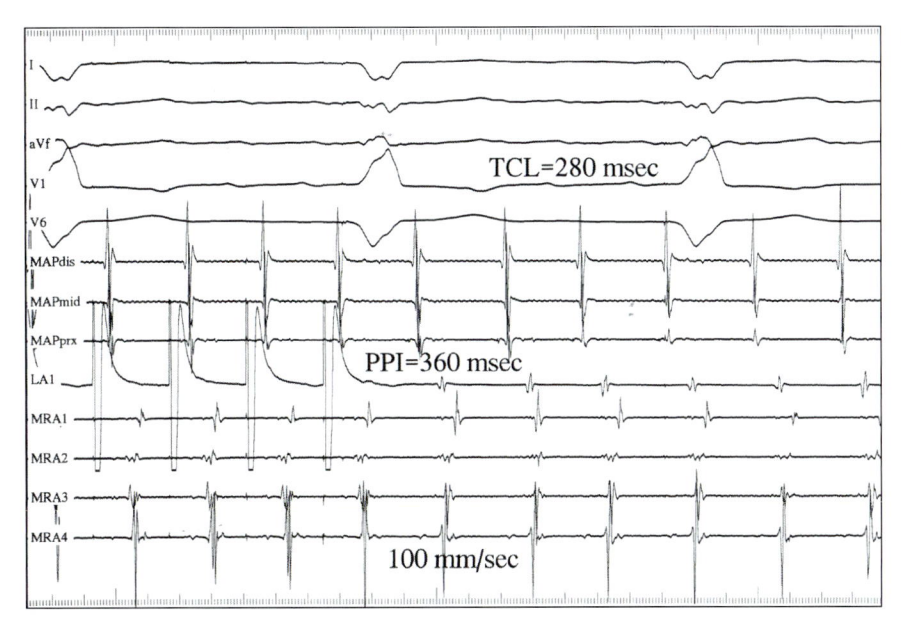

Figure 3.3 Intracardiac and surface ECG recordings during intra-atrial reentry tachycardia, in same patient as Figure 3.2, demonstrating the entrainment response from the roof of the LA (systemic venous atrium in the Senning anatomy). Tachycardia cycle length (TCL) is 280 ms, the paced cycle length is 240 ms, and the PPI measured on the LA electrode pair is 360 ms, indicating that this site is not in the circuit. Abbreviations: MAP: mapping/ablation catheter. MRA: mid-RA catheter, placed in the systemic venous atrium. dis: distal electrode pair. mid: middle electrode pair. prx: proximal electrode pair. (Reproduced with permission from Balaji S, Gillette PC, Case CL. *Cardiac Arrhythmias after Surgery for Congenital Heart Disease.* London: Arnold; 2001:314.)

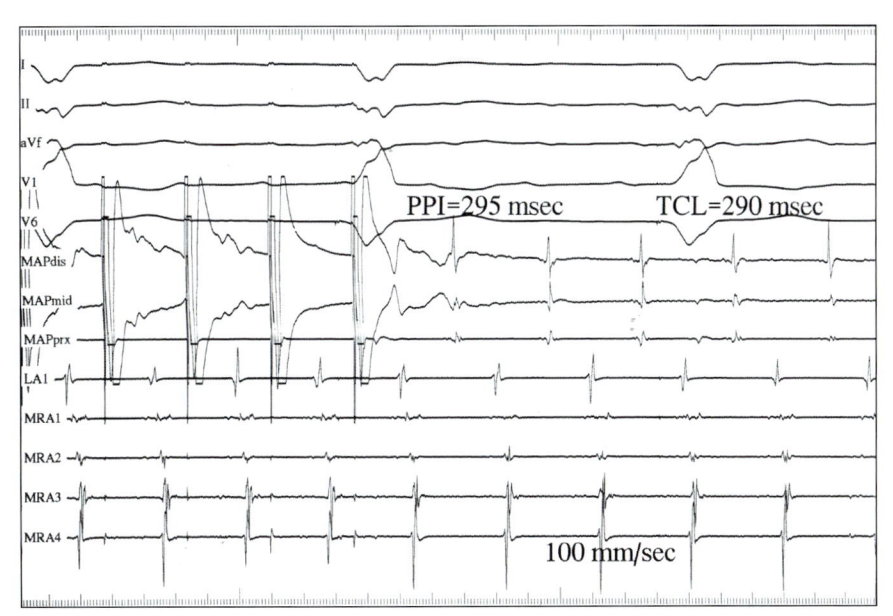

Figure 3.4 Intracardiac and surface ECG recordings during intra-atrial reentry tachycardia, in same patient as Figure 3.2, demonstrating the entrainment response from the mapping catheter placed in the "flutter isthmus" after the catheter was introduced to the pulmonary venous atrium in a retrograde fashion. Note that PPI and TCL are nearly equivalent, indicating that this site is in the circuit. Abbreviations: MAP: mapping/ablation catheter. MRA: mid-RA catheter, placed in the systemic venous atrium. dis: distal electrode pair. mid: middle electrode pair. prx: proximal electrode pair. (Reproduced with permission from Balaji S, Gillette PC, Case CL. *Cardiac Arrhythmias after Surgery for Congenital Heart Disease.* London: Arnold; 2001:314.)

anatomy and the superimposed surgical details in that particular patient. Having a copy of the original operative report in the laboratory during the procedure is always useful. It is also helpful to understand the details of the patient's likely conduction system anatomic location.

Preliminary Mapping

Next, it is helpful to get a rough idea, from roving and/or simultaneous multisite maps during tachycardia, of which areas are likely to be early in relation to the P wave and therefore may be candidate protected slow zones. In most laboratories, this is done by the use of electroanatomic mapping, in which the entire RA is traced in 3 dimensions and both an isochronal map during tachycardia, as well as a voltage map, are constructed. Such a map should identify the major anatomic landmarks (IVC, SVC, tricuspid annulus) as well as identifiable lines of block due to prior atriotomies or patch/scar areas (**Figure 3.5**).

Assessment of Entrainment Response

While the creation of an electroanatomic map may be considered sufficient to proceed with ablation, as discussed above, simple timing information from the isochronal map may be misleading due the possible areas of blind channels that are not part of the circuit. Therefore, one studies the map and identifies a number of candidate ablation target sites that make sense anatomically. Such sites are usually narrow isthmuses between areas of block or anatomic obstacles. The most important of these is, of course, the CTI in patients with normal tricuspid valve anatomy, as this site is more often than not involved in the AFL circuit. In practice, it makes sense to always start with entrainment pacing from this site to establish quickly whether one is dealing with CTI-based flutter versus incisional reentry. This can often be done simply by pacing from the proximal CS electrode pair, positioned close to the mouth of the CS (**Figure 3.6**). Other common sites include the gap between the lower end of an atriotomy and either the IVC or the tricuspid annulus. One tests each of these candidate sites using entrainment pacing, determining whether these sites are "in" or "out" of the circuit. Only candidate sites that are in the circuit are reasonable ablation targets.

Ablation

Once a candidate ablation target site is determined, a series of lesions is then placed in the atrial myocardium to sever the protected isthmus of atrial tissue in order to connect, by means of the RF lesions, 2 anatomic and/or surgical barriers. This may be performed during tachycardia until termination of tachycardia is observed. One may also employ a technique for continuously monitoring conduction across the isthmus, as is commonly done in typical AFL, using pacing from the CS and recording RA lateral wall activation patterns (**Figures 3.7** and **3.8**). Lateral wall activation may also be assessed using electroanatomic mapping (**Figure 3.9**). Following establishment of isthmus block, retesting is carried out to test for inducibility, and additional lesions are placed as necessary.

Endocardial Lesion Creation

Unfortunately, lesion formation in patients who have postoperative arrhythmias is not as straightforward as in those whose hearts are otherwise normal. Patients who have AFL in the setting of the modified Fontan procedure (atriopulmonary connection) often have a dilated, capacious RA, which interferes with energy delivery due to difficulty in achieving excellent catheter contact, as well as to the probable high convective heat loss associated with the large chamber volume. On the other hand, at times, the

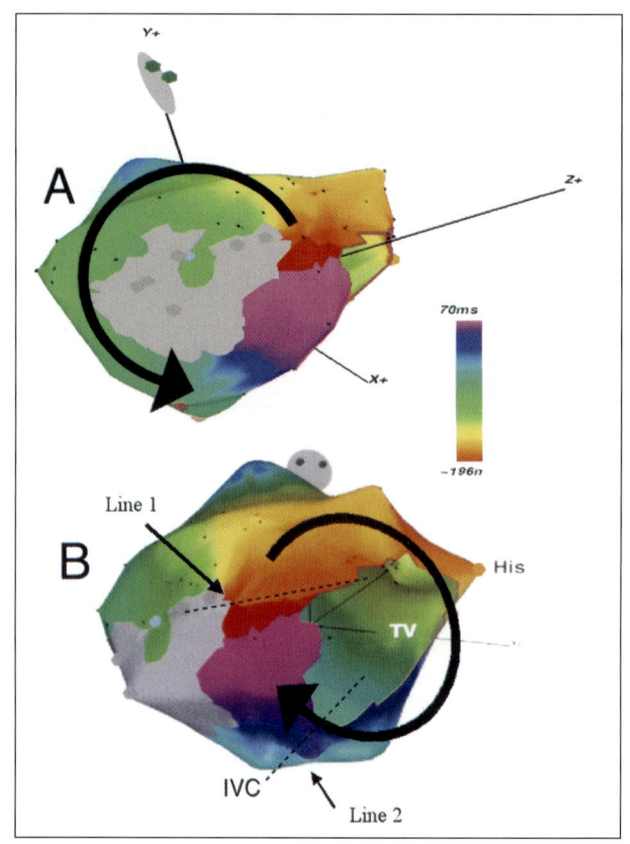

Figure 3.5 Three-dimensional electroanatomic activation maps of both scar-related and cavotricuspid isthmus (CTI)-dependent flutters in a single patient. In this patient, electroanatomic mapping using the CARTO system demonstrated that the clinical flutter involved a reentry circuit moving circumferentially around the incisional scar (A). The arrow in A indicates the direction of movement of activation from earliest to latest for this scar-related flutter. This flutter was successfully ablated by creating an ablation line from the scar to the tricuspid annulus (B, line 1). However, a second, cavotricuspid isthmus-dependent flutter was induced moving in a clockwise direction as indicated by the arrow in B. This flutter required a second isthmus ablation line to be created from the tricuspid annulus to the IVC (B, line 2). TV = tricuspid valve. (Reproduced with permission from Verma A, et al, *J Am Coll Cardiol* 2004;44:409–414.)

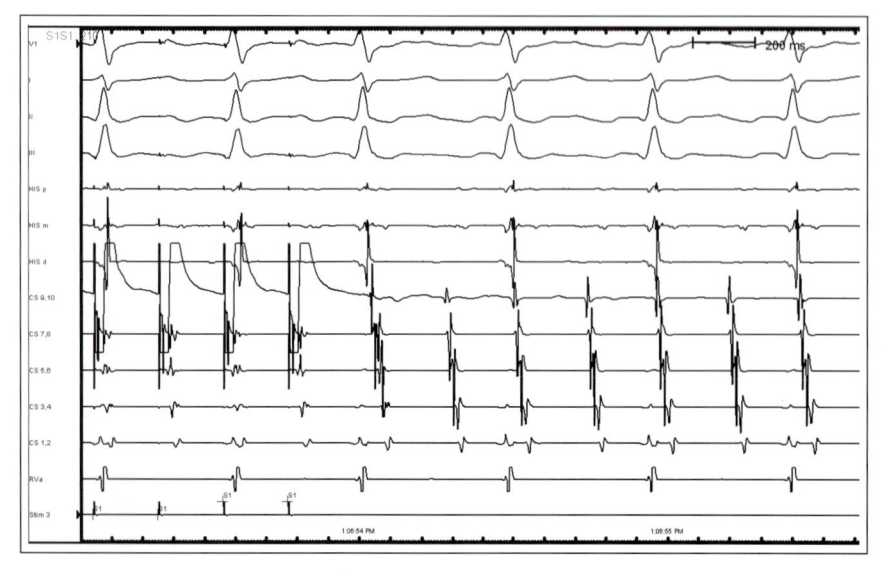

Figure 3.6 Intracardiac and surface ECG recordings in a 16-year-old patient with AFL and 2:1 conduction, who is s/p transatrial repair of a ventricular septal defect. Entrainment pacing at a cycle length of 210 ms is carried out from the proximal CS electrode pair (CS 9,10), which has been positioned fluoroscopically at a site close to the mouth of the CS os. The postpacing interval (240 ms) is within 20 ms of the tachycardia cycle length (230 ms), indicating the likely involvement of the CTI in the AFL circuit. Abbreviations: CS: coronary sinus. RVa: right ventricular apex. Stim: stimulus channel.

target chosen for ablation turns out to be in an area of very low flow and, as such, target temperature may be achieved at very low generator outputs with consequent limited energy delivery. For macroreentrant rhythms, it is likely that larger lesions will be necessary to completely transect an isthmus of myocardium between 2 barriers, which increases the difficulty of the procedure. Finally, it is apparent that some types of cardiac repair (eg, atriopulmonary connection) are associated with significant myocardial hypertrophy and wall thickening, making the achievement of a transmural lesion difficult or impossible. Newer technology, involving the use of catheter tip irrigation for cooling and long linear lesion creation, may influence the efficacy of these ablation procedures, and in fact have been employed in such patients.[18]

Assessment of Ablation Endpoint

Although it may seems like a simple matter to determine whether AFL has been successfully ablated, in practice, the assessment of ablation endpoint is not at all straightforward in the postoperative patient. As will be seen, this problem stems from the large variability of macroreentrant circuits that may be seen in the EP laboratory.

In practice, there are 3 points of evidence that one may use to document a successful ablation. These are, in order of increasing reliability: (1) termination of tachycardia during RF energy application; (2) lack of tachycardia inducibility following ablation; and (3) documentation of block at a critical isthmus of conduction. These points are discussed below.

Termination of Tachycardia During RF Energy Application

The sudden termination of an incessant tachycardia during application of RF energy is a dramatic event, which strongly suggests that the lesion placed at the particular site

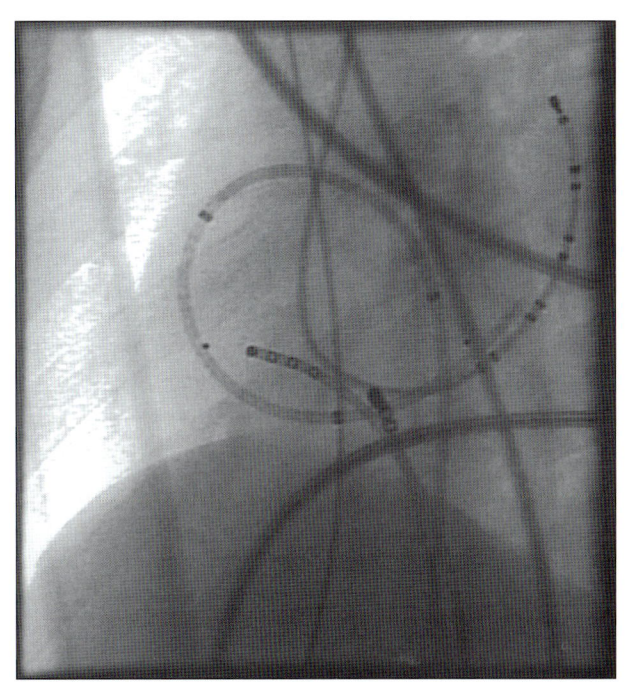

Figure 3.7 Fluoroscopy image in left anterior oblique view of catheter positions in a 7-year-old patient who was s/p repair of total anomalous pulmonary venous return. Despite the LA surgery, the patient was found to have CTI-based AFL, most likely due to the right atriotomy that was used for the repair. Note that the CS is entered with a decapolar catheter, and a Halo catheter is deployed in the RA with the tip entering the CS. (Reproduced with permission from Balaji S, Gillette PC, Case CL. *Cardiac Arrhythmias after Surgery for Congenital Heart Disease*. London: Arnold; 2001:321.)

has severed a critical isthmus of conducting tissue. However, reliance upon RF termination as the sole criterion of a successful ablation is questionable. Such tachycardias may terminate spontaneously or in response to spontaneous premature atrial contractions. More commonly, RF application may cause transient but not permanent block in the targeted isthmus of conducting tissue. Such block may last

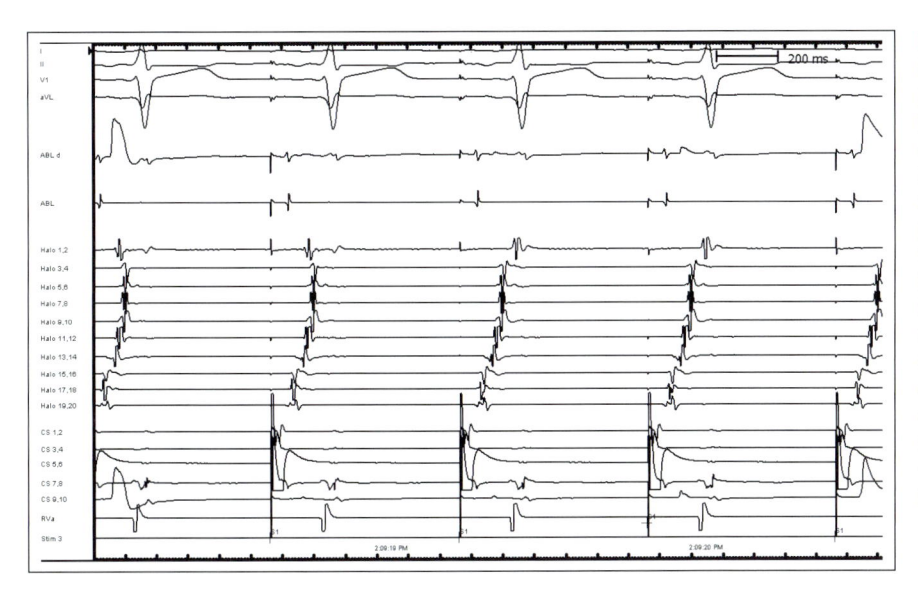

Figure 3.8 Intracardiac and surface ECG recordings during pacing of the proximal CS, in the same patient as in Figure 3.7, during RF ablation at the cavotricuspid isthmus. For the first 2 beats of the tracing, there is early activation of both the distal and the proximal Halo catheter electrode pairs, with later activation of the middle pairs, indicating intact conduction across the flutter isthmus. With the third and subsequent beats, there is early activation of only the proximal Halo catheter electrode pairs, with later activation of the distal pairs, indicating absent conduction across the CTI. Abbreviations: ABL: ablation catheter. d: distal electrode pair. RVa: right ventricular apex.

long enough to terminate the tachycardia by preventing conduction in a critical portion of the circuit but may resolve after several seconds or minutes. The observance of sudden termination may be very useful, however, in the course of a mapping procedure. Should the termination occur without premature beats, which might be responsible for the termination, this finding provides additional evidence (beyond entrainment response) that the site is indeed critical to the maintenance of the tachycardia and therefore should be targeted for additional lesions.

Lack of Tachycardia Inducibility Following Ablation

Unfortunately, postoperative arrhythmias are not always easily inducible at EP study despite clearly being clinically symptomatic. Therefore, the inability to induce an arrhythmia after a possibly successful ablation is not as helpful as one would like, particularly if the initial induction was difficult or inconsistent. If one proposes to use the lack of inducibility as the primary criterion of success, it is important to spend a significant amount of time prior to the ablation documenting the best method of induction and demonstrating repeatedly that the tachycardia can be induced. For patients with AFL/intra-atrial reentry, attempts at induction must include prolonged cycles of ramp pacing, consisting of atrial overdrive pacing at progressively shortening cycle lengths. Provided that such a complete and careful assessment of inducibility is performed prior to ablation, one considers the lack of inducibility following ablation, in the setting of easy inducibility prior to ablation, to be a better criterion of success than termination of tachycardia with RF ablation.

Documentation of Block at a Critical Isthmus of Conduction

A major advance in the treatment of common, "type 1" AFL, with counterclockwise rotation around the tricuspid annulus, was the recognition that it was possible to assess the conduction patterns in the RA in the absence of AFL, allowing assessment of the conduction through the critical isthmus between the tricuspid annulus and IVC.[19,20] This meant that one no longer needed to rely on the above imperfect criteria (termination during RF application, lack of inducibility) for documentation of success. Instead, one may now document bidirectional conduction in the isthmus before ablation, observe the development of isthmus block during RF application, and, finally, demonstrate persisting bidirectional block following ablation. In this way, ablation of AFL became technically similar to the ablation of, for example, an accessory pathway, in which signs of bidirectional accessory pathway block can be documented without necessarily needing to rely on lack of tachycardia inducibility as the sole criterion of success.

The use of these various maneuvers for assessing block in the flutter isthmus makes the ablation procedure smoother, as one does not need to repeatedly induce AFL

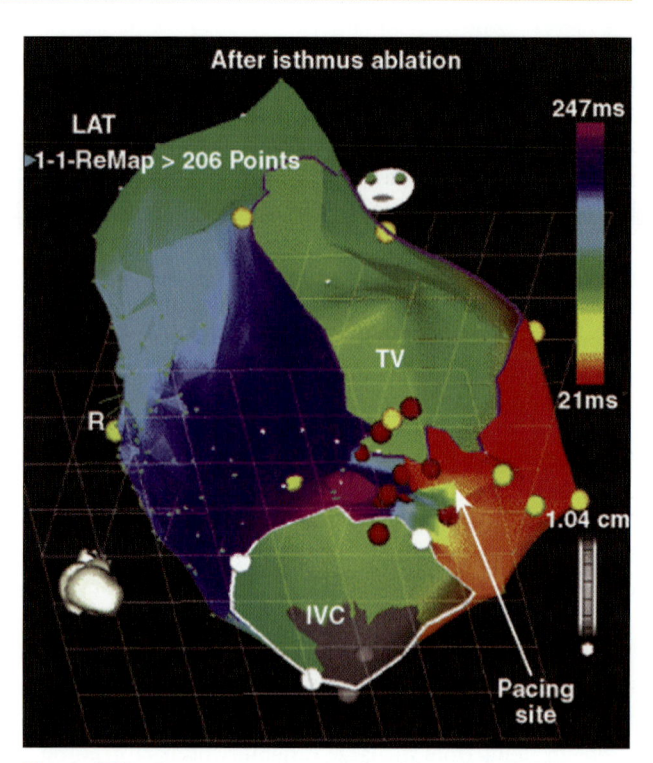

Figure 3.9 Electroanatomic map of atrial activation while pacing near the mouth of the CS in a patient who had just undergone successful interruption of conduction through the cavotricuspid isthmus. The *red dots* mark the sites of RF applications. The late electrogram times *(blue and purple)* recorded just on the other side of the ablation line suggest that propagation of atrial activation away from the pacing site had to occur in a counterclockwise manner all the way around the tricuspid valve ring rather than across the isthmus. Abbreviations: IVC, inferior vena cava; TV, tricuspid valve. (Reproduced with permission from Walsh EP. Ablation of postoperative atrial tachycardia in patients with congenital heart disease. In SKS Huang, MA Wood, eds. *Catheter Ablation of Cardiac Arrhythmias*, 2nd edition. Philadelphia, PA: Elsevier Saunders; 2011:230.)

after each lesion, and therefore avoids the risk of inducing atrial fibrillation inadvertently. One may continuously observe conduction via the isthmus during RF application and be able to observe when block occurs in the isthmus (eg, by pacing the low lateral RA and watching P-wave morphology during RF application).

The adaptation of these techniques to the situation of the postoperative heart is challenging. As stated earlier, many patients with intra-atrial reentry essentially have the same circuit as patients with typical counterclockwise AFL, proceeding either counterclockwise or clockwise.[12] Once the importance of the flutter isthmus is documented in such a patient, all of the above techniques can be employed to assess conduction in the isthmus. This is straightforward in patients with atriopulmonary connections and those with simple defects such as atrial or ventricular septal defects, in which there is normal access to the RA structures. It is not as straightforward in patients in whom the morphologically RA structures are in the pulmonary venous atrium, such as patients who have undergone the Senning, Mustard, or lateral tunnel Fontan procedures. In such patients, it is unlikely that a multipolar catheter can be deployed in the pulmonary venous atrium. However, the morphology of paced P waves from the low lateral RA, as well as bidirectional conduction times through the isthmus, can certainly be assessed. Although laborious, documentation of bidirectional block may also be established by rebuilding an electroanatomic map with critical site pacing to demonstrate bidirectional block in unusual or difficult-to-access isthmuses (**Figure 3.9**).[21]

Postprocedure Care

Catheter ablation for postoperative AFL is a somewhat more challenging procedure than for routine supraventricular arrhythmias, but not excessively. More important issues for postoperative care include the patient's baseline hemodynamic status, which, if compromised with ventricular dysfunction, may mandate postprocedure monitoring in an ICU setting. If AFL has been long-standing, after successful ablation, the clinician may choose to initiate a period of systemic anticoagulation.[22]

Procedural Complications

Ablation of postoperative AFL is safe in general, and the risks are similar to those for more routine ablations. One area of particular concern, however, is the potential for inadvertent AV block. In cavotricuspid isthmus-based flutter, the compact AV node is not far from the ablation site, and so care must be exercised, of course (**Figure 3.10**). In patients with AFL in the setting of prior surgery for AV canal defect, including ostium primum atrial septal defect, it should be remembered that in this anatomy, the AV conducting tissue is located more inferior and posterior, and in fact is quite close to the mouth of the CS.[23] In this situation, AV block is more likely as the CTI is targeted, and cryoablation should be considered.

Although rare, right phrenic palsy is another possible complication if the lateral wall of the atrium is targeted. One may attempt to avoid this complication by testing high-output pacing at proposed lateral RA sites, observing for diaphragm movement.

Advantages and Limitations

There are clear advantages, of course, to definitive therapy by ablation as opposed to long-term antiarrhythmic medication or to surgical ablation. Limitations exist primarily related to the lack of 100% efficacy of the techniques as they currently exist.[24] In addition, the more complex the anatomy, in general, the more likely it is that the clinician will encounter multiple tachycardia circuits. In addition to the sometimes disappointing initial results, there is also a rather high incidence of recurrence, prompting the need for repeat ablation. Another issue to consider is the anatomic setting of the arrhythmia. In some cases, the appearance of AFL is an indication of worsening hemodynamic status, and in such cases, catheter ablation may contribute to clinical improvement but not provide the entire answer.

Conclusions

It is clear that the field of catheter-based cardiac ablation has evolved rapidly. In most cases, definitive treatment by ablation should be preferable to long-term antiarrhythmic therapy, especially when one considers the numerous potential side effects of antiarrhythmic medication in this patient population. The results of catheter ablation, unfortunately, are not as good as ablation of more routine arrhythmias in the population of patients with otherwise

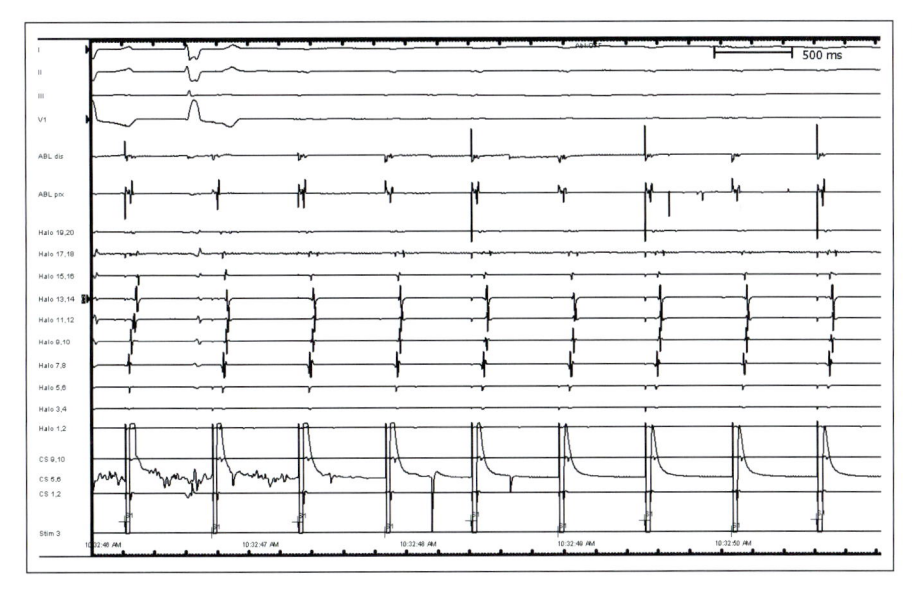

Figure 3.10 Intracardiac and surface ECG recordings in a 13-year-old girl who is s/p repair of tetralogy of Fallot with absent pulmonary valve and a mitral valve cleft. AFL was inducible and mapped to the cavotricuspid isthmus using entrainment mapping. RF ablation was carried out using pacing from the mid-CS, monitoring lateral RA wall activation via a 20-electrode Halo catheter. Complete AV block was observed during this lesion, despite the inferior location of the ablation catheter, suggesting a more posterior and inferior location of the compact AV node in this particular patient. AV conduction returned and ablation attempt was abandoned at this site. Abbreviations: CS: coronary sinus. ABL: ablation catheter. prx: proximal electrode pair. dis: distal electrode pair. Stim: stimulus channel.

normal hearts. While this may partly be due to a lack of understanding of the exact macroreentrant circuits that exist in each patient, it is more likely that the ability to make long linear and transmural lesions is limited. Future progress in catheter and lesion formation technology may allow more such patients to benefit from the advantages of definitive cure.

References

1. Waldo AL, MacLean WA, Karp RB, Kouchoukos NT, James TN. Entrainment and interruption of atrial flutter with atrial pacing: Studies in man following open heart surgery. *Circulation.* 1977;56:737–745.
2. Kalman JM, Olgin JE, Saxon LA, Fisher WG, Lee RJ, Lesh MD. Activation and entrainment mapping defines the tricuspid annulus as the anterior barrier in typical atrial flutter [see comments]. *Circulation.* 1996;94:398–406.
3. Lesh MD, Van Hare GF, Fitzpatrick AP, Griffin JC, Chu E. Curing reentrant atrial arrhythmias. Targeting protected zones of slow conduction by catheter ablation. *J Electrocardiol.* 1993;26:194–203.
4. Olgin JE, Kalman JM, Fitzpatrick AP, Lesh MD. Role of right atrial endocardial structures as barriers to conduction during human type I atrial flutter. Activation and entrainment mapping guided by intracardiac echocardiography. *Circulation.* 1995;92:1839–1848.
5. Triedman JK, Bergau DM, Saul JP, Epstein MR, Walsh EP. Efficacy of ablation for control of intraatrial reentrant tachycardia in patients with congenital heart disease. *J Am Coll Cardiol.* 1997;30:1032–1038.
6. Triedman JK, Saul JP, Weindling SN, Walsh EP. Ablation of intra-atrial reentrant tachycardia after surgical palliation of congenital heart disease. *Circulation.* 1995;91:707–714.
7. Van Hare GF, Lesh MD, Ross BA, Perry JC, Dorostkar PC. Mapping and ablation of intraatrial reentrant tachycardia after the Senning or mustard procedure for transposition of the great arteries. *Am J Cardiol.* 1996;77:985–991.
8. Van Hare GF, Lesh MD, Stanger P. Catheter ablation of supraventricular arrhythmias in patients with congenital heart disease: Results and technical considerations. *J Am Coll Cardiol.* 1993;22:883–890.
9. Olshansky B, Okumura K, Hess PG, Waldo AL. Demonstration of an area of slow conduction in human atrial flutter. *J Am Coll Cardiol.* 1990;16:1634–1648.
10. Feld GK. Catheter ablation for the treatment of atrial tachycardia. *Progress Cardiovasc Dis.* 1995;37:205–224.
11. Rodefeld MD, Bromberg BI, Schuessler RB, Boineau JP, Cox JL, Huddleston CB. Atrial flutter after lateral tunnel construction in the modified fontan operation: A canine model. *J Thorac Cardiovasc Surg.* 1996;111:514–526.
12. Chan DP, Van Hare GF, Mackall JA, Carlson MD, Waldo AL. Importance of atrial flutter isthmus in postoperative intra-atrial reentrant tachycardia. *Circulation.* 2000;102:1283–1289.
13. Kalman JM, VanHare GF, Olgin JE, Saxon LA, Stark SI, Lesh MD. Ablation of "incisional" reentrant atrial tachycardia complicating surgery for congenital heart disease. Use of entrainment to define a critical isthmus of conduction. *Circulation.* 1996;93:502–512.
14. Nakagawa H, Shah N, Matsudaira K, Overholt E, Chandrasekaran K, Beckman KJ, Spector P, Calame JD, Rao A, Hasdemir C, Otomo K, Wang Z, Lazzara R, Jackman WM. Characterization of reentrant circuit in macroreentrant right atrial tachycardia after surgical repair of congenital heart disease: Isolated channels between scars allow "focal" ablation. *Circulation.* 2001;103:699–709.
15. Mines GR. On circulating excitation in heart muscles and their possible relations to tachycardia and fibrillation. *Trans R Soc Can.* 1914;8 (ser III, sec IV):43–52.
16. Henthorn RW, Okumura K, Olshansky B, Plumb VJ, Hess PG, Waldo AL. A fourth criterion for transient entrainment: The electrogram equivalent of progressive fusion. *Circulation.* 1988;77:1003–1012.
17. Stevenson WG, Khan H, Sager P, Saxon LA, Middlekauff HR, Natterson PD, Wiener I. Identification of reentry circuit sites during catheter mapping and ablation of ventricular tachycardia late after myocardial infarction. *Circulation.* 1993;88:1647–1670.
18. Triedman JK, DeLucca JM, Alexander ME, Berul CI, Cecchin F, Walsh EP. Prospective trial of electroanatomically guided, irrigated catheter ablation of atrial tachycardia in patients with congenital heart disease. *Heart Rhythm.* 2005;2:700–705.
19. Cauchemez B, Haïssaguerre M, Fischer B, Thomas O, Clementy J, Coumel P. Electrophysiological effects of catheter ablation of tricuspid annulus isthmus in common atrial flutter. *Circulation.* 1996;93:284–294.
20. Poty H, Saoudi N, Abdel Aziz A, Nair M, Letac B. Catheter ablation of type 1 atrial flutter. Prediction of late success by electrophysiological criteria. *Circulation.* 1995;92:1389–1392.
21. El Yaman MM, Asirvatham SJ, Kapa S, Barrett RA, Packer DL, Porter CB. Methods to access the surgically excluded cavotricuspid isthmus for complete ablation of typical atrial flutter in patients with congenital heart defects. *Heart Rhythm.* 2009;6:949–956.
22. Feltes TF, Friedman RA. Transesophageal echocardiographic detection of atrial thrombi in patients with nonfibrillation atrial tachyarrhythmias and congenital heart disease. *J Am Coll Cardiol.* 1994;24:1365–1370.
23. Pillai R, Ho SY, Anderson RH, Lincoln C. Ostium primum atrioventricular septal defect: An anatomical and surgical review. *Ann Thorac Surg.* 1986;41:458–461.
24. Papagiannis J, Maounis T, Laskari C, Theodorakis GN, Rammos S. Ablation of atrial tachycardias with current after surgical repair of complex congenital heart defects. *Hellenic J Cardiol.* 2007;48:268–277.

CHAPTER 4

THE ABLATION OF ATRIAL TACHYCARDIA

Patrick M. Heck, BM, BCh, DM; Peter M. Kistler, MBBS, PhD;
Andrew W. Teh, MBBS, PhD; Jonathan M. Kalman, MBBS, PhD

Introduction

Atrial tachycardias (AT) can be either focal or macroreentrant arrhythmias, with the latter often being referred to as AFLs. In 2001, a joint expert working group established the current consensus for the classification of AT according to the underlying EP mechanism. In this classification, focal AT was defined as atrial activation originating from a discrete focus, arbitrarily defined as < 2 cm in diameter, radiating centrifugally. Macroreentrant AT, on the other hand, is due to activation encircling a "large" central obstacle, typically several centimeters in diameter, which may be functional or fixed. Activation mapping of macroreentrant AT defines continuous activity as 100% of tachycardia cycle length, as opposed to a maximum of 75% recorded in focal AT.

Catheter ablation for AF is rapidly becoming the most commonly performed ablation procedure worldwide, and more centers are tackling persistent long-standing AF. To achieve higher success rates in patients with persistent AF, a more extensive biatrial ablation strategy is adopted, often involving a combination of linear ablation and the targeting of CFAE. This can result in areas of slowed conduction and scar, which may create an EP milieu for both focal (microreentrant) and macroreentrant AT. It is becoming increasingly apparent that the incidence of postablation AT is becoming more common and is determined by the duration of AF and extent of ablation during the index procedure.

This chapter will deal exclusively with mapping and ablation of focal ATs.

Focal Atrial Tachycardia

Focal AT is the least common type of SVT, accounting for approximately 10 to 15% of patients referred for EP evaluation of SVT. Focal AT occurs equally in men and women.[1] The EP mechanisms underlying focal AT include abnormal automaticity, triggered activity, and microreentry. Elucidating the mechanism underlying a focal AT in the EP laboratory is often difficult and of limited practical value for the ablation of these arrhythmias.

Confirming the Diagnosis

Typically, the diagnosis of focal AT can be made based upon the clinical characteristics of the arrhythmia and the surface ECG. Differential diagnoses include sinus tachycardia, AVNRT, AVRT, and macroreentrant AT. The ECG of a focal AT is normally that of a long R-P tachycardia, but not universally so. Unlike both typical AVNRT and

AVRT, where the R-P relationship is fixed, in focal AT, there may be a variable or unhooked R-P relationship, and at rapid rates, decremental AV nodal conduction may result in an apparent short R-P tachycardia. Distinguishing focal AT from sinus tachycardia is straightforward when the P-wave morphology is different. AT arising from the superior crista terminalis may have a morphology indistinguishable from that of sinus tachycardia. In this setting the presence of a "warm-up" over 3 to 4 beats at onset and "cool down" over 3 to 4 beats at termination supports a diagnosis of AT over sinus tachycardia, which typically accelerates and decelerates over more than 30 seconds.[2] The ECG of a macroreentrant AT is distinct in that it typically shows an undulating baseline with no clear isoelectric segment. The same can be true for focal ATs when the cycle length is very short or the atria are heavily scarred with slowed conduction, but this is less common.

Anatomic Locations

It is now well recognized that de novo focal ATs do not occur randomly throughout the atria but cluster at specific anatomic sites.[3] In the RA, common locations include the crista terminalis, tricuspid annulus, CS ostium, RAA, and perinodal region. In the LA, the PV ostia,[4] the aortomitral continuity, and the LAA[3] are frequent locations (**Figures 4.1** and **4.2**).

The anatomic location of ATs occurring after AF ablation is largely determined by the index ablation strategy. When prior ablation was limited to PV isolation, then postablation ATs are uncommon and typically arise from one or more reconnected PV. The addition of linear and/or CFAE ablation further increases the incidence of postablation AT, with the majority of focal ATs arising close to sites previously targeted for ablation.[5] Detailed knowledge of the sites of prior ablation is of great assistance to the electrophysiologist attempting to localize the likely site of origin of a postablation AT.

Surface ECG and P-Wave Morphology

The surface ECG can provide a useful guide to the likely anatomic site of origin for de novo focal AT. Kistler et al published an algorithm (**Figure 4.3**) for the localization of ATs based on surface ECG P-wave morphology that was able to identify the correct anatomic location with an accuracy of 93%.[3] However, it should be remembered that the spatial resolution of P-wave morphology has been estimated at 17 mm. Distinguishing left and right atrial foci is

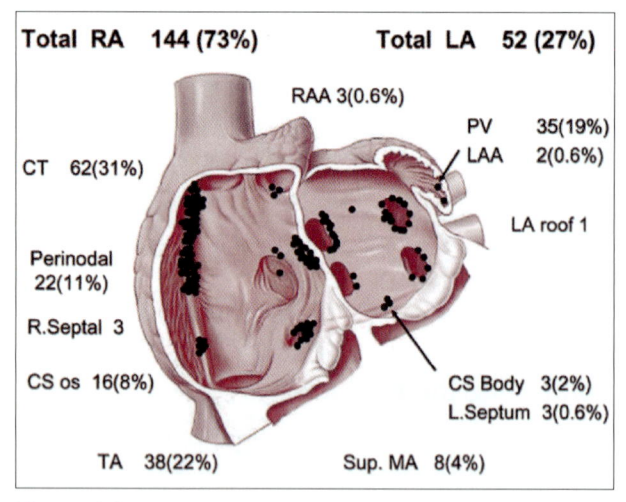

Figure 4.1 Anatomical distribution of de novo focal ATs in the left and right atria. The atrioventricular valves have been removed from this view and are shown in Figure 4.2. RA = right atrium; LA = left atrium; RAA = right atrial appendage; LAA = left atrial appendage; CT = crista terminalis; CS = coronary sinus; PV = pulmonary veins; TA = tricuspid annulus; MA = mitral annulus. (Reprinted with permission from Kistler et al., *J Am Coll Cardiol.* 2006;48;1010-1017.)

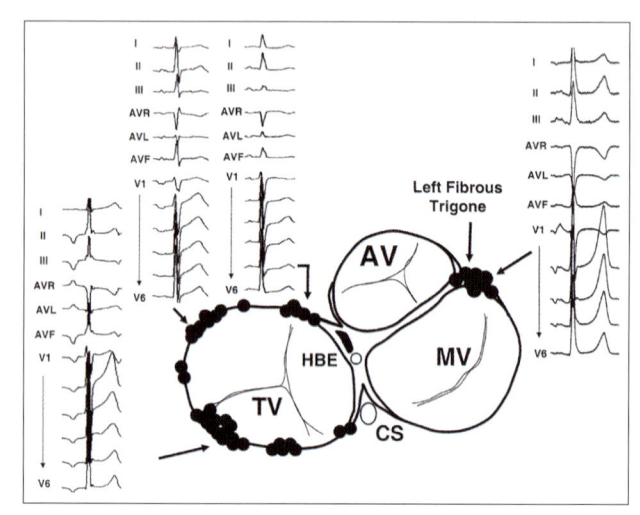

Figure 4.2 Anatomical distribution and representative P-wave morphologies of focal ATs arising from the tricuspid and mitral annuli. TV = tricuspid valve; MV = mitral valve; HBE = His bundle EGM. (Reprinted with permission from Kistler et al., *J Am Coll Cardiol.* 2006;48;1010-1017.)

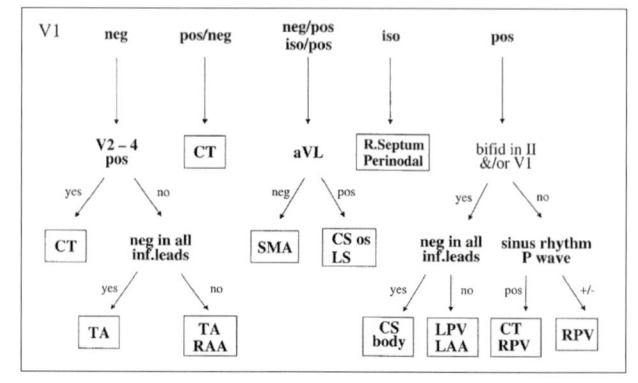

Figure 4.3 An algorithm for using P-wave morphology of an AT to localize the focus. Abbreviations as in figures 1 and 2. LS = left septum; SMA = superior mitral annulus; LPV = left pulmonary veins; RPV = right pulmonary veins. (Reprinted with permission from Kistler et al., *J Am Coll Cardiol.* 2006;48;1010–1017.)

of particular importance when planning an ablation procedure, as transseptal access may be anticipated based on the P-wave morphology. A left-sided focus is suggested by a positive P wave in V_1 and negative P wave in I and aVL. Successful analysis of P-wave morphology is contingent on the P wave being clearly visible and unencumbered from the preceding T wave. Prior to EP study, vagal maneuvers or adenosine may be useful in separating the P wave from the preceding T wave. Within the EP lab this is readily achieved by ventricular pacing at a faster cycle length than the AT (**Figure 4.4**). Examples of P-wave morphology of focal ATs are shown in **Figures 4.5** and **4.6**.

The major determinant of P-wave morphology is septal and LA activation. Therefore, prior ablation for AF with extensive substrate modification with consequent scar and altered conduction renders the P wave less reliable in localizing the responsible focus.

Indications for Ablation

Focal atrial ectopy is common, is rarely symptomatic, and typically requires no treatment. Frequent ectopy and sustained AT are often symptomatic and respond poorly to pharmacologic therapy, making catheter ablation an increasingly utilised procedure. The clinical course of focal AT is typically benign, although incessant tachycardia can occur and may result in cardiomyopathy.[6] Catheter ablation of focal AT in patients with incessant tachycardia or recurrent symptoms has a class I recommendation from the consensus ACC/AHA/ESC guidelines published in 2003.[1]

The Electrophysiological Study

Although the surface ECG may have provided a likely diagnosis, it is often the role of the invasive electrophysiological study to confirm the diagnosis.

Intracardiac Catheters

The typical intracardiac recording catheters used will vary slightly depending on the likely origin of the AT. The most basic setup required to perform the diagnostic study should include a quadripolar catheter placed at the His location to enable right ventricular pacing and recording and a decapolar catheter within the CS.

Once the diagnosis of focal AT is confirmed, additional multipolar catheters may facilitate the mapping of the AT, although they are not essential. For ATs arising from the RA, 20-pole catheters designed to be placed against the tricuspid annulus or along the crista terminalis can be used (example in **Figure 4.7**). Similarly, for ATs arising within the LA, a PV circular mapping catheter can be used, although this may necessitate the placement of 2 transseptal sheaths.

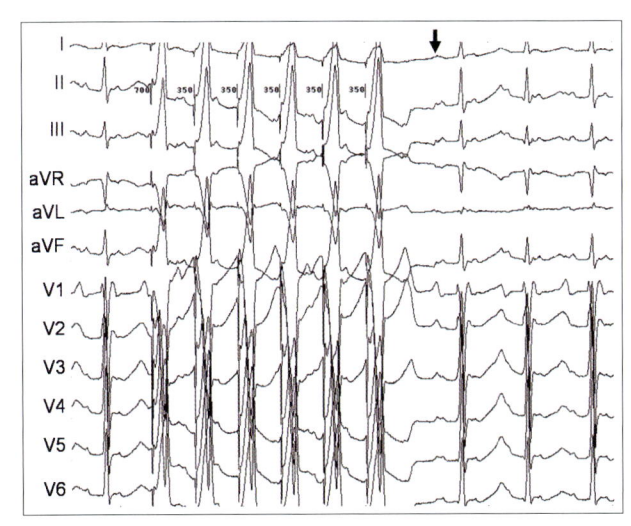

Figure 4.4 A 12-lead ECG showing ventricular pacing during sustained AT in order to unencumber the P wave (indicated by the arrow) from the preceding T wave, allowing analysis of the P-wave morphology and its onset.

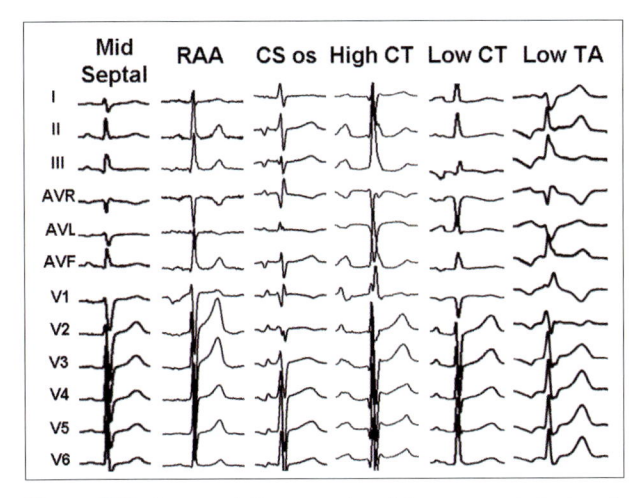

Figure 4.5 Representative examples of P-wave morphologies of focal ATs arising from structures within the RA. Abbreviations as per Figure 4.1.

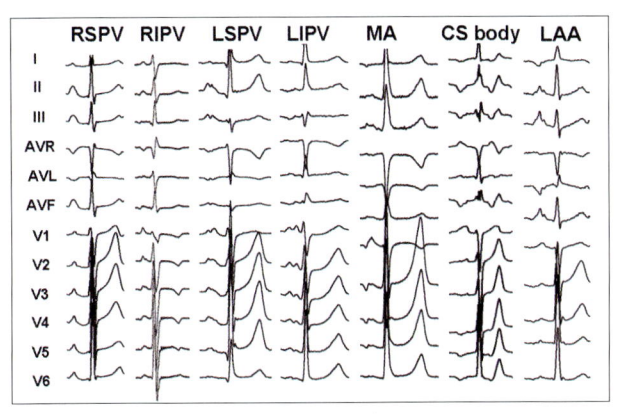

Figure 4.6 Representative examples of P-wave morphologies of focal ATs arising from structures within the LA. Abbreviations as per Figure 4.1. LSPV = left superior pulmonary vein; LIPV = left inferior pulmonary vein; RSPV = right superior pulmonary vein; RIPV = right inferior pulmonary vein.

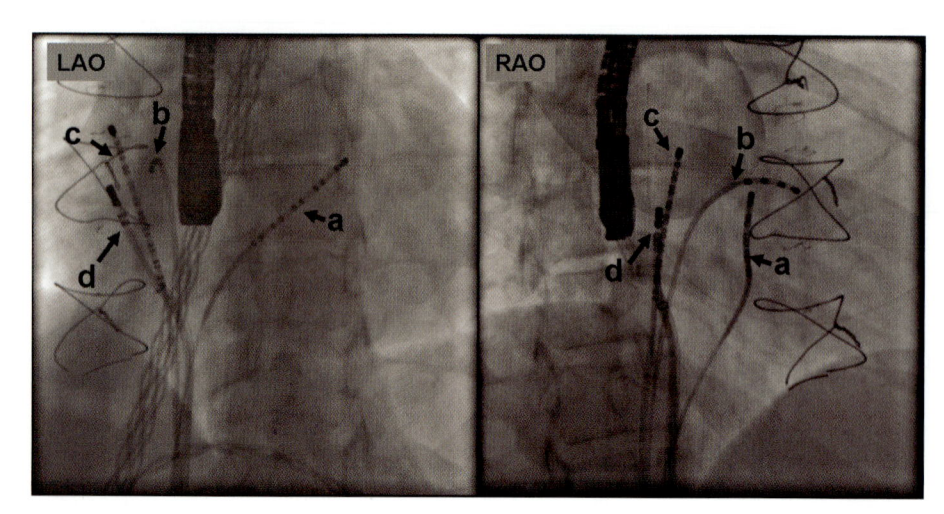

Figure 4.7 Left anterior oblique (LAO, left image) and right anterior oblique (RAO, right image) fluroscopic views of a typical catheter setup used for mapping a cristal AT. Four intracardiac catheters are used: a = decapolar catheter in the CS; b = quadripolar catheter at the His bundle/RV location; c = duodecapolar catheter placed along the crista terminalis; d = mapping/ablation catheter in a long vascular sheath.

Inducing Focal AT

Noninducibility of the AT is by far the most common reason planned mapping and ablation procedures fail. In cases in which the tachycardia is not incessant, care must be taken with the level of sedation given to the patient, as this may render some focal ATs impossible to induce. Burst atrial pacing and programmed atrial extrastimulation may be successful in inducing the focal AT, particularly if the underlying mechanism is microreentry or triggered activity. High doses of isoproterenol may be needed in the induction of automatic focal AT. Despite all of these measures, it is not uncommon for the AT to be noninducible or the ectopy too infrequent to enable mapping and the procedure may have to be rescheduled.

Confirming the Diagnosis

Once the arrhythmia is induced, the diagnosis can be confirmed on the basis of several observations and pacing maneuvers. The 3 main differential diagnoses at this stage are AVRT, AVNRT, and macroreentrant AT. On examination of the intracardiac recordings, the relationship between the ventricular and atrial EGMs (VA relationship) is fixed or "hooked" in AVNRT and AVRT but variable in AT. Various pacing maneuvers may facilitate the observation of VA unhooking. Following termination of atrial overdrive pacing at a cycle length just below the tachycardia cycle length, the VA relationship remains fixed in both AVNRT and AVRT, but VA unhooking is observed when the mechanism is focal AT.[7] The response after entrainment of the tachycardia by ventricular pacing is also helpful provided the entrainment of the atrium is achieved and tachycardia persists after pacing. If the first EGM of the tachycardia recorded after the final entrained atrial EGM is ventricular, termed a "V-A-V" response, this is characteristic of AVRT or AVNRT. If the first recorded EGM of tachycardia is atrial, termed a "V-A-A-V" response, this is observed in AT.

The distinction between focal and macroreentrant AT is best made using atrial entrainment maneuvers. Demonstration of entrainment from within the circuit, defined as PPI minus TCL of less than 20 ms (PPI-TCL< 20 ms), from 2 sites more than 2 cm apart or the ability to record activity throughout the entire tachycardia cycle length are both definitive for macroreentrant AT.[1]

Conventional Mapping

Successful endocardial activation mapping of focal AT is achieved by identifying a focal site of early activation with centrifugal spread. A local activation time at least 20 to 30 ms ahead of the surface ECG P-wave onset (**Figure 4.8**) is desired to indicate a potential site for successful ablation.[2] It is important to correctly identify the P-wave onset, which can then be referenced against a stable intracardiac reference point, such as the proximal bipole on the CS catheter. In cases in which atrial ectopy is infrequent, then pace-mapping may also be used to complement activation sequence mapping, although as noted above, the spatial resolution of the P-wave morphology is only approximately 17 mm.

The first critical step in mapping focal AT is determining whether the focus is in the LA or RA. The surface P-wave morphology will have provided some clues, but it can be unreliable if there has been significant prior ablation. In general, an LA focus should be expected when earliest activation in the RA occurs over a relatively large region on the septal aspect. In this setting, earliest activation timing with respect to P-wave onset will not be less than −10 ms at RA septal sites and later further away from the septum. For certain focal ATs, notably perinodal AT, it may be necessary to perform both LA and RA mapping and to map the aortic root.

3-dimensional Electroanatomic Mapping Systems

The development and more widespread use of 3-dimensional mapping systems has improved the ability of clinicians to successfully locate and ablate focal arrhythmias. The technologies in the various systems differ, but

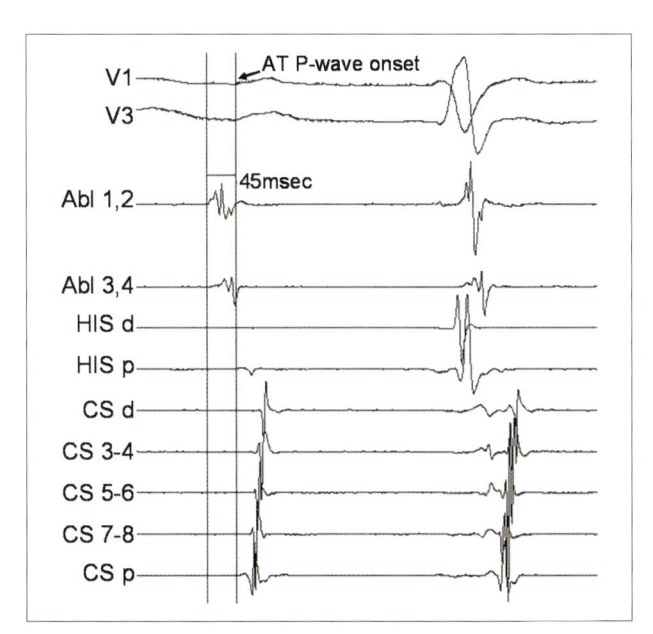

Figure 4.8 Intracardiac EGMs of the successful ablation site of a focal AT. The local EGM on the ablation catheter is recorded 45 ms before the onset of the surface P wave. A local activation time at least 20 to 30 ms ahead of the surface ECG P-wave onset is desired to indicate a potential site for successful ablation. Abl = ablation/mapping catheter electrodes; HIS = His catheter electrodes; CS = coronary sinus catheter electrodes.

essentially they all enable the registration of a mapping/ablation catheter position in 3-dimensional space relative to a fiducial point. This enables the electrophysiologist to acquire both anatomical and EGM data at multiple sites, resulting in the construction of 3-dimensional chamber geometry combined with activation sequence mapping (traditionally color-coded). These systems also have the facility to superimpose the acquired data onto images of the atria taken by either computed tomography or MRI, allowing a more detailed and accurate correlation of the atrial anatomy with intracardiac EGMs (**Figure 4.9**). The systems can potentially enhance success rates and reduce radiation doses, but they are still reliant upon the presence of sufficient atrial ectopy to create an activation map.

The Successful Site

There are a number of features of the EGM that make a site more likely to be successful. First and foremost, it should be the earliest recorded intracardiac activation point and be at least 20 ms ahead of the surface P wave. The EGM may be fractionated, but this is not a universal finding in de novo focal AT and is likely to be specific to certain anatomical sites, such as the crista terminalis.[2] At these sites, it is hypothesized that the fractionation represents underlying slow conduction, making microreentry possible. In the setting of postablation focal AT, then, it is far more likely that the successful site will have a fractionated EGM, as the majority of these arrhythmias are thought to be due to microreentry around prior ablation sites.[5]

The unipolar EGM can also be useful in locating the focus of the AT. The characteristic QS pattern recorded from the unipolar EGM on the distal tip of the ablation catheter is a good predictor of a successful site.[8]

The use of catheter tip pressure to terminate a sustained AT has been reported to improve on the specificity and positive predictive value of identifying an AT focus.[9] However, it has been our experience that once a tachycardia has been terminated by catheter pressure, it is difficult to judge whether ablation has been truly successful or if the mechanical pressure has simply stunned the AT focus transiently and it will potentially recover hours or days later.

Characteristic acceleration ("speeding") of the tachycardia prior to abrupt termination may also be seen at sites of successful ablation (**Figure 4.10**).

Ablation

The majority of focal AT can be successfully ablated with standard RF ablation catheters, often with the use of long vascular sheaths to improve catheter stability. Irrigation may be useful when the AT focus is in an area of the atrium where blood flow is slow due to trabeculation, or within the CS. For AT foci in the perinodal region, cryoablation may be a preferable ablation energy source, as potential sites can be tested for any effect on the AV node with a "reversible" lesion at −30°C before applying a full lesion at −80°C.[10]

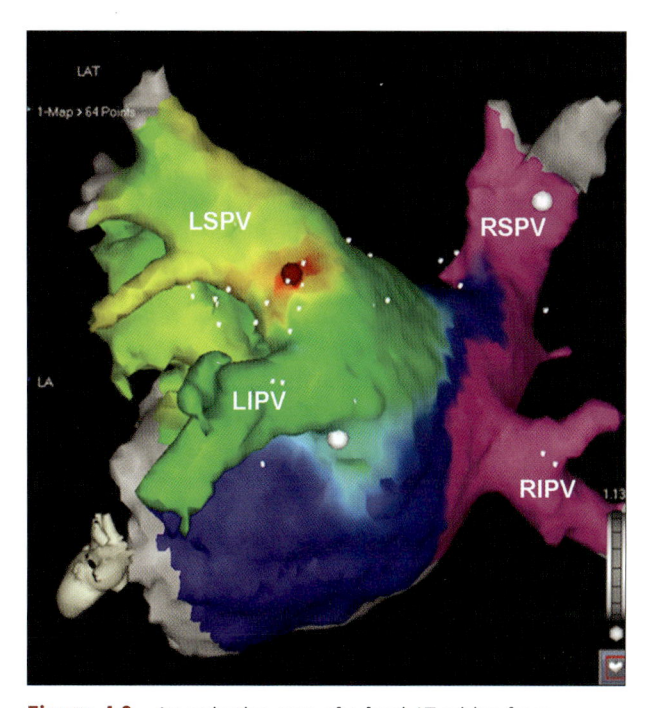

Figure 4.9 An activation map of a focal AT arising from the ostium of the left superior pulmonary vein created with a 3-dimensional anatomical mapping system and coregistered with a CT of the LA. The earliest activation signals are color-coded red, with the latest in purple. The red circle indicates the site of successful ablation of the arrhythmia. Abbreviations as in Figure 4.6.

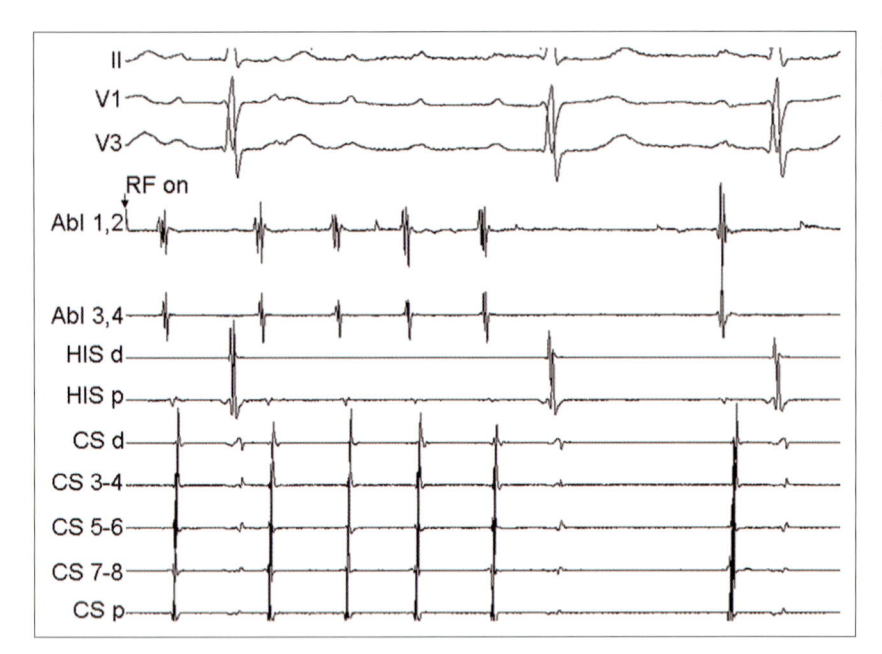

Figure 4.10 RF ablation of a focal AT showing the characteristic speeding and then termination of the arrhythmia at the successful site. Abbreviations as in Figure 4.7.

Endpoint

Focal arrhythmias, especially when difficult to induce, often pose a problem when trying to judge when enough ablation has been performed. Incessant focal AT provides the most definitive endpoint, namely noninducibility, but the endpoint for infrequent ectopy is much harder to assess. Following the delivery of ablation to the presumptive AT focus repeat inducibility testing, with both isoproterenol infusion and burst atrial pacing, may help to determine whether the ablation has been successful.

Despite the not infrequent problem posed by noninducibility, the success rates for the ablation of ATs are excellent. Reported series quote between 69% and 100% cure rates[2] with recurrence rates around 7%.[11] RA foci were found to have a lower recurrence rate, while male gender, multiple foci, older patients, and those with coexisting cardiac pathology were all factors that predicted recurrence.

References

1. Blomstrom-Lundqvist C, Scheinman MM, Aliot EM, et al. ACC/AHA/ESC guidelines for the management of patients with supraventricular arrhythmias—executive summary: a report of the American College of Cardiology/American Heart Association Task Force on Practice Guidelines and the European Society of Cardiology Committee for Practice Guidelines (Writing Committee to Develop Guidelines for the Management of Patients With Supraventricular Arrhythmias). *Circulation.* 2003;108:1871–1909.
2. Roberts-Thomson KC, Kistler PM, Kalman JM. Focal atrial tachycardia II: management. *Pacing Clin Electrophysiol.* 2006;29:769–778.
3. Kistler PM, Roberts-Thomson KC, Haqqani HM, et al. P-wave morphology in focal atrial tachycardia: development of an algorithm to predict the anatomic site of origin. *J Am Coll Cardiol.* 2006;48:1010–1017.
4. Kistler PM, Sanders P, Fynn SP, et al. Electrophysiological and electrocardiographic characteristics of focal atrial tachycardia originating from the pulmonary veins: acute and long-term outcomes of radiofrequency ablation. *Circulation.* 2003;108:1968–1975.
5. Jaïs P, Matsuo S, Knecht S, et al. A deductive mapping strategy for atrial tachycardia following atrial fibrillation ablation: importance of localized reentry. *J Cardiovasc Electrophysiol.* 2009;20:480–491.
6. Medi C, Kalman JM, Haqqani H, et al. Tachycardia-mediated cardiomyopathy secondary to focal atrial tachycardia: long-term outcome after catheter ablation. *J Am Coll Cardiol.* 2009;53:1791–1797.
7. Knight BP, Ebinger M, Oral H, et al. Diagnostic value of tachycardia features and pacing maneuvers during paroxysmal supraventricular tachycardia. *J Am Coll Cardiol.* 2000; 36:574–582.
8. Tang K, Ma J, Zhang S, et al. Unipolar electrogram in identification of successful targets for radiofrequency catheter ablation of focal atrial tachycardia. *Chin Med J (Engl).* 2003;116:1455–1458.
9. Pappone C, Stabile G, De Simone A, et al. Role of catheter-induced mechanical trauma in localization of target sites of radiofrequency ablation in automatic atrial tachycardia. *J Am Coll Cardiol.* 1996;27:1090–1097.
10. Wong T, Segal OR, Markides V, Davies DW, Peters NS. Cryoablation of focal atrial tachycardia originating close to the atrioventricular node. *J Cardiovasc Electrophysiol.* 2004; 15:838.
11. Chen SA, Tai CT, Chiang CE, Ding YA, Chang MS. Focal atrial tachycardia: reanalysis of the clinical and electrophysiologic characteristics and prediction of successful radiofrequency ablation. *J Cardiovasc Electrophysiol.* 1998;9: 355–365.

CHAPTER 5

How to Ablate Atrial Tachycardias in Patients with Congenital Heart Disease

John K. Triedman, MD

Introduction

Patients who have undergone palliative surgery for congenital heart disease (CHD) have a high prevalence of both sinus node dysfunction and AT as they age into adult life, due to fibrosis, surgical scarring, and abnormal anatomy. Within 10 to 20 years of initial surgery, half or more of these patients will have such findings, causing significant morbidity in the young adult population with CHD.[1] Unfortunately, these ATs tend to be quite refractory to medical management. For this reason, many centers have adopted an interventional approach to treatment and prophylaxis of ATs in CHD patients, either by catheter ablation or, in some cases, by adaptation of surgical maze procedures. Because these arrhythmias are most commonly macroreentrant and often highly organized by anatomy and scarring, they are extremely well suited to targeted, catheter-based approaches to mapping and ablation. Although the recurrence rate after ablation of these arrhythmias is relatively high, advances in mapping and lesion generation, in combination with effective approaches to vascular access and improved understanding of the electroanatomical relationships that underlie these arrhythmia circuits, have been improving long-term outcomes.

Preprocedural Planning

Anatomical and Surgical Review

Review of the underlying anatomy of the patient's congenital heart defect and the surgical modifications to this anatomy that the patient has experienced in the course of treatment are of critical importance to the operator. Although the variety of congenital heart defects is daunting, from the perspective of the ablating electrophysiologist, most patients can be characterized in one of 3 general types. The first group consists of patients with simple valvar and/or septal defects who have undergone a biventricular repair, such as tetralogy of Fallot, atrial and ventricular septal defects, and repair of anomalous pulmonary veins. These patients have cardiac anatomy that approximates normal and have atrial arrhythmias that principally reflect cardiac fibrosis and scarring. A second group includes patients who have undergone extensive intra-atrial baffling procedures, most notably those who have had a Mustard or Senning procedure for transposition of the great vessels. Although these patients may also have a physiologically biventricular repair, the postoperative anatomy of their atria presents special challenges for ablative intervention. The final group includes patients who have had a spectrum of palliative surgeries for functionally single ventricular physiology, typically varieties of the Fontan procedure. These patients often have highly complex atrial substrates that are highly arrhythmogenic (**Figure 5.1**).

ECG Review

In patients with ATs status postrepair of congenital heart defect, it is commonly the case that a variety of organized tachycardias can be induced by programmed stimulation, with varying CLs and P-wave morphologies (**Figure 5.2**). Ideally, after ablation, the tachycardia will be rendered noninducible. However, given the complexity of some atrial substrates in these patients, it is helpful to be able to identify and target clinically occurring ATs when possible based on review of prior electrocardiograms. The prior occurrence of AF should also be noted, as this identifies a subgroup of patients who may be more likely to have recurrences after successful targeted ablation of organized ATs and who might be considered as candidates for catheter-based or surgical maze procedures if recurrence occurs.

It is also important to note whether the patient has sinus node dysfunction, a concomitant finding in many CHD patients with AT. Both antibradycardia and antitachycardia pacing may be useful adjunct therapies for arrhythmia control in such patients. Those patients with a pacemaker in situ, either epicardial or transvenous, must be ablated with attention to the locations of the implanted leads to avoid causing exit block by ablation of underlying myocardium.

Imaging

Prior to ablation, thorough evaluation should be performed with a focus on the identification of any hemodynamically significant lesions that should be investigated or addressed

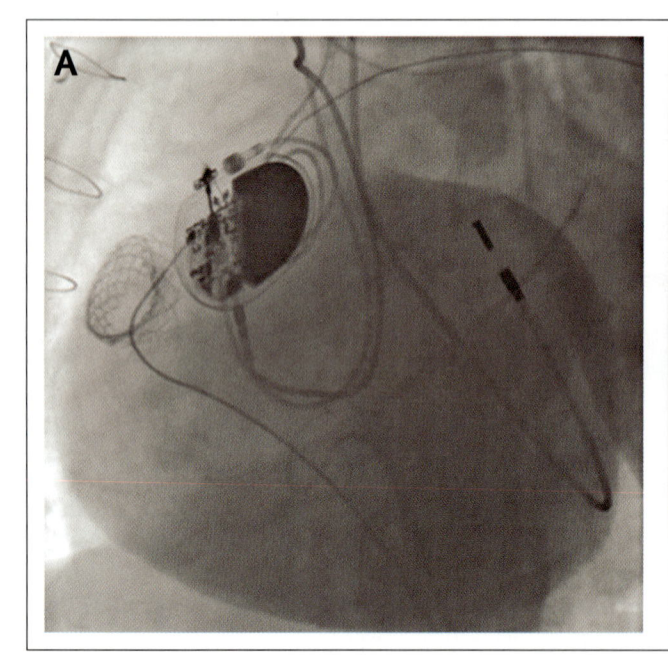

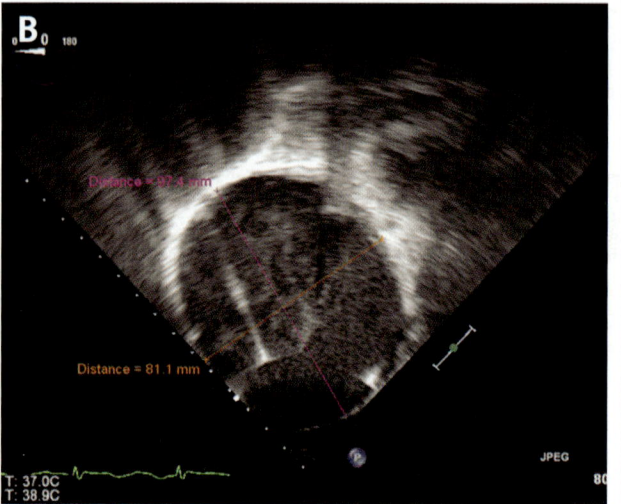

Figure 5.1 Massively enlarged RA anatomy in a patient with an older variant of the Fontan procedure. **A.** Angiographic view in left lateral projection. **B.** Transesophageal echocardiographic view.

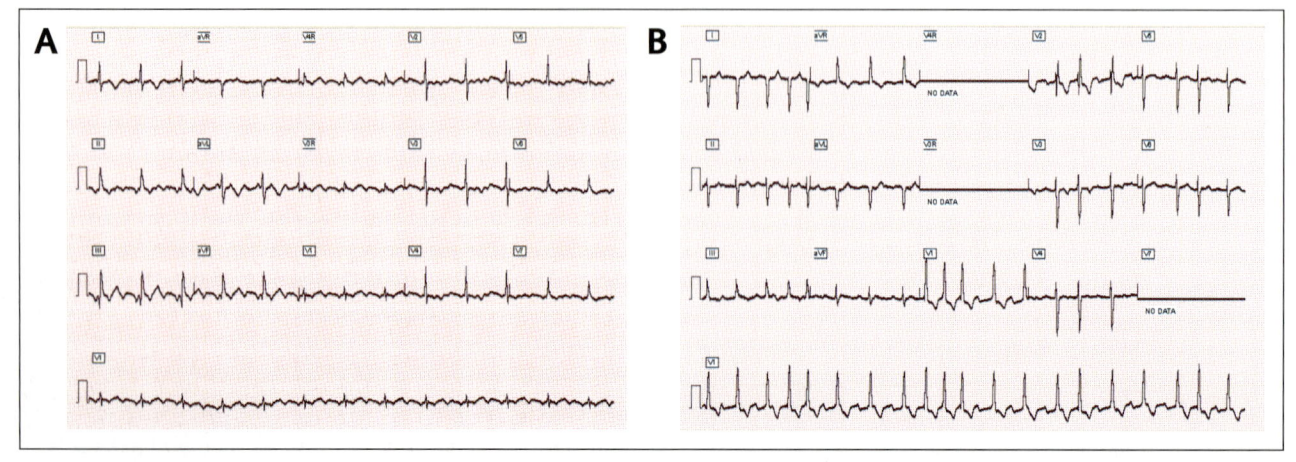

Figure 5.2 Exemplary clinical ECGs of ATs in patients with complex congenital diagnosis. **A.** AT with well-delineated P-wave morphology, clear diastolic interval and regular AV relation. **B.** AT with low-amplitude P waves and variable AV conduction.

at the time of catheterization. In patients managed at an adult EP center, this may involve consultation with a pediatric or adult congenital cardiologist. A standard 2-dimensional echocardiogram should be performed, and consideration may be given in many patients to imaging using CT or MRI. In addition to often providing superior views of intracardiac anatomical and functional properties, these data sets may be utilized in conjunction with electroanatomical mapping systems to guide catheter navigation and ablation planning.[2]

During ablation, standard electroanatomical mapping is often supplemented by incorporation of 3-dimensional data sets obtained during preoperative evaluation (**Figures 5.3** and **5.4**). In the case of the former, it is of significant value for the operating physician to participate directly in image segmentation and model construction of the CT or MRI datasets (▶ **Videos 5.1** and **5.2**). This is because the postoperative anatomy observed in these patients is frequently quite abnormal, and the imaging is sometimes difficult to interpret without specific anatomical knowledge of the patient. Additionally, it is the observation of the author that time spent in meticulous anatomical review of the data is usually of significant benefit to the operator in procedure planning. Specific anatomical features that may be of value include the specific anatomy of atrial baffles in relation to the native atrial septum, the ostium of the CS and the AV valves, the presence of unusual venous connections, the anatomy of the atrial septum or baffle with respect to possible need for transseptal access, the presence of intracardiac thrombus and the relationships of the great vessels and semilunar valves with regard to possible need for retrograde catheterization.

Anticoagulation

Acute intracardiac thrombosis has been anecdotally observed in atrial ablation in CHD patients, but concern for cerebrovascular events is considerably lower than for patients undergoing catheter-based procedures for AF. This is because the majority of intervention is typically performed on the systemic venous atrium, and the arrhythmias themselves appear to have somewhat lower thrombotic potential. Nevertheless, many patients are maintained chronically on warfarin, and while it is rare for bleeding to be an issue, it is generally considered prudent to interrupt chronic anticoagulation therapy for a period of days and ensure that the INR is not excessive prior to the procedure. Heparin "bridging" is rarely necessary, although for a patient with chronic arrhythmia and a history of thrombosis, this may be appropriate. During the procedure, heparinization is appropriate, with most laboratories targeting an ACT of 250 to 300 seconds as an indicator of adequate anticoagulation. Our laboratory protocol is an initial bolus dose of heparin of 100 U/kg, with assessment of the ACT hourly or more frequently, with intermittent follow-up dosing as necessary.

Procedure

Patient Preparation

Because AT ablation in these patients is often a long procedure, patients in our lab are placed under general anesthesia. A urinary catheter is also placed in all patients both to monitor renal function and to balance intake and output over the course of the procedure, as the frequent use of irrigated-tip catheter may result in administration of 1 to 3 liters of excess fluid.

Vascular Access

In general, AT ablations in congenital heart patients can be performed using a limited number of catheters—one catheter for mapping and ablation (usually requiring an 8-Fr sheath to allow for use of an irrigated-tip catheter) and a second for placement of a reference catheter in the atrium or CS. At times, it is useful to place an esophageal lead as

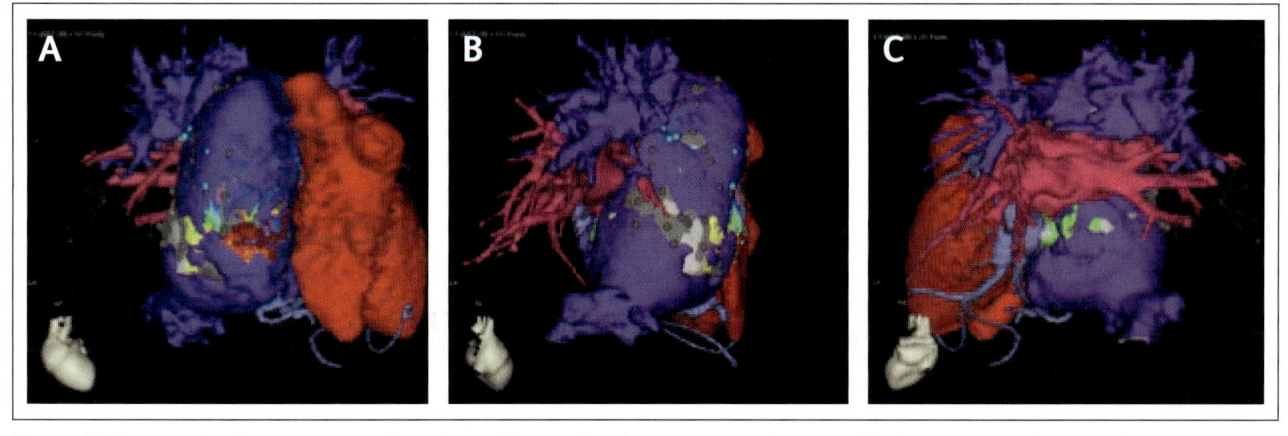

Figure 5.3 Segmented MRI anatomy of a patient with an atriopulmonary connection ("modified Fontan procedure"), which was commonly performed in the 1980s and 1990s as the preferred palliation for single-ventricle physiology. This procedure commonly resulted in massively enlarged right atria as seen in Figure 5.1. **A.** AP view. **B.** Right lateral view. **C.** PA view.

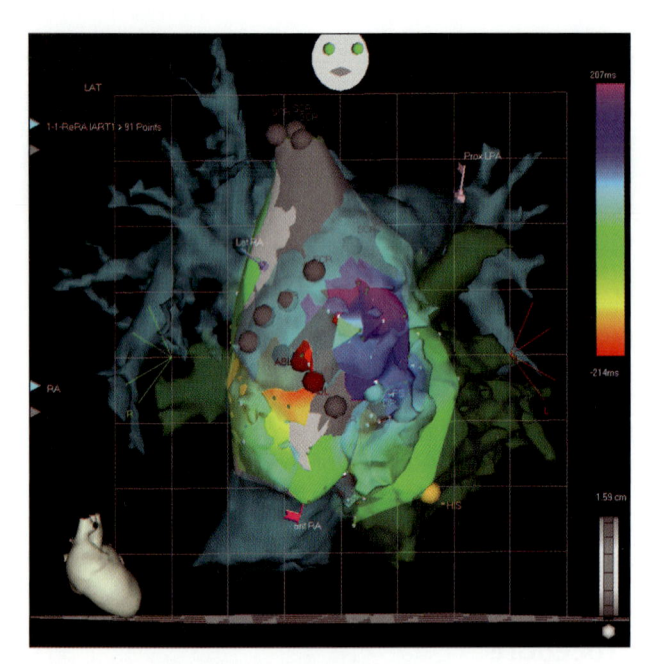

Figure 5.4 Combined electroanatomical map and coregistered Fontan right atrium in a patient with atrial tachycardia.

a reference EGM, but the atrial signal obtained from these catheters is sometimes of such low amplitude and frequency content as to be of limited use. If it is desired to use ICE, an adjunct imaging modality that we have increasingly found to be of value in these procedures, an additional 8- or 10-Fr sheath, is necessary.

Given these requirements, vascular capacitance is not often a limiting issue, although we typically divide sheaths between right and left femoral veins for organization of the field and ease of catheter manipulation. A much more important issue in congenital heart patients who have undergone many prior catheterizations, surgeries, and intensive care stays is whether a given femoral vein is open. Examination of prior catheterization notes may reveal that a femoral vein is occluded, or in the case of heterotaxy patients, that the IVC is interrupted and drains via an azygos connection to the SVC. Observation of the patient's groin may reveal prior cutdown scars, especially if they were catheterized in the 1960s or 1970s or were ever placed on peripheral cardiopulmonary bypass. If it is possible to access a vessel percutaneously but not to easily pass a guide wire to the IVC and atrium, it is useful to perform an angiogram of the pelvis by hand injection and document the patency of the femoral and iliac vessels for future operators. If the femoral veins are obstructed, it is possible to catheterize these patients via the internal jugular approach. In rare cases, transhepatic puncture may be indicated.

Long Vascular Sheaths and Transseptal Puncture

In patients with extremely dilated right atria, the use of long vascular sheaths may be critical to augmenting the reach of the mapping and ablation catheter and ensuring that adequate endocardial contact is being made (▶ Videos 5.3 and 5.4). This is especially true in patients with older-style atriopulmonary Fontan anastomoses and in patients with severe Ebstein's anomaly. The use of these sheaths is often particularly important to reach the anterior wall of the RA.

Transseptal puncture is often not necessary in ablation of AT in congenital heart patients, as the substrate for ablation is often located in the systemic venous atrium. The most common scenario in which transseptal puncture is indicated is with patients who have portions of the native RA that contain the AT substrate baffled to the pulmonary venous atrial chamber.[3] This includes patients who have undergone a Mustard or Senning procedure and some forms of the Fontan procedure, which involve RA baffling ("lateral tunnel" procedures and RA baffles designed to direct blood from an atrial septal defect to a right-sided AV valve). In these patients, the CTI must usually be ablated from the pulmonary venous atrium, necessitating a transseptal puncture. Other transseptal puncture indications include patients who have clear evidence of left ATs, a relatively rare finding, and patients in whom AF is the primary ablation target and in whom a maze procedure is planned.

It is generally wise to consider and search for any native or postoperative interatrial communication, which might be used for transseptal access prior to performance of a puncture. When transseptal puncture must be performed, care must be taken, as they often involve passage through prosthetic and/or thickened septae, and the anatomy of the systemic and pulmonary venous atria is almost always unique. ICE imaging may be a valuable adjunct in crossing a septum safely (**Figure 5.5**), but at present in our laboratory, we use fluoroscopy and angiography as primary tools to understand the geometry of the procedure. Performance of a levophase angiogram of the pulmonary venous atrium is often useful in defining the transseptal course (▶ Videos 5.5 and 5.6). Although transseptal sheath and dilator will sometimes pass easily into the LA with mild pressure, it is common that considerable force may still not result in passage of the sheath. In these cases, the best strategy for safe puncture may be to search for a better spot to apply pressure, with moves of as little as a millimeter or two sometimes revealing a much easier spot to pass the sheath. Valuable adjunct techniques include use of the RF transseptal needle[4] (Baylis transseptal needle, Baylis Medical, Montreal, Canada) and/or placement of a fine exchange wire through the transseptal needle lumen and use of a coronary balloon to dilate the hole.

Successful transseptal puncture can be confirmed with visualization of contrast (▶ Video 5.7). Attention must be paid to careful removal of the dilator and wire, lest air become entrained in the sheath and subsequently embolized when a catheter is introduced.

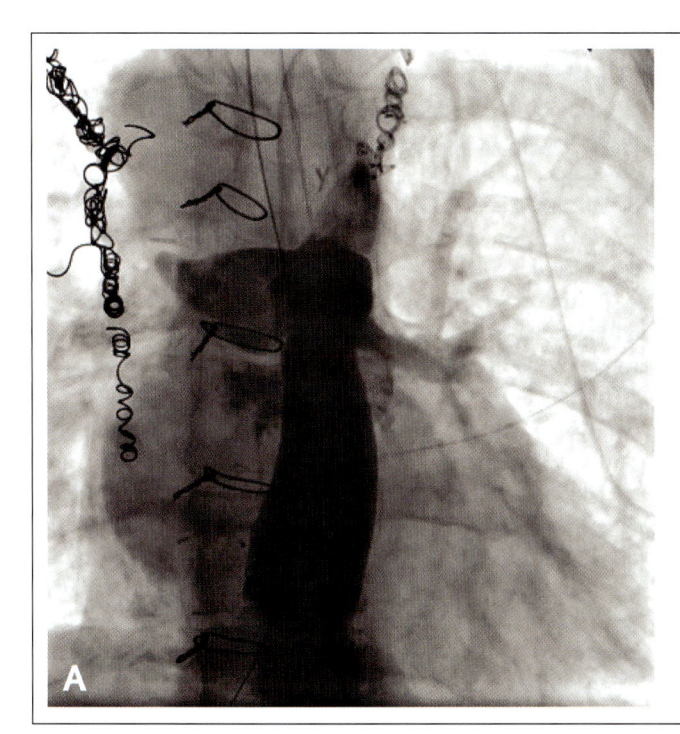

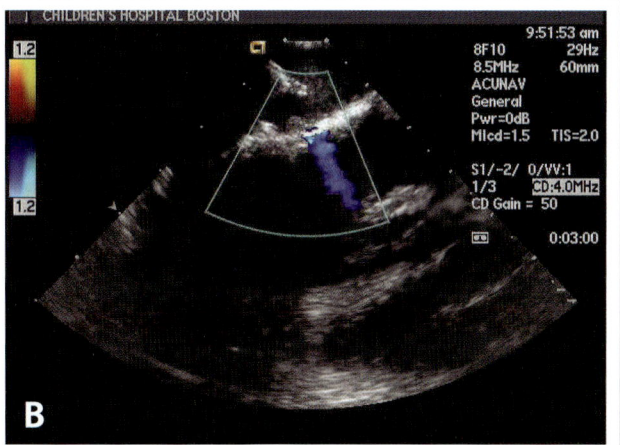

Figure 5.5 Use of ICE from within the intra-atrial baffle of a patient with a Fontan procedure to assist with transbaffle access. **A.** Angiography of the systemic venous pathway. Note that a prior surgical fenestration has been closed by placement of a transcatheter device, and a small residual defect is present at its superior margin. **B.** Echocardiographic identification of a small baffle leak adjacent to the closure device using Doppler imaging. Note the tip of the transseptal sheath aligned with the defect.

Catheter Selection

We routinely use RF for energy delivery for performing AT ablation and, most commonly, RF catheters enhanced by open irrigation. This allows for increased power delivery in atrial chambers, which are frequently large and have low local blood-flow velocities. Under these conditions, normal temperature-controlled catheters are frequently quite limited with respect to power. It has been our and others' observation that irrigated ablation in these patients has not increased the incidence of adverse events, and the increased efficacy of ablation using this technology has been demonstrated in patient series specific to CHD.[5,6] A modest disadvantage of irrigated ablation is that the open-system irrigation that we most commonly use (ThermoCool, Biosense Webster Inc, Diamond Bar, CA) results in a significant volume load over longer procedures, not infrequently 1 to 3 liters. This is management by placement of a Foley catheter, monitoring of urinary output and administration of IV diuresis as needed.

Mapping

During ablation of APs, the AV annulus may be effectively located by analysis of the EGM itself, in combination with fluoroscopic support. In contrast, mapping of a macroreentrant circuit that may involve many areas of the atrial surface requires a technique for recording and integrated display of that entire surface. Although attempts to ablate AT in complex congenital heart patients were initiated prior to the availability of electroanatomical mapping tools such as CARTO (Biosense Webster, Inc, Diamond Bar, CA) and NavX (St. Jude Medical, Sunnyvale, CA), rapid and effective interpretation of activation sequences was exceedingly difficult and success rates relatively low. It is fair to say that 3-dimensional mapping is an enabling technology for these ablation procedures.[7]

The process of mapping in ablation of ATs thus involves creation of an anatomical shell for mapping and superimposition of an electrical activation pattern onto this model. The original versions of 3-dimensional mapping tools collected anatomical and electrical information entirely from the recorded movements of the catheter tip; as the mapping electrode moved through the cardiac chamber and recorded electrical signals from the endocardium, a shell representing the endocardial surface was sequentially built. Successful efforts have been made to integrate anatomical imaging with electroanatomical mapping, either by import, segmentation, and registration of cardiac MRI or CT data sets[2] or by real-time integration of navigated ICE (**Figures 5.6** and **5.7**).[8] Each of these techniques has been demonstrated to be of great potential value in understanding the often complex anatomy of patients with congenital heart defects and complex atrial surgical palliation, and each ensures that important anatomical detail is not overlooked in the mapping and ablation process.

Targeted Ablation

In determining an appropriate strategy for ablation, it is important to recognize that the mechanisms of atrial reentrant arrhythmias common in patients with CHD constitute a spectrum ranging from the common form of AFL to AF. Within this spectrum, a very large number of

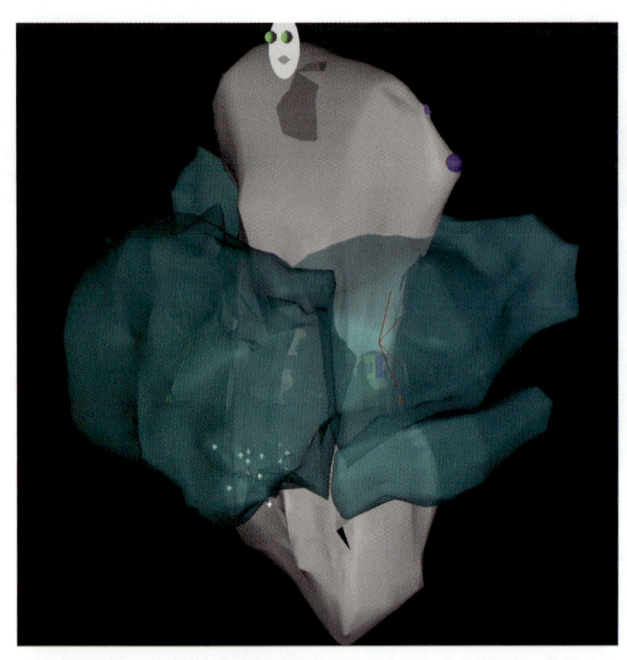

Figure 5.6 Construction of a patient Fontan anatomy prior to mapping on an arrhythmia, using navigated ICE, created by segmentation of many echocardiographic frames and assignment of contours to appropriate chambers. This patient example is also seen in Video 5.8. The systemic venous baffle is shown in gray, while the pulmonary venous structures (LA, pulmonary venous RA and CS) are colored in green.

patients display atypical forms of macroreentry, sometimes many in a single patient, which are based on myocardial features that are sometimes difficult to ascertain. Most of these patients have clinical and inducible tachycardias that are of fixed CL and P-wave morphology, ranging in CL generally from 200 to 400 ms, and thus are suitable for electroanatomical mapping and targeted attempts at ablation (**Figure 5.8**; also see **Figure 5.2**).

The specific ablative approach that is most commonly applied in our laboratory is the careful creation of an anatomical shell, followed by mapping of a stable AT. Attention is paid to covering the entire RA surface and observing that the entire CL of the tachycardia has been sampled. Although it is often the case that the entry into the anatomical LA is not necessary in these cases (because of the relative rarity of LA tachycardias in CHD patients), it is critical to recognize that in patients who have undergone surgical placement of atrial baffles and patches, major components of the RA may actually be located on the pulmonary venous side of the circulation. Those pulmonary venous but anatomically RA locations are often critical components of clinical arrhythmia circuits, and they are only accessible by either retrograde placement of a catheter in the pulmonary venous side of the RA or puncture of the surgically placed baffle as described above (**Figures 5.9** and **5.10**, ▶ **Video 5.8**).

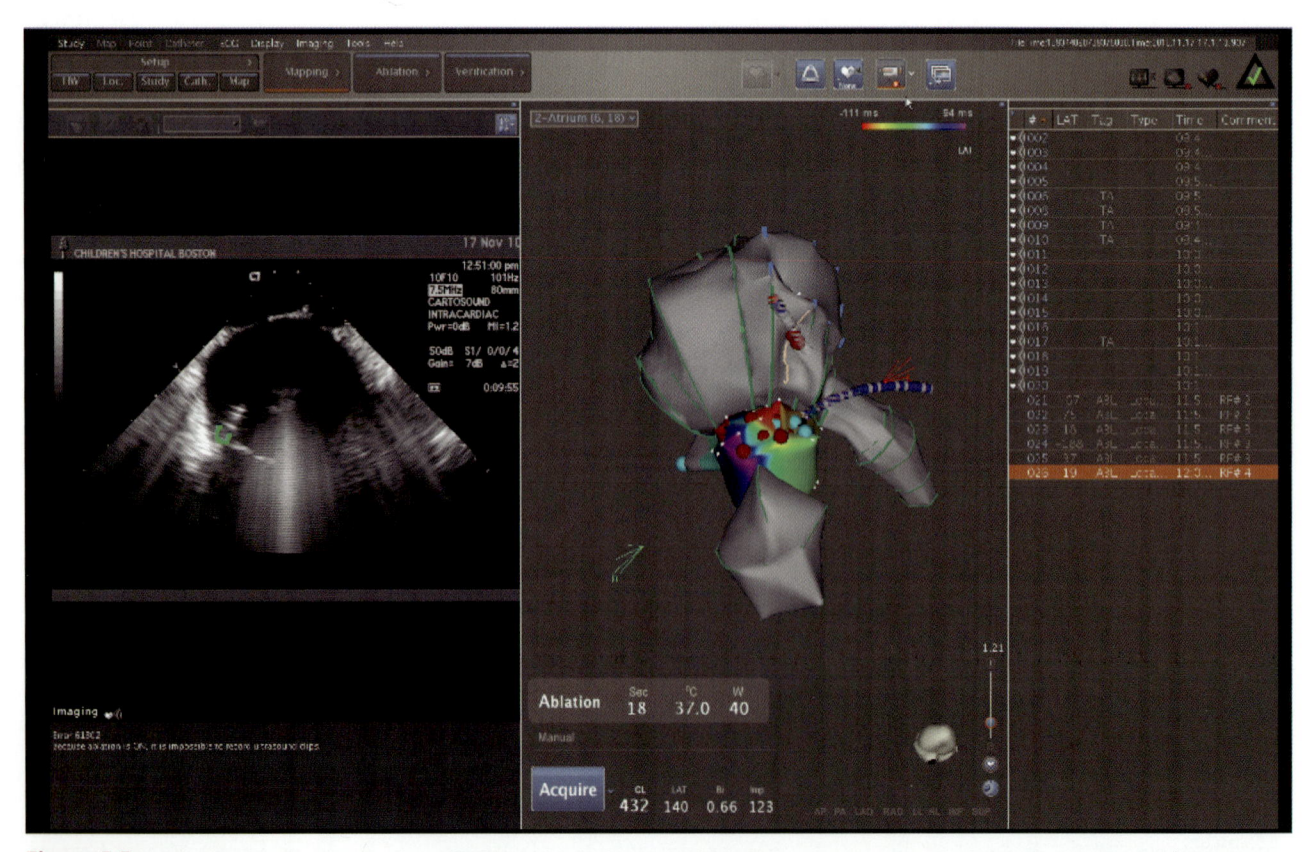

Figure 5.7 User interface for construction of integrated mapping and echo-based real-time anatomical views in CartoSOUND™ (Biosense Webster, Inc, Diamond Bar, CA). Panel on left shows 2-dimensional echo image, with catheter tip located by green annotation. Center frame portrays combination of echo- and mapping-based anatomy and activation sequence, anatomical structures, location of other catheters, and ablation lesions.

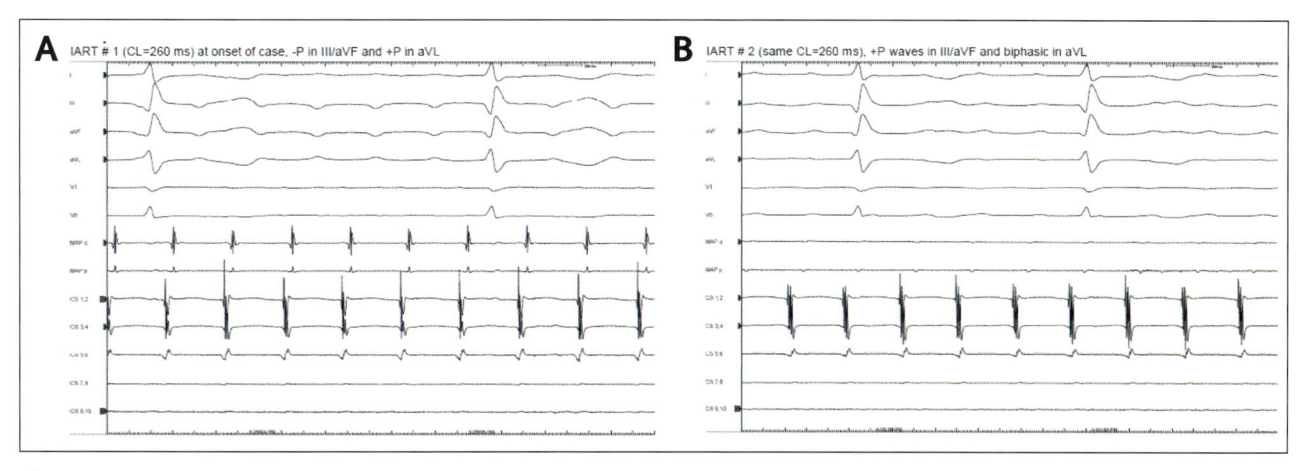

Figure 5.8 Typical appearance of atrial EGMs recorded during intracardiac study of complex congenital patients in AT. **A** and **B** represent 2 distinct activation sequences seen in one patient, both of which mapped to the same anatomical pathway. Even though surface P waves may be indistinct in some cases (see Figure 5.2), intracardiac recording usually proves the presence of a sTable and relatively monomorphic AT. Rapid atrial conduction during mapping and ablation can usually be managed by judicious use of short-acting calcium channel blockers. AF is observed in the minority of cases.

Efforts are made to carefully delineate all potential central obstacles to a macroreentrant circuit when and to indicate their anatomical locations accurately. These features include the ostia of the caval veins, the AV valves, areas of surgically created scar (e.g., atriotomies, patches) and areas of patchy fibrosis. Scarred atrium is identified by the annotation of double potential EGMs, which indicates a fixed line of block, and by definition of areas in which endocardial electrode contact results in EGMs that are absent or of extremely low voltage (**Figure 5.11**). The specific voltage that is considered to represent "scar" is a topic for debate, and few pathological correlations have been performed to inform this point, but most authors have found that voltage thresholds of 0.1 to 0.5 mV are useful in creating electroanatomical maps when the mechanism of the arrhythmia, the scar location and the effect of ablation are aligned (**Figure 5.12**).[9] These putative areas of scarring can be identified using automated features of the mapping system or by manual adjustment of color scale parameters in voltage-mapping modes.

It is not infrequent in these cases that the tachycardia mechanism changes before a complete map has been created. This must be recognized immediately to avoid entry of incorrect and confusing data into an active map and can be detected by observation of abrupt changes in CL, P-wave morphology, and activation sequence and morphologies of other reference atrial EGMs. In these cases, it

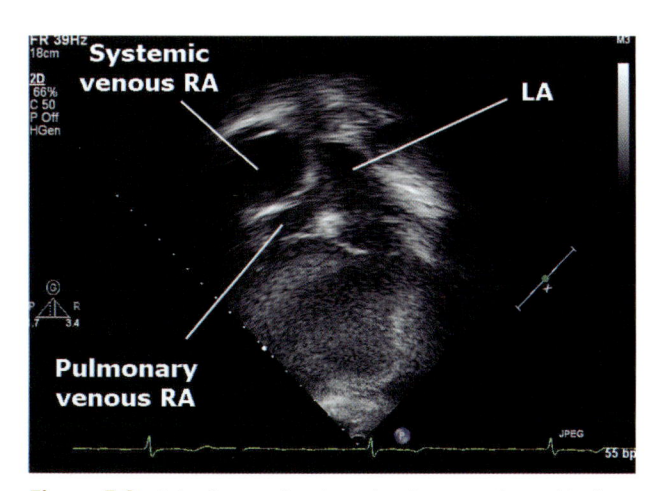

Figure 5.9 Echo frame of patient also shown angiographically in Video 5.8 and Figure 5.10. The Fontan has been surgically constructed by insertion of an intra-atrial baffle patch, which directs blood flowing through a large ASD to the right-sided AV valve. A small, pulmonary venous supravalvar RA chamber is seen, corresponding to the anatomical location (in a patient with normal anatomy) of the CTI.

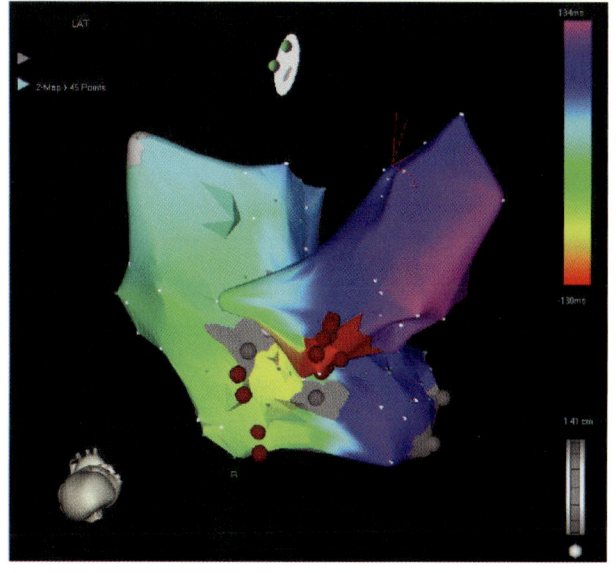

Figure 5.10 Companion to Figure 5.9. This electroanatomical map shows an inferior view of the activation map, with successful interruption of a periannular flutter from ablation within this small supravalvar chamber.

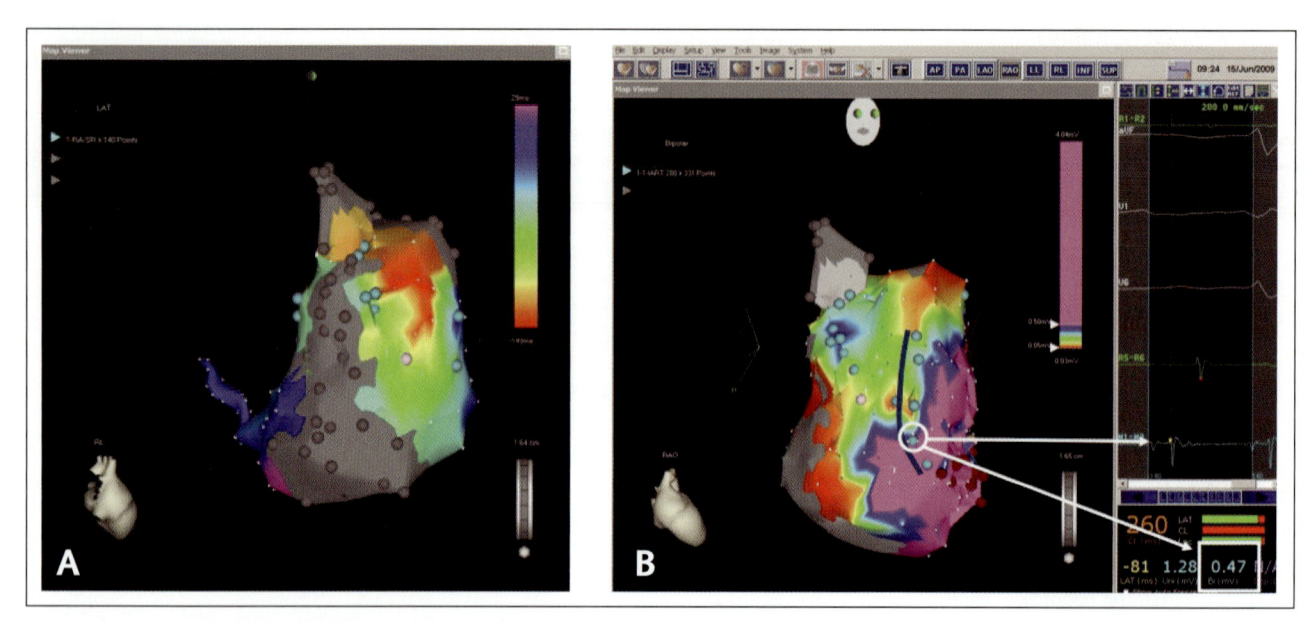

Figure 5.11 Identification of diffuse and discrete scarring in the atria of patients with congenital heart defects. **A.** Areas of diffuse fibrosis and scarring can be generally identified by annotation of mapped areas with EGMs below a threshold voltage amplitude as "scar" (grey dots and areas). In this map, the threshold has been set to be 0.1 mV. Use of higher or lower thresholds will result in smaller or larger areas being selected. **B.** A discrete line of double potentials is constructed to identify fixed barriers to conduction, in this case a likely site of prior surgical atriotomy.

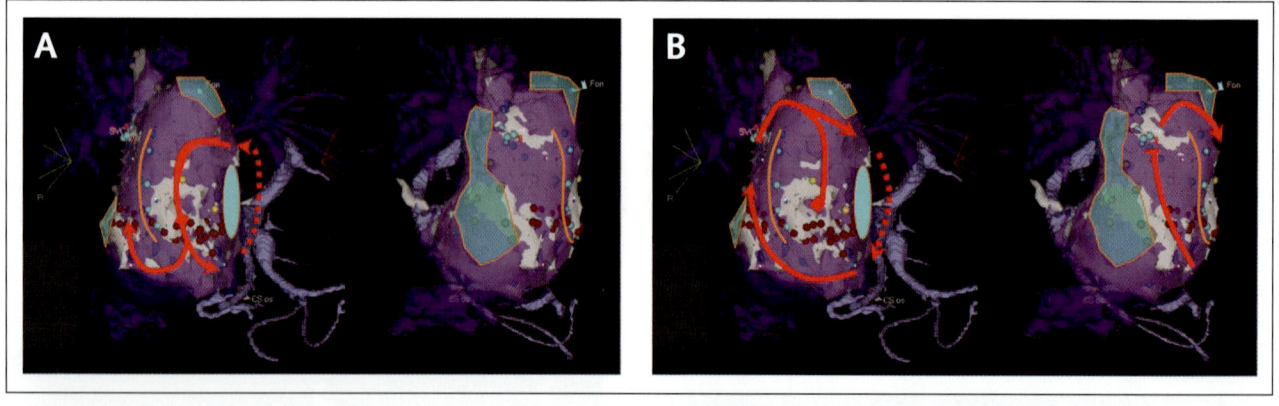

Figure 5.12 Integration of anatomy, scar location, activation sequence and ablation site in a complex AT circuit. This patient is also shown in Figures 5.3 and 5.11. Surgical scarring (heavy orange line) and areas of fibrosis (blue shading outlined in orange), as well as the hypoplastic and surgically closed ostium of the right AV valve (blue oval) create a complex arrhythmia substrate with demonstration of 2 of the potential circuits ("dual-loop tachycardia," represented by heavy red arrows). **A.** Initial periannular circuit, terminated by ablation between lateral border of the AV groove and the surgical atriotomy. **B.** Slower tachycardia inducible after ablation of the first circuit, requiring additional closure of a more lateral corridor of activation.

is our practice to open up a new map, utilizing the preexisting atrial anatomy that we have already acquired. In some cases an entire sequence of partially completed maps is simultaneously active, and close attention to working in the correct map is important.

Once an arrhythmia circuit has been mapped and related to the underlying atrial anatomy, a decision must be made as to whether to move on to ablation or to confirm the mechanism of the circuit using entrainment pacing. Entrainment pacing is often very useful for confirmation of arrhythmia mechanism in cases in which there is no initial response of the tachycardia to ablation.[10] A potential drawback to routine entrainment pacing is that it has the potential to terminate the mapped arrhythmia. To minimize the likelihood of this, we tend to limit entrainment pacing to cases in which we have a specific unanswered question, and we pace only slightly faster (~10 ms) than the TCL (**Figure 5.13**).

As mentioned above, we currently use irrigated ablation catheters for most macroreentrant AT ablations in patients with CHD. We begin with 30 W of energy and titrate to a maximum of 50 W, with a maximum temperature of 42°C. If the area that we are targeting appears to be a broad isthmus (eg, the isthmus between the IVC and the right AV valve), we will place lesions in a sequential linear manner. In arrhythmias in which there is a narrow channel of

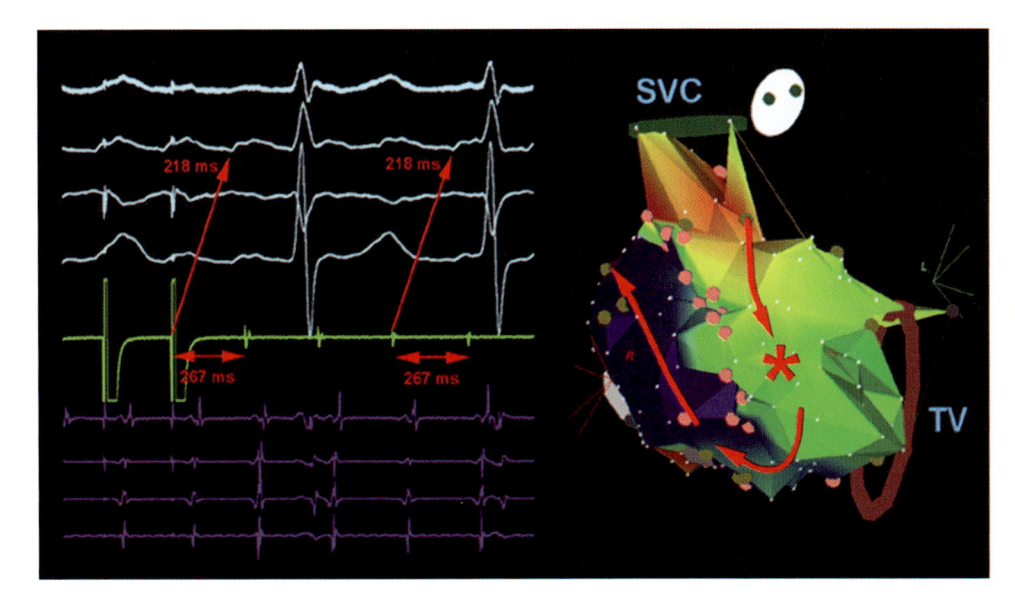

Figure 5.13 Demonstration of entrainment pacing in a patient with incisional right AT after a biventricular repair of tetralogy of Fallot. A line of double potentials indicating a discrete atriotomy scar is represented as pink dots and the putative activation pattern by the red arrow. Pacing just faster than the CL within the circuit results in acceleration of the rhythm, followed by a first PPI at the pacing site, which is approximately equal to the TCL measured in subsequent beats.

activation and an exit point, delivery of energy is more focused. Assuring excellent endocardial contact of the ablation catheter is critical in effective ablation. Although this can be determined fluoroscopically by catheter deflection or motion during the cardiac cycle, it can be difficult to determine in some volumes of very enlarged or abnormal atrial chambers. Additional criteria for contact include recording of sharp atrial EGMs, concordance of catheter position with the atrial endocardial surface as determined by electroanatomical mapping, and, more recently, by direct visualization of the catheter tip in relation to the endocardium by ICE (see **Figure 5.7**, ▶ **Videos 5.3** and **5.4**).

Immediate feedback that indicates an appropriate target during ablation includes termination or abrupt slowing of the tachycardia. In the case of termination, it is important to ensure that the tachycardia was not interrupted by an atrial extrasystole; conversely, we believe that slowing of the tachycardia prior to termination is a positive sign reflecting the effect of ablation in a critical conduction corridor. In cases in which the tachycardia abruptly slows but does not terminate, it is important to determine whether the mechanism has changed. Because of the complex nature of the atrial substrate, it is not uncommon to reveal "dual-loop" reentries by the successful ablation of one loop prior to recognition of the second potential circuit. If this is suspected, a new activation map should be performed.

Lesion Confirmation

It is desirable, if possible, to prove after ablation that conduction through the ablated area has been completely blocked. In the relatively large number of patients who require ablation of the isthmus between the IVC and the right AV valve, this is relatively easy to do using pacing in the mouth of the CS or at the lateral margin of the isthmus. "Gaps," when they are identified, are often at the actual hinge point of the AV valve or posterior to the Eustachian ridge, as they are for the common varieties of AFL.

Arrhythmia circuits that are ablated elsewhere in the atrium can be considerably more problematic to test in this way, as it can be difficult to establish and maintain appropriate pacing sites and to record the novel activation patterns thoroughly enough to prove conduction block. A general principle that should be applied to this type of testing is that the pacing electrode should be placed as close as possible to the ablated zone, and the recorded map should demonstrate that the opposite end of the ablated corridor shows no sign whatsoever of activation through the ablated tissue.

Empiric Ablation Strategies

Although targeted ablation is generally appropriate for organized ATs in CHD patients, in some situations it is appropriate to consider empiric ablation strategies. The first such group consists of the great majority of patients who have an identifiable isthmus of tissue between the IVC and the right AV valve, whether it is a tricuspid or mitral valve. Almost all patients with this anatomy have the potential for periannular AFL. In patients with biventricular repairs and those with postoperative Mustard/Senning anatomy, the CTI should always be considered as an important target for ablation, as it is the substrate most commonly associated with clinical arrhythmia. Thus, it is generally prudent and indicated in these patients to ablate the isthmus, even if other arrhythmias are also present (**Figure 5.14** and ▶ **Video 5.9**).

The second such group consists of patients who have AF or such complex and rapidly changing ATs that they are effectively impossible to map. These patients are more commonly those with massive atrial enlargement, often older variants of the Fontan procedure. The use of RA and

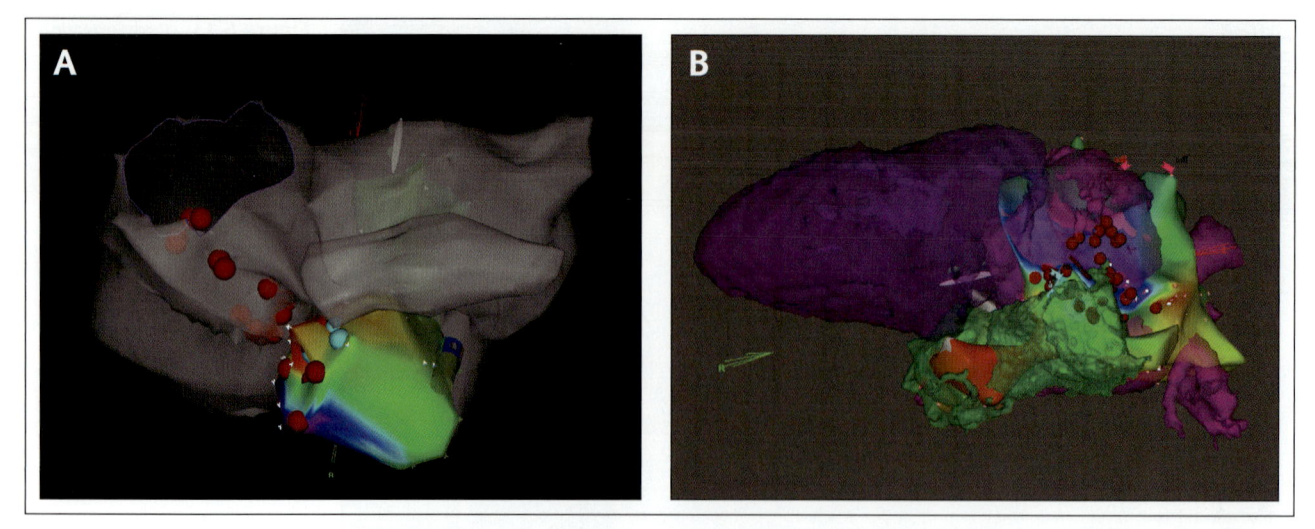

Figure 5.14 Examples of isthmus lines in congenital heart lesions with intra-atrial baffling resulting in pulmonary venous location of the CTI. **A.** Patient with a lateral tunnel Fontan, also shown in Figure 5.6 and Video 5.10, showing inferior view of transbaffle ablation line from right-sided AV groove to intra-atrial baffle. Additional lesions have been placed on the systemic venous side of the baffle down to the IVC. **B.** Patient with dextrocardia, situs inversus and a Mustard procedure also shown in Videos 5.1 and 5.2, showing an ablation line formed from the AV groove (in this case, the anterior mitral valve), again on both pulmonary venous and systemic venous sides of the intra-atrial baffle.

biatrial catheter maze procedures in these CHD patients is anecdotal to date, as these patients are relatively rare, present unique technical challenges, and are more often considered to be candidates for surgical maze procedures, often in conjunction with repair of other concomitant hemodynamic issues. We have on occasion performed these types of procedures, modeling our interventions on the creation of long ablative lines as performed intraoperatively. Arrhythmia control after these procedures is variable; although there have been some successful procedures, this is an area in development that will benefit from more research and innovation.

Postprocedure Care

Follow-Up, Recurrence, and Repeat Ablation

The specific follow-up for patients with CHD undergoing ablation of AT varies with respect to the acute success of the procedure, the severity of their underlying heart disease, and, since most of these procedures are performed at regional referral centers, their geographical location relative to the center. In the opinion of the author, minimal follow-up for these patients should include clinical evaluation at 2 and 12 months with evaluation of symptoms and events and some form of noninvasive monitoring (either 24-hour ambulatory ECG or pacemaker telemetry).

Long-term recurrence of ATs is not uncommon in patients with acutely successful ablation procedures.[11,12] This is most commonly observed in patients with very complex atrial arrhythmias, often older patients with variants of the Fontan procedure[13] who have extreme atrial enlargement and diffuse scarring. Recurrences may be due to incomplete ablation of existing arrhythmia substrates or clinical emergence of arrhythmia patterns not detected on initial EP study.[14] Because they are relatively frequent, it is often reasonable to leave patients on their preablation antiarrhythmic medications for a period of months after ablation. Repeat ablation is a practical alternative, particularly in patients who were noted to have a relatively simple arrhythmia substrate and in whom recurrence appears to reflect the same clinical tachycardia previously ablated. This is often a sign that the specific reason for that recurrence was incomplete ablation.

Procedural Complications

Because it is relatively less common that CHD patients require extensive LA ablation, some of the more significant adverse event concerns relating to ablation of AF are of less concern in these patients. In particular, the rate of postprocedural thromboembolism appears to be lower in CHD patients, and to the author's knowledge, atrioesophageal fistula has not been reported. However, these are often sick patients with relatively fragile hemodynamic physiology, and considerable care must be taken to provide them with a safe ablation procedure. During ablation, rapid conduction of AT may result in hypotension and limit ability to perform mapping. This may be addressed in many patients by judicious administration of calcium-channel blocking agents, sometimes prior to tachycardia induction, but may also require inotropic support and, in rare cases, limit the ablation to an empiric strategy.

Attention must be paid to cardiac injury, which can be sustained secondary to ablation in the RA. Most important, all operators must constantly be aware that the location of the AV node and specialized conduction tissues may be anatomically unpredictable and not always detectable by endocardial mapping. Iatrogenic AV block has the potential to be disastrous for CHD patients, both acutely (as they may have no easy access for ventricular pacing) and chronically, and must be carefully avoided. The locations of previously implanted atrial pacing leads, either transvenous or epicardial, should be clearly marked on the electroanatomical maps and noted during ablation, as these existing leads can be rendered useless by ablation lesions.

Diaphragmatic paresis can also occur after ablation, although evidence from surgical series suggests that this is usually a transient and reversible injury. The operator should also maintain a level of awareness as to the possible location of the phrenic nerve when ablating in the posterolateral RA. If proximity is suspected, it is sometimes useful to perform pacing at relatively high outputs from the ablation catheter to determine whether that structure immediately underlies the planned ablation site.

On the first postcatheterization day, we commonly use low-dose intravenous heparin to anticoagulate all patients who have undergone ablation on the pulmonary venous side of their circulation following the procedure and, barring specific contraindications, most patients who have undergone extensive right-sided ablation. Patients are rapidly returned to their preablation anticoagulation regimen, and if they were on no such medication prior to ablation, will typically be placed on aspirin for 2 to 3 months.

Advantages and Limitations

Acute success rates for ablation of CHD patients with AT are quite center dependent but have generally improved over the past 15 years, in conjunction with greater capabilities of mapping and ablative technology and increasing expertise of centers performing this procedure. In general, procedural success is reported to range from 80 to 90% in recent case series. Long-term freedom from recurrence is less well documented, and because recurrence is more likely in complex patients, this parameter is also likely to vary considerably depending on the case-mix of CHD patients that are ablated in a given center.

It is widely believed, without strong clinical studies to support it, that medical and pacing therapies for these arrhythmias are at most adjunctive, and while they may suppress clinical arrhythmia in some selected patients, they are not reliably effective treatment modalities. The comparator for catheter ablation therapies is the surgical maze procedure, but no direct comparison between these therapy modalities has been made in a single study. Review of case series published in both areas suggests that compared to arrhythmia surgery, catheter ablation may have a lower long-term efficacy, but it is also less likely to be complicated by procedural mortality. Arrhythmia surgery would appear to have a significant therapeutic advantage in those patients with AF who may be difficult to address even acutely with catheter-based approaches.

Conclusions

Ablation of AT in patients with CHD is a complex procedure that requires an understanding of the underlying anatomy, advanced technological support, and a variety of specific catheter-manipulation and vascular-access skills. Ablation in this patient group presents a very distinct set of challenges to those encountered in ablation of AF, although the two procedures do share some common techniques. While acute procedural success rates are quite high, patients with more complex anatomy are at significant risk for recurrence. Good follow-up is important, and repeat ablation attempts may be necessary.

References

1. Triedman JK. Arrhythmias in adults with congenital heart disease. *Heart.* 2002;87(4):383–389.
2. Pflaumer A, Deisenhofer I, Hausleiter J, Zrenner B. Mapping and ablation of atypical flutter in congenital heart disease with a novel three-dimensional mapping system (Carto Merge). *Europace.* 2006;8(2):138–139.
3. Perry JC, Boramanand NK, Ing FF. "Transseptal" technique through atrial baffles for 3-dimensional mapping and ablation of atrial tachycardia in patients with d-transposition of the great arteries. *J Interv Card Electrophysiol.* 2003;9(3):365–369.
4. Smelley MP, Shah DP, Weisberg I, Kim SS, Lin AC, Beshai JF, Burke MC, Knight BP. Initial experience using a radiofrequency powered transseptal needle. *J Cardiovasc Electrophysiol.* 2010;21(4):423–427.
5. Tanner H, Lukac P, Schwick N, Fuhrer J, Pedersen AK, Hansen PS, Delacretaz E. Irrigated-tip catheter ablation of intraatrial reentrant tachycardia in patients late after surgery of congenital heart disease. *Heart Rhythm.* 2004;1(3):268–275.
6. Triedman JK, DeLucca JM, Alexander ME, Berul CI, Cecchin F, Walsh EP. Prospective trial of electroanatomically guided, irrigated catheter ablation of atrial tachycardia in patients with congenital heart disease. *Heart Rhythm.* 2005;2(7):700–705.
7. Triedman JK, Alexander ME, Love BA, Collins KK, Berul CI, Bevilacqua LM, Walsh EP. Influence of patient factors and ablative technologies on outcomes of radiofrequency ablation of intra-atrial re-entrant tachycardia in patients with congenital heart disease. *J Am Coll Cardiol.* 2002;39(11):1827–1835.
8. Kean AC, Gelehrter SK, Shetty I, Dick M, 2nd, Bradley DJ. Experience with CartoSound for arrhythmia ablation in pediatric and congenital heart disease patients. *J Interv Card Electrophysiol.* 2010;29(2):139–145.
9. De Groot NM, Kuijper AF, Blom NA, Bootsma M, Schalij MJ. Three-dimensional distribution of bipolar atrial electrogram voltages in patients with congenital heart disease. *Pacing Clin Electrophysiol.* 2001;24(9 Pt 1):1334–1342.

10. Delacretaz E, Ganz LI, Soejima K, Friedman PL, Walsh EP, Triedman JK, Sloss LJ, Landzberg MJ, Stevenson WG. Multi atrial macro-reentry circuits in adults with repaired congenital heart disease: entrainment mapping combined with three-dimensional electroanatomic mapping. *J Am Coll Cardiol.* 2001;37(6):1665–1676.
11. de Groot NM, Atary JZ, Blom NA, Schalij MJ. Long-term outcome after ablative therapy of postoperative atrial tachyarrhythmia in patients with congenital heart disease and characteristics of atrial tachyarrhythmia recurrences. *Circ Arrhythm Electrophysiol.* 2010;3(2):148–154.
12. Kannankeril PJ, Anderson ME, Rottman JN, Wathen MS, Fish FA. Frequency of late recurrence of intra-atrial reentry tachycardia after radiofrequency catheter ablation in patients with congenital heart disease. *Am J Cardiol.* 2003;92(7):879–881.
13. Yap SC, Harris L, Silversides CK, Downar E, Chauhan VS. Outcome of intra-atrial re-entrant tachycardia catheter ablation in adults with congenital heart disease: negative impact of age and complex atrial surgery. *J Am Coll Cardiol.* 2010;56(19):1589–1596.
14. De Groot NM, Blom N, Vd Wall EE, Schalij MJ. Different mechanisms underlying consecutive, postoperative atrial tachyarrhythmias in a Fontan patient. *Pacing Clin Electrophysiol.* 2009;32(11):e18–e20.

Video Descriptions

Video 5.1 Segmentation of a patient with complex anatomy prior to ablation procedure. This patient has corrected transposition in situs inversus and has undergone a "double switch" procedure (arterial switch procedure and intra-atrial Mustard baffle). The posterior right ventricle and enlarged pulmonary arteries are removed first, followed by the anterior left ventricle. The green posterior chamber is the systemic venous atrium, consisting of baffles from the left-sided vena cavae to the right subpulmonary atrium. The purple chamber is the pulmonary venous atrium, which wraps around the "crotch" of the baffles and directs blood to the anterior mitral valve. A brief angiogram of this patient is presented in Video 5.2, and the ablation line for her AT appears in Figure 5.14, Panel B.

Video 5.2 Angiographic companion to Video 5.1 showing the systemic venous pathway.

Video 5.3 ICE in a patient with massively enlarged RA, showing irrigated catheter during ineffective ablation with catheter tip ~1 cm from endocardial surface, undetected without use of imaging.

Video 5.4 Same patient as Video 5.3, with long vascular sheath used to advance catheter tip further to anterior RA endocardial surface. ICE now shows good tissue contact, and ablation was effective and resulted in tachycardia termination.

Video 5.5 Patient with transposition of the great arteries who has undergone a Senning procedure, a form of intra-atrial baffling similar to the Mustard procedure described above and diagrammatically illustrated in Figure 5.7 (different patient). In this video, an angiogram is performed in the pulmonary artery, and levophase clearly demonstrates the pulmonary venous atrium, which is the target for "transbaffle" puncture, shown in Video 5.6.

Video 5.6 Companion video to Video 5.5. In the same patient, a transseptal catheter is poised with proper trajectory to pierce the baffle and enter the pulmonary venous atrium. A small amount of angiographic contrast demonstrates that the needle is tenting the baffle material.

Video 5.7 Demonstration of pulmonary venous atrial anatomy with an angiographic contrast injection through a transbaffle sheath. This angiogram was performed in the same patient shown in Figure 5.6.

Video 5.8 Companion to Figures 5.9 and 5.10. This patient with an intra-atrial baffle has undergone transbaffle puncture, and a sheath is placed into the pulmonary venous atrium. A small angiographic catheter has been advanced into the supravalvar RA on the pulmonary venous side of the baffle.

Video 5.9 Propagation sequence of periannular AT in a lateral tunnel Fontan, companion to Figures 5.6 and 5.14 (Panel A). Mapping has only been performed in the systemic venous side of the baffle but shows that the circuit must implicitly traverse the pulmonary venous portion of the atrium located between the right-sided AV groove and the margin of the intra-atrial baffle.

CHAPTER 6

How to Perform Radiofrequency and Cryoablation Ablation for AV Nodal Reentrant Tachycardia

Paul J. Wang, MD; Zhongwei Cheng, MD

Introduction

AVNRT is the most common paroxysmal SVT, affecting women twice as frequently as men.[1-3] Catheter-based RF ablation[1-23] and cryoablation[24-28] are now well established as the definitive treatments for most patients, with excellent success rates (> 90–97% cure) and a low incidence of serious complications.[4,5] AVNRT occurs in patients with dual AV nodal physiology. The fast pathway is anteriorly situated along septal portion of the tricuspid annulus. The slow pathway is posteriorly situated close to the CS ostium. Discontinuous, nonuniform anisotropy within the triangle of Koch is a substrate that can support functional, anisotropic reentry, a condition that can exhibit dual-pathway physiological characteristics.

There are 3 types of AVNRT: slow-fast (SF), also called "typical"; fast-slow (FS) and slow-slow (SS) type. In the common or "typical" form of AVNRT, which accounts for about 90% of cases, the antegrade limb of the reentrant circuit usually conducts slowly, whereas the retrograde limb conduction is fast.

The 2 major energy sources used for AVNRT therapy include RF energy and cryoablation. Lesion formation with RF energy is more rapid, occurring within 30 seconds and resulting in junctional beats, which provide a marker of ablation. Cryoablation lesions are longer, usually 4 minutes in duration, but provide a safety margin of reversibility, essentially eliminating the risk of AV block.[2]

Preprocedural Preparation

There are very limited tests required before catheter ablation of AVNRT. It may be useful to have an echocardiogram to exclude any coexisting abnormalities of the tricuspid valve and annulus.

It is quite useful to have an ECG recording of the SVT, since in most cases the diagnosis of mechanism of the tachycardia is not known and an ECG of the rhythm may provide clues. Atrial activity 80 ms or less after the onset of the QRS complex is most consistent with AVNRT. There may a somewhat inverted P wave in the inferior leads and an rSr in lead V_1. Occasionally the P wave may be later after the termination of the QRS complex. In atypical AVNRT, the P wave is usually before the QRS complex. A P-wave morphology that is upright in the inferior leads effectively excludes AVNRT.

Having a recording of the SVT prior to the ablation procedure also provides a greater degree of certainty that a patient's palpitations are not due to sinus tachycardia. If no SVT is induced during EP testing, the decision will need to be made how to proceed. Some electrophysiologists will perform an empiric ablation of the slow AV nodal pathway if the patient has dual AV nodal pathways and a documented SVT consistent with AVNRT despite the noninducibility of the tachycardia.

An ECG at the spontaneous initiation of the SVT is particularly helpful, since it provides a potential clue to the mechanism. An abrupt prolongation of the PR interval with the first beat of the tachycardia would be highly suggestive of AVNRT as the mechanism. Similarly, spontaneous termination of the tachycardia may provide clues regarding the mechanism. Termination with a P wave that is not premature would be most consistent with an AVNRT or AV reciprocating tachycardia.

The baseline ECG should be examined for PR prolongation. Preexisting prolongation of the PR is not a contraindication to slow pathway ablation, but one will need to characterize the fast pathway refractory period to determine that adequate AV conduction will remain after slow pathway ablation.

Any ECG monitoring should be examined for clues regarding AV nodal refractory period such as blocked premature atrial complexes. Medications, including AV nodal blocking agents and antiarrhythmic agents, are usually stopped 5 or more half-lives before the procedure to increase the likelihood of inducibility of the supraventricular tachycardia. Written informed consent, including the success rate and possible complications, must be obtained from every patient before the procedure.

Procedure

Patient Preparation

The patients undergoing RF ablation or cryoablation most commonly receive conscious sedation, but selected patients may request or require general anesthesia. In some patients, general anesthesia or a deep level of sedation may make the AVNRT less inducible, and occasionally these patients may need to receive less sedation or have termination of anesthesia to permit assessment of inducibility as a procedural endpoint.

The number of access and introducers placed for EP testing and catheter ablation varies from laboratory to laboratory. In our laboratory, we routinely place a CS catheter in all SVT studies. Access for the CS catheter may be femoral venous, usually on the right side, or via the right internal jugular. A 6-Fr sheath is used if a decapolar catheter is used, and a 7-Fr sheath is used if a duodecapolar catheter is used. The left femoral vein accommodates two 6-Fr sheaths for the placement of two 4-pole catheters—one placed in the RA, the other in the right ventricle. The right vein accommodates one 6-Fr sheath and one 8-Fr sheath. The 6-Fr sheath is used for the placement of a 4-pole catheter in the His region, while the 8-Fr sheath is used for the placement of the ablation catheter.

Anticoagulation with IV heparin is not routinely used. Individuals with an increased risk of deep vein thrombosis, such as women taking oral contraceptives or patients with known Factor V Leiden deficiency or a history of deep vein thrombosis, may be exceptions.

Electrophysiological Testing and Assessment: Pathophysiology of Dual AV Nodal Pathways

An important part of the AVNRT procedure is the baseline characterization of AV and VA conduction. Ventricular drive pacing and premature stimulation are used to characterize VA conduction and to exclude the existence of a retrograde conducting accessory pathway. In atypical AVNRT, ventricular stimulation may be needed for induction. Atrial drive pacing and atrial premature stimulation are performed to characterize AV conduction. The atrial drive cycle length at which AV Wenckebach occurs is determined. During atrial premature stimulation, the AV nodal effective refractory period is determined. Dual AV nodal pathways, usually defined as an increase in the A2H2 interval of 50 ms or more for a 10- to 15-ms decrease in the A1A2, is noted (**Figure 6.1**). Initiation of AVNRT is noted. In some cases, isoproterenol infusion, usually from 1 to 4 mcg per minute IV, is required to induce AVNRT. Double atrial stimuli in sinus rhythm sometimes may be more effective than atrial premature stimulation alone.

Moe et al[6] was first to demonstrate the existence of 2 AV nodal pathways underlying AVNRT. The fast pathway was found to have a longer refractory period than the slow pathway. These different EP properties facilitate the onset and maintenance of AVNRT. Dual AV nodal physiology is a normal behavior of the human AV node. The presence of dual AV nodal physiology in itself does not imply the presence of AVNRT. **Table 6.1** summarizes the diagnostic criteria for dual AV nodal physiology.

Mapping and Diagnosis

An initial careful baseline EP study is required before the ablation procedure. This is especially relevant for AVNRT because other supraventricular or ventricular arrhythmias may mimic or coexist with this arrhythmia. The presence of a concealed accessory AV pathway should be ruled out before induction of the tachycardia by performing parahisian and differential ventricular pacing. The baseline study will demonstrate dual AV nodal physiology in about 85% of patients with AVNRT, but dual AV nodal physiology can also be observed in patients without AVNRT. Conversely, the absence of verifiable dual AV nodal physiology does not rule out AVNRT.

Three main forms of AVNRT are found: slow-fast, slow-slow, and fast-slow AVNRT. There is no EP finding that alone is diagnostic of AVNRT; the diagnosis is made based on the typical features and the exclusion of atrial tachycardias, junctional tachycardia, and septal accessory AV pathways. **Table 6.2** summarizes the diagnostic criteria of AVNRT and left-sided variants.

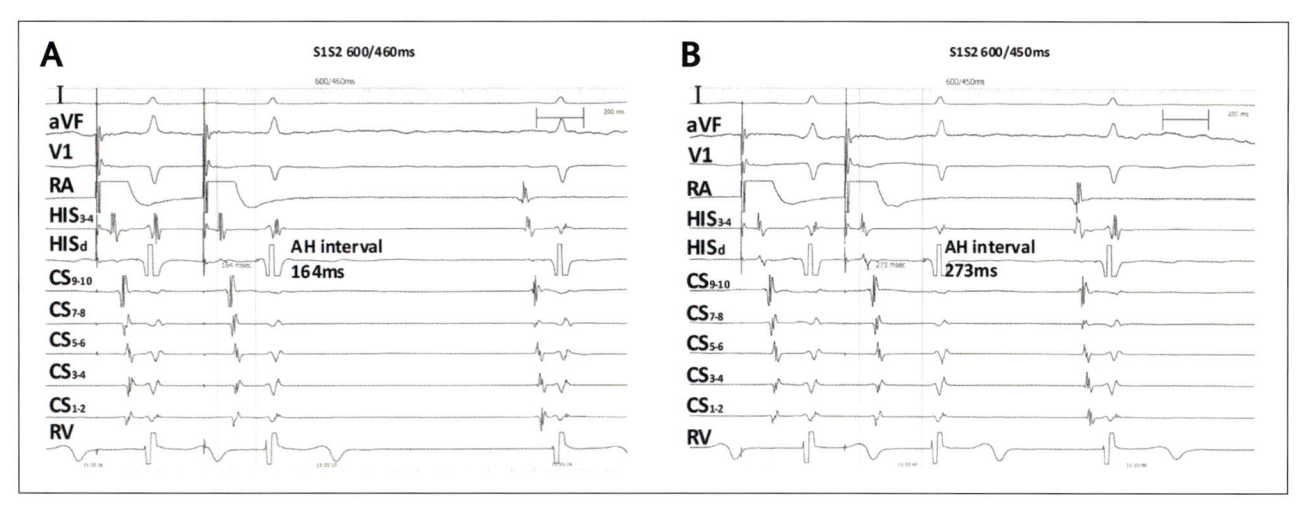

Figure 6.1 The A2H2 interval was 164 ms at S1S2 600/460ms (**A**), and A2H2 interval became 273 ms at S1S2 600/450 ms (**B**); the AH "jump" was 109ms (273 − 164 = 109), consistent with dual AV nodal physiology. The channels from top to bottom were lead I, lead aVF, lead V1, RA, HIS_{3-4}, HIS_d, CS_{9-10}, CS_{8-9}, CS_{7-8}, CS_{5-6}, CS_{3-4}, CS_{1-2} and RV.

Induction of AVNRT is dependent on achieving a critical AH interval for typical slow-fast AVNRT. This requires exclusive antegrade slow pathway conduction, which can be achieved by atrial extrastimulus or atrial burst pacing near the Wenckebach cycle length. If antegrade slow pathway conduction cannot be achieved because short antegrade fast pathway refractoriness, S3 stimulation, burst atrial pacing, or ventricular stimulation with or without isoproterenol may be required. If retrograde fast pathway conduction is absent during ventricular pacing (VA block or earliest retrograde atrial activation at proximal CS) or by lack of echoes or AVNRT following antegrade slow pathway conduction, isoproterenol infusion should be given.

Slow-Fast

The ECG obtained during tachycardia can suggest the diagnosis when the retrograde P wave is superimposed on the terminal portion of the QRS. The antegrade limb of the tachycardia is the slow pathway, with an AH interval longer than 180 ms. A short VA (measured from the surface QRS to the earliest intracardiac atrial electrogram) time of < 60 ms excludes the concealed accessory pathway tachycardias.[7] Adrenergic stimulation (isoproterenol, 1–4 mcg/min) may be used for AVNRT induction. Induction of slow-fast AVNRT from the atrium requires antegrade block over the fast AV nodal pathway, with antegrade conduction over the slow AV nodal pathway allowing retrograde conduction over the fast AV nodal pathway. The site of earliest retrograde atrial activation is critical to differentiate slow-fast from slow-slow AVNRT. About 6% of patients demonstrate early retrograde atrial activation in the CS (so-called eccentric atrial activation) because of muscular connections between the LA and the CS.[8]

Slow-Slow

In this form of reentry, a slow AV nodal pathway is used as the antegrade limb and another slow AV nodal pathway as the retrograde limb. The ECG during tachycardia may show characteristic negative P waves in inferior and

Table 6.1 Features of dual atrioventricular nodal physiology and slow pathway conduction

Dual AV Nodal Physiology
>50 ms increase in A2H2 interval with 10 ms decrease in A1A2 interval
>50 ms increase in AH interval with 10 ms decrease in atrial pacing CL
Double response (2 ventricular responses to a single atrial activation due to simultaneous fast and slow pathway conduction)
Slow Pathway Conduction
AH interval > 180 ms
Stable PR interval > paced PP interval in absence of isoproterenol
Stable VA interval > RR interval with ventricular pacing (retrograde slow pathway)
Earliest retrograde atrial activation near CS ostium (exclude accessory pathway)

A1A2, coupling interval of a single atrial extrastimulus after a basic atrial pacing; AH, atrium–His bundle interval; A2H2, AH interval following the atrial extrastimulus; AV, atrioventricular; VA, ventricular-atrial interval.

Gonzalez MD, Banchs JE, Rivera J. Ablation of atrioventricular nodal reentrant tachycardia and variants. In: Huang SKS, Wood MA, eds. *Catheter Ablation of Cardiac Arrhythmias*. 2ed. Philadelphia, PA: Elsevier; 2011:318–350. With permission.

Table 6.2 Diagnostic criteria of AVNRT and left-sided variants

Slow-Fast
Dual AV nodal physiology in most (85%) cases
Long AH interval (>180 ms) during tachycardia
Initiation of tachycardia dependent on critical AH interval during antegrade slow pathway conduction
Earliest retrograde atrial activation in tachycardia posterior to the tendon of Todaro, near apex of triangle of Koch
Ventricular postpacing interval > 115 ms longer than TCL
VA interval during ventricular pacing at TCL minus VA interval during tachycardia > 85 ms
Late ventricular extrastimuli that advance His bundle activation also advance retrograde atrial activation and reset the tachycardia
Exclude atrial tachycardia and AV reciprocating tachycardia

Slow-Slow
Same as for slow-fast except for early retrograde atrial activation near the CS ostium
Initiation dependent on critical HA interval during retrograde slow pathway conduction
At identical cycle length, the HA interval during ventricular pacing is usually longer than that observed during tachycardia (lower common pathway)

Fast-Slow
Short AH interval during tachycardia (<180 ms)
Inverted P waves in inferior leads during long RP tachycardia
Initiation dependent on critical HA interval during retrograde slow pathway conduction
Early retrograde atrial activation near the CS ostium or in the proximal portion of the CS
At identical cycle length, the HA interval during ventricular pacing is usually longer than that observed during tachycardia (lower common pathway)
Exclude atrial tachycardia and reciprocating tachycardia

Left-Sided
Same as for slow-fast variant except for the following:
Inability to eliminate 1:1 slow pathway conduction from RA or CS

AH, atrium–His bundle; AV, atrioventricular; CS, coronary sinus; HA, His bundle–atrium; TCL, tachycardia cycle length.

Gonzalez MD, Banchs JE, Rivera J. Ablation of atrioventricular nodal reentrant tachycardia and variants. In: Huang SKS, Wood MA, eds. *Catheter Ablation of Cardiac Arrhythmias*. 2ed. Philadelphia, PA: Elsevier; 2011:318–350. With permission.

precordial leads, typical of earliest retrograde atrial activation in the proximal CS. This tachycardia can be induced by atrial or ventricular stimulation and frequently requires administration of isoproterenol. The earliest site of retrograde atrial activation was found near the anterior edge of the CS ostium or just inside the CS. The earliest site of retrograde atrial activation near the CS ostium is what characterizes slow-slow AVNRT. Neither the antegrade nor the retrograde fast pathway is necessary for this reentrant circuit and therefore the fast pathway may be absent. Characteristic of the slow-slow form of AVNRT is the presence of a lower common pathway.[9]

Fast-Slow

In fast-slow AVNRT, it is assumed that the fast AV nodal pathway is used as the antegrade limb and the slow AV nodal pathways as the retrograde limb. The ECG during tachycardia may show a PR interval that is shorter than the RP interval (long RP tachycardia). The AH interval is less than 180 ms, with P waves inverted in inferior leads. The HA interval is longer than the AH interval because of retrograde conduction over the slow AV nodal pathway. Similar to the slow-slow form, fast-slow AVNRT can be induced by atrial or ventricular stimulation, frequently during administration of isoproterenol. In addition, the presence of a lower common pathway results in an HA interval during tachycardia that is shorter than that observed during ventricular stimulation. Earliest retrograde atrial activation is close to the CS ostium.

Left-Sided Variant

The left-sided variant occurs in up to 1.5% of patients undergoing ablation for AVNRT.[10,11] The activation pattern is usually that of slow-fast AVNRT. The diagnosis is confirmed by EP findings consistent with AVNRT but with successful slow pathway ablation from the LA after failure of RA ablation. The presence of a short HA interval (≤ 15 ms) and the occurrence of antegrade double response to atrial pacing are sometimes noted in patients with this AVNRT variant. The AH intervals and TCLs are shorter in the left-sided variant than in "right-sided" slow-fast AVNRT.

Ablation

Elimination of 1:1 conduction over the slow pathway is the target for ablation in all forms of AVNRT.[1,2,12] Once slow pathway conduction can be reproducibly demonstrated and the diagnosis of AVNRT is confirmed, the ablation catheter is positioned along the tricuspid annulus immediately anterior to the CS ostium. The RAO view is especially useful for positioning catheters because it displays Koch's triangle en face. The angle of the left anterior oblique view should be adjusted so that the His catheter is perpendicular to the fluoroscopic plane. The initial target zone for slow pathway ablation is the isthmus of tissue

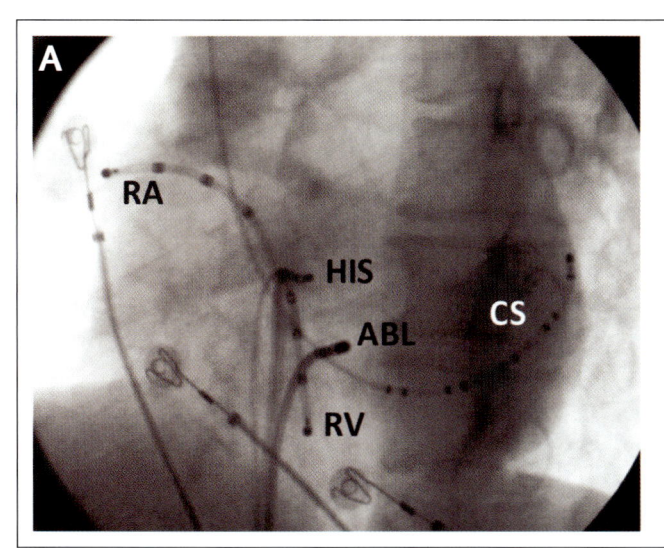

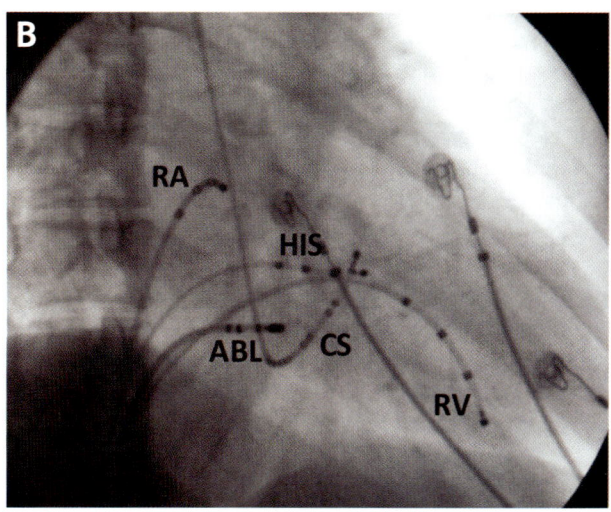

Figure 6.2 Locations of the mapping and ablation catheters for AVNRT in LAO 45° (**A**) and RAO 30° (**B**). RA, right atrial mapping catheter; RV, right ventricular mapping catheter; HIS, His bundle mapping catheter; CS, coronary sinus mapping catheter; ABL, ablation catheter.

between the tricuspid valve annulus and ostium of the CS. **Figure 6.2** shows the locations of the mapping and ablation catheters. The targets for slow pathway ablation are given in **Table 6.3**.

Anatomic Approach

The anatomic approach targets the area near the tricuspid annulus just outside the CS os in the inferior paraseptal region or at the os of CS. These locations contain the musculature that is in continuity with the right and LA extensions of the AV node. The ablation catheter is advanced into the right ventricle, moved inferiorly and medially so that it lies anterior to the ostium of the CS, and then withdrawn until the distal pair of electrodes records an atrial deflection in addition to the ventricular deflection. Clockwise torque will move the sheath and catheter toward the septum.

In RF ablation, the A/V ratio recorded from the distal electrode pair in sinus rhythm may range from about 1:2 to 1:3. In cryoablation, an A/V ratio of about 1:1 to 1:2 is achieved. There are 2 commonly used techniques for positioning the cryoablation catheter. Some operators start by positioning the tip of the cryoablation one-third of the distance from the level of the CS os to the level of the His bundle catheter in the left anterior oblique view. Other operators perform cryoablation in a manner more similar to RF ablation by first entering the right ventricle, withdrawing the catheter while deflecting the tip caudally. The cryoablation catheter tip is usually at the level of the CS ostium.

The deflecting segment of the RF ablation catheter in the range of 2.0 to 3.0 inches (D-F curves) has proven quite effective. For cryoablation, a medium curve with 55 mm curvature is most commonly used.

The use of a long sheath with slight distal septal angulation (eg, Daig SR0, St. Jude Medical, St. Paul, MN) often enhances catheter reach and stability. When using a sheath, it is important to keep the curves of the sheath and catheter coaxial. The atrial electrogram at successful sites may show multiple components.

Energy Application

RF current is delivered from the distal 4-mm-tip electrode of the mapping-ablation catheter toward a pair of dispersive electrode pads. Impedance is carefully monitored, and RF energy is halted for any sudden drop or rise in impedance or any evidence of AV or VA block. Catheter position is continuously monitored by fluoroscopy or real-time

Table 6.3 Targets for slow pathway ablation

Anatomic Guidance
Location between CS ostium and tricuspid annulus at the level of CS ostium
Proximal CS musculature (connection with leftward inferior input via LA-CS connections)
Increased risk for AV block: area triangle of Koch, superior to the CS ostium
Electrogram Guidance
Slow pathway activation potentials
Earliest retrograde atrial activation near CS (slow-slow and fast-slow AVNRT only)

AV, atrioventricular; AVNRT, atrioventricular nodal reentrant tachycardia; CS, coronary sinus; LA, left atrium.

Gonzalez MD, Banchs JE, Rivera J. Ablation of atrioventricular nodal reentrant tachycardia and variants. In: Huang SKS, Wood MA, eds. *Catheter Ablation of Cardiac Arrhythmias*. 2ed. Philadelphia, PA: Elsevier; 2011:318–350. With permission.

3-dimensional catheter localization. RF ablation is usually performed in the temperature mode with a target temperature of 60°C for 30 to 60 seconds. Some operators initially use low power (20 to 30 W) to test for unwanted effects such as prolongation of the AH interval, and after 15 seconds, they gradually increase the maximum power to 50 W. During RF delivery, the impedance is continuously monitored, because a drop in impedance is a better indicator of tissue temperature than is the tip electrode temperature. A few RF lesions are usually sufficient to eliminate AVNRT induction. During catheter ablation of the slow AV nodal pathway, a junctional rhythm is induced. Although a junctional rhythm is not specific for eliminating AVNRT, it is more commonly elicited at successful than at unsuccessful sites. Energy delivery must be rapidly interrupted if a junctional beat fails to conduct retrograde through the fast AV nodal pathway to the atrium, because this may reflect damage to the compact AV node. In a few cases, successful ablation of slow AV nodal pathway conduction can be achieved in the absence of junctional beats during RF energy application.[13] More frequently, however, successful ablation is heralded by a junctional rhythm that gradually subsides during ablation.[14] After RF energy has been delivered, programmed atrial stimulation, rapid atrial pacing, or both are performed to determine the presence or absence of slow pathway conduction or inducible AVNRT. If AVNRT remains inducible, the catheter is repositioned, and RF current is applied at a different position.

Catheter cryoablation is performed with either an 8-mm tip or a 6-mm tip. The 8-mm-tip catheter requires a larger sheath. During cryoablation, the AH is carefully monitored. In some cases the AH prolongs but rapidly becomes constant and is usually not greater than 200 ms. More commonly, AH prolongation progressively increases to the point of high-grade or complete AV block. Cryoablation is rapidly discontinued when the AV block becomes progressive or results in high-grade or complete AV block. Usually the AH rapidly returns to normal after cessation of cryoablation. However, it is possible that there may be some residual AH prolongation but persistent AV block is extremely rare and almost impossible to achieve using this approach.

Cryoablation is typically performed for 4-minute lesions. To increase the lesion size, sometimes a "freeze-thaw-freeze" is performed by completing the 4-minute lesion, allowing the temperature to rise, and then immediately freezing again for an additional 4 minutes. Testing inducibility of AVNRT during the cryoablation lesion may improve success of the process.

Endpoints for Ablation

Ablation is considered successful if the tachycardia cannot be reinduced, even during administration of isoproterenol.[3,10,15] Elimination of 1:1 conduction over the slow AV nodal pathway may be used as surrogate endpoint in cases of unreliable inducibility at baseline. Not uncommonly, AH interval jumps and slow-fast AV nodal echo beats may still be inducible after successful ablation. The presence of residual AH jumps with or without single-echo beats in the absence of tachycardia inducibility are an endpoint for ablation.[16,17] It is important to test for noninducibility in the presence of isoproterenol after ablation even if this agent was not necessary for induction at baseline. Table 6.4 summarizes the endpoints for ablation.

Efficacy

The acute success rate for slow pathway ablation for AVNRT is 97% to 100%; postprocedure recurrences of AVNRT are reported in 0.7% to 5.2%.[18-22] The absence of junctional tachycardia during RF application and younger age are associated with higher recurrence rates.[22]

Complication

Complications are relatively uncommon during ablation for AVNRT. For RF ablation, heart block represents the greatest risk and is reported to occur in less than 0.5%. The risk for acute heart block is increased in those with absent antegrade fast pathway function, ablation superior to the CS os, greater numbers of delivered RF lesions, and junctional rhythm with retrograde block. Late heart block is greatest in patients with transient AV block during the procedure and in those with baseline PR prolongation who undergo complete slow pathway ablation.

AV block is the major complication of RF catheter ablation for AVNRT; therefore, preventing AV block during catheter ablation is the most important safety issue. AV block from slow pathway ablation may occur because of direct injury to the compact AV node or fast pathway, especially if it is inferiorly displaced as an anatomic variant.

Table 6.4 Endpoints for ablation

Anatomic Guidance
Tachycardia rendered noninducible with and without isoproterenol
Elimination or modification of slow pathway function
• Elimination of atrium–His bundle (AH) interval jumps
• Elimination of 1:1 antegrade conduction over the slow atrioventricular (AV) nodal pathway
• Retrograde ventricular-atrial block through the slow AV nodal pathway (fast-slow and slow-slow)
AH interval jump with single echoes only (previously inducible)

Gonzalez MD, Banchs JE, Rivera J. Ablation of atrioventricular nodal reentrant tachycardia and variants. In: Huang SKS, Wood MA, eds. *Catheter Ablation of Cardiac Arrhythmias*. 2ed. Philadelphia, PA: Elsevier; 2011:318–350. With permission.

In addition, damage to the AV nodal artery or preexisting fast pathway dysfunction (intrinsic or from previous ablation) may be unrecognized before slow pathway ablation. Several strategies have been suggested to minimize the risk for ablation-induced AV block. The most important method is close attention to retrograde conduction during RF ablation and immediate discontinuation in the event of any VA block. Delivery of RF energy during atrial pacing faster than the junctional rhythm rate allows for continuous assessment of antegrade conduction in cases of doubt. Rapid junctional rhythm (cycle length, < 350 ms) has been described as an indicator of impending AV block.[23] AV block is unlikely at sites at or below the middle level of the CS os. The risk for block increases with more superior ablation sites. Table 6.5 summarizes the measurements for preventing AV block.

As mentioned previously, the reversibility of cryoablation permits the monitoring of gradual AH prolongation and the near elimination of the risk of permanent high-grade or complete AV block.

The success with catheter cryoablation is similar to that of RF ablation. However, there are some data supporting the conclusion that cryoablation has a higher recurrence rate.

Postprocedural Care

The patient will stay in the bed for 4 to 6 hours. Patients may be observed overnight or discharged the same day.

Conclusions

AVNRT is reentry involving fast and slow AV nodal pathways. The typical slow-fast form of AVNRT is diagnosed by the presence of a long AH interval (>180 ms) during tachycardia, with the earliest retrograde atrial activation localized at the level of the superior part of the triangle of Koch, just behind the tendon of Todaro. The fast-slow variant has a short AH interval during tachycardia (<180 ms), and early retrograde atrial activation is localized near the CS ostium or in the proximal portion of the CS. The slow-slow variant has a long AH interval (>180 ms), with early retrograde atrial activation near the CS ostium or in the proximal portion of the CS similar to the fast-slow form of AVNRT. The left-sided variant is similar to the slow-fast type, but slow pathway conduction cannot be eliminated from the RA or proximal CS. The ablation target for all variants is the antegrade or retrograde slow pathway. The acute success rate is high, almost 100%, with a higher recurrence rate for cryoablation compared to RF. The rate of complications (AV block) is ≤ 0.5% for RF energy and nearly 0% for cryoablation.

References

1. Jackman WM, Beckman KJ, McClelland JH, et al. Treatment of supraventricular tachycardia due to atrioventricular nodal reentry, by radiofrequency catheter ablation of slow-pathway conduction. *N Engl J Med.* 1992;327:313–318.
2. Haïssaguerre M, Gaita F, Fischer B, Commenges D, Montserrat P, d'Ivernois C, Lemetayer P, Warin JF. Elimination of atrioventricular nodal reentrant tachycardia using discrete slow potentials to guide application of radiofrequency energy. *Circulation.* 1992;85:2162–2175.
3. Kay GN, Epstein AE, Dailey SM, Plumb VJ. Selective radiofrequency ablation of the slow pathway for the treatment of atrioventricular reentrant tachycardia: Evidence for involvement of perinodal myocardium within the reentrant circuit. *Circulation.* 1992;85:1675–1688.
4. Calkins H, Yong P, Miller JM, et al. Catheter ablation of accessory pathways, atrioventricular nodal reentrant tachycardia, and the atrioventricular junction: Final results of a prospective, multicenter clinical trial. The Atakr Multicenter Investigators Group. *Circulation.* 1999;99:262–270.
5. Clague JR, Dagres N, Kottkamp H, Breithardt G, Borggrefe M. Targeting the slow pathway for atrioventricular nodal reentrant tachycardia: Initial results and long term follow-up in 379 consecutive patients. *Eur Heart J.* 2001;22:82–88.
6. Moe GK, Preston JB, Burlington H. Physiologic evidence for a dual A-V transmission system. *Circ Res.* 1956; 4: 357–375.
7. Josephson ME. Supraventricular tachycardias. In: Josephson ME, ed. *Clinical Cardiac Electrophysiology*, 4th ed. Philadelphia: Wolters Kluwer/Lippincott Williams & Wilkins; 2008:175–284.
8. Hwang C, Martin DJ, Goodman JS, Gang ES, Mandel WJ, Swerdlow CD, Peter CT, Chen PS. Atypical atrioventricular node reciprocating tachycardia masquerading as tachycardia using a left-sided accessory pathway. *J Am Coll Cardiol.* 1997; 30:218–225.
9. Heidbuchel H, Jackman WM. Characterization of subforms of AV nodal reentrant tachycardia. *Europace.* 2004; 4:316–329.
10. Lockwood D, Otomo K, Wang Z, et al. Electrophysiologic characteristics of atrioventricular nodal reentrant tachycardia: implications for the reentrant circuits. In: Zipes DP, Jalife J, eds. *Cardiac Electrophysiology: From Cell to Bedside.* Philadelphia, PA: Saunders; 2004:537–557.

Table 6.5 Measurements for preventing AV block using RF energy

Measurement	Description
Ablation sites below triangle of Koch	Inferior to level of CS roof
Monitor retrograde junctional conduction	Discontinue RF for loss of 1:1 retrograde conduction
Monitor for rapid junctional rhythm	Discontinue RF for junctional rhythm < 350 ms
Overdrive atrial pacing	Pace atrium faster than junctional rate to monitor antegrade conduction

CS, coronary sinus; RF, radiofrequency.

11. Kilic A, Amasyali B, Kose S, et al. Atrioventricular nodal reentrant tachycardia ablated from left atrial septum: clinical and electrophysiological characteristics and long-term follow-up results as compared to conventional right-sided ablation. *Int Heart J.* 2005;46:1023–1031.
12. Jazayeri MR, Hempe SL, Sra JS, et al. Selective transcatheter ablation of the fast and slow pathways using radiofrequency energy in patients with atrioventricular nodal reentrant tachycardia. *Circulation.* 1992;85:1318–1328.
13. Hsieh MH, Chen SA, Tai CT, Yu WC, Chen YJ, Chang MS. Absence of junctional rhythm during successful slow-pathway ablation in patients with atrioventricular nodal reentrant tachycardia. *Circulation.* 1998;98:2296–2300.
14. Wagshal AB, Crystal E, Katz A. Patterns of accelerated junctional rhythm during slow pathway catheter ablation for atrioventricular nodal tachycardia: temperature dependence, prognostic value, and insights into the nature of the slow pathway. *J Cardiovasc Electrophysiol.* 2000;11:244–254.
15. McElderry HT, Kay GN. Ablation of atrioventricular nodal reentry by the anatomic approach. In: Huang SKS, Wood MA, eds. *Catheter Ablation of Cardiac Arrhythmias.* Philadelphia, PA: Saunders; 2006:325–346.
16. Lindsay BD, Chung MK, Gamache MC, Luke RA, Schechtman KB, Osborn JL, Cain ME. Therapeutic end points for the treatment of atrioventricular node reentrant tachycardia by catheter-guided radiofrequency current. *J Am Coll Cardiol.* 1993;22:733–740.
17. Manolis AS, Wang PJ, Estes 3rd NA. Radiofrequency ablation of slow pathway in patients with atrioventricular nodal reentrant tachycardia: do arrhythmia recurrences correlate with persistent slow pathway conduction or site of successful ablation? *Circulation.* 1994;90:2815–2819.
18. Topilski I, Rogowski O, Glick A, Viskin S, Eldar M, Belhassen B. Radiofrequency ablation of atrioventricular nodal reentry tachycardia: a 14-year experience with 901 patients at the Tel Aviv Sourasky Medical Center. *Isr Med Assoc J.* 2006;8:455–459.
19. Kihel J, Da Costa A, Kihel A, Roméyer-Bouchard C, Thévenin J, Gonthier R, Samuel B, Isaaz K. Long-term efficacy and safety of radio-frequency ablation in elderly patients with atrioventricular nodal re-entrant tachycardia. *Europace.* 2006;8:416–420.
20. Rostock T, Risius T, Ventura R, Klemm HU, Weiss C, Keitel A, Meinertz T, Willems S. Efficacy and safety of radiofrequency catheter ablation of atrioventricular nodal reentrant tachycardia in the elderly. *J Cardiovasc Electrophysiol.* 2005;16:608–610.
21. Efremidis M, Sideris A, Letsas KP, Alexanian IP, Pappas LK, Mihas CC, Manolatos D, Xydonas S, Gavrielatos G, Filippatos GS, Kardaras F. Potential-guided versus anatomic-guided approach for slow pathway ablation of the common type atrioventricular nodal reentry tachycardia: a randomized study. *Acta Cardiol.* 2009;64:477–483.
22. Estner HL, Ndrepepa G, Dong J, et al. Acute and long-term results of slow pathway ablation in patients with atrioventricular nodal reentrant tachycardia: an analysis of the predictive factors for arrhythmia recurrence. *Pacing Clin Electrophysiol.* 2005;28:102–110.
23. Thakur RK, Klein GJ, Yee R. Junctional tachycardia: a useful marker during radiofrequency ablation for AV node reentrant tachycardia. *J Am Coll Cardiol.* 1993;22:1706–1710.
24. Bastani H, Schwieler J, Insulander P, et al. Acute and long-term outcome of cryoablation therapy of typical atrioventricular nodal reentrant tachycardia. *Europace.* 2009;11:1077–1082.
25. Chan NY, Mok NS, Lau CL, et al. Treatment of atrioventricular nodal re-entrant tachycardia by cryoablation with a 6 mm-tip catheter vs. radiofrequency ablation. *Europace.* 2009;11:1065–1070.
26. Chanani NK, Chiesa NA, Dubin AM, Avasarala K, Van Hare GF, Collins KK. Cryoablation for atrioventricular nodal reentrant tachycardia in young patients: predictors of recurrence. *Pacing Clin Electrophysiol.* 2008;31:1152–1159.
27. Deisenhofer I, Zrenner B, Yin Y-H, et al. Cryoablation versus radiofrequency energy for the ablation of atrioventricular nodal reentrant tachycardia (the CYRANO Study): results from a large multicenter prospective randomized trial. *Circulation.* 2010;122(22):2239–2245.
28. Rivard L, Dubuc M, Guerra PG, et al. Cryoablation outcomes for AV nodal reentrant tachycardia comparing 4-mm versus 6-mm electrode-tip catheters. *Heart Rhythm.* 2008;5:230–234.

CHAPTER 7

Ablation of Left-Lateral Accessory Pathways

Abram Mozes, MD; Mark S. Link, MD; Ann C. Garlitski, MD;
Jonathan Weinstock, MD; Munther Homoud, MD;
N. A. Mark Estes III, MD

Introduction

Left-lateral AP ablation is a common procedure that becomes necessitated often as the unforeseen result of a comprehensive EP evaluation of a SVT. At other times, it is a procedure that can be suspected long in advance, based on a preexcited surface ECG pattern in patients with WPW. In either situation, the target of ablation is a tract of myocardial tissue that crosses the atrioventricular groove, allowing the propagation of arrhythmias in a circuitous motion between the atria and ventricles.

Preprocedural Planning

Patients with predetermined evidence of accessory pathways are routinely referred for trans-thoracic 2-D echocardiography, to exclude conditions often associated with WPW, including Ebstein's Anomaly, Tetralogy of Fallot, MVP, and atrial-septal defect. The presence of underlying structural heart disease may influence the selection of equipment to be used and may altogether preclude a transseptal approach to ablation. In asymptomatic patients referred to our attention based on a preexcited surface ECG, extended mobile cardiac outpatient telemetry is occasionally arranged to determine (1) the presence of asymptomatic SVT, and (2) the presence of an intermittent preexcitation pattern, suggesting a pathway associated with a low risk of sudden death. In those with minimal preexcitation (so-called "inapparent" preexcitation) or in those in whom the diagnosis is altogether questioned, an adenosine challenge is performed to search for AV conduction during complete blockade through the AV node.

Patients referred for ablation are universally referred for routine labs prior to the procedure, including CBC, chemistries, and coagulation parameters, including PTT and PT/INR. Those patients on warfarin for thrombophilia are usually not instructed to discontinue this medication, as our experience suggests that it is not associated with an increased risk of periprocedural bleeding complications. Furthermore, avoiding interruption of warfarin therapy allows for an earlier discharge and obviates the need for bridging with anticoagulant agents that may increase bleeding risk.

Based on the need for ablating concealed left-lateral APs that become apparent following comprehensive EP evaluation of SVTs, our lab is equipped with a Siemens Acuson Sequoia 512 Ultrasound Apparatus (Siemens AG, Berlin, Germany) and Siemens Accunav 8-Fr ICE probes to guide puncture across the IAS.

Procedure

Patient Preparation

After informed consent is obtained and all requisite lab work drawn, patients are brought to the EP lab in a fasting state. As with a standard EP study, R2 pads are applied to the chest and back, as are standard 12-lead ECG electrodes. Conscious sedation is administered by the nursing staff through the duration of the procedure. Three femoral sheaths (9-Fr, 7-Fr, and 6-Fr) are introduced into the LFV to accommodate quadripolar catheters advanced to the HRA, the bundle of His, and the RVA. One of these venous sheaths is primed with isuprel to facilitate induction of SVT. From the contralateral groin, a 7-Fr and an 8-Fr sheath are each introduced into the RFV; the former is used to accommodate a deflectable decapolar catheter advanced into the CS, and the other permits exchange for a transseptal sheath. Prior to proceeding with transseptal puncture, a baseline ACT is measured.

Transseptal Puncture

For ablation of left-lateral APs, our preferred guiding sheaths include the Medtronic Mullins (Medtronic, Minneapolis, MN) and Swartz SL1 (St. Jude, St. Paul, MN). The selected sheath is first advanced to the superior vena cava over a wire and then engaged with a blunted, radiofrequency-powered needle (Baylis Medical, Montreal, QC, Canada) all the way to the tip of the dilator. The selection of sheath usually influences the choice of needle: for sheaths with more curvature at the tip, a less curved needle such as the Baylis C0 61-cm transseptal needle is used, whereas a more curved needle is selected for use with those sheaths bearing less curve. The quadripolar catheter in the HRA is usually exchanged for the ICE probe to facilitate visualization of the IAS and guide transseptal crossing.

Transseptal puncture is performed under biplane fluoroscopic and ICE guidance. Once adequate visualization of the IAS under ICE is obtained, the sheath-needle complex is slowly pulled down from the SVC until it engages the fossa ovalis. The trajectory of the needle is checked under RAO and LAO projections and adjusted to ensure that the needle does not course too anteriorly in an RAO projection. In the LAO projection, the sheath and needle should appear to point leftward. The sheath and needle are then advanced together and cinched up against the IAS until adequate tenting of the latter is visualized. The needle is then advanced out beyond the dilator tip and a 3-second RF burst is delivered through the tip of the Baylis needle. This approach is usually successful in crossing the septum. Occasionally, the sheath and needle tend to "ride up" the septum when efforts are made to better engage it, in which case the needle is removed from the sheath and more curve is introduced into it. The exchange-length wire sometimes must be reintroduced through the dilator and the sheath readvanced into the SVC before being re-engaged with the needle.

Once the tip of the needle has crossed, LA position must be confirmed before advancing the dilator and sheath. First, an O_2 saturation is measured on a sample of blood aspirated from the tip of the needle. Next, pressure is transduced through the needle to ensure that the LA and not the aorta has been penetrated. Finally, a small injection of agitated, heparinized saline is injected through the needle while the ICE image is inspected for echo contrast in the LA. After these steps are taken, the sheath, dilator and needle are advanced slightly further into the LA to avoid losing transseptal position before the dilator and then the sheath are gradually "telescoped" into the LA. Clockwise or posterior torque is sometimes applied to the sheath and dilator while advancing over the septum to avoid coursing too laterally in the LA and perforating the appendage.

Once the sheath has entered the LA, the needle and dilator are withdrawn while aspirating through the side-arm of the sheath to avoid introducing air. Weight-based heparin (usually 100 U/kg of body weight) is then immediately injected and flushed through and a heparinized saline infusion of 50 U/hr is run through the sheath. ACT is then checked, and heparin titrated to maintain ACT above 350 seconds. Finally, the mapping/ablation catheter is introduced through the sheath.

Mapping

With manifest preexcitation of the ventricles, as in WPW, confirmation of a left-lateral AP is usually suspected based on surface ECG delta wave morphology and confirmed at the time of invasive EP evaluation.

Ablation of a left-lateral AP can be achieved by targeting either its atrial or ventricular insertion along the mitral valve annulus. During sinus rhythm or atrial pacing with maximal ventricular preexcitation, the AP's approximate location may be estimated by examination of the earliest ventricular EGM in the CS in relation to the delta wave. This approach is of particular importance, as our lab has recently come across patients with exclusively antegrade conduction over the AP, precluding the ability to map during retrograde activation. It is important to note, however, that APs often traverse the atrioventricular groove in an oblique fashion[1] so that the atrial and ventricular insertions may be separated by some distance along the annulus. Further confounding matters is that CS recordings give only an approximation of transannular activation sequence, as the CS is an epicardial structure and is itself superiorly displaced from the AV groove.

Our lab's practice has been to ablate the LA insertion of the AP, usually identified during orthodromic AVRT (**Figure 7.1**) or via pacing from the RVA. Assuming the ERP of the AV node is longer than that of the AP's, mapping of its atrial insertion is achieved during pacing from

Chapter 7: Ablation of Left-Lateral APs • 61

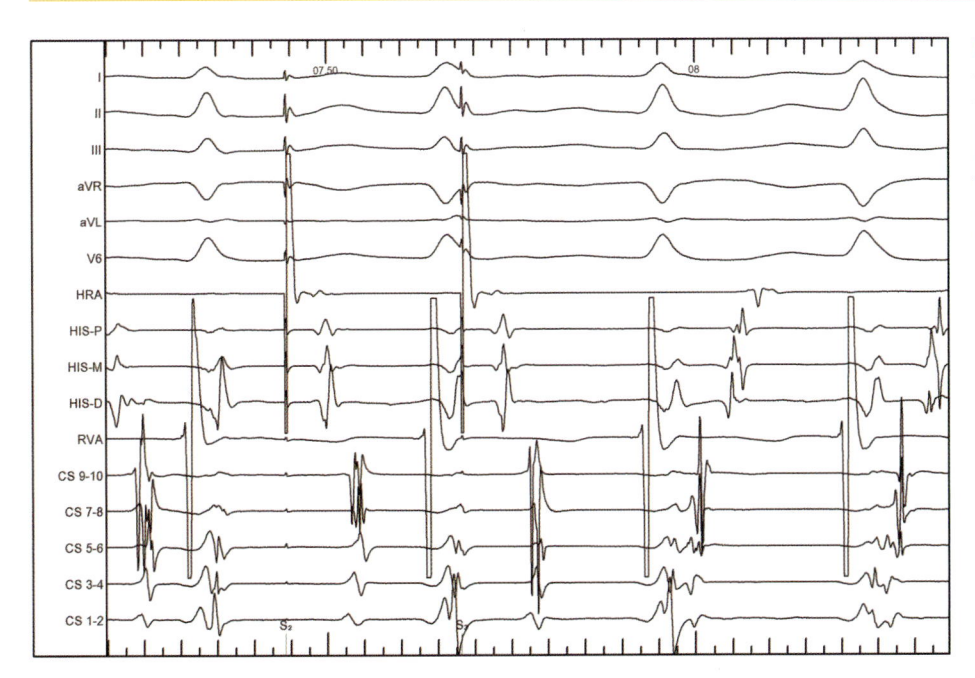

Figure 7.1 Induction of orthodromic AVRT with sensed double atrial extrastimuli in a patient with a concealed left lateral accessory pathway. Note the "bracketing" of earliest atrial activation during tachycardia in CS 5–6.

the RVA at a cycle length shorter than the AV node's ERP so that retrograde atrial activation while mapping is exclusively via the AP. In rare instances, the ERP of the AP is longer than or equal to that of the AV node, which can make mapping extremely difficult unless tachycardia may be readily induced and sustained.

Ablation

Catheter selection for ablating a left-lateral AP hinges on the decision of whether electroanatomic mapping is used to localize the pathway's insertion. In situations in which electroanatomic mapping is deemed unnecessary, our lab has had success using the Boston Scientific EPT Blazer 4-mm RF catheter (Boston Scientific, St. Paul, MN). When more advanced mapping is called for, our preference has been to use a NaviStar® enabled catheter such as the Biosense Webster 4-mm Carto catheter (Biosense Webster, Diamond Bar, CA) for use with the Carto-XP system. After crossing the IAS, the catheter is directed inferiorly toward the mitral valve annulus.

The annulus is mapped during ORT or during ventricular pacing. Mapping during tachycardia has the advantage of eliminating retrograde fusion through the AV

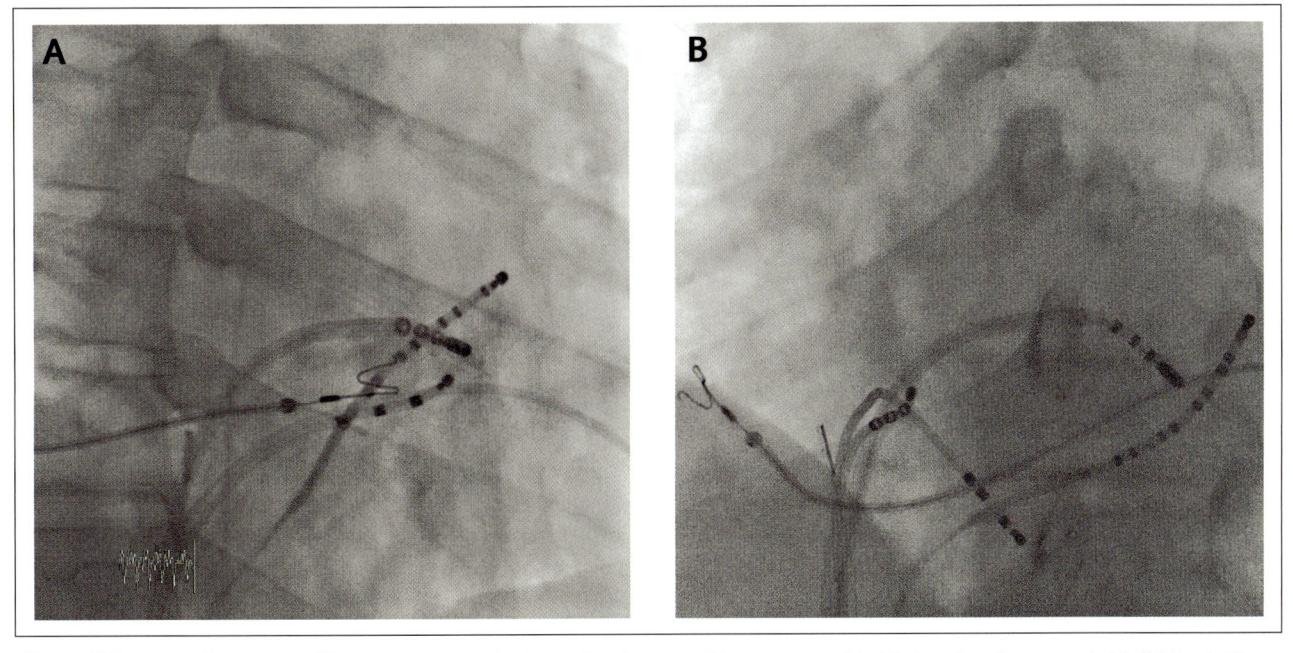

Figure 7.2 RAO (**A**) and LAO (**B**) fluoroscopic projections of catheter position at successful ablation site of a concealed left-lateral AP.

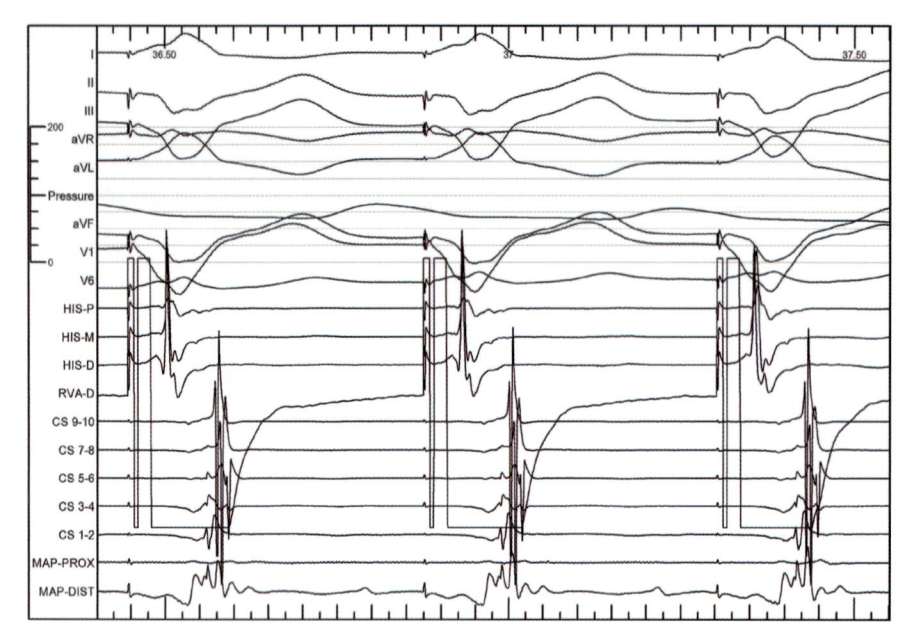

Figure 7.3 Continuous electrical activity and an AP potential on the mapping catheter during right ventricular pacing at the successful ablation site immediately prior to ablation.

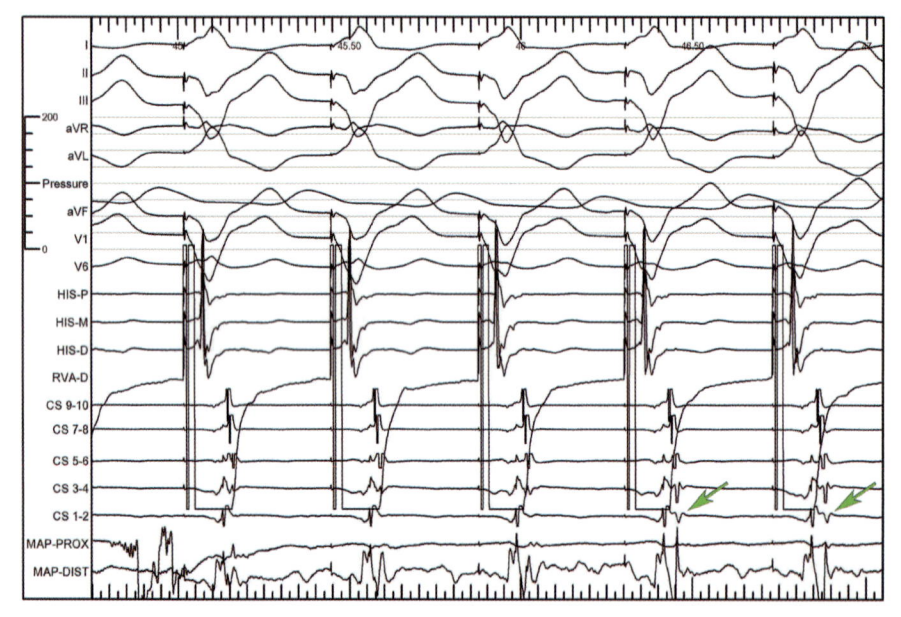

Figure 7.4 Change of atrial activation sequence during right ventricular pacing during application of a successful lesion delivered to a concealed retrograde AP. Arrowheads indicate the change in retrograde activation.

node, but comes at the expense of losing catheter stability. The catheter is gently advanced and withdrawn until the atrial EGM on the mapping catheter precedes or coincides with the earliest activation along the CS catheter (**Figure 7.2**). Particular attention is paid to searching for continuous electrical activity (a "W" sign[2]) (**Figure 7.3**) or for an AP potential.[3]

Once a satisfactory position is reached, RF energy is delivered during sinus rhythm or during ventricular pacing. We typically begin with 50 W of energy delivered for 30 seconds, with a temperature limit of 60°C. A successful lesion is defined by loss of preexcitation if the AP is ablated during sinus rhythm or a change in retrograde activation if the pathway is ablated during ventricular pacing (**Figure 7.4**). If the initial lesion is successful, we generally deliver one or two "bonus" lesions of 30 seconds' duration. On rare occasions, ablation of the atrial insertion of the AP is unsuccessful, in which case a decision to pursue ablation of the ventricular insertion via a retrograde aortic approach is considered.

Following successful elimination of AP conduction, an EP evaluation of the modified conduction system is performed. First, "new" baseline intervals, including AH and HV intervals, are obtained. Next, decremental atrial pacing is performed in an effort to document Wenkebach periodicity in patients having undergone AP ablation for the WPW syndrome. Antegrade and retrograde refractory determinations are then made to search for AH jumps that may suggest dual AV nodal physiology. Isoproterenol, at a dose of 1 to 5 mcg/min, is sometimes infused to determine further inducibility of macroreentrant tachycardia. Finally, when there is no evidence of resumption of AP conduction after a 30-minute wait period, transseptal sheaths and catheters are pulled back to the right side, and heparin infusion is discontinued.

Postprocedure Care

Recovery

Sheaths and catheters are typically removed when the ACT declines to the patient's baseline or below 180 seconds. Protamine is sometimes administered to reverse the anticoagulant effect, and ACT is rechecked at 15- to 20-minute intervals until such time. While waiting for the ACT to decline, the ICE probe is repositioned to evaluate for pericardial effusion. Following achievement of hemostasis, patients are transferred to a telemetry unit for 6 hours of monitored bed rest. Heparin infusion is restarted 6 hours after sheath removal and continued for a minimum of 12 hours. In addition, full-dose aspirin (325 mg) is administered for a period of 3 months following the procedure. Patients are usually discharged home the next day.

Follow-Up

Follow-up visits are routinely scheduled for 4 to 6 weeks. Patients are instructed to notify the physician of any discomfort, swelling, or bleeding at the venotomy sites or of any chest discomfort, palpitations, or difficulty breathing.

Procedural Success and Complications

Ablation of left-lateral APs via the transseptal approach is associated with a high success rate, with a low rate of complications and a low rate of recurrence. Though there is an upfront time cost associated with gaining transseptal access, manipulation of the ablation catheter during mapping from the atrial side of the AV groove is not encumbered by obstruction from the mitral valve apparatus.[4] Results of the ATAKR prospective, multicenter clinical trial reported a success rate of 95% with a single ablation procedure for left-lateral APs, with a recurrence rate of only 3%.[5] In the same analysis, only 1 of 270 patients who underwent left free-wall AP ablation developed heart block, and 1 patient with a transseptal approach suffered a stroke.

Our experiences with left-lateral AP ablation are in keeping with these results in regards to the low risks of death, heart block, and stroke. Minor complications such as groin hematomas are not uncommon, particularly with our practice of administering heparin following the procedure. In addition, arteriovenous fistulas or pseudoaneurysms may occur. To ensure early discovery of pericardial effusions, our practice has been to maintain the ICE probe in a neutral position (following transseptal puncture), thereby visualizing the right heart (and pericardial space) in a short axis view. Sudden changes in hemodynamics or any patient report of chest discomfort or shortness of breath is aggressively pursued and investigated with ECG and echocardiography intra- or postprocedurally. There exists a risk of air embolism with the transseptal approach due to the use of long intravascular sheaths accompanied by frequent exchanges of needles and catheters, but this complication is, fortunately, uncommon. Avoidance of arterial complications such as coronary artery dissection, peripheral embolization, and valve trauma is inherent to the transseptal approach to left-lateral AP ablation.

References

1. Otomo K, Gonzalez MD, Beckman KJ, et al. Reversing the direction of paced ventricular and atrial wavefronts reveals an oblique course in accessory AV pathways and improves localization. *Circulation*. 2001;104:550–556.
2. Manolis A, Wang P, Estes NA. Radiofrequency ablation of atrial insertion of left-sided accessory pathways guided by the "W Sign." *J Cardiovasc Electrophysiol*. 1995;6:1068–1076.
3. Jackman WM, Wang X, Friday KJ et al. Catheter ablation of accessory atrioventricular pathways (Wolff-Parkinson-White Syndrome) by radiofrequency current. *N Engl J Med*. 1991;324(23):1605–1611.
4. Lesh MD, Van Hare GF, Scheinman MM, Ports TA, Epstein LA. Comparison of the retrograde and transseptal methods for ablation of left free-wall accessory pathways. *J Am Coll Cardiol*. 1993;22(2):542–549.
5. Calkins H, Yong P, Miller JM, et al. Catheter ablation of accessory pathways, atrioventricular nodal reentrant tachycardia, and the atrioventricular junction: final results of a prospective, multicenter clinical trial: the Atakr Multicenter Investigators Group. *Circulation*. 1999;99(2):262–270.

CHAPTER 8

CATHETER ABLATION OF ACCESSORY PATHWAYS

Hiroshi Nakagawa, MD, PhD; Warren M. Jackman, MD

Introduction

A number of different approaches have been developed for catheter ablation of accessory AV pathways.[1-6] The high success rate (> 90%) and low incidence of complication (< 5%) in catheter ablation have let this modality become first-line therapy for arrhythmia associated with accessory pathways. In this chapter, we describe our current approach for mapping and ablation of accessory pathways.[2,7-9]

Catheter Mapping of Accessory Pathways

We perform decremental atrial pacing from 2 widely separate sites, usually at the RAA and posterolateral CS, since one atrial pacing site far from the AP may not present clear preexcitation. A change in the morphology of the preexcited QRS or the ventricular activation sequence by changing the atrial pacing site indicates the presence of 2 or more APs.

The presence of retrograde AP conduction is indicated by a retrograde atrial activation sequence. However, the retrograde activation sequence for anteroseptal and posteroseptal APs is similar to the activation sequence during retrograde conduction over the fast and slow AV nodal pathways, respectively. The presence of more than one V-A connection is manifested by ventricular pacing at 2 widely separate sites close to the base. Confirmation of retrograde AP conduction can be obtained by parahisian ventricular pacing (with intermittent HB capture)[10,11] and by advancing atrial activation during AVRT using a late ventricular extrastimulus delivered close to the site of earliest atrial activation.

Our approach to localize APs for ablation is based on the possibilities that: (1) an AP often has an oblique course (atrial and ventricular insertions are located at different sites along the AV groove)[8,12]; and (2) multiple pathways may be present. We map the annulus during antegrade AP conduction with atrial pacing as well as during retrograde AP conduction with ventricular pacing. We perform differential atrial pacing (atrial pacing at 2 separate sites close to the annulus on opposite sides of the site of earliest antegrade ventricular activation) and differential ventricular pacing (ventricular pacing at 2 separate sites close to the annulus on opposite sides of the site of earliest retrograde atrial activation) to identify an oblique course of a single AP and presence of more than one AP connection.

For a single AP with an oblique course, differential ventricular pacing produces 2 different local V-A intervals (≥ 15 ms difference) measured at the site of earliest retrograde atrial activation (**Figure 8.1**).[7,8] The ventricular pacing site that produces a ventricular wavefront propagating from the direction of the ventricular end of the AP (concurrent direction, **Figure 8.1A**) results in an artificially short local V-A interval at the site of earliest atrial activation (**Figure 8.1C**). Because ventricular activation and AP activation are propagating simultaneously in the same direction, the ventricular potential overlaps the AP activation potential (AP potential) and may mask the atrial potential (**Figure 8.1, A, C, and E**). In contrast, pacing from the opposite side (reversing the direction of the ventricular wavefront: countercurrent direction) produces the ventricular wavefront propagating away from the AP shortly after activation of its ventricular end (**Figure 8.1B**). This pacing results in an increase of the local V-A interval along the length of the AP, exposing the AP potential and the atrial activation sequence (**Figure 8.1, D and F**).[7,8,13,14]

For an AP with an oblique course, differential atrial pacing produces 2 different local A-V intervals (≥ 15 ms difference), measured at the site of earliest ventricular activation (**Figure 8.2**). Atrial pacing from the direction of the atrial insertion (concurrent atrial wavefront) shortens the local A-V interval at the site of earliest ventricular activation and results in overlapping atrial and AP potentials, masking the AP potential and often masking the site of earliest ventricular activation (**Figure 8.2, A and C**). Pacing from the opposite side reverses the direction of the atrial wavefront (countercurrent direction), resulting in the atrial wavefront propagating away from the AP shortly after activating its atrial end (**Figure 8.2B**). The A-V interval all along the AP is increased, unmasking the AP potential and the ventricular activation sequence (**Figure 8.2D**).[7,8,13,14]

During AP conduction, the ability to record an isolated AP potential indicates an oblique course of AP. The absence of an oblique course should produce fusion between the atrial, AP and ventricular potentials unless the atrial or ventricular insertion of the AP is located far from the annulus, such as in Ebstein's anomaly.

Differential atrial and ventricular pacing was performed in 114 consecutive patients with a single AP (left free-wall AP in 65 patients, right free-wall AP in 22 patients, posteroseptal AP in 21 patients, and anteroseptal AP in 6 patients).[8] Reversing the direction of ventricular or atrial activation increased the local V-A or local A-V interval by ≥ 15 ms in 99 (87%) of the 114 patients, indicating that the majority of APs have an oblique course. Separating the atrial and ventricular potentials by differential pacing exposed an AP potential in 102 of 114 (89%) patients. Ablation was attempted in 111 of the 114 patients, and an

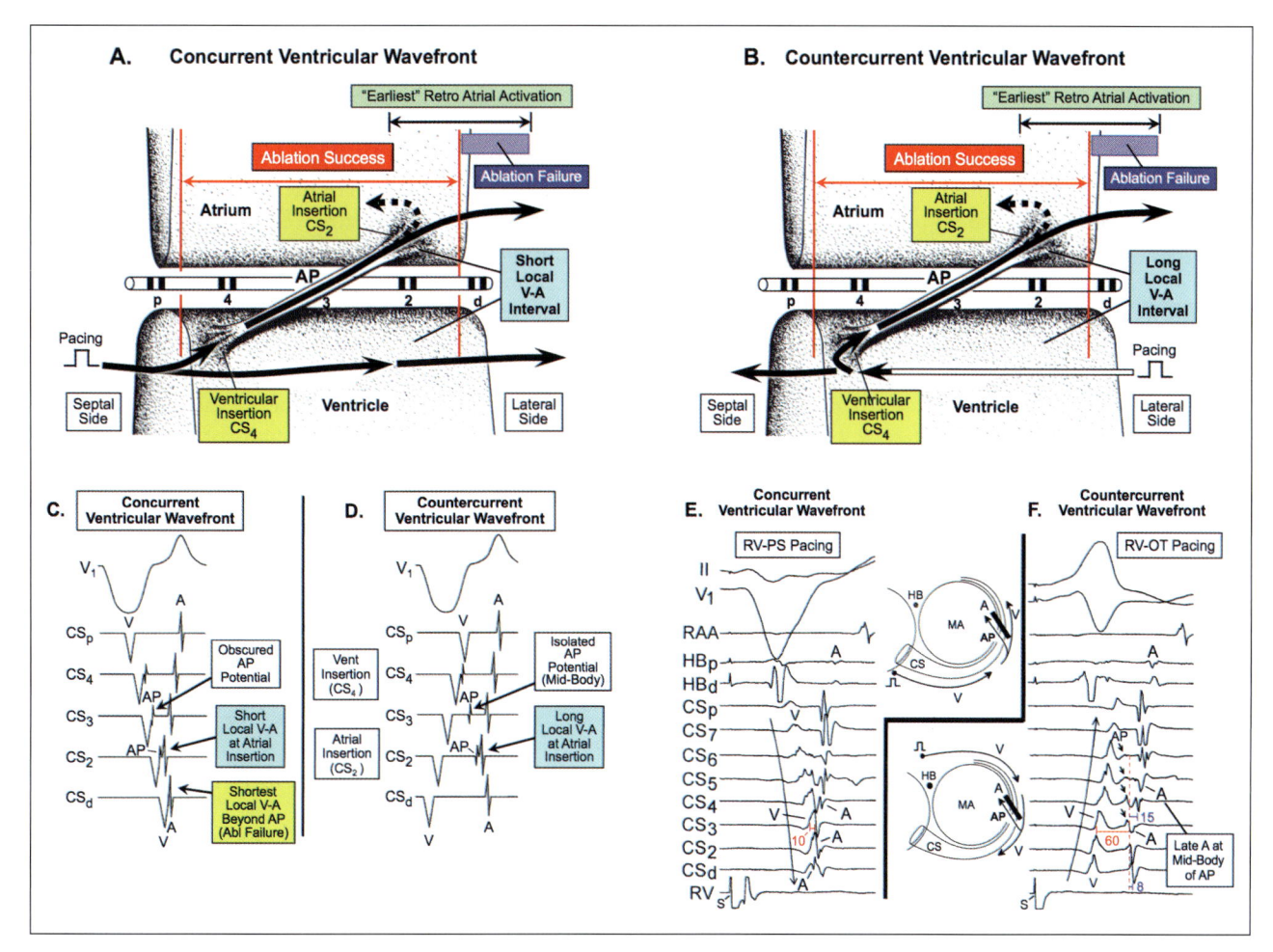

Figure 8.1 Effects of the oblique course in a left free-wall AP on the timing of ventricular (V), atrial (A), and AP potentials (AP) by reversing the direction of the ventricular wavefront. (See text; modified with permission from reference 7.)

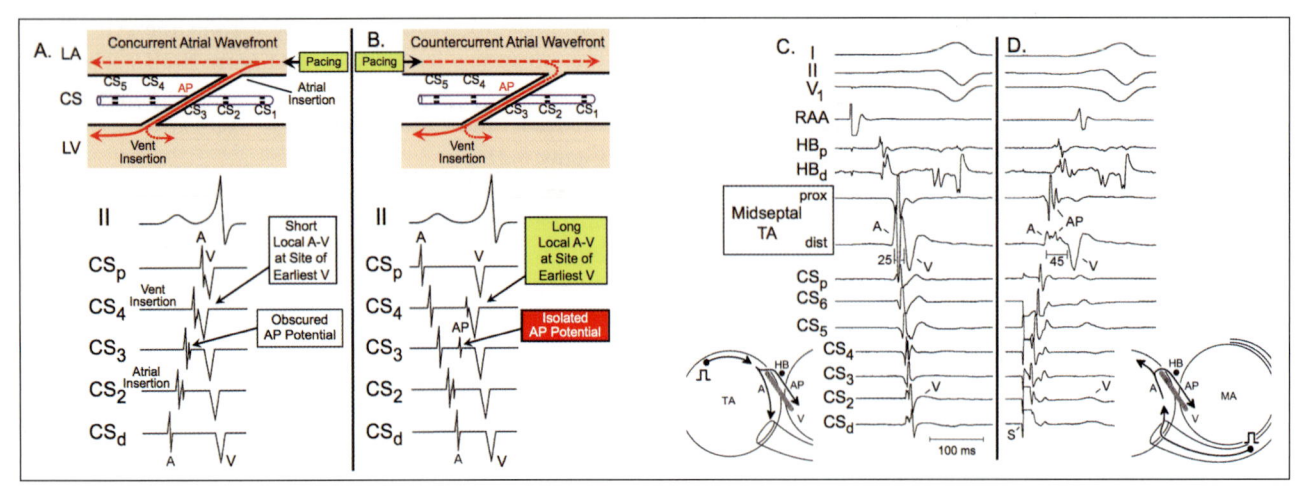

Figure 8.2 Effects of the oblique course in a left free-wall AP on the timing of atrial (A), ventricular (V), and AP(AP) potentials by reversing the direction of the atrial wavefront. (See text; modified with permission from reference 8.)

AP potential was recorded in 99 of these 111 patients. By targeting the AP potential in these 99 patients, AP conduction was eliminated with a median of only 1 RF application (range 1–11 applications). In contrast, a median of 4.5 RF applications (range 1–18 applications) was required in the 12 patients in whom an AP potential was not recorded, despite separating the atrial and ventricular potentials using differential pacing.[8] These data strongly support the AP potential as the optimal target for ablation.

In the same study, 60 of the 111 patients had 1 to 3 prior failed ablation procedures. The number of RF applications required to eliminate AP conduction was not significantly greater for the 60 patients who had a prior failed ablation than the 51 patients undergoing their first ablation procedure (median 1 RF application for both groups).[8] AP conduction was eliminated by only 1 to 2 RF applications in 41 of the 60 patients with prior failed ablation. In these 41 patients, differential pacing demonstrated an oblique course and exposed an AP potential for the ablation target. In most cases, there were low-amplitude fractionated atrial potentials located 2 to 10 mm beyond the atrial insertion of the AP (blue hatched box in **Figure 8.1, A and B**), suggesting the location of previous ablation sites. These findings suggest that an oblique AP course may lead to placing unsuccessful RF applications beyond the atrial insertion of the AP when using other approaches for localizing APs (ie, the site of earliest retrograde atrial activation and the shortest local V-A interval).[15-18] During retrograde AP conduction, atrial activation propagates rapidly in the same direction as the AP due to the parallel atrial fiber orientation (**Figure 8.1F**). This rapid atrial propagation may cause bipolar intracardiac EGMs to identify "earliest" retrograde atrial activation over a wide range, extending beyond the atrial insertion of the AP (black arrow, *"Earliest" Retro Atrial Activation* in **Figure 8.1, A and B**). RF applications in the distal half of this region (blue hatched area in **Figure 8.1, A and B**) are likely to fail to eliminate AP conduction.[7,8,13,14]

The shortest local V-A interval for selecting an ablation site may be misleading in the presence of an oblique course. With a concurrent ventricular wavefront, ventricular activation initially precedes the atrial activation near the atrial insertion of the AP (CS_2 EGM in **Figure 8.1, A and C**). However, the velocity of the atrial wavefront parallel to the annulus is greater than the velocity of the ventricular wavefront. The local V-A interval shortens progressively beyond the atrial insertion of the AP as the atrial wavefront catches the ventricular wavefront (CS_d EGM in **Figure 8.1, A, C and E**). The shorter local V-A interval beyond the atrial insertion of the AP may explain the location of the fractionated atrial EGMs in the majority of patients with a prior failed ablation procedure.

For most APs along the mitral annulus (posteroseptal and left free-wall pathways), the direction from ventricular insertion to atrial insertion follows a counterclockwise orientation (as viewed in the left anterior oblique projection, **Figure 8.3**).[7,8,12] For many of the APs along the tricuspid annulus (especially anteroseptal pathways), the direction from ventricular insertion to atrial insertion follows a clockwise orientation (as viewed in the left anterior oblique projection, **Figure 8.3**). Therefore, for anteroseptal and right anterior paraseptal APs, the ventricular insertion is often located toward the right free-wall, allowing ablation away from the septum to reduce the risk of AV block.

To acquire optimal ventricular pacing sites close to the annulus for reversing the direction of the ventricular wavefront, we use a deflectable pacing catheter. For left anterolateral and lateral pathways, a counterclockwise ventricular wavefront can be achieved by pacing from the inferobasal RV septum (close to the tricuspid annulus) or from the middle cardiac vein. A clockwise LV waveform can be achieved either by pacing at the RVOT or the anterior aspect of the great cardiac vein (or anterior interventricular vein). For posteroseptal APs, the counterclockwise ventricular wavefront is obtained by pacing at the inferobasal RV septum. The clockwise ventricular

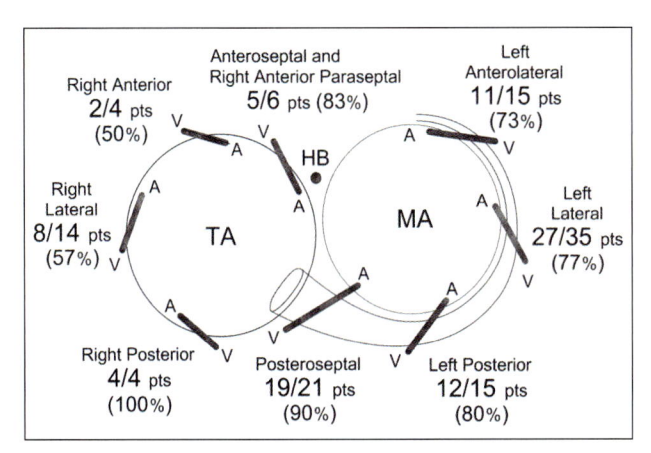

Figure 8.3 Orientation of oblique course of 114 APs in 8 anatomical regions. A, atrial end; V, ventricular end; TA, tricuspid annulus; MA, mitral annulus. (Modified with permission from reference 8.)

wavefront is obtained by pacing from the posterior or lateral coronary vein. For right free-wall APs, the counterclockwise ventricular wavefront is obtained by pacing at the inferobasal RV septum. The clockwise ventricular wavefront is obtained by pacing the basal RV free-wall anterior to the AP. For anteroseptal and right anterior paraseptal APs, the counterclockwise ventricular wavefront is obtained by pacing the basal anterior RV septum, similar to the site used for parahisian pacing.[10,11] The clockwise ventricular wavefront is obtained by pacing the basal anterolateral RV free-wall.

The AP potential can be validated by dissociating the AP potential from the local atrial and ventricular potentials. An antegrade AP potential is validated during atrial pacing using ventricular extrastimuli, gradually shortening the coupling intervals. Advancing the local ventricular potential without affecting the timing or morphology of the AP potential, dissociates the AP potential from the local ventricular potential (**Figure 8.4A**).[7,13,14] With an earlier ventricular extrastimulus, advancing the AP potential without affecting the timing or morphology of the atrial potential in the mapping EGM and any surrounding EGMs (such as the adjacent coronary sinus EGMs) dissociates the AP potential from the local atrial potential (**Figure 8.4B**).[7,13,14] A retrograde AP potential is validated during ventricular pacing using atrial extrastimuli. Advancing the local atrial potential without affecting the timing or morphology of the AP potential, dissociates the AP potential from the local atrial potential. With an earlier atrial extrastimulus, advancing the AP potential without affecting the timing or morphology of the ventricular potential, dissociates the AP potential from the local ventricular potential.

Catheter Ablation of APs

We generally prefer ablation during ventricular or atrial pacing, rather than during AVRT. When ablation is performed during AVRT, the catheter often may be dislodged when AVRT terminates after only a few seconds into the RF application due to the enhanced contraction of the first posttachycardia beat. The incomplete RF lesion may lead to a recurrence of AP conduction.

After localizing the isolated AP potential, the ablation catheter is positioned to record a large, sharp AP potential on the unipolar EGM from the ablation-tip electrode (**Figure 8.5**). Localization using just a bipolar EGM may be misleading, because a sharp AP potential may be recorded from the second (ring) electrode (**Figure 8.5**).[7]

RF energy is delivered at 30 to 40 W for 60 seconds (usually using a saline irrigated electrode), but terminating the RF application immediately with a 5- to 10-ohm increase in impedance above the lowest value. If AP

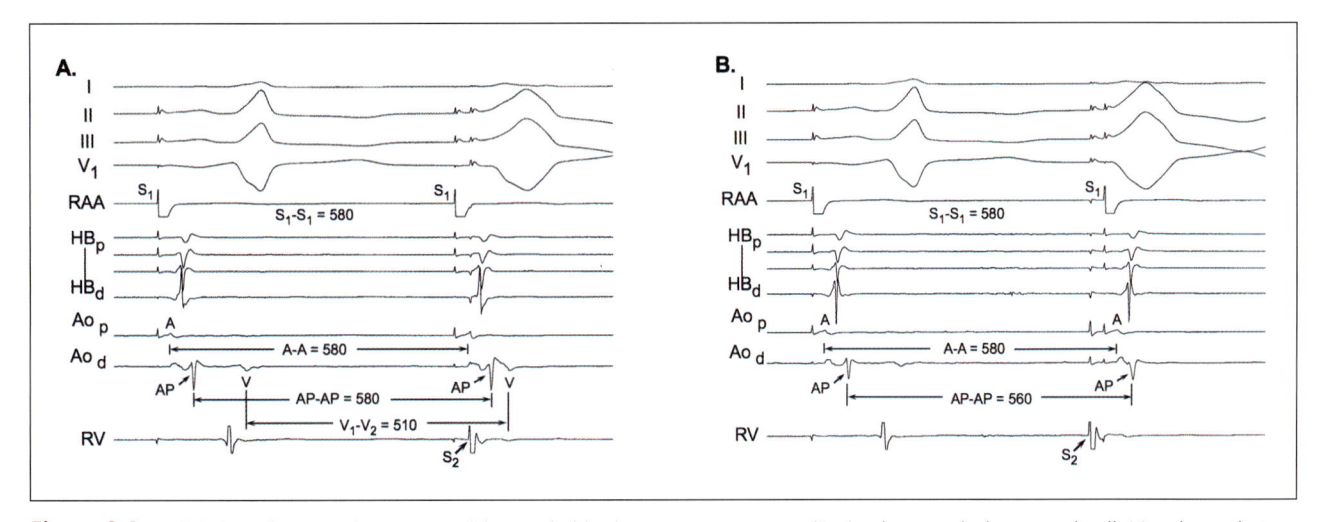

Figure 8.4 Validation of antegrade AP potential recorded in the noncoronary cusp (Ao$_d$) using ventricular extrastimuli. Mapping catheter in the noncoronary cusp of the aortic valve (Ao$_d$) recorded a large, sharp AP potential. A single RF application in the noncoronary cusp at site recording a large, sharp AP potential from the tip unipolar EGM eliminates AP conduction without affecting AV nodal conduction. (See text; modified with permission from reference 7.)

conduction is not eliminated, we still continue the RF application for the full 60 seconds, because the AP potential that was recorded before the RF application may have represented activation of a branch of the AP. Earlier termination of the RF application may lead to late recovery of AP conduction and long-term ablation failure.

In the event that an AP potential is not identified during mapping, we target earliest antegrade ventricular activation (QS pattern on the unipolar EGM at the site of earliest activation) or earliest retrograde atrial activation.[6,7] These pathways are often atypical anatomically and may require more extensive ablation.

For 30 to 60 minutes following ablation, programmed atrial and ventricular stimulation is performed to confirm the absence of antegrade and retrograde AP conduction and elimination of the inducibility of AVRT. To confirm the absence of retrograde AP conduction, it is best to perform ventricular stimulation at a basal ventricular site (near the annulus) close to the location of the AP. For anteroseptal, right anterior, and posteroseptal APs, the parahisian site (basal anterior RV septum) is optimal. Parahisian pacing with intermittent HB capture differentiates between retrograde fast AV nodal pathway conduction and retrograde conduction over an anteroseptal or right anterior AP and differentiates between retrograde conduction over the slow AV nodal pathways and retrograde conduction over a posteroseptal AP.[10,11]

Epicardial Posteroseptal APs

The true CS is located between the CS ostium and the Veussen's valve. The true CS is a muscular chamber with extensive muscular connections to the LA (**Figure 8.6**).[7,9,19,20] The CS myocardium occasionally extends onto the MCV, posterior coronary vein or other veins entering the true CS.[19] A myocardial (and electrical) connection forms between the epicardial surface of the left ventricle and the myocardial extension along the veins (CS myocardial–ventricular connection), forming an "epicardial posteroseptal AP (**Figures 8.6A–C**)."[9] These connections also result from CS diverticula, which are muscular chambers attached to the epicardial surface of the left ventricle and connected to the true CS through a neck.[9] This complex anatomy is a frequent cause for ablation failure of posteroseptal APs.[9,21] We found this anatomy in 42 (20%) of 212 patients with a posteroseptal or left posterior AP and no prior attempt at ablation but in 144 (47%) of 306 patients with a one or more previous failed ablation procedures.[9] The finding of a steep negative delta wave in ECG lead II in a patient with a posteroseptal AP (V_1–V_2 transition and negative delta wave in lead aVF) is specific but only moderately sensitive (70%) for an epicardial AP location.[22]

During antegrade conduction (**Figure 8.6B**), earliest endocardial ventricular activation (downstroke of the unfiltered unipolar EGM) is usually recorded more than

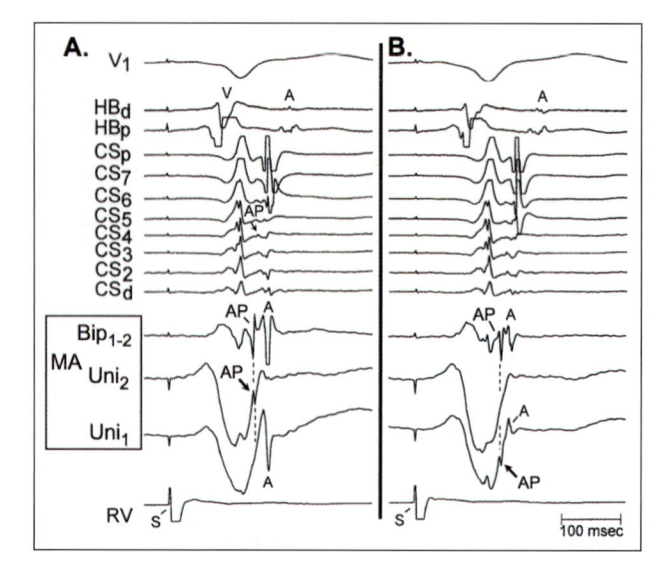

Figure 8.5 AP potential recorded in the unipolar and bipolar EGMs from the distal 2 electrodes on an ablation catheter positioned across the mitral annulus (MA) using the retrograde transaortic approach in a patient with a left posterolateral AP. **A.** During RV pacing, the sharp bipolar AP potential (Bip_{1-2}) was generated by the second electrode (Uni_2). **B.** The catheter was withdrawn toward the ventricle. The bipolar AP potential was then generated from the tip electrode (Uni_1). One RF application there eliminated AP conduction. A, atrial potential; V, ventricular potential; HB, His bundle; CS, coronary sinus. (Modified with permission from reference 7.)

25 ms after the onset of far-field activation and 1 to 3 cm apical to the mitral annulus. When the AP is formed by a CS myocardial extension along the MCV, endocardial activation is recorded nearly simultaneously on the right and left sides of the interventricular septum. Earliest ventricular activation (usually ≤ 15 ms after the onset of far-field activation) is recorded from the middle cardiac vein, other coronary vein, or neck of a CS diverticulum and is preceded by a distinct potential (similar to an AP potential) resulting from antegrade activation of the CS myocardial extension.[7,9]

During retrograde conduction over epicardial posteroseptal APs (**Figure 8.6C**), a characteristic pattern of 3 distinct potentials is recorded from the coronary venous system.[27] The first potential (#1 *CS Extn* in **Figure 8.6D**), similar to an AP potential, is recorded from the MCV (or other coronary vein or CS diverticulum) and is generated by retrograde activation of the CS myocardial extension. The second potential (#2 *CS Myo* in **Figure 8.6D**) is often smaller and is recorded along the floor of the proximal CS. This potential begins over the orifice of the MCV (or other vein or diverticulum) and propagates leftward due to the fiber orientation in the CS.[19,20] As another result of fiber orientation, the CS myocardium activates the LA at a location 2 to 4 cm leftward of the MCV (or other) orifice. The parallel orientation of the CS myocardium and the LA results in rapid LA activation in the leftward direction (**Figure 8.6C**). The third potential (#3 *LA* in **Figure 8.6D**) is generated by the late LA activation recorded near the

Chapter 8: Catheter Ablation of APs • 69

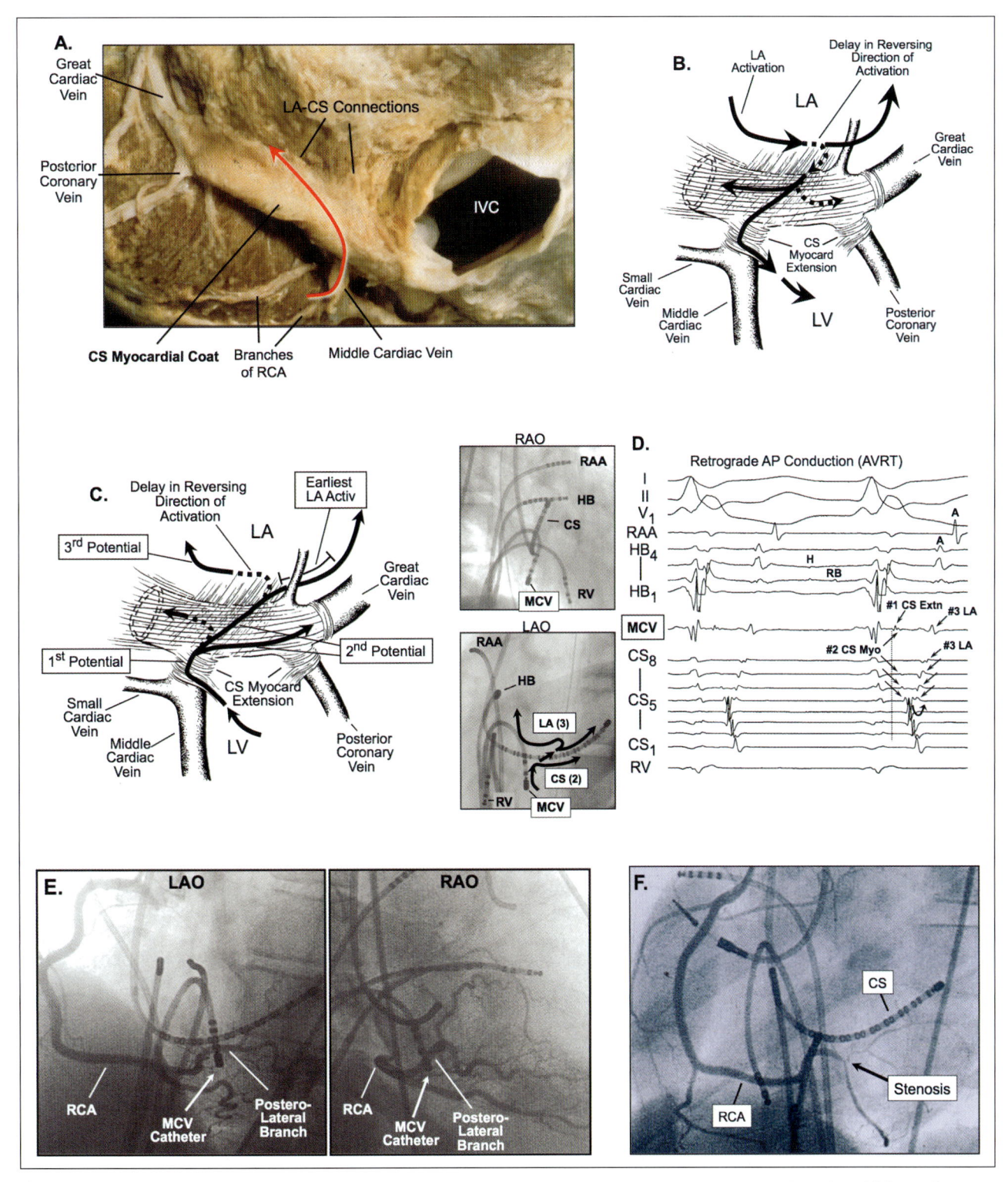

Figure 8.6 Epicardial posteroseptal AP resulting from connection between an extension of CS myocardium along the middle cardiac vein (MCV) and epicardial left ventricle (LV). **A.** Photograph showing CS myocardial coat, LA-CS connections, and relationship between MCV and distal branches of right coronary artery (RCA). (Modified with permission from reference 7.) **B.** Schematic (LAO projection) of antegrade conduction of epicardial epicardial posteroseptal AP. **C-D.** Schematic (LAO projection) and recordings of retrograde conduction, demonstrating characteristic pattern of 3 potentials. See text. **E.** Right coronary arteriography with an ablation catheter positioned in the MCV. The ablation electrode (AP recording site) is located very close to (< 2 mm) the posterolateral branch of the right coronary artery. Cryoablation was performed from the MCV to avoid arterial injury, eliminating AP conduction. **F.** Significant stenosis of distal right coronary artery in a 14-year-old male who underwent RF ablation at the floor of the CS ostium 5 years earlier at another hospital.

orifice of the MCV. LA activation in the rightward (septal) direction is delayed due to slowing of conduction during the reversal in direction of activation (**Figure 8.6C**).[7,9]

CS angiography using a balloon occlusion technique is useful to delineate the coronary venous anatomy associated with an epicardial posteroseptal AP. CS diverticula are also visualized due to their contraction, which fill the diverticula with blood from the CS. CS angiography reveals totally normal venous anatomy in 70% of the patients with a CS myocardial–ventricular connection.[9] A CS diverticulum is found in only 20% of patients, and a distorted coronary vein (associated with the AP) is identified in the remaining 10% of patients.

In the majority of patients who had a failed ablation procedure of epicardial posteroseptal APs, RF energy had been delivered endocardially to the site of earliest retrograde atrial activation at the posterolateral mitral annulus. Due to the extensive connections between the CS myocardium and the LA (**Figure 8.6A**), ablation at the posterolateral mitral annulus resulted only in a shift in the site of earliest retrograde atrial activation toward the septum (rightward shift). At the end of the failed ablation procedure, many of these patients were incorrectly thought to have had 2 different APs, a left posterolateral pathway (successfully ablated) and a posteroseptal pathway (failed ablation). Because of the extensive CS-LA connections, the optimal ablation site is within the MCV (or other coronary vein or neck of CS diverticulum) at the site recording the largest, sharpest potential generated by the CS myocardial extension on the unipolar ablation tip EGM. Before ablation, we perform coronary arteriography to determine the proximity of any significant coronary artery to the ideal ablation site within the MCV, other coronary vein, or neck of a CS diverticulum (**Figure 8.6E**). RF ablation is safe when coronary arteriography shows that the site recording the largest, sharpest CS myocardial extension potential is located at least 4 to 5 mm from the closest significant coronary artery. Saline irrigated RF electrodes are recommended to provide adequate electrode cooling within the small vein. We start the RF application at 10 to 15 W and increase power as required up to 25 W. It is important to terminate the RF application as quickly as possible when an impedance rise occurs, even a very small rise (3- to 5-ohm increase above the lowest value), to prevent adherence of the electrode to the vein. AP conduction is usually eliminated by 1 or 2 RF applications, with a low long-term recurrence, when ablation is performed at the site of a sharp unipolar CS extension potential.[7]

We found that an RF application in a coronary vein located within 2 mm of a coronary artery is associated with a high risk (> 50%) of arterial stenosis or occlusion (**Figure 8.6F**).[7,23-26] When the optimal ablation site in the vein is located within 3 to 4 mm of a significant coronary artery, cryoablation is recommended.[24,27]

References

1. Borggrefe M, Budde T, Podzeck A, Breithardt G. High frequency alternating current ablation of an accessory pathway in humans. *J Am Coll Cardiol*. 1987;10:576–582.
2. Jackman WM, Wang X, Friday KJ, et al. Catheter ablation of accessory atrioventricular pathways (Wolff-Parkinson-White syndrome) by radiofrequency current. *N Engl J Med*. 1991;324:1605–1611.
3. Calkins H, Sousa J, Rosenheck S, de Buitleir M, Kou WH, Kadish AH, Langberg JJ, Morady F. Diagnosis and cure of the Wolff-Parkinson-White syndrome or paroxysmal supraventricular tachycardias during a single electrophysiologic test. *N Engl J Med*. 1991;324:1612–1618.
4. Kuck KH, Schluter M, Geiger M, Siebels J, Duckeck W. Radiofrequency current catheter ablation of accessory atrioventricular pathways. *Lancet*. 1991;337:1557–1561.
5. Lesh MD, Van Hare GF, Schamp DJ, et al. Curative percutaneous catheter ablation using radiofrequency energy for accessory pathway in all locations: results in 100 consecutive patients. *J Am Coll Cardiol*. 1992;19:1303–1309.
6. Haïssaguerre M, Dartigues JF, Warin JF, Le Metayer P, Montserrat P, Salamon R. Electrogram patterns predictive of successful catheter ablation of accessory pathways: value of unipolar recording mode. *Circulation*. 1991;84:188–202.
7. Nakagawa H, Jackman WM. Catheter ablation of paroxysmal supraventricular tachycardia. *Circulation*. 2007;116: 2465–2478.
8. Otomo K, Gonzakez MD, Beckman KJ, et al. Reversing the direction of paced ventricular and atrial wavefronts reveals an oblique course in accessory AV pathways and improves localization for catheter ablation. *Circulation*. 2001;104: 550–556.
9. Sun Y, Arruda MS, Otomo K, et al. Coronary sinus-ventricular accessory connections producing posteroseptal and left posterior accessory pathways: incidence and electrophysiological identification. *Circulation*. 2002;106:1362–1367.
10. Hirao K, Otomo K, Wang X, et al. Para-Hisian pacing: New method for differentiating between retrograde conduction over an accessory AV pathway and the AV node. *Circulation*. 1996;94:1027–1035.
11. Nakagawa H, Jackman WM. Para-Hisian pacing: Useful clinical technique to differentiate retrograde conduction between accessory atrioventricular pathways and atrioventricular nodal pathways. *Heart Rhythm*. 2005;2:667–672.
12. Becker AE, Anderson RH, Durrer D, Wellens HJ. The anatomical substrates of Wolff-Parkinson-White syndrome: a clinicopathologic correlation in seven patients. *Circulation*. 1978;57:870–879.
13. Jackman WM, Friday KJ, Scherlag BJ, et al. Direct endocardial recording from an accessory atrioventricular pathway: localization of the site of block, effect of antiarrhythmic drugs, and attempt at nonsurgical ablation. *Circulation*. 1983;68:906–916.
14. Jackman WM, Friday KJ, Yeung Lai Wah, Fitzgerald DM, Beck B, Stelzer P, Harrison L, Lazzara R. New catheter technique for recording left free-wall accessory AV pathway activation: identification of pathway fiber orientation. *Circulation*. 1988;78:598–611.

15. Calkins H, Kim YN, Schmaltz S, Sousa J, el-Atassi R, Leon A, Kadish A, Langberg JJ, Morady F. Electrogram criteria for identification of appropriate target sites for radiofrequency catheter ablation of accessory atrioventricular connections. *Circulation.* 1992;85:565–573.
16. Silka MJ, Kron J, Halperin BD, Griffith K, Crandall B, Oliver RP, Walance CG, McAnulty JH. Analysis of local electrogram characteristics correlated with successful radiofrequency catheter ablation of accessory atrioventricular pathways. *Pacing Clin Electrophysiol.* 1992;15:1000–1007.
17. Swartz JF, Tracy CM, Fletcher RD. Radiofrequency endocardial catheter ablation of accessory atrioventricular pathway atrial insertion sites. *Circulation.* 1993;87:487–499.
18. Cappato R, Schuter M, Mont L, Kuck KH. Anatomic, electrical and mechanical factors affecting bipolar endocardial electrograms: impact on catheter ablation of manifest left free-wall accessory pathway. *Circulation.* 1994;90:884–894.
19. von Ludinghausen M, Schott C. Microanatomy of the human coronary sinus and its major tributary. In: Meerbaum S, ed. *Myocardial perfusion, reperfusion, coronary venous retroperfusion.* Darmstadt: Steinkopff Verlag;1990:93–122.
20. Chauvin M, Shah DC, Haïssaguerre M, Marcellin L, Brechenmacher C. The anatomical basis of connections between the coronary sinus musculature and the left atrium in humans. *Circulation.* 2000;101:647–652.
21. Schweikert RA, Saliba WI, Tomassoni G, et al. Percutaneous pericardial instrumentation for endo-epicardial mapping of previously failed ablation. *Circulation.* 2003;108:1329–1335.
22. Arruda MS, McClelland JH, Wang X, et al. Development and validation of an ECG algorithm for identifying accessory pathway ablation site in Wolff-Parkinson-White syndrome. *J Cardiovasc Electrophysiol.* 1998:9:2–12.
23. Sun Y, Po S, Arruda M, Beckman K, Nakagawa H, Spector P, Lustgarten D, Calame J, Lazzara R, Jackman WM. Risk of coronary artery stenosis with venous ablation for epicardial accessory pathways. *Pacing Clin Electrophysiol.* 2001;24:266 (Abstract).
24. Aoyama H, Nakagawa H, Pitha JV, et al. Comparison of cryothermia and radiofrequency current in safety and efficacy of catheter ablation within the canine coronary sinus close to the left circumferential coronary artery. *J Cardiovasc Electrophysiol.* 2005;16:1–9.
25. Paul T, Kakavand B, Blaufox AD, Saul JP. Complete occlusion of the left circumflex coronary artery after radiofrequency catheter ablation in an infant. *J Cardiovasc Electrophysiol.* 2003;14:1004–1006.
26. Takahashi Y, Jaïs P, Hocini M, et al. Acute occlusion of the left circumflex coronary artery during mitral isthmus linear ablation. *J Cardiovasc Electrophysiol.* 2005;16:1104–1107.
27. Friedman PL, Dubuc M, Green MS, et al. Catheter cryoablation of supraventricular tachycardia: results of the multicenter prospective "frosty" trial. *Heart Rhythm.* 2004;1:129–138.

CHAPTER 9

RIGHT-SIDED ACCESSORY PATHWAYS

Anne M. Dubin, MD

Introduction

Right-sided APs account for a minority of accessory connections but can be some of the most difficult pathways to eliminate, with ablation success rates usually reported in the 90% range.[1] Catheter stability placement is often cited as a major issue in right free-wall pathways and can be quite challenging. Posteroseptal pathways can be difficult to eliminate, as the pathway can straddle the septum and/or involve the CS. Anteroseptal and midseptal pathways have a higher incidence of complete heart block associated with ablation.[2] Decremental pathways are more commonly found on the right side of the heart and can add an additional layer of complexity. This chapter will address each of these issues and potential techniques used when encountering the right-sided pathway.

Classifications

Right-sided pathways can be classified according to position as well as by pathway characteristics (decremental vs. nondecremental conduction). Anatomically, APs are divided into free-wall, anteroseptal, midseptal, and posteroseptal locations (**Figure 9.1**). The distribution of these pathways is not equal, with free-wall and posteroseptal being the most common and midseptal the least.[1]

Most right-sided pathways exhibit nondecremental conduction and have a discrete conduction velocity and refractory period. The majority of right-sided APs can conduct in both directions, while right free-wall pathways are more likely than septal pathways to conduct only in the antegrade direction.[3]

Some right-sided pathways can exhibit decremental conduction (conduction that slows as the frequency of excitation increases). These pathways often have unidirectional conduction. As both limbs of tachycardia (the AVN and AP) can have varying conduction velocities, tachycardia can often be frequent and incessant in these situations. These pathways tend to be sensitive to adenosine, which can complicate diagnosis. Many of these connections may not be atrioventricular but can also be atriofacicular, nodofascicular, or even fascicular-ventricular (**Figure 9.2**).

General Considerations

Right-sided APs can be obliquely oriented, branched, or have multiple insertion points.[4] Thus, it is important to use both antegrade and retrograde mapping when faced with a right-sided pathway. Oblique pathways may require mapping from a retrograde approach when attempted from the atrial side and an antegrade approach when attempted from the ventricular side. Branching may require multiple ablation lesions at different sites. It is important to perform a full EP study before and after ablation to ensure that no additional pathways remain.

Right Free-Wall Pathways

Catheter ablation of right free-wall pathways is the least successful, with a success rate averaging only about 90%.[1] The difficulty with these may be attributed to the tricuspid valve anatomy as opposed to the MV anatomy. The MV

Figure 9.1 Schematic localization and prevalence of accessory pathway. (Courtesy of ECGpedia.org)

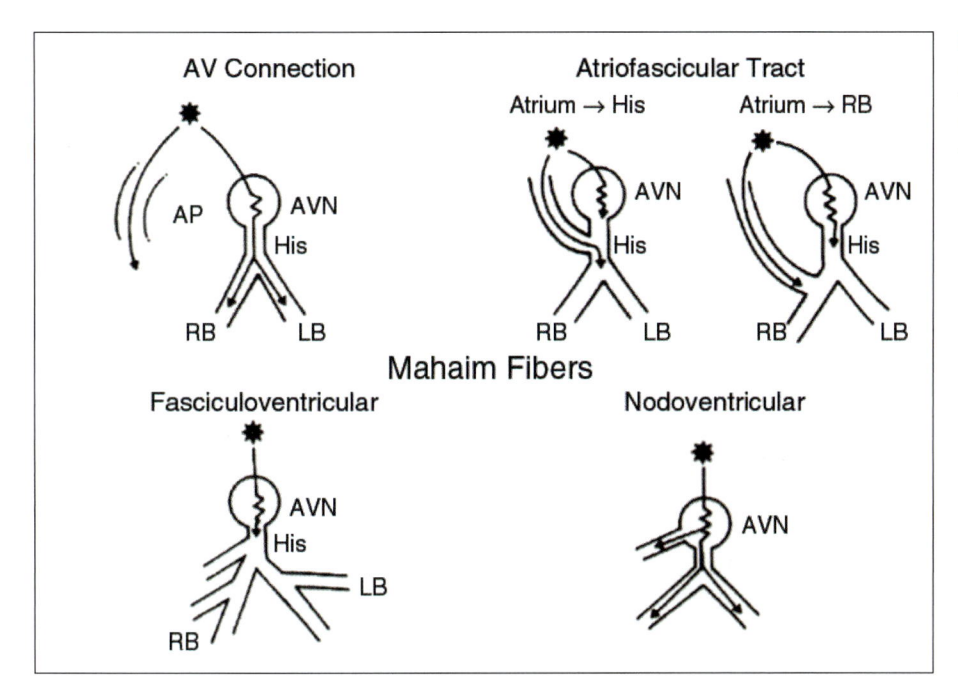

Figure 9.2 Schematic of accessory pathways: AV, atriofascicular, fasciculoventricular, and nodoventricular pathways. (Courtesy of Medscape.)

tends to be smaller, and the mitral–aortic fibrous continuity is an area that is devoid of AP connections. Right-sided pathways may be several millimeters from the fibrous annulus and have been associated with a higher prevalence of branching pathways. Finally, the right AV groove is not as easily seen on fluoroscopy, as the CS typically outlines the left AV groove. Several possible approaches and techniques have been advocated to try and improve success rates with these pathways.

Multiple approaches have been advocated when faced with a right free-wall pathway. In general, a typical IVC approach to the atrial side of the tricuspid valve is useful when faced with a right posterior or posterolateral pathway. However, if the pathway is anterior or anteroseptal, many authors have found an SVC approach more useful, as the catheter can be more easily stabilized (**Figure 9.3**).[5] Right lateral and anterolateral pathways are often the most difficult pathways to ablate and tend to have the highest recurrence rates.[6] There are several possible reasons for this, but it is often difficult to achieve catheter stability and adequate temperatures in this location.

One important way to stabilize and improve success in right-sided pathways is to use a long sheath (**Figure 9.4**). These sheaths (Daig, Minnetonka, MN; Agilis, St. Jude Medical, St. Paul, MN) come in a variety of preformed or steerable curves, which relate to areas on the tricuspid valve annulus. The reduced-radius series allows these sheaths to be used in smaller children as well. The sheath can provide catheter stability and improve torque transmission to the tip. These sheaths were judged to contribute directly to success in 43% of pathways in one pediatric study.[7]

One of the major issues with catheter ablation along the right free wall is difficulties with the tricuspid valve anatomy. The RCA runs along the ventricular aspect of the right epicardial AV groove, and RCA mapping has been reported as an aid to precise mapping and ablation of right free-wall pathways. This technique has been shown to be extremely helpful in pediatric ablation, resulting in 100% success in the two studies in which it has been used.[8,9] The RCA was visualized using angiography. A 6-F guiding catheter was advanced to the RCA where the os was engaged. A 2.3- to 2.5-Fr quadripolar or octapolar microcatheter (Pathfinder,

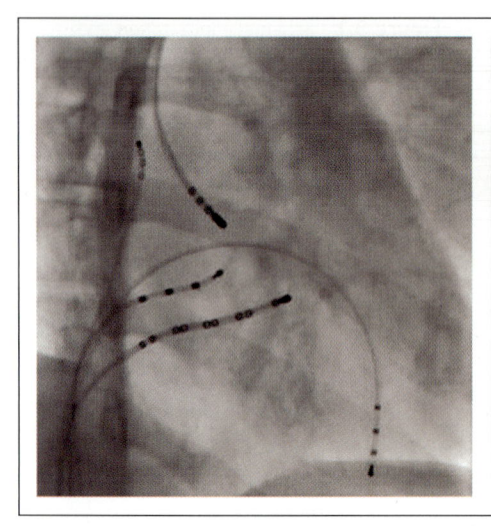

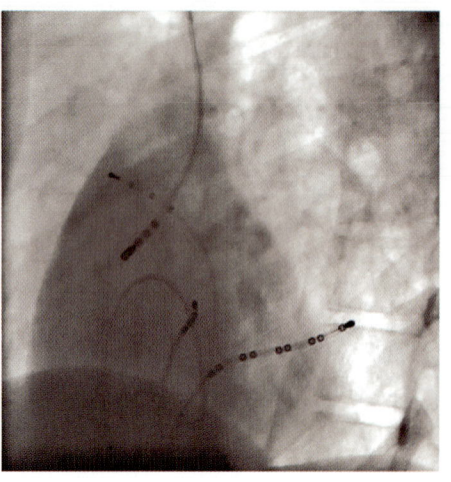

Figure 9.3 Right and left anterior oblique fluoroscopic views of superior approach to ablation of a right anterolateral pathway. RF ablation catheter is advanced from the right internal jugular through the SVC to the site of the pathway.

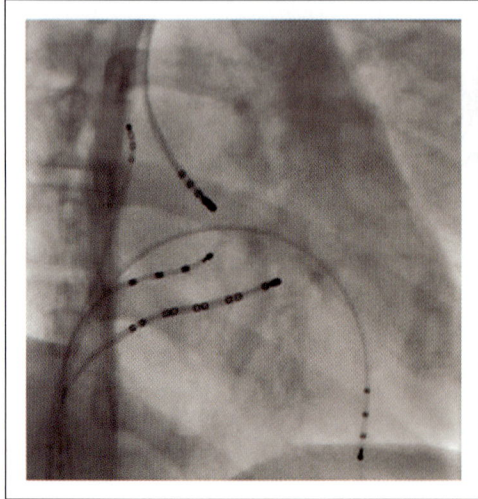

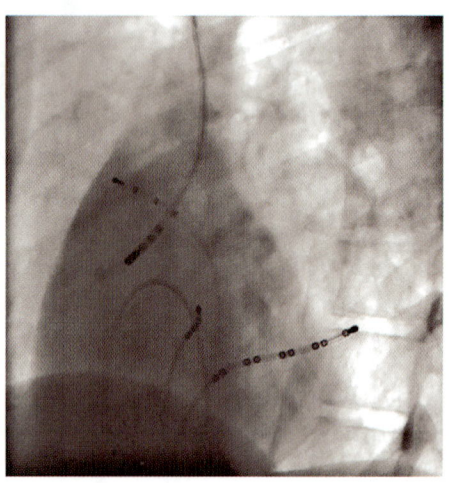

Figure 9.4 Right and left anterior oblique fluoroscopic view of a right lateral pathway ablation site. A long steerable sheath is in place to provide stability during ablation.

Cardima, Fresno, CA) was then advanced into the RCA to follow the tricuspid valve annulus (**Figure 9.5**). This allowed for earliest activation either retrograde or antegrade and easy recognition of the AV annulus. No complications were reported in either study. Follow-up coronary artery angiography demonstrated no abnormalities in any of these patients. Unfortunately, at the time of writing this chapter, these wires are no longer available. Renewed production is anticipated in early 2013.

Another method for improved mapping of the tricuspid valve uses a 20-pole Halo catheter (Biosense-Webster, Diamond Bar, CA). This catheter is commonly used to map the tricuspid valve annulus to guide ablation of the CTI for AFL; however, it has also been useful in right-sided APs. Use of this catheter has allowed for successful ablation in 100% of patients following a prior failed ablation in one study.[10]

Anteroseptal Pathways

Pathways are classified as anteroseptal if an AP potential as well as a HB potential is simultaneously recorded from a catheter placed at the HB region. These pathways tend to run anteriorly along the central fibrous body, along the right anterior free-wall. Ablation of these pathways can be difficult, as there is a risk of AV block. Optimally, the ablation catheter should be placed where only a tiny HB potential is seen. This can be accomplished with an approach from the right internal jugular (the superior approach as mentioned in Figure 9.3). The catheter is usually advanced into the right ventricle and then curved back to ablate the pathways from the ventricular aspect of the tricuspid annulus. Some authors feel that this superior approach allows for a more stable position and suggest that higher success rates can be found using this method.

Anteroseptal pathways may require an approach from the noncoronary cusp of the aortic valve.[11] The aortic valve is quite central and is anatomically related to both the atria and the ventricles. The noncoronary cusp lies directly adjacent to the atrial septum. Electrically active myocardial sleeves, which can constitute an AP, have been described that cross the aortic valve plane and extend into the cusp.[12] Thus, APs can extend into the cusp itself. Several subtle differences in the surface ECG preexcitation pattern have been suggested to help differentiate AP found in the noncoronary cusp from a conventional right anteroseptal pathway.[11] Typically, a right anteroseptal pathway can be characterized by an isoelectric or negative delta wave in lead V_1 with transition to a positive delta wave in lead V_2 and a strongly positive delta wave in the inferior surface leads (II, II, aVF). In patients in whom a noncoronary cusp location was found, a small positive delta wave already was seen in lead V_1 and an isoelectric delta wave in lead III (**Figure 9.6**).[11]

Midseptal Pathways

Midseptal pathways are defined as pathways located along the septum between the His position and the CS. As the AV node is in close proximity to this area, it can be difficult to ablate here safely. The catheter should therefore be positioned closer to the ventricular aspect of the AV annulus, with the local V potential amplitude being greater than the local atrial amplitude.

An important technique, which can be crucial when trying to differentiate between retrograde conduction across a septal AP and the AV node, is parahisian pacing.[13] This technique consists of pacing the RV close to the HB. When pacing output is increased, it is often possible to capture the HB and directly stimulate the HPS; this should result in a relatively narrow QRS complex. As the output is decreased, the insulated His is no longer excited, and the local ventricle is stimulated instead. This results in a wider QRS pattern. The presence or absence of a change in the atrial activation sequence and VA timing identifies whether retrograde conduction uses an AP or the AV node (or both) (**Figure 9.7**).

One problem with the above technique is that it is not possible to differentiate a bystander AP from orthodromic AVRT using the pathway. A variation of this concept is used when trying to differentiate orthodromic AVRT from AVNRT. Entrainment or resetting of SVT from the parahisian position can help define the retrograde limb of conduction during tachycardia and help differentiate between an AP used in a tachycardia versus one that is a bystander.[14] A longer VA time during tachycardia (> 40 ms) was seen with AVNRT, while (< 40 ms) was consistent with an AVRT.

Posteroseptal Pathways

Posteroseptal pathways are often considered some of the most difficult to ablate, with longer procedure times and more radiofrequency lesions than other pathways.[15] This is directly related to the anatomy of the posteroseptal region. The posteroseptal region has been defined as the space posterior to the septum and thus can involve both the left and right side of the heart. This anatomic issue can complicate the ablation of these pathways, and often what appears to be a right posteroseptal pathway needs to be approached from the left side. Many times these pathways will take a course close to the terminal portion of the CS and may be in a subepicardial site around the CS mouth or

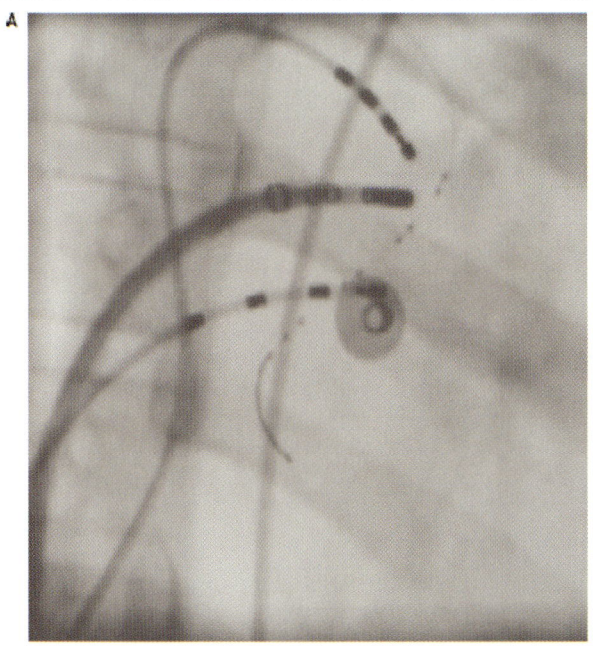

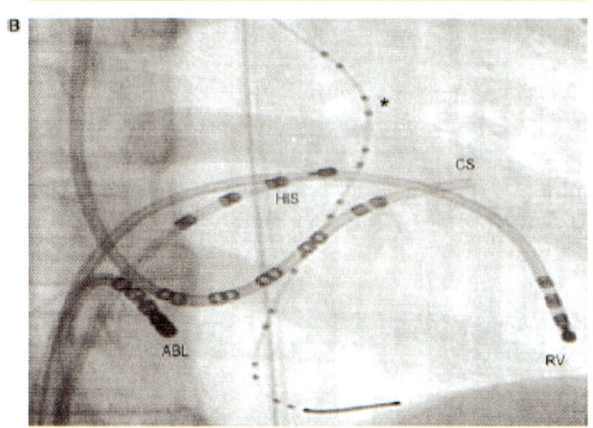

Figure 9.5 Coronary artery microcatheter mapping **A.** Magnified fluoroscopic view of a 2.3-Fr microcatheter in the RCA for mapping of a right anterior accessory pathway. Two quadripolar catheters are seen in the high right atrium and His position. An ablation catheter is positioned using a long sheath at the site of the pathway. **B.** Right anterior oblique projection of the microcatheter advanced to the posterior region of the right AV groove. ABL = ablation catheter, CS = coronary catheter, HIS = His bundle, RV = right ventricle. (Used with permission from Shah et al., *J Cardiovasc Electrophysiol* 2004;15(11):1238–1243; reference 8.)

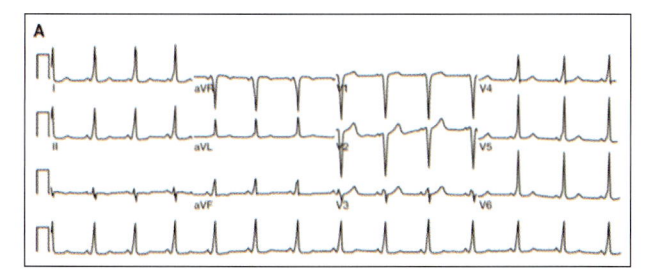

Figure 9.6 ECG of noncoronary cusp anteroseptal pathway. A small positive delta wave is seen in lead V_1 and an isoelectric delta wave is seen in lead III. (Used with permission from Suleiman et al., *J Cardiovasc Electrophysiol* 2011;22(2):203–209; reference 11.)

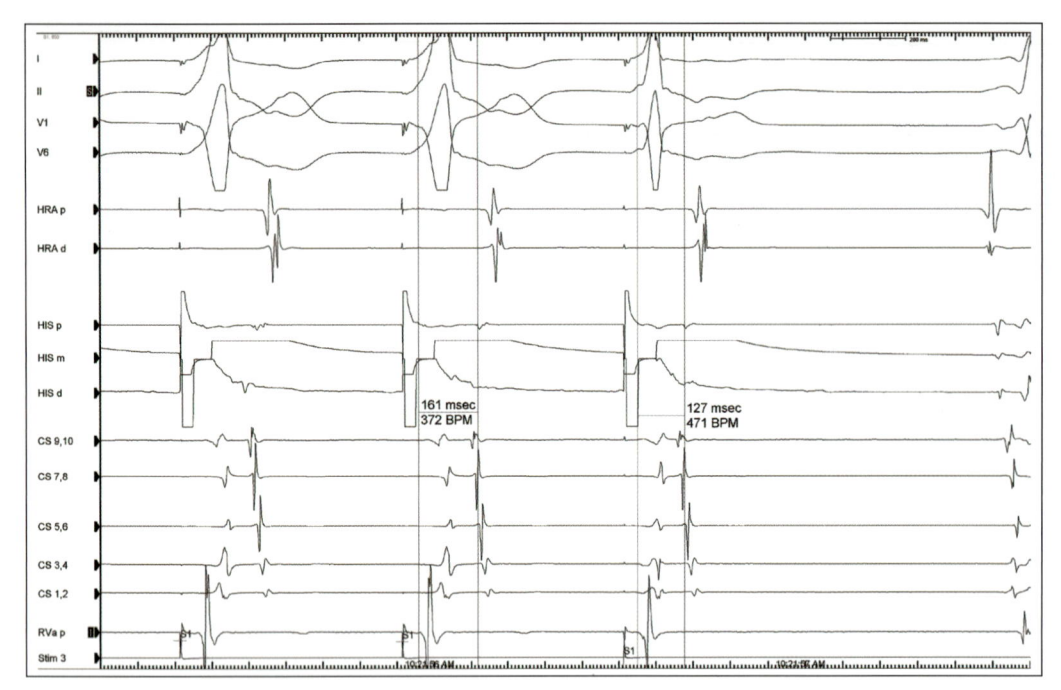

Figure 9.7 Example of parahisian pacing in a patient without a midseptal pathway. Pacing at normal output captures the ventricular tissues (note the wide QRS) with a VA time of 161 ms. With high output, the HB is captures (QRS is narrower) and the VA time shortens to 127 ms as conduction is directly from the HB to the atrium.

within the middle cardiac vein. Thus, these pathways can often only be ablated within the mouth or in a vein of the CS.[16] Difficulty in determining the best area for ablation has led to algorithms to help differentiate right-sided pathways from pathways within the CS or on the left side of the heart (**Figure 9.8**).[17] Mapping with the ablation catheter along the floor of the CS can often identify a large AP potential. The ablation catheter may drop into a diverticulum or cardiac vein during this process. A CS angiogram can be quite helpful to fully understand the anatomy of this region and to aid in ablation (**Figure 9.9**). Caution must be taken when ablating in this region, as perforation and coronary damage have been reported with these ablations.[3] This can be especially problematic when using RF energy. Impedances tend to be higher in coronary veins, which can lead to excess heating, and perforation. Thus, power should be set initially low (3-10 W). Cryoablation has also been considered in these pathways, but difficulty in manipulating the cryocatheter within the CS may limit its utility.

Mahaim Tachycardias

Over time, investigators have realized that there are several different types of APs besides AV pathways: these include nodoventricular, fasciculoventricular, and, most commonly, atriofascicular pathways. Most Mahaim tachycardias (which have a characteristic LBBB pattern) originate from atriofascicular pathways. These atriofascicular pathways most commonly arise from the anterior RA and insert into the right ventricle close to the RBBB. Mahaim pathways tend to conduct in the antegrade direction only and tend to have decremental conduction. The baseline ECG tends to have poor or no preexcitation. An atriofascicular pathway can be differentiated from a nodal or fascicular originating pathway when one or more of the following criteria is met: an RA extrastimulus (delivered as late as 40 ms after onset) of the RA septal electrogram advances ventricular activation during tachycardia without affecting atrial activation at the low RA; the tachycardia can be entrained with atrial fusion during right atrial pacing; or ventricular preexcitation is more easily seen when pacing from the right atrium than from the CS.[18]

Atriofascicular pathways constitute 80% of Mahaim fibers.[4] They tend to have a long intracardiac course and insert into the distal right bundle or the right ventricle near the apex. It can be difficult to map these pathways, as they tend not to be ablatable in the usual AV position. Several strategies for mapping and ablating have been successfully employed when these pathways are encountered. Targeting the distal insertion site is problematic, as patients often are left with an RBBB, and can develop incessant tachycardia as the circuit is often lengthened. Thus, ablation tends to be successful when the atrial insertion site is identified. These pathways do not conduct in the retrograde direction; thus, it is not possible to map the proximal insertion site using ventricular pacing. There have been several methods proposed for mapping the atrial site. These include recording of a Mahaim potential along the right AV junction; induction of mechanical conduction block in the AP with catheter manipulation; or stimuli to delta-wave mapping.

The most commonly used technique is identifying a local action potential (Mahaim potential) along the tricuspid valve annulus (**Figure 9.10**).[4] The site of the potential coincides with the atrial insertion of the pathway. It is important to realize that a fused A and V signal will not be seen even with maximal preexcitation, as the conduction along these pathways is decremental and the Mahaim potential will be evident on the isoelectric baseline between the 2 potentials (**Figure 9.11**).

Figure 9.8 Algorithm to differentiate right and left posteroseptal pathways. SVT = supraventricular tachycardia, LPS = left posteroseptal pathway, RPS = right posteroseptal pathway. (Adapted from Chiang et al., *Circulation* 1996, 93:982–991; reference 17.)

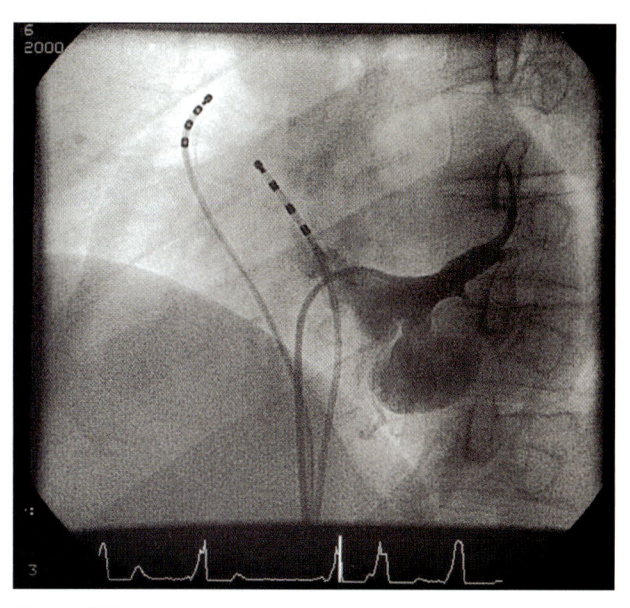

Figure 9.9 Left anterior oblique view of CS angiogram, which reveals a large diverticulum. (Reproduced with permission from Bennett DH, Hall MC. Coronary sinus diverticulum containing posteroseptal accessory pathway. *Heart* 2001;85(5):539.)

Catheter manipulation can easily cause mechanical conduction block. This is probably secondary to the subendocardial course of these fibers. Light pressure on the area of interest commonly results in conduction block. Ablation in this area has been shown to be successful.[19] However, recurrence after acutely successfully ablation is more likely for Mahaim fibers than for typical pathways, most likely because of the difficult factor of mechanically induced Mahaim block.[19]

The third technique for identifying the atrial insertion requires atrial stimulation, and measuring the stimulus to QRS complex. This is not as successful as the prior 2 techniques for several reasons.[19] There can be difficulty in maintaining a stable catheter position at the tricuspid valve annulus when atrial pacing as well as an inability to completely understand the atrial-AP interface. It is often the case that an identical or shorter interval can be recorded from regions distal to the atrial insertion site.[19]

Ablation is more likely to be acutely and permanently successful at the ventricular side of the tricuspid annulus than either the atrial side or the typical ventricular insertion along the right bundle.[19] Often with application of RF energy, Mahaim automaticity is seen, with initiation of a slow accelerated Mahaim rhythm that disappears after

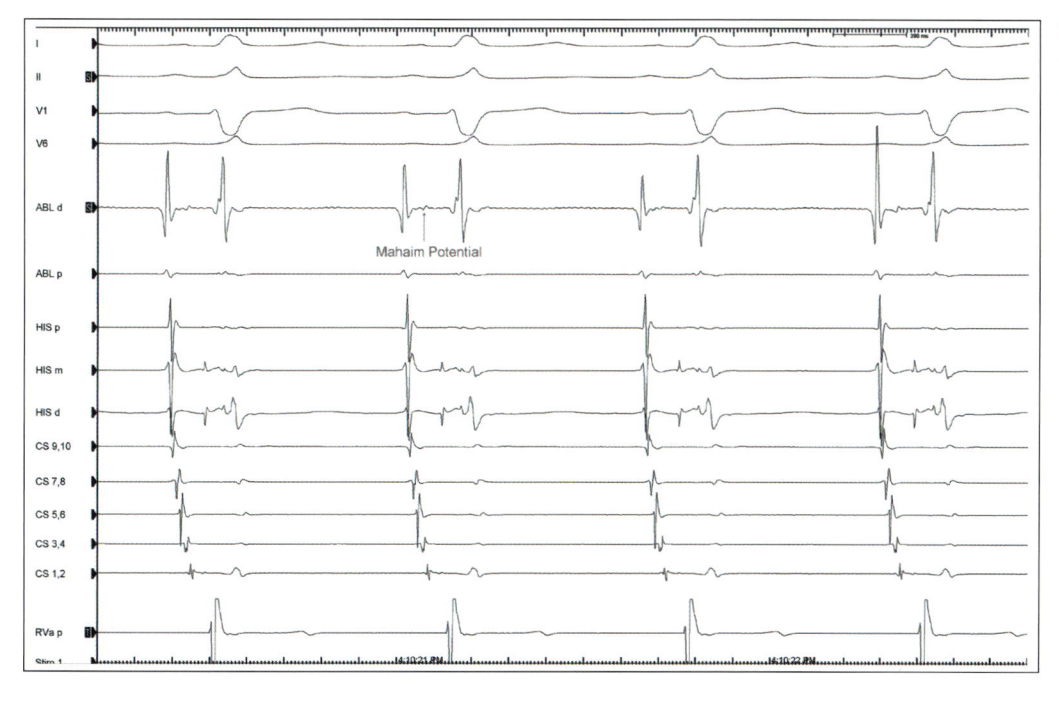

Figure 9.10 Example of Mahaim potential seen at successful ablation site.

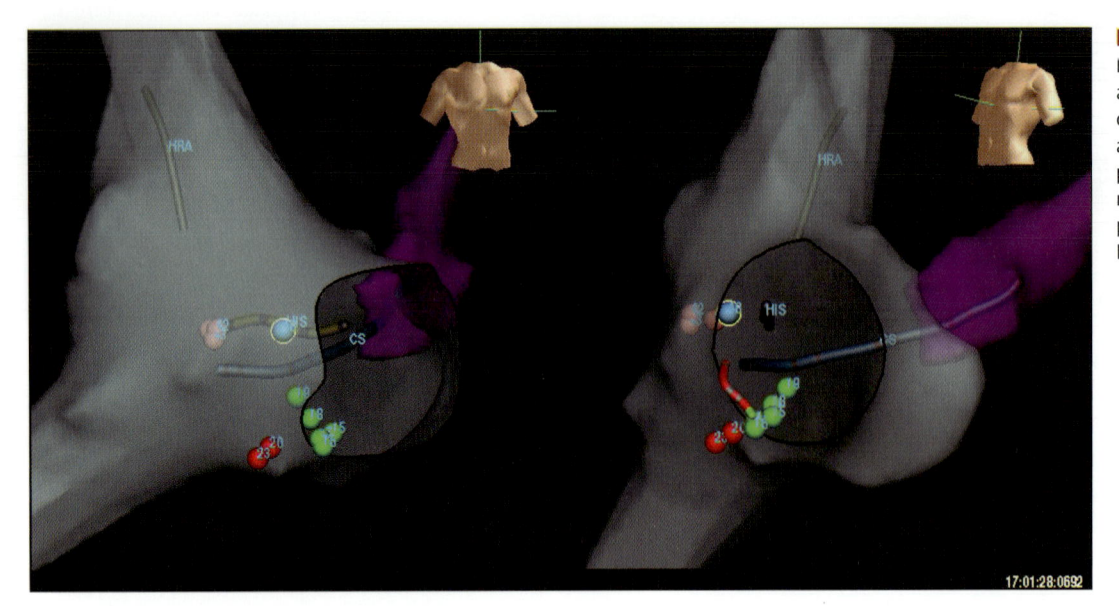

Figure 9.11 NavX image of RAO and LAO view of catheter position and ablation sites in patient with both a right posteroseptal pathway and a Mahaim tachycardia.

the first few seconds of RF energy application.[20] This automaticity can also be used as a marker of successful catheter positioning.

Permanent Junctional Reciprocating Tachycardia (PJRT)

The permanent form of junctional reciprocating tachycardia (or PJRT) is a nearly incessant tachycardia that often leads to tachycardia-induced cardiomyopathy and severe left ventricular dysfunction.[21] It is characterized by a narrow QRS complex, an RP interval longer than the PR interval, and retrograde P waves in surface leads II, III, and aVF. It is most commonly seen in children, but it has been identified in adult patients as well.[22] PJRT is caused by a concealed decremental AP, which classically has been described as being in a posteroseptal location. However, it has been shown that these decremental incessant tachycardias can originate elsewhere, including the CS os, midseptum, and left posteroseptal and lateral regions.[23] It can be quite difficult to control medically, and ablation has become the treatment of choice.

These pathways provide their own challenges, as mapping is somewhat different than when faced with a decremental pathway. It is often impossible to use standard techniques of atrial preexcitation by a ventricular premature beat while the His is refractory in these situations. Retrograde conduction is decremental, and often no atrial preexcitation is seen. VA fusion is not seen at the site of the pathway; the VA interval is generally long, with a long isoelectric segment between the ventricular and atrial signals. It is often difficult to obtain pure retrograde conduction across the AP, and fusion with retrograde AVN conduction is often seen. Thus, mapping is best conducted in tachycardia.

It is also important to distinguish PJRT for the atypical form of AVNRT. Three criteria have been used to help distinguish the 2 using a timed ventricular premature beat while the His is refractory. If this (1) produces advancement of the retrograde atrial potentials (though with decremental conduction it may not), (2) terminates the tachycardia without retrograde atrial activation, or (3) results in significant prolongation (> 50 ms) of the local VA interval, the tachycardia can be classified as PJRT.[24]

Ablation can also be a challenge, as many of these patients are in incessant tachycardia during the study. This can lead to difficulties with catheter stability, especially if the tachycardia abruptly breaks with ablation. Several investigators have suggested techniques to aid with this problem. Ventricular pacing and entrainment at slightly higher than TCL during ablation can help stabilize the catheter while ablating. Cryoablation has also been advocated in this situation; cryoadhesion keeps the catheter stable despite a rapid change of rhythm. Cryotherapy has the added benefit of reversibility, thus decreasing any potential risk of AV block.

Despite the challenges, a success rate of more than 95% is found, though recurrences are higher, and patients may require more than one procedure.[25] Risk of AV block is minimal.[26] As medical therapy is often ineffectual in this disease, the low morbidity and high success rate makes ablation a first-line therapy in this condition.[27]

New Techniques

Several new techniques have recently become available for mapping and ablation and have been shown to be successful when faced with a right-sided pathway. Electroanatomic mapping (CARTO system, Biosense Webster, Diamond Bar, CA and EnSite NavX, St. Jude Medical, St. Paul, MN) can reduce the number of catheters needed (thus decreasing vascular access) and reduce fluoroscopy times (**Figure 9.12**).[28] This technique may also be useful to help map difficult right free-wall pathways as well as to assess catheter stability during ablation.

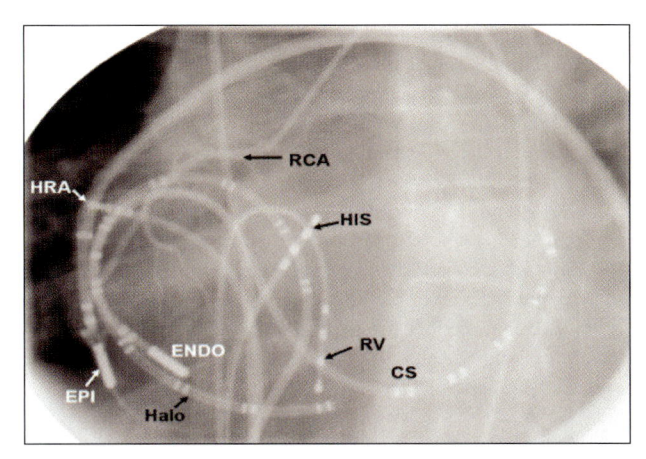

Figure 9.12 Epicardial ablation site in a right lateral pathway. Left anterior oblique fluoroscopic view of catheters. CS = coronary sinus, ENDO = endocardial catheter, EPI = epicardial catheter through an SL1 sheath, Halo = halo catheter around the tricuspic annulus, HIS = His-bundle catheter, HRA = high right atrium, RCA = right coronary artery, RV = right ventricular catheter (Used with permission from Valderrabano M, Cesario DA, Ji S, et al. Percutaneous epicardial mapping during ablation of difficult accessory pathways as an alternative to cardiac surgery. *Heart Rhythm*. 2004 Sep;1(3):311–316.)

The recently introduced Niobe system (Sterotaxis Inc, St. Louis, MO) allows a soft ablation catheter to be positioned by magnetic fields within the cardiac chambers.[29] This technology has been used in parahisian and anteroseptal pathways and theoretically can help decrease the risk of AV block during ablation. Robotic positioning of the catheter has also been shown to result in more stable catheter position.[30]

Percutaneous epicardial mapping has been used in select patients who have had multiple failed attempts at conventional ablation with some success.[31] Specifically, this technique has been used in the unusual AV pathway connecting the right atrial appendage to the right ventricle.[32] Unfortunately, most right-sided APs, even epicardial pathways, lie within the AV groove, which is usually embedded within fatty tissue. This positioning can preclude ablation from an epicardial approach.[33]

How We Approach Right-Sided Pathways

In a patient with a structurally normal heart and a right-sided AP, we start with a 4-catheter study, including a CS catheter from the internal jugular vein. We place our catheters and map with the aid of an electroanatomic mapping system to minimize fluoroscopy exposure. We prefer to map retrograde using either SVT or echo beats as opposed to ventricular pacing. However, in situations in which neither SVT nor echo beats can be elicited, we use ventricular pacing to assess retrograde conduction. In patients with Wolff-Parkinson-White syndrome, we map both the antegrade and retrograde sequence, as many right-sided pathways are obliquely oriented. We often use adenosine, both in sinus rhythm and with ventricular pacing, to assess for APs when we encounter a slick AV node. Finally, we always retest after ablation, as it is common to find multiple right-sided pathways, which can become more evident after the ablation of the dominant pathway.

Free-wall Pathways

If a right free-wall pathway is found, we carefully map with our ablation catheter to find the earliest retrograde activation in tachycardia or with echo beats as outlined above. We will quickly move to a long sheath to aid with catheter stability, as adequate temperatures are often an issue in these locations.

Midseptal

If we suspect a right midseptal pathway, we proceed with parahisian pacing to attempt to differentiate between a midseptal pathway and AV nodal conduction. If a midseptal pathway is found, we use cryoablation to protect AV nodal conduction.

Anterolateral and Anteroseptal

We often approach a right anteroseptal and anterolateral pathway from above, as this approach tends to provide better catheter stability in these locations.

Posteroseptal

We use a luminal CS catheter in the majority of our cases. This allows us to image the CS completely and assess for CS diverticulum. This can be useful when approaching the posteroseptal pathway. We also do not hesitate to approach a posteroseptal pathway from the left side if unsuccessful on the right side of the heart.

References

1. Calkins H, Yong P, Miller JM, et al. Catheter ablation of accessory pathways, atrioventricular nodal reentrant tachycardia, and the atrioventricular junction: final results of a prospective, multicenter clinical trial. The Atakr Multicenter Investigators Group. *Circulation*. 1999;99(2):262–270.
2. Schaffer MS, Silka MJ, Ross BA, Kugler JD. Inadvertent atrioventricular block during radiofrequency catheter ablation. Results of the Pediatric Radiofrequency Ablation Registry. Pediatric Electrophysiology Society. *Circulation*. 1996;94(12):3214–3220.
3. Jackman WM, Wang XZ, Friday KJ, Roman CA, Moulton KP, Beckman KJ, et al. Catheter ablation of accessory atrioventricular pathways (Wolff-Parkinson-White syndrome) by radiofrequency current. *N Engl J Med*. 1991;324(23):1605–1611.
4. Haïssaguerre M, Cauchemez B, Marcus F, et al. Characteristics of the ventricular insertion sites of accessory pathways with anterograde decremental conduction properties. *Circulation*. 1995;91(4):1077–1085.

5. Schluter M, Kuck KH. Radiofrequency current for catheter ablation of accessory atrioventricular connections in children and adolescents. Emphasis on the single-catheter technique. *Pediatrics*. 1992;89(5 Pt 1):930–935.
6. Calkins H, Prystowsky E, Berger RD, et al. Recurrence of conduction following radiofrequency catheter ablation procedures: relationship to ablation target and electrode temperature. The Atakr Multicenter Investigators Group. *J Cardiovasc Electrophysiol*. 1996;7(8):704–712.
7. Saul JP, Hulse JE, De W, et al. Catheter ablation of accessory atrioventricular pathways in young patients: use of long vascular sheaths, the transseptal approach and a retrograde left posterior parallel approach. *J Am Coll Cardiol*. 1993;21(3):571–583.
8. Shah MJ, Jones TK, Cecchin F. Improved localization of right-sided accessory pathways with microcatheter-assisted right coronary artery mapping in children. *J Cardiovasc Electrophysiol*. 2004;15(11):1238–1243.
9. Olgun H, Karagoz T, Celiker A. Coronary microcatheter mapping of coronary arteries during radiofrequency ablation in children. *J Interv Card Electrophysiol*. 2010;27(1):75–79.
10. Wong T, Hussain W, Markides V, Gorog DA, Wright I, Peters NS, et al. Ablation of difficult right-sided accessory pathways aided by mapping of tricuspid annular activation using a Halo catheter: Halo-mapping of right-sided accessory pathways. *J Interv Card Electrophysiol*. 2006;16(3):175–182.
11. Suleiman M, Brady PA, Asirvatham SJ, Friedman PA, Munger TM. The noncoronary cusp as a site for successful ablation of accessory pathways: electrogram characteristics in three cases. *J Cardiovasc Electrophysiol*. 2011;22(2):203–209.
12. Hasdemir C, Aktas S, Govsa F, et al. Demonstration of ventricular myocardial extensions into the pulmonary artery and aorta beyond the ventriculo-arterial junction. *Pacing Clin Electrophysiol*. 2007;30(4):534–539.
13. Hirao K, Otomo K, Wang X, et al. Para-Hisian pacing. A new method for differentiating retrograde conduction over an accessory AV pathway from conduction over the AV node. *Circulation*. 1996;94(5):1027–1035.
14. Reddy VY, Jongnarangsin K, Albert CM, et al. Para-Hisian entrainment: a novel pacing maneuver to differentiate orthodromic atrioventricular reentrant tachycardia from atrioventricular nodal reentrant tachycardia. *J Cardiovasc Electrophysiol*. 2003;14(12):1321–1328.
15. Schluter M, Geiger M, Siebels J, Duckeck W, Kuck KH. Catheter ablation using radiofrequency current to cure symptomatic patients with tachyarrhythmias related to an accessory atrioventricular pathway. *Circulation*. 1991;84(4):1644–1661.
16. Haïssaguerre M, Gaita F, Fischer B, Egloff P, Lemetayer P, Warin JF. Radiofrequency catheter ablation of left lateral accessory pathways via the coronary sinus. *Circulation*. 1992;86(5):1464–1468.
17. Chiang CE, Chen SA, Tai CT, et al. Prediction of successful ablation site of concealed posteroseptal accessory pathways by a novel algorithm using baseline electrophysiological parameters: implication for an abbreviated ablation procedure. *Circulation*. 1996;93(5):982–991.
18. Klein GJ, Guiraudon GM, Kerr CR, et al. "Nodoventricular" accessory pathway: evidence for a distinct accessory atrioventricular pathway with atrioventricular node-like properties. *J Am Coll Cardiol*. 1988;11(5):1035–1040.
19. Cappato R, Schluter M, Weiss C, et al. Catheter-induced mechanical conduction block of right-sided accessory fibers with Mahaim-type preexcitation to guide radiofrequency ablation. *Circulation*. 1994;90(1):282–290.
20. Sternick EB. Automaticity in a Mahaim fiber. *Heart Rhythm*. 2005;2(4):453.
21. Dorostkar PC, Silka MJ, Morady F, Dick M, 2nd. Clinical course of persistent junctional reciprocating tachycardia. *J Am Coll Cardiol*. 1999;33(2):366–375.
22. Meiltz A, Weber R, Halimi F, et al. Permanent form of junctional reciprocating tachycardia in adults: peculiar features and results of radiofrequency catheter ablation. *Europace*. 2006;8(1):21–28.
23. Ticho BS, Saul JP, Hulse JE, De W, Lulu J, Walsh EP. Variable location of accessory pathways associated with the permanent form of junctional reciprocating tachycardia and confirmation with radiofrequency ablation. *Am J Cardiol*. 1992;70(20):1559–1564.
24. Cappato R, Schulter, M., Kuck, KH. Catheter ablation of atrioventricular reentry. In: Zipes DP, Jalife J, eds. *Cardiac Electrophysiology from Cell to Bedside*. Philadelphia, PA: W.B. Saunders Company; 2000:1035–1049.
25. Tanel RE, Walsh EP, Triedman JK, Epstein MR, Bergau DM, Saul JP. Five-year experience with radiofrequency catheter ablation: implications for management of arrhythmias in pediatric and young adult patients. *J Pediatr*. 1997;131(6):878–887.
26. Gaita F, Haïssaguerre M, Giustetto C, Fischer B, Riccardi R, Richiardi E, et al. Catheter ablation of permanent junctional reciprocating tachycardia with radiofrequency current. *J Am Coll Cardiol*. 1995;25(3):648–654.
27. Boyce K, Henjum S, Helmer G, Chen PS. Radiofrequency catheter ablation of the accessory pathway in the permanent form of junctional reciprocating tachycardia. *Am Heart J*. 1993;126(3 Pt 1):716–719.
28. Miyake CY, Mah DY, Atallah J, et al. Nonfluoroscopic imaging systems reduce radiation exposure in children undergoing ablation of supraventricular tachycardia. *Heart Rhythm*. 2011;8(4):519–525.
29. Faddis MN, Blume W, Finney J, et al. Novel, magnetically guided catheter for endocardial mapping and radiofrequency catheter ablation. *Circulation*. 2002;106(23):2980–2985.
30. Ernst S, Hachiya H, Chun JK, Ouyang F. Remote catheter ablation of parahisian accessory pathways using a novel magnetic navigation system—a report of two cases. *J Cardiovasc Electrophysiol*. 2005;16(6):659–662.
31. Valderrabano M, Cesario DA, Ji S, et al. Percutaneous epicardial mapping during ablation of difficult accessory pathways as an alternative to cardiac surgery. *Heart Rhythm*. 2004;1(3):311–316.
32. Lam C, Schweikert R, Kanagaratnam L, Natale A. Radiofrequency ablation of a right atrial appendage-ventricular accessory pathway by transcutaneous epicardial instrumentation. *J Cardiovasc Electrophysiol*. 2000;11(10):1170–1173.
33. Schweikert RA, Saliba WI, Tomassoni G, et al. Percutaneous pericardial instrumentation for endo-epicardial mapping of previously failed ablations. *Circulation*. 2003;108(11):1329–1335.

CHAPTER 10

How to Diagnose, Map, and Ablate AVRT Due to Atriofascicular Conduction Fibers

Melvin M. Scheinman, MD; David S. Kwon, MD, PhD

Introduction

In 1938, Ivan Mahaim presented the first description of specialized conduction fibers connecting the AVN or His bundle to ventricular myocardium.[1] These connections have since become known as nodoventricular (NV) or fasciculoventricular (FV) fibers. In 1971, H. J. J. Wellens presented the first electrophysiologic characterization of these tracts,[2] describing decremental conduction properties associated with these fibers. Several years later, Becker et al[3] identified an AVN-like structure in the tricuspid valve annulus, from which emerged an accessory connection to the anterior right ventricle in a patient with Ebstein's anomaly. We now understand that fibers may originate from the AVN proper and insert into ventricular muscle (NV) or into either the left or right fascicles (NF) (true Mahaim tracts). However, atriofascicular fibers usually arise from the lateral tricuspid annulus and insert into or are adjacent to the right bundle branch at the right ventricular apex (**Figure 10.1**). Independently, the Jackman and Haïssaguerre labs have defined these pathways with meticulous mapping studies, following the fibers from their atrial origin to the ultimate ventricular insertion.[4,5] An understanding of these connections, the diagnostic criteria, and EP ablation techniques will be the focus of this chapter.

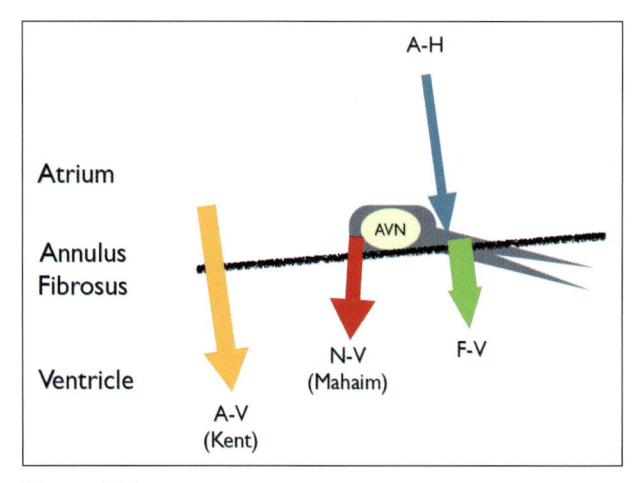

Figure 10.1 Diagram of an atriofascicular fiber emanating from the lateral tricuspid annulus and inserting into or adjacent to the right bundle branch on the anterior right ventricular wall.

Surface Electrocardiogram

The ECG for atriofascicular tachycardias typically reveals a left bundle morphology with a late transition and leftward axis (**Figure 10.2**). In sinus rhythm, the ECG may exhibit only minimal preexcitation. In 2004, Sternick et al noted a consistent rS or rsR' pattern in lead III among patients

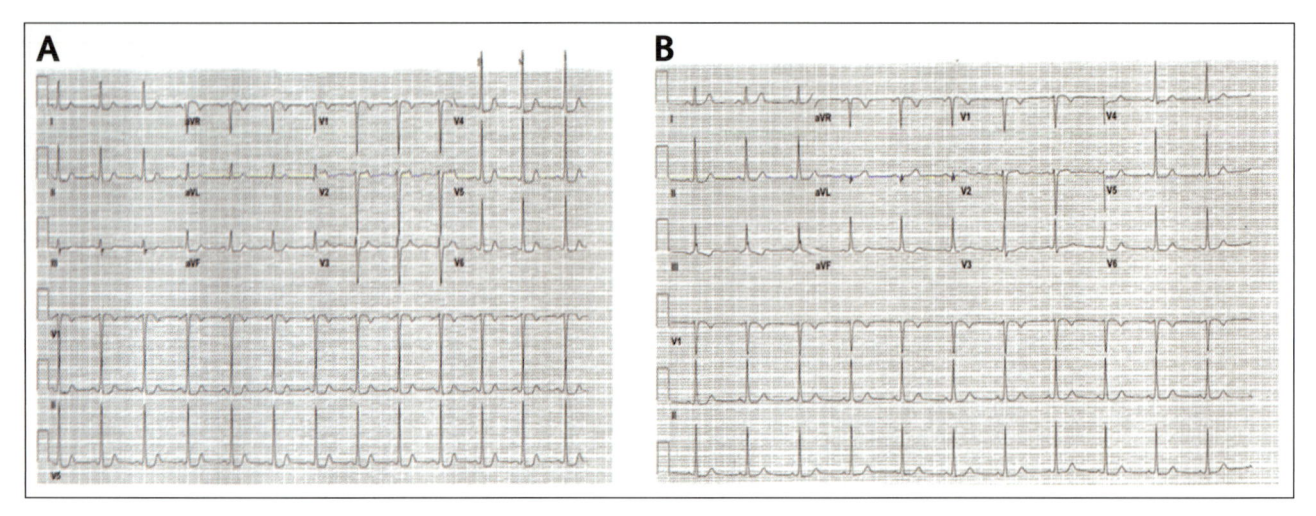

Figure 10.2 **A.** Example of a 12-lead ECG from a patient with an atriofascicular pathway prior to ablation. Note the RS pattern of the QRS complex in lead III. **B.** A 12-lead ECG from the same patient following ablation of the atriofascicular pathway. Note the absence of the RS pattern of the QRS complex in lead III.

diagnosed with atriofascicular tachycardias (**Figure 10.3**).[6] Although this pattern may be present in some normal ECGs, the atriofascicular tachycardias were never associated with a Q wave in lead I, where subtle preexcitation may be observed. Moreover, the rS pattern changed after successful ablation of the atriofascicular pathway.

Electrophysiology Study

Atriofascicular pathways have special properties. These tracts have decremental conduction properties, and they respond to vagal stimulation and to adenosine administration like the AVN. In fact, dual conduction through these pathways has also been reported.[7] Atriofascicular pathways are unidirectional and, thus, support only antidromic AVRT.

An understanding of these particular properties of atriofascicular pathways is required to correctly diagnose and treat the arrhythmia. In sinus rhythm, the 12-lead ECG manifestation depends on the relative conduction properties between the atriofascicular pathway and the AVN. Consequently, with atrial pacing at faster rates, especially on the lateral RA wall closer to the pathway, a greater degree of preexcitation will emerge with a LBBB pattern. Depending on the relation between the AVN and the atriofascicular pathway conduction and refractory characteristics, preexcitation is accomplished by simple overdrive pacing and also with single atrial extrastimuli. During the transition from AVN conduction to AP conduction, the AH-AV interval lengthens while the HV interval shortens. Once antidromic tachycardia is initiated, the H-V relationship is reversed, and the His bundle recording may be found after the QRS with a constant VH interval.[6] In addition, there is reversal of the normal His-to-right bundle branch activation. During preexcitation over the atriofascicular pathway, the right bundle branch precedes the His depolarization, and it is this change in the electrogram that proves conduction over the atriofascicular (or NF) pathway.

Interestingly, tachycardia variations have been noted. Sternick et al have also reported 2 distinct CLs of atriofascicular tachycardias eliminated by ablation at a single point.[8] Their findings were explained by either retrograde conduction via dual AVN pathways or by retrograde block in the right bundle branch. Changes in the VH interval explain the mechanism of variation in TCL.

An important maneuver for patients with antidromic APs is to introduce a premature atrial stimulus on the lateral tricuspid annulus at a time when the septal atrium has been depolarized.[9] Analogous to the His-refractory ventricular extrastimulus, an APC delivered when the septal A is committed would be expected to advance the ensuing ventricular depolarization and reset the tachycardia. If this maneuver results in ventricular capture and consequent resetting of the tachycardia, then an atriofascicular

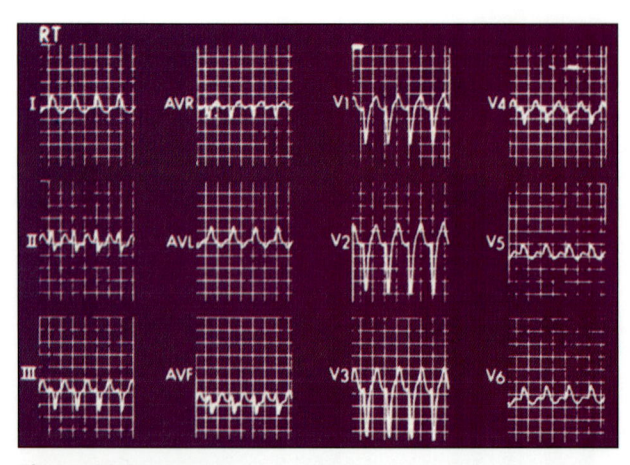

Figure 10.3 Example of an atriofascicular tachycardia exhibiting the typical left bundle branch block pattern with left axis deviation and rS pattern in lead III.

pathway is present and participates in the tachycardia (**Figure 10.4**). Once established, the retrograde limb must be confirmed, whether retrograde via the normal conduction pathway or utilizing a different septal AP. For such a determination, parahisian pacing would reveal the presence of such a septal pathway.

Techniques for Mapping and Ablation

The key to localization of the atriofascicular pathways is the ability to finely map along the tricuspid annulus. Various catheters are available, but using a 20-pole recording catheter offers rapid localization around the annulus. It is critical to avoid injury to the pathway due to catheter manipulation while placing this type of catheter, as well as during fine mapping with an ablation catheter. Searching for atriofascicular potentials requires careful attention to the details of mapping, as these sharp electrograms may show low voltage (**Figure 10.5**). They may be mapped either from the atrial or ventricular aspect of the tricuspid annulus.

Alternatively, the pathway may be eliminated at the ventricular insertion point at or near the right bundle branch. With this approach, the electrophysiologist must be cautious to avoid damage to the right bundle branch by clearly identifying these atriofascicular potentials preceding the ventricular electrogram, often very sharp and of large voltage compared to the annular potentials (**Figure 10.6**). Block of the right bundle branch may result in an incessant tachycardia with retrograde VA conduction via the left bundle branch system and an increased path length of the circuit. Typically, the VA time increases by 85 to 100 ms.[10]

Once the atriofascicular potential is recorded, great care must be used to avoid approaching the atriofascicular tract in a perpendicular fashion, as this technique may result in trauma and subsequent disappearance of the atriofascicular potential. Rather, the ablation catheter should be positioned parallel to the presumptive ablation site before energy delivery. Application of RF energy in standard fashion is appropriate with careful monitoring of the QRS complex to detect any evidence of damage to the right coronary artery. A flurry of complexes from the atriofascicular pathway is pathognomonic of successful ablation.

Associated Findings

The presence of atriofascicular pathways may not occur in isolation, and with any type of AP-mediated arrhythmia, the electrophysiologist must be watchful for additional findings. Other APs might participate as the retrograde limb of the circuit. Also, congenital diseases such as Ebstein's anomaly may be present.

In the face of finding a preexcited tachycardia, one must discern whether the atriofascicular pathway is a necessary component of the circuit or a bystander pathway incident

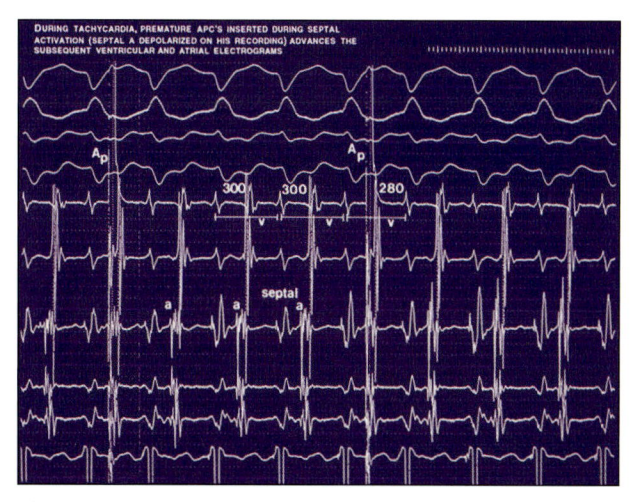

Figure 10.4 A premature atrial complex given once the septal atrium has been depolarized advances the tachycardia by 20 ms.

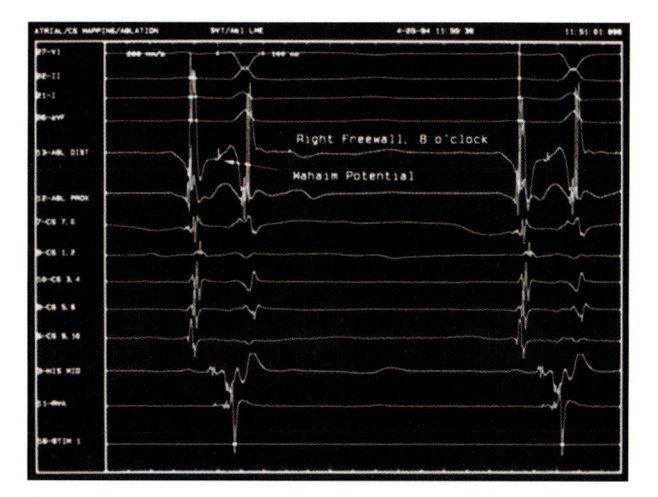

Figure 10.5 Atriofascicular pathway potential on the lateral tricuspid annulus.

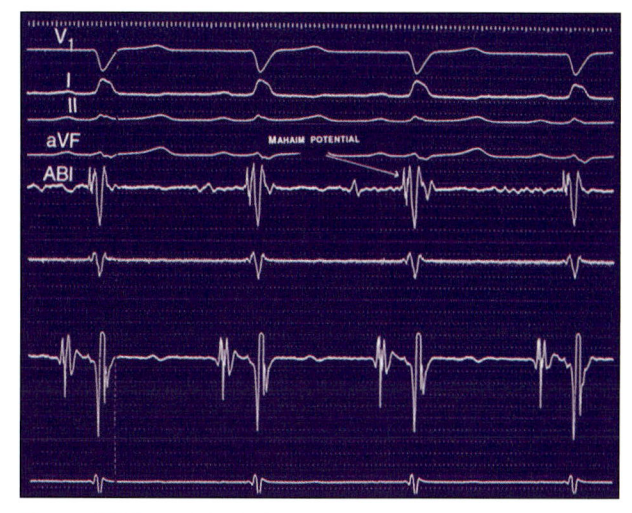

Figure 10.6 Atriofascicular pathway potential in the right ventricle precedes the QRS complex.

to associated atrial tachycardia or AV nodal reentry. The key maneuver (as discussed earlier) is insertion of an atrial premature beat when the septal A is refractory. If this maneuver resets the tachycardia, then the atrium and atriofascicular pathway are part of the circuit and constitute strong evidence for an atriofascicular tract. In contrast, maneuvers showing that the atrium is not part of the circuit point to the presence of a true NV (Mahaim) tract.

Conclusions

Atriofascicular APs are distinct anatomical pathways that arise from the lateral tricuspid annulus and insert into or near the right bundle branch. These pathways are rare and exhibit decremental conduction properties due to the AVN-like cells at their origin. Care must be taken to correctly diagnose the arrhythmia circuit and even greater attention must be given during the ablation procedure to avoid inadvertent damage to the pathway. Atriofascicular pathways are unique APs that are extremely challenging to diagnose and ablate.

References

1. Mahaim I, Benatt A. Nouvelles recherches sur les connexions superieures de la branche gauche du faisceau de His-Tawara avec cloison interventriculaire. *Cardiologia*. 1938;1:61.
2. Wellens HJJ. *Electrical Stimulation of the Heart in the Study and Treatment of Tachycardias*. Baltimore, MD: University Park Press; 1971.
3. Becker AE, Anderson RH, Durrer D, & Wellends HJ. The anatomical substrates of Wolff-Parkinson-White syndrome. A clinicopathologic correlation in seven patients. *Circulation*. 1978;57:870–879.
4. McClelland JH, Wang X, Beckman KJ, Hazlitt HA, Prior MI, Nakagawa H, Lazzara R, Jackman WM. Radiofrequency catheter ablation of right atriofascicular (Mahaim) accessory pathways guided by accessory pathway activation potentials. *Circulation*. 1994;89:2655–2666.
5. Haïssaguerre M, Cauchemez B, Marcus F, Le Metayer P, Lauribe P, Poquet F, Gencel L, Clementy J. Characteristics of the ventricular insertion sites of accessory pathways with anterograde decremental conduction properties. *Circulation*. 1995;91(4):1077–1085.
6. Sternick EB, Timmermans C, Sosa E, Cruz FES, Rodriguez LM, Fagundes M, Gerken LM, Wellens HJJ. The electrocardiogram during sinus rhythm and tachycardia in patients with Mahaim fibers: The importance of an "rS" pattern in lead III. *J Am Coll Cardiol*. 2004;44(8):1626–1635.
7. Sternick EB, Sosa EA, Scanavacca MI, Wellens HJ. Dual conduction in a Mahaim fiber. *J Cardiovasc Electrophysiol*. 2004;15(10):1212–1215.
8. Sternick EB, Rodriguez LM, Timmermans C, Sosa E, Cruz FE, Gerken LM, Fagundes M, Scanavacca M, Wellens HJ. Effects of right bundle branch block on the antidromic circus movement tachycardia in patients with presumed atriofascicular pathways. *J Cardiovasc Electrophysiol*. 2006;17(3):256–260.
9. Mahmud R, Denker ST, Tchou PJ, Jazayeri M, Akhtar M. Modulation of conduction and refractoriness in atrioventricular junctional reentrant circuit. Effect on reentry initiated by atrial extrastimulus. *J Clin Invest*. 1988;81(1):39–46.
10. Sternick EB, Lokhandwala Y, Timmermans C, Rodriguez LM, Gerken LM, Scarpelli R, Soares F, Wellens HJ. The atrioventricular interval during pre-excited tachycardia: A simple way to distinguish between decrementally or rapidly conducting accessory pathways. *Heart Rhythm*. 2009;9:1351–1358.

CHAPTER 11

How to Ablate Accessory Pathways in Patients with Ebstein's Syndrome

Christina Y. Miyake, MD

Introduction

The highest incidence of APs and arrhythmias among patients with congenital heart disease occurs among those with Ebstein's anomaly. Catheter ablation in this group of patients tends to be more difficult than in those with structurally normal hearts, and although cases may be straightforward, they can make for a long and difficult day. Hemodynamic instability during tachycardia, low-frequency and fragmented signals, difficulty locating and maintaining stability on the tricuspid annulus, and multiple pathways are just some of the challenges that may arise.

A survey of experts across the country who have been performing ablations in Ebstein's patients for years revealed there is no single best approach to these patients. However, all would agree that despite advances in technology and imaging capabilities, success is dependent on a good understanding of basic electrophysiology and the ability to interpret intracardiac signals. This chapter will briefly review Ebstein's anatomy, its effects on the conduction system, and helpful techniques when bringing a patient to the lab for ablation.

Anatomy of Ebstein's Anomaly

Ebstein's anomaly is due to failure of the septal and posterior leaflets of the tricuspid valve to delaminate from the RV endocardium. This results in apical displacement of the effective valve opening or hinge point and a relative decrease in the size of the functional RV (**Video 11.1, Figure 11.1**). The area between the true tricuspid valve annulus, which remains in the normal position at the atrioventricular groove, and the displaced tricuspid valve is referred to as the "atrialized" portion of the RV (**Figure 11.2**). This atrialized RV myocardium becomes relatively thin walled under atrial- rather than ventricular-level pressures. While the septal and posterior leaflets may be dysplastic or deficient, the anterior leaflet is often large and "sail-like" and may cause obstruction of the RVOT (**Figure 11.3**). Patients may have other coexisting cardiac anomalies, most commonly ventricular septal defects and pulmonary stenosis.

The hemodynamic effect of Ebstein's anomaly varies depending on the severity of tricuspid valve displacement and the competency of the tricuspid valve. Although some infants require early surgical intervention, a majority of individuals do not require any intervention for years. Over time, however, tricuspid regurgitation leads to atrial and ventricular enlargement, widening of the tricuspid valve annulus, and possible right-to-left shunting (a majority of patients will have an atrial-level communication consisting of a patent foramen ovale or a secundum atrial septal defect). The reduced functional RV cavity along with tricuspid regurgitation results in retardation of forward blood flow and cyanosis, which can lead to hemodynamic instability and even syncope in patients who develop arrhythmias.

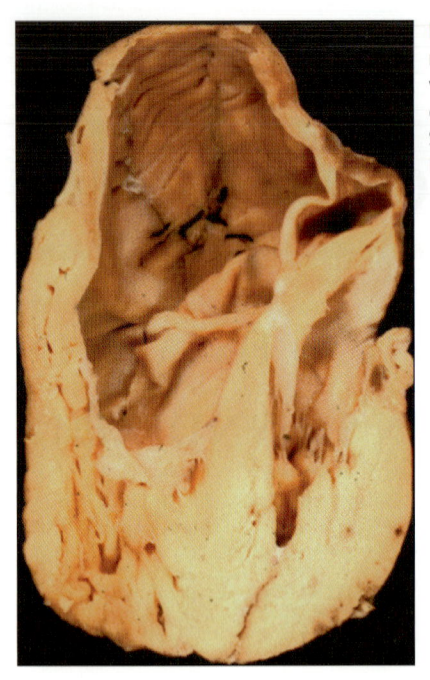

Figure 11.1 Displacement of the tricuspid valve leaflets. (Image courtesy of Dr. Norman Silverman and Dr. Robert H. Anderson.)

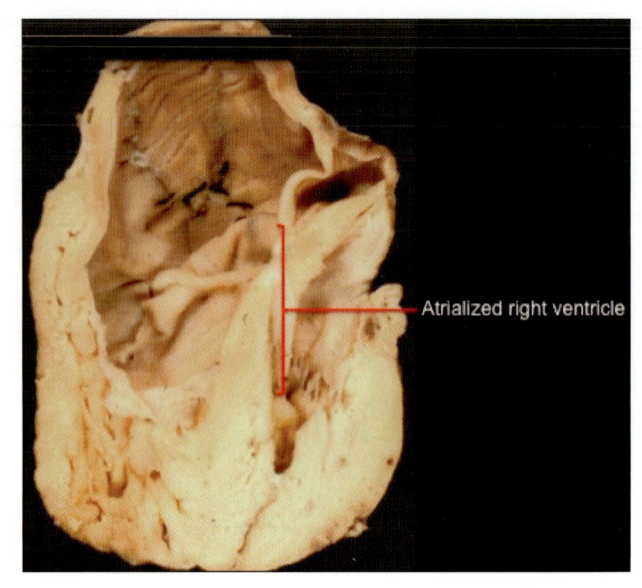

Figure 11.2 Displacement of the tricuspid valve results in an atrialized portion of the RV. (Image courtesy of Dr. Norman Silverman and Dr. Robert H. Anderson.)

Effects of Valve Displacement on the Conduction System and Associated Arrhythmias

Displacement of the tricuspid valve leads to separation of the valve hinge point from the AV node. While conduction through the AV node is generally maintained, this displacement may lead to bridging myocardium and an increased incidence of atrioventricular APs. It is thought that approximately 30% of Ebstein's patients have paroxysmal SVT, with 20% having manifest bypass tracts; however, the true incidence of APs is unknown.[1,2] Among those with APs, 30 to 50% will have multiple pathways.[3,4] Nearly all APs found in Ebstein's patients will be right sided, with a majority located in the posterolateral to posteroseptal location. The exception is the congenitally corrected transposition with an Ebsteinoid left-sided systemic tricuspid valve. The APs have typical nondecremental, "all or none" conduction properties; however, the presence of intra-atrial, infranodal, and atrialized RV conduction delays can result in (1) minimal preexcitation patterns on ECG, and (2) longer PR/AV or VA times at baseline and during tachycardia. Atriofasicular pathways (so called Mahaim fibers) can also be seen in this population but are less common.

SVT can occur for several reasons. Younger patients with SVT most commonly have AP-mediated tachycardia. With age, atrial dilation can lead to AFL, IART, and AF. VTs can also occur in this population.

Displacement of the tricuspid valve also results in fibrosis of the right-sided HPS, resulting in 75 to 80% of Ebstein's patients with an RBBB pattern on their ECG.

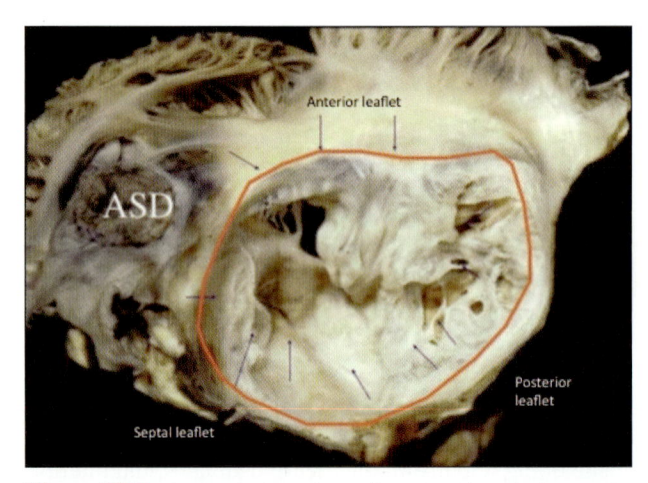

Figure 11.3 Anatomical specimen demonstrating displacement of the septal and posterior leaflets of the tricuspid valve. The septal leaflet is deficient. The anterior leaflet hinges at the annulus but is large and "sail-like." (Image courtesy of Dr. Norman Silverman and Dr. Robert H. Anderson.)

How to Decide Which Patients to Bring to the EP Laboratory

There are no specific guidelines to determine which patients require an EP study. However, there is high morbidity and mortality due to arrhythmias in the postoperative period. Furthermore, surgery on the tricuspid valve can result in future inability to access the annulus or isthmus by transcatheter approach. Patients who are scheduled for surgery with Ebstein's anomaly and any history of palpitations or concern for a possible AP should be evaluated with a formal EP study. In some centers, including our own, patients with no evidence of preexcitation or concern for SVT will be referred for an EP study to rule out the possibility of a concealed AP prior to surgical repair.

The general consensus suggests that the following patients should be evaluated by an EP study:

1. All patients undergoing surgical repair
2. Patients with manifest preexcitation on ECG
3. Symptomatic patients

Preprocedural Planning

Patients should have a complete preprocedural evaluation, including an ECG, echocardiogram, and a full physical exam, including oxygen saturation and an evaluation by a cardiac anesthesiologist. Previous records should be reviewed, including any prior cardiac surgeries, catheterizations, and imaging studies. Further imaging, such as CT or MRI scan, is not required; however, if the patient has had a recent study, prior review of these images is generally helpful. Operative notes should be reviewed for sites of surgical incisions and procedures performed on the tricuspid valve. Vessel occlusions noted on imaging studies or prior catheterizations should be identified. At our center, we generally perform a right-sided hemodynamic catheterization on all Ebstein's patients coming in for an EP study.

An informed consent should be obtained from patients for angiography, including selective coronary injection, in addition to the EP study. Risks of possible injury to the coronary artery should be discussed. If assistance is required by a catheterization interventionalist, this should be arranged in preparation for the procedure. Patients should be instructed to discontinue any antiarrhythmic medication for 5 half-lives prior to the procedure.

Most patients can be discharged home the same day. However, patients with severe disease, baseline cyanosis, polycythemia, and poor hemodynamics may not tolerate prolonged anesthesia, contrast injections, and long periods of tachyarrhythmia. Consideration for postprocedural care in an intensive care unit should be given.

ECG

Patients with right atrial enlargement may demonstrate tall P waves or first-degree AV block. The ECG should be examined for evidence of a manifest AP. Conduction delays both through the HBs and through the atrialized RV may lead to very subtle preexcitation patterns, making this difficult. However, a majority of patients, regardless of the degree of tricuspid valve displacement, have an incomplete or complete RBBB pattern (**Figure 11.4**). The lack of an RBBB pattern is not diagnostic but should raise suspicion for a manifest pathway, particularly if there is a short PR interval (**Figure 11.5, A–C**).[5] A symptomatic patient with a normal PR interval may have a concealed pathway or a Mahaim fiber (particularly if there is an LBBB). ECG preexcitation patterns can be helpful to determine right- versus left-sidedness[6] but should not be used to determine definitive pathway location; however, negative delta waves in the inferior leads generally correspond to bypass tracts in the posteroseptal location.

Echocardiogram

An echocardiogram is obtained in all patients as part of the preoperative evaluation. Visualization of the degree of tricuspid valve displacement, amount of tricuspid regurgitation, presence of outflow tract obstruction, size of the RA and RV, and the presence and size of atrial septal communications can be helpful prior to mapping. Overall ventricular systolic function should also be assessed.

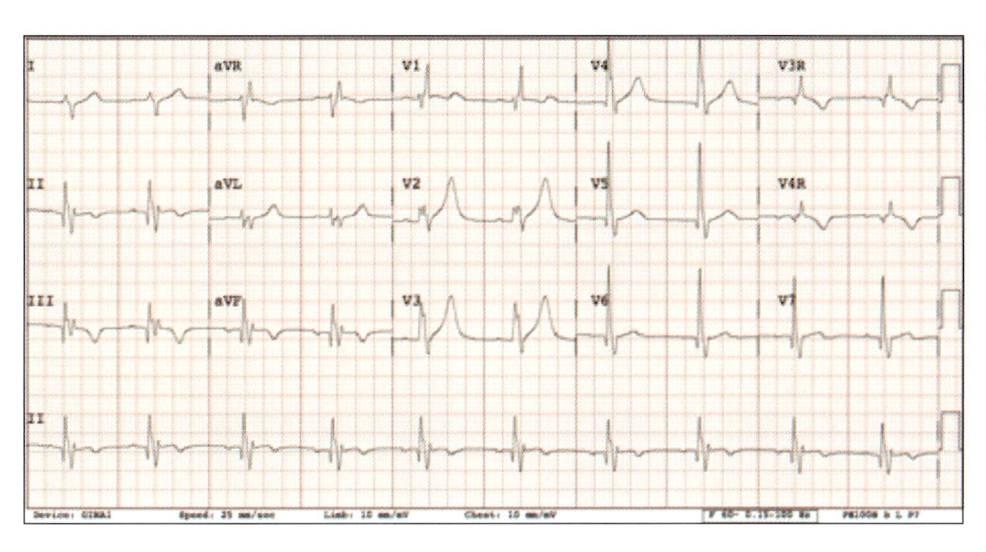

Figure 11.4 Example of typical ECG seen in patients with Ebstein's anomaly. There is an RBBB pattern.

88 • Ablation of SVT

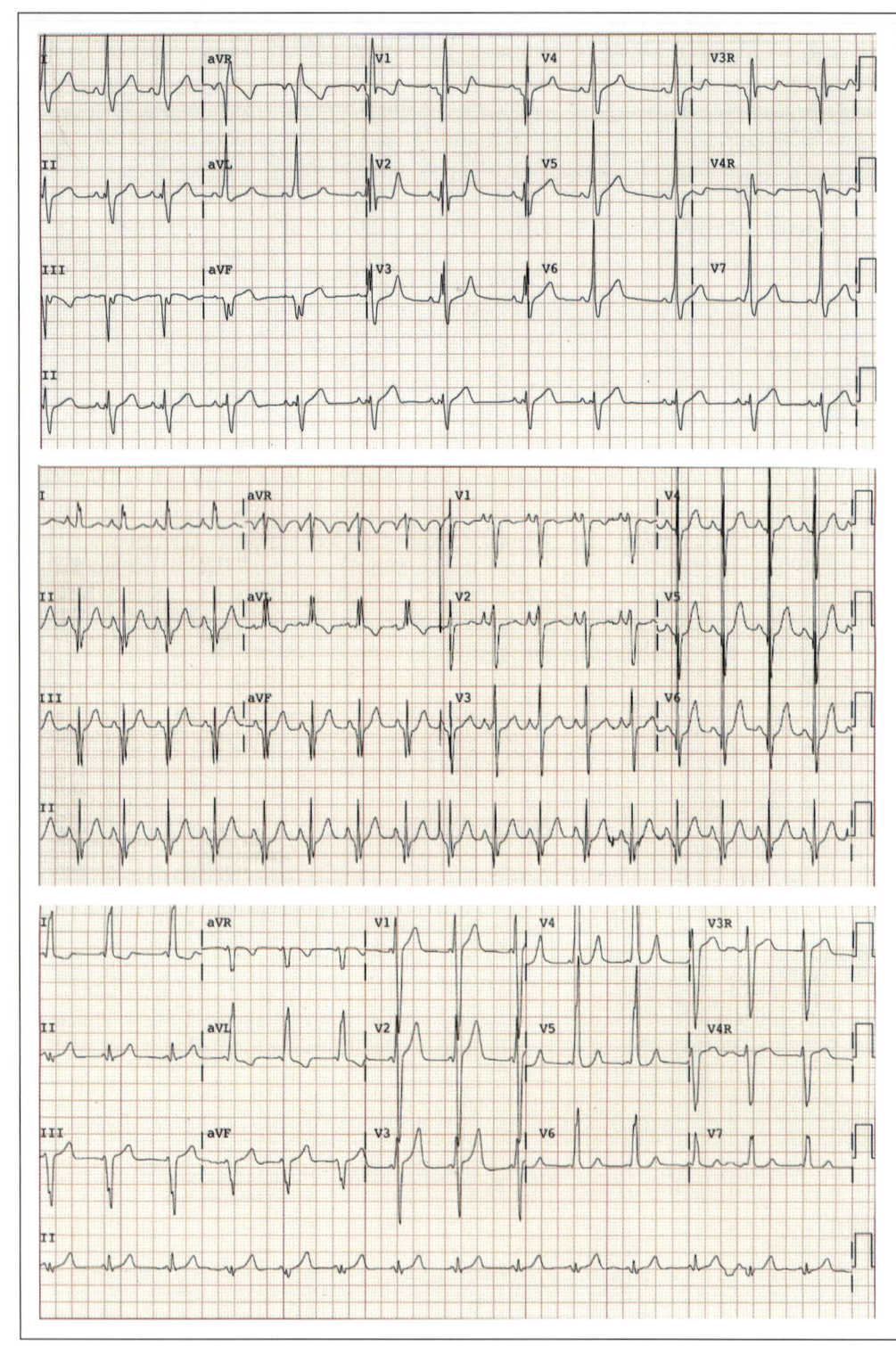

Figure 11.5 Examples of ECGs demonstrating manifest accessory pathways. Note the lack of an RBBB pattern on each of these ECGs.

Physical Exam

A patient's hemodynamic status is important to assess prior to the procedure. A full physical exam should be performed. Elevated jugular venous pressures, hepatomegaly, and peripheral edema are signs of right-sided heart failure and should be taken into account, as some patients may not hemodynamically tolerate the procedure. Baseline desaturation, creatinine, and evidence of polycythemia should also be noted.

Procedure

Patient Preparation

At our center, all patients, regardless of age, are placed under general anesthesia by cardiac anesthesiologists. Particularly in the younger patients, where cardiac structures are small and ablation catheters are relatively large, it is important to eliminate the risk of sudden catheter movement.

Access

Known vessel occlusions should be determined prior to the patient entering the lab. Patients with Glenn procedures will not have access via the SVC. At least 4 sheaths should be placed for standard recording catheters, to be initially located in the HRA, HB position, RVA, and CS. Consideration should be given for placement of a 4-Fr sheath into a femoral artery prior to heparin administration. This sheath can be used to monitor hemodynamic status during the case and can be used to take coronary angiography if needed later in the case. In patients with manifest preexcitation, it can be helpful to have a HRA pacing catheter during mapping and ablation, but this requires an additional venous sheath.

Anticoagulation

The use of heparin varies between centers and individual operators. At our center, due to the high incidence of atrial-level communications and relatively higher risk of right-to-left shunting in this population, we give all patients heparin (100 U/kg, maximum 5000 U) prior to insertion of any catheters and maintain the ACT > 200 seconds. Patients are also discharged on 2 to 3 months of baby aspirin daily.

Selection of Guiding Sheaths and Catheters

If catheter stabilization is a problem, long sheaths should be used. In particular, Swartz sheaths (St. Jude Medical Inc., St. Paul, MN) for the posteroseptal (SR0), lateral (SR4), anterolateral (SR3), and anterior (SR2) positions can be helpful. For posterior or posterolateral, try a Mullins Introducer Sheath (Medtronic Inc., Minneapolis, MN). The Agilis steerable sheath (St. Jude Medical Inc., St. Paul, MN) can be used for any position. For pediatric patients, a limited selection of reduced-radius Swartz sheaths are available but generally target only the anterolateral (SRR3) and lateral (SRR4) positions.

Tricuspid Valve Anatomy

The tricuspid annulus is thinner than the left AV groove and is often incomplete. The annulus may also be dilated, and tricuspid regurgitation can be severe. This can make catheter stabilization and tissue contact a challenge. Although annular signals can sometimes be normal, often these signals are low frequency and fragmented, making it difficult to differentiate between atrial and ventricular EGMs (**Figure 11.6**). If locating the tricuspid valve annulus becomes an issue, there are several things that can be attempted (**Table 11.1**).

The RCA runs within the epicardial fat next to the ventricular side of the right epicardial AV groove. Anatomically, it always runs along the true AV groove regardless of where the displaced tricuspid valves are located. Locating the epicardial fat pad by fluoroscopy can be a helpful start to locating the AV groove.

An angiogram taken in the RA can help demonstrate the epicardial fat pad and the tricuspid valve annulus.

A good aortic root angiogram using power injection through a pigtail catheter will often delineate the RCA.

If the aortic root injection is not helpful, a selective right coronary angiogram can be taken (**Figure 11.7**).

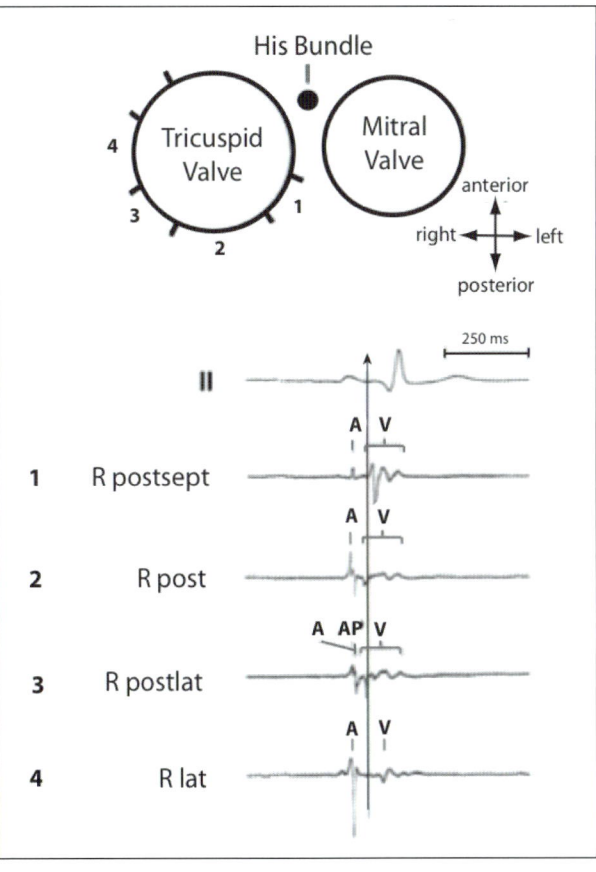

Figure 11.6 Preablation recordings during sinus rhythm in a patient with Ebstein's anomaly and a manifest right posterolateral AP. Surface ECG lead II and local EGMs from 4 sites along the tricuspid annulus can be seen. Note abnormal ventricular (V) EGMs extending from the posteroseptal (R postsept) to the posterior (R post) and posterolateral (R postlat) regions. Normalization of V EGM is observed in the lateral (R lat) region. A indicates atrial EGM; AP, presumed AP activation potential; and Δ, onset of delta wave. (Reprinted with permission from Cappato R, et al. *Circulation*. 1996;94:376–383.)

Table 11.1 Tips for locating the tricuspid valve annulus

1. Locate the epicardial fat pad.
2. Take a right atrial angiogram.
3. Use a 3-dimensional mapping system to mark the annulus.
4. Take an aortic root angiogram to delineate the right coronary artery.
5. Take a selective right coronary artery angiogram.
6. Use a microcatheter (if available) within the right coronary artery.

Table 11.2 Tips for mapping

1. Atrial pace from different locations within the atrium or CS to augment single pathways or elicit different activation patterns.
2. Take advantage of atrial and ventricular pacing maneuvers and ORT to distinguish between atrial and ventricular electrograms of different pathways.
3. Use atrial fibrillation to elicit different activation patterns in the presence of multiple accessory pathways.
4. Use a duodecapolar catheter along the tricuspid valve annulus.
5. Use a decapolar catheter within the atrialized right venticle to help differentiate fractionated ventricular signals.
6. Use a long sheath if needed to maintain stability on the annulus.
7. Use a 3-dimensional mapping system to help mark areas of ablation or successful lesion sites.

In select cases, a recording catheter can be placed into the RCA (see further details in mapping section that follows).

EP Study and Mapping

We begin each study by performing standard atrial and ventricular stimulation protocols (at twice diastolic threshold), as we would in any patient with SVT. The baseline rhythm and intervals should be documented. AV nodal and AP conduction properties and characteristics should be assessed. If the patient is preexcited, the presence of multiple pathways should be assessed. The presence of multiple pathways should be suspected if there are changes in preexcitation morphology, even if subtle. Up to 50% of patients who have APs will have multiple pathways and/or mechanisms. There are several ways to identify multiple pathways (**Table 11.2**). Atrial pacing at differing locations near sites of suspected APs can augment preexcitation or elicit variations in activation patterns that can be helpful when dealing with several pathways (**Figure 11.8**). Similarly, one can look for variable atrial activation sites during ventricular pacing or during ORT. During AF, variable preexcitation and ventricular activation patterns can also be a clue. Tachycardia that switches from antidromic to ORT is another clue. While care should be taken to try and determine whether one or more pathways exist, it can get quite confusing. Sometimes it is impossible to determine the total number of pathways until ablation of one uncovers coexisting pathways. Also, note the presence of dual AV nodal physiology, because patients can have AVNRT.

Due to the possible presence of multiple pathways and dual AV nodes, tachyarrhythmia mechanisms can be complex. ORTs tend to demonstrate long VA timing due to delay in both infranodal conduction as well as delayed conduction through the atrialized RV. Average VA times in Ebstein's patients during ORT have been reported to be 192 ms.[7] Using standard timing criteria for ablation in these patients may not work, and one should instead seek the earliest sites of activation.

Precision mapping can be difficult due to the low-frequency and fragmented EGMs in approximately 50% of patients. APs connecting AV myocardium also tend to be broader in this patient population. In the presence of manifest preexcitation, use of atrial extrastimuli to

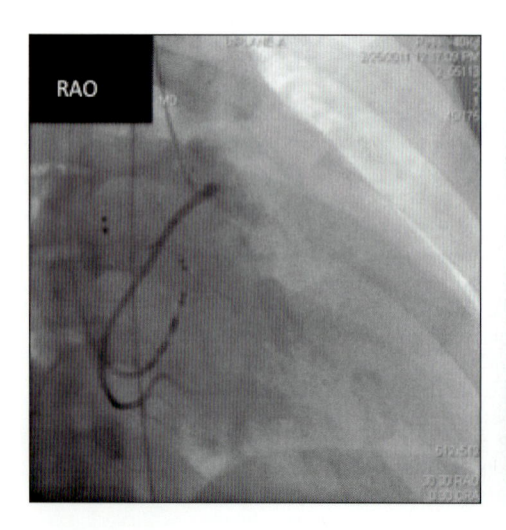

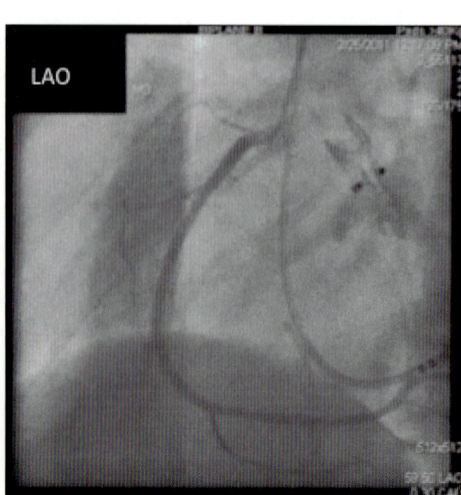

Figure 11.7 Cine images of selective RCA injections (RAO and LAO projections). These images can be stored and used to help guide mapping of the tricuspid annulus.

differentiate between atrial and ventricular EGMs can be very helpful (**Figure 11.9**). Similarly in concealed pathways, ventricular extrastimuli or echo beats can be used to differentiate atrial and ventricular signals. Another strategy is to place a duodecapolar catheter along the tricuspid valve annulus (**Figures 11.10, 11.11,** and **11.12**). The use of a duodecapolar catheter can be particularly helpful in cases in which the patient has had previous ablation attempts. In these cases, prior lesion sites will also contribute to low-amplitude signals.

Staying on the tricuspid valve annulus and using both atrial and ventricular extrastimuli to differentiate between atrial and ventricular signals is helpful. Do not be afraid to use long sheaths. Even with good catheter stability, differentiating between atrial and ventricular signals and earliest sites of activation can be difficult. Therefore, mapping should be performed using multiple approaches. If the AP is bidirectional, then mapping can be performed antegrade, retrograde, and in SVT. When fractionated ventricular signals become confusing, it can sometimes be helpful to place a decapolar catheter within the atrialized RV to differentiate far-field ventricular signals. This catheter can also be used to stimulate the ventricle closer to the atrial insertion site(s). Care should be taken during mapping;

Figure 11.8 **A.** Pacing from the HRA demonstrates a different manifest AP than that seen at baseline. **B.** In the same patient, pacing from the CS demonstrates the same preexcitation pattern seen at baseline.

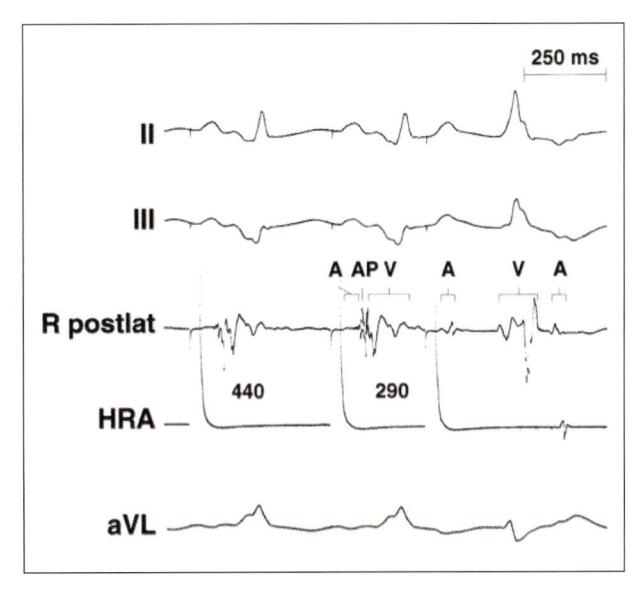

Figure 11.9 Surface ECG leads II, III, and aVL, and 2 intracardiac EGMs recorded during pacing (basic drive cycle, 440 ms) at the HRA in same patient as in Figure 11.6. An atrial extrastimulus is delivered with a coupling interval of 290 ms. In response to this extrastimulus, preexcitation disappears (third beat) and separation of the local atrial (A) and ventricular (V) activation potentials can be appreciated in the electrogram recorded at the right posterolateral (R postlat) tricuspid annulus. During this beat, also note the disappearance of the high-frequency component—suggestive of an AP potential (AP)—immediately after the A potential in the preexcited beats. (Reprinted with permission from Cappato R, et al. *Circulation.* 1996;94:376–383.)

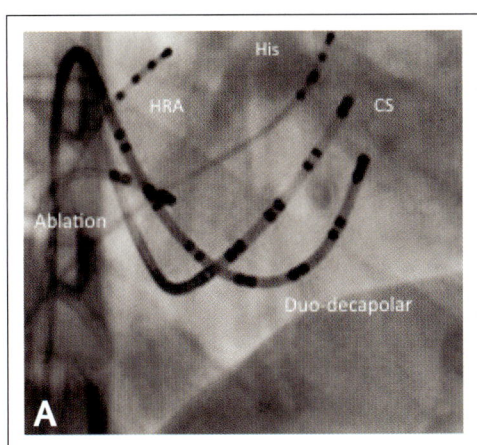

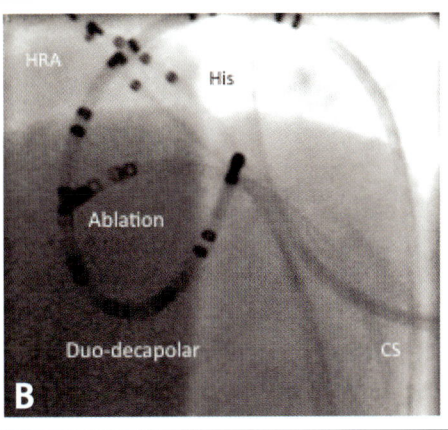

Figure 11.10 **A.** An RAO fluoroscopic projection of a duodecapolar catheter being used to help during a case with multiple APs. The ablation catheter is at the site of successful ablation of a right lateral bypass tract. **B.** LAO projection of the catheters at the site of successful ablation.

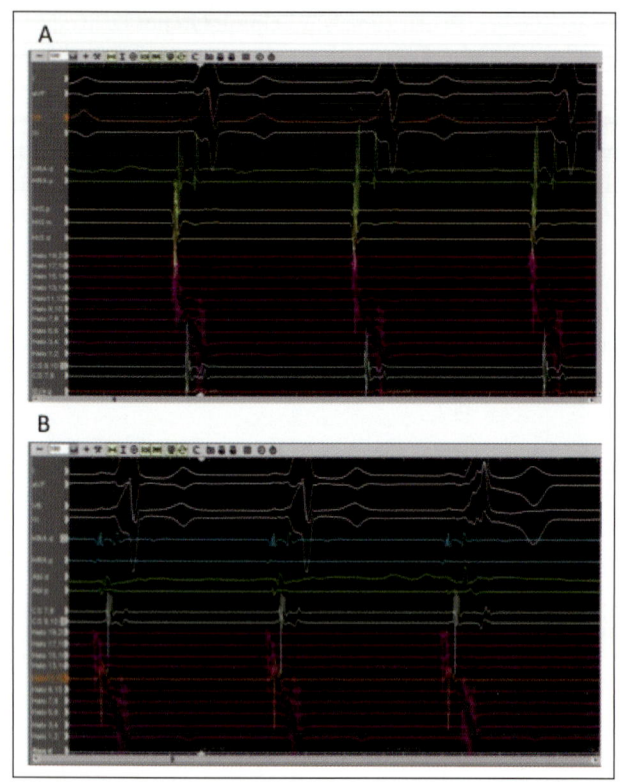

Figure 11.11 **A.** In sinus rhythm, use of a duodecapolar catheter (labeled "Halo") demonstrates earliest ventricular activation near the poles 7,8 and 9,10. **B.** Ablation at this site 7,8 results in immediate shift in preexcitation pattern, demonstrating loss of one of the manifest bypass tracts and emergence of a second manifest AP. Note the low-amplitude signals on the ablation catheter (labeled Abl d), loss of local preexcitation at poles 7,8 and new pattern of preexcitation on poles duo-decapolar ("Halo" 11,12).

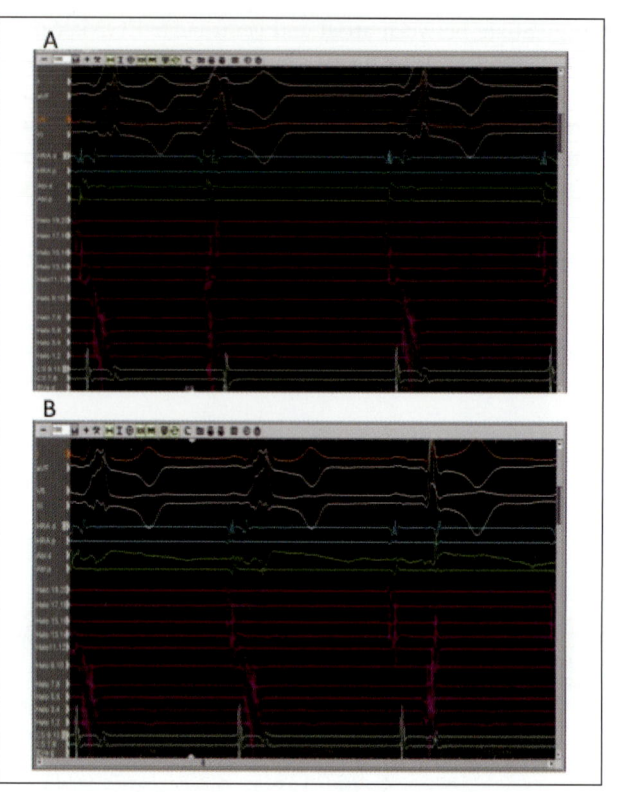

Figure 11.12 **A.** Tracing from the same patient in Figures 11.10 and 11.11. During ventricular pacing, earliest retrograde atrial activation is seen on duodecapolar ("Halo" 11,12) consistent with a bidirectional manifest pathway at this right lateral location. **B.** Ablation in sinus rhythm demonstrates loss of delta wave, with emergence of a nonpreexcited sinus rhythm. Note that there is not a typical RBBB pattern. Further testing did not demonstrate any bypass tracts.

induction of VT is not uncommon, particularly with catheter manipulation within the atrialized RV, and mechanical trauma to the pathway is also not uncommon.

There are several 3-dimensional mapping systems available for use. Although none are necessary, in these complex cases, if you have experience using them, they may be helpful in marking the true AV annulus and pathway location in instances where there is mechanical trauma and loss of pathway conduction. Use of nonfluoroscopic imaging systems may also be helpful in decreasing fluoroscopy times.[8]

Coronary Artery Mapping

In select patients, particularly those with life-threatening arrhythmias, mapping of the tricuspid valve can be performed by inserting a microcatheter into the RCA (**Figure 11.13**). A selective coronary angiogram should first be obtained and the caliber of the RCA evaluated for catheter insertion. The RCA should be imaged using both the 30° RAO and 60° LAO projection. Patients with small RCAs or those with left-dominant systems should be excluded. For pediatric patients, a 6-Fr Judkins 3.5-cm catheter (Cook Inc, Bloomington, IN) is helpful to enter the RCA. Heparin levels should be titrated to maintain a level > 300 seconds. The RCA catheter should be connected to a rotating hemostatic valve and the entire system flushed with saline to eliminate air, followed by a continuous saline infusion through the catheter. The RCA os should be cannulated and the microcatheter inserted as distally as possible. Bipolar EGMs with a filter set between 30 and 250 Hz should be recorded.[9] Note that availability of microcatheters may be an issue. At the time of printing, production of microcatheters had been discontinued.

Ablation

Standard 4-mm tip RF catheters are generally adequate for ablation. Temperatures > 50°C to 55°C should be achieved at a minimum, with a target temperature closer to 60°C for the RA free-wall. A 5- to 10-ohm impedance drop signifies adequate tissue heating. While atrial tissue can become quite thickened, the atrialized RV muscle can be very thin and consideration should be given before using larger-tip catheters due to risk of injury to the coronary artery or perforation.

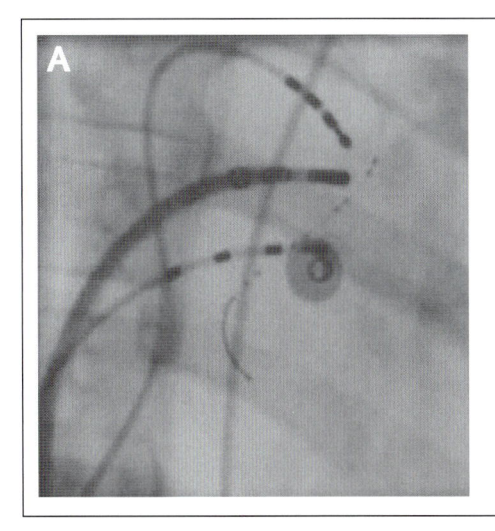

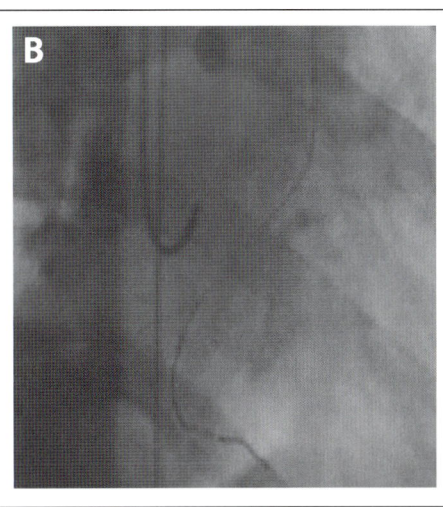

Figure 11.13 A. An RAO fluoroscopic projection of a 2.3-Fr octapolar microcatheter (2-6-2 mm) in the right coronary artery. An ablation catheter within a long sheath is positioned at the site of an anterior AP. Diagnostic catheters in the high right atrium and His bundle position can also be seen. **B.** RAO fluoroscopic projection of a 2.5-Fr microcatheter with eight electrode pairs (2-6-2 mm) advanced to the posterior region of the right atrioventricular groove. (Figure 11.13A reprinted with permission from Shah MJ, et al. *J Cardiovasc Electrophysiol.* 2004;15:1238–1243. Figure 11.13B courtesy of Dr. Frank Cecchin.)

Standard ablation techniques used in ablation of AVRT should be used. The difficulty with these pathways is that they often tend to be broader in this population, rendering the typical 10-second test lesion strategy inadequate. If you are convinced that your signals are correct and that you are in the right spot, it may require staying on "test" lesions longer or creating multiple linear lesions while paying close attention to minute changes in local signals (also pay attention to your proximal ablation signals) as well as surface ECG morphology, which may suggest that you are making a change in the AP. In some cases, if AP conduction is not lost quickly and you have been previously limiting maximum temperature to 60°C, you can consider increasing the maximum temperature to 70°C while watching the impedance closely. If there is significant respiratory variation and the patient is intubated, performing a "breath-hold" during the ablation can be helpful. If adequate temperatures or power are an issue, try a long sheath first to make sure you have good tissue contact. If lesions continue to be inadequate, try a different approach. Particularly for right anterolateral to anteroseptal locations, sometimes approaching from the internal jugular vein can be successful when the femoral vein approach fails. One other approach that can be attempted, particularly if catheter stability is an issue and RF fails, is cryoablation. Cryoablation may help by "sticking" to the lesion site and creating a deeper lesion.

Postprocedure Care

Recovery

Patients should have continuous cardiac monitoring after the study, and a postprocedural ECG should be obtained in all patients. Complaints of chest pain accompanied by ST changes in the ECG, particularly if consistent with ischemic changes, or any other catheter-related complications should be evaluated promptly. For those patients with manifest preexcitation and a successful ablation, ECG changes generally demonstrate the emergence of an RBBB pattern.

Prior to discharge, patients should be evaluated for (1) presence of rubs to suggest a pericardial effusion, (2) gross neurologic exam, and (3) groin complications. A stethoscope should be placed over all access sites, particularly where both artery and vein were punctured. Bruits or murmurs should alert to the possible presence of an AV fistula. Although groin complications are rare, in the CHD patient where access can be difficult, we have a lower threshold to evaluate for complications. We also examine the lower extremities for venous congestion, presence of arterial pulses, and neuropathies, which can develop from pressure during long cases.

We discharge patients on baby aspirin for 2 months.

Follow-Up

Follow-up should be arranged within 1 month from the procedure. In the general pediatric population, recurrence of APs typically occurs within the first few months. Among patients with Ebstein's disease, the risk of recurrence is much higher and is thought to be approximately 25% within 1 year.[3,4] Due to this high recurrence risk, we recommend follow-up at 1 month, 6 months, and 1 year after ablation, followed by yearly routine follow-up.

Repeat Ablations

Unfortunately, success rates in Ebstein's patients are lower than those with structurally normal hearts. Acute success rates in adults are approximately 76%.[4] In pediatric patients with Ebstein's disease, acute success rates for right free-wall pathways are approximately 79% and right posteroseptal pathways 89%.[3] Recurrence of APs after successful ablation is approximately 20 to 25%.[3,4] We counsel patients prior to the procedure that more than one procedure may be necessary.

Procedural Complications

Patients with Ebstein's anomaly have variable hemodynamic responses to tachyarrhythmias, which may be exacerbated by general anesthesia. Patients should be monitored for signs of hemodynamic compromise, including acute drops in blood pressure and cyanosis. Although complications are generally rare, acute coronary artery stenosis in pediatric patients has been reported. The atrialized RV can become extremely thin, and several reports of catheter manipulation within this area resulting in VT or VF have been reported. Ablation within the atrialized RV (instead of the annulus) can also risk potential perforation.

Advantages and Limitations

There have been no randomized studies performed evaluating the use of RF catheter ablation in Ebstein's patients. Some studies have demonstrated a 100% success rate with surgical ablation of APs in Ebstein's[10]; however, long-term follow-up is needed, and surgical morbidity and mortality are not insignificant. Retrospective data on catheter ablation have demonstrated a lower overall acute success rate and higher risk of recurrence; despite this, catheter ablation offers a viable treatment option, particularly in those patients who are not scheduled for surgical intervention.

Conclusions

In summary, APs in Ebstein's patients are common, and catheter ablation offers a safe and effective treatment in a majority of patients. From both an EP standpoint in terms of interpreting signals and arrhythmias, as well as technical standpoint in terms of maintaining catheter stability and tissue contact, these cases can pose challenges. Nevertheless, both immediate and long-term success are achievable and can not only significantly impact the lives of these patients but can also prevent sudden cardiac death.

Acknowledgments

I would like to thank Drs. Frank Cecchin, Anne Dubin, Ron Kanter, John Kugler, George Van Hare, and Edward Walsh for their invaluable input and expertise in helping write this chapter.

References

1. Watson H. Natural history of Ebstein's anomaly of tricuspid valve in childhood and adolescence. An international cooperative study of 505 cases. *Br Heart J*. 1974;36:417–427.
2. Attenhofer CH, Jost CH, Edwards WD, Hayes D, Warnes CA, Danielson GK. Ebstein's anomaly: review of a multifaceted congenital cardiac condition. *Swiss Med Wkly*. 2005;135:269–281.
3. Reich JD, Auld D, Hulse E, Sullivan K, Campbell R. The Pediatric Radiofrequency Ablation Registry's experience with Ebstein's anomaly. Pediatric Electrophysiology Society. *J Cardiovasc Electrophysiol*. 1998;9:1370–1377.
4. Cappato R, Schluter M, Weiss C, et al. Radiofrequency current catheter ablation of accessory atrioventricular pathways in Ebstein's anomaly. *Circulation*. 1996;94:376–383.
5. Iturralde P, Nava S, Salica G, et al. Electrocardiographic characteristics of patients with Ebstein's anomaly before and after ablation of an accessory atrioventricular pathway. *J Cardiovasc Electrophysiol*. 2006;17:1332–1336.
6. Bar-Cohen Y, Khairy P, Morwood J, Alexander ME, Cecchin F, Berul CI. Inaccuracy of Wolff-Parkinson-White accessory pathway localization algorithms in children and patients with congenital heart defects. *J Cardiovasc Electrophysiol*. 2006;17:712–716.
7. Kastor JA, Goldreyer BN, Josephson ME, et al. Electrophysiologic characteristics of Ebstein's anomal of the tricuspid valve. *Circulation*. 1975;52:987–995.
8. Miyake CY, Mah DY, Atallah J, et al. Nonfluoroscopic imaging systems reduce radiation exposure in children undergoing ablation of supraventricular tachycardia. *Heart Rhythm*. 2011;8:519–525.
9. Shah MJ, Jones TK, Cecchin F. Improved localization of right-sided accessory pathways with microcatheter-assisted right coronary artery mapping in children. *J Cardiovasc Electrophysiol*. 2004;15:1238–1243.
10. Khositseth A, Danielson GK, Dearani JA, Munger TM, Porter CJ. Supraventricular tachyarrhythmias in Ebstein anomaly: management and outcome. *J Thorac Cardiovasc Surg*. 2004;128:826–833.

Video Description

Video 11.1 Apical view of right and left ventricle. The tricuspid valve leaflets are displaced inferiorly with adhesions preventing normal coaptation. The TV annulus can still be seen in its normal position. The area between the normal TV annulus and the point of TV leaflet coaptation is called the atrialized right ventricle. The right atrium and right ventricle are dilated and the functional RV size is decreased.

SECTION II

ABLATION OF ATRIAL FIBRILLATION

CHAPTER 12

How to Perform a Transseptal Puncture

Gregory E. Supple, MD; David J. Callans, MD

Introduction

Transseptal catheterization of the LA was initially developed in 1958 and has facilitated a variety of interventional cardiac procedures. For the electrophysiologist, this technique is essential, as it allows for endocardial mapping and ablation of left-sided bypass tracts, LA tachycardia, AF, and ventricular tachycardia. There are, of course, significant complications that can arise when performing transseptal puncture, but newer technologies have made this procedure increasingly safe when performed by an experienced operator.

Preprocedure Planning

Patients should have cardiac imaging prior to the procedure, generally with transthoracic ECG, or with TEE if there is any risk of LA thrombus. Patients may also have had cardiac CT or MRI performed, depending upon the ablation procedure being performed. Any of these allow for the evaluation of the LA size and the IAS for abnormalities such as aneurysm (**Figures 12.1** and **12.2**; ▶ **Videos 12.1** and **12.2**) or lipomatous hypertrophy (**Figure 12.3**, ▶ **Video 12.3**), which can make transseptal puncture more challenging. If the patient has previously had a transseptal puncture performed, resultant scarring can also make crossing the septum more difficult. Prior surgical or percutaneous repair of an ASD or PFO can also make transseptal puncture difficult or even impossible, depending on the materials used for the repair.

In addition, the patient's anticoagulation status should be assessed prior to transseptal puncture. We routinely perform transseptal punctures for the ablation of AF in patients with therapeutic INR values; however, we avoid doing the procedure if the INR is greater than 3.

Table 12.1 provides a description of the required equipment and personnel that should be available in order to perform a transseptal puncture.

Procedure

Initial Sheath and Catheter Placement

Access is first obtained with short sheaths in the femoral veins. If 2 transseptal punctures are planned, 2 8 French short sheaths are place in the right femoral veins, to be exchanged later for the transseptal sheaths. Additional diagnostic catheters are useful to denote fluoroscopic landmarks, and we routinely place a CS catheter through the left femoral vein. The course taken by the CS catheter helps to define the patient's cardiac rotation, and the site of transseptal puncture is superior and slightly posterior to the CS ostium in the RAO projection. The course of the transseptal sheath should be roughly parallel to the CS,

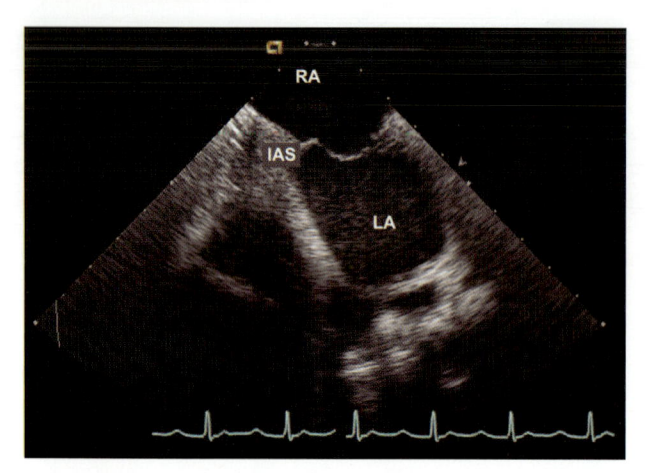

Figure 12.1 ICE image from the RA showing a mildly aneurysmal IAS bowing slightly into the LA.

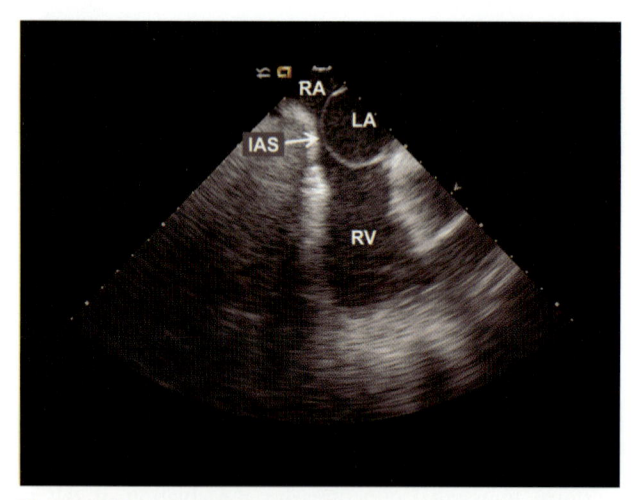

Figure 12.2 ICE image from the right atrium (RA) showing a severely aneurysmal septum bowing across the tricuspid valve annulus to touch the RA free wall.

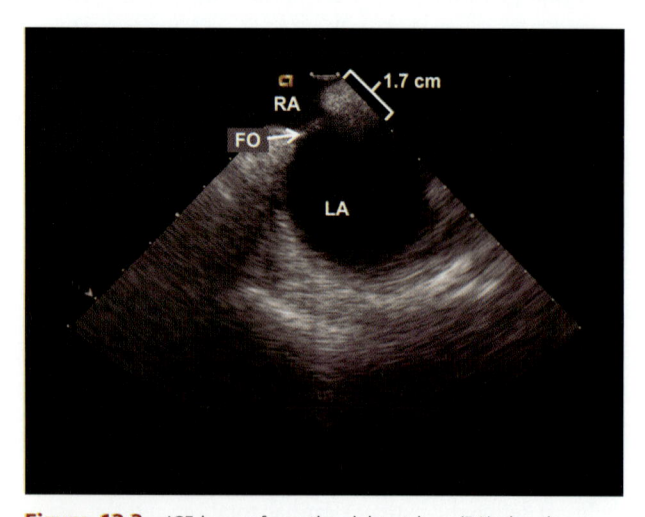

Figure 12.3 ICE image from the right atrium (RA) showing an IAS with lipomatous hypertrophy thickening the septum to 1.7 cm. The fossa ovalis (FO) to the left side has a normal thickness and can serve as a target (albeit smaller than usual) for the transseptal puncture.

Table 12.1 Required equipment and personnel

Specific Task	Adaptation
Imaging	Fluoroscopy
	Optional: radiopaque contrast
	Optional: intracardiac ultrasound catheter
Sheaths	8 French short sheath (to be exchanged for transseptal sheath)
	Additional short sheaths for ICE, CS, etc.
	Transseptal sheath and dilator (Mullins, SL series, LAMP, Agilis, etc.)
	Brockenbrough needle
	Long J-curve-tipped 0.0032-inch wire
Catheters	CS catheter
	Optional: His catheter, aortic pigtail catheter
Additional equipment	Flush syringes (3 20-ml)
	Pressure transducer
	Heparinized saline flush lines
Personnel	Physician performing transseptal puncture
	Secondary operator to steer ICE, aid with sheath exchanges
	Nurse/anesthetist to provide sedation and hemodynamic monitoring
	Circulator to provide equipment and assistance

and the CS catheter can define the LA border in the LAO projection (**Figure 12.4**) and thus indicate how far the dilator should be advanced into the LA after crossing the septum.

Baseline Imaging Prior to Transseptal Puncture

Transseptal puncture can be performed with fluoroscopic guidance alone, but the use of ICE has been shown to reduce the incidence of complications.[1-3] We routinely use ICE guidance for transseptal punctures, and a second operator is usually present to steer the ICE catheter and assist with the sheath exchanges during the procedure.

A 9 French sheath is placed in the left femoral vein through which an 8 French ICE catheter is advanced. We use a phased-array catheter with a frequency range of 5.0 to 10.0 MHz, with a tip deflectable in 160 degrees in anterior/posterior and left/right directions (ACUSON AcuNAV Catheter, Siemens Medical Solutions USA, Inc., Malvern, PA). This catheter allows for real-time 2D intracardiac imaging, as well as color Doppler, continuous, and pulse-wave Doppler. The ICE catheter is advanced into the heart and baseline images are obtained. From the RA,

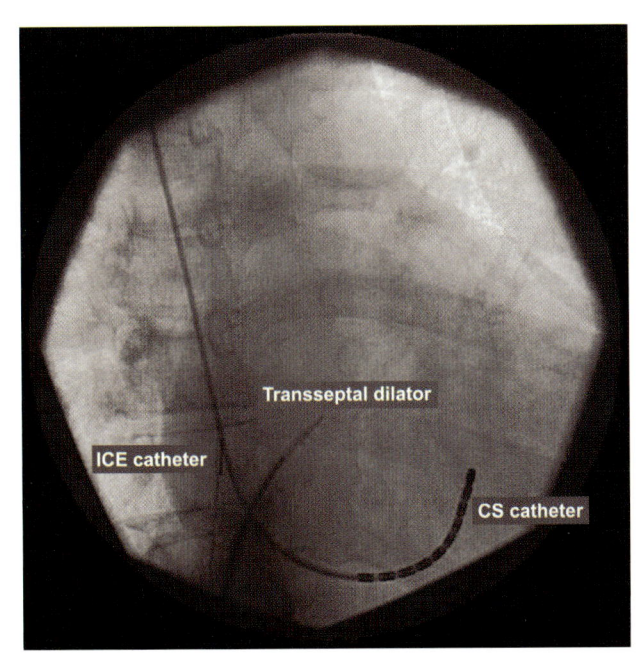

Figure 12.4 Fluoroscopy AP view of the transseptal dilator with the tip at the fossa ovalis. The CS (CS) catheter demonstrates the AV groove, which helps indicate the position of the LA free wall—in this case directly superior to the distal tip of the CS catheter.

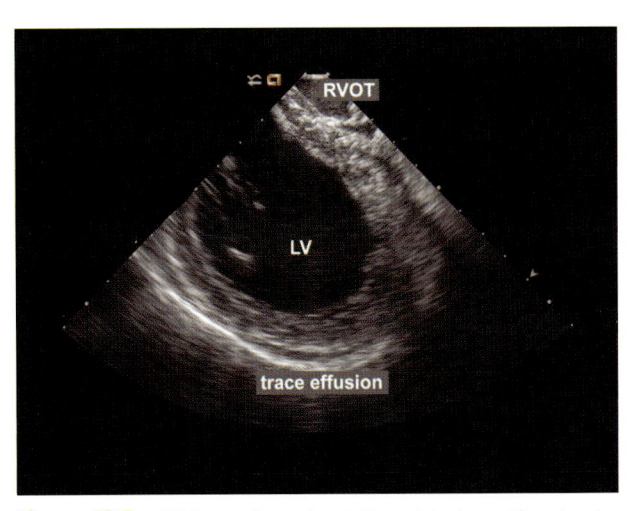

Figure 12.5 ICE image from the right ventricular outflow tract (RVOT) of the LV (LV) showing a very small effusion or region of pericardial fat along the inferior wall during baseline imaging prior to performing a transseptal puncture.

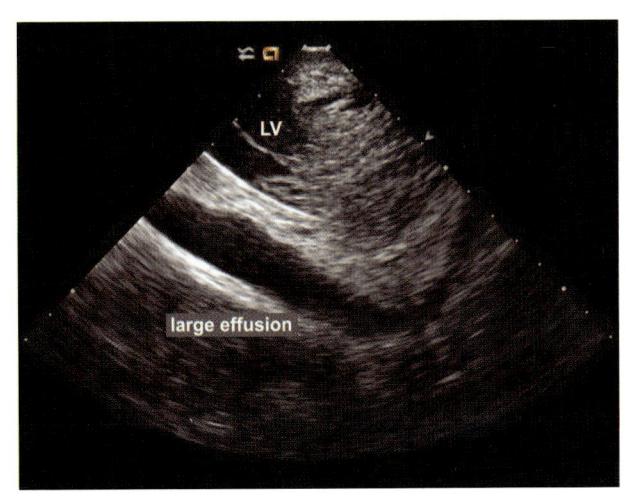

Figure 12.6 ICE image from the RVOT of the LV showing a large pericardial effusion after a transseptal puncture.

the IAS is imaged to determine the location and anatomy of the fossa ovalis. Slight posteroflexion of the ICE catheter is often helpful in bringing the fossa into view. By rotating the ICE catheter clockwise, the LA can be imaged to identify the LA appendage, the left and right pulmonary veins, and the aorta. Typically the ostium of the left pulmonary veins provides a target toward which the transseptal puncture will be oriented; however, for transseptal ventricular ablation or for balloon-based ablation of AF, a more anterior transseptal target may be helpful. The pericardial space is imaged as well, first from the RA, then from within the RV, to enable better analysis of the pericardium inferior and posterior to the LV (**Figure 12.5**, ▶ **Video 12.4**). These baseline images allow for rapid identification of a pericardial effusion should it develop after a transseptal puncture or later in the ablation procedure (**Figure 12.6**, ▶ **Video 12.5**). To image the LV and its pericardial space from the RV, the ICE probe is rotated until the tricuspid valve is imaged. The catheter is anteflexed while keeping the tricuspid valve in view until the RV apex is seen and then advanced through the tricuspid valve into the mid RV. The anteflexion is released, leaving the catheter tip in the proximal RV outflow tract. From this position, the RV free wall and anterior pericardial space is imaged. The catheter is rotated clockwise, allowing imaging of the interventricular septum, and, with further rotation, the LV and its adjacent pericardial space. The ICE catheter is then withdrawn back into the RA in preparation for the transseptal puncture.

Anticoagulation Prior to the Transseptal Puncture

To minimize the risk of thrombus formation on catheters or at ablation sites in the left heart, patients are anticoagulated with intravenous heparin prior to the transseptal puncture. Once all the sheaths have been placed, a bolus of heparin (80–100 U/kg) is given and a drip started (18 U/kg/h) and titrated to maintain the ACT between 350 and 400 seconds for the duration of the procedure. ACT values are checked 15 minutes after the bolus and every subsequent half-hour.

Transseptal Puncture

The right femoral vein short sheath is exchanged using a long 0.032-inch J-curve-tipped wire which is first advanced into the SVC. The short sheath is removed over the wire, and the transseptal sheath and dilator are advanced over the wire under fluoroscopic guidance until the tip of the dilator is in the SVC, at the level of the tracheal carina. The side port on the sheath aligns with its major curvature and is used to orient the tip of the dilator. The wire is withdrawn and blood is aspirated from the dilator with a syringe to remove any bubbles, which is then flushed with saline. Occasionally, the dilator presses against the wall of the SVC, preventing aspiration; in this case, a small rotation of the sheath and dilator can free the tip from the wall to allow aspiration.

Next the stylet is removed from the transseptal needle, which is then connected to a flush line with a pressure transducer. The needle is flushed rapidly during insertion into the dilator (to avoid introducing bubbles) and is advanced into the dilator under fluoroscopic guidance until the tip is just inside the end of the dilator, when the hub of the needle is one to two fingers' breadths from the hub of the sheath. The base of the needle has a flat metal hub with an arrow that points in the direction of the curvature of the needle. As the needle is advanced into the dilator, the arrow is gently aligned with the side port on the sheath to ensure that the curvature of the needle and sheath are oriented in the same direction once the needle is fully inserted (**Figure 12.7**). RA pressure is recorded through the transducer on the needle at this point, and the scale is set to 20 to 40 mmHg in preparation for measurement of the LA pressure (if the tip of the dilator is against the vessel wall, RA pressure may not be seen until the dilator is being withdrawn into the RA).

With the left hand on the dilator and sheath and the right hand on the needle to maintain needle position just inside the dilator, the assembly is withdrawn as one under fluoroscopic guidance. The assembly is withdrawn primarily under the LAO view (▶ Video 12.6), and by turning the assembly to about a 4 o'clock position, the curve of the needle and sheath is oriented in a left posterior direction. The second operator adjusts the ICE image to keep the IAS and fossa ovalis in view. As the assembly is withdrawn under fluoroscopy, the tip can be seen to have two distinct "jumps" to the left. The first corresponds to the tip dropping from the SVC into the RA, and the second corresponds to the tip dropping over the superior limbus into the fossa ovalis (▶ Videos 12.7 and 12.8). ICE imaging at this point is used to confirm that the tip is in contact with the IAS in the center of the fossa ovalis—the assembly can be withdrawn a little more if need be to ensure that it is at the correct height (▶ Videos 12.9 and 12.10), after which gentle forward pressure on the entire assembly is applied to ensure tenting of the septum. The ICE probe is rotated slightly clockwise and counterclockwise to ensure that the tip is visualized and that it is oriented toward the left pulmonary veins (**Figure 12.8**, ▶ Video 12.11). On fluoroscopy, this correlates with a course parallel to the CS catheter (away from the imager in an RAO view). We feel

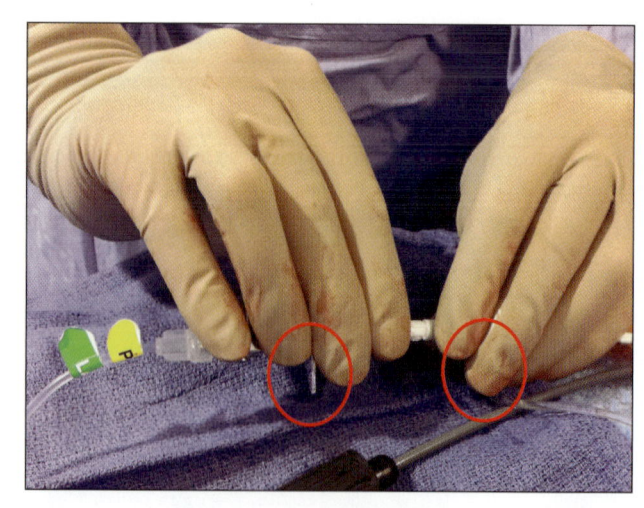

Figure 12.7 Holding the transseptal needle with the hub 2 fingers-breadths back from the hub of the dilator. The metal arrow on the needle hub is oriented in the same direction as the side port on the sheath (red circles), indicating the orientation of the curvature of the needle.

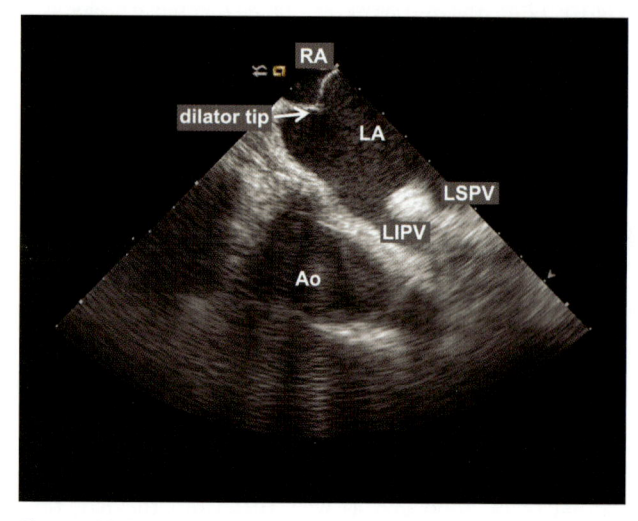

Figure 12.8 ICE image from the RA of the dilator tip tenting the IAS toward the pulmonary veins, an appropriate orientation for a transseptal puncture. (Ao = descending thoracic aorta seen posterior to the LA.)

that this is the perfect positioning for transseptal puncture. More anterior positions are either dangerous (aortic perforation) or result in subsequent difficulty delivering catheters to posterior targets such as the pulmonary veins. More posterior positions are dangerous as there is less room in the atrium, increasing the risk of posterior wall perforation. If the dilator tip is visualized in too anterior a view on ICE—such as toward the LA appendage, mitral valve, or even the ascending aorta (▶ Video 12.12)—the assembly is rotated clockwise to a more posterior orientation. Similarly, if the dilator tip is visualized in too posterior a view on ICE—toward the posterior LA wall (▶ Video 12.13) or right pulmonary veins—the assembly is rotated counterclockwise to bring it more anterior.

Once the appropriate orientation has been confirmed with ICE and fluoroscopy, the needle is advanced under fluoroscopic visualization in the LAO view. A "pop" is often felt as the needle crosses the septum (▶ Video 12.14). The pressure tracing (which is usually damped during pressure against the septum) now displays LA pressure. The second operator can adjust the ICE to visualize the needle tip entering the LA. Saline bubbles from the flush line on the needle can be seen in the LA on ICE (▶ Video 12.15) to confirm the correct location of the needle tip. Once the needle is across the septum, its position is fixed and the dilator and sheath are advanced over the needle under fluoroscopic guidance in an LAO view to ensure that the dilator is not advanced beyond the cardiac border. The second operator adjusts the ICE to visualize the tip of the dilator advancing towards the left pulmonary veins, again with slight rotation clockwise and counterclockwise to ensure that the tip is being visualized. Once the dilator has crossed the septum and the needle is just inside the dilator tip, some of the septal tenting on ICE is seen to relax (▶ Video 12.16). Next, the dilator position is fixed, and the sheath is advanced over the dilator into the LA. The leading edge of the sheath will often catch the septum, again causing tenting of the septum on ICE. This can be especially challenging with larger steerable sheaths such as the Agilis NxT Steerable Introducer (St. Jude Medical, Inc., St. Paul, MN), as the outer diameter of this sheath is significantly larger than the diameter of the dilator. Slight rotation back and forth of the sheath can help the transition across the septum, often associated again with a tactile "pop," at which point the tenting on ICE relaxes (▶ Video 12.17). The aiding operator at this point uses a syringe to provide gentle back-pressure through the side port on the sheath, while the primary operator withdraws the dilator and needle from the sheath. The sheath is then flushed and connected to an air-filtered heparinized saline flush line for the remainder of the case.

Immediately after the transseptal sheath and catheter have been placed, the ICE catheter is again advanced into the RV and rotated to evaluate for the development of any pericardial effusion. See Video 12.6 and ▶ Video 12.18 for fluoroscopy of transseptal punctures and Video 12.16 and ▶ Video 12.19 for ICE of transseptal punctures.

Second Transseptal Puncture

If a second transseptal sheath is to be placed, the first sheath is usually stabilized well inside the LA, either by orienting it toward the mitral annulus (**Figure 12.9**, ▶ Video 12.20) or with the ablation catheter advanced through the sheath and placed in the left superior pulmonary vein (**Figure 12.10**).

The second transseptal sheath can be placed through the same initial transseptal puncture site by first

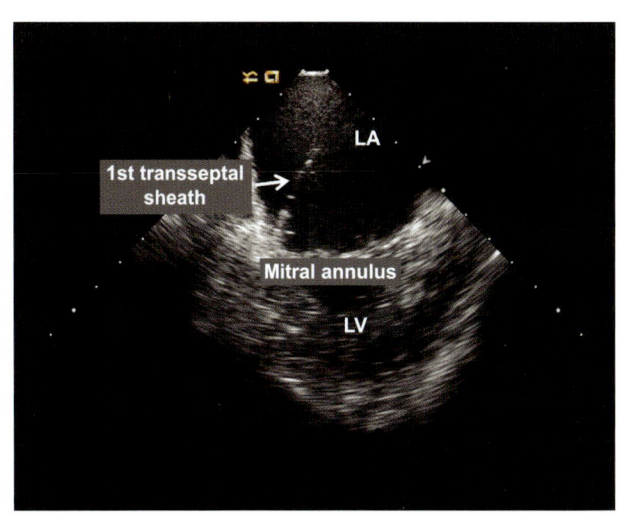

Figure 12.9 ICE image from the RA of a transseptal sheath that has already been placed. The tip of the sheath has been curved and pointed toward the mitral annulus as preparations are made for the second transseptal puncture.

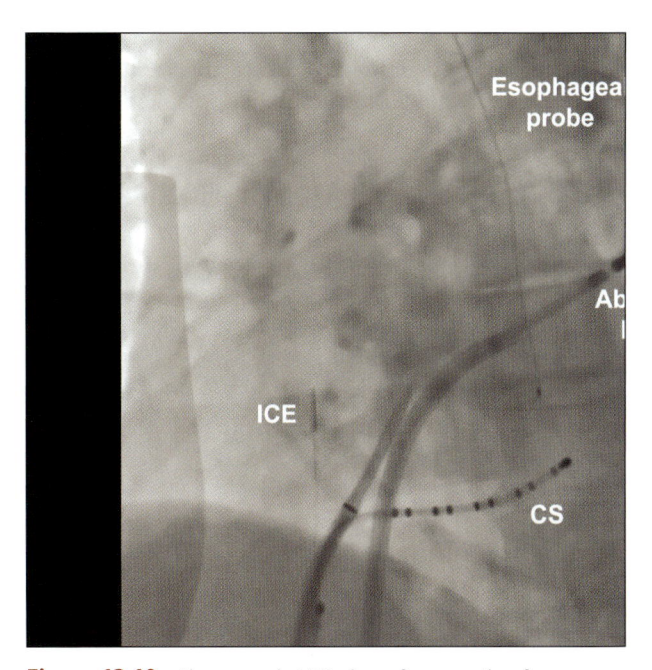

Figure 12.10 Fluoroscopic LAO view of preparation for a second transseptal puncture. An ablation catheter has been advanced through the first transseptal sheath into the left superior pulmonary vein (LSPV), advanced beyond the LA border as denoted by the CS catheter tip (CS). The ICE catheter is visible in the RA on the left of the screen. An esophageal temperature probe is seen coursing behind the LSPV. The second transseptal sheath is tenting the IAS just superior to where the first transseptal sheath crosses the septum.

withdrawing the initial sheath over a retained wire in the LA and advancing a dilator and sheath bluntly (without a needle) through the puncture site next to the retained wire.

Alternatively, a second transseptal puncture procedure can be performed using the same steps outlined above. We routinely use the latter approach and perform a second transseptal puncture. This approach allows for some separation in the fossa ovalis between the two puncture sites (▶ Videos 12.21 and 12.22), which in turn generally permits better independent steering and manipulation of the two transseptal sheaths with minimal interaction. In addition, the double puncture technique has been shown to result in a reduced risk of persistent iatrogenic ASDs.[4-7]

Alternative Techniques

While we routinely use ICE to guide our transseptal punctures, the procedure was performed for decades without the assistance of ICE. In this setting, there are alternative steps that can help to better define the cardiac anatomy. With arterial access, a pigtail catheter can be placed at the aortic root with the course of the catheter defining the inferior and posterior border of the aorta. Under fluoroscopy, the transseptal puncture is therefore performed below the pigtail to prevent puncturing the aorta. Alternatively, using only venous access, a catheter can be placed at the His bundle, which can then be used fluoroscopically to indirectly define the most inferior aspect of the aortic valve (noncoronary cusp).

Radiopaque contrast can also be used to stain the fossa ovalis and localize it fluoroscopically if ICE is not used. Once the dilator has been withdrawn into the RA, a small injection of contrast through the needle will stain the adjacent tissue and allow visualization of the IAS. Similarly, after the needle has been advanced into the LA, a contrast injection can confirm the location of the needle tip.

Additional Tools for Abnormal IAS

Crossing the septum with the Brockenbrough needle can sometimes be difficult, especially in cases of anatomic abnormalities such as an atrial septal aneurysm or lipomatous hypertrophy or in patients with a septum that is scarred from prior puncture or surgical repair. In these situations, crossing with the standard needle can require additional force, which increases the risk of perforation of the far wall of the LA when the needle or dilator jumps across the septum. There are a variety of tools that can be used in these situations.

Steerable sheaths have been designed to assist catheter stability and placement in a variety of locations in the heart. An example that we use commonly is the Agilis NxT Steerable Introducer (St. Jude Medical, Inc., St. Paul, MN). Such sheaths are also stiffer and can therefore be helpful to provide more support for advancing the needle across the septum in the desired location and orientation.

Cautery can also be helpful when applied to the tip of the needle to cross a thickened or scarred septum. This can be done by applying Bovie electrocautery to the hub of the needle when the tip is tenting the septum. Alternatively, there is a dedicated system that uses RF on a rounded catheter tip, the Toronto Transseptal Catheter (Baylis Medical Company, Inc., Montreal, Canada). This system does not require much mechanical force to cross the septum and allows for more controlled crossing of a difficult septum.

In the setting of a significantly aneurysmal septum, it can be difficult to advance the needle across the septum before getting close to the LA border (**Figure 12.11**, ▶ Video 12.23), thereby increasing the risk of LA perforation. The SafeSept Transseptal Guidewire (Pressure Products, Inc., San Pedro, CA) is a long 0.014-inch-diameter nitinol guidewire tipped with a flexible J-curve needle. Once this needle is across the septum and out of the dilator, it forms a J-curve and the blunt edge serves as the leading edge (**Figure 12.12**, ▶ Videos 12.24, 12.25, and 12.26). This wire can be advanced through the usual sheath and dilators used for transseptal puncture.

Pitfalls to Avoid

Placing a CS catheter helps to define the rotation of a patient's heart, and the course of the CS catheter can be used to guide the direction that the transseptal sheath should take as it crosses the septum. It is important, therefore, to ensure that the distal tip of the CS catheter is in the true CS rather than a branch, which could mislead the operator about the cardiac orientation. Examination of the atrial and ventricular signals on the electrograms from the length of the CS catheter should help confirm the correct position.

ICE is helpful in allowing real-time visualization of the position of the needle and dilator tip in relation to the cardiac structures. It is important, however, to realize the

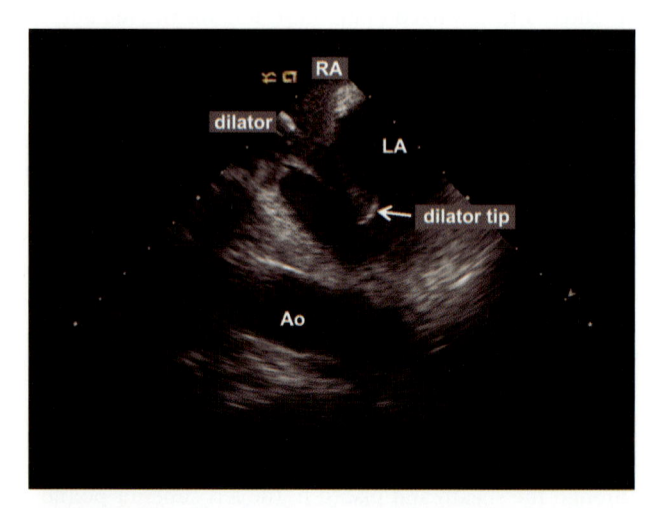

Figure 12.11 ICE image from the RA of a patient with a very aneurysmal septum. The dilator is tenting the septum very far into the LA, near the ostium of the left pulmonary veins. (Ao = descending thoracic aorta)

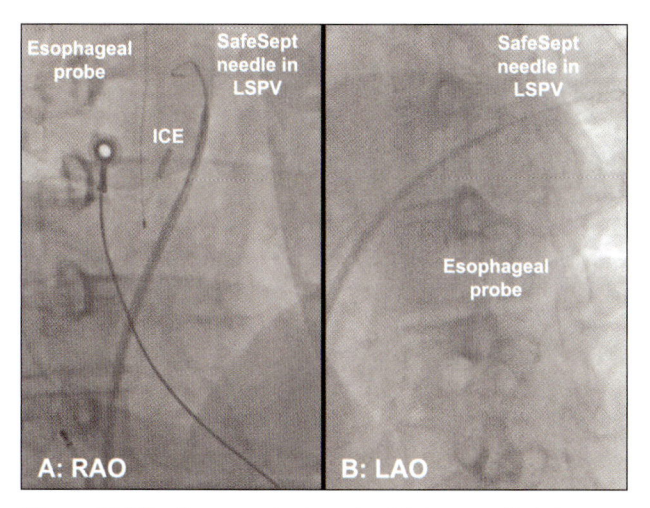

Figure 12.12 Fluoroscopic view of a SafeSept needle being used for transseptal puncture in a patient with a very aneurysmal septum (Figure 12.10). The needle is out of the dilator and across the septum and has advanced into the LSPV. **A.** Right anterior oblique view. **B.** Left anterior oblique view.

limitations of ICE so it does not provide false reassurance. ICE is very good at imaging structures close to the probe, but image quality is degraded as distance from the probe increases. This can result in poor visualization of the back wall of the LA in some patients. A TEE probe may provide better imaging of the posterior LA wall in some patients (particularly those with lipomatous hypertrophy) and can therefore be helpful to avoid advancing the needle or dilator and perforating the posterior LA. Some centers use TEE routinely for transseptal puncture for this reason.

We commonly place two different transseptal sheaths for procedures such as AF ablation. These sheaths may come with Brockenbrough needles of different lengths depending on the sheath lengths, and we generally have both sheaths prepared for use ahead of time on our equipment table. It is therefore important to ensure that the correct needle-and-sheath pair is used to prevent advancing a long needle out through a shorter sheath and lacerating the SVC or RA.

The Brockenbrough needles come packaged with internal stylets. Our practice is to remove the stylet and actively flush the needle through a line while it is being advanced into the dilator to prevent the introduction of air through the needle. In the past, some needle designs could shear slivers of plastic off the inside of dilators when advanced, and it was recommended that the needle be advanced into the dilator with the stylet in place to avoid this.[8,9] The needles that we currently use no longer have this problem; however, it is worth verifying that a particular needle-and-dilator combination does not have this problem when it is being used for the first time by advancing the needle into the dilator outside the patient and checking for shearing.

Postprocedure Care

After the transseptal puncture has been performed and the sheath is in place, ICE is used to assess for the presence of a pericardial effusion. Hemodynamics are monitored continuously during the case to assess for tachycardia, hypotension, or other signs of pericardial tamponade. Repeat ICE imaging is done periodically during the case, especially if there is evidence of hemodynamic compromise. At the end of the case after all other sheaths and catheters are removed from the heart, ICE images are again taken. A transseptal sheath placed too superiorly or posteriorly can potentially enter the pericardial space before reentering the LA. In this setting, bleeding into the pericardial space may not become apparent until after the transseptal sheath has been removed.

After catheters and sheaths have been withdrawn across the septum, heparin is stopped and the ACT is checked. Protamine can be given if needed to hasten the reversal of heparin and allow sheaths to be removed.

Patients are monitored overnight on a telemetry unit to assess for any evidence of tamponade, in addition to the routine post–cardiac catheterization monitoring. We frequently perform a transthoracic echocardiogram on the day following the procedure to again assess for the presence of a pericardial effusion.

Procedural Complications

The complications associated with performing transseptal puncture can be life threatening. They include the risks of perforation of the SVC, RA free wall, or the posterior or lateral LA, which can result in pericarditis and tamponade; or of the aorta, which can result in mediastinal exsanguination or hemodynamic collapse of the right heart. In addition, accessing the LA results in a risk of systemic thrombo- or air embolism, causing stroke or ST segment elevation MI. Historically, transseptal puncture was performed by interventional cardiologists with fluoroscopic guidance. A large series of transseptal punctures performed in this setting reported a major complication rate of 1.3%, with a 1.2% risk of tamponade, a 0.1% risk of systemic embolism, and a 0.08% risk of death.[10]

Since 2000, with the advent of technologies to facilitate ablation of AF, there has been a dramatic increase in the number of transseptal catheterizations performed, which are now being done primarily by electrophysiologists. With the use of adjunctive tools such as pressure transducers, catheter placement to denote anatomical boundaries (aortic pigtail, CS catheters), and ICE, the complication rates have decreased despite the relatively reduced duration of experience in the average operator performing transseptal puncture. A large multicenter series of 5520 transseptal punctures performed up to 2003 reported a risk of major complications of less than 0.8%, with a risk of tamponade of less than 0.1%, aortic perforation of less than 0.1%, a risk of systemic embolism of 0.1% (▶ Video 12.27), and a risk of death of 0.02%.[11] The risk of life-threatening bleeding is reduced somewhat (but not completely) if needle perforation is recognized before the dilator or sheath is advanced into the pericardium or aorta. If a pericardial effusion is noted on ICE imaging, the procedure is immediately halted and anticoagulation is reversed. The size of the effusion and hemodynamics are carefully monitored. These steps are often all that is needed in the setting of perforation. If, however, the effusion expands rapidly, the patient may require urgent pericardiocentesis to prevent or treat pericardial tamponade and, rarely, may require surgical repair if pericardial bleeding persists.

There is also a risk of persistent ASD after transseptal catheterization. Small studies have shown that the risk of a persistent ASD after a double transseptal puncture is significantly smaller than if two catheters are passed through a single puncture.[4] In addition, the majority of ASDs have been shown to have only left-to-right shunting. Most of these iatrogenic ASDs will spontaneously close after about 3 months and have not been shown to have an increased risk of paradoxical embolism.[5]

Advantages and Limitations

Transseptal puncture is an indispensible technique for electrophysiologists who perform ablations in the LA and frequently the LV. To perform the technique safely, we rely on additional tools such as intracardiac catheters to denote cardiac landmarks on fluoroscopy, pressure monitoring to determine if the correct chamber has been entered with the transseptal needle, and ICE to provide real-time imaging of catheters as they are maneuvered in the heart. These adjunctive tools have made transseptal puncture safer and shortened the time required for the practitioner to master this technique but have also increased the expense. Currently ICE is widely used in AF ablations not only to guide transseptal puncture but also to assess pulmonary venous anatomy, guide ablation catheter placement, and evaluate pulmonary vein flow velocities during the procedure. However, in cases of left-sided bypass tracts with normal cardiac anatomy, the cost of ICE may not be justified for a practitioner experienced in transseptal puncture with fluoroscopic guidance alone.

Abnormal atrial septal anatomy can rarely prevent successful transseptal puncture, and similarly patients with percutaneous or surgical repair of a PFO or ASD can prove difficult. However, with ICE guidance and additional tools such as RF-tipped catheters or the J-curve needle, we have been able to successfully perform transseptal puncture in patients with profoundly aneurysmal atrial septa, lipomatous hypertrophy, and ASD repair devices. While it may not be possible to cross a large Gore-Tex (W.L. Gore & Associates, Flagstaff, AZ) patch, pericardial or Dacron patches can generally be punctured, and even patients with percutaneous closure devices can have transseptal puncture performed if there is enough space on the IAS inferior and posterior to the patch or closure device.[12]

The presence of a LA thrombus should be considered an absolute contraindication to performing transseptal puncture. In addition, profound coagulopathy that is not reversed should be considered a contraindication, although we now routinely perform transseptal puncture on patients with an INR between 2 and 3.

Conclusions

Transseptal puncture has become a routine and essential tool in the electrophysiology lab for a variety of left heart procedures. It is a technically demanding procedure, and experience and understanding of the cardiac anatomy are important factors in performing transseptal puncture safely. The use of ICE has helped by providing additional real-time imaging of the transseptal catheter's position in the heart and has reduced the risk of complications. ICE also allows the prompt recognition of complications should they occur. Newer devices and technologies have also emerged to allow transseptal puncture in patients with abnormal anatomy, expanding the patient population in whom this technique can be performed safely.

References

1. Hahn K, Gal R, Sarnoski J, Kubota J, Schmidt DH, Bajwa TK. Transesophageal echocardiographically guided atrial transseptal catheterization in patients with normal-sized atria: Incidence of complications. *Clin Cardiol.* 1995;18: 217–220.
2. Szili-Torok T, Kimman G, Theuns D, Res J, Roelandt JR, Jordaens LJ. Transseptal left heart catheterisation guided by intracardiac echocardiography. *Heart.* 2001;86:E11.
3. Daoud EG, Kalbfleisch SJ, Hummel JD. Intracardiac echocardiography to guide transseptal left heart catheterization for radiofrequency catheter ablation. *J Cardiovasc Electrophysiol.* 1999;10:358–363.
4. Hammerstingl C, Lickfett L, Jeong KM, et al. Persistence of iatrogenic atrial septal defect after pulmonary vein isolation—an underestimated risk? *Am Heart J.* 2006;152:362. e1–e5.
5. Rillig A, Meyerfeldt U, Birkemeyer R, Treusch F, Kunze M, Jung W. Persistent iatrogenic atrial septal defect after

pulmonary vein isolation: Incidence and clinical implications. *J Interv Card Electrophysiol.* 2008;22:177–181.
6. Obel O, Mansour M, Picard M, Ruskin J, Keane D. Persistence of septal defects after transseptal puncture for pulmonary vein isolation procedures. *Pacing Clin Electrophysiol.* 2004;27:1411–1414.
7. Fagundes RL, Mantica M, De Luca L, et al. Safety of single transseptal puncture for ablation of atrial fibrillation: Retrospective study from a large cohort of patients. *J Cardiovasc Electrophysiol.* 2007;18:1277–1281.
8. Leong-Sit P, Callans D. Equipment for Transseptal Punctures. In: Thakur R, Natale A (Eds.). *Transseptal Catheterization and Interventions.* Minneapolis, MN: Cardiotext Publishing, 2010:55–64.
9. Fisher WG, Ro AS. Trans-septal Catheterization. In: Huang SKS, Wood MA (Eds.). *Catheter Ablation of Cardiac Arrhythmias.* Philadelphia, PA: Saunders Elsevier, 2006: 635–648.
10. Roelke M, Smith AJ, Palacios IF. The technique and safety of transseptal left heart catheterization: the Massachusetts General Hospital experience with 1,279 procedures. *Cathet Cardiovasc Diagn.* 1994;32(4):332–339.
11. De Ponti R, Cappato R, Curnis A, Della Bella P, Padeletti L, Raviele A, Santini M, Salerno-Uriarte JA. Trans-septal catheterization in the electrophysiology laboratory: data from a multicenter survey spanning 12 years. *J Am Coll Cardiol.* 2006;47(5):1037–1042. Epub 2006 Feb 9.
12. Lakkireddy D, Rangisetty U, Prasad S, et al. Intracardiac echo-guided radiofrequency catheter ablation of atrial fibrillation in patients with atrial septal defect or patent foramen ovale repair: a feasibility, safety, and efficacy study. *J Cardiovasc Electrophysiol.* 2008;19(11):1137–1142. Epub 2008 Jul 25.

Video Descriptions

Video 12.1   ICE from the RA of an aneurysmal IAS. (Image oriented so caudal is to the right, cranial is to the left)

Video 12.2   ICE from the RA of an extremely aneurysmal septum, bowed into the right atrium across the tricuspid valve. (Image oriented so caudal is to the right, cranial is to the left)

Video 12.3   ICE from the RA of a lipomatous septum, over 1.5 cm thick. (Image oriented so caudal is to the left, cranial is to the right) The presence of significant lipomatous hypertrophy often degrades the ability to visualize LA structures by ICE.

Video 12.4   ICE from the RV of the LV, showing a pericardial fat posterior to the LV prior to performing a transseptal puncture. (Image oriented so caudal is to the right, cranial is to the left)

Video 12.5   ICE from the RV of the LV showing a large pericardial effusion after performing a transseptal puncture. (Image oriented so caudal is to the right, cranial is to the left)

Video 12.6   LAO fluoroscopic video of two transseptal punctures being performed. The dilator is first withdrawn from the SVC into the RA, where it falls against the fossa. The dilator is advanced slightly to tent against the septum, and the needle is advanced across. The dilator is then advanced over the needle. The sheath is next advanced over the dilator, with some difficulty initially before it eventually jumps across the septum. The dilator is withdrawn. This process is repeated for the second puncture, after placing the ablation catheter in the LSPV through the first sheath.

Video 12.7   LAO fluoroscopic video of a single transseptal puncture being performed, with similar steps as described in Video 12.6.

Video 12.8   RAO fluoroscopic video of a single transseptal puncture being performed, with similar steps as described in Video 12.6.

Video 12.9   ICE from the RA of the dilator tenting at the top of the fossa—too high on the septum. (Image oriented so caudal is to the right, cranial is to the left)

Video 12.10   ICE from the RA of the dilator tenting at the bottom of the fossa—too low on the septum. (Image oriented so caudal is to the right, cranial is to the left)

Video 12.11   ICE from the RA of the dilator tenting at a good position, oriented toward the left pulmonary veins (LPVs). The second half of the video shows color Doppler of the venous inflow from the LPVs. (Image oriented so caudal is to the left, cranial is to the right)

Video 12.12   ICE from the RA of the dilator tenting at a mid-fossa location, but oriented too anteriorly—toward the mitral valve. As the ICE probe is panned counterclockwise from the LPVs to the mitral valve, the dilator tip is seen. (Image oriented so caudal is to the left, cranial is to the right)

Video 12.13   ICE from the RA of the dilator tenting at a mid-fossa location, but oriented too posteriorly—toward the posterior LA wall with the descending thoracic aorta seen behind it. (Image oriented so caudal is to the left, cranial is to the right)

Video 12.14   ICE from the RA of the dilator tenting toward the LPVs, while the needle is advanced across the septum. (Image oriented so caudal is to the left, cranial is to the right)

Video 12.15   ICE from the RA of saline bubbles seen in the LA when the sheath is flushed. (Image oriented so caudal is to the right, cranial is to the left)

Video 12.16   A series of ICE clips from the RA of the dilator being withdrawn down to the mid-fossa, oriented toward the LVPs. The needle is advanced across (0:26), then the dilator is advanced over it and the septal tenting is seen to relax (0:32). (Image oriented so caudal is to the right, cranial is to the left)

Video 12.17   ICE from the RA of the sheath being advanced over the dilator. Tenting of the septum is seen until the sheath jumps across the septum. (Image oriented so caudal is to the right, cranial is to the left)

Video 12.18 RAO fluoroscopic video of two transseptal punctures being performed. The dilator is first withdrawn from the SVC into the RA, where it falls against the fossa. The dilator is advanced slightly to tent against the septum, and the needle is advanced across. The dilator is then advanced over the needle. The sheath is next advanced over the dilator, with some difficulty initially before it eventually jumps across the septum. The dilator is withdrawn. This process is repeated for the second puncture after placing the ablation catheter in the LSPV through the first sheath.

Video 12.19 A series of ICE clips from the RA of the dilator being withdrawn down to the mid-fossa, oriented toward the LVPs. The needle is advanced across (0:16), then the dilator is advanced over it (0:21), and finally the sheath across over the dilator (0:28). (Image oriented so caudal is to the right, cranial is to the left)

Video 12.20 ICE from the RA of the steerable sheath oriented toward the mitral annulus in preparation for performing the second transseptal puncture. (Image oriented so caudal is to the right, cranial is to the left)

Video 12.21 ICE from the RA of a second transseptal puncture. The dilator is seen tenting the septum below the first sheath, oriented toward the LVPs. Saline bubbles from the flush on the first sheath can be seen circulating in the LA. (Image oriented so caudal is to the left, cranial is to the right)

Video 12.22 ICE from the RA of a second transseptal puncture. The dilator is tenting the fossa below the first sheath, and the needle is advanced across the septum. (Image oriented so caudal is to the left, cranial is to the right)

Video 12.23 ICE from the RA of a dilator tenting a very aneurysmal septum. (Image oriented so caudal is to the right, cranial is to the left)

Video 12.24 LAO fluoroscopic video of the SafeSept needle being used for transseptal puncture. The needle is advanced into the LSPV, with the dilator following. The sheath tents the septum and finally jumps across following the wire into the LSPV at 0:19.

Video 12.25 LAO fluoroscopic video of the SafeSept needle being used for a second transseptal puncture. The needle is advanced into the LSPV, with the dilator following. The sheath tents the septum and jumps across following the wire and pushing the dilator into the LSPV at 0:24.

Video 12.26 ICE video from the RA of a SafeSept needle being used for a second transseptal puncture in a patient with a moderately aneurysmal septum. (Image oriented so caudal is to the right, cranial is to the left)

Video 12.27 ICE video from the RA of a sheath in the LA with a mobile thrombus that has formed on the sheath. (Image oriented so caudal is to the left, cranial is to the right)

CHAPTER 13

How to Utilize ICE for Optimal Safety and Efficacy with AF Ablation

Mathew D. Hutchinson, MD

Introduction

The inherent complexity of catheter-based ablation for AF necessitates multimodality image integration. ICE provides dynamic, real-time images that are uniquely suited to complex ablation procedures. In fact, ICE satisfies all of the requirements of image-guided AF ablation: the delineation of pulmonary venous anatomy and its variants, the facilitation of intracardiac catheter positioning relative to potential ablation targets, the real-time characterization of catheter-tissue contact, the assessment of intracardiac lesion formation, and the early detection of procedural complications.

There are two commercially available types of ICE transducers: radial and phased-array systems. The radial ICE transducer is mounted on a 9-Fr, nonsteerable catheter and emits an imaging beam at a 15° forward angle, perpendicular to the long axis of the catheter. The transducer rotates at 1800 rpm, thus producing a 360° imaging plane. The fixed, 9-MHz transducer frequency provides excellent near-field resolution; however, far-field structures are poorly visualized with radial ICE, necessitating imaging proximate to the structure of interest (**Figure 13.1**).

The phased-array ICE transducer contains 64 elements with frequencies ranging from 5 to 10 MHz. This provides more flexibility in imaging either adjacent or distant structures with a potential imaging depth of up to 15 cm (**Figure 13.1**). The transducer is mounted on an 8- or 10-Fr catheter that can be deflected in four directions (anterior, posterior, right, and left) in addition to 360° axial rotation. Its steerability and low profile allow the imaging transducer to be navigated throughout any cardiac chamber of interest. The phased-array transducer is also capable of full spectral and color Doppler measurements, greatly enhancing the physiologic data achievable. The most commonly used phased-array ICE transducer is the AcuNav™ system (Siemens Medical, Mountain View, CA). Unless otherwise indicated, the remainder of this article will describe imaging with the phased-array ICE system.

Preprocedure Planning

Anatomical Characterization

PVI procedures are often performed with preacquired tomographic reconstructions of the LA. Image integration has been shown to facilitate ablation in areas with complex 3-dimensional structure, such as the ridge separating the LAA and LPVs, and is particularly useful in patients who have pulmonary venous anatomical variants.[1] Unfortunately, CT imaging incurs the additional risks of radiation and iodinated contrast exposure, which may render it unsuitable in selected patients. Likewise, gated MRI quality is

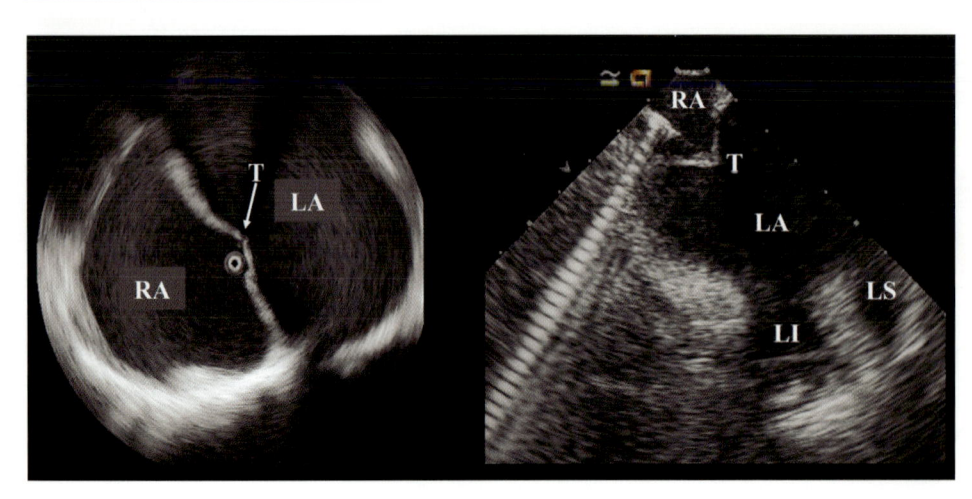

Figure 13.1 Transseptal puncture visualized with radial (left) and phased-array (right) ICE systems. Note the improved resolution of the far-field pulmonary venous structures with the phased-array catheter. Tenting (T) of the IAS is shown in both panels.

often limited by the rapid and irregular ventricular rates encountered in many preablation patients.

Like with tomographic imaging, complex anatomical relationships can also be clearly defined with phased-array ICE imaging (**Figure 13.2**). In a similar manner to tomographic reconstructions, 3-dimensional ICE contours can also be precisely integrated with electroanatomic mapping systems (**Figure 13.3**). These reconstructions have been shown to correlate well when coregistered with tomographic LA reconstructions.[2]

Left Atrial Thrombus Detection

It is our practice to obtain TEEs before AF ablation in patients with either nonparoxysmal forms of AF or inadequate preoperative anticoagulation. Some patients have either a contraindication to TEE or equivocal findings on serial examinations, which are misinterpreted as thrombus. In these cases, a secondary imaging study is required to adjudicate the presence of thrombus. We can reliably image the LAA with ICE by placing the imaging transducer into the RVOT or LPA (**Figure 13.4**).[3] Imaging from other proximate structures such as the CS has also been described.[4]

Procedural Imaging

Vascular Access

The phased-array ICE catheter is advanced through a standard vascular access sheath. We routinely upsize the access sheath one French size to allow unencumbered intravenous infusion through the sheath while the ICE catheter is in place. In patients with limited femoral venous access, we often place static diagnostic catheters (eg, CS) via the internal jugular vein, thus allowing the ICE catheter to be inserted via the femoral vein. This permits the operator to easily manipulate the echo imaging planes throughout the procedure.

Navigating the Phased-Array ICE Catheter

Passing the imaging catheter from the femoral vein to the heart can be easily performed without fluoroscopy in the majority of patients. The catheter is rotated axially and/or deflected in order to maintain the tip of the imaging transducer within the long axis of the vein (**Figure 13.5**; ▶ **Video 13.1**). The cardinal rule in safely maneuvering the phased-array catheter without fluoroscopic guidance is to always maintain an echocardiographic clear space between the transducer tip and the wall of the structure being imaged.

Imaging with ICE requires a modest learning curve but is a logical extension for operators with basic catheter manipulation and echocardiography skills. The phased-array catheter has eight degrees of freedom: (1) deflection: anterior, posterior, left, and right; (2) axial rotation: clockwise and counterclockwise; and (3) translational movement: advancement or withdrawal. Given that the imaging planes obtained with ICE vary relative to the position of the catheter, there are infinite potential imaging planes. As a result, any single 2-dimensional view taken out of anatomic context can be disorienting to the operator. If, however, the catheter is manipulated from a fiducial imaging plane, then the resulting anatomic relationships are intuitive.

Baseline ICE Imaging in AF Ablation

The phased-array catheter is initially placed in the mid-RA. The "home" view in the preablation survey, a long-axis view of the right ventricle and tricuspid valve, is easily obtained without any catheter deflection (**Figure 13.6**; ▶ **Video 13.2**). The home view allows the assessment of tricuspid valve structure and function, as well as the estimation of pulmonary arterial pressure with continuous-wave Doppler. Most of the subsequent imaging planes can be obtained by careful clockwise rotation of the imaging catheter from the home view. Whenever an unfamiliar imaging plane is encountered at any point during the study, we return the catheter to the home view by

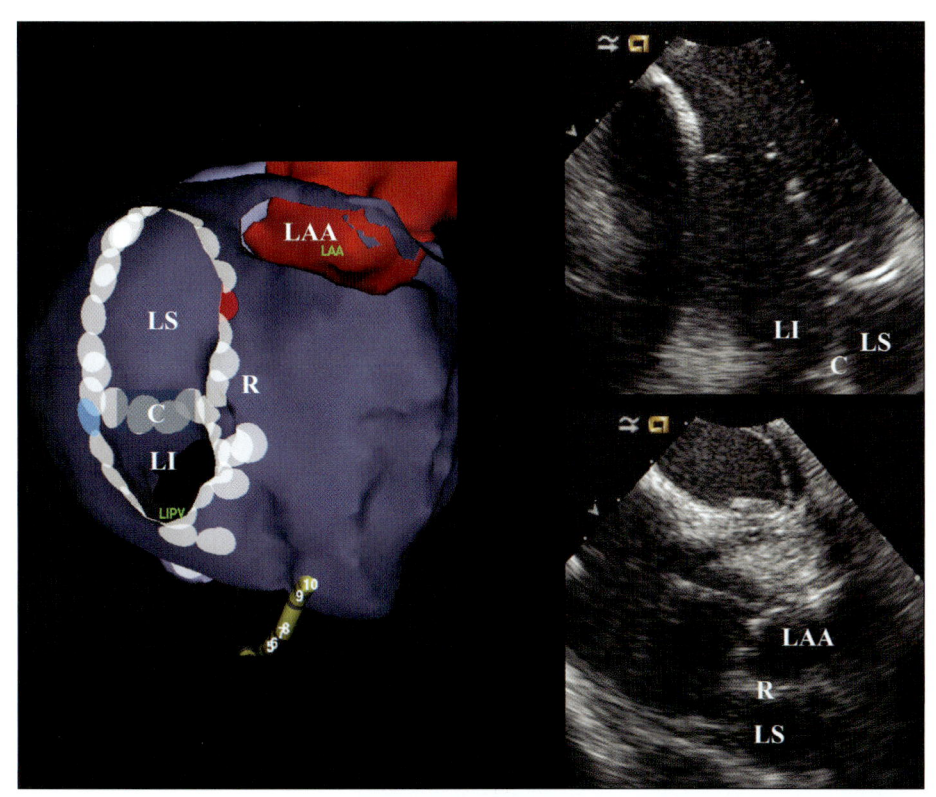

Figure 13.2 Left: A 3-dimensional CT reconstruction is displayed using an endoscopic perspective and demonstrates circumferential ablation of the LPVs. Top Right: An ICE image taken from the RA septum shows the common ostium of the LPVs with a recessed carina (C); a circular mapping catheter is present in the left superior vein (LS). Bottom Right: An ICE image taken from the RVOT shows the prominent ridge (R) separating the LS vein and left atrial appendage (LAA).

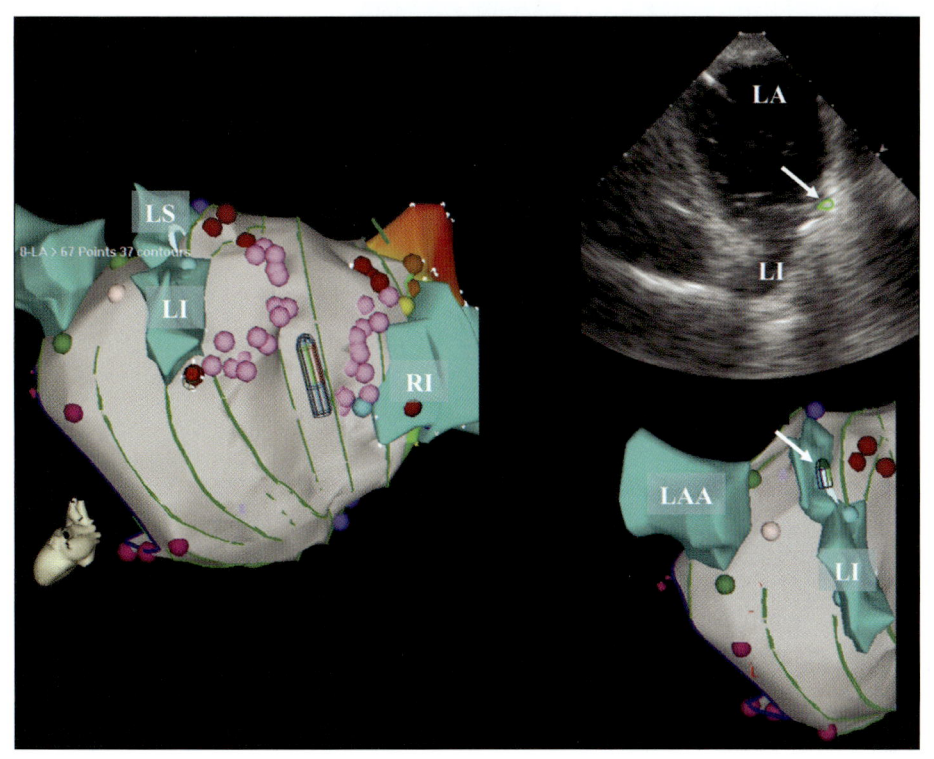

Figure 13.3 Integration of ICE with electroanatomic mapping with the CARTO Sound™ system. A 3-dimensional shell of the LA is created by combining multiple two-dimensional ultrasound contours (left). The tip of the ablation catheter (arrow) is located at the top of the LS vein and is projected onto the live echo image (top right). The corresponding location of the catheter tip (arrow) is shown on the 3-dimensional map (bottom right).

removing all catheter deflection and gently rotating the imaging catheter in a clockwise direction until the tricuspid valve is visualized.

With clockwise rotation from the home view, the imaging plane is directed posteriorly and leftward. At 45° CW rotation, a long-axis view of the aortic root is seen; the assessment of aortic valve structure and function, as well as the presence of aortic atheroma, is possible from this view (**Figure 13.6**). Continued clockwise rotation of the ICE catheter (90° from the home view) brings the

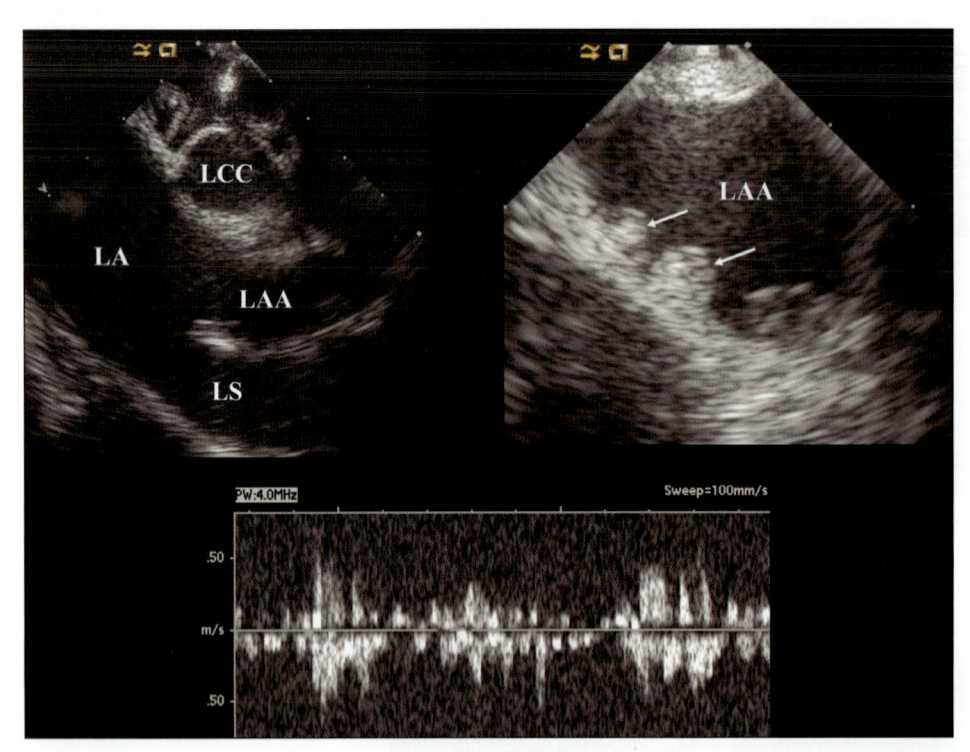

Figure 13.4 The LAA is viewed in the far-field from the RVOT (upper left) and in the near-field from the LPA (upper right). Pulsed-wave Doppler flow in the LAA is also shown (bottom center). See text for discussion.

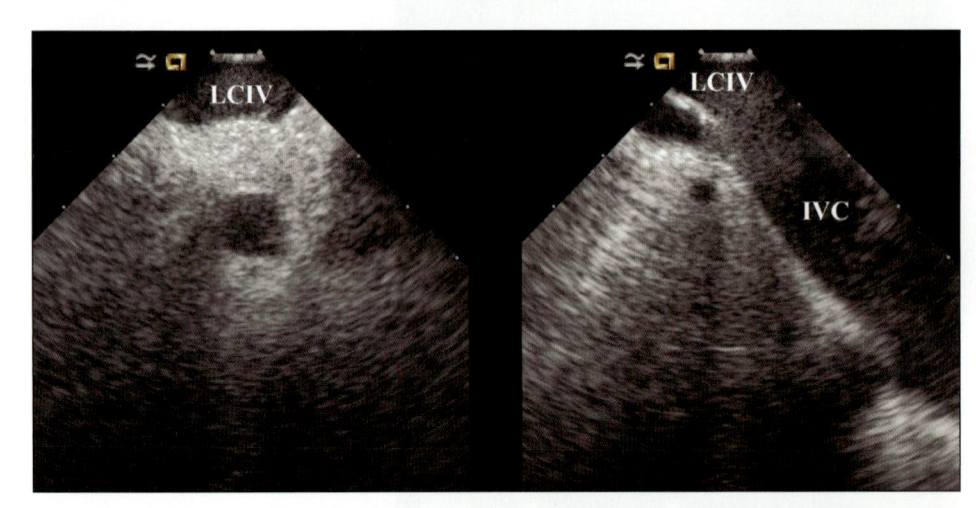

Figure 13.5 Nonfluoroscopic navigation of the phased-array ICE catheter through the lower-extremity veins. The acute angle between the left common iliac vein (LCIV) and the IVC is visible in the left panel as a loss of echo clear space at the tip of the imaging transducer. With gentle flexion and clockwise rotation of the catheter, a long-axis view (right) of the IVC is seen.

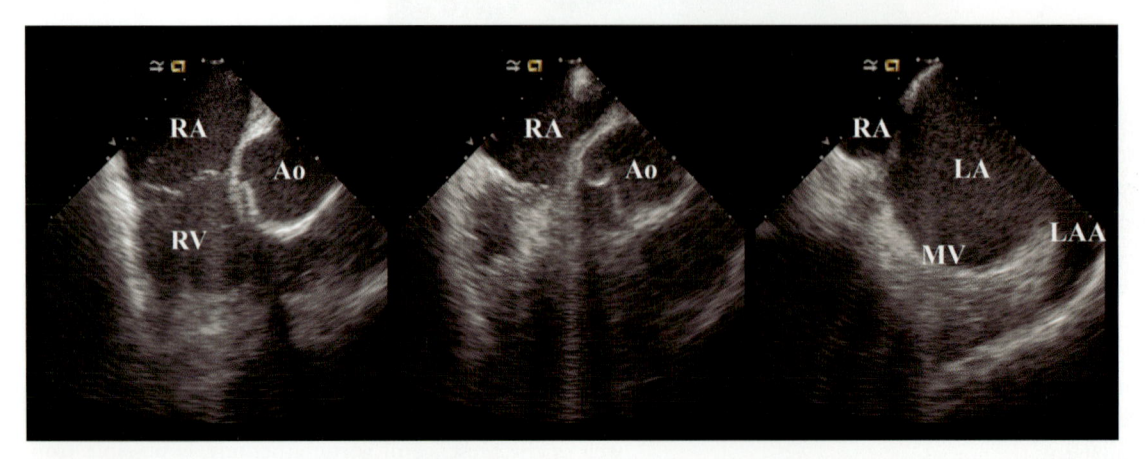

Figure 13.6 The baseline ICE survey begins with the "home" view, a long-axis view through the tricuspid valve (left). With gentle clockwise rotation of the catheter, the imaging plane is directed leftward and posterior, revealing a long-axis view of the aortic valve (middle). Further clockwise rotation directs the imaging plane through the fossa ovalis to reveal the mitral annulus (MV) and LAA.

mitral annulus and LAA into view (Figure 13.6; ▶ Video 13.3). Since the lateral mitral annulus and LAA are obligately present in the echo far-field, it may be necessary to decrease the imaging frequency to improve imaging resolution of these distal structures. As previously mentioned, the LAA is better visualized from more proximate structures such as the LPA or the distal CS.

Further clockwise rotation from the mitral valve plane brings the LPVs into view (▶ Video 13.4). This view is extremely useful to characterize the size and morphology of the LPVs. The LPVs often share a common ostium; however, the carina between the veins may be quite prominent and require ablation to achieve PVI. The dimensions of the individual LPVs and the common ostium are recorded from this view (**Figure 13.7**). PV color and pulse-wave Doppler flow velocities are also recorded in the baseline state (Figure 13.7; ▶ Video 13.5). The esophagus may lie in closer proximity to the posterior aspect of the LPV or the RPV and can be imaged longitudinally with further clockwise rotation of the ICE catheter (**Figure 13.8**). At this point, the imaging transducer has been rotated 180° from the original home view.

With slight additional clockwise rotation along the posterior wall, the RIPV is visualized. The RPVs often have separate ostia and the RSPV characteristically originates near the IAS and courses rightward. As a result, the RSPV and RIPV are uncommonly seen in the same 2-dimensional imaging plane (**Figure 13.9**; ▶ Video 13.6). The RSPV is usually the most difficult to visualize, since the imaging plane is often directed through the thick, superior limbus of the IAS. This anatomical constraint is overcome either by deflecting the imaging catheter posteriorly toward the tricuspid annulus or by wedging the transducer tip under the superior limbus of the fossa ovalis. When using the latter technique, the imaging catheter will often migrate into the LA via a PFO; this is

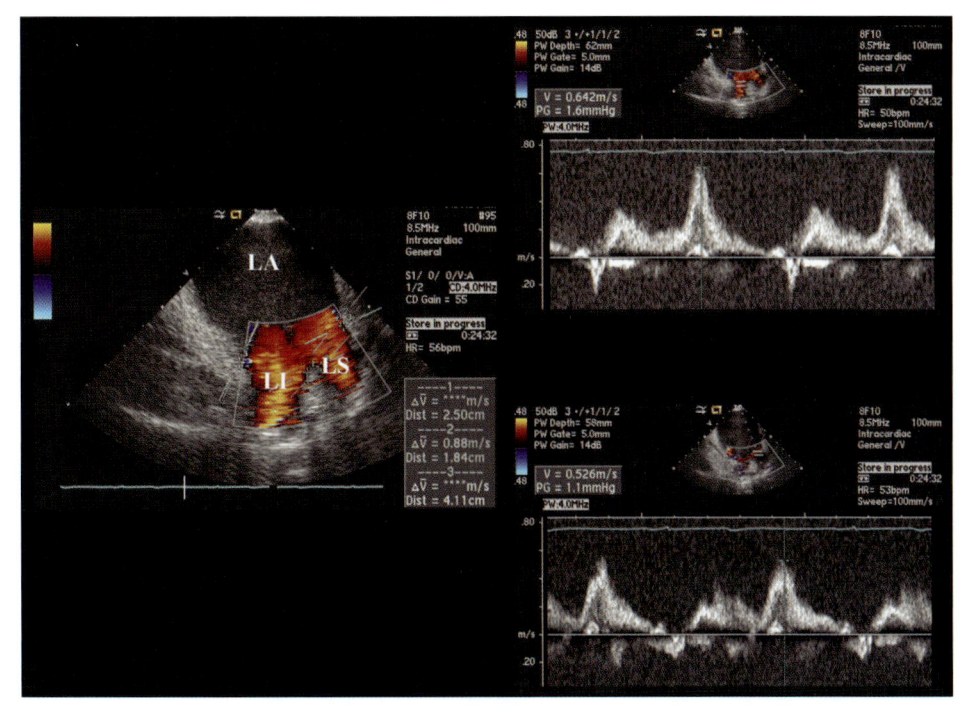

Figure 13.7 The LPVs (LS, LI) are shown with color Doppler flow (left). The diameters of the individual left veins as well as the common ostium are measured in this view. Pulsed-wave Doppler flow velocities are shown for the LS (top right) and LI (bottom right) pulmonary veins.

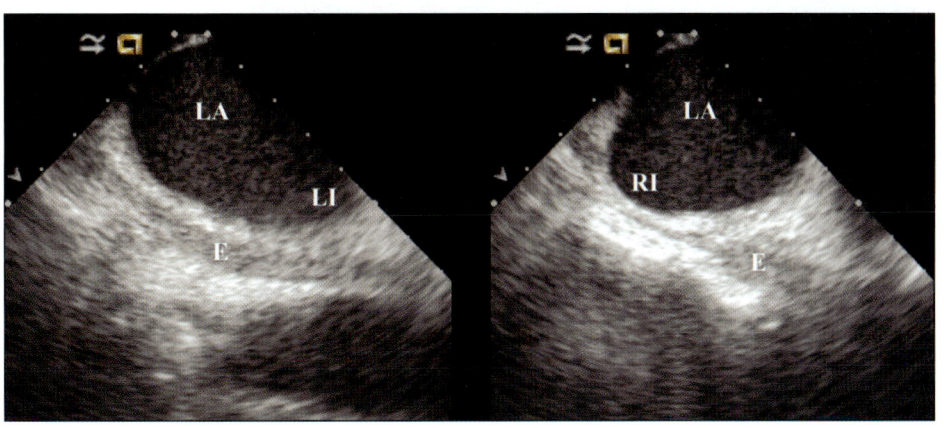

Figure 13.8 The location of the esophagus (E) can vary considerably within an individual, and often has an oblique course. The left panel shows the esophagus in its long axis. Taken from the same patient, the right panel shows the esophagus in close proximity to the posterior aspect of RIPV (RI).

recognized by a lack of atrial septal tissue interposed between the catheter tip and the LA (▶ Video 13.6). Direct LA imaging provides spectacular visualization of the RPVs. Careful assessment of the RPVs will often identify a separate middle PV ostium, allowing the operator both to incorporate this vein in an antral ablation strategy and to avoid inadvertently ablating inside it (**Figure 13.10**; ▶ **Video 13.7**).

Following detailed characterization of the LA and PVs, we assess the baseline left ventricular function and the presence of a preexisting pericardial effusion. This is achieved by placing the ICE catheter within the right ventricle and imaging through the interventricular septum. Beginning from the home view, the imaging catheter is deflected anteriorly and advanced through the tricuspid valve (▶ **Video 13.8**). Once the tip of the catheter passes through the valve, the anterior deflection is released. From this initial view of the inferior right ventricle, the catheter is rotated clockwise 90°, which brings the lateral wall of the left ventricle into view (**Figure 13.11**; ▶ **Video 13.9**). This view is easy to obtain, and we use it numerous times during the ablation procedure to monitor for pericardial fluid accumulation. Further 45° clockwise rotation of the catheter displays the aortic root in short axis. Below the aortic root, the LAA, LSPV, and separating ridge are visualized (▶ **Video 13.10**).

The integration of ICE and electroanatomical mapping with the CARTO Sound™ system (Biosense Webster, Diamond Bar, CA) allows the operator to create a 3-dimensional LA geometry without the use of fluoroscopy. This is done by tracing individual 2-dimensional LA endocardial contours and assembling them into a 3-dimensional geometry (Figure 13.3). Individual PVs can be traced independently and important anatomical structures (eg, PV ostium, ridge, mitral annulus) can be individually tagged. We often use a combination of imaging planes from the RA and the RVOT to fully model the LA. It is important to avoid obtaining multiple overlapping contours, which may distort the LA geometry.

Transseptal Puncture

After experiencing the exquisite detail afforded by ICE during transseptal puncture, it is difficult to imagine performing the procedure without it. With the catheter in the mid-RA position, ICE provides immediate feedback about the presence of abnormalities of the IAS such as lipomatous hypertrophy or aneurysms (**Figure 13.12**; ▶ **Video 13.11**). It is not uncommon for aneurysmal septa to tent across the entire LA diameter, even into the LPVs; seeing this may persuade the operator to use specialized transseptal equipment such as atraumatic guidewire-based systems.

ICE also gives insight into the directionality of the transseptal needle during tenting. Gentle axial rotation of the catheter at the fossa ovalis displays the relationship of the transseptal sheath to the adjacent structure; this feature virtually eliminates the possibility of inadvertent aortic

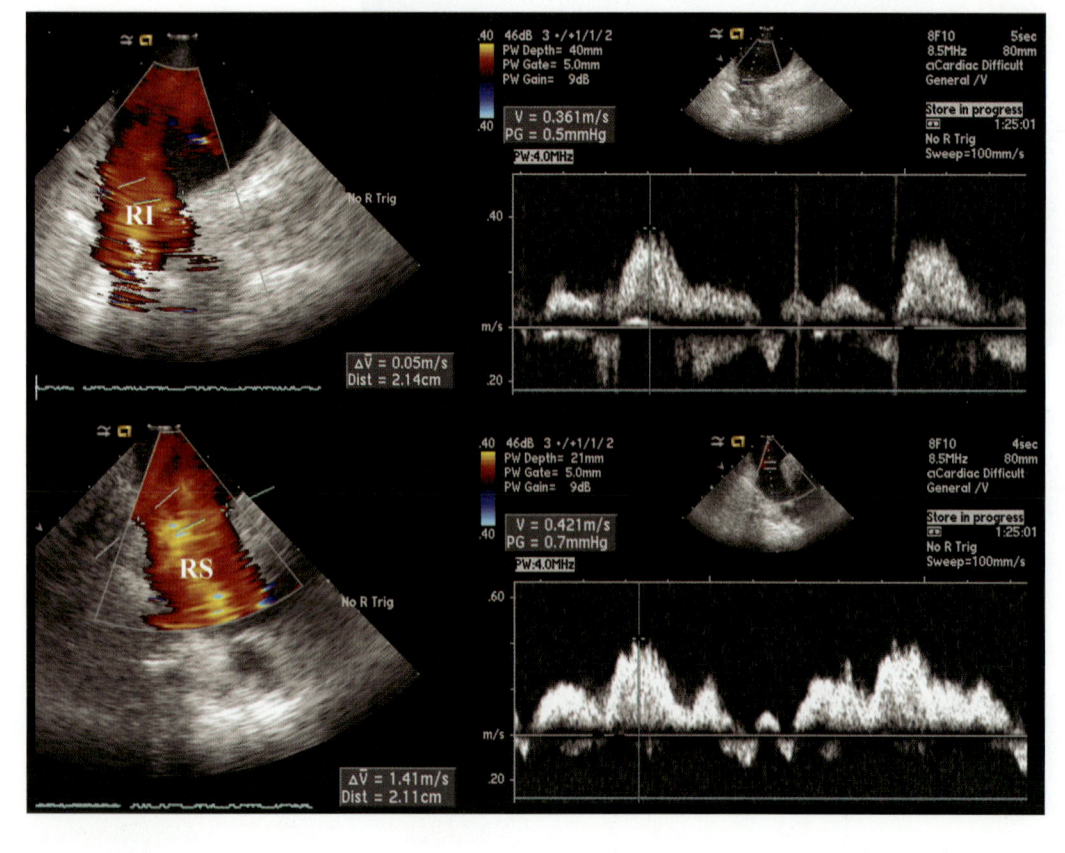

Figure 13.9 We routinely image the right and left ventricles in the baseline state to assess both biventricular function and the presence of a pericardial effusion. The RV is imaged directly by passing the ICE probe just past the tricuspid valve (left). Clockwise rotation of the ICE catheter directs the imaging plane through the interventricular septum and brings the LV into view (right). The arrows demarcate the pericardial space; in supine patients, these dependent regions are often the first to display early pericardial effusions.

Chapter 13: Using ICE for AF Ablation • 113

Figure 13.10 The RPVs (RS, RI) are shown with color Doppler flow (left upper and lower). The diameters of the individual right veins are measured in this view. Pulsed-wave Doppler flow velocities are shown for the RS (top right) and RI (bottom right) pulmonary veins.

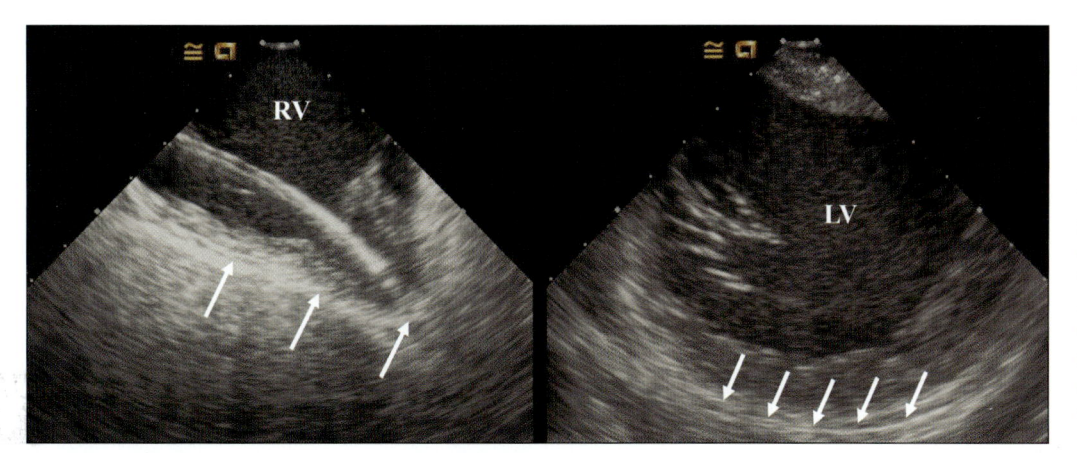

Figure 13.11 Anatomical variations of the RPVs are commonly encountered. The left panel shows a separate right middle (RM) PV. The right panel shows an anomalous PV originating posterior to the right superior (RS) vein ostium. If not visualized, these veins may be inadvertently damaged during ablation.

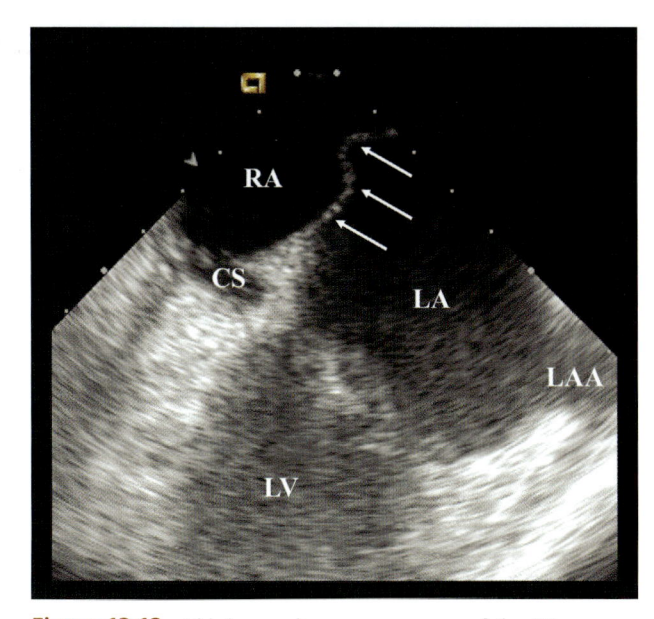

Figure 13.12 This image shows an aneurysm of the IAS (arrows). We find ICE of particular benefit during transseptal catheterization in these cases. These aneurysms often stretch across the entire LA diameter during needle tenting, increasing the risk of inadvertent puncture of the atrial wall. Fluoroscopic imaging fails to display these important relationships.

puncture. Often imperceptible changes in the orientation of the transseptal sheath can result in dramatic alterations of the trajectory of crossing; these subtle changes are often difficult to appreciate with fluoroscopy alone (**Figure 13.13**; ▶ Videos **13.12** and **13.13**).

We typically use ICE to direct the transseptal sheath toward the LPVs. In some patients, the right inferior PV often originates quite low in the LA; in these cases, we use ICE to direct the transseptal puncture site to the inferior margin of the fossa ovalis to facilitate intubation of the vein with the circular mapping catheter. In patients with small LA diameters or in whom magnetic navigation is used, we prefer a more anterior puncture (directed toward the LAA) to allow a safer dimension for sheath crossing and more space for catheter manipulation.

Catheter Positioning and Contact

PVI requires clear delineation of the PV anatomy. Preoperative assessment of PV diameters facilitates the selection of an appropriately sized circular mapping catheter. Using ICE, the circular mapping catheter can be placed at either the PV ostium or antrum (**Figure 13.14**).

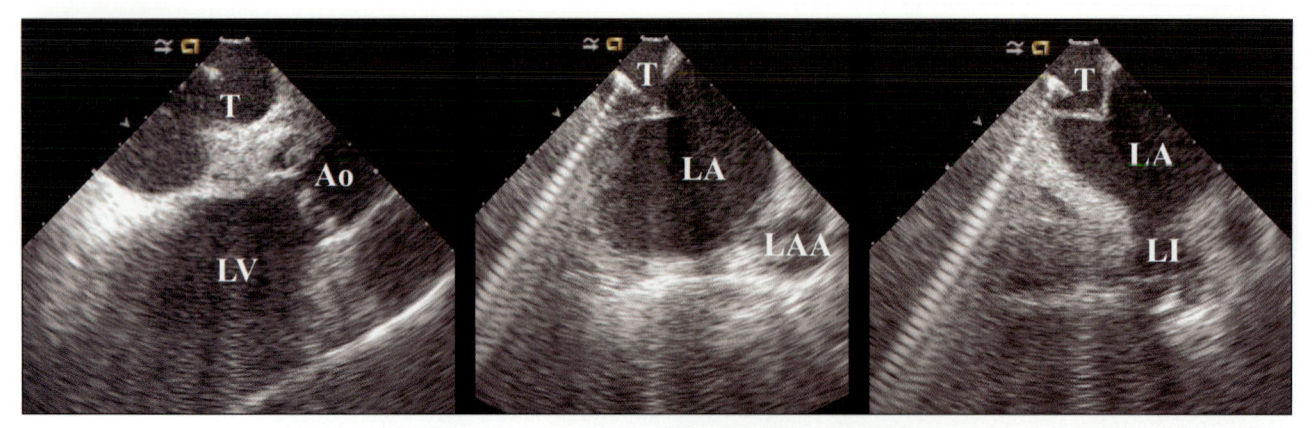

Figure 13.13 Phased-array ICE provides important perspective about the orientation of the transseptal needle and sheath before puncture. This technique eliminates the possibility of inadvertent aortic puncture (left). In patients with small atrial diameters or in whom magnetic navigation is used, we elect a more anterior puncture site (middle) toward the LAA. In most patients, we direct the transseptal puncture toward the LPVs (right).

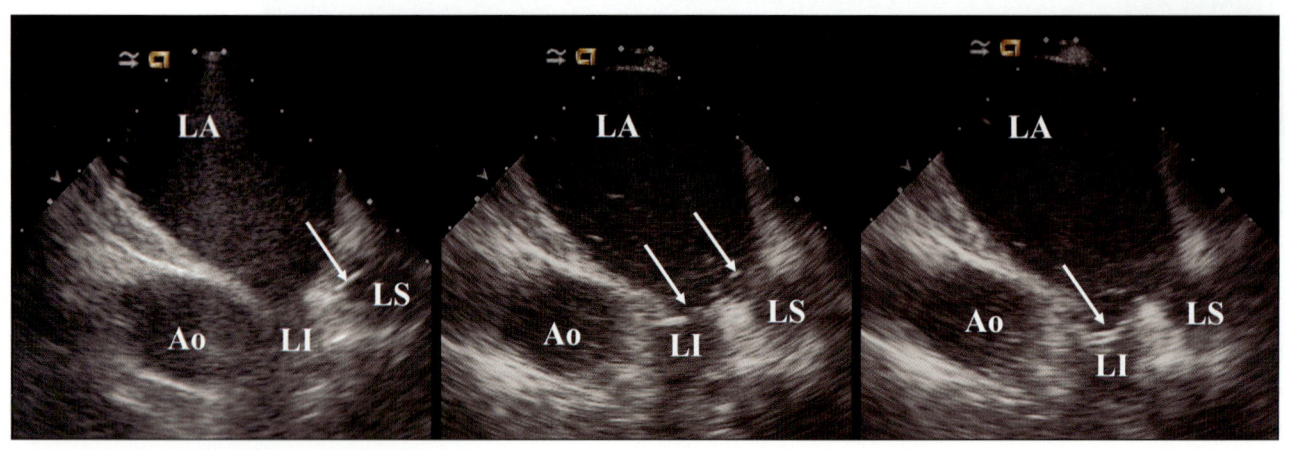

Figure 13.14 Positioning the circular mapping catheter is easily accomplished with ICE. We use ICE to define the ostium of each PV; these positions can be stored as reference locations on electroanatomic maps. Arrows denote the position of the circular mapping catheter at the ostium of the LS (left), L common (middle), and LI (right) pulmonary veins.

It is often useful to selectively intubate individual PVs to assess for entrance and exit block, and this is difficult to achieve with an oversized circular catheter. Tissue edema around the PV after ablation may also narrow the PV ostial diameter, making it difficult to fully engage the vein. Thus, for patients with small PV diameters we commonly use a 15-mm fixed-diameter circular catheter; this can be particularly useful for patients undergoing repeat ablation procedures who have ostial PV narrowing.

Ablation of the ridge between the LAA and LPVs is critically important and often difficult, due in part to its complex 3-dimensional geometry and relative thickness. We often use ICE to define this anatomical structure and facilitate its ablation. This complex anatomical relationship is easily visualized with the ICE catheter placed in the RVOT (▶ **Video 13.14**).

The confirmation of ablation catheter contact using fluoroscopy and electroanatomic mapping can be misleading; ICE allows this assessment in real time. In some cases, localized tissue edema during ablation is heralded by increasing tissue echodensity at the catheter tip (**Figure 13.15**; ▶ **Videos 13.15** and **13.16**).

ICE can also be useful in selected patients undergoing cavotricuspid isthmus ablation for right AFL. The home view can provide insight into the length of the CTI, as well as the presence of anatomical variants (eg, RA diverticulum or "pouch") (**Figure 13.16**).

Monitoring for Complications

The continuous monitoring capability afforded by ICE provides maximal sensitivity for the early detection and treatment of procedural complications, including pericardial effusion/tamponade, intracardiac thrombus, and PV stenosis.

The development of a hemodynamically significant pericardial effusion during AF ablation can occur quickly, and ICE can rapidly confirm the diagnosis and facilitate immediate treatment (▶ **Video 13.17**). This is particularly true in patients undergoing ablation on concurrent warfarin therapy. In patients without prior cardiac surgery, the pericardial fluid usually collects circumferentially but often appears first in the dependent segments. Imaging from the RV septum clearly delineates the posterior and lateral LA

Chapter 13: Using ICE for AF Ablation • 115

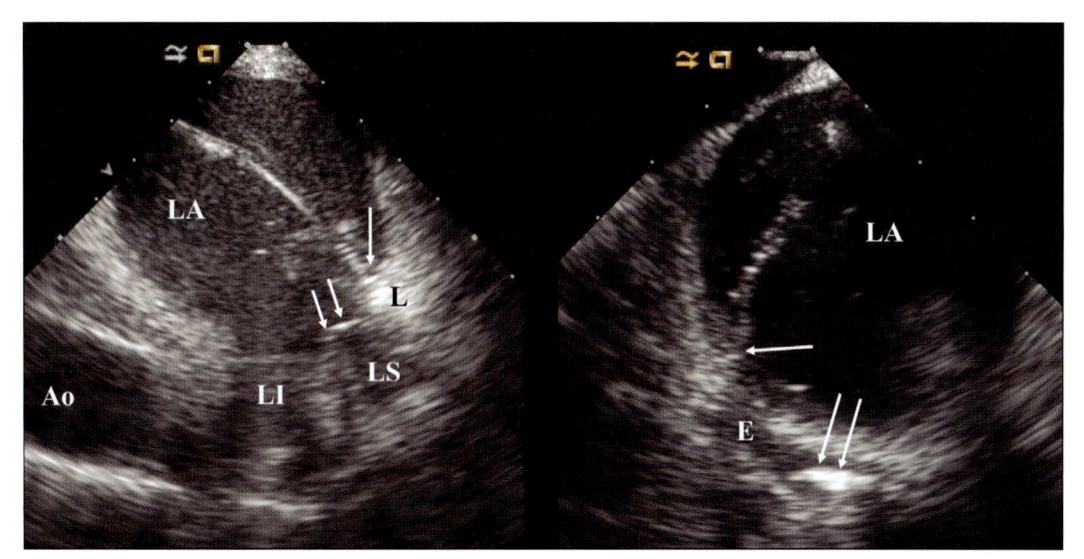

Figure 13.15 ICE provides real-time monitoring during ablation. The left panel shows an echo bright ablation lesion (L) on the LA roof above the LSPV. Also seen are the circular mapping catheter (two arrows) at the LSPV ostium and the ablation catheter tip (single arrow) more proximally at the LA roof. The right panel is taken from a different patient during ablation at the posterior aspect of the RIPV. The tip of the ablation catheter (single arrow) is seen in close proximity to the esophagus (E). When ablating near the esophagus, we routinely reduce power settings and monitor esophageal temperature with a probe (two arrows).

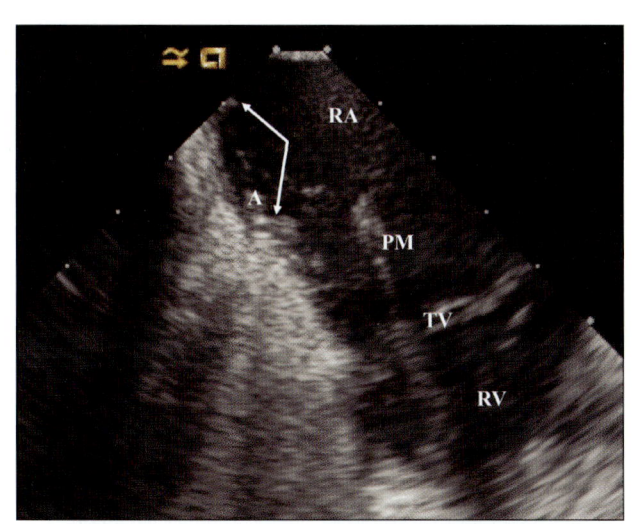

Figure 13.16 An image taken from a CTI ablation after multiple lesions failed to produce bidirectional conduction block. There is a large atrial diverticulum or pouch present (arrows). The ablation catheter tip (A) was subsequently wedged into the apical recess of the pouch; ablation at this spot resulted in bidirectional conduction block across the CTI. A pacemaker lead (PM) is also seen traversing the tricuspid valve.

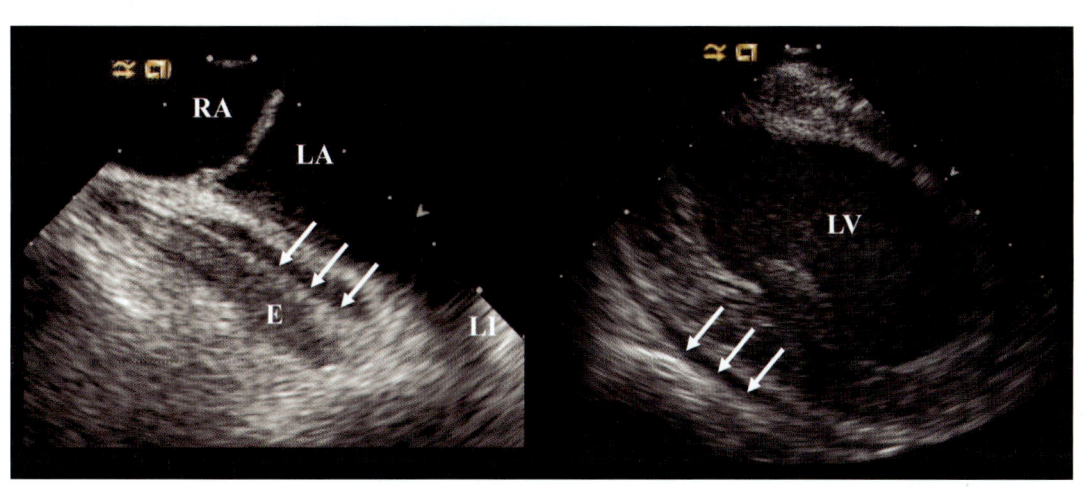

Figure 13.17 ICE allows the rapid detection and treatment of traumatic pericardial effusions. The left panel shows a small fluid collection (arrows) producing an echo clear space between the posterior LA wall and the esophagus. The right panel reveals a 4-mm fluid collection layering along the posterolateral LV (arrows) in a different patient. Both effusions were thought to be related to local endocardial disruption during ablation; neither patient required percutaneous drainage after rapid diagnosis and reversal of anticoagulation.

and LV, the regions where traumatic effusions commonly originate during AF ablation. For patients with previous cardiac surgery, we take care to use multiple imaging planes to exclude a loculated fluid collection (**Figure 13.17**). Of course, significant hemodynamic compromise is a late finding of pericardial effusion, so we will reflexively screen for an effusion with any significant decrease in systolic blood pressure. We also find it useful to periodically screen for an effusion in the absence of clinical signs; we will routinely do this at the time of ACT checks.

The evaluation of other causes of hypotension during ablation can also be aided by ICE imaging. Occult air embolism can occur either through the transseptal sheaths or through the systemic venous sheaths with paradoxical septal passage. The right coronary artery is most commonly affected, and transient inferior wall motion abnormalities can be seen with the ICE catheter positioned in the RVOT (**Figure 13.18**). There are always associated ST segment elevations; however, these changes can be difficult to detect on EP recording systems with sweep speeds often set to 100 mm/sec. Hypotension during isoproterenol infusion is quite common and is typically due to systemic arterial vasodilation. This can be overcome in most patients by coadministration of alpha-agonists such as phenylephrine. Particular care should be given to patients with fixed or dynamic LVOT obstruction, since significant hypotension can occur.

Intracardiac thrombus forms most commonly on the transseptal sheath but can also occur on intracardiac catheters or in situ on ablated myocardium (**Figure 13.19**; ▶ **Video 13.18**).[5] Asymptomatic clots are likely quite common, and experience suggests that the diagnostic yield is directly proportional to the intensity of monitoring. Many of these clots likely embolize without apparent clinical sequelae. Sheath-associated thrombus within the LA can often be aspirated into the transseptal sheath or "trapped" against the IAS and withdrawn into the RA.

The increasing utilization of ICE has been instrumental in reducing the incidence of PV stenosis. Significant elevations above baseline in pulse Doppler PV flow measurements (> 120 cm/sec) may predict long-term PV stenosis and should prompt repeat PV imaging several months postprocedure (**Figure 13.20**). With true antral PVI, significant elevations in PV flow velocities are exceedingly uncommon. The pulse Doppler measurements can be confounded by concomitant catecholamine administration, so we routinely obtain these measurements prior to isoproterenol infusion.

Postprocedural Care

A repeat ICE survey is performed after all intracardiac catheters are removed to exclude a pericardial effusion. We have noted rare episodes of postprocedure tamponade, which are thought to result from occult catheter perforations (eg, distal CS) that are unmasked after catheter removal. We partially reverse intravenous heparin with low-dose protamine (10–15 mg infused over 10 minutes). Patients often develop systemic hypotension during

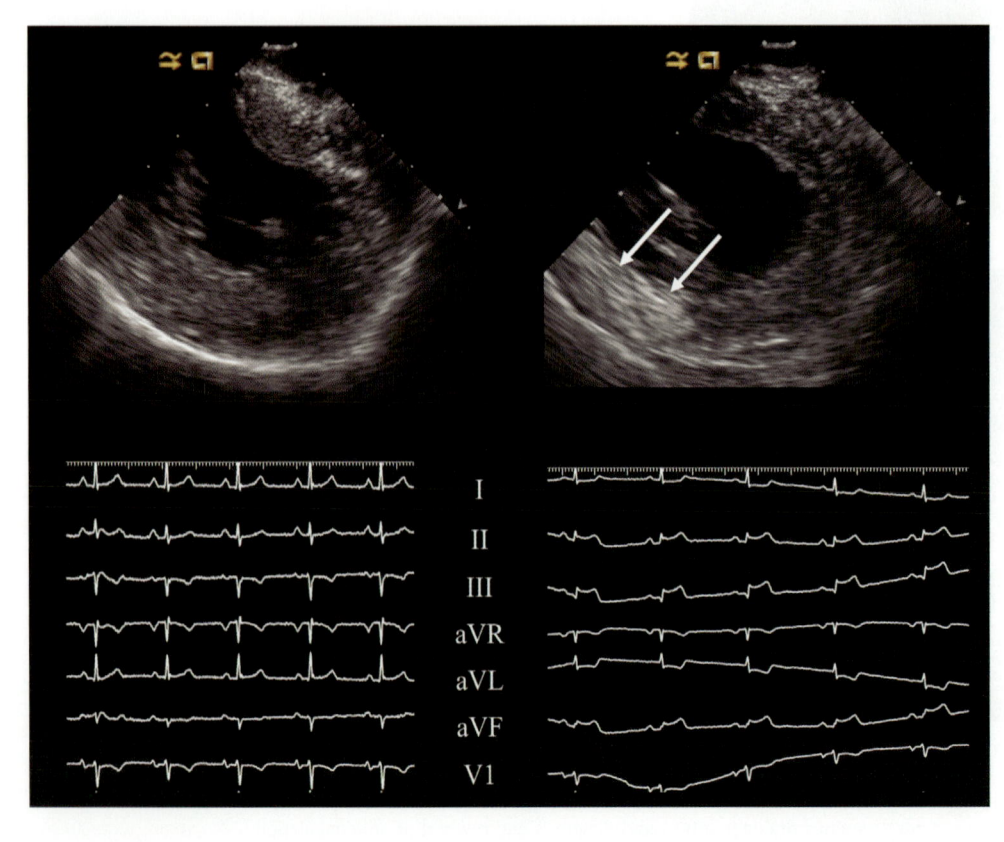

Figure 13.18 These images were taken from a patient who suffered an air embolism during AF ablation. The baseline echo image taken at end systole is shown along with the ECG (left top and bottom). After occult air embolism, there is reduced systolic thickening of the posterolateral LV walls (arrows) coincident with marked ST segment elevation in the inferior leads (right top and bottom). See text for discussion.

Figure 13.19 ICE can detect mural or catheter-associated intracardiac thrombi. The left panel reveals a large thrombus (arrow) attached to a transseptal sheath during transseptal catheterization. This thrombus formed in this patient despite an ACT of 380 seconds and an INR of 3.5. The right panel shows a small thrombus (arrow) attached to the LA roof above the RSPV in an area of recent ablation. Neither thrombus resulted in clinical sequelae.

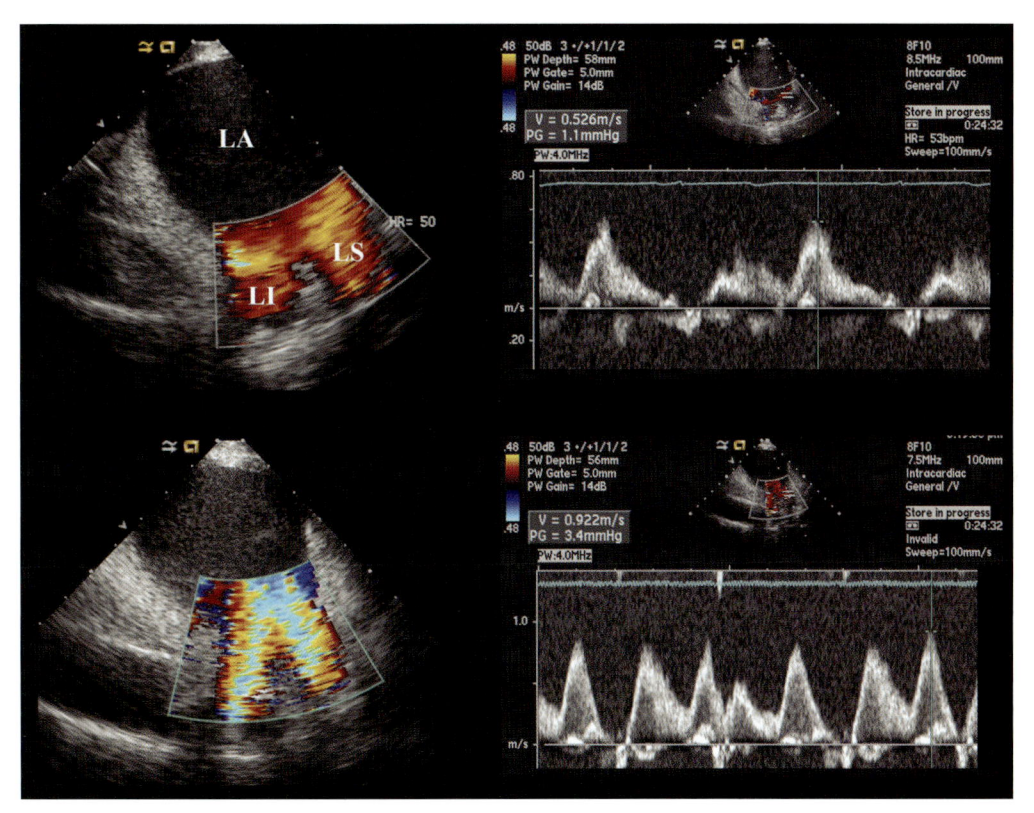

Figure 13.20 Pulmonary venous narrowing after ablation produces an increase in measured Doppler flow velocity and turbulent color Doppler flow. Compared to the baseline state (left top), this patient has mild narrowing of the LPVs and turbulence of the color Doppler flow post ablation (left bottom). The LSPV flow velocity increased from 53 cm/s at baseline (right top) to 92 cm/s post ablation (right bottom). See text for discussion.

protamine infusion, which may persist for up to an hour. We remove venous sheaths when the ACT falls below 200 seconds. Patients remain flat for 4 hours after the procedure.

Procedural Complications

The procedural risk associated with ICE imaging is largely driven by the requirement of vascular access and right heart catheterization; this risk should be < 2%. Inadvertent arterial puncture confers a risk of AV fistula or pseudoaneurysm. An unexplained decrease in serum hemoglobin, often associated with unexplained hypotension during or postprocedure, should prompt an evaluation for an occult retroperitoneal or thigh hematoma. There is always a risk of vascular or cardiac perforation by the ICE catheter; this risk is minimized by never advancing the catheter against resistance and always maintaining an echo clear space at the tip of the imaging transducer.

Advantages and Limitations

There are numerous advantages that ICE confers during AF ablation procedures. It provides real-time assessment of: (1) LA and PV structure; (2) intracardiac catheter positioning and contact; and (3) early detection of complications. The facilitation of transseptal puncture is also invaluable, and in our experience, eliminates traumatic needle perforations. The use of ICE can also substantially reduce fluoroscopic exposure to both the patient and the operator.[6]

In addition to the requirement of intravenous access, the main disadvantage of ICE is cost. High-volume laboratories will need a dedicated ultrasound machine, which can cost $50,000 to $200,000. The cost of a single, new phased-array ICE catheter averages $2,100. The catheter can be safely reprocessed and reused, at a substantial cost savings. Our experience with reprocessed catheters has been mixed, with occasional loss of imaging quality noted.

Conclusions

The use of ICE to guide AF ablation has substantially improved both procedural safety and efficiency. Despite a modest learning curve to obtain the standard ICE imaging planes, most operators with basic echocardiography experience will become rapidly proficient. In addition to 2-dimensional imaging, phased-array catheters add valuable physiologic data, including full color and spectral Doppler capabilities. The early detection of complications and the limitation of procedural fluoroscopy provide immediate benefit to patients. In our experience, the increased procedural cost associated with ICE is easily justified by the peace of mind afforded by its real-time imaging capability.

References

1. Dong J, Dickfeld T, Dalal D, et al. Initial experience in the use of integrated electroanatomic mapping with 3-dimensional MR/CT images to guide catheter ablation of atrial fibrillation. *J Cardiovasc Electrophysiol*. 2006;17(5):459–466.
2. Singh SM, Heist EK, Donaldson DM, et al. Image integration using intracardiac ultrasound to guide catheter ablation of atrial fibrillation. *Heart Rhythm*. 2008;5(11):1548–1555.
3. Reddy VY, Neuzil P, Ruskin JN. Intracardiac echocardiographic imaging of the left atrial appendage. *Heart Rhythm*. 2005;2(11):1272–1273.
4. Hutchinson MD, Jacobson JT, Michele JJ, Silvestry FE, Callans DJ. A comparison of intracardiac and transesophageal echocardiography to detect left atrial appendage thrombus in a swine model. *J Interv Card Electrophysiol*. 2010;27(1):3–7.
5. Ren JF, Marchlinski FE, Callans DJ. Left atrial thrombus associated with ablation for atrial fibrillation: identification with intracardiac echocardiography. *J Am Coll Cardiol*. 2004;43(10):1861–1867.
6. Reddy VY, Morales G, Ahmed H, et al. Catheter ablation of atrial fibrillation without the use of fluoroscopy. *Heart Rhythm*. 2010;7(11):1644–1653.

Video Descriptions

Video 13.1 Nonfluoroscopic navigation of the phased-array ICE catheter through the lower-extremity veins. The acute angle between the left common iliac vein (LCIV) and the inferior vena cava (IVC) is initially evident as a loss of echo clear space at the tip of the imaging transducer. With gentle anterior flexion and clockwise rotation of the catheter, a long-axis view of the IVC is seen and the imaging catheter is advanced.

Video 13.2 This long-axis view through the tricuspid valve, the "home view," is easily obtained from the mid-RA. Most basic intracardiac views can be obtained with clockwise rotation of the ICE catheter from this imaging plane.

Video 13.3 This clip was obtained with clockwise rotation of the imaging catheter from the home view; this directs the imaging plane leftward and posterior. The tricuspid valve gives way to a long-axis view of the aortic root (45° CW). The mitral annulus and LAA are then seen (90° CW). Thereafter, the LPVs, the posterior LA/esophagus (180° CW), and the RPVs are seen sequentially.

Video 13.4 The LPVs are visualized. The inferior vein (left) and superior vein (right) are separated by a prominent carina.

Video 13.5 Laminar color Doppler flow from the LPVs is visualized. The inferior vein (left) and superior vein (right) are separated by a prominent carina.

Video 13.6 This clip opens with color Doppler flow from the right inferior PV. After clockwise rotation of the ICE catheter, the right superior vein is visualized. The RPVs are not often seen in the same imaging plane.

Video 13.7 This clip shows a common anatomical variation of the RPVs with a separate middle vein ostium. The right inferior vein is seen to the left and the right superior vein to the right of the middle branch in the clip.

Video 13.8 From the home view, the ICE catheter is deflected anteriorly and advanced through the tricuspid valve into the right ventricle.

Video 13.9 After the ICE catheter is placed into the right ventricle, clockwise rotation of the imaging plane through the interventricular septum brings the left ventricle into view. This important view allows the operator to rapidly assess both the LV function and the presence of a pericardial effusion.

Video 13.10 The ICE catheter is rotated clockwise in the right ventricular outflow to view the aortic root in short axis. This is an important view to differentiate the ostium of the left superior vein from the LAA.

Video 13.11 The fossa ovalis is directly visualized from the mid RA. This patient has a large interatrial septal aneurysm which is deviated toward the RA. The aneurysm is more prominent along the anterior aspect of the fossa, and becomes less prominent with posterior (clockwise) rotation of the imaging catheter.

Video 13.12 The transseptal needle tents the IAS toward the LPVs. A prior transseptal sheath is seen crossing the IAS inferior to the needle.

Video 13.13 After the needle punctures the septum, relief of tenting is noted. The transseptal dilator extends just past the end of the transseptal sheath in the LA. A second sheath is seen more inferiorly, extending across the atrial septum.

Video 13.14 We routinely use a circular mapping catheter to create the LA geometry with electroanatomical mapping. ICE is extremely valuable in defining spatially complex 3-dimensional structures such as the ridge between the left veins and the LAA. In this view, obtained from the RVOT, the circular mapping catheter is seen sweeping across the ridge.

Video 13.15 The tissue edema from acute ablation lesions can often be visualized as tissue brightening adjacent to the ablation catheter. This clip shows an expanding ablation lesion above the LSPV. The circular mapping catheter is also seen at the ostium of the left superior vein.

Video 13.16 When ablating near the esophagus, we routinely reduce power settings and monitor esophageal temperature with a probe. This clip is taken during ablation at the posterior aspect of the right inferior vein. The tip of the ablation catheter is seen in close proximity to the esophagus. A temperature probe is also seen within the esophageal lumen.

Video 13.17 ICE allows rapid detection and treatment of pericardial effusions. This view of the LV is obtained with the ICE catheter in the RV. There is a large, circumferential pericardial effusion noted.

Video 13.18 This clip reveals a large thrombus attached to a transseptal sheath during transseptal catheterization. The transseptal dilator is tenting the IAS; however, the thrombus is attached more proximally to the tip of the sheath. This thrombus formed in this patient despite an ACT of 380 seconds and an INR of 3.5.

CHAPTER 14

How to Perform Pulmonary Vein Antrum Isolation for Atrial Fibrillation

Marco V. Perez, MD; Amin Al-Ahmad, MD; Andrea Natale, MD

Introduction

Pulmonary vein antrum isolation (PVAI) is the achievement of PV electrical isolation through ablation of the posterior wall of the LA and the circumferential regions of the PV ostia. During early embryonic development, the PV smooth muscle extends over the posterior wall as well as some aspects of the roof of the LA and areas anterior to the right-sided PVs.[1] These areas are considered the antrum of the PVs. Antral isolation targets many of the arrhythmogenic targets in the LA and potentially modifies other factor such as neural inputs into the LA. This approach for ablation of AF has gained acceptance, as it has been associated with improved long-term outcomes as well as an acceptably low rate of complications.[2]

Preprocedural Planning

Left Atrial Imaging

All patients undergo cardiac evaluation with imaging pre-procedure. A standard 2-dimensional echocardiogram is most commonly used. LA dimensions, a thickened or aneurysmal atrial septum and other abnormalities seen on echocardiography are important to note for the procedure (▶ Video 14.1). In some individuals, additional LA imaging with either computerized tomography (CT) or magnetic resonance imaging (MRI) is also utilized. On cardiac CT scan or MRI, the antrum appears to be a funnel-like structure (**Figure 14.1**). These images also yield valuable information regarding the anatomic features of the PVs and appendage (**Figure 14.2**, ▶ Video 14.2) or abnormalities such as a common PV trunk or anomalous PV return.

When an electroanatomical mapping system is used, the CT scan can either be placed for a side-to-side comparison (**Figure 14.3**) or superimposed on the electroanatomical map. While preoperative cardiac CT and MRI are useful in defining the antrum, they are not required to perform the procedure, in part due to the utility of intracardiac echocardiography (ICE).

Use of ICE immediately before and during ablation is helpful for anatomic orientation. ICE helps define where the tubular part of the PV enters the LA and during the procedure can define the location of the catheters in the antrum relative to the PVs (**Figure 14.4**, ▶ Video 14.3).

Stroke Prevention

Patients in AF undergoing PVAI will either convert to sinus rhythm during ablation or will be electrically cardioverted immediately following ablation. To minimize embolic risk, TEE prior to the procedure is primarily used

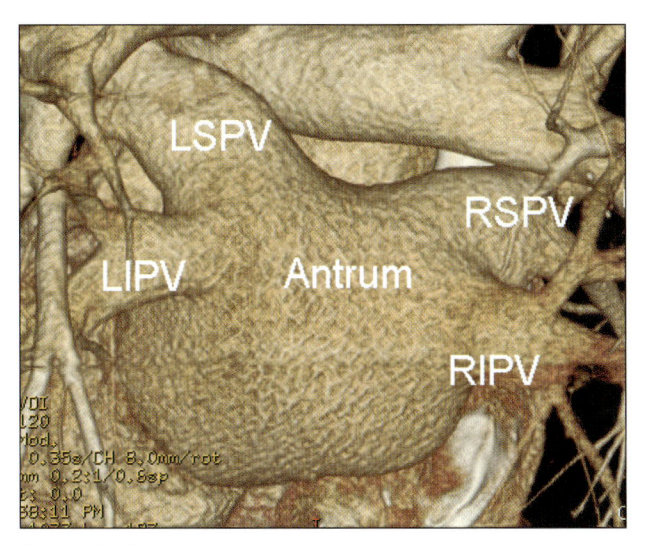

Figure 14.1 Three-dimensional CT reconstruction of the LA.

to rule out presence of atrial clot. This is usually done the morning of the procedure or, preferentially, the day prior. Patients with a $CHADS_2$ score of 0 or 1 will undergo TEE only if in AF for greater than 48 hours, but all patients with a $CHADS_2$ score of 2 or greater will undergo a TEE regardless of their rhythm. Patients are asked to use a home loop monitor and transmit their rhythm on the days prior to the ablation.

Most patients in our practice are asked to discontinue warfarin prior to the procedure, using low-molecular-weight heparin as a bridge. This has traditionally been the practice to minimize excessive bleeding complications, such as cardiac tamponade and groin hematomas. However, recent experience from our group suggests that patients can safely undergo the procedure while on therapeutic levels of warfarin. We have recently observed that ablation on therapeutic warfarin can reduce the risk of stroke.[3]

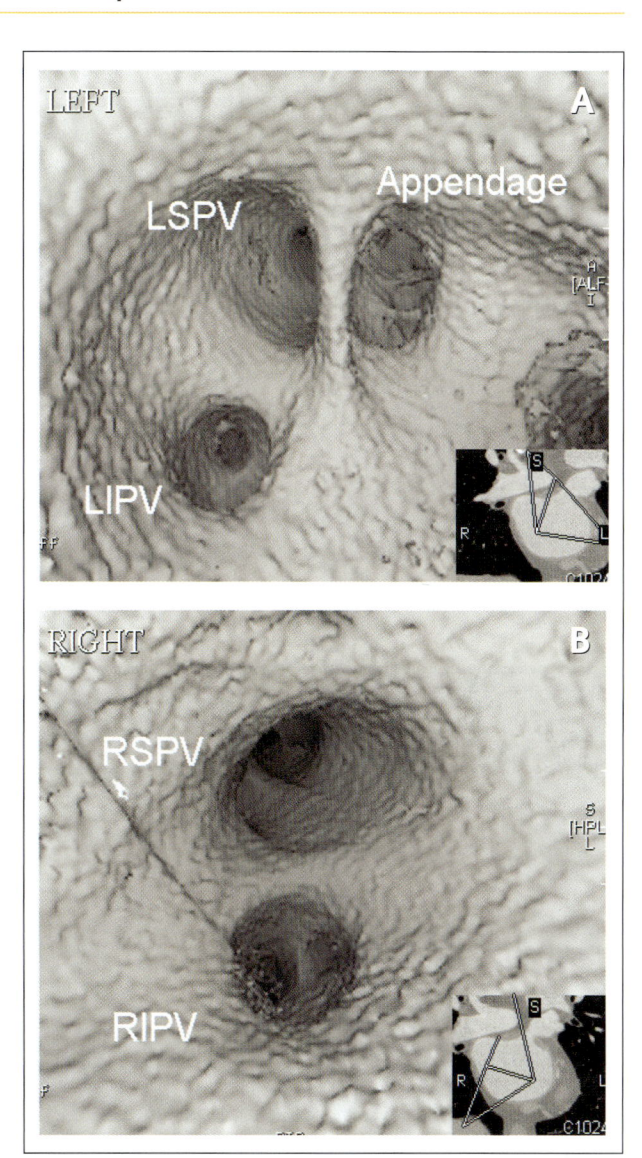

Figure 14.2 Three-dimensional reconstruction of CT scan viewed from inside the LA. **A.** Left pulmonary veins and appendage. **B.** Right pulmonary veins.

Procedure

Patient Preparation

The majority of our patients undergo PVAI under general anesthesia. General anesthesia has many advantages, but the most important in this context is that it helps control respiration by eliminating deep breathing that may result in sudden catheter movement. Pain thresholds and response to sedation may vary significantly. A Foley urinary catheter is placed in all patients after sedation since the volume of fluid given during the procedure with an irrigated-tip catheter is typically 2 to 4 liters. A temperature probe is also placed into the esophagus after sedation for monitoring of the esophageal position and temperature.

Two 8-Fr sheaths are placed in the right femoral vein and later replaced with the trans-spetal sheaths. An 11-Fr sheath is placed in the left femoral vein for placement of a phased-array ICE catheter. An arterial line is often placed in the left femoral artery for hemodynamic monitoring. Right internal jugular access is used to pass a 20-pole deflectable catheter. This catheter is placed in the CS such that the distal 10 poles are in the CS and the proximal 10 poles are in the RA (**Figure 14.5**).

A heparin bolus of 100 to 150 U/kg is typically given before transseptal puncture, but it can be given immediately after the first puncture. Another heparin bolus of 50 U/kg is given after the second transseptal puncture and a heparin drip at approximately 14 U/kg/min is initiated. The goal ACT is 350 to 400 seconds. The ACT is checked every 10 to 15 minutes during the procedure. Repeat boluses and titration of the heparin drip are necessary to keep the ACT at goal.

122 • *Ablation of AF*

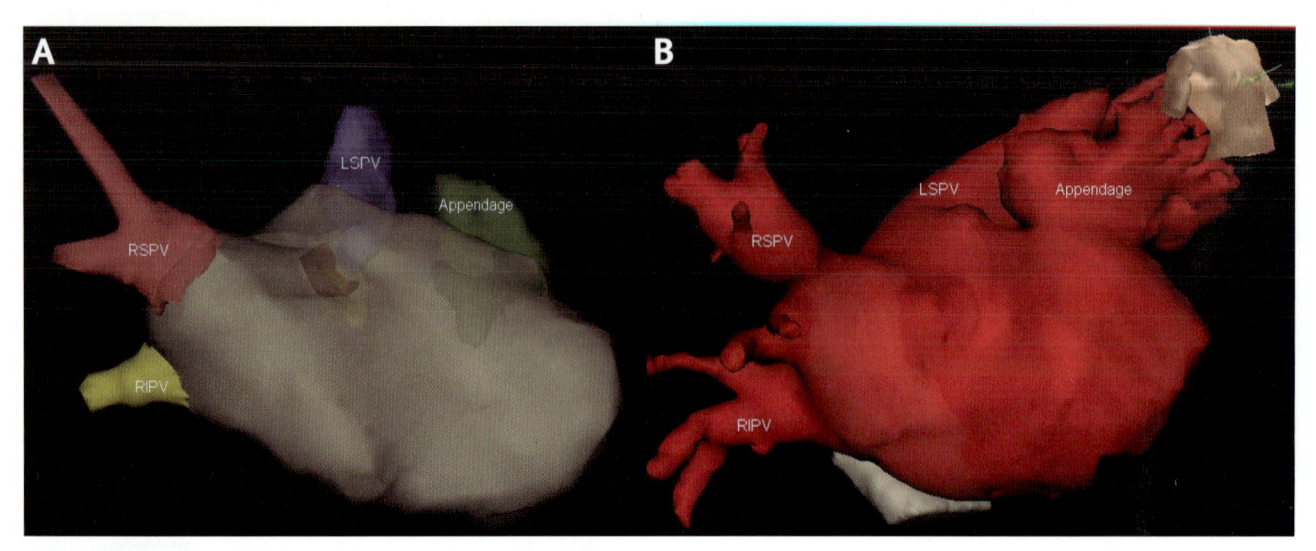

Figure 14.3 RAO view of an electroanatomic map (**A**) merged with a three dimensional CT image (**B**).

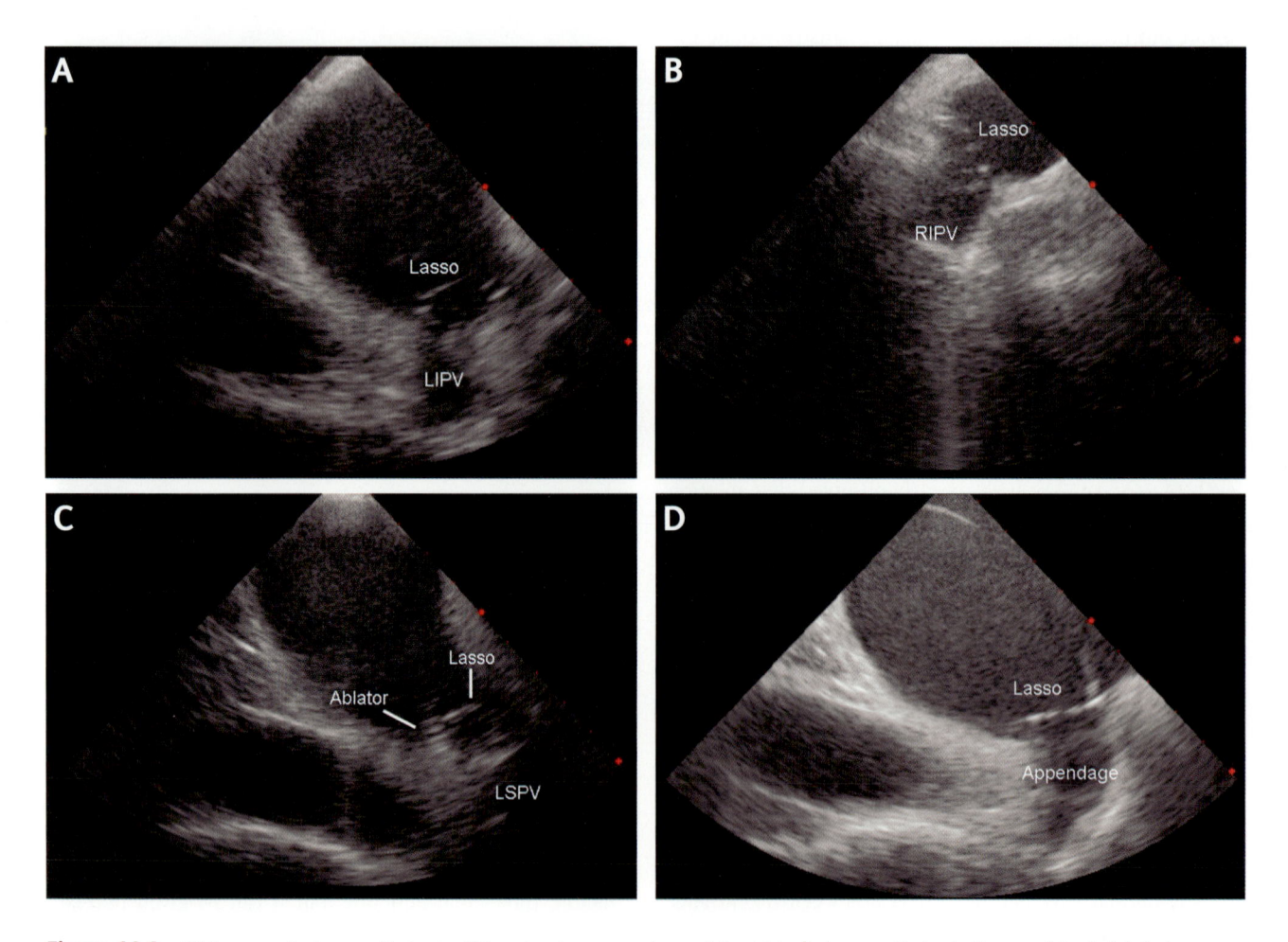

Figure 14.4 ICE images of a lasso catheter in different pulmonary veins and the LAA. **A.** Lasso catheter in the os of the left inferior pulmonary vein. **B.** Lasso catheter in the os of the RIPV. **C.** Lasso catheter and ablator in the os of the LSPV. **D.** Lasso catheter in the os of the LAA.

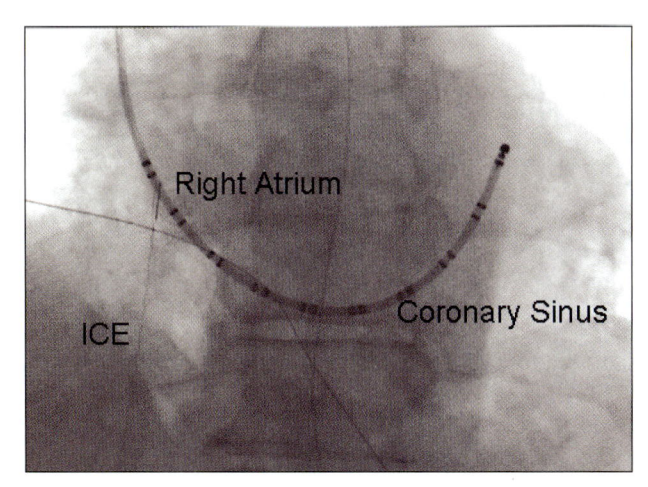

Figure 14.5 Positioning of the duodecapolar catheter and ICE catheter.

Transseptal Puncture

Two transseptal punctures are performed using ICE guidance. Care is taken to cross into the LA in a posterior direction along the septum such that the left-sided PVs are in clear view using ICE imaging during tenting and prior to crossing the septum (**Figure 14.6**, ▶ **Videos 14.4 and 14.5**). Manual pressure can be used to advance a mechanical transseptal needle within the guiding sheath and dilator into the LA. In our recent experience, a blunted, RF-powered transseptal needle (Baylis transseptal needle, Baylis Medical Company Inc., Montreal, QC, Canada) requires less force and permits crossing into the LA with more control. Successful transseptal puncture can be confirmed with visualization of contrast or of bubbles in the LA on fluoroscopy or echocardiography, respectively. Transduction of LA pressure can be used to check for aortic puncture. After the first transseptal puncture, the lasso catheter is advanced through the transseptal sheath and fixed in one of the PVs during the second transseptal puncture. Although a second transseptal sheath can be introduced via wire exchange, we find that a separate transseptal puncture minimizes sheath-to-sheath interaction.

Selection of Guiding Sheaths and Catheters

LA access can be obtained using a variety of guiding sheaths. We have found that guiding sheaths with a moderate primary curve and no secondary curve, such as the Daig SL-0 (St. Jude Medical, St. Paul, MN) for the ablation catheter and a LAMP-90 for the circular mapping catheter, allow for easier guidance to the posterior aspect of the LA.

A lasso catheter is used as a roving catheter for mapping and directing the ablation catheter. The catheter should be small enough to move within the chamber easily but of a large enough diameter that it does not readily fall deep inside the PVs. In most adults, a 20-mm, 10-pole lasso catheter provides a balance between maneuverability and size. Although the procedure may be performed without a lasso catheter, lasso-guided ablation allows for much more efficient targeting of electrical potentials. One can check for electrical signal reduction in real time during the ablation procedure with lasso guidance.

The use of RF for energy delivery has become standard in performing PVAI. Compared to passively cooled catheters, open irrigated catheters allow for delivery of greater power without significant temperature rise or clot formation, enabling more efficient delivery of larger lesion sets.[4] There are two main disadvantages to using open irrigation catheters. The first is a higher risk of "pops," pericardial effusions, and gastrointestinal complaints with the open-irrigation catheters. These can be minimized with appropriate titration of energy delivery. The second is a small drop in hematocrit that we frequently note after the procedure in the absence of blood loss. This drop is likely due to irrigation, an infusion of 2 to 4 liters in each case. Our catheter of choice is a Thermocool 3.5-mm tip catheter with an F curve (Biosense Webster Inc, Diamond Bar, CA). A smaller curve may be considered in the minority of patients with very small atria, and a J curve for patients with large atria.

Mapping

The use of 3-dimensional mapping systems has facilitated PVAI significantly. Although not necessary, they do permit efficient registration of ablation sites and documentation of the extent of antral ablation. Any electroanatomic mapping system may be used, but currently only the EnSite NavX Navigation & Visualization Technology (St. Jude Medical, St. Paul, MN) and the Carto-3 System (Biosense Webster, Diamond Bar, CA) allow real-time display of any cardiac catheter during ablation. The ability to display a lasso catheter allows for very rapid creation of a LA map and direction of the ablation catheter toward the desired poles on the lasso catheter.

Early and accurate identification and mapping of the PVs and LAA also facilitate the procedure. We have found that the use of ICE during mapping of the PVs with the lasso catheter helps confirm the location of each of the PVs (**Figure 14.4**). On ICE, the left-sided PVs can be found a few degrees after the appendage on clockwise rotation of the ICE catheter. To image the right PVs, the ICE catheter must first be advanced slightly and further rotated clockwise. The appendage can be recognized by a high amplitude signal on the superior-anterior aspect of the LA.

Ablation

The goals of PVAI are to achieve PVI and to eliminate electrical signals in the antrum of the LA. Using lasso guidance, lesions are delivered throughout the antral

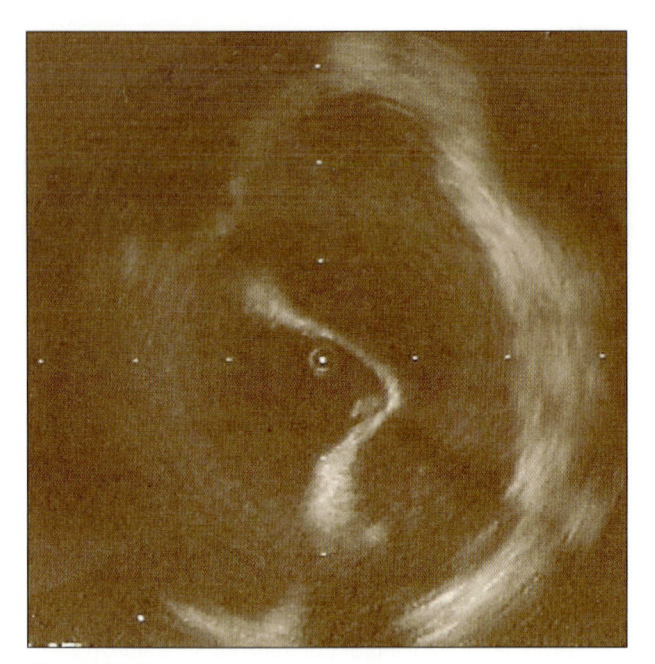

Figure 14.6 Tenting of the atrial septum before transseptal puncture.

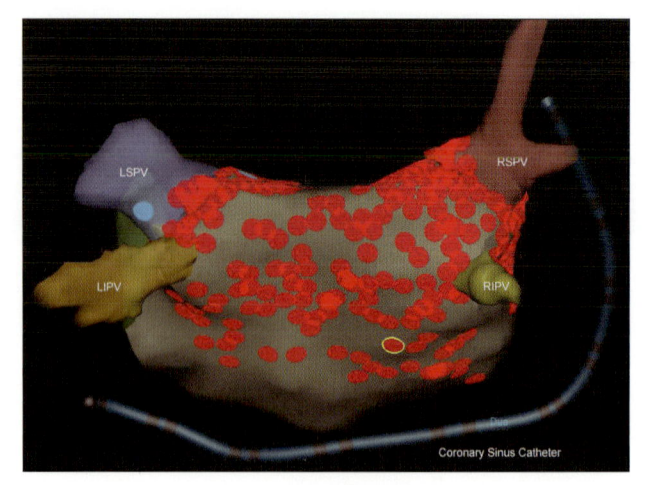

Figure 14.7 Lesions delivered with PV antral isolation.

surface, including the areas between and around the PVs and the roof of the atrium (**Figure 14.7**). Electrical potentials are identified on the roving lasso catheter, and the ablation catheter is maneuvered to these targets.

Using an irrigated-tip catheter, we begin with 30 W of energy and titrate to a maximum of 40 W, with a maximum temperature of 42°C. Occasionally, a higher wattage is needed, but we generally do not exceed 45 W. Our approach is to deliver energy in a continuous manner, maneuvering the ablation catheter to different sites on the lasso catheter until the electrical signals are eliminated.

Contact with the lasso catheter can be seen with fluoroscopy (**Figure 14.8**) and with 3-dimensional imaging (**Figure 14.9**) and can be confirmed by observing electrical interaction between the two catheters. Assuring catheter contact also helps avoid ablation deep inside the PVs. We perform most of our procedures in the AP or RAO view; however, an orthogonal view is often helpful when lasso-ablator contact is not clear. The LAO view can also be helpful when ablating around the right-sided PVs.

Once lasso contact is confirmed, energy is delivered for approximately 20 seconds per lesion site or until the electrical signals have diminished. In areas near the esophagus, we typically deliver energy for 15 to 20 seconds per lesion site, taking care to move the catheter during ablation to different areas and returning at a later time once the esophagus has cooled. We monitor esophageal temperatures closely and will frequently readjust the esophageal

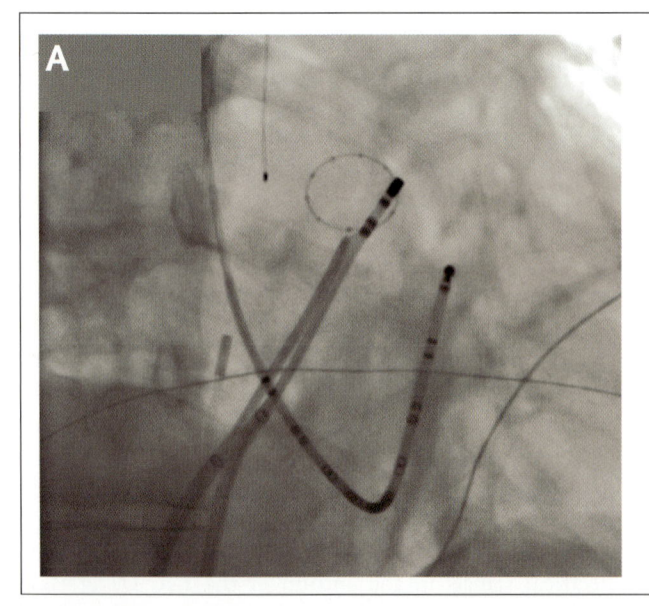

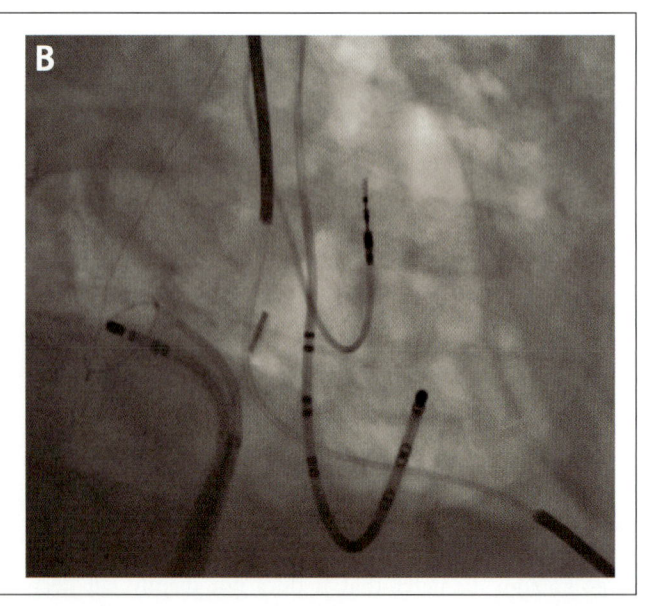

Figure 14.8 Fluoroscopic RAO view of the ablation catheter in contact with the lasso catheter at different PV ostea. **A.** Lasso at the LSPV os. **B.** Lasso at the RSPV os in a patient with a dual-chamber defibrillator.

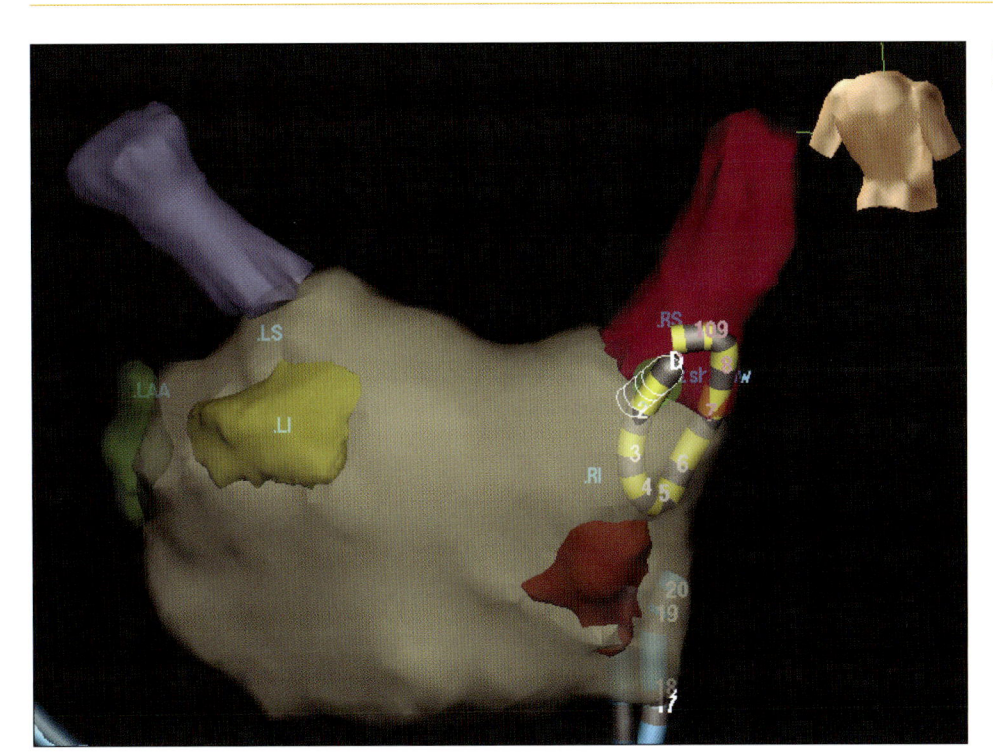

Figure 14.9 Lasso-directed ablation near the RSPV ostium.

probe close to the ablation area. A rapid rise in temperature is often noted, and when this happens, the ablation catheter should be moved away immediately. Despite movement of the catheter, delayed rise in esophageal temperatures is often observed. Esophageal temperatures greater than 38° to 39°C should be avoided to minimize the risk of deep tissue injury.

We usually begin with lasso-guided ablation of electrical potentials surrounding each PV. PV electrical isolation can be confirmed by entrance and exit block. The lasso catheter can be placed in each of the PVs, and entrance block can be confirmed by the absence of electrical signals where these signals had been previously observed. Occasionally, dissociated PV potentials can be recorded (**Figure 14.10**) to confirm exit block. In addition, pacing from within the PV to confirm exit block can be performed, although we do not confirm exit block routinely.

Once PVI is achieved, we focus on the remaining antral areas. The lasso catheter is particularly useful for identifying additional electrical potentials along the posterior wall and roof of the LA. As before, the ablator is maneuvered to the lasso poles, where the potentials are observed and energy is delivered.

We have observed a high degree of variation in the effort required to eliminate electrical signals. Some patients have a rapid reduction in electrical amplitude, and others require extensive energy delivery. We try to eliminate all electrical activity, whether or not it is believed to be a driver of AF, in the antrum and roof of the LA. The procedure can be done while the patient is in either AF or sinus rhythm.

We often complete ablation in approximately 2 hours for most patients with AF who require PVAI. After the catheter is withdrawn into the right atrium, the lasso catheter is advanced into the SVC at the site of entry into the right atrium. Potentials in this area are then targeted for ablation as well. Care is taken to deliver pacing stimuli at a high output along the lateral wall of the SVC to delineate the course of the right phrenic nerve and to avoid ablation near the nerve.

When patients remain in AF at the end of the procedure, cardioversion is performed and electrical signals that remain in the antrum, which can be larger during sinus rhythm, are targeted. When patients are in sinus rhythm at the end of the procedure, 20 to 30 mcg/kg/min of isoproterenol are infused and further sites are ablated if they appear to trigger either consistent PACs or atrial arrhythmias.

Adjunctive Ablation Sites

In young patients with paroxysmal atrial fibrillation, elimination of PV and antral triggers may be sufficient for success. In patients with more primary structural disease, extension of the ablation to other sites in the atria may prove beneficial, though most of these approaches have not been well studied. Additional ablation along the septum just anterior to the right PV antrum may improve success rates. Isolation of the SVC and CS may also be beneficial in select populations with permanent AF. Ablation of CFAE as an adjunct to PVAI often helps organize the atrial rhythm into AT or AFL. In PVAI, aggressive ablation with the goal of termination of AF and associated

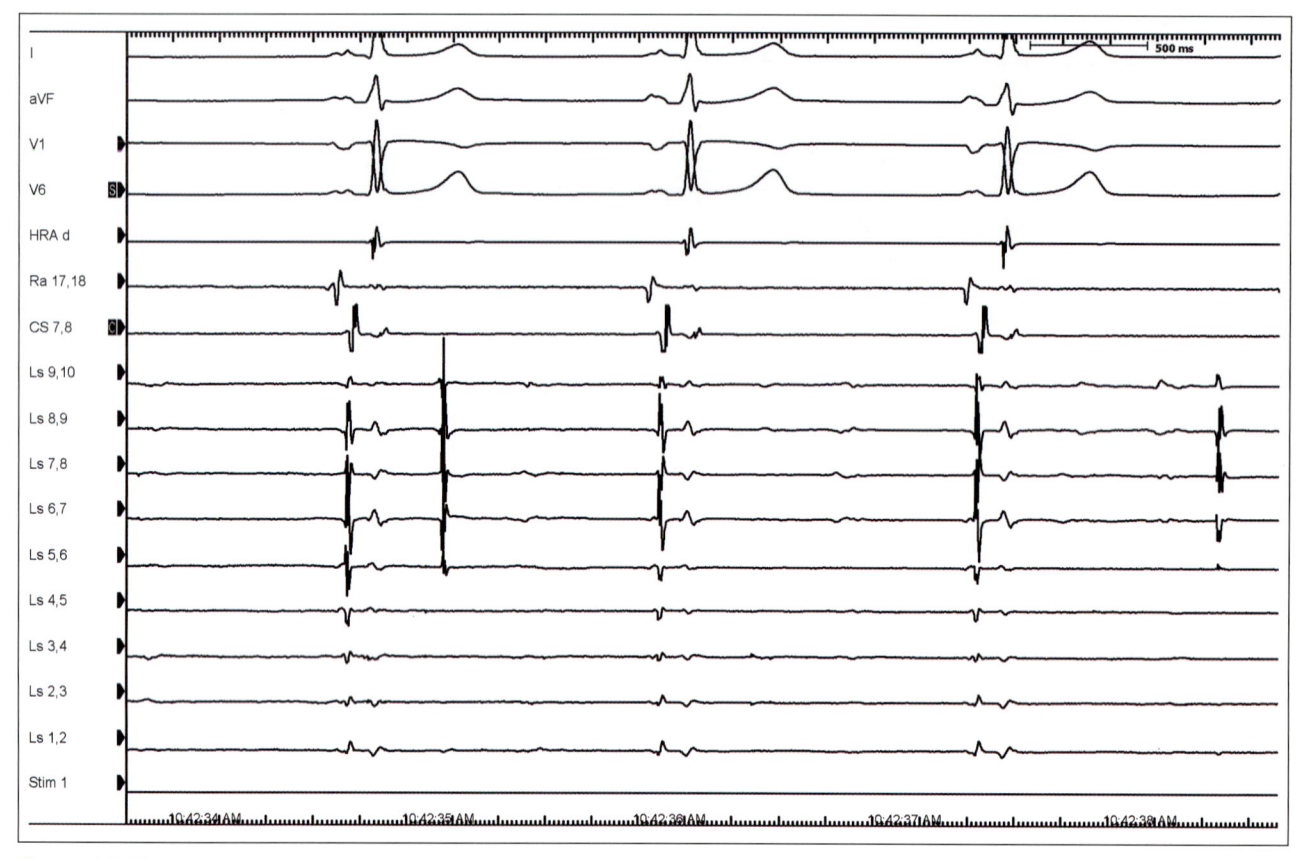

Figure 14.10 Dissociated PV potentials. The lasso catheter is in the LIPV.

organized tachycardias does not correlate with long-term success of ablation.[5] Patients with documented typical AFL will undergo concomitant CTI ablation immediately following PVAI. Ablation of the antrum may also result in ablation of the ganglionic plexi, which are believed to play a role in the triggering and maintenance of AF.[6] The extension of the ablation to further areas of the LA, such as the floor or anterior wall, may also prove beneficial, particularly in patients who have previously undergone ablation and are found to have an electrically silent antrum. In this group, electrical isolation of the LAA might be required to cure AF.

Postprocedure Care

Recovery

Following ablation, the guiding sheaths are pulled out of the LA and heparin is stopped. Protamine can be given to help reverse the heparin, and access sheaths can be pulled once the activated clotting time is less than 180 seconds. Many patients will have a large net positive fluid balance when irrigated-tip catheters are used, and diuretics can be administered accordingly. Patients will typically lie flat for 6 hours after sheaths are pulled due to the large sheaths used. We also begin anticoagulation 6 hours after sheaths are pulled.

All patients are treated with warfarin after ablation. Patients for whom warfarin was discontinued prior to the procedure are given an i.v. heparin bridge overnight, without a bolus, and then transitioned to low-molecular-weight heparin the following morning. There is no need for a heparin bridge for patients whose warfarin was not discontinued. We administer half of a full dose of enoxaparin (0.5mg/kg twice a day) to maintain stroke prophylaxis and minimize bleeding complications until the warfarin is therapeutic. Patients are usually discharged the following day. For patients who undergo the procedure with a therapeutic INR, low-molecular-weight heparin is not needed.

Follow-Up

Patients are followed closely for the year following a PVAI ablation procedure. We typically see our patients in clinic 3, 6, and 12 months afterward, having routine outpatient multiday event monitoring take place before each visit. We typically do not change a patient's antiarrhythmic regimen during the first 2 to 3 months, and the decision to discontinue, continue, or change antiarrhythmics depends on the burden of AF. All patients, regardless of stroke risk, are anticoagulated with warfarin for the first 3 months.

The choice of long-term anticoagulation depends heavily on the CHADS$_2$ score. Patients with a score of 0 or 1 can be comfortably taken off warfarin after 3 months. The long-term stroke risk of patients with a score of 2 or greater following PVAI ablation is not well studied, but those with lower risk and without recurrence of AF may be considered for discontinuation.

Repeat Ablations

Success rates as high as 67% in persistent/permanent AF and 77% in paroxismal AF with a single PVAI have been reported.[1] We explain to patients up front, however, that second and sometimes third procedures could be necessary. In patients with recurrent AF, the burden of the disease and symptoms are often mitigated. Many conditions that could not previously be controlled by medication can now be controlled with antiarrhythmic agents. In some patients, particularly those with permanent AF, PVAI may serve as a modifier of the underlying disease substrate, making AF more manageable.

When patients have symptomatic AF or a high burden of recurrence after at least a 3-month window, despite antiarrhythmic therapy, we discuss repeat ablation with them. The procedural approach to a second PVAI is similar to the first procedure. Most patients, to varying degrees, have recurrence of PV conduction and return of antral electrical signals. During repeat ablations, we isolate the PVs again and more aggressively target antral areas near the esophagus that may have been avoided during the first ablation due to esophageal heating. This often takes several short applications of energy with intervening periods of cooling.

Procedural Complications

Careful hemodynamic and temperature monitoring during the ablation procedure allows avoidance or early detection of potential complications. During ablation, sudden drops in blood pressure or oxygen saturation should be evaluated carefully. Although a vagal response to ablation near ganglionic plexi may result in transient hypotension and bradycardia, evaluation of cardiac tamponade should be made if there is no immediate recovery. Suspicion should be higher after a difficult transseptal puncture or an inadvertent application of excess pressure in the appendage or the roof of the atrium. Assessment for pericardial effusion causing tamponade can be performed initially with ICE, but TTE is necessary for a more comprehensive evaluation.

Since patients are anticoagulated following the procedure, the most common complications are vascular, including hematomas and arteriovenous fistulas, occurring in approximately 1 to 2% of patients. Less than 0.5% of patients suffer from a cerebrovascular accident. Since PVAI involves extensive burning near the esophagus, esophageal-atrial fistulas can present in the weeks following ablation, though these are exceedingly rare. Phrenic nerve paralysis can also occur but is often reversible. Patients presenting with shortness of breath should be evaluated for phrenic nerve paralysis and PV stenosis, both of which are usually reversible. Effusions without hemodynamic compromise are sometimes noted following the procedure. Most asymptomatic effusions can be managed conservatively.

Advantages and Limitations

Few randomized, long-term studies have been performed comparing PVAI to other AF ablation approaches. Although concerns of impairment in atrial function have been raised with such an extensive ablation set, no significant functional impairment has been observed on follow-up imaging.[7] Small studies have shown significantly higher success rates of PVAI when compared with CFAE.[8] In patients with permanent AF, PVAI has been shown to be superior to wide-area circumferential ablation alone.[9]

New onset of atypical AFL is often observed in patients who undergo wide-area circumferential PVI with addition of adjunctive lines, such as those along the roof or mitral isthmus. It has been our experience, however, that these tachycardias are highly unusual after PVAI, possibly because the substrate for reentry has been ablated.

The PVAI approach, particularly when lasso guidance and electroanatomical mapping are used, can cut down AF ablation time considerably. The total procedural time is typically reduced to approximately 3 hours. Although the procedure can be performed by a single operator, using two operators—one controlling the lasso and the other controlling the ablator—can expedite the procedure further.

Conclusions

In summary, PVAI is an approach to PVI that targets the tissue around the PV as well as the posterior LA and roof that encompass extensions of the PV smooth musculature and may function as triggers of AF. This approach to AF ablation may result in higher success rates compared to others, such as CFAE, and may result in a lower incidence of AT, but large comparative studies are lacking. The approach has been facilitated greatly by preoperative imaging, ICE, lasso guidance, and 3-dimensional electroanatomic mapping. In experienced hands, the procedure time using these tools can be cut down to an average of 3 to 4 hours.

Although it is generally agreed that PVI is necessary during AF ablation, there has not been consensus regarding the extent and location of additional ablative lesions. Further studies are necessary to determine if ablation in the floor of the LA or other areas should be targeted in addition to PVAI. Technological advances may also permit further improvement in the efficiency of the procedure. Our early experience with robotic catheter manipulation to perform PVAI has resulted in a diminished need for energy output and also increased comfort and protection from radiation for the primary operator. Future studies will be necessary to assess the advantages and success rates of remotely operated catheter control systems. AF ablation has progressed significantly, and further studies will help us determine the optimal strategy to cure this disease.

References

1. Mommersteeg MT, Christoffels VM, Anderson RH, Moorman AF. Atrial fibrillation: a developmental point of view. *Heart Rhythm.* 2009;6(12):1818–1824.
2. Bhargava M, Di Biase L, Mohanty P, et al. Impact of type of atrial fibrillation and repeat catheter ablation on long-term freedom from atrial fibrillation: results from a multicenter study. *Heart Rhythm.* 2009;6(10):1403–1412.
3. Di Biase L, Burkhardt JD, Mohanty P, et al. Periprocedural stroke and management of major bleeding complications in patients undergoing catheter ablation of atrial fibrillation: the impact of periprocedural therapeutic international normalized ratio. *Circulation.* 2011;121(23):2550–2556.
4. Kanj MH, Wazni O, Fahmy T, et al. Pulmonary vein antral isolation using an open irrigation ablation catheter for the treatment of atrial fibrillation: a randomized pilot study. *J Am Coll Cardiol.* Apr 17 2007;49(15):1634–1641.
5. Elayi CS, Di Biase L, Barrett C, et al. Atrial fibrillation termination as a procedural endpoint during ablation in long-standing persistent atrial fibrillation. *Heart Rhythm.* 2010;7(9):1216–1223.
6. Hou Y, Scherlag BJ, Lin J, et al. Ganglionated plexi modulate extrinsic cardiac autonomic nerve input: effects on sinus rate, atrioventricular conduction, refractoriness, and inducibility of atrial fibrillation. *J Am Coll Cardiol.* 2007;50(1):61–68.
7. Verma A, Kilicaslan F, Adams JR, et al. Extensive ablation during pulmonary vein antrum isolation has no adverse impact on left atrial function: an echocardiography and cine computed tomography analysis. *J Cardiovasc Electrophysiol.* 2006;17(7):741–746.
8. Di Biase L, Elayi CS, Fahmy TS, et al. Atrial fibrillation ablation strategies for paroxysmal patients: randomized comparison between different techniques. *Circ Arrhythm Electrophysiol.* 2009;2(2):113–119.
9. Elayi CS, Verma A, Di Biase L, et al. Ablation for long-standing permanent atrial fibrillation: results from a randomized study comparing three different strategies. *Heart Rhythm.* 2008;5(12):1658-1664.

Video Descriptions

Video 14.1 Thickened atrial septum seen on echo.

Video 14.2 A "fly-through" left atrium CT reconstruction.

Video 14.3 ICE video, panning from the MV to the right PVs.

Video 14.4 ICE video, transseptal puncture.

Video 14.5 Fluoroscopy, transseptal puncture.

CHAPTER 15

How to Perform Circumferential Ablation for Atrial Fibrillation

Carlo Pappone, MD, PhD; Vincenzo Santinelli, MD

Introduction

Currently, atrial fibrillation is considered to be one of the key factors in the cardiovascular epidemic of the 21st century. Its increased morbidity and mortality are alarming. Currently, the most effective therapy for paroxysmal or persistent AF is catheter ablation rather than chronic antiarrhythmic drug therapy. At present, 20 years after transcutaneous catheter ablation of APs, catheter ablation of AF is the most commonly performed ablation procedure worldwide in most major hospitals without serious complications, and the progress made is indeed remarkable. Successful ablation of AF also prevents the occurrence and progression of electrical, structural, and mechanical myocardium remodelling, improves function of the left ventricle in patients with heart failure, and prevents the risk of thrombembolism. Onset of sinus rhythm activates the reversal of remodelling, leading to wall reconstruction and atrial size reduction. Therefore, catheter ablation of AF has become a widely accepted and practiced therapeutic strategy. In many laboratories worldwide, ablation techniques have evolved over the years, particularly for the two distinct forms of paroxysmal and persistent AF, from PVI alone[1] to additional ablation, as initially performed by circumferential pulmonary vein ablation (CPVA).[2] In patients with paroxysmal AF but without LA enlargment and structural heart disease or with minimal atrial enlargment, PVI alone may be sufficient, particularly in the initial phase of the arrhythmia.[1] The possibility that rapidly discharging atrial foci frequently located in the PVs could serve as a driver also for AF perpetuation led to several attempts to treat more complex AF forms by PVI alone, which resulted in insufficient and repeated procedures were frequently required. Additional linear lesions led to higher success rates with a single ablation procedure and without serious complications in patients with paroxysmal AF and LA enlargement as well as in those with persistent AF. It is conceivable that further ablation eliminates more atrial substrates and partially compartmentalizes the atria with the purpose of preventing macroreentrant circuits, which have been postulated to sustain AF. Currently, PVI plus linear ablation is the most common ablation strategy to treat patients with AF; higher success rates are reported, but repeat procedures are frequently required. Over the next few years, it is likely that with technological advancement and newer tools, single-procedure success rates will dramatically increase in many EP laboratories worldwide, avoiding repeated procedures with potential complications.

Technological Advances and New Tools

Although great progress has been made in improving the safety and efficacy of AF ablation strategy, much research is still needed. New technologies such as multi-image integration with mapping systems, rotational angiography, and remote magnetic navigation systems are being developed to address many of the limitations preventing this procedure from being more commonplace with higher success rate after a single procedure.[3,4] With the expected increase in the prevalence of AF and expanding indications for ablation, new technologies are welcome additions to the current tools in delivering optimal therapies. At present, new tools, technologies, and techniques are under investigation in our EP laboratory in order to improve safety and efficacy of a single ablation procedure, particularly for patients with long-standing persistent AF. These technologies include irrigated remote magnetic catheters and systems to better address the technological demands of the remote procedure, improved imaging and electrical mapping systems including rotational angiography, and MRI-guided ablation strategies. In inexperienced centers, it may be challenging to achieve complete electrical isolation of the PVs and additional contiguous transmural linear lesions while avoiding gaps on the lesion line. Imaging integration enables electroanatomic guidance during mapping and ablation by showing 3-dimensional, preacquired computed tomography or magnetic resonance images and the relative real-time position of the ablation catheter on the screens of these systems. Recently, we have developed a new imaging technology using "rotational angiography" integrated with electroanatomic systems such as CARTO or NavX systems, which uses standard fluoroscopy to obtain multiple images while rotating around the patient. The contrast is injected into the pulmonary artery or directly into the LA itself by transseptal puncture. The C arm is rapidly rotated, and images are immediately acquired during rotation while contrast fills the LA. If the contrast is injected into the pulmonary artery, a timing bolus is performed to evaluate how long until the LA fills and how long it remains opacified to assess the optimal timing of image acquisition. All images are processed by a dedicated software to produce 3-dimensional CT-quality images, which can be used during the same procedure (**Figures 15.1** and **15.2**). Since CT-type images are acquired during the procedure, they represent a real anatomy rather than a remotely acquired image. Like CT, the images can be viewed or integrated into the imaging

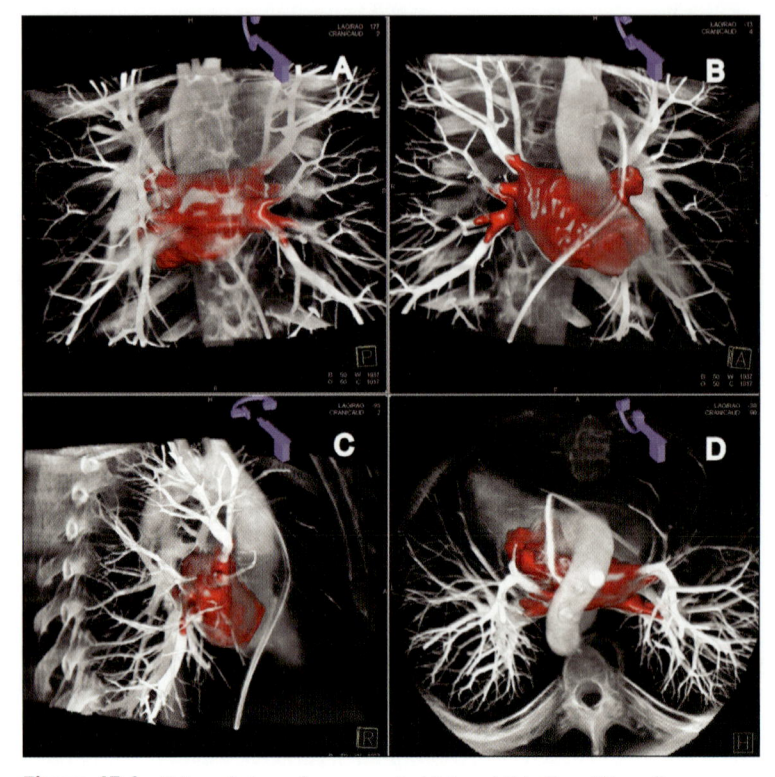

Figure 15.1 External view of a segmented LA and PVs. DynaCT cardiac segmentation surface of the LA and PVs (red). Panels show (**A**) posterior-anterior, (**B**) anterior-posterior, and (**C**) latero-lateral projections as well as (**D**) superior tilted view.

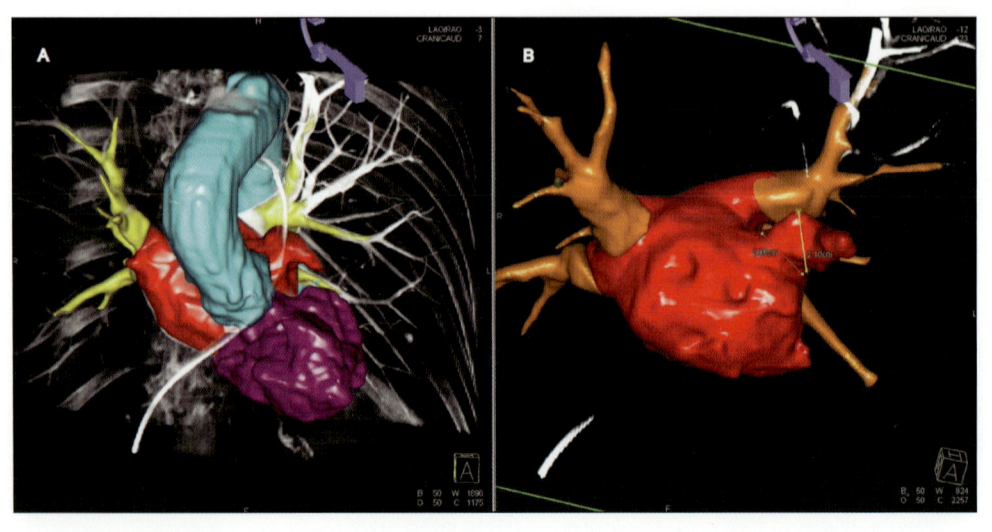

Figure 15.2 Three-dimensional reconstruction from DynaCT and rotational angiography of the LA (red) and adjacent structures in anterior-posterior view. (Panels **A** and **B**).

system or electroanatomical mapping system (**Figure 15.3**). In our laboratory, we use the Artis zeego (Siemens, Medical Erlangen, Germany), which is a car-manufacturing type of robotic arm able to manipulate the fluoroscopic C arm (**Figure 15.4A**). This permits a greater freedom of movement of the C arm and a platform for very rapid rotation. The robotic arm can move up and down the table and in any rotational axis because it is not fixed in space. This technology increases image quality and makes acquisition much easier. In our experience, rotational imaging integration provides accurate visual information with improvement in the procedure parameters, and its anatomical accuracy is comparable to that of CT with lower radiation dose, shorter time, and more cost effectiveness. Now that AF ablation represents the preferred treatment strategy, technological innovation is strongly required so that the procedure can be safely and effectively performed by many operators in a short period of time with high success rates and low complication rates, particularly for patients with long-standing persistent AF.

Remote Ablation

Remote technologies have been developed in our laboratory to allow optimal catheter stability and reproducible catheter movements with the aim of achieving contiguous and transmural lesion delivery.[3,4] A novel system for remote navigation of catheters within the heart has been developed in our laboratory; this is based on a magnetic navigation system (Niobe®, Stereotaxis, St. Louis, MO), which has proven to be feasible for performing ablation of complex arrhythmias, such as AF. The robotic magnetic catheter navigation system consists of two

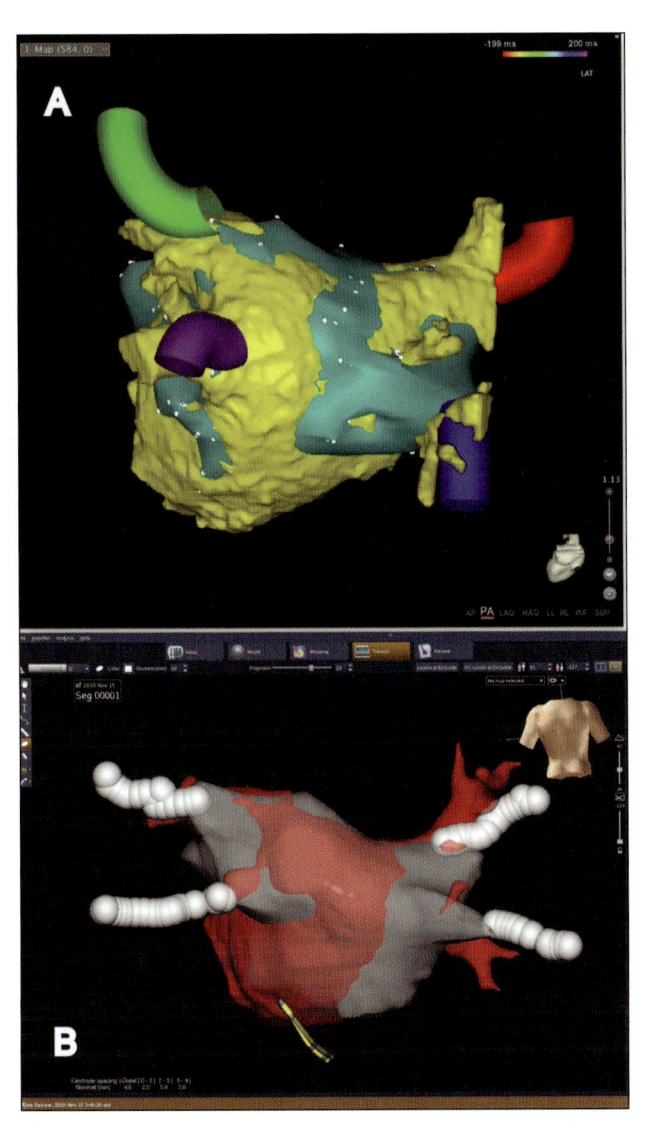

Figure 15.3 Cardiac segmentation surface of LA and PVs by rotational angiography integrated into 2 electroanatomic mapping systems. CartoMerge, Biosense Webster Inc. (**A**) and Ensite Velocity, St. Jude Medical (**B**).

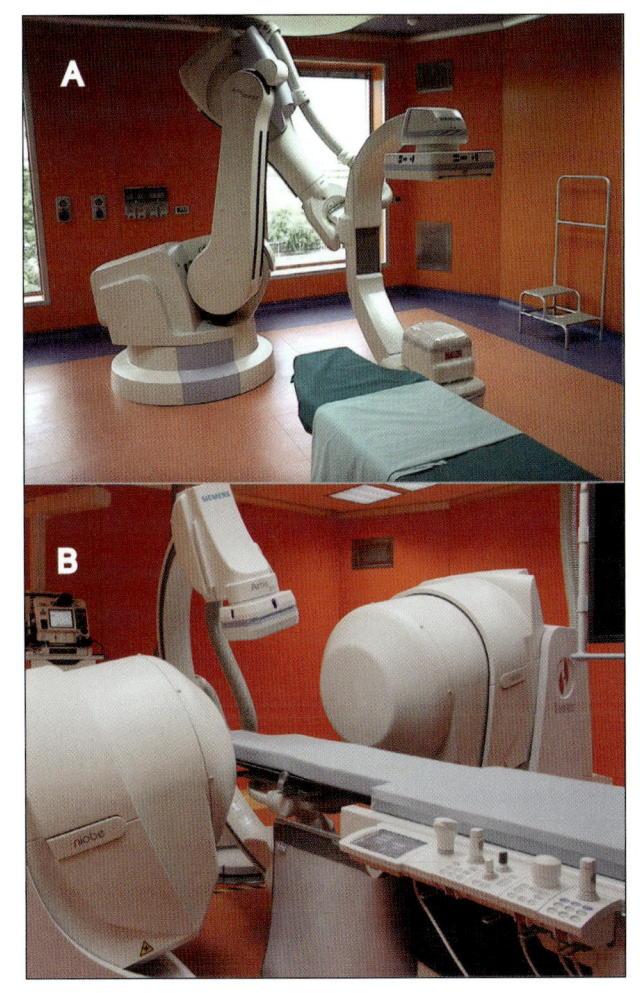

Figure 15.4 **A.** The "Artis zeego" system (Siemens, Medical Erlangen, Germany). **B.** The remote magnetic ablation system (Niobe, Stereotaxis, St. Louis, MO).

computer-controlled, focused-field, permanent magnets placed on either side of the patient (**Figure 15.4B**). The magnetic field creates a spherical navigation volume of 20 cm, in which a catheter containing 3 magnets is introduced and manipulated via the magnetic field vectors. The operator navigates the catheter using a joystick and keyboard commands from a separate control room (**Figure 15.5**). Our experience has shown similar single-procedure success rates for AF ablation compared to that of manual ablation, with reduction in fluoroscopy times.[4] The early learning curve demonstrated longer procedure times, mainly due to additional setup times. However, by performing increasing numbers of remote ablation procedures, fluoroscopy times have been lower than manual ablation. As the demand for catheter ablation for arrhythmias such as AF increases and the number of centers performing these ablations increases, the demand for systems that reduce the hand-skill requirement and improve the comfort of the operator will also increase. Until recently, irrigated ablation catheters were not available for use in conjunction with the Niobe system. However, this important limitation was overcome when irrigated ablation catheters were released, and they are now being used for AF ablation procedures at the many sites with a Niobe system. Currently, a novel-tip irrigated magnetic catheter is available for remote ablation.[4] The magnetic irrigated ablation produces deeper and effective lesions without char formation as for the first series of solid magnetic catheters.[3] At present, the safety and effectiveness of the Niobe system appear to be similar to conventional ablation tools.

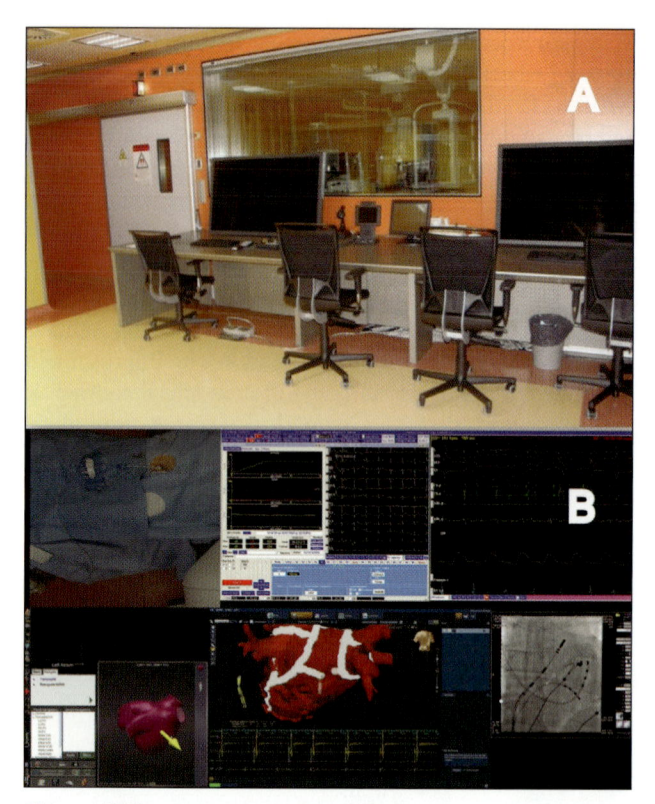

Figure 15.5 The operating room (**A**) for remote mapping and ablation with Odyssey (Stereotaxis, St. Louis, MO) screen, which combines disparate systems into a single content management solution (**B**).

Catheter Ablation of Atrial Fibrillation

Since 1999, we have performed standard CPVA guided by 3-dimensional electroanatomic systems in order to disconnect all PV as well as to eliminate or limit potentially arrhythmogenic substrates in patients with AF.[2] As initially proposed by our group, CPVA has been successfully applied over the years to a broad range of patients with AF, including the paroxysmal and persistent forms with or without LA enlargment, with or without structural heart diseases or comorbidities, all of which are commonly found in the vast majority of patients with AF. The high single-procedure success rates without serious complications, both in the short- (1 year) and long-term follow-up, suggest that CPVA is perhaps the most appropriate strategy to cure the vast majority of patients with AF. By contrast, the ablation technique of PVI alone, as initially proposed by the Bordeaux group,[1] was limited to patients with paroxysmal AF without LA enlargement and without structural heart disease. Unfortunately, for patients with LA enlargement and/or structural heart disease or with comorbidities, as well as for those with persistent AF, the PVI-alone strategy was insufficient to obtain a good outcome. Therefore, it is now widely accepted that in such patient populations, which represent the vast majority of patients with AF, additional linear lesions targeting the substrate for arrhythmia maintenance are required beyond PVI alone.[2]

CPVA Procedure

The circumferential PV ablation is the standard procedure for patients with AF. Currently, mapping and ablation are guided by new specially designed 3-dimensional electroanatomic systems (CARTO, NavX), including but not limited to rotational angiography (Figures 15.1–15.3). The procedure is performed by a single transseptal puncture and usually with manual tip-irrigated catheters or remotely by magnetic tip-irrigated catheters. The technique consists of large circumferential lesions to perform a point-by-point tailored electrical isolation of PVs with additional linear lesion lines, all of which are usually validated by pacing maneuvers (**Figure 15.6**). Noninducibility of both AF and AT at the end of the procedure is required and, if after achieving sinus rhythm AF/AT are still inducible, all lesion lines and encircled areas are accurately revisited for potentially residual gaps and eliminated if necessary. Data from our laboratory show that among patients with AF and minimally enlarged atria, a single CPVA procedure results in success rates up to 90%. However, patients with long-standing persistent AF (> 1 year of duration) may require further bi-atrial ablation in a stepwise fashion in order to achieve a stable sinus rhythm with noninducibility of AF/AT by a single but prolonged procedure (> 3 hours). This time-consuming stepwise lesion strategy consists of a sequential ablation of structures that are supposed to be critical for maintenance of AF, all of which are essentially identified by the effect of their ablation on the AF CL and inducibility of AF/AT. The order and extent in which the extra–CPVA standard lesion set is applied may be variable from patient to patient based upon clinical characteristics.

Endpoints of CPVA

Step 1: PV electrical isolation.

Electrical isolation of the PVs is the first step of CPVA and consists of a series of point-by-point RF lesions, which are performed outside the ostium of the PVs, an area usually termed as antra. Linear lesions encircle both left and right PVs individually or in pairs to electrically disconnect all PVs (**Figure 15.7**). Validation by Lasso catheter is not routinely performed since we have demonstrated a true distal electrical isolation by potential abatement (> 90% reduction of EGM amplitude or < 0.1 mV) even within the encircled areas.[5] PV disconnection is obtained by good catheter stability and optimal wall contact, which results in rapid attenuation of atrial EGMs during each RF energy application up to complete elimination for up to 50 seconds, usually within a few seconds, depending on the local effect. Partially ablated signals require further RF applications before ablating the next ablation site.

Figure 15.6 The standard set of lesions (red points) as performed in CPVA in different views guided by anatomical CartoMerge maps.

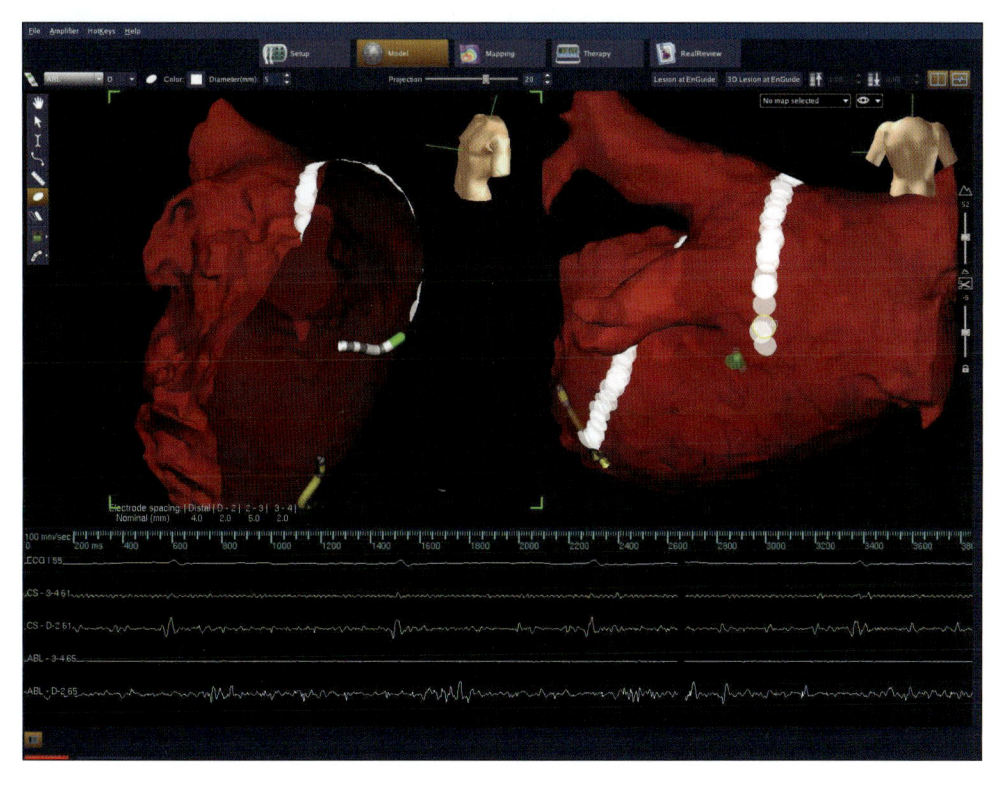

Figure 15.7 LA and PVs anatomical map (red) obtained by Ensite Velocity System integrated by DynaCT. The mitral isthmus line and an ongoing circumferential lesion line encircling the left PVs in pairs are shown. Ablation points are marked as white dots.

Step 2: Vagal denervation.

The relationship between AF and the autonomic nervous system is an area of intense research. Our group was the first to report a link between stimulation of the autonomic nervous system during AF ablation and ablation outcome.[6] We reported that one-third of patients undergoing AF ablation develop a vagal reflex during AF ablation. Therefore, during any procedure, an important endpoint is termination of vagal reflexes, followed by sinus tachycardia or AF. Failure to reproduce baseline reflexes despite repeat RF applications is considered as confirmation of denervation. This observation was associated with a 99% success rate as compared with an 85% success rate among patients in whom a vagal reflex was not observed.[6] These results have stimulated several groups to further explore the potential role of targeting autonomic ganglia as a stand-alone or adjunctive AF ablation strategy. Detailed "autonomic maps" of the LA as a target for ablation have been reported by our group.[6] We believe that more research is needed to better define the role of catheter ablation of autonomic ganglia in the treatment of patients with AF.

Steps 3 and 4: Posterior lines connecting the superior and inferior PVs and the mitral isthmus lines.

In the standard CPVA, additional ablation lines are deployed along the back and the roof of LA between the two sets of PVs connecting the superior and inferior PVs (**Figure 15.8**) and the mitral valve annulus (**Figure 15.9**). The roof line requires a few minutes of RF delivery without use of fluoroscopy. The mitral isthmus line is performed to prevent postablation macroreentrant LA tachycardias[7-9] and to further reduce the substrate for arrhythmia perpetuation. A complete LA roof line may be demonstrated by activation progressing in a caudocranial direction on the posterior wall during LAA pacing. Validation of the mitral isthmus line represents a crucial endpoint and is performed during CS pacing by endocardial and CS mapping, looking for widely spaced double potentials across the line of block and confirmed by differential pacing.[7] We demonstrated that the minimum double-potential interval at the mitral isthmus during CS pacing after block is achieved is 150 ms, depending on the atrial dimensions and the extent of lesion creation.[7]

Step 5: Coronary sinus disconnection.

If necessary, further linear ablation (usually the septum or the base of LAA) is performed before CS isolation, which is the last target. Conduction block is assessed by the presence of a corridor of double potentials and demonstration of activation moving toward the line of block on both sides. Rapid atrial activity from the musculature of the CS may be a driver for long-lasting or persistent AF. Electrical disconnection of the CS from the atrium is performed by endocardial or epicardial ablation (**Figure 15.10**). Total elimination of CS activity is the ideal endpoint, but organization of CS activity and/or slowing of local rate with dissociation between CS and LA potential activity is also considered as proof of CS isolation. Endocardial and/or epicardial CS ablation is frequently required in patients with long-standing AF and enlarged atria.

Step 6: Cavotricuspid isthmus line.

Patients with long-standing AF undergo ablation of the cavotricuspid isthmus line.

Postablation Remapping

Once AF/AT noninducibility has been achieved, the LA is remapped, and preablation and postablation activation

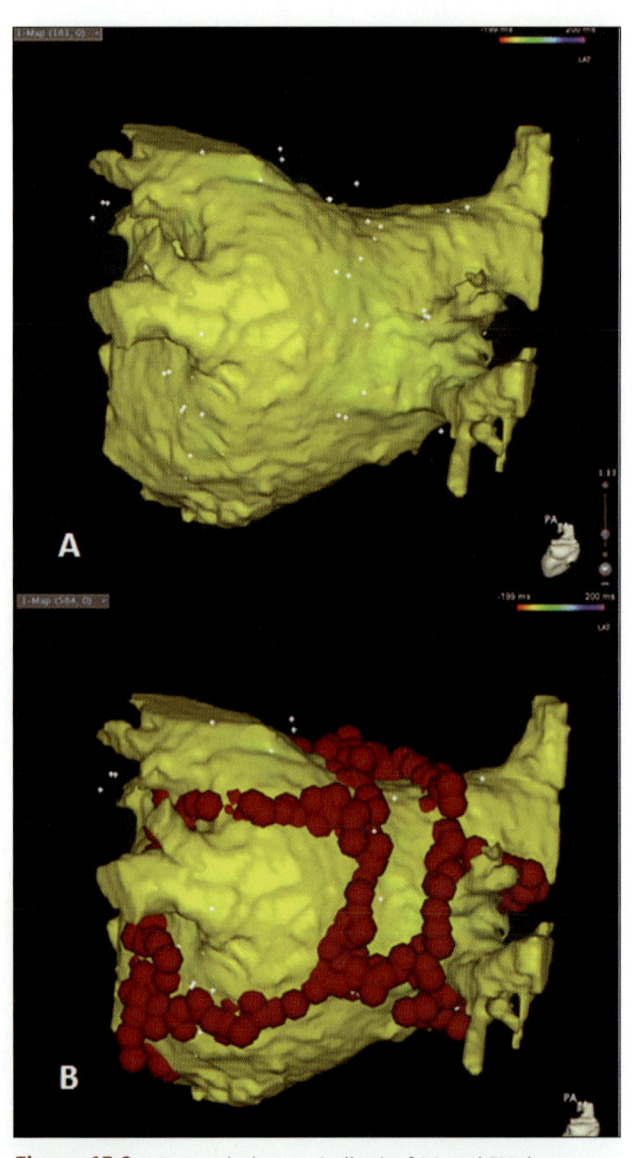

Figure 15.8 Anatomical maps (yellow) of LA and PVs by CartoMerge System in posterior-anterior view before (**A**) and after ablation (**B**).

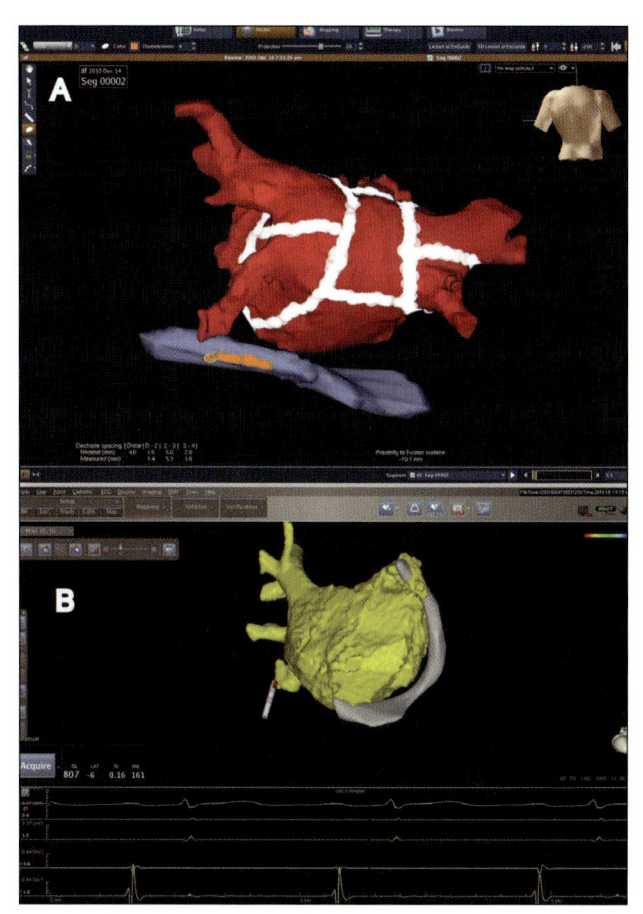

Figure 15.9 Anatomical maps of LA and PVs by Ensite Velocity System in latero-lateral projection (**A**) and tilted lateral view (**B**). The mitral isthmus line is depicted as a white line and white dots represent ablation points.

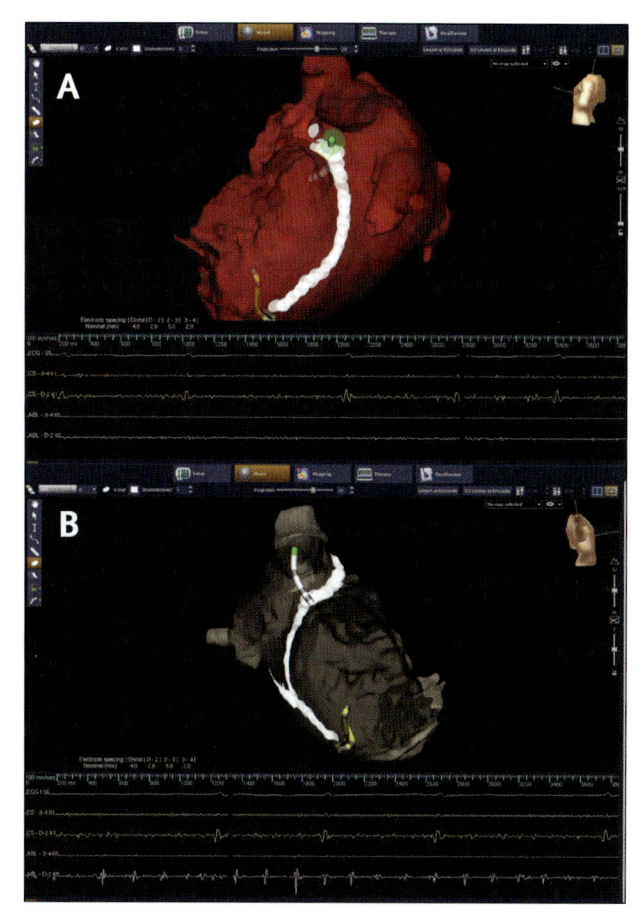

Figure 15.10 A. Anatomical reconstruction of LA, PVs, and CS after ablation. Standard set of lesions is depicted in white dots, while orange dots represent ablation points within the CS. **B.** Anatomical reconstruction of LA, PVs (yellow), and CS (gray) by CARTO 3 system and fast anatomical mapping.

maps are compared. In patients in sinus rhythm, postablation remapping of the LA is done using preablation map for acquisition of new points to compare pre and postablation bipolar voltage maps (**Figure 15.11**). In patients in AF, after sinus rhythm restoration, postablation remapping is performed using the anatomic map acquired during AF for accurate lesion validation. Incomplete block is revealed by impulse propagation across the line and requires further RF applications for completeness of the line despite noninducibility.

Identification of Ablation Targets

Accurate target identification and ablation in a relatively short period of time to avoid major complications is essential to successfully achieve all endpoints and an excellent long-term outcome. Currently, this is facilitated using 3-dimensional navigation and mapping systems, which provide accurate anatomical and electrophysiologic guidance. CPVA is being performed within 1 hour, but it may be longer (up to 3 hours) in patients with permanent AF and enlarged atria to achieve all endpoints including CS disconnection and AF/AT noninducibility. We do not use routinely intracardiac echocardiography and Lasso catheter.

Challenging Ablation Targets

Achievement of all endpoints is crucial, but it may be challenging in specific areas.[8] Usually, repeat RF applications of short duration, greater power, and higher irrigation rates are necessary around the LSPV where atrial EGM potentials may be difficult to eliminate. Complete abatement of atrial potentials in the ridge between the LSPV and LAA also requires repeat and longer RF applications with higher-power delivery settings. If the ridge is too narrow, the ablation line is performed at the base of LAA (**Figure 15.12**). The right-sided PV area and the mitral isthmus also represent 2 difficult sites for both mapping and ablation, requiring continuous adjustment of delivery settings and irrigation rates to achieve the desired endpoint. Incomplete lesion lines, particularly the mitral isthmus line, may result in residual gaps and postablation incessant left atrial tachycardia. In patients with mitral and/or aortic metallic prosthetic valves, mapping and ablation in the mitral area may be challenging, but no case of catheter entrapment in the mitral valve has ever occurred in our laboratory. The mitral isthmus line requires validation of disconnection with pacing maneuvers and, in a majority of patients, further RF applications within CS are required. Ablation of connection sites between CS and atrial musculature requires strict attention by lower energy settings and lower irrigation rates to avoid perforation and cardiac tamponade. Usually we deliver two short, low-energy sequential RF applications (usually between 15 and 30 W) by dragging the catheter in a distal to proximal direction, instead of performing a single application, in order to keep the temperature down and avoid potential complications. The posterior wall also represents a vulnerable area for possible complications such as cardiac perforation and esophageal injury with tip-irrigated catheters. It is well known that the posterior wall not only is the thinnest area of the LA, but it lies in close proximity to the esophagus as well. While applying RF energy on this region, we use lower-energy delivery settings, shorter RF applications, and lower irrigation rates whenever ablation is performed.

Rhythm Outcome

The absence of symptoms may not correspond to stable restoration of sinus rhythm, and the accuracy of evaluating postablation recurrences depends mostly on the duration of ECG recording. Usually, after ablation we schedule 24- to 48-hour Holter recordings at 1, 3, 6, and 12 months and daily transtelephonic ECG monitoring, supplemented by ECG transmission, up to 1 year after the index procedure to assess the asymptomatic recurrences burden.[10-12]

Efficacy

The success of CPVA is defined as freedom from symptomatic or asymptomatic AF, AT, or AFL lasting 30 seconds or longer at least 12 months following AF ablation. We consider a 3-month "blanking period" in which recurrences of AF or AFL are not counted as failures of the procedure. Therefore, early recurrences of AF after the index procedure usually occur within the first 3 months,[7,10,11] but in half of cases they are a transient phenomenon not requiring a repeat procedure. Long-term efficacy of CPVA is > 90% for patients with paroxysmal AF and about 85% for persistent AF once AF/AT noninducibility has been achieved at the end of the procedure. In patients with paroxysmal AF and local vagal denervation, the long-term success rate is higher. If recurrence of persistent AF or monthly episodes of symptomatic paroxysmal AF occur beyond the

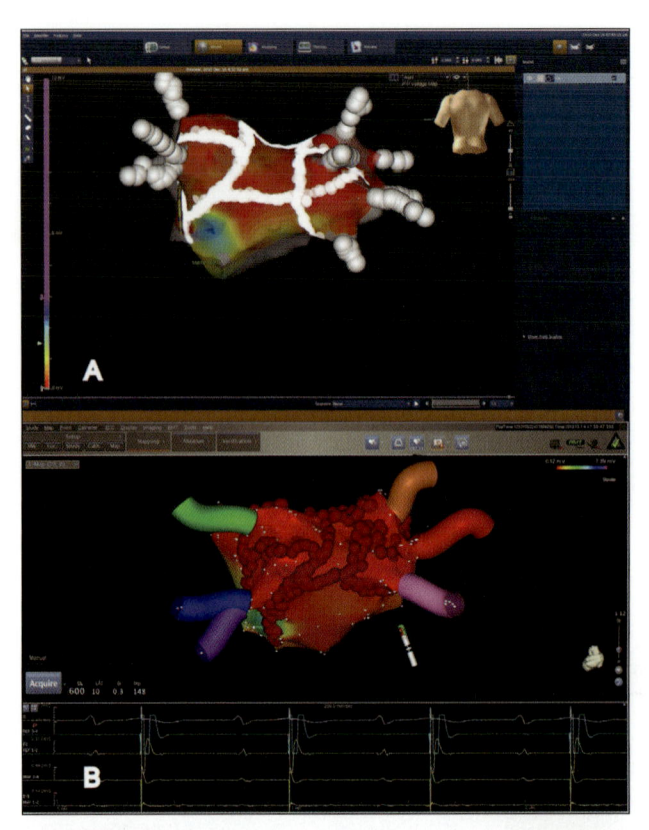

Figure 15.11 Postablation 3-dimensional electroanatomical voltage maps by Ensite Velocity (**A**) and CARTO 3 (**B**). Red color indicates voltage abatement (< 0.1 mV).

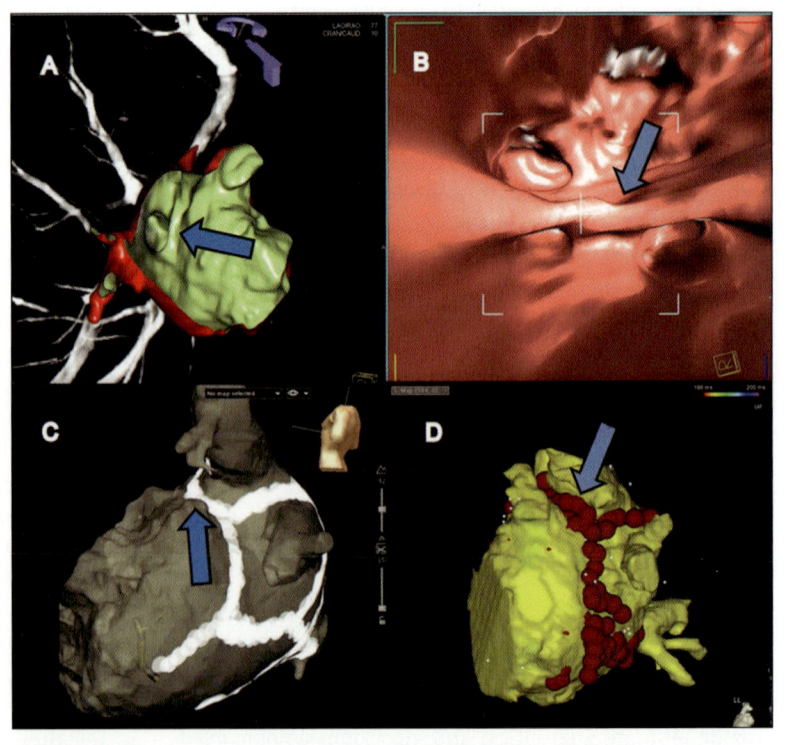

Figure 15.12 **A.** A clipping plane of a DynaCT cardiac segmentation of the LA toward the left superior PV before ablation showing the ridge (arrow). The outer surface is in red color while the inner one is in green. **B.** Internal view of the ridge (arrow). **C** and **D.** Ablation of the ridge (arrows) as guided by Ensite Velocity (**C**) or by CartoMerge (**D**).

blanking period or incessant highly symptomatic left or right atrial flutter is present, then a second procedure is scheduled at 6 months after the index procedure. A maximum of 3 ablation procedures per patient is allowed.

Atrial Remodeling

The assessment of potential consequences of RF ablation on the LA contractility is important for a potential relationship to thromboembolic risk. After ablation, we evaluate carefully the LA transport function before and after the procedure and serially during the long-term follow-up. In our experience, after ablation, the LA diameters decrease and LA contractile function is improved, but the magnitude of this benefit mainly depends on the atrial dimensions before ablation.[6,13] In patients without recurrences and with improved atrial transport and function (reverse atrial remodeling), we discontinue chronic anticoagulation therapy.

Postablation AT

If endpoints are successfully achieved in the index procedure, postablation ATs may develop in less than 5% of patients[7] and usually are macro- or microreentrant gap related rather than focal tachycardias (**Figure 15.13**). In our extensive experience, these ATs should initially be treated conservatively, with medical therapy and cardioversion. Only incessant ATs in symptomatic patients require a repeated procedure to optimize ablation therapy, which will lead to a cure in most case.[7-11] Ablation should be tailored to the arrhythmia mechanism rather than performing empiric lesion lines. Close inspection of the 12-lead ECG with P-wave morphology and axis evaluation should be done initially, since continuous activation suggests a macroreentrant mechanism, whereas a clear isoelectric baseline between P waves suggests a focal mechanism. We routinely perform both activation and voltage maps combined with entrainment pacing maneuvers to optimize the ablation therapy. Usually, the activation map reveals earliest and latest activations in different colors relative to the reference site within a time window equal to the TCL. The most common postablation AT is macroreentrant (> 80% of the CL) mitral annular tachycardia. Entrainment with PPI ≈ TCL from ≥ 3 sites around the superior and inferior mitral annulus, with an activation time around the mitral annulus ≈ to the AT CL, strongly suggests a mitral annular AT. Like the RA isthmus-dependent flutter, the narrowest area of the circuit is between the LIPV and the mitral annulus and the most appropriate approach is to perform reablation of the mitral isthmus looking for residual gaps. For focal microreentrant

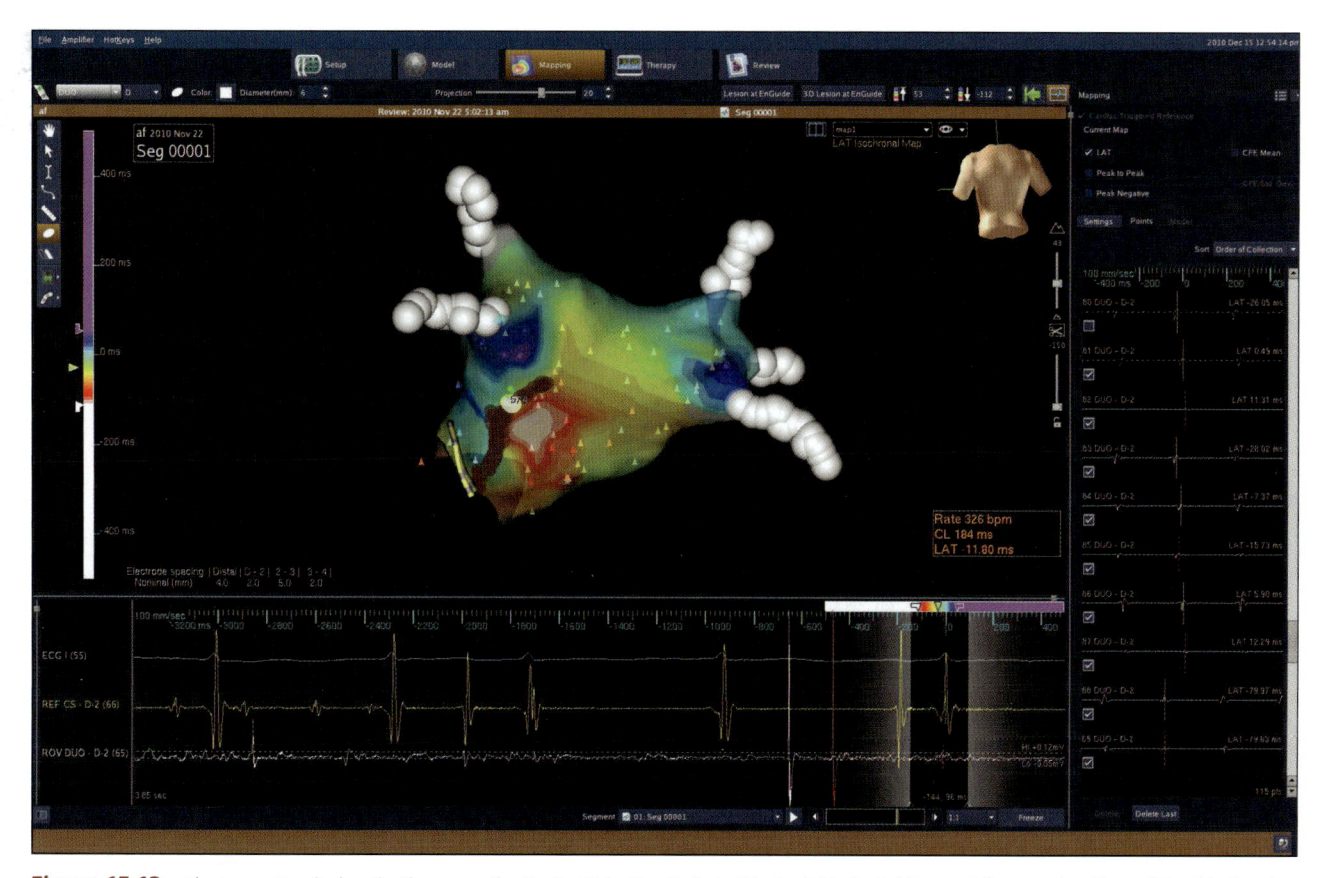

Figure 15.13 Electroanatomical activation map (by Ensite Velocity, St. Jude Medical, St. Paul, Minnesota) reconstruction of the LA showing a centrifugal atrial activation from the mitral isthmus area. Ablation at this site resulted in immediate termination of AT followed by sinus rhytm, as demonstrated by intracardiac recordings.

ATs (<80% of the CL) originating from reconnected PV ostia, ablation of sites with earliest activation that demonstrate concealed entrainment will usually be successful. Frequently, voltage maps show areas of preserved voltage at the site of earliest activation, suggesting areas not previously targeted or incompletely ablated during the index procedure. Reentry around left or right PVs can be demonstrated by proximal and distal CS, LA roof, and septal pacing. Their management requires the use of 3-dimensional activation maps for delineating the tachycardia course and for deploying a lesion line connecting anatomic obstacles to interrupt AT circuits. RF applications are delivered after critical isthmuses have been identified by detailed electroanatomic maps and concealed entrainment. Usually, few RF applications on the critical isthmus are sufficient to eliminate such tachycardias and their inducibility, but in some cases a further ablation line is required. Successful ablation is defined as termination of tachycardia during ablation and noninducibility of the same tachycardia morphology with burst pacing and/or programmed pacing.

Conclusion

It has become increasingly apparent that in patients with AF, particularly in those with long-standing persistent AF,[14] maintenance of a stable sinus rhythm by a single procedure is an important endpoint, since AF ablation seems to be an effective therapy and a realistic alternative to current pharmacologic therapy. However, in order to have the maximum long-term success of single-procedure catheter ablation avoiding serious complications, all acute endpoints should be safely achieved. In our opinion, single-procedure success rates can and will increase dramatically over the next years up to 90% by technological advances, new tools, and better understanding of the AF pathophysiology. At present, many AF ablation strategies are effective as CPVA, but in most cases, repeat procedures are required, which may increase the risk of major complications.

References

1. Haïssaguerre M, Jaïs P, Shah DC, et al. Spontaneous initiation of atrial fibrillation by ectopic beats originating in the pulmonary veins. *N Engl J Med.* 1998;339:659–666.
2. Pappone C, Oreto G, Rosanio S, et al. Atrial electroanatomic remodeling after circumferential RF pulmonary vein ablation: efficacy of an anatomic approach in a large cohort of patients with atrial fibrillation. *Circulation.* 2001;104:2539–2544.
3. Pappone C, Vicedomini G, Manguso F, et al. Robotic magnetic navigation for atrial fibrillation ablation. *J Am Coll Cardiol.* 2006;47:1390–1400.
4. Pappone C, Vicedomini G, Frigoli E, et al. Irrigated-tip magnetic catheter ablation of AF: a long-term prospective study in 130 patients. *Heart Rhythm.* 2011;8(1):8–15.
5. Augello G, Vicedomini G, Saviano M, et al. Pulmonary vein isolation after circumferential pulmonary vein ablation: comparison between Lasso and 3-dimensional electroanatomical assessment of complete electrical disconnection. *Heart Rhythm.* 2009;6:1706–1713.
6. Pappone C, Santinelli V, Manguso F, et al. Pulmonary vein denervation enhances long-term benefit after circumferential ablation for paroxysmal atrial fibrillation. *Circulation.* 2004;109:327–334.
7. Pappone C, Manguso F, Vicedomini G, et al. Prevention of iatrogenic atrial tachycardia after ablation of atrial fibrillation: a prospective randomized study comparing circumferential pulmonary vein ablation with a modified approach. *Circulation.* 2004;110:3036–3042.
8. Pappone C, Santinelli V. How to perform encircling ablation of the left atrium. *Heart Rhythm.* 2006;3:1105–1109.
9. Mesas CE, Pappone C, Lang CE, et al. Left atrial tachycardia after circumferential pulmonary vein ablation for atrial fibrillation. *J Am Coll Cardiol.* 2004;44:1071–1079.
10. Pappone C, Augello G, Sala S, et al. A randomized trial of circumferential pulmonary vein ablation versus antiarrhythmic drug therapy in paroxysmal atrial fibrillation: the APAF Study. *J Am Coll Cardiol.* 2006;48:2340–2347.
11. Oral H, Pappone C, Chugh A, et al. Circumferential pulmonary-vein ablation for chronic atrial fibrillation. *N Engl J Med.* 2006;354:934–994.
12. Oral H, Scharf C, Chugh A, et al. Catheter ablation for paroxysmal atrial fibrillation: segmental pulmonary vein ostial ablation versus left atrial ablation. *Circulation.* 2003;108:2355–2360.
13. Pappone C, Rosanio S, Augello G, et al. Mortality, morbidity, and quality of life after circumferential pulmonary vein ablation for atrial fibrillation: outcomes from a controlled nonrandomized long-term study. *J Am Coll Cardiol.* 2003;42:185–197.
14. Haïssaguerre M, Sanders P, Hocini M, et al. Catheter ablation of long-lasting persistent atrial fibrillation: critical structures for termination. *J Cardiovasc Electrophysiol.* 2005;11:1125–1137.

CHAPTER 16

How to Perform Ablation of Atrial Fibrillation by Targeting Complex Fractionated Atrial Electrograms

Koonlawee Nademanee, MD; Montawatt Amnueypol, MD

Introduction

Pulmonary vein isolation (PVI) has been recommended to be a cornerstone of catheter ablation of the AF, and most laboratories perform PVI as the primary approach for patients with paroxysmal AF. Its success rate in the paroxysmal AF subset ranges from 38 to 70% after a single procedure and 65 to 90% after repeated procedures.[1]

However, PVI alone is not effective for treating patients with persistent and permanent AF. As a result, there is a strong trend to add ablation lines in the LA and ablate in the CS and the RA over and above traditional PVI. These developments demonstrate the importance of AF substrate ablations, which should be an integral part of successful ablation strategies.

Logically, the best approach to identify target sites of AF ablation would be to find substrates that perpetuate the arrhythmia. In the past, it was believed that AF substrates could not be mapped because reentrant circuits underlying the substrate are random and not amenable for point-to-point or endocardial mapping. However, our recent observational studies have demonstrated that substrates serving as "AF perpetuators" can be identified by searching for areas that have complex fractionated atrial electrograms (CFAE). During sustained AF, CFAE are often recorded in specific areas of the atria and exhibit surprisingly remarkable temporal and spatial stability. By ablating areas that have persistent CFAE recording, our studies showed that AF was terminated in over 85% of patients, and more importantly, the procedure yielded a very good long-term outcome in both paroxysmal and chronic AF patients.[2,3] In this chapter, we will explain how we perform AF ablation guided solely by targeting CFAE areas.

Preprocedural Planning

All patients undergo cardiac evaluation, including 2-dimensional echocardiography. LA imaging with either CT or MRI is not usually required for CFAE ablation except for research purposes. All patients must have thyroid function test to rule out thyroid disorder, especially hyperthyroidism. All antiarrhythmic agents are discontinued at least 5 half-lives before the procedure (1 month, in the case of amiodarone). However, we do not stop anticoagulation treatment for the procedure. For patients who have not been on anticoagulation at the time of preprocedural evaluation, warfarin (target INR 2–3) or dabigatran is initiated at least 2 to 3 weeks before the procedure. Since the practice of continuing anticoagulation for the procedure was begun approximately 3 years ago, we have found that both major bleeding and embolic complications occur far less often than using the conventional approach of warfarin discontinuation with low-molecular-weight heparin bridging prior to the procedure.

In the past, TEE was routinely performed in all patients with persistent and long-standing AF and high-risk patients with paroxysmal AF. However, since the advent of 2-dimensional real-time integrated ICE, we substitute ICE for evaluation of clot in the LA. Additionally, real-time 2-dimensional integrated ICE images provide invaluable information about all intracardiac structures, including PV antrum, location of esophagus, etc., that could be dovetailed seamlessly into the CFAE electroanatomical map (CARTO).

Procedure

Patient Preparation

The majority of our patients undergo ablation procedures under conscious sedation with midazolam, fentanyl, and occasionally hydromorphone. Rarely, in selected cases (eg, those with advanced heart disease, pulmonary disease, or marked obesity), patients will undergo the procedure under general anesthesia. In general, our average procedure duration is between 2 and 3 hours and poses no major challenge to keep patients under adequate sedation without pain or bad memory of the procedure. Less than 5% of the patients generate difficulty in providing smooth sedation that may result in excess movement by the patient and, eventually, a need for general anesthesia. We believe that keeping procedure time relatively short without general anesthesia provides many advantages, especially when treating elderly patients, because of concerns about cognitive function after general anesthesia. A Foley urinary catheter is not routinely placed in our patients. We do not place a temperature probe into the esophagus for monitoring of the esophageal position and temperature.

Access in the right femoral vein is obtained using 2 venous sheaths (7-Fr and 8-Fr); the 8-Fr sheath is later replaced with a transseptal sheath. Occasionally another 8-Fr venous sheath is also placed in the right femoral vein for right atrial and CS mapping and ablation unless we decide to perform 2-dimensional real time ICE imaging with a SoundStar ICE catheter (Biosense Webster, Diamond Bar, CA). In that case, the LFV is entered with an 11-Fr sheath for accommodating the SoundStar ICE catheter that could also be used for mapping and ablation of the RA and CS. The SoundStar and the mapping and ablation catheter can be interchanged via this sheath. Noninvasive blood pressure monitoring is routinely utilized and occasionally an arterial line for arterial pressure monitoring is performed. A decapolar catheter (BARD) is advanced via the 7-Fr venous sheath in the CS.

Transseptal Puncture

One transseptal puncture is performed without ICE guidance; however, in rare cases with unusual septal anatomy or thick septum that require force to get through the fossa ovalis (ie, patients who had previous multiple transseptal ablative procedures), a pigtail catheter positioned at the aortic valve and/or ICE are used to ensure the location of the needle, giving the operator confidence to force the needle through the septum. We continuously monitor the atrial pressure; the typical waveform of the LA pressure is seen once the needle is successfully advanced into the LA. Contrast injection is also routinely performed to confirm successful entry into the LA. It is our practice to continuously monitor LA pressure throughout the procedure. A heparin bolus of 3500 to 5000 U is given for patients whose INR is in the therapeutic range (2–3) during the procedure. The goal ACT is 300 to 350 seconds. The ACT is checked every 15 minutes during the procedure. Repeat boluses and titration of the heparin drip are necessary to keep the ACT at goal.

Selection of Guiding Sheaths and Catheters

LA access can be obtained using a variety of guiding sheaths. We predominantly use the Daig SL-0 (St. Jude Medical, St. Paul, MN) and occasionally SL-1 sheath.

We use a Thermocool 3.5-mm-tip catheter with an F curve (Biosense Webster Inc, Diamond Bar, CA) in patients with relatively normal-size LA and a J curve for patients with large LA.

Mapping

The cornerstone of our approach in identifying substrates of AF is to thoroughly look for areas that harbor CFAE. Thus, it is of paramount importance for anyone who wish to employ this technique in their approach in ablating AF to understand what kind of atrial EGMs are ideal as targets for the ablation and recognize their regional distribution and possible underlying mechanisms of CFAE.

Atrial EGMs during sustained AF have three distinct patterns: single potential, double potential, and complex fractionated potential. The distribution of these atrial EGMs during AF has a propensity to localize in specific areas of the atria and not meander; in other words, these atrial EGMs exhibit surprisingly remarkable temporal and spatial stability. CFAEs are perhaps the most interesting EGMs because they may represent AF substrates. Hence, sites that harbor CFAE should be important target sites for ablation of AF substrate. Indeed, by ablating such areas that have persistent CFAE recordings, one eliminates AF and usually renders AF noninducible. With this observation, over the past 10 years, CFAE mapping has become our approach for guiding successful ablation of AF substrate with excellent long-term outcomes.

We define CFAE as follows: (1) atrial EGMs that have fractionated EGMs composed of 2 deflections or more and/or have a perturbation of the baseline with continuous deflection of a prolonged activation complex, as shown in **Figure 16.1**, or (2) atrial EGMs with a very short cycle length (≤ 120 ms), as shown along the LA roof in Figure 16.1. However, it is important to recognize that not all CFAE is the same. We are mostly interested in CFAEs that localize in specific areas of the atria and do not meander, exhibiting surprisingly remarkable temporal and spatial stability as well as usually low-voltage multiple potential signals between 0.05 and 0.25 mV that have a much shorter cycle length when compared to the other part of the atria. In some AF patients, CFAEs may exhibit signals of a very short cycle length (< 100 ms) without clear-cut multiple prolonged potentials. However, when compared to the rest of the atria, this site has the shortest CL that drives the rest of the atria.

Electrophysiologic Mechanisms Underlying CFAEs

The underlying etiology of CFAE has not yet been elucidated, but several theories are being investigated. Pioneering work by Wells et al[4] identified four types of atrial EGMs that may be present in AF:

- Type I: Discrete complexes separated by an isoelectric baseline free of perturbation.
- Type II: Discrete complexes, but with perturbations of the baseline between complexes.
- Type III: Fractionated EGMs that fail to demonstrate either discrete complexes or isoelectric intervals.
- Type IV: EGMs of Type III alternating with periods characteristic of Type I and/or Type II EGMs.

Konings et al[5] applied this knowledge during intra-operative studies and identified three types of AF based on their mechanism of propagation:

- Type I: Single broad-wave fronts propagating without significant conduction delay, exhibiting only short arcs of conduction block or small areas of slow conduction not disturbing the main course of propagation.
- Type II: Activation patterns characterized either by single waves associated with a considerable amount of conduction block and/or slow conduction or the presence of two wavelets.

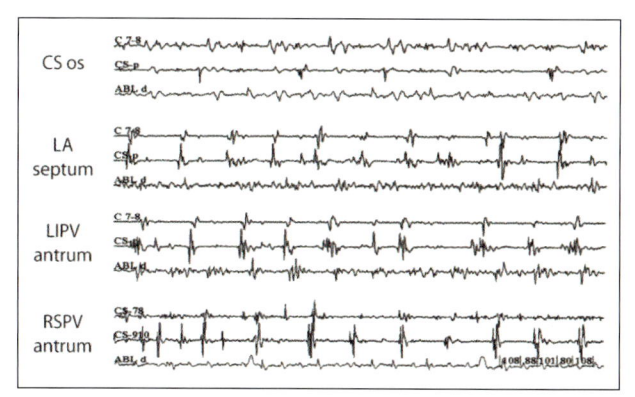

Figure 16.1 Various examples of CFAE that were recorded from the ablation catheter (*ABL d*) from different sites. The figure illustrates 4 trace panels showing CFAE recorded from CS ostium (CS os), LA septum, LIPV antrum, and RIPV antrum. Each panel also shows recordings from reference site in the proximal CS (CS-7,8 and CS-9,10 [CSp]). The most highly fractionated EGMs can be seen in this example to exist on the LA septal wall, although they still exist in the CS ostia and LIPV antrum. The local EGMs at the RSPV antrum are less fractionated but have a very short cycle length, and this may represent a "driver." CS = coronary sinus; LA = left atrium; LIPV = left anterior pulmonary vein; RSPV = right superior pulmonary vein.

- Type III: Presence of three or more wavelets associated with areas of slow conduction (10 cm/s) and multiple arcs of conduction block.

Kalifa et al[6] identified a key relationship between areas of dominant frequency and areas of fractionation in sheep. The investigators were able to localize areas with regular, fast, spatiotemporally organized activity and map the regions around them. Waves propagating from these areas were found to break and change direction recurrently at a boundary zone and demonstrate fractionation of local EGMs. Their findings suggested that one of the possible electrophysiologic mechanisms for AF relating to the hypothesis that high-frequency reentry at the boundary zones is responsible for the fractionation.

The most prominent theory underlying the occurrence of CFAE involves the complex interplay of the intrinsic cardiac nervous system on atrial tissues. The cardiac ganglionic plexi are a collection of autonomic nervous tissues with afferent and efferent sympathetic and parasympathetic fibers.[7-10] Six major ganglionic plexi that may exert influence on the atria (**Figure 16.2**) are:

Superior LA

Posterolateral LA

Posteromedial LA

Anterior descending

Posterior RA

Superior RA

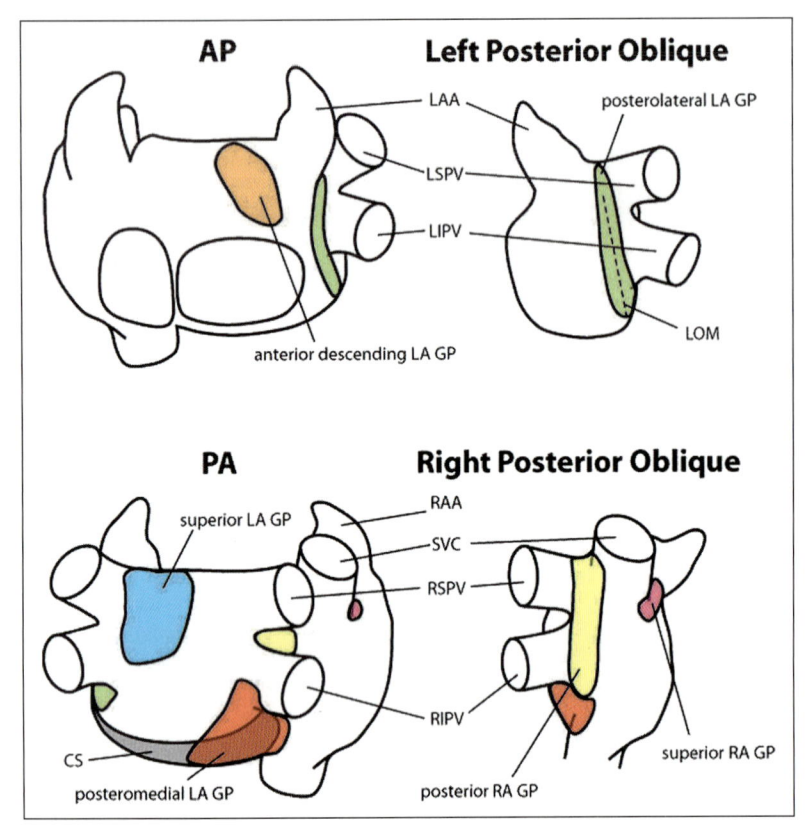

Figure 16.2 Six cardiac ganglionic plexi are located on or near the left and right atria and have been shown to exhibit influence on the initiation and perpetuation of AF: superior left atrial ganglionic plexi, posterolateral left atrial ganglionic plexi, posteromedial left atrial ganglionic plexi, left anterior descending ganglionic plexi, posterior right atrial ganglionic plexi, and superior right atrial ganglionic plexi. AP = anteroposterior; PA = posterior-anterior; LAA = left atrial appendage; RAA = right atrial appendage; CS = coronary sinus; LOM = ligament of Marshall; SVC = superior vena cava; LSPV = left superior pulmonary vein; LIPV = left inferior pulmonary vein; RSPV = right superior pulmonary vein; RIPV = right inferior pulmonary vein. (Adapted from Armour JA, Murphy DA, Yuan BX, Macdonald S, Hopkins DA. Gross and microscopic anatomy of the human intrinsic cardiac nervous system. *Anat Rec.* 1997;247:289–298; and Pauza DH, Skripka V, Pauziene N, Stropus R. Morphology, distribution, and variability of the epicardiac neural ganglionated subplexuses in the human heart. *Anat Rec.* 2000;259:353–382.)

In animal models, the stimulation of parasympathetic fibers within the ganglionic plexi has been shown to decrease atrial ERPs and allow AF to perpetuate. Simultaneously, stimulation of sympathetic fibers may occur in similar areas, which can initiate PV ectopy. Unfortunately, mapping and ablating the ganglionic plexi is time consuming and difficult.

Ongoing research has identified a close relationship between the location of CFAE and the ganglionic plexi in animal models. CFAE-targeted ablation may provide a surrogate for modification of the ganglionic plexi if this relationship can be confirmed in humans. Certainly, ablation in areas that have resulted in a vagal response has shown excellent results in the treatment of AF.

Regional Distribution of CFAE

Each individual has temporal and special stability of CFAE, which facilitates accurate mapping. These regions are not symmetrically located within the atria but can be predictably sought in certain places during mapping. The following key areas have demonstrated a predominance of CFAE within our cohort: (1) the proximal CS, (2) SVC-RA junction, (3) septal wall anterior to the RSPV and IPVs, (4) anterior wall medial to the LAA, (5) area between the LAA and LSPV, and (6) posterosuperior wall medial to the LSPV (**Figure 16.3**). Typically, patients with persistent or permanent AF have greater numbers and locations of sites with CFAE than those with paroxysmal AF.[1]

The distribution of CFAEs in the right and left atria is vastly different from one area to another. Despite regional differences in the distribution of these atrial EGMs, CFAEs are surprisingly stationary, exhibiting relative spatial and temporal stability. Thus, one can perform point-to-point mapping of these CFAE areas and associate them into the electroanatomical map.

CFAE Mapping and Ablation

Mapping is always performed during AF by point-to-point mapping; detailed mapping of the LA, CS, and occasionally RA are required. Patients who are not in AF at the onset of the procedure undergo an aggressive induction protocol utilizing burst pacing in the CS and atria at a lower limit of 1:1 capture or at cycle length ≥ 170 ms with additional intravenous isoproterenol (1–20 mcg/min) as required. AF is considered stable for mapping if it can be sustained for more than 60 seconds. The special and temporal stability of CFAE allows the precise localization of these EGMs.

In our institution, we usually create a map with a minimum of 100 data points, especially in high-density areas commonly known to have CFAE. Additionally, we usually create a detailed map of the proximal CS and occasionally the RA. We identify locations with stable CFAE, and these are "tagged" to create targets for ablation. Areas with fleeting CFAE are not sought as a primary target. A highly reliable map allows for minimal use of fluoroscopy. We

Figure 16.3 The most common locations of CFAE are identified (darkest shading) on a grid representing the regions of the right and left atria. LA = left atrium; LAA = left atrial appendage; RA = right atrium; CS = coronary sinus; FO = fossa ovalis; LSPV = left superior pulmonary vein; LIPV = left inferior pulmonary vein; RSPV = right superior pulmonary vein; RIPV = right inferior pulmonary vein.

routinely use less than 10 minutes during an average procedure duration of 113 to 150 minutes.

Recently, we developed and tested a customized software package to assist in the process of mapping (CFAE software module, CARTO, Biosense Webster, Diamond Bar, CA).[3] The software analyzes data on atrial EGMs collected from the ablation catheter over a 2.5-second recording window and interprets it according to two variables: (1) shortest complex interval (SCL) minus the shortest interval found (in milliseconds), out of all intervals identified between consecutive CFAE complexes; and (2) interval confidence level (ICL) minus the number of intervals identified between consecutive complexes identified as CFAE, where the assumption is that the more complex intervals that are recorded—that is, the more repetitions in a given time duration—the more confident the categorization of CFAE. Information from these variables is projected on the 3-dimensional electroanatomic shell according to a color-coded scale. This allows targeting and retargeting of areas of significant CFAE (see ▶ **Video 16.1**).

The advent of real-time 2-dimensional integrated ICE imaging is invaluable and provides us a tool to evaluate thoracic and cardiac structures such as esophagus, LAA, and PV ostium in real time. Real time ICE images give us very useful information and allow us to titrate power of RF applications to avoid injury to esophagus or pulmonary veins. We use an open-irrigation 3.5-mm-tip ablation catheter with a large or extra-large curve (Thermocool F or J curve, Biosense Webster) irrigating at 30 ml/min during lesion creation. Power settings are 35 to 50 W throughout the atria except for the posterior wall (15–30 W) that is in juxtaposition to the esophagus (seeing in real-time 2D-ICE integrated map and CS (10–25 W) (**Figure 16.4**). Careful

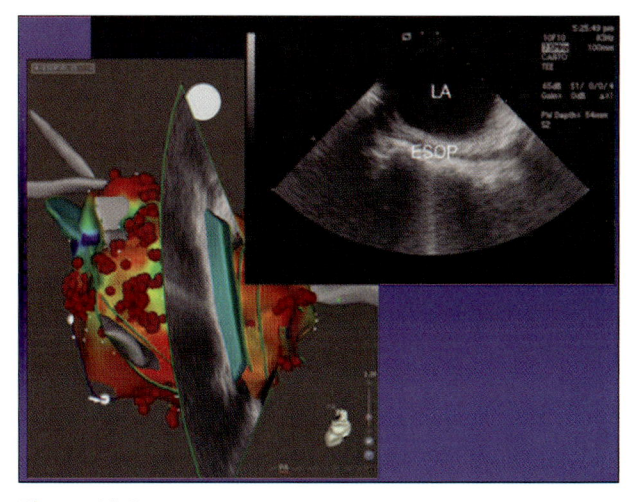

Figure 16.4 A posterior-anterior view of an integrated real-time 2-dimensional imaging contour with electroanatomical map of the LA. The figure shows a location of esophagus in the middle of the LA away from ablations around the posterior aspect of the LSPV antrum. The inset shows 2-dimensional ultrasound image of the esophagus (ESOP) and the left atrium (LA).

power titration is required during RF to ensure complete lesion creation. RF duration is usually 10 to 60 seconds and is halted because of patient discomfort or elimination of CFAE. Because of occasional noise on the ablation catheter during RF, multiple short (15- to 30-second) applications may be used.

One of the most important aspects of CFAE ablation (and one of the most common challenges early in the learning curve of this technique) is to revisit areas that were initially ablated to ensure that there has been no recovery of electrical activity. If the patient remains in AF despite elimination of all visible CFAE, intravenous ibutilide (1 mg over 10 minutes; may repeat once to a maximum of 2 mg) is used to increase the cycle length of the arrhythmia in "nondriver" atrial tissue and thus highlight the remaining areas of greatest significance (eg, CFAE associated with perpetuating AF).

Alternatively, an intravenous dose of procainamide at 1000 mg given as 20 mg/min may be used. Often during CFAE-targeted AF ablation, the arrhythmia evolves into an atrial tachyarrhythmia. Using the CS catheter as a reference, the atrial tachyarrhythmia is subsequently mapped and ablated. Most often the sites of origin of the atrial tachyarrhythmia are at the same locations as the CFAE, which were targeted during the initial part of the procedure. The endpoints employed are either: (1) termination of AF (and if the presenting rhythm was paroxysmal AF, it must not be reinducible); or (2) elimination of all CFAE.

Occasionally, a patient will remain in AF or atrial tachyarrhythmia after an extensive ablation eliminating all CFAE and despite the use of ibutilide. In this small group of patients, an external cardioversion is required.

Postprocedure Care

Recovery

Following ablation, all sheaths are pulled out immediately in the procedure room without reversing heparin effects with protamine. Interestingly, over the past year we began to remove the sheath and maintain hemostasis with manual compression regardless of ACT. While the duration of manual compression to achieve hemostasis often could last up to 30 minutes, we found that incidence of groin complication rate is very much lower than that of the past experience, when we did not pull sheaths for several hours until ACT come down below 200 seconds.

Since we always monitor LA pressure, we will give furosemide intravenously (20–40 mg) if LA pressure is > 20 mmHg at the end of the procedure. Patients will typically lie flat for 4 hours after sheath removal. The majority of our patients undergo the procedure without stopping anticoagulant, which is continued immediately after the procedure. Patients are usually discharged the following day. For patients who undergo the procedure with a therapeutic INR, low-molecular-weight heparin is not needed.

Follow-Up

Patients are followed closely after the procedure. We typically see our patients in clinic within 2 weeks after ablation, then 3, 6, and 12 months afterward, having routine outpatient multiday event monitoring at 6 months and yearly thereafter. We typically do not resume patient's antiarrhythmic regimen during the first 2 to 3 months. All patients, regardless of stroke risk, are anticoagulated with warfarin for the first 3 months. Based on our study in high-risk AF patients, if the patients stay in NSR 3 months after the ablation, warfarin is discontinued and aspirin, clopidrogrel, or both are prescribed. Patients who developed recurrent AF were restarted on warfarin if their AF episodes lasted longer than 12 hours or their estimated cumulative AF duration of all episodes is greater than 12 hours per week. The above practice is undoubtedly controversial. However, our recently published data clearly indicate that our patients who have maintained sinus rhythm after ablation have a significantly reduced stroke risk and do not require a long-term anticoagulation. Patients who had recurrent AF or atrial tachyarrhythmias 3 months after the ablation will be offered a repeat ablation.

Procedural Complications

In recent years, considerable progress has been made in making AF ablation procedure much safer. Using an irrigated-tip catheter, maintaining adequate anticoagulation before, during, and after procedure, careful hemodynamic monitoring, using 2-dimensional real-time imaging in identifying important structure such as esophagus, PV antrum, and atrial appendage so that one can avoid potential injury to these organs are all important advances. In our center, we do not use temperature-monitoring probes, and we have not yet encountered esophageal fistula complication in over 5000 procedures performed. Over the past 2 years, we have been utilizing 2-dimensional integrated ICE imaging to identify esophagus location in real time so that RF power during an ablation on the posterior wall of the LA could be titrated to avoid injury to the esophagus. During the past the past 3 years and over 1000 cases, our complication rate has been quite low; we have witnessed no ischemic strokes, but one patient had intracranial hemorrhage 2 days after discharge home while on low-molecular-weight heparin (Lovenox) for bridging due to subtherapeutic INR. Our incidence of cardiac tamponade, despite using high-power RF energy, is less than 1%. Assessment for pericardial effusion, causing tamponade, can be performed initially with ICE, and pericardiocentesis could be executed in the timely manner.

Advantages and Limitations

Our introduction of CFAE mapping to guide AF ablation as an alternative to the anatomical approach of PVI—either alone for paroxysmal AF or with linear lesions for chronic AF—has spurred other investigators to follow our approach.[1,2,11] Unfortunately, our results were not fully emulated by others. Most studies failed to replicate our acute termination of AF to sinus rhythm and a long-term good outcome.

Although the factors underlying the differences in both acute and long-term outcomes and between these studies and ours are unclear, as discussed in detail previously,[12] it seems more likely that one or more of the following key variables may help explain the differences among these studies:

1. *RA ablation.* We found that 15% of our patients required RA ablation. The common sites are right posteroseptum, CTI, tricuspid annulus, and rarely posterior wall of the RA and SVC-RA junction.

2. *Power and duration of RF energy applications.* Our power of RF applications is significantly higher than those published in the literature.

3. *Ablation endpoint.* Perhaps this variable is the most significant factor influencing the outcomes. We believe that CFAEs are low-voltage atrial signals usually ranging from 0.05 to 0.25 mV, and the areas with the very low-voltage signals (between 0.05–0.1 mV) are often the most desirable. By contrast, most investigators defined successful lesion creation as a voltage reduction to <0.1 mV or decreased by ≤ 80% reduction. This single factor may explain why the investigators did not have a high success rate of acute termination. In our experience, the ablation sites where AF terminated are often the sites that we had applied RF before, and often the voltage of atrial signals at these successful sites were in the range of 0.5 to 0.8 mV.

4. *Procedure endpoint.* The procedure endpoint between other studies and our study is also different. After elimination of CFAE site ablations, we deliberately attempt to ablate all "new" arrhythmias, including pleomorphic forms of atrial tachyarrhythmias, to achieve conversion to sinus rhythm. Furthermore, we did not use ibutilide solely for converting the arrhythmias to sinus rhythm, but rather as an aid to assist in mapping the tachycardia after CFAE ablations. Often after ibutilide, we found that we had to go back to the areas that we had previously ablated and reapply RF applications to terminate tachycardia. CFAE mapping in the LA requires a deliberate and painstaking effort to explore all areas of the atria.

5. *Comprehensive mapping.* Last, the electroanatomic map for CFAE should have high density of evenly spread mapping points. It was unclear whether other investigators committed to detailed mapping of the CFAE, but there is no question that the key to the success of AF ablation guided by CFAE is that all areas of the atria and CS must be explored.

Ablation of CFAE as an Adjuvant to Pulmonary Vein Isolation and Linear Ablations

Recently, ablation of CFAE areas during AF has been adopted as part of the hybrid approaches for AF ablation, especially for nonparoxysmal AF. This is because PVI alone is not highly effective in the majority of patients with long-lasting persistent AF. Thus, many investigators continue to search for a better technique for AF treatment for this subset. Many centers presently incorporate CFAE ablation as an adjuvant to their approach. Using PVI as a cornerstone of their AF ablation, many investigators have added CFAE ablations in their strategies with variable success. In one study in paroxysmal AF,[13] investigators performed ablation initially targeting CFAE and resulting in AF termination in 88% of the patients, and the investigators then proceeded to perform PVI in these patients, yielding 90% long-term success in these PAF patients after a single procedure. These results are quite impressive and clearly suggest the need for further evaluations of the role of combined PVI and CFAE ablations in treating patients with AF.

Conclusions

In conclusion, data from the technique of substrate ablation guided by CFAE mapping, in contrast with previous studies in AF ablation that included largely a young paroxysmal AF population, show greater benefits to the elderly and high-risk populations with structural heart disease. Clearly, more studies are needed before recommending catheter ablation as the first-line therapy for all high-risk AF patients. In the meantime, our research demonstrates that the catheter-based ablative approach is a promising modality for many symptomatic AF patients and has great potential to become the mainstay for AF treatment.

Finally, one must recognize that AF ablation, regardless of the technique used, is a challenging task that requires operator skills in manipulating catheters in the atrial chambers, understanding all facets of clinical electrophysiology, early recognition, and treating procedure-related complications. Many of these skills can be achieved with proper training and hands-on experience after exposure to an adequate number of the procedures.

Advances in technologies and development of new tools such as robotic navigation of catheters, which are being introduced at an impressive pace, will undoubtedly help electrophysiologists to become more proficient to the task. Similarly, it is imperative that the AF ablation procedures be done in centers that are well equipped with an advanced EP mapping system and ancillary equipment, along with an experienced team, to ensure the best possible patient outcomes.

References

1. Calkins H, Brugada J, Packer DL, et al. HRS/EHRA/ECAS expert Consensus Statement on catheter and surgical ablation of atrial fibrillation: recommendations for personnel, policy, procedures and follow-up. A report of the Heart Rhythm Society (HRS) Task Force on catheter and surgical ablation of atrial fibrillation. *Heart Rhythm.* 2007;4:816–861.
2. Nademanee K, McKenzie J, Kosar E, et al. A new approach for catheter ablation of atrial fibrillation: mapping of the electrophysiologic substrate. *J Am Coll Cardiol.* 2004;43: 2044–2053.
3. Nademanee K, Schwab M, Porath J, Abbo A. How to perform electrogram-guided atrial fibrillation ablation. *Heart Rhythm.* 2006;3:981–984.
4. Wells JL Jr, Karp RB, Kouchoukos NT, MacLean WA, James TN, Waldo AL. Characterization of atrial fibrillation in man: studies following open heart surgery. *Pacing Clin Electrophysiol.* 1978;1:426–438.
5. Konings KT, Smeets JL, Penn OC, Wellens HJ, Allessie MA. Configuration of unipolar atrial electrograms during electrically induced atrial fibrillation in humans. *Circulation.* 1997;95:1231–1241.
6. Kalifa J, Tanaka K, Zaitsev AV, et al. Mechanisms of wave fractionation at boundaries of high-frequency excitation in the posterior left atrium of the isolated sheep heart during atrial fibrillation. *Circulation.* 2006;113:626–633.
7. Armour JA, Murphy DA, Yuan BX, Macdonald S, Hopkins DA. Gross and microscopic anatomy of the human intrinsic cardiac nervous system. *Anat Rec.* 1997;247:289–298.
8. Scherlag BJ, Yamanashi W, Patel U, Lazzara R, Jackman WM. Autonomically induced conversion of pulmonary vein focal firing into atrial fibrillation. *J Am Coll Cardiol.* 2005;45:1878–1886.
9. Patterson E, Po SS, Scherlag BJ, Lazzara R. Triggered firing in pulmonary veins initiated by in vitro autonomic nerve stimulation. *Heart Rhythm.* 2005;2:624–631.
10. Scherlag BJ, Nakagawa H, Jackman WM, et al. Electrical stimulation to identify neural elements on the heart: their role in atrial fibrillation. *J Interv Card Electrophysiol.* 2005; 13:37–42.
11. Nademanee K, Schwab MC, Kosar EM, et al. Clinical outcomes of catheter substrate ablation for high-risk patients with atrial fibrillation. *J Am Coll Cardiol.* 2008;51:843–849.
12. Nademanee K. Trials and travails of electrogram-guided ablation of chronic atrial fibrillation. *Circulation.* 2007; 115:2592–2594.
13. Porter M, Spear W, Akar JG, et al. Prospective study of atrial fibrillation termination during ablation guided by automated detection of fractionated electrograms. *J Cardiovasc Electrophysiol.* 2008;19:613–620.

Video Descriptions

Video 16.1 CFAE mapping and ablation: The maps are displayed in both electroanatomical maps only and with CT-CARTO merge maps. Ablations, fluoroscopic locations of the catheter and corresponding EGMs are shown periodically.

CHAPTER 17

How to Ablate Long-Standing Persistent Atrial Fibrillation Using a Stepwise Approach (The Bordeaux Approach)

Daniel Scherr, MD, PD; Michala Pedersen, MD; Ashok J. Shah, MD; Sébastien Knecht, MD, PhD; Pierre Jaïs, MD

Introduction

Persistent AF is a complex arrhythmia and represents the sum of multiple profibrillatory elements, all of which need to be considered for ablation in an individual patient to restore sinus rhythm. The stepwise approach for catheter ablation of persistent AF includes PVI, electrogram-based ablation (CFAE ablation) in the LA and in the CS, linear lesions at the LA roof, the mitral isthmus, and the CTI, and RA ablation if necessary. Therefore, this technique focuses on the elimination of mechanisms involved in the initiation and maintenance of AF, which are essentially represented by triggers and substrate, using the least amount of ablation necessary.

As the procedure progresses, AF is gradually converted from a chaotic process to one which is slower and more organized. The cumulative effect of each step can be visualized in **Figure 17.1**. The endpoint of this sequential ablation strategy is termination of AF at any step of the ablation procedure. This can be achieved either by passing directly from AF to sinus rhythm or, more commonly, to atrial tachycardia (AT) that is then mapped and ablated.

This article will go through each step of the ablation approach. AT mapping and ablation will be described in a separate chapter.

Preprocedural Planning

Patient Selection

By definition, persistent AF is defined as AF which is sustained beyond 7 days or lasting less than 7 days but necessitating pharmacologic or electrical cardioversion. Included within the category of persistent AF is "long-standing persistent AF," which is defined as continuous AF of greater than 1 year's duration.[1] Patients with symptomatic persistent AF who are refractory to antiarrhythmic drug therapy are candidates for the ablation procedure if they accept the benefits and risks, as well as a > 50% chance of requiring a second procedure. Catheter ablation of AF is a demanding procedure that may result in severe complications. We emphasize that patients should only undergo AF ablation after carefully weighing the risks and benefits of the procedure.

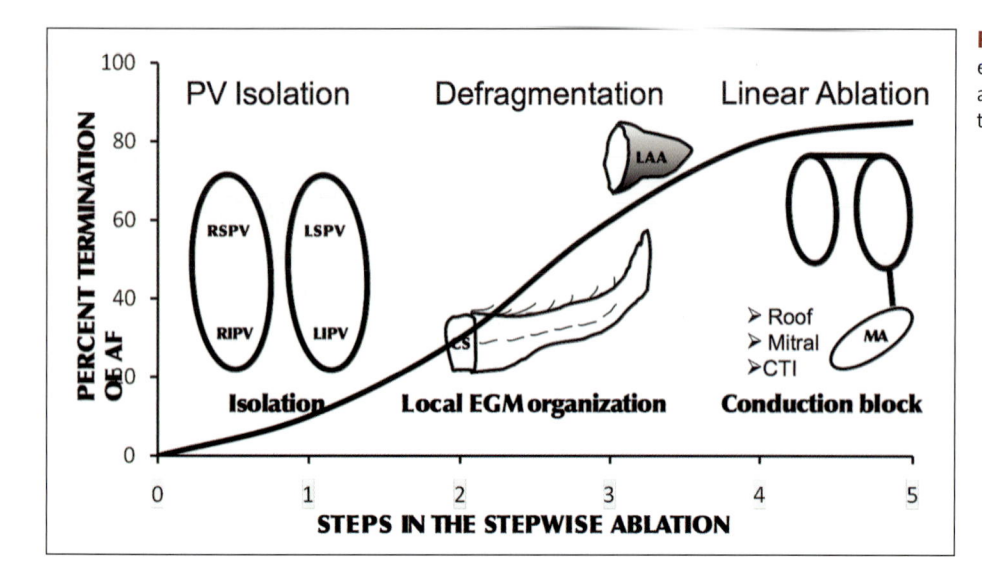

Figure 17.1 Cumulative effect of the stepwise ablation of atrial fibrillation (AF) leading to termination of AF.

Patients are not excluded on the basis of LA size or the presence of concomitant structural heart disease. On the contrary, selected patients with heart failure and/or reduced ejection fraction especially seem to benefit from sinus rhythm restoration. All antiarrhythmic drugs are stopped for at least 5 half-lives prior to ablation except in the case of amiodarone, which is continued.

Left Atrial Imaging

All patients undergo preprocedural evaluation, including cardiac imaging. A standard 2-dimensional echocardiogram is most commonly used. Besides standard parameters such as atrial dimensions and ventricular function, other abnormalities, such as an IAS aneurysm or a persistent foramen ovale, are actively sought by the echocardiographer.

A TEE is performed in all patients prior to the procedure to exclude LA thrombus, which is present in approximately 1% of cases despite appropriate anticoagulation and irrespective of the patients' CHADS$_2$ score.[2] The TEE is usually performed the day prior to the procedure. CT and MRI may be used preprocedurally in order to gain more detailed atrial anatomical and structural information as well as for possible merging with 3-dimensional electroanatomical mapping systems. However, we do not routinely use preprocedural 3-dimensional imaging and/or 3-dimensional electroanatomic mapping for every AF ablation procedure.

Stroke Prevention

Patients are treated with warfarin to maintain an INR between 2 and 3 for at least 4 weeks leading up to the ablation, with cessation of warfarin 48 hours prior to the procedure. Patients routinely receive bridging therapy with low-molecular-weight heparin between the cessation of warfarin and the procedure.

Procedural Aspects

Patient Preparation

All of our patients undergo the AF ablation procedure under conscious sedation and not under general anesthesia. Sedation is accomplished with midazolam and morphine and additional anesthetist-guided sufentanil if required. Arterial lines, urinary catheters, or esophageal temperature probes are not routinely used.

One 6-Fr sheath and two 8-Fr sheaths (one of which is later replaced with the transseptal sheath) are placed in the right common femoral vein, and a decapolar steerable catheter is placed in the CS such that its tip is at the 3 o'clock position in the 30° LAO view.

Transseptal Puncture

Several different techniques are used to obtain a safe transseptal puncture. Here we suggest one way of proceeding: An anteroposterior x-ray position is used for the pulldown (usually started with a 4 to 5 o'clock needle position) and for the transseptal puncture. Before crossing the septum with the needle, the monoplane fluoroscopy system is briefly positioned in a left-lateral position to check for needle position in the anteroposterior plane (ideal position usually between 12 and 1 o'clock). A single transseptal puncture is performed with pressure monitoring and with contrast injection to confirm LA access prior to advancing the dilator and sheath assembly. A guidewire is advanced to a left PV, and the dilator and sheath (SL-0, St. Jude Medical, St. Paul, MN) are pulled back into the RA to allow passage of the ablation catheter through the single puncture site. The dilator and sheath are then advanced over the guidewire into the LA alongside the ablation catheter. Immediately after LA access, a bolus of heparin (50 U/kg) is administered. The long sheath is continuously flushed with heparinized saline at 200 ml/hr. The ACT is checked every 30 to 60 minutes during the procedure and repeat boluses of heparin are administered to achieve a constant ACT between 250 to 300 seconds.

Sheaths and Catheters

A 10-pole, 20-mm circular decapolar catheter is advanced via a transeptal sheath and positioned just distal to the PV ostia to map the PV perimeter during PVI. An irrigated-tip mapping/ablation catheter (Thermocool 3.5-mm–tip catheter, Biosense Webster Inc, Diamond Bar, CA) is used for ablation.

Radiofrquency Delivery

RF energy is delivered using a Stockert generator (Biosense Webster) with the power settings shown in **Figure 17.2**. These power settings have been determined to provide effective lesions while also minimizing the risks of PV stenosis, steam pops, cardiac tamponade, and collateral damage to the phrenic nerve, esophagus, and circumflex coronary artery. Target temperatures of 42°C are achieved (maximum temp 45°C) by manual titration of irrigation rates ranging from 5 to 60 ml/min (0.9% saline via CoolFlow pump, Biosense Webster).

Signal Processing

During AF ablation procedures, 12-lead surface ECGs and bipolar endocardial ECGs are continuously monitored and stored using a digital amplifier and computer recording system (LabSystem Pro, Bard Electrophysiology, Lowell, MA). All signals are sampled at 1 kHz with filter settings from 30 to 250 Hz for intracardiac signals and 0.1 to 50 Hz for surface ECGs. Intracardiac signals are displayed at an amplification of 0.1 mV/cm and with a gain of 16× for the mapping/ablation catheter, 0.2 mV/cm with 8× gain for the CS as well as the Pentaray and the Lasso catheters.

Ablation site	Power (Watts)	Usual duration of radiofrequency delivery (mins)
Coronary sinus	20	4–8
Posterior wall LA	25	3–6
Anterior wall LA	30	3–6
Inferior LA	30	5–10
Roof LA	30	10–15
PVs (if posterior 25W)	30	25–35
Septum LA	30	3–6
Right atrium	30	0–20
Mitral isthmus	35	10–20

Figure 17.2 Power settings during AF ablation.

3-Dimensional Mapping

Various 3-dimensional electroanatomic mapping technologies (EnSite NavX Navigation & Visualization Technology, St. Jude Medical, St. Paul, MN; CARTO System, Biosense Webster, Diamond Bar, CA), may be used for assessment of anatomy, EGM analysis, and quantification of the impact of ablation on LA and RA voltages. These technologies are also useful for mapping ATs that may arise after AF termination or during subsequent procedures. Electroanatomic mapping systems allow real-time display of intracardiac catheter(s) during ablation. The ability to display a lasso catheter allows for very rapid creation of a LA map and direction of the ablation catheter toward the desired poles on the lasso catheter.

Pulmonary Vein Angiography

Before starting the ablation, angiography of the pulmonary veins is performed. This is done by selectively engaging each of the four PV ostia with an over-the-wire multipurpose angiography catheter or an NIH catheter and injecting contrast media into each vein. This gives very useful acute and precise anatomical definition of the ostia and hence helps guide the ablation to minimize complications such as pulmonary vein stenosis, which result from ablation inside the vein.

Atrial Fibrillation Cycle Length (AFCL)

Assessment of the AFCL is an important tool in guiding the ablation procedure. EGMs in persistent AF are complex and the CL cannot be reliably measured, except in the RAA and LAA (**Figure 17.3**). Throughout the stepwise ablation, the AFCL will gradually prolong until AF terminates either to sinus rhythm or, as in the majority of cases, to AT that can then be mapped and ablated conventionally.

Atrial Fibrillation Ablation

Pulmonary Vein Isolation

Ablation strategies that target the PVs are the cornerstone for all AF ablation procedures. If the PVs are targeted, electrical isolation and elimination of all electrical near-field signals around the PVs should be the goal.[1] Careful identification of the PV ostia is mandatory to avoid ablation within the PVs. The circumferential lasso catheter can provide guidance for mapping and ablation around the PVs.

Ablation should be performed 1 to 2 cm away from the PV ostia. We typically start the ablation on the posterior wall toward the LSPV. We ablate in a continuous manner, delivering energy at any given site for 30 to 60 seconds or until the local electrical signals have diminished, before we

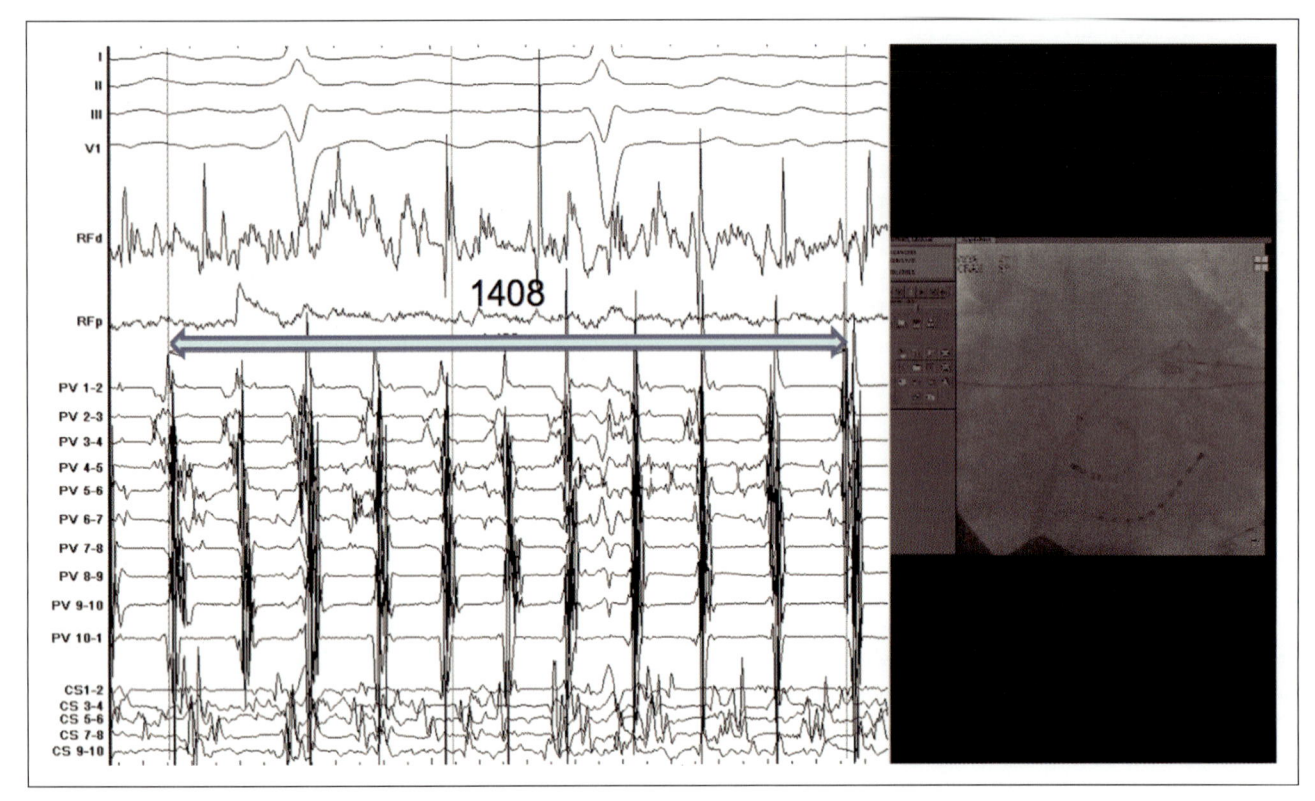

Figure 17.3 Surface ECG leads I, II, III, and V_1. The RF catheter in the inferior LA. A circumferential catheter is in the LAA. CS 1–10 displays a decapolar catheter in the CS. The AFCL cannot be measured on the surface ECG or in the CS. However, the circumferential catheter in the LAA enables measurement of a more exact AFCL. Here, 10 cycles are counted, giving an AFCL of 141 ms.

move on to the next site in a continuous fashion, creating a posterior ablation line (vertical line from high to low) on the left side, followed by ablation to target anterior parts of the left PV ostia. Circumferential ablation can also be performed around the right PVs with a continuous circular lesion. Additional ablation targeting the earliest PV activity or sites of reverse PV polarity may be required. Absence or dissociation of PV potentials recorded distal to the ablation lesions by the circumferential catheter is considered proof of electrical isolation (**Figures 17.4** and **17.5**).

During ongoing AF, the sequence of PV activation is incessantly changing. A consistent activation sequence usually means discrete sites of breakthrough, either spontaneous or following prior ablation. Delivery of RF narrows the width or number of LA-PV connections, resulting in progressive consistency of the PV activation sequence.

In AF, far field potentials can be distinguished from PV potentials using the following methods:

- Consistent prolongation of PV CL may be observed due to reduction of LA to PV connections with ablation.

- PV potentials represent local myocardial activation and therefore display sharper and larger EGMs than the far-field potentials.

- If doubt remains, far-field potentials can be unmasked by putting a recording catheter in the suspected structure, in particular the LAA. Synchronous activity between LAA and PV potentials confirms an external origin of potentials recorded on the circumferential catheter (not impossible, but difficult in AF).

As previously explained, long-standing persistent AF will terminate after PVI alone only in a small minority of patients. Once sinus rhythm is restored, it is important to confirm the complete PVI. This is best done by reinserting the circumferential lasso catheter into each vein.

Electrogram-Based Ablation

The next step in this approach is EGM-based ablation, also colloquially called defragmentation or CFAE ablation. Following PVI, LA activity is usually chaotic, with disorganized sites everywhere, and the overall activity is too complex to map in terms of activation, morphology, or local CL. The aim is to ablate favorable areas that result in slowing and organization of global LA activity.

Favorable areas in the LA that are targets for ablation are continuous EGMs, complex fractionated potentials, sites with a gradient of activation (significant EGM offset

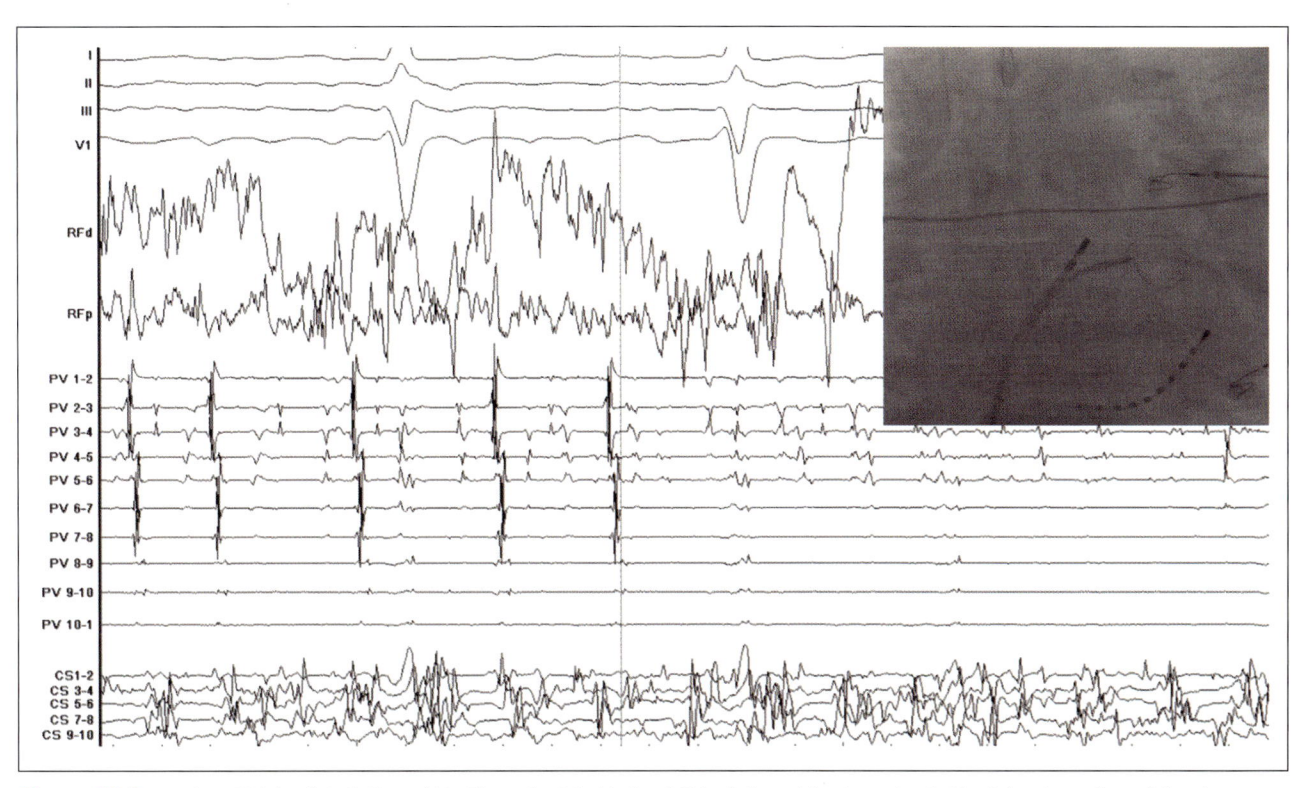

Figure 17.4 Surface ECG leads I, II, III, and V$_1$. Then, the RF ablation EGMs, followed by the poles 1–10 of the circumferential catheter and the lowest 5 EGMs, are the bipoles of the decapolar catheter in the CS. There is 2:1 entry block into the vein prior to isolation. The fluoroscopy image shows the decapolar catheter in the CS, the circumferential catheter in the left superior pulmonary vein, and the RF catheter ablating just proximal to the ostium of the left inferior pulmonary vein.

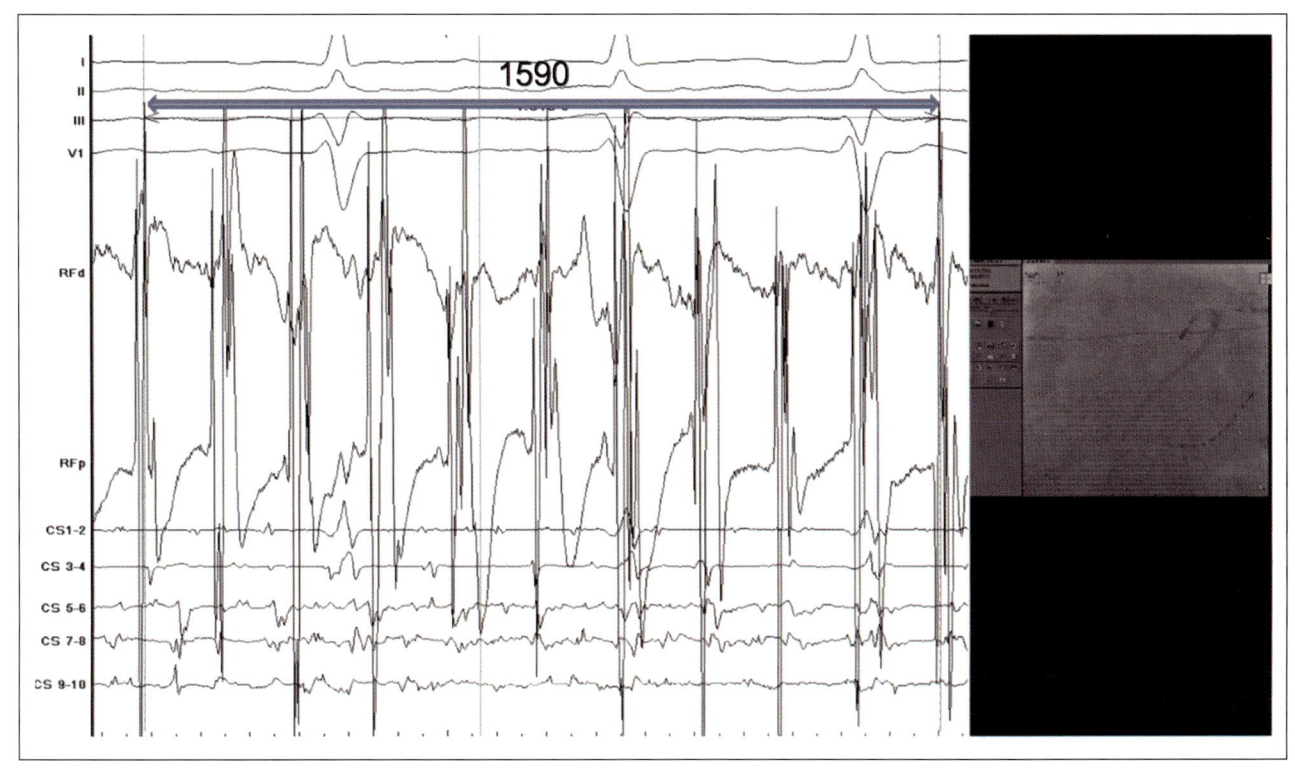

Figure 17.5 AFCL prolongation achieved following pulmonary vein isolation. This tracing is from the same patient who had an AFCL of 141 ms in Figure 17.2 and who underwent PVI as shown in Figure 17.3. His LA AFCL has now prolonged from 141 ms to 159 ms.

between the distal and proximal recording bipoles on the map electrode), or regions with a CL that are shorter that the mean LAA cycle length.[3,4] A recent study found that ablation of areas with continuous activity had the greater impact on AFCL prolongation and AF termination than ablation of areas with high fractionation index, EGM voltages, and local CL.[5]

The various zones of CFAEs may be explained by several different underlying etiologies. They may represent areas of colliding wave fronts, pivot points of moving wavelets, or collision with barriers such as scars or existing structures, for instance, valves or appendages. Complex EGMs are seen in the periphery of sites of rapid activity, often with a frequency gradient to surrounding tissue. **Figure 17.6** shows examples of complex EGMs that are targeted for ablation.

The base of the LAA, the IAS, the inferior LA, and the anterior LA are specifically targeted. The aim of LA ablation is to organize local activity; that is, convert complex, fractionated, rapid, or continuous EGMs into more regular, organized activity with synchronous activation at distal and proximal bipoles (indicating passive activation of this local site). This would abolish local fibrillatory conduction and facilitate conversion to AT or sinus rhythm. **Figure 17.7** is an example of ablation of chaotic EGMs at the inferior LA. Throughout the defragmentation process, the AFCL should be repetitively assessed in the LAA (**Figure 17.8**).

Linear Ablation

If the patient is still in AF after the previous steps, the next stride in the ablation procedure is linear ablation, which is an important tool in the stepwise ablation procedure.[6]

The LA roof and the lateral mitral isthmus are the most common sites for linear ablation. Such linear ablation is often done during AF, but assessment of bidirectional block can only be done in sinus rhythm. It is possible that the previous steps have rendered the patient in an AT. In this case the lines are ablated (if appropriate) during the AT as part of the conventional mapping and ablation procedure (see below).

In general, linear ablation is the last step in the stepwise approach. This is because it can be very difficult, and it may require not only a long time but also a large amount of RF to successfully achieve bidirectional block. This alone increases the risk for complications such as perforation and tamponade, but in addition, incomplete lines are associated with pro-arrhythmic effects.[7] The 2 LA lines will be discussed separately.

Linear Ablation at the LA Roof

The LA roof line is relatively short, forming a continuous line between the already isolated LSPV and RSPV. In the majority of patients, this step is done during AF and the endpoint (during AF) is abolition of all local EGMs along the line. The line is performed as cranially as possible to avoid ablating the posterior LA, hence aiming to avoid complications such as damage to the esophagus.[8]

This lesion is delivered using the ablation catheter inserted into the LA through the long sheath. This combination is important and allows adjusting the orientation of the RF catheter to fit with the variable anatomy of the LA roof. The ablation catheter is curved and dragged along the line with the tip of the irrigated catheter positioned parallel to the roof, either from right to left or left to right. A large loop in the LA is often helpful (**Figure 17.9**). If the orientation of the catheter tip is perpendicular to the roof, power settings should be reduced (to 25 W) to lessen the possibility of steam pops and perforation.

The EP endpoint of roof ablation is the creation of a complete line of conduction block between the SPVs. Following a complete roof line, pacing of the LAA captures the anterior LA. In the presence of a completed roof line, the activation of the posterior LA is from inferior to superior, as the activation can no longer pass over the roof (**Figure 17.10**).

Linear Ablation at the Mitral Isthmus

Ablation of the mitral isthmus further increases the success rate of catheter ablation in persistent AF.[9] In general, this ablation step is only carried out if deemed necessary, that is, if the previous steps have not terminated the AF or if the patient now is in mitral isthmus-dependent AT. If carried out during AF, the goal is abolition or 90% diminution of all local EGMs, usually with the creation of double potentials along the line (**Figure 17.11**). If carried out during AT (eg, mitral isthmus-dependent flutter), the goal is arrhythmia termination. Again, it is likely that more ablation is needed in sinus rhythm to achieve bidirectional block.

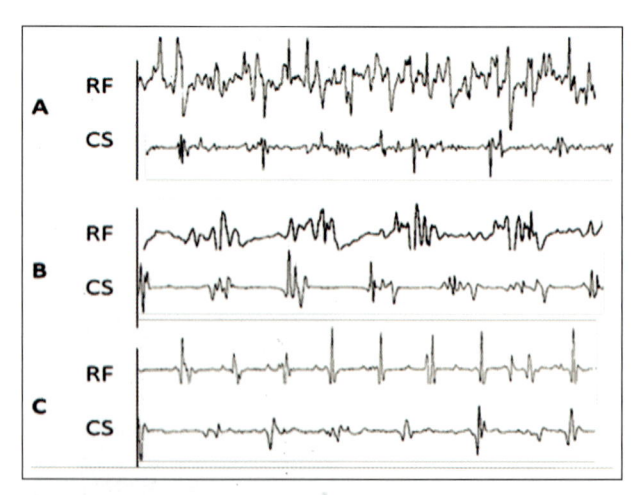

Figure 17.6 Simultaneous recordings from the ablation (RF) and CS catheters, both in the LA. **A.** A recording of continuous activity on the RF catheter without a return to baseline. **B.** A fractionated potential on the RF catheter with an interposed isoelectric interval. **C.** An example of rapid activity recorded on the RF catheter with a frequency gradient to the CS.

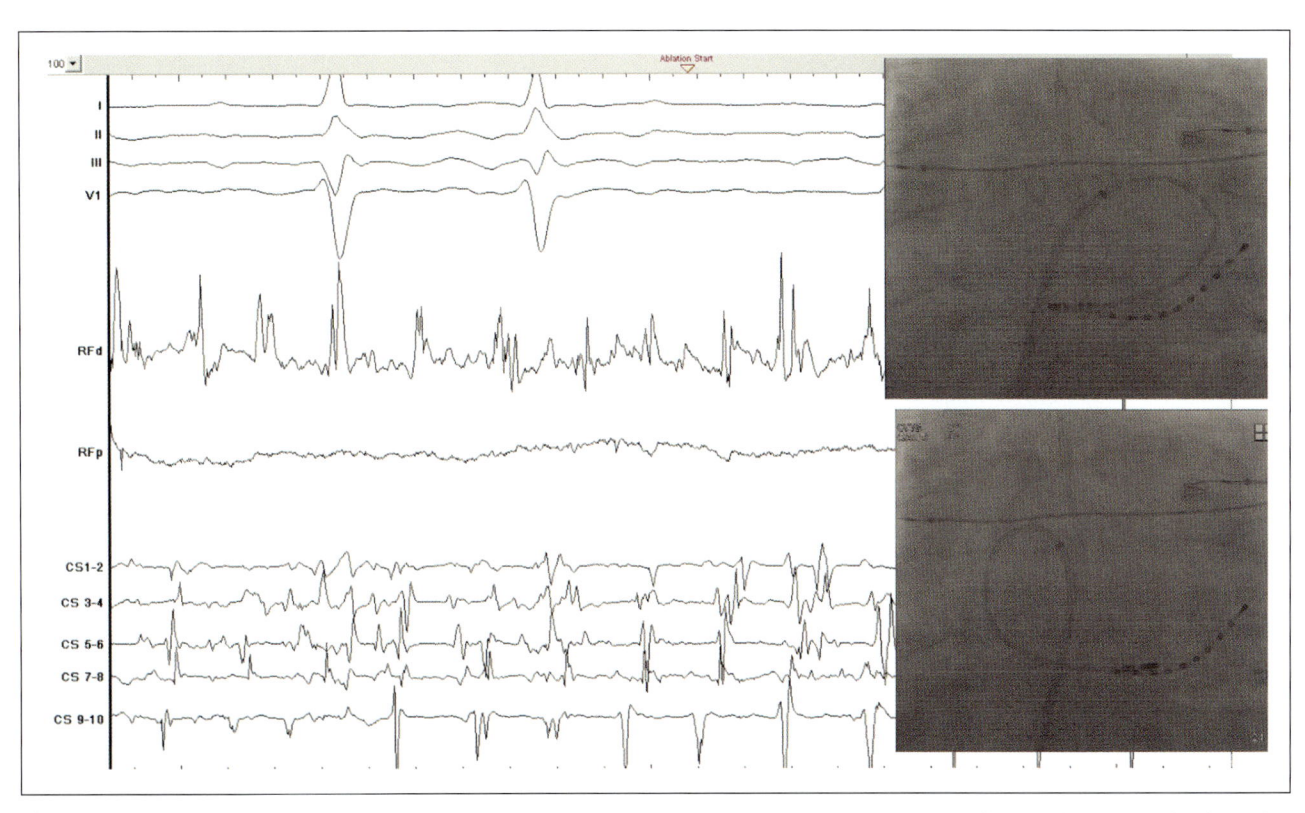

Figure 17.7 Upper panel shows leads I, II, III, and V₁ of the surface ECG. The RF catheter shows EGMs of a complex nature. The decapolar catheter in the CS confirms AF. Ablating in the inferior LA can be done by dragging the catheter along the floor of the atrium, either from left to right (upper insert) or from right to left (lower insert).

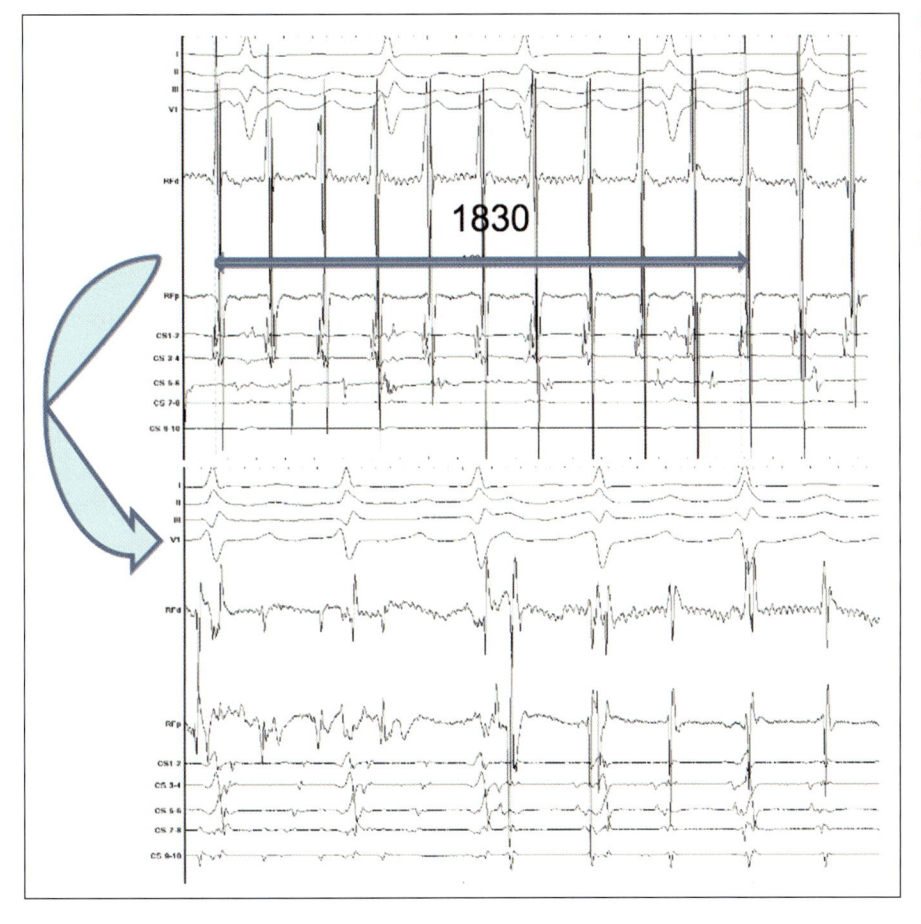

Figure 17.8 Both panels show surface leads I, II, III, V₁, and a decapolar catheter in the CS. In the upper panel the RF catheter is in the LAA and the AFCL is measured over 10 cycles (183 ms). With further ablation, the AF can no longer be sustained and converts to an atrial tachycardia. Same patient as in Figure 17.4.

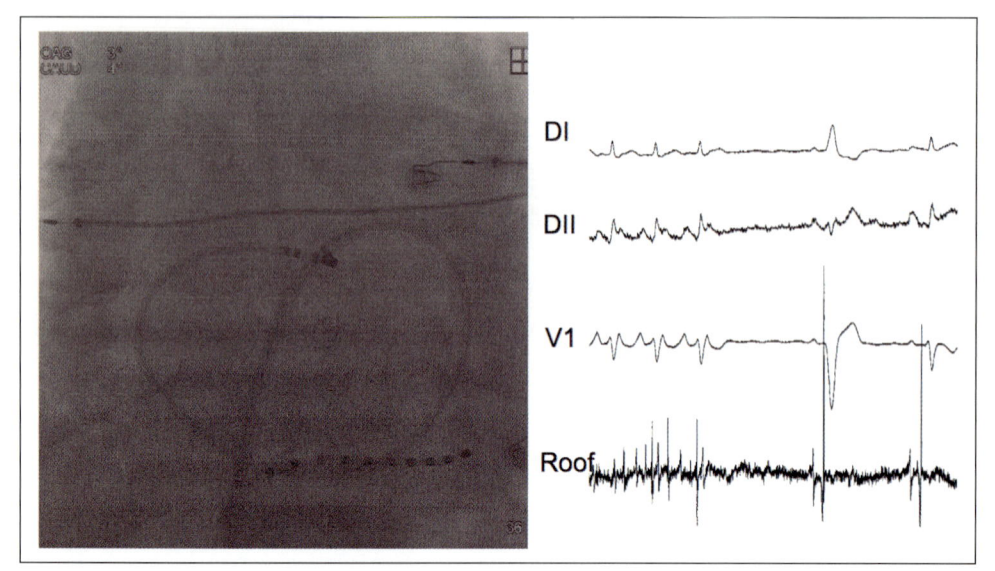

Figure 17.9 The left panel is an example of catheter position during linear ablation of the roof. The right panel shows surface lead I, II, and V$_1$ together with the EGMs from the RF catheter. This roof line is carried out during roof-dependent atrial tachycardia; complex and fractionated EGMs can be seen on the RF catheter prior to conversion to sinus rhythm.

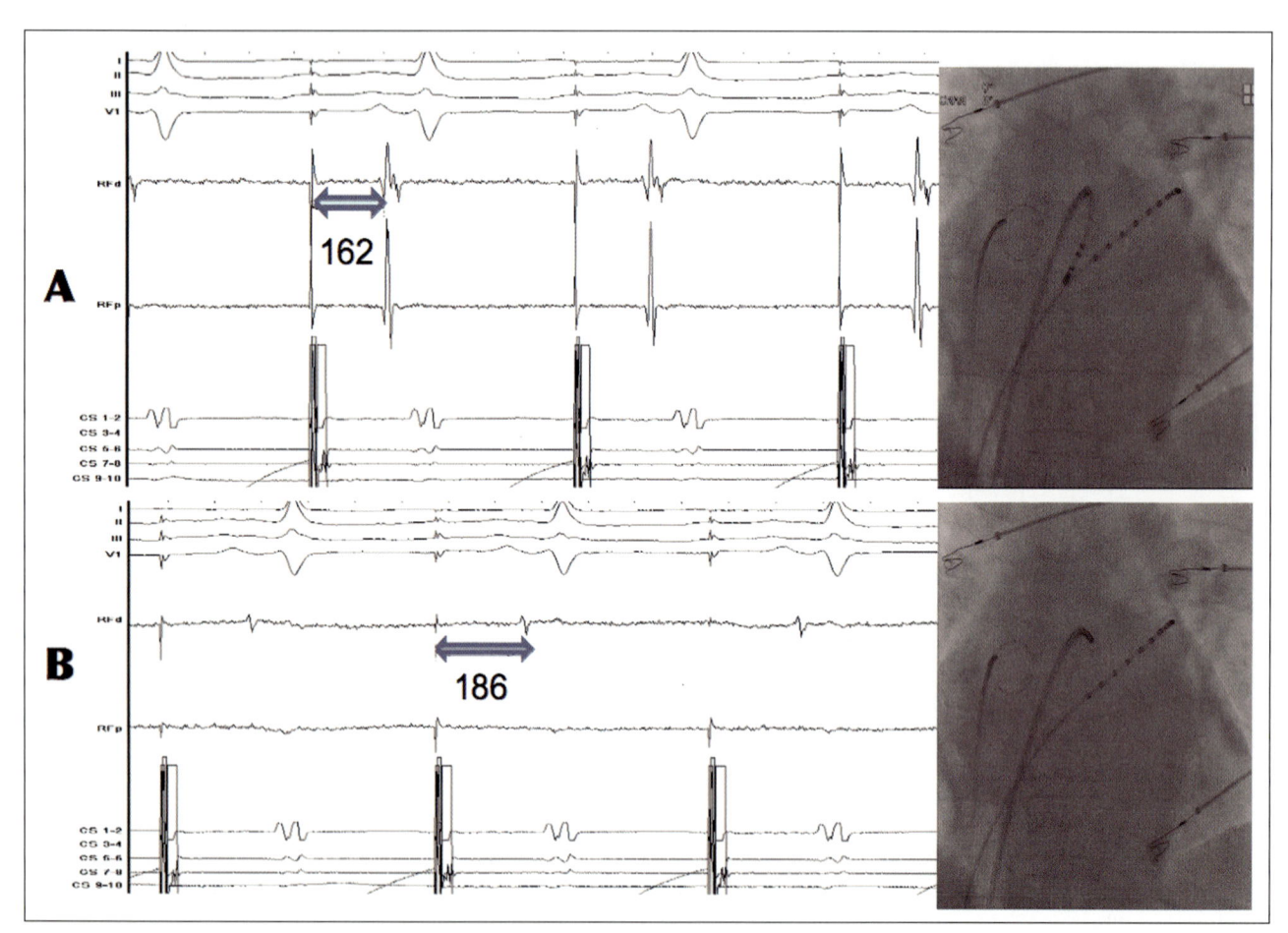

Figure 17.10 The left panels show the surface ECG leads I, II, III, and V$_1$. Then the EGMs of the RF catheter and lowest 5 bipoles of the decapolar catheter, now positioned though the transseptal hole to the LAA. Pacing is done from the distal CS (LAA). In **A**, the RF catheter is placed low on the posterior wall; in **B**, it is placed high on the posterior wall. During pacing from the LAA, the time to low posterior wall is 162 ms and to high posterior wall 184 ms, demonstrating a low-to-high conduction posteriorly and thereby confirming LA roof block.

The mitral isthmus is short, 2 to 4 cm from the mitral annulus to the LIPV ostium (or the LAA). It is often necessary to extend to line from the ostium of the inferior PV to the base of the LAA in order to achieve block; similarly, it is necessary in up to 80% to ablate within in CS to achieve block.[9] The mitral isthmus line is begun at the ventricular aspect of the mitral annulus. With clockwise rotation on the sheath and catheter, the lesion is extended

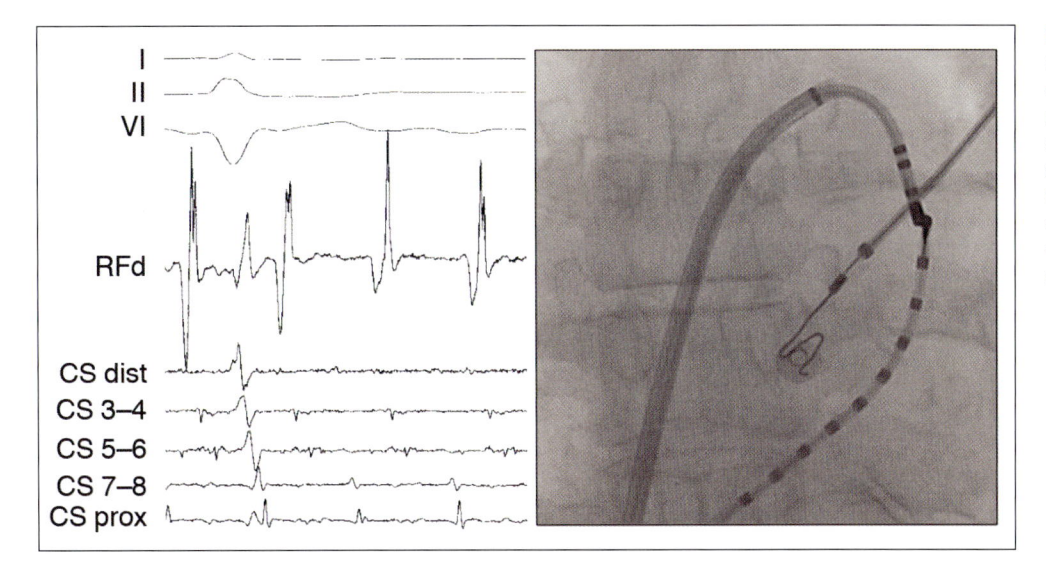

Figure 17.11 The RF catheter at the beginning of the linear ablation of the mitral isthmus. The left panel shows surface ECG leads I, II, and V_1, the RF catheter, and the poles of the decapolar catheter in the CS. Large-voltage EGMs are seen at the mitral isthmus preablation.

to the LIPV and further to the base of the LAA if needed. If mitral isthmus block is not achieved by this, the ablation is extended to the epicardial aspect of the mitral isthmus via the CS. Powers up to 35 W with irrigation rates up to 60 ml/min are needed to achieve transmural lesions during endocardial ablation.

Following a mitral isthmus line, block is confirmed using differential CS pacing and pacing from the RF catheter at the lateral LA just anterior to the mitral line or in the LAA. In the presence of block, the activation front moves along the anterior wall to the septum and then along the posterior wall, septal to laterally, during LAA pacing. This gives a proximal to distal activation sequence of the CS (**Figure 17.12A**). In the other direction, block is assessed by pacing the first the distal poles of the CS catheter, which is near the mitral line, and measuring the delay to LAA. The pacing is then changed to a more proximal pole, from which the delay to the LAA should be shorter in the presence of blocked linear lesion (**Figure 17.12B**).

Right Atrial Ablation

In 15% of patients with persistent AF, sinus rhythm cannot be restored by ablation in the LA, and the presence of perpetuators in the RA should be considered.[10] This state of affairs should be suspected when the AFCL in the RAA prolongs less than the AFCL in the LAA during ablation; a shorter AFCL in the RAA compared to LAA by more than 10 to 20 ms can be due to the drivers of AF originating in the RA. Similarly, pauses in activity in the LA EGMs without corresponding pauses in the RA EGMs would suggest the RA as the driving chamber. The approach to mapping (ie, each step of the ablation), and the EGM targets within the RA are as for the LA. Preferential anatomical areas at which there is a higher incidence of AF termination during ablation of complex fractionated atrial EGMs are the RAA, the intercaval region, the SVC, and the CS ostium. Also, CTI ablation is routinely part of our stepwise ablation approach.

Atrial Tachycardia in the Context of Atrial Fibrillation Ablation

Atrial tachycardia may occur at any point throughout the stepwise ablation of AF. As described, the endpoint of the stepwise ablation is restoration of sinus rhythm, and this may occur via ablation of one or more atrial tachycardias.[11,12] In addition, atrial tachycardia is the dominant mode of arrhythmia recurrence in patients in whom AF was terminated during the index procedure.[13]

Postprocedural Care

The immediate postprocedural management consists of continuing and maintaining anticoagulation, maintaining hemostasis at puncture sites, and supportive treatment.

Following ablation, the guiding sheaths are pulled out of the LA and heparin is stopped. Patients will typically lie flat for 6 hours after sheaths are pulled due to the large sheaths used. All patients are treated with warfarin after ablation. Patients receive low-molecular-weight heparin injections beginning on the evening of the ablation and continuing until the INR is therapeutic. Patients are usually subjected to echocardiography postprocedure.

Patients are followed closely for the year following an ablation procedure. At 3, 6, and 12 months, patients are admitted to hospital for 24 hours and undergo clinical evaluation including Holter monitoring and TTE. After the procedure, warfarin is continued for at least 6 months and guided thereafter by the presence or absence of conventional risk factors for thromboembolism and maintenance of sinus rhythm. Patients with a $CHADS_2$ score ≥ 2 are usually kept on warfarin regardless of their rhythm outcome. All antiarrhythmic drugs are discontinued by 3 to 6

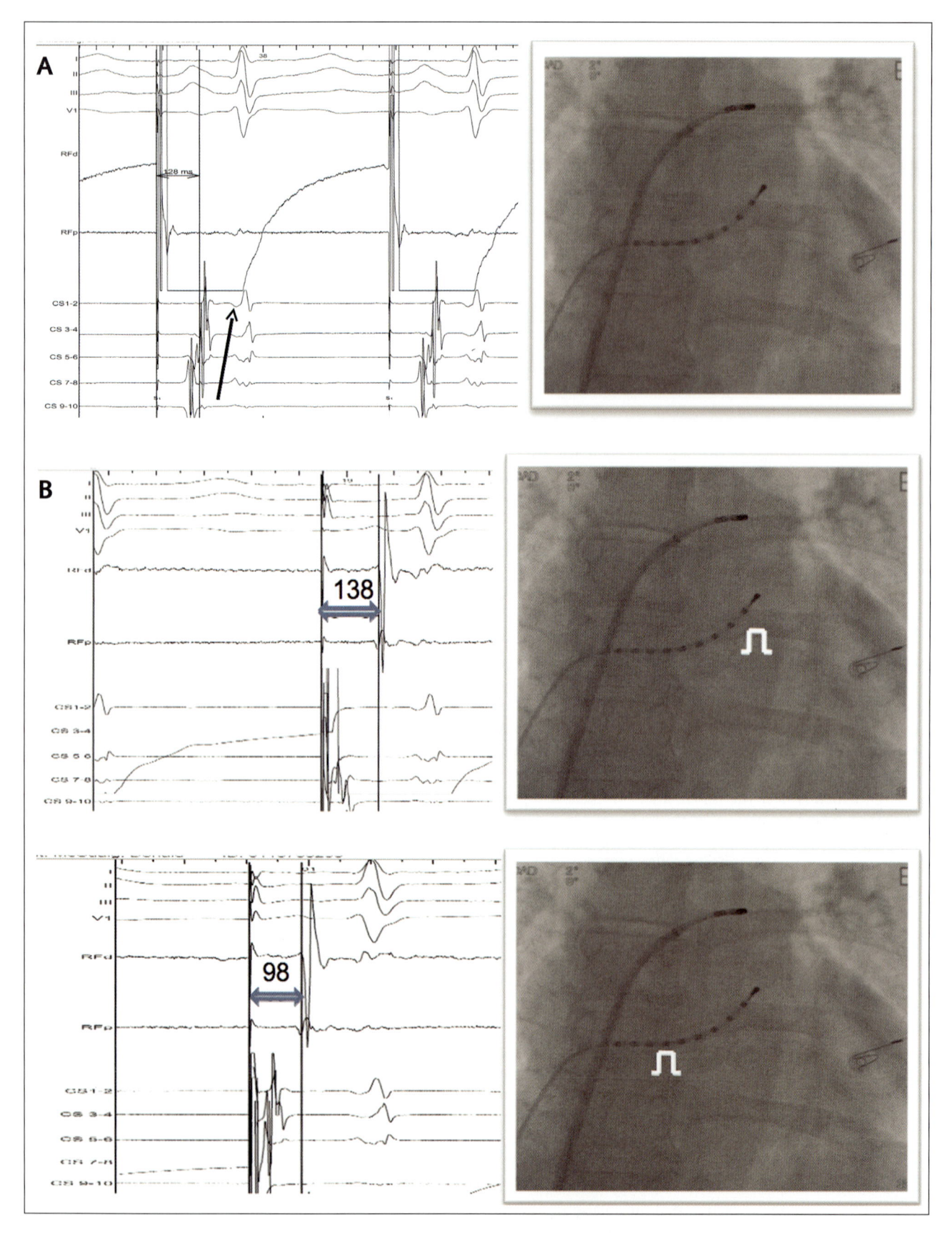

Figure 17.12 The left panels show surface ECG leads I, II, III, and V$_1$, then the RF catheter placed just anterior to the mitral line. Lowest are the EGMs of the bipoles of the decapolar catheter in the CS. In **A**, pacing from the RF catheter confirms clockwise block over the mitral line by activating the CS catheter in a proximal to distal manner. **B** confirms counterclockwise block by differential pacing. The interval measured from stim to RF is longer (138 ms) when pacing the distal CS than when pacing the more proximal CS (98 ms).

months except in case of recurrence. In such case, patients are offered a repeat procedure.

Procedural Complications

Serious complications can occur during an ablation for permanent AF, and it is important that these (and their rate of occurrence) are carefully discussed with the patients prior to him or her signing the consent form. The major complications are described in detail in the *HRS/EHRA/ECAS Guidelines on AF Ablation*; any providers or institutions carrying out these ablations should familiarize themselves with this document.[1] Overall, tamponade, pulmonary vein stenosis, atrioesophageal fistula and/or death, air emboli, and cerebrovascular or peripheral-vascular complications comprise a cumulative 2 to 4% complication rate. Two specific complications, cardiac tamponade and phrenic nerve paralysis, are discussed in some detail below.

Cardiac Tamponade

While we do not routinely perform an arterial line for blood pressure (RR) monitoring, we will noninvasively measure the RR every 10 minutes. Sudden drops in systolic blood pressure > 10 to 20 mmHg will alert us to exclude cardiac tamponade. We pay careful attention to any change in the cardiac silhouette on fluoroscopy and we have a low threshold to use TTE for the exclusion of tamponade. The competence and experience to perform emergency needle pericardiocentesis must be present or promptly available.

Phrenic Nerve Paralysis

Phrenic nerve paralysis can especially occur in the context of RA ablation. The right phrenic nerve has a close anatomic relationship to the RSPV and SVC and is vulnerable to collateral injury during endocardial RF delivery at or close to these structures. We attempt to identify the phrenic nerve location with high-output pacing prior to RA or RSPV RF delivery and will pay attention to diaphragmatic contraction during ablation at these sites.

Procedural Outcomes

The stepwise ablation of persistent AF leads to procedural termination of AF in up to 87% of patients. After repeat ablations, sinus rhythm can be maintained medium-term in up to 95% of all patients in whom AF terminated by ablation. On the contrary, if AF termination is not achieved by ablation during the index procedure, stable sinus rhythm was only found in 52% of patients during follow-up.[11,13] Subsequent studies from our group as well as studies published from other groups have reported similar findings, and also supported the finding that of AF termination by ablation is strongly predictive of long-term success.[10,14]

Duration of continuous AF and also AFCL are independent predictors of AF termination.[13,15] If the duration of AF is < 12 months, there is a 90% chance of AF termination. This success rate gradually decreases to 54% with a duration of AF > 48 months. Similarly, the AFCL is a predictor of success, with a likelihood of AF termination of 95% if the AFCL is > 161 ms, gradually decreasing to 50% likelihood of success with a very short AFCL < 120 ms.

Conclusion

The stepwise ablation of persistent AF is a hybrid approach of partly predetermined lesion sets and partly EGM guided ablation steps.[16] It is a patient-tailored approach that is guided by EP endpoints. The method can lead to termination of AF in up to 85% of patients and render them arrhythmia free at least in the medium term. However, 50% of patients need more than one procedure to achieve sustained sinus rhythm. Termination of AF by ablation is associated with a better long-term clinical outcome then when AF cannot be terminated by ablation.

Acknowledgments

We would like to thank Professor Michel Haïssaguerre as well as current and recent members of the EP team at our division for their inspiration and vital contributions to this book chapter.

References

1. Calkins H, Kuck KH, Cappato R, et al. 2012 HRS/EHRA/ECAS Expert Consensus Statement on catheter and surgical ablation of atrial fibrillation: recommendations for patient selection, procedural techniques, patient management and follow-up, definitions, endpoints, and research trial design. A report of the Heart Rhythm Society (HRS) Task Force on catheter and surgical ablation of atrial fibrillation. *Heart Rhythm.* 2012;9:632–696.
3. Scherr D, Sharma K, Dalal D, et al. Incidence and predictors of periprocedural cerebrovascular accident in patients undergoing catheter ablation of atrial fibrillation. *J Cardiovasc Electrophysiol.* 2009;20:1357–1363.
4. Nademanee K, McKenzie J, Kosar E, et al. A new approach for catheter ablation of atrial fibrillation: mapping of the electrophysiologic substrate. *J Am Coll Cardiol.* 2004;43:2044–2053.
5. Haïssaguerre M, Sanders P, Hocini M, et al. Catheter ablation of long-lasting persistent atrial fibrillation. critical structures for termination. *J Cardiovasc Electrophysiol.* 2005;16:1125–1137.
6. Takahashi Y, O'Neill MD, Hocini M, et al. Characterization of electrograms associated with termination of chronic atrial

fibrillation by catheter ablation. *J Am Coll Cardiol.* 2008;51: 1003–1010.
7. Knecht S, Hocini M, Wright M, et al. Left atrial linear lesions are required for successful treatment of persistent atrial fibrillation. *Eur Heart J.* 2008;19:2359–2366.
8. Chugh A, Oral H, Lemola K, et al. Prevalence, mechanisms, and clinical significance of macroreentrant atrial tachycardia during and following left atrial ablation for atrial fibrillation. *Heart Rhythm.* 2005;2:464–471.
9. Hocini M, Jaïs P, Sanders P, et al. Techniques, evaluation, and consequences of linear block at the left atrial roof in paroxysmal atrial fibrillation: A prospective randomized study. *Circulation.* 2005;112:3688–3696.
10. Jaïs P, Hocini M, Hsu LF, et al. Technique and results of linear ablation at the mitral isthmus. *Circulation.* 2004;110: 2996–3002.
11. Hocini M, Nault I, Wright M, et al. Disparate evolution of right and left atrial rate during ablation of long-lasting persistent atrial fibrillation. *J Am Coll Cardiol.* 2010;55: 1007–1016.
12. Haïssaguerre M, Hocini M, Sanders P, et al. Catheter ablation of long-lasting persistent atrial fibrillation. Clinical outcome and mechanisms of subsequent arrhythmias. *J Cardiovasc Electrophysiol.* 2005;16:1138-47.
13. Jaïs P, Matsuo S, Knecht S, et al. A deductive mapping strategy for atrial tachycardia following atrial fibrillation ablation: importance of localized reentry. *J Cardiovasc Electrophysiol.* 2009;20:480–491.
14. O'Neill MD, Wright M, Knecht S, et al. Long-term follow-up of persistent atrial fibrillation ablation using termination as a procedural endpoint. *Eur Heart J.* 2009;30: 1105–1112.
15. Rostock T, Salukhe TV, Steven D, et al. Long-term single- and multiple-procedure outcome and predictors of success after catheter ablation for persistent atrial fibrillation. *Heart Rhythm.* 2011;8(9):1391–1397.
16. Matsuo S, Lellouche N, Wright M, et al. Clinical predictors of termination and clinical outcome of catheter ablation for persistent atrial fibrillation. *J Am Coll Cardiol.* 2009;54:788–795.
17. O'Neill M, Jaïs P, Takahashi Y, Jönsson A, Sacher F, Hocini M, Sanders P, Rostock T, Rotter M, Pernat A, Clémenty J, Haïssaguerre M. The stepwise ablation approach for chronic atrial fibrillation—evidence for a cumulative effect. *J Interv Card Electrophysiol.* 2006;16:153–167.

CHAPTER 18

How to Ablate Long-Standing Persistent Atrial Fibrillation Using a Stepwise Approach (The Natale Approach)

Luigi Di Biase, MD, PhD; Pasquale Santangeli, MD; Andrea Natale, MD[1]

Introduction

Long-standing persistent AF is the most difficult arrhythmia to treat. Results are not yet satisfactory, although the outcomes improve after repeat procedures. The approach utilized may influence the outcome. This chapter describes our approach for the treatment of long-standing persistent AF, which we have named the "Natale approach" because it reflects the approach followed by Dr. Natale and his partners.

Preprocedural Management

All patients are required to undergo at least 2 months of effective thromboprophylaxis with oral anticoagulant therapy. Warfarin is initiated in an outpatient setting; all patients receive weekly INR monitoring during the 4 to 6 weeks preceding the procedure with a target INR of 2 to 3. We do not discontinue warfarin before the procedure and we do not bridge with low-weight heparin.[1]

Preprocedural TEE is not routinely performed unless patients cannot show a history of therapeutic INR in the 4 to 6 weeks preceding the procedure or are subtherapeutic on the day of the procedure. All patients are type and cross-matched, and packed red blood cells and fresh frozen plasma are made available for infusion in case of hemorrhagic complications. If the preprocedural INR is above 3.5, we partially reverse the anticoagulant effect with one or two units of fresh frozen plasma. In a large cohort study including patients with persistent and long-standing persistent AF, this approach has been proven to significantly decrease the risk of bleeding and thromboembolic complications when compared to warfarin discontinuation and bridging with low-molecular-weight heparin.[1–3]

Antiarrhythmic drugs are discontinued 3 to 5 days prior to the ablation.[1–3] Amiodarone is discontinued 4 to 6 months prior to the procedure; patients are usually switched to dofetilide, which is discontinued 5 days before the procedure.

Preoperative CT scan or MRI for imaging of PVs is generally performed only in patients undergoing "redo" procedures unless a history of congenital heart disease is known. Postoperative CT or MRI scan is performed in all patients at the 3 months follow-up.[4,5]

All the authors contributed equally to the drafting and editing of this chapter.

1. Disclosure/Conflict of Interest: Dr. Di Biase is a consultant for Hansen Medical and Biosense Webster. Dr. Natale is a consultant for Biosense Webster and has also received a research grant from St. Jude Medical and received speaker honoraria from St. Jude Medical, Medtronic, Boston Scientific, Biotronik, and Biosense Webster.

Anesthesia Protocol

All patients undergo ablation under general anesthesia. Anesthesia is initiated with propofol (2 mg/kg) and fentanyl (1 to 2 mg/kg), followed by a neuromuscular blocking agent (usually rocuronium 0.6 to 1 mg/kg) and by endotracheal intubation with intermittent positive pressure ventilation. An esophageal probe is inserted in all patients to monitor esophageal temperature during ablation.[6]

Instrumentation for Electrophysiological Study

After anesthesia induction, 4 venous accesses are obtained via the Seldinger technique: two in the right femoral vein, one in the left femoral vein, and one in the right internal jugular vein. For the physicians who are concerned about the risk of vascular injury while inserting sheaths under full anticoagulation, ultrasound guidance might be useful. In addition, cannulation of the right internal jugular vein can be performed with the use of a mapping catheter or a wire advanced into the superior vena cava as a marker for the vein access during fluoroscopy (**Figure 18.1**).

Right internal jugular vein access is used to place a 20-pole catheter in the CS. The distal 10 poles are positioned in the CS along the mitral annulus and the proximal 10 poles along the HRA and/or crista terminalis, depending on the RA size.

Left femoral venous access is obtained with an 11-Fr venous sheath to insert a 10-Fr 64-element phased-array ultrasound imaging catheter (AcuNav, Acuson, Mountain View, CA, USA) in the right atrium under fluoroscopic guidance. The ICE catheter is positioned in the mid-right atrium. Clockwise rotation of the ICE catheter provides posteriorly directed views. Therefore, clockwise torque to the ICE catheter brings into sequential view the aortic arch (more anterior), followed by the anterior LA, mitral valve and LAA, the left PVs, the posterior wall, and the right PVs. The IAS is always visualized in the near-field; if the septum is too close to the probe, gentle bending of the transducer toward the RA free wall moves the imaging plane of the septum toward the mid-field of view (**Figure 18.2**).

LA access is obtained with a double transseptal puncture (see Chapter 12). The technique employed for the transseptal puncture is the same as when performed under fluoroscopic guidance. Briefly, a long 0.032-inch J guide wire is advanced via the right groin venous access to the SVC at the level of the tracheal carina under fluoroscopic guidance. A long transseptal sheath (LAMP 90° 8.5 Fr, St. Jude Medical, St. Paul, MN, for the first transseptal and SLO 50° 8.5 Fr, St. Jude Medical, St. Paul, MN, for the second transseptal) is advanced over the wire to reach the tracheal carina; the long wire is withdrawn and the sheaths are continuously flushed with heparinized saline. During this stage, we usually administer an unfractioned heparin bolus of 10,000 U in males and 8,000 U in females. To maintain an ACT > 300 seconds, an additional heparin bolus may be administered. It is imperative for our approach that the heparin bolus is administered before the transseptal access is performed.

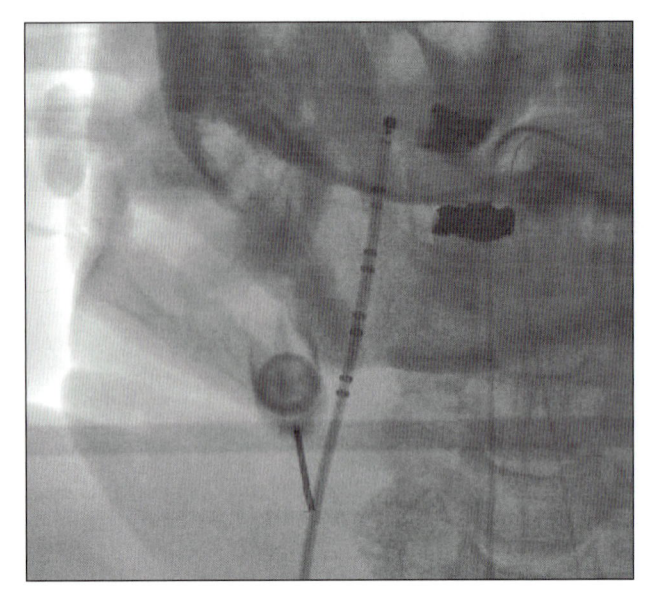

Figure 18.1 Antero-posterior fluoroscopy view of the 20-pole catheter advanced in the right internal jugular vein to be a marker for the jugular vein access during fluoroscopy.

A flushed Brockenbrough transseptal needle armed with its stylet is then introduced into the sheath and advanced to within 2 to 4 cm of the tip of the dilator. The stylet is removed and the needle is flushed with heparinized saline and radiopaque contrast. The entire system is gently withdrawn under fluoroscopic LAO or anteroposterior views, with the arrow-shaped handle of the needle usually oriented at between 4 and 6 o'clock. Correct positioning of the tip of the apparatus in the fossa ovalis for puncture is assessed by fluoroscopic visualization of a "jump" to the septum (most easily assessed in the LAO projection), and definitely confirmed by ICE imaging. Once the correct trajectory is confirmed, the dilator is gently advanced to obtain tenting of the fossa ovalis; therefore, the needle is advanced to further tent the IAS (Figure 18.2).[7] Usually, the needle crosses the fossa ovalis applying a gentle pressure, and a small injection of contrast is sufficient to confirm the LA access at ICE. In cases of thickened or hypertrophied IAS resistant to transseptal puncture (such as the cases of lipomatous degeneration or postcardiac surgery patients), RF energy application to the external end of the needle during septum tenting is of invaluable aid to access the LA. This is usually performed applying energy at the hub of the needle through an electrocautery in the "cut" modality, setting the RF power up to 30 W (▶ Video 18.1).

Once LA access has been confirmed by ICE imaging (1 second after RF energy application), the dilator is advanced over the needle and the sheath is advanced over the dilator to finally reach the LA. At this stage, the needle and dilator are removed, and the sheath is accurately aspirated and flushed with heparinized saline.

Figure 18.2 **A.** The RF "Bovie" touches the proximal end of the needle on the transseptal apparatus. The "Bovie" is activated as the needle is advanced out of the dilator with a cut power of 30 W and 0 W of coag. **B.** ICE showing the tenting of the needle on the right septum just before RF with the "Bovie." **C.** Anteroposterior fluoroscopy view of the transseptal apparatus tenting the fossa ovalis at the same level as shown in panel **B**.

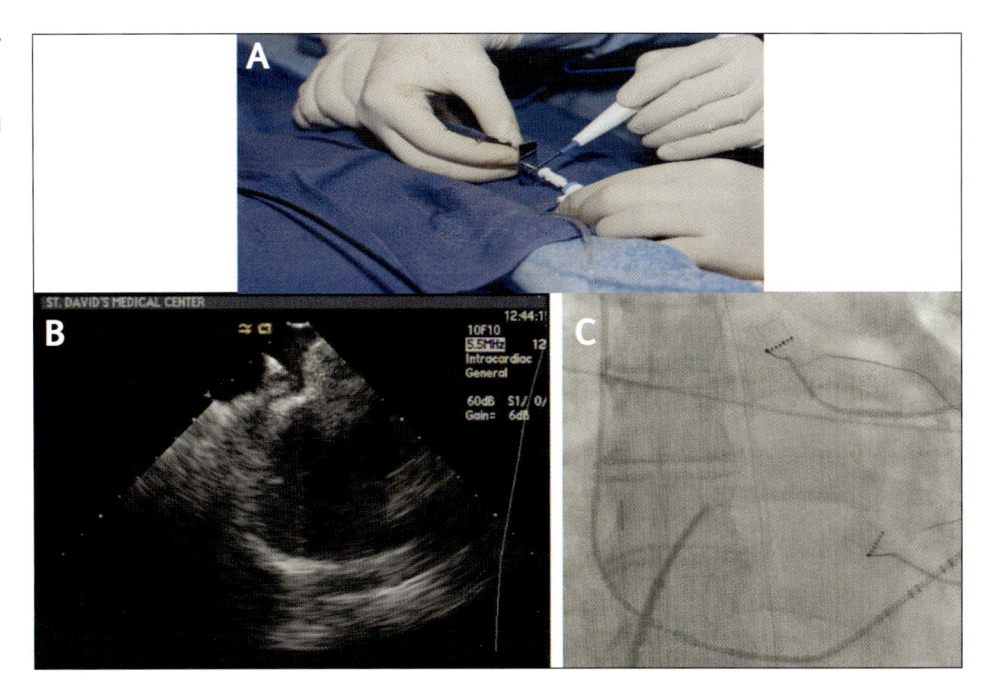

The best sites for transseptal puncture can only be assessed with ICE guidance to facilitate catheter maneuverability in the LA. A more anterior stick is usually performed for the first transseptal access (LAMP sheath), in which the circular mapping catheter is inserted; a more posterior stick, facing the left PVs where the distance from the aortic root and the posterior LA wall is maximal, is performed for the second stick, in which the open irrigated ablation catheter is inserted (SLO sheath).

PVAI and Isolation of the SVC

The circular mapping catheter is positioned under fluoroscopic and ICE guidance at the antrum of each PV. PV antrum potentials are identified by the circular mapping catheter, and RF energy is applied to achieve abolition of all PV antrum electrograms, targeting the left PVs first and then the right PVs. Since the PV antrum has usually a cross-sectional diameter larger than the circular mapping catheter, multiple movements of the circular mapping catheter around each PV antrum are needed to achieve complete isolation. The circular mapping catheter is dragged around each vein, creating small microloops. Entry block is verified when no PV potentials can be recorded along the antrum or inside the vein by the circular mapping catheter. When present, dissociated firing of the PV from the LA confirms exit block as well.

The PV antra include the entire posterior wall between the PVs and extend anteriorly to the right PVs along the left side of the IAS. Given that, the endpoint of the procedure is the complete elimination of local potentials that can be assessed only by means of circular catheter mapping (**Figures 18.3** and **18.4**). RF energy is delivered with a maximum temperature setting of 41°C and a power of 40 to 45 W with a

Figure 18.3 Different fluoroscopy views showing the dragging of the circular mapping catheter in different areas of the posterior wall and left septum. From right to left and from top to bottom, the roof and the low septum are shown.

flow rate of 30 cc/min. When ablating the posterior wall between the PVs, the power is decreased to 35 W. At the posterior site close to the esophagus, energy delivery is discontinued when the esophageal temperature probe has a rapid increase and reaches 39°C, while the power is reduced if the temperature increase is slow. Importantly, we limit each RF application per ablation site to 20 seconds.

Continuous impedance monitoring and catheter tip temperature are also employed to minimize the risk of steam pops. At the end of these steps, all four PV antra are extensively remapped to check the presence of any residual PV potentials and deliver further ablation in case of PV reconnection or residual recordings.

After PV antrum remapping and ablation of persistent breakthrough conduction gaps, and after the ablation of the posterior wall is complete, the ablation is extended to the endocardial aspect of the coronary sinus and to the left side of the septum. Ablation of complex fractionated atrial electrograms (CFAEs) in the left atrium and in the endocardial and epicardial aspect of the coronary sinus is also performed. If AF termination is unsuccessful after these steps, cardioversion is performed to restore sinus rhythm. At this time, patients receive a challenge with isoproterenol infusion up to 30 mg/min for 15 minutes to increase the chance of disclosing early PV reconnection or latent non-PV triggers of AF. Mapping during isoproterenol is performed positioning the circular mapping catheter in the left superior pulmonary vein and the ablation catheter in the right superior PV (**Figure 18.5**).

In this way, the site of origin of any significant ectopic atrial activity can be mapped and targeted for ablation by looking at the activation sequence in comparison to sinus beats. Differential activation between the distal CS and the circular mapping catheter can distinguish LAA versus left PV firing. In the presence of rapid conduction through the Bachmann bundle, the circular mapping catheter positioned at the ostium of the LAA is of invaluable aid in correctly detecting LAA firing, which in this case is usually associated with rapid septal-RA activation. If we see triggers from either the CS or the LAA, isolation of these structures is the best endpoint (**Figures 18.6, 18.7, and 18.8**).

In case of right-sided atrial ectopy, the site of origin can be detected analyzing the differential activation occurring at the ablation catheter tip and at the crista terminalis and CS recording poles.

Once the LA ablation is completed, heparin is stopped and catheters and sheaths are pulled back in the RA. The circular mapping catheter is positioned at the junction between the SVC and the HRA under ICE guidance and ablation to isolate the SVC is performed. We usually begin targeting potentials at the septal aspect of the SVC. High-voltage pacing (at least 30 mA) is used to check for phrenic nerve stimulation prior to isolating the lateral portion of the SVC. In the case of phrenic nerve capture, the lateral SVC is not isolated (**Figure 18.9**).[7–9]

At the end of the procedure, systemic anticoagulation with heparin is partially reversed with up to 40 mg of

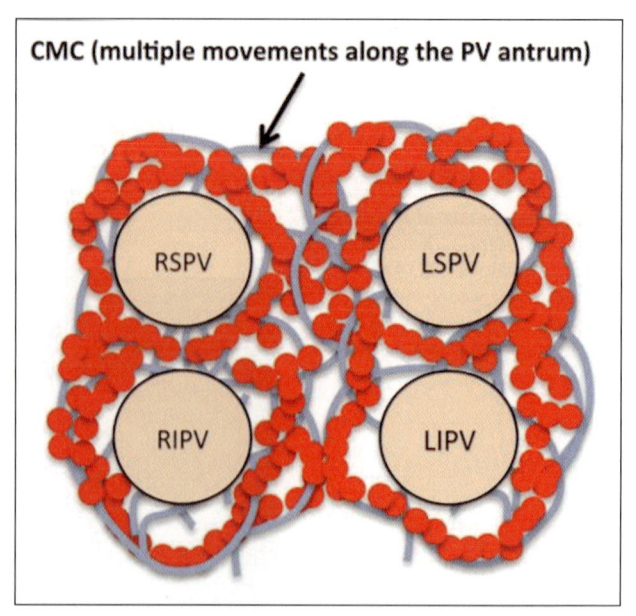

Figure 18.4 Diagram showing the lesion set performed while dragging the ablation catheter along the PV antrum and the posterior wall with the extension of the low septum. The black arrow points to the circular mapping catheter that is continuously dragged.

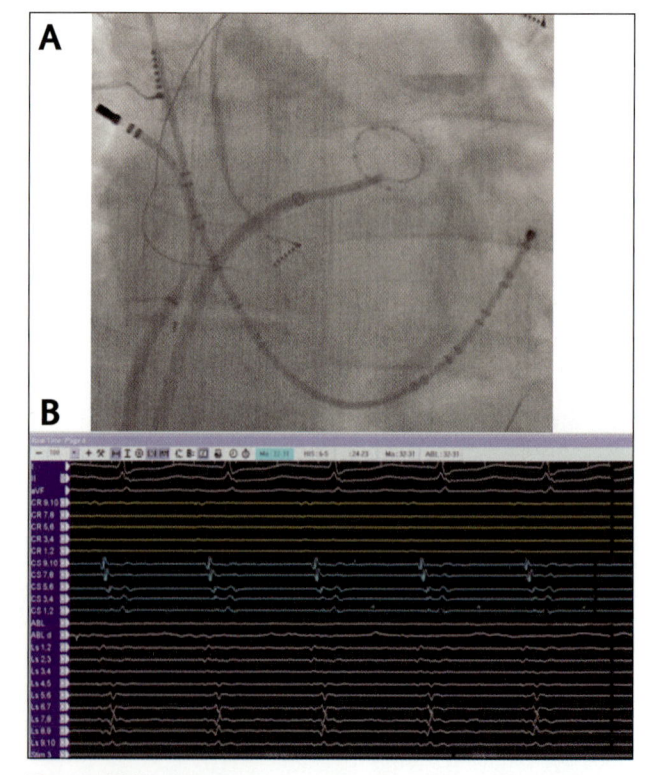

Figure 18.5 **A.** RAO fluoroscopy view showing the circular mapping catheter in the left superior pulmonary vein, the ablation catheter in the right SPV, and the 20 poles catheter along the right crista and the distal CS. The circular mapping catheter records far-field potentials from the LAA. **B.** Sinus tachycardia during isoproterenol infusion at 20 mcg/min. From top to bottom:
- Surface ECG leads: I, II, aVF
- Right atrium crista (RA) from proximal (9–10) to distal (1–2)
- CS catheter (CS) from proximal (9–10) to distal (1–2)
- Ablation catheter (ABL) from proximal (p) to distal (d)
- Circular catheter (LS) from 1-2 to 9-10 of the LAA.

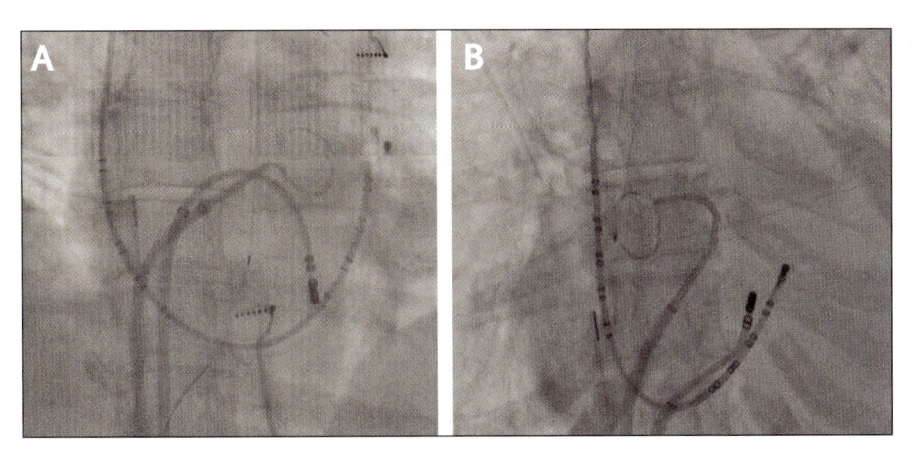

Figure 18.6 A. AP fluoroscopy view of the ablation catheter positioned at the level of the endocardial mid-CS to achieve CS isolation. **B.** AP fluoroscopy view of the ablation catheter positioned at the level of the epicardial distal CS.

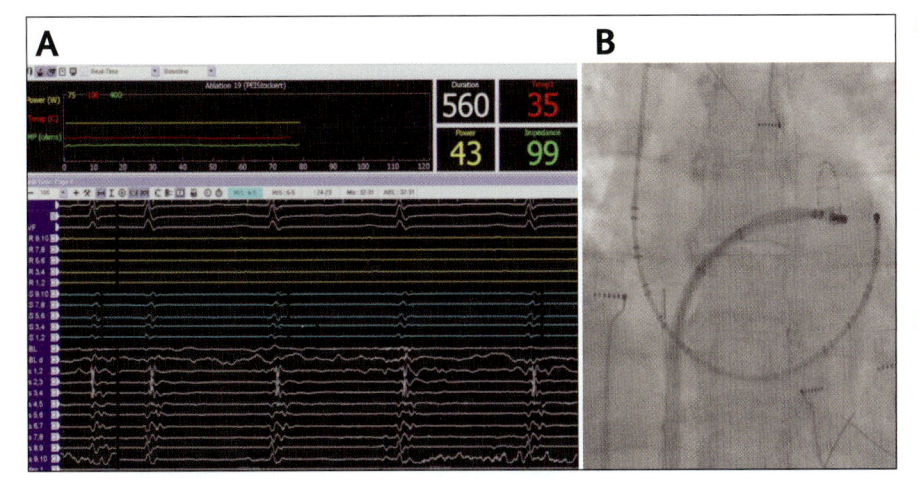

Figure 18.7 A. Intracardiac electrograms. The circular catheter is positioned at the base of the LAA. Top to bottom:
- Surface ECG leads: I, II, aVF
- RA crista proximal (9-10) to distal (1-2)
- CS catheter (CS) from proximal (9-10) to distal (1-2)
- Ablation catheter (ABL) from proximal (p) to distal (d)
- Circular catheter (LS) from 1-2 to 9-10 of the LAA.

B. AP fluoroscopy view of the circular mapping catheter at the base of the LAA. The ablation catheter is positioned at the site of the earliest activation on the circular mapping catheter while attempting LAA isolation.

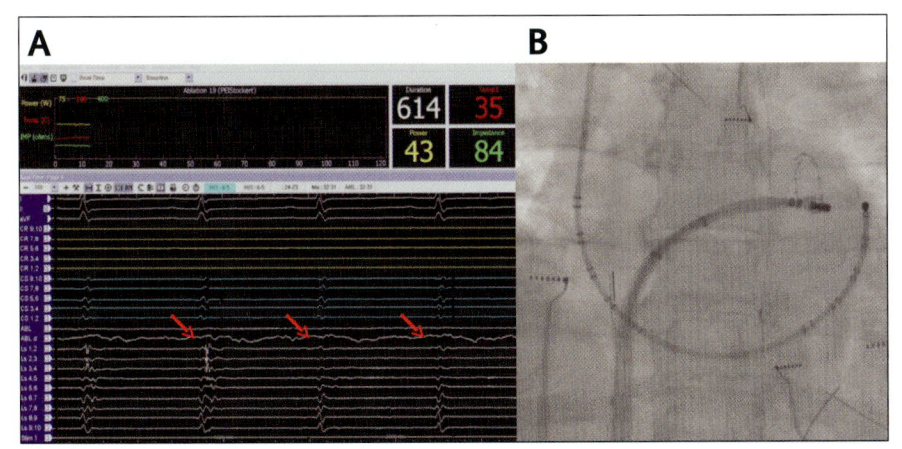

Figure 18.8 Intracardiac electrograms (**A**) and fluroscopy (**B**) while attempting LAA isolation. Red arrows indicate the LAA achieved isolation. From top to bottom:
- Surface ECG leads: I, II, aVF;
- Right atrium crista (RA) from proximal (9-10) to distal (1-2)
- CS catheter (CS) from proximal (9-10) to distal (1-2)
- Ablation catheter (ABL) from proximal (p) to distal (d)
- Circular catheter (LS) from 1-2 to 9-10 at the level of the LAA.

protamine guided by the ACT, and the sheaths are removed when the ACT is less than 250 seconds.

An example of a standard lesion set with the "Natale approach" in patients with long standing persistent AF is shown in **Figures 18.10** and **18.11**.

Other Targets

In adjunct to PVAI, the ablation is extended to the entire LA posterior wall down to the CS and to the entire left side of the septum. CFAE in the LA and within the CS are targeted as well.[10,11]

We have abandoned RA CFAE ablation. The technique implemented for completing ablation in the posterior LA wall down to the CS is similar to that of PVAI. In brief, the circular mapping catheter is positioned at the posterior wall and ablation is delivered to abolish potentials recorded by the mapping catheter. As previously mentioned, we decrease the RF power to 35 W when ablating the posterior wall and discontinue ablation when the esophageal temperature probe suddenly increases and reaches 39°C.

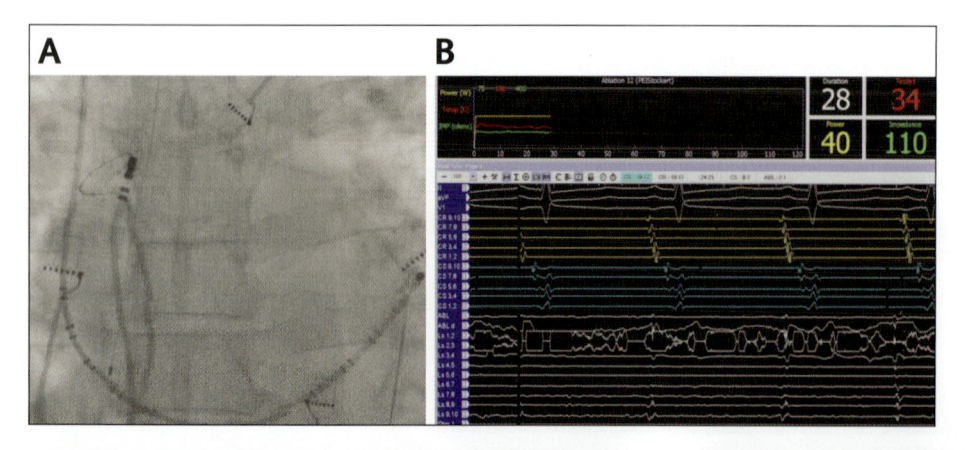

Figure 18.9 Fluroscopy (**A**) and intracardiac electrograms (**B**) while attempting SVC isolation. From top to bottom:
- Surface ECG leads: I, II, aVF;
- Right atrium crista (RA) from proximal (9-10) to distal (1-2)
- CS catheter (CS) from proximal (9-10) to distal (1-2)
- Ablation catheter (ABL) from proximal (p) to distal (d)
- Circular catheter (LS) from 1-2 to 9-10 at the level of the SVC.

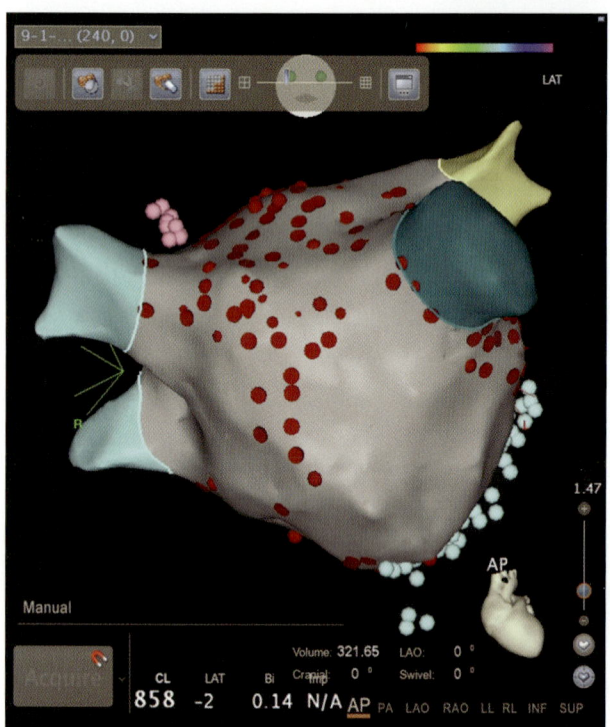

Figure 18.10 Antero-posterior view of a 3D electroanatomic LA map (CARTO-3™). Red dots indicate lesions at the level of the PV antra and the left septum. Lesions within the CS are depicted as blue. Pink dots indicate ablation lesions at the level of the SVC.

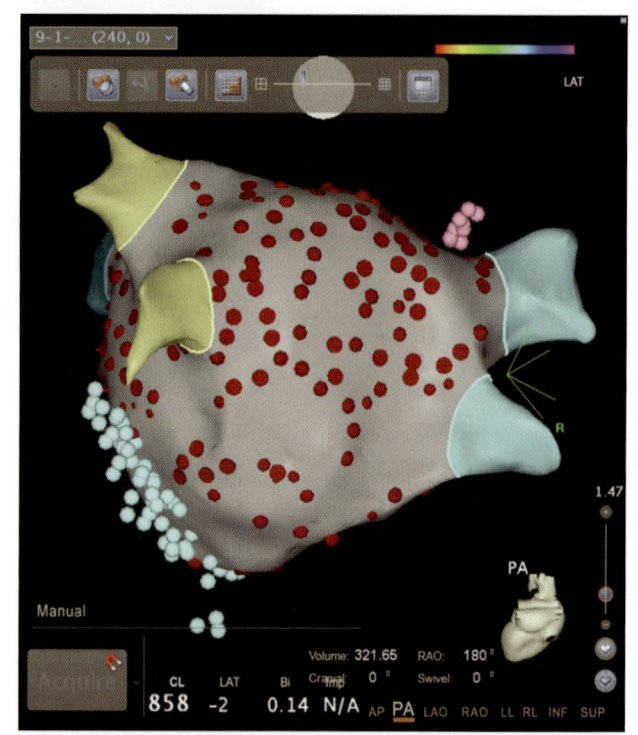

Figure 18.11 Postero-anterior view of a 3D electroanatomic LA map (CARTO-3™). Red dots indicate lesions at the level of the PV antra and the entire posterior wall down to the CS. Lesions within the CS are depicted as blue. Pink dots indicate ablation lesions at the level of the SVC.

CFAE ablation follows PVAI. CFAE criteria are defined as: (1) atrial electrograms with fractionation and composed of two defections or more and/or with continuous activity of the baseline or (2) atrial electrograms with a CL ≤ 120 ms.[10] The ablation catheter must be in a stable position for at least 10 seconds when recording these electrograms in order to avoid artifacts due to instability of the catheter. The intracardiac bipolar electrograms filter ranged from 30 to 500 Hz and the CFAE detection and ablation are guided by visual inspection. Nonfluoroscopic mapping systems are of particular aid during CFAE ablation to assist catheter navigation.

Isolation of the CS is usually performed first along the endocardial aspect (Figure 18.6A) and then completed within the vessel (Figure 18.6B). From the endocardial aspect, we usually begin ablation from the distal CS (lateral LA at about 4 o'clock in the LAO projection), progressing to the septal area anterior to the right PVs. A correct positioning of the ablation catheter to target the endocardial aspect of the CS is usually accomplished advancing the sheath and looping the ablation catheter in the antero-superior LA in order to direct the tip toward the posterior mitral annulus. A 90° to 180° loop is often necessary to complete endocardial ablation of the CS (Figure 18.6A). Continuous monitoring of the PR interval is warranted during ablation along the proximal CS and the low LA septum, since lesion of leftward extensions of AV nodal tissue may result in PR prolongation and occasionally into AV block.

After endocardial ablation, CS isolation is completed delivering RF energy from within the coronary sinus.

Ablation is started distally and continued along the vein to reach the vessel ostium. The endpoint is the complete abolition of all CS potentials (Figure 18.6B). Monitoring of the PR interval is crucial in this phase, and RF energy is prompted discontinued in case of PR prolongation. The power setting is 30 W up to 35 W at this location.

The importance of extending the ablation to structures other than the PV antra and the SVC in these patients has been highlighted by several clinical studies. Persistent and long-standing persistent AF is characterized by significant changes in atrial structure and EP function, which take the name of "atrial remodeling." In this setting, non-PV sites play a significant role in triggering and maintaining the arrhythmia, which supports the inadequacy of PV isolation alone as an effective ablation strategy.[10,11]

Procedural termination of AF is not sought as an endpoint at our institution.[11] In a prospective study on 306 patients with long-standing persistent AF undergoing the first procedure of PVAI plus CFAE ablation, only 6 (2%) patients converted directly to sinus rhythm during ablation, while 172 (56%) organized into atrial tachycardia, which was mapped and ablated, and 128 (42%) patients remained in AF and were cardioverted at the end of the procedure.

Interestingly, after a mean follow-up of 25 ± 6.9 months, 69% of patients remained in sinus rhythm without significant differences between those who had procedural termination/organization of AF and those who remained in AF and received cardioversion. Of note, procedural organization of AF predicted the mode of recurrence, with a significant association with recurrence of atrial tachycardia ($P = 0.022$).[11]

In conclusion, we deliver an extensive set of ablation lesions in patients with persistent and long-standing persistent AF. PVAI and SVC isolation is associated with ablation of the entire LA posterior wall, CS, and LA ablation of CFAE. Our approach is supported by clinical evidence.

Considerations for Patients Presenting for Repeat Procedure

In a recent study, we reported the prevalence of AF triggers from the LAA in a series of 987 patients (29% paroxysmal AF, 71% nonparoxysmal AF) referred for repeat catheter ablation.[14] LAA firing was assessed only after all the potential sites of reconnection, including the PV antra, the posterior wall, and the septum were checked and targeted if reconnected.

Overall, 266 (27%) patients showed firing from the LAA at baseline or after administration of isoproterenol, and in 8.7% of patients, the LAA was found to be the only source of arrhythmia. LAA firing was defined as consistent atrial premature contractions with the earliest activation in the LAA, or as AF/atrial tachyarrhythmia originating from the LAA. In these cases, a complete isolation of the LAA is the ablation strategy that provides the best long-term outcome.

Of the 266 patients presenting LAA firing, 43 were not ablated (Group 1), 56 received a focal ablation (Group 2), and 167 underwent LAA isolation guided by a circular mapping catheter and ICE (Group 3). After a mean follow-up of 1 year, AF recurred in 74% of Group 1 patients, as compared to 68% of Group 2 and 15% of Group 3 ($P < 0.001$ for multiple comparison).[12]

The technique employed for LAA isolation is similar to that adopted for PVAI, although the procedure requires more ablation time. Moreover, since the LAA has a very thin wall and may be prone to perforation, particular caution should be taken into account when isolating this structure (Figures 18.7 and 18.8). Of interest, LAA isolation does not appear to significantly alter the mechanical function. We found a preserved contractility at TEE 6 months after the ablation in about 60 to 65% of patients.

On the other hand, further prospective studies are necessary to disclose the clinical relevance of LAA and its consequences with respect to potential complications. The "BELIEF" study (Effect of Empirical LAA Isolation on Long-term Procedure Outcome in Patients With Persistent or Long-standing Persistent AF Undergoing Catheter Ablation [NCT01362738 on www.clinicaltrial.gov]), a randomized controlled trial comparing the ablation outcome in patients with long-standing persistent AF undergoing LAA isolation plus our standard approach, versus our standard approach alone, will probably answer this issue. Importantly, after reporting on triggers from LAA, we currently perform LAA isolation if trigger from this site is demonstrated even during the initial procedure.

Postprocedural Care and Follow-Up

All patients receive a single dose of aspirin (325 mg) before leaving the EP laboratory and continue their warfarin dosage regimens to maintain a target INR of 2 to 3.

Use of the open-irrigation-tip catheter may results in fluid overload and/or pulmonary congestion, since up to 4L of fluid can be administered in a case of long-standing persistent AF. We routinely monitor the fluid intake and the diuresis during the procedure. Between 40 and 60 mg of furosemide are used immediately after the procedure. In addition, the morning after the ablation, all patients receive additional 80 mg of IV furosemide and 40 mg of potassium and are discharged with a regimen of 80 mg of furosemide twice a day for 2 or 3 days. Each patient is advised to check body weight and to call in if this does not drop to the preprocedure value.

All patients are strictly monitored for outcome and complications during overnight hospital stay, and on the following day prior to discharge using symptom assessment, serial neurological examinations, and puncture site checks. All patients undergo an Echocardiogram to rule out pericardial effusion in the 6 hours following the procedure. Patients are discharged after overnight observation.

Patients are usually discharged on their previously ineffective antiarrhythmic drugs, which are continued during the blanking period (12 weeks). After the blanking period, antiarrhythmic drugs are discontinued. In cases of recurrences after the blanking period, patients resume antiarrhythmic drugs.

Follow-up is performed at 3, 6, 9, 12 and then every 6 months after the procedure, with a 12-lead ECG and 7-day Holter monitoring. Patients are given event recorder for 5 months after ablation and are asked to transmit their rhythm every time they have symptoms compatible with arrhythmias and at least twice a week even if asymptomatic. Any episode of AF/AT longer than 30 seconds is considered to be a recurrence.

Progress of recovery and symptoms are assessed by dedicated nurses. In case of symptoms or suspected complications, patients are asked to seek medical attention at either a local emergency department or our emergency department, or to follow up with their primary physician. All documentations from these visits are collected by our AF center. With regard to the out-of-hospital long-term anticoagulation management, patients are referred to dedicated anticoagulation clinics with the aim of maintaining a stable therapeutic INR level. We follow a standard, uniform, and validated protocol of long-term postprocedural anticoagulation management. Briefly, oral anticoagulation is discontinued, regardless of the $CHADS_2$ score, if patients do not experience any recurrence of atrial tachyarrhythmias, severe PV stenosis (PV narrowing > 70%), and severe LA mechanical dysfunction, as assessed by TTE and TEE.

Patients with a $CHADS_2$ score ≥ 1 experiencing early recurrence of AF are maintained on warfarin for at least 6 months. In these patients, warfarin is discontinued if there is no AF recurrence in the last 3 months without antiarrhythmic drugs, and aspirin (81 to 325 mg) is started. In the case of a new AF recurrence after warfarin discontinuation in patients with a $CHADS_2$ score ≥ 1, oral anticoagulation is restarted.

In addition to the above criteria, patients who have undergone LAA isolation are assessed with a TEE 6 months after the procedure to decide anticoagulation discontinuation. If the LAA contractility is deemed preserved and the flow velocity is normal (> 0.3 m/s), warfarin is discontinued. If the LAA contractility is not preserved, patients are maintained on warfarin or a LAA closure device might be considered to achieve warfarin discontinuation.

With our approach, which utilizes general anesthesia to gain catheter stability and an open irrigated catheter with high power (up to 45 W), recovery of conduction around the PV antrum is seldom seen in patients with recurrence of AF either at the mid-term or at the long-term follow up. The presence of extra PV firings from the CS, the LA roof, and the LAA are often the only sites of reconnection. At long-term follow up, new extra PV sites or reconnected extra PVs firing previously ablated are the most common cause of arrhythmias.[6]

References

1. Di Biase L, Burkhardt JD, Mohanty P, et al. Periprocedural stroke and management of major bleeding complications in patients undergoing catheter ablation of AF: the impact of periprocedural therapeutic international normalized ratio. *Circulation.* 2010;121:2550–2556.
2. Santangeli P, Di Biase L, Sanchez JE, Horton R, Natale A. AF ablation without interruption of anticoagulation. *Cardiol Res Pract.* 2011;2011:837–841.
3. Gopinath D, Lewis WR, Di Biase LD, Natale A. Pulmonary vein antrum isolation for AF on therapeutic coumadin: special considerations. *J Cardiovasc Electrophysiol.* 2011; 22:236–239.
4. Di Biase L, Fahmy TS, Wazni OM, et al. Pulmonary vein total occlusion following catheter ablation for AF: clinical implications after long-term follow-up. *J Am Coll Cardiol.* 2006;48:2493–2499.
5. Barrett CD, Di Biase L, Natale A. How to identify and treat patients with pulmonary vein stenosis post AF ablation. *Curr Opin Cardiol.* 2009;24:42–49.
6. Di Biase L, Conti S, Mohanty P, et al. General anesthesia reduces the prevalence of pulmonary vein reconnection during repeat ablation when compared with conscious sedation: results from a randomized study. *Heart Rhythm.* 2011;8: 368–372.
7. Bhargava M, Di Biase L, Mohanty P, et al. Impact of type of AF and repeat catheter ablation on long-term freedom from AF: results from a multicenter study. *Heart Rhythm.* 2009;6:1403–1412.
8. Arruda M, Mlcochova H, Prasad SK, et al. Electrical isolation of the superior vena cava: an adjunctive strategy to pulmonary vein antrum isolation improving the outcome of AF ablation. *Cardiovasc Electrophysiol.* 2007;18:1261–1266.
9. Corrado A, Bonso A, Madalosso M, Rossillo A, Themistoclakis S, Di Biase L, Natale A, Raviele A. Impact of systematic isolation of superior vena cava in addition to pulmonary vein antrum isolation on the outcome of paroxysmal, persistent, and permanent AF ablation: results from a randomized study. *J Cardiovasc Electrophysiol.* 2010;21:1–5.
10. Elayi CS, Verma A, Di Biase L, et al. Ablation for long-standing permanent AF: results from a randomized study comparing three different strategies. *Heart Rhythm.* 2008;5: 1658–1664.
11. Elayi CS, Di Biase L, Barrett C, et al. AF termination as a procedural endpoint during ablation in long-standing persistent AF. *Heart Rhythm.* 2010;7:1216–1223.
12. Di Biase L, Burkhardt JD, Mohanty P, et al. Left atrial appendage: an underrecognized trigger site of AF. *Circulation.* 2010;122:109–118.
13. Themistoclakis S, Corrado A, Marchlinski FE, et al. The risk of thromboembolism and need for oral anticoagulation after successful AF ablation. *J Am Coll Cardiol.* 2010; 55:735–743.

Video Descriptions

Video 18.1 The movie shows the tenting of the transseptal apparatus over the fossa and the instrumentation of the LA (note the bubbles) after the RF application with the "bovie" over the external end of the needle, as shown in Figure 18.2.

CHAPTER 19

How to Use Balloon Cryoablation for Ablation of Atrial Fibrillation

Pipin Kojodjojo, MRCP, PhD; D. Wyn Davies, MD

Introduction

Electrical isolation of pulmonary veins is the cornerstone of all AF ablation procedures. One such procedure is successful in preventing recurrence of paroxysmal AF in 60 to 77% of patients.[1,2] In ablation of persistent AF, PVI is usually the first step in a stepwise approach to terminate AF.[3]

Achieving PVI using conventional point-by-point ablation lesions remains technically challenging with a shallow learning curve, mostly due to the highly variable anatomy of the posterior LA and difficulty in maintaining good, stable catheter tip-tissue contact during ablation.[4] PVI at the antral level is preferred to minimize the risk of PV stenosis and to include arrhythmogenic antral foci within the level of isolation. To this extent, antral ablation has been shown to be more effective than ostial segmental ablation in preventing AF recurrence.[5] With these considerations in mind, ablation technology that can deliver circumferential ablation centered on the PV antra should facilitate successful AF ablation.

Although a range of different ablation energy sources such as RF energy, laser, and cryotherapy are available, cryoablation offers theoretical advantages in that it does not disrupt target tissue architecture and could thus reduce the overall incidence of procedural complications such as pulmonary venous stenosis, LA perforation, and atrioesophageal fistulation.[6] Symptomatic pulmonary venous stenosis is rare after cryoballoon ablation but has been reported for the first time in the recently presented STOP-AF trial.[7] Atrioesophageal fistulation and coronary occlusion have not been reported in association with cryoablation for AF. Despite recognizing the benefits of cryoablation, an efficient delivery platform to deliver contiguous lesions around PV antra had been lacking until the introduction of the cryoablation balloon catheter system. PVI using earlier delivery platforms, such as 6-mm tipped and expandable circular cryoablation catheters, required lengthy procedures of more than 6 hours and were associated with unsatisfactory clinical outcomes.[8-10] This was thought to be due to the effects of competitive warming by blood flowing past the catheter, thus reducing lesion sizes. The cryoablation balloon catheter obstructs blood flow from the PV being treated, thereby removing this limitation.

In the following sections, we will describe our local protocol and experience with the use of a balloon cryoablation catheter for treatment of AF.

Preprocedure Planning

Patients with symptomatic AF refractory to 2 or more antiarrhythmic agents are offered the choice of undergoing cryoablation. In our practice, balloon cryoablation is reserved for patients undergoing their first AF ablation procedure, for reasons that will be discussed below. These subjects have either paroxysmal AF (defined as self-terminating AF episodes lasting less than 7 days) or early persistent AF (defined as episodes of AF that lasted greater than 7 days, requiring direct current cardioversion to restore sinus rhythm and transition from a clinical pattern of paroxysmal AF within the previous 12 months). So far, we have subselected our persistent AF patients for cryoablation because patients with a longer history of persistent AF are known to have larger, more diseased atria. These patients are therefore much more likely to require adjunctive atrial ablation either at sites with fractionated electrograms and/or to create linear lesions to increase chances of maintaining sinus rhythm. These additional ablation strategies cannot easily be achieved by the cryoballoon.

Informed consent is obtained from all patients prior to the procedure. All antiarrhythmic agents except amiodarone are stopped at least 5 half-lives before the procedure. Patients with a CHADS2 score of greater than 1 will receive anticoagulation with warfarin for at least 1 month before the procedure. Warfarin was stopped 5 days prior to the procedure with a low-molecular-weight heparin bridge until and including the day before the procedure. Patients with a CHADS2 score of 0 to 1 will usually be on 75mg of aspirin for stroke prophylaxis and will not receive warfarin either before or after the procedure. All patients will receive a transthoracic echocardiogram as part of the outpatient cardiovascular assessment. No other preprocedural imaging such as MRI or CT is routinely performed to assess LA and pulmonary venous anatomy. On the day of the procedure, TEE will be performed on every patient to exclude intracardiac thrombus. For those patients undergoing balloon cryoablation under general anesthesia, the TEE will be performed after induction and the probe kept in the esophagus to guide transseptal punctures.

Procedure

Two 8-Fr short sheaths are placed in the right femoral vein and are exchanged for 2 8-Fr transseptal sheaths (SR0 sheath, St. Jude Medical, St. Paul, MN) These are, in turn, introduced into the LA by 2 separate transseptal punctures. A 6-Fr arterial sheath is placed in the left femoral artery for continuous monitoring of systemic arterial pressure and to allow placement of a pigtail catheter to mark the position of the aortic valve and the ascending aorta during the transseptal puncture in patients who are receiving conscious sedation rather than general anesthesia. A 7-Fr sheath is also inserted into the LFV. Successful entry into the LA is confirmed by the appearance of LA pressure waveforms measured through the transseptal needle (BRK needle, St. Jude Medical, St. Paul, MN) and the visualization of contrast and bubbles in the LA on fluoroscopy or echocardiography respectively (▶ **Video 19.1**). A bolus of 10,000 U of unfractionated heparin is given, and repeated boluses are given during the procedure to maintain ACTs of greater than 300 seconds, with measurements made every 30 minutes. An alternative approach to balloon cryoablation with a single trans-septal puncture has also been used successfully.[11]

Contrast pulmonary venography is performed with a 7-Fr NIH catheter via one of the transseptal sheaths. This is then replaced with a curvilinear, 20-pole, deflectable, variable-diameter mapping catheter (Inquiry Optima, St. Jude Medical, St. Paul, MN, or Lasso, Biosense Webster, Diamond Bar, CA) to map each PV ostium. (▶ **Videos 19.2, 19.3, 19.4,** and **19.5**). Over a 300-cm exchange-length 0.035-inch J-tipped guidewire (Cook Medical, Bloomington, IN) usually positioned into the left superior PV, the second 8-Fr transseptal sheath is exchanged for a 15-Fr deflectable sheath (Flexcath, Medtronic, Minneapolis, MN) to allow introduction of a 28-mm cryoablation balloon (Arctic Front, Medtronic, Minneapolis, MN) (▶ **Video 19.6**). The Arctic Front balloon is available in 2 sizes, 23-mm and 28-mm, but the 28-mm is the cryoballoon used in virtually all our cases, as the larger balloon results in electrical isolation at a more antral level and is less likely to injure the right phrenic nerve during applications to the right pulmonary veins.[11,12]

The Arctic Front cryoballoon is a deflectable "balloon within a balloon" catheter whereby refrigerant (nitrous oxide) is delivered into the inner balloon (**Figure 19.1**). A constant vacuum applied between the inner and outer balloon prevents the leakage of refrigerant into the circulation in the event of a defect in the inner balloon. An extra-support, standard-length 0.035-inch J-tipped guide wire (Cook Medical, Bloomington, IN) is placed within the central lumen of the Arctic Front before the catheter is introduced into the Flexcath sheath. When inside the sheath, this is then advanced, ensuring that the J-tip is always outside the tip of the balloon catheter for safety. Using the deflectable sheath, the assembly is placed at the PV ostia and the guide wire introduced under fluoroscopy, sequentially into each targeted PV. The cryoballoon is inflated in the body of the LA before it is advanced over the wire into the PV antrum (**Figure 19.2**). Fifty percent contrast is injected distally via the central lumen of the catheter (which is wide enough to allow for contrast injection without removing the guidewire) to confirm a good seal between the balloon and the PV antra (▶ **Videos 19.7, 19.8, 19.9,** and **19.10**; **Figure 19.3**) Ideally, the injected contrast is completely trapped within the PV, indicating perfect balloon-to-antral contact around the entire circumference of the PV antrum. However, at this stage, delayed emptying of contrast from the PV or evidence of a localized leak of contrast is acceptable, as there is some balloon expansion when the freeze begins, which may improve the seal. If a good seal cannot be achieved, the orientation of the Arctic Front catheter is adjusted by either deflecting the Flexcath sheath, manipulating the

Chapter 19: Balloon Cryoablation for AF • 169

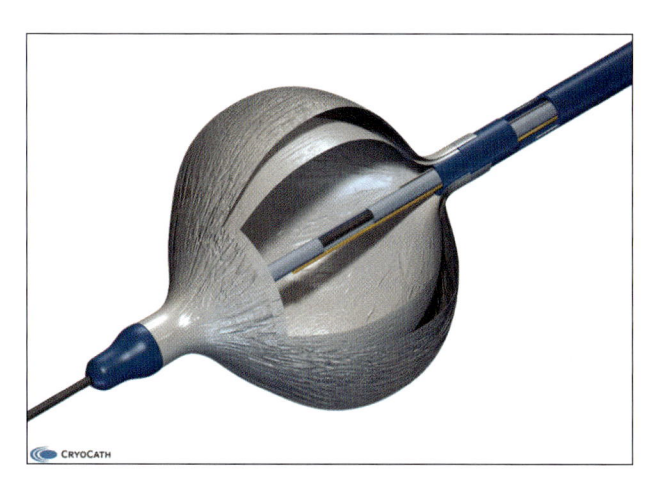

Figure 19.1 Construction of the cryoablation balloon (Arctic Front, Medtronic, Minneapolis, MN).

guidewire into a different branch of the PV to change the orientation of the balloon in relation to the PV antrum, or a combination of these maneuvers. Once a good seal is achieved, 2 separate 5-minute cryoballoon applications are applied to each PV, aiming for a trough temperature of less than −40°C during each application (**Figure 19.4**). A lower trough temperature during cryoballoon application as well as a tighter occlusion of the PV by the balloon is associated with an increased likelihood of achieving pulmonary venous isolation. Once cryoablation is commenced, any point of contact between the endothelium and balloon will be ablated (**Figure 19.5**). If the seal and trough temperature during the first freeze are not optimal, the balloon is reoriented as described above to achieve better contact and temperatures for the second freeze.

Forward pressure is applied to the balloon catheter to ensure maximal contact between the cryoballoon and the PV antra until cryoadherence occurs. This attribute is especially helpful to aid cryoablation of the RIPV. This PV is the most difficult to achieve a good seal with the cryoballoon. A helpful technique is to first establish good contact between the superior margin of the RIPV and the cryoballoon. Once the cryoballoon becomes adherent to

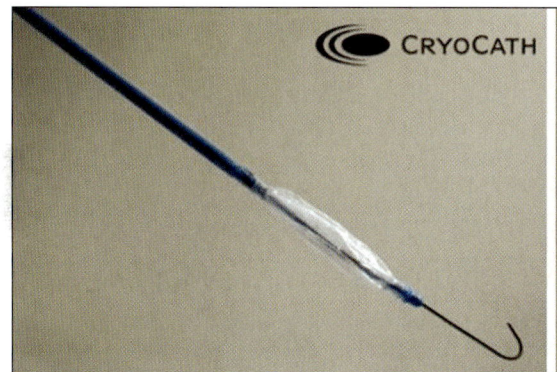

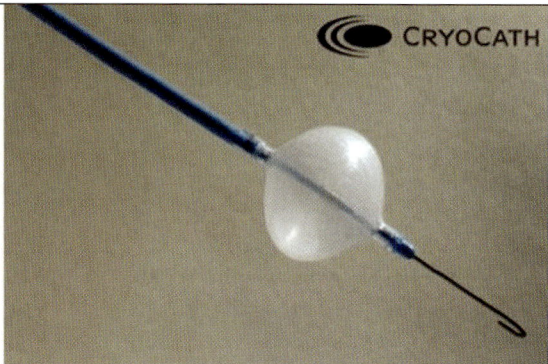

Figure 19.2 Deflated and inflated cryoablation balloon (Arctic Front, Medtronic, Minneapolis, MN)

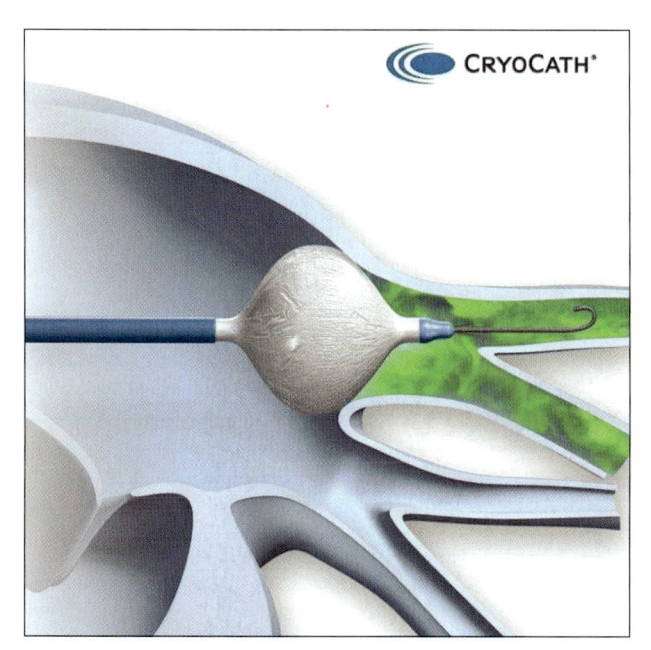

Figure 19.3 Schematic representation of an inflated cryoablation balloon (Arctic Front, Medtronic, Minneapolis, MN) with a good seal around a PV.

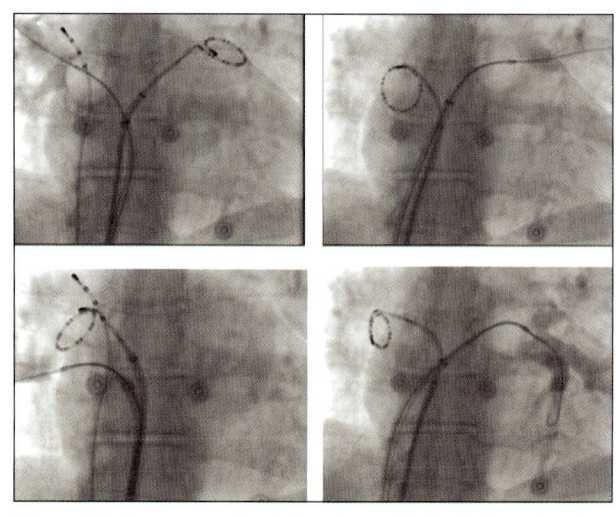

Figure 19.4 Images of an inflated cryoablation balloon (Arctic Front, Medtronic, Minneapolis, MN) positioned at the antra of all 4 pulmonary veins in a patient with paroxysmal AF.

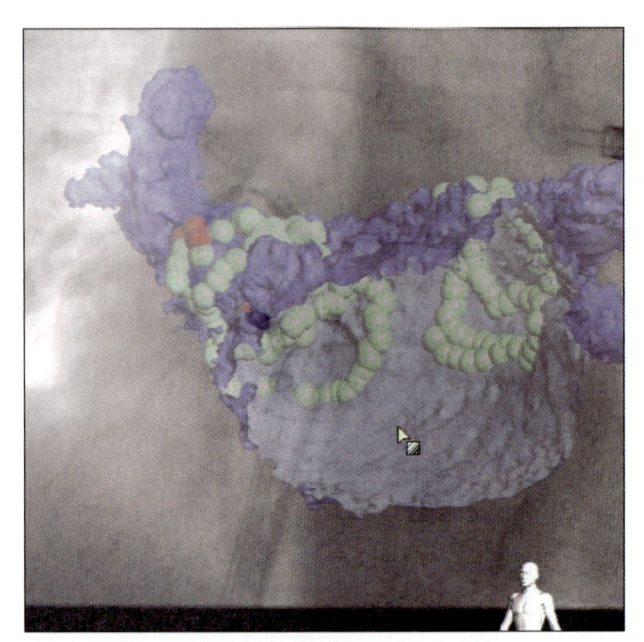

Figure 19.5 The points of contact between the inflated cryoballoon and pulmonary antra (green and red dots) are marked using the Philips EP Navigator system. Note the antral level of isolation. As a result, only the mid-posterior wall is not included within the cryoablation lesion set.

the endocardium, after approximately 1 minute of freezing, the balloon and sheath are pulled down to seal the inferior margin of the PV (▶ **Video 19.11**). This and similar maneuvers, such as torquing the balloon catheter during a freeze, may be used to improve contact and therefore temperatures. An alternative technique to enter the RIPV is to loop the Flexcath in the LA body before advancing the cryoballoon over the guidewire into the RIPV.

We have observed an interesting phenomenon of transient periods of hypotension and bradycardia lasting for up to 30 seconds, commonly described as a vagal response to ablation and thought to be due to injury to neural elements in the posterior LA. Although this phenomenon is seen typically with the onset of RF energy delivery, with cryoballoon ablation, it develops during the rewarming period, after the cessation of cryoballoon therapy. This phenomenon is most commonly seen with treatment of the LSPV.

Typically during the second freeze to the LIPV, a deflectable quadripolar catheter is introduced via the LFV for pacing in the SVC to capture the right phrenic nerve. When necessary, it can also be used for differential atrial pacing. During cryoballoon applications to the right-sided PVs, the right phrenic nerve is stimulated by pacing (1500 ms CL, 20 mA output) in the SVC to detect early signs of right phrenic nerve palsy, a complication that is seen more frequently during treatment of the right PVs using any balloon-based ablation. The operator monitors the strength of right hemi-diaphragmatic contractions during right phrenic nerve pacing by palpating the abdomen. Cryoballoon applications are immediately terminated when any reduction in the strength of right hemi-diaphragmatic contractions is felt, a finding that heralds the onset of right phrenic nerve palsy (▶ **Video 19.12**).

The EP endpoint sought is pulmonary venous isolation, as determined by the presence of entrance block from LA to each PV. After each PV antrum has been treated with two 5-minute cryoballoon applications, the PV antra are remapped with the curvilinear mapping catheter and entrance block is confirmed by the absence of local PV electrical signals where these signals were previously observed pre-ablation. Frequently, dissociated PV firing can be recorded confirming the presence of exit block.

With just 2 cryoballoon applications per vein, 83% of targeted PVs are isolated.[13] Based on early clinical experience with another balloon ablation system, we found that any PV that has not been isolated by 2 energy applications could be difficult to isolate with repeat balloon applications, with additional risk of phrenic nerve injury during right-sided ablation and extending procedural time in the LA. We have therefore taken a pragmatic approach that, after 2 cryoballoon applications, any remaining connection to a PV will be eliminated by ostial, map-guided focal cryoablation using the 8-mm-tipped 9-Fr Freezor Max catheter (Medtronic, Minneapolis, MN). If additional cavo-tricuspid isthmus (CTI) ablation is planned, such "touch-up" ablation is performed with an externally irrigated tip ablation catheter (Thermocool, Biosense Webster, Diamond Bar, CA), which is then used to ablate the CTI. In other experienced centers, with unrestricted number of cryoballoon applications to each vein, up to 89% of PVs are isolated, although, in some cases, both the 23-mm and 28-mm cryoballoon had to be used.[11,14]

We usually find after applying just 2 cryoballoon application with the larger 28-mm balloon, provided there were good PV-balloon seals and trough temperatures of at least −40°C, any residual LA–PV connections will consist of only 1 to 2 discrete sleeves, which are easily treated by map-guided ostial focal cryoablation or RF ablation (**Figure 19.6**). The EP endpoint of entrance block into the PVs is reconfirmed at the end of the procedure. In persistent AF patients, direct current cardioversion is usually necessary to restore sinus rhythm.

Other than the cavo-tricuspid ablation line to eliminate typical atrial flutter, no other ablation lines are created. The mean procedural time for our protocol is 108 minutes, with a mean fluoroscopic time of 27 minutes.[13]

Postprocedure Care

Recovery

Following ablation, 50 to 100 mg of protamine is given to reverse heparinization before venous sheaths are removed and manual compression applied. The femoral arterial puncture is closed with an Angioseal closure device (St. Jude Medical, St. Paul, MN) when possible. Patients

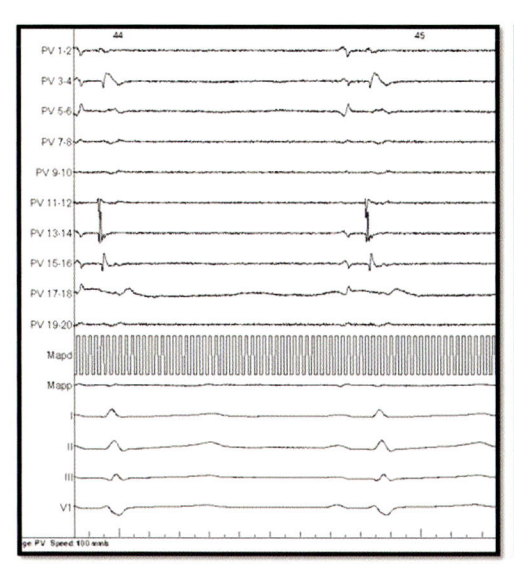

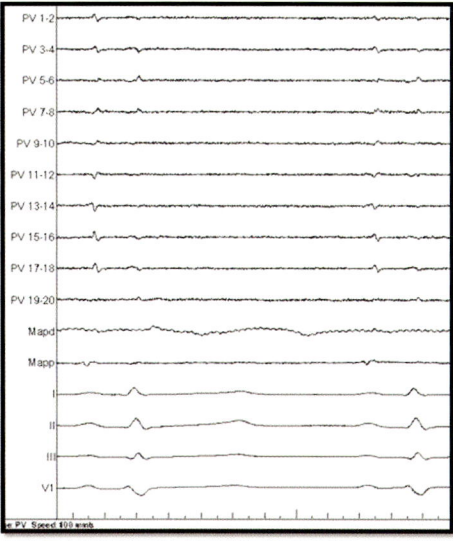

Figure 19.6 Left panel: Evidence of residual but delayed LA-PV conduction after two 5-minute cryoballoon applications to the LUPV. Note the artefact generated on the Freezor Max (Medtronic, Minneapolis, MN) catheter during ostial focal "touch-up" cryoablation. Right panel: The same PV was isolated with a single application of focal cryoablation.

are advised to lie flat for at least 4 hours after sheath removal. Should hemostasis be maintained after 4 hours, and if it is indicated by the patient's CHADS2 score, oral anticoagulation with warfarin with bridging low-molecular-weight heparin is recommenced until the INRs is above 2.0. All patients are kept overnight for observation and discharged the following day after a repeat transthoracic echocardiogram to exclude pericardial effusion. All antiarrhythmic agents that were discontinued prior to the procedure are recommenced, with a view to stopping all antiarrhythmic agents after a 3-month blanking period if patients remained free from AF.

Follow-Up

Follow-up is performed by clinic visits at 1, 3, 6 months and subsequently at 6-month intervals for at least 2 years with repeated 24-hour Holter monitoring and event recorders. Recurrence is defined as any documented episode of AF or atrial tachycardia (either symptomatic or asymptomatic) lasting for more than 30 seconds. In the absence of any reliable data to guide clinical practice, the decision to keep patients with CHADS2 scores of greater than 1 on warfarin after maintaining sinus rhythm for more than 12 months is a highly individualized one, based on patients' preferences, ongoing risk of thromboembolism balanced against the risk of hemorrhagic complications.

Repeat Ablation

With our protoccol, 77% of paroxysmal AF patients and 48% of early persistent AF patients are free from AF recurrence at 12 months after a single procedure (**Figure 19.7**).[13] Of these patients, 87% of paroxysmal AF

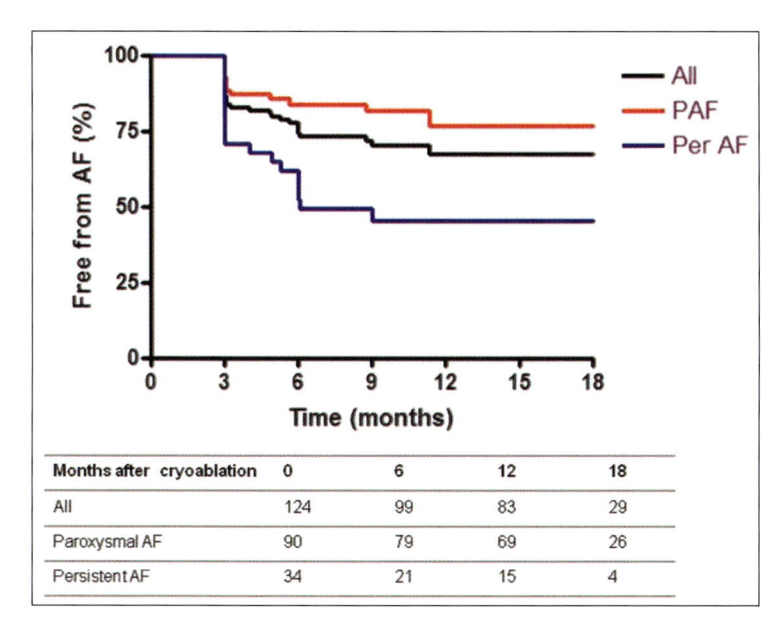

Figure 19.7 Kaplan-Meier survival curves of patients with paroxysmal and persistent AF, demonstrating freedom from AF after a single cryoballoon ablation procedure. (Kojodjojo P, O'Neill MD, Lim PB, et al. Pulmonary venous isolation by antral ablation with a large cryoballoon for treatment of paroxysmal and persistent atrial fibrillation: medium-term outcomes and non-randomised comparison with pulmonary venous isolation by radiofrequency ablation. *Heart*. 2010 Sept;96(17):1370–1384.)

Months after cryoablation	0	6	12	18
All	124	99	83	29
Paroxysmal AF	90	79	69	26
Persistent AF	34	21	15	4

and 86% of persistent AF subjects were no longer taking any antiarrhythmic agents. In the majority of patients with AF recurrence, AF burden, as measured by frequency and duration of paroxysms, is significantly reduced such that symptoms become tolerable or controlled by previously ineffective antiarrhythmic agents. This is consistent with the experiences of patients developing AF recurrence after conventional RF ablation.

AF is the dominant recurrent arrhythmia documented during follow-up. A few cases of typical atrial flutter have been seen in patients without a prior cavotricuspid isthmus ablation and 2 patients have developed probable LA flutter, which spontaneously resolved in both patients. Patients who continue to have symptomatic AF after at least 3 months following their first procedure are offered the choice to have repeat ablation. For the second procedure, cryoballoon therapy is not repeated. The majority of patients will have reconnection of previously isolated pulmonary veins. In a small series of patients undergoing a second procedure after cryoballoon therapy, 73% of previously isolated PVs had reconnected. This compares to 77% of PVs isolated by RF ablation in a separate group of patients who had conventional PVI.[13] In both groups, the veins are easier to isolate with recurrence of electrical conduction occurring via a few narrow sleeves, which can be easily treated with cooled-tipped RF ablation. Depending on the patient's response to their first procedure of only antral PVI and the pattern of their recurrent AF, patients with recurrent persistent AF will receive additional ablation lesions such as linear ablation or targeting regions of complex fractionated electrograms during the second procedure in order to increase the likelihood of maintaining long-term sinus rhythm.

Procedural Complications

Procedural complications can be grouped into those related to vascular access, transseptal puncture, LA ablation, and specifically phrenic nerve palsy. The complication rates described below are aggregated from interventions on 611 patients reported in the 3 large series of patients who underwent balloon cryoablation at 5 different European hospitals.[11,13,15] Similar to conventional AF ablation, complications at sites of vascular access such as groin hematoma and arterial pseudoaneurysm occurred in 1.6% of patients. Eleven of 611 (1.8%) patients developed pericardial effusions requiring drainage but no surgery. This should be considered in the event of any unexpected deterioration in hemodynamic status, and we would strongly advise that any laboratory performing transseptal procedures should have echocardiography machines available at all times in the room. To date, no case of atrioesophageal fistulation has been described in patients undergoing cryoablation. The probability of cerebrovascular accident during RF ablation of AF is about 0.9%. In the combined European series, there was no transient ischaemic attack nor stroke.[11,13,15] Symptomatic, severe pulmonary venous stenosis also did not occur in these studies.

In contrast, the recently reported STOP-AF trial reported 5 strokes, 5 transient ischaemic attacks, and 2 cases of symptomatic, severe pulmonary venous stenosis out of 163 patients undergoing cryoballoon therapy.[7] This disparity in complication rates may be in part due to the fact that participants in this study were treated as the initial experience of 26 recruiting centers, and even the most experienced operators in this trial had only performed between 12 to 23 cryoballoon ablations. Consequently, procedure success rates varied between 90% in the most experienced centers, compared to 56% at centers doing their first cryoablation. Post-hoc analysis showed that operator experience was an independent predictor of treatment success, and with each additional procedure performed, there was a 9% increase in the odds of treatment success.

The incidence of right phrenic nerve palsy is higher with any balloon-based therapy for AF compared to conventional RF ablation. Neumann et al reported a 7.5% rate of right phrenic nerve palsy among 346 patients treated at 3 German hospitals, and van Belle et al had a lower rate of 2.8% after treating 141 patients.[11,15] In the STOP-AF trial, phrenic nerve palsy occurred after 11.2% of ablation cases.[7] Phrenic nerve palsy was more common with the use of the 23-mm balloon, which resulted in more distal PV cryoablation.[11] In our institution, the incidence of phrenic nerve palsy is less than 1.6%, and we believe that injury to the right phrenic nerve can be minimized by our protocol of only using the 28-mm cryoballoon, limiting cryoballoon applications to 2 per vein, pacing the right phrenic nerve at a higher frequency of 40 contractions per minute during cryoablation of both the right superior and inferior veins, and by palpating the abdomen for a reduction in the strength of diaphragmatic contraction which, in our experience, heralds the onset of complete phrenic nerve palsy. All cases of right phrenic nerve palsies in these 3 European series resolved within 14 months.[11,13,15]

Advantages and Limitations

The STOP-AF trial is the only randomized study that compared treatment efficacy of cryoballoon ablation versus antiarrhythmic agents for paroxysmal AF. Two hundred and forty-five paroxysmal AF patients were randomized across 26 U.S. centers in a 2:1 ratio to receive either balloon cryoablation with a 23- or 28-mm balloon or antiarrhythmic agents respectively. After 12 months, 69.9% of patients treated with the cryoballoon remained free from AF compared to only 7.3% on drug therapy.[7] The superiority of

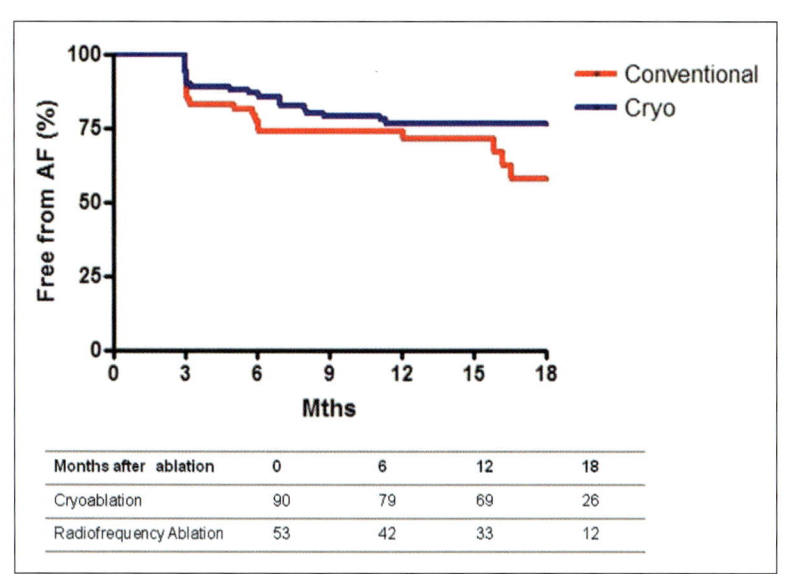

Figure 19.8 Kaplan-Meier survival curves comparing paroxysmal AF subjects undergoing either balloon cryoablation or conventional RF ablation, with no statistically significant differences in freedom from AF at 12 months postoperative. (Kojodjojo P, O'Neill MD, Lim PB, et al. Pulmonary venous isolation by antral ablation with a large cryoballoon for treatment of paroxysmal and persistent atrial fibrillation: medium-term outcomes and non-randomised comparison with pulmonary venous isolation by radiofrequency ablation. *Heart.* 2010 Sept;96(17):1370–1384.)

Months after ablation	0	6	12	18
Cryoablation	90	79	69	26
Radiofrequency Ablation	53	42	33	12

cryoballoon ablation over antiarrhythmic therapy was probably exaggerated by large numbers of subjects in the medical therapy arm crossing over to receive cryoballoon ablation. By the end of the study, 79% of medical therapy patients had crossed over as early as 3.5 months after entering the trial.

To our knowledge, there is no randomized study comparing cryoballoon versus RF therapies for AF. In a nonrandomized comparison of consecutive subjects undergoing their first AF ablation procedure using either balloon cryoablation ($n = 90$) or RF ablation ($n = 53$) for paroxysmal AF at our institution, there was no difference in arrhythmia-free survival after 12 months with a single procedure (77% versus 72% respectively, P = NS) (**Figure 19.8**).[13] The main advantages of using this system to isolate PVs is its ease of use, the ability to achieve isolation of all veins in less than 2 hours with our protocol, clinical results comparable to conventional RF ablation, and an almost painless procedure for patients under conscious sedation, although some complain of an "ice-cream headache" during cryotherapy.

The disadvantages of cryoballoon therapy are the need for a 15-Fr sheath, the additional costs of catheters incurred if the cryoballoon alone could not achieve PVI, inability to perform ablation beyond the PV antra, and the higher risk of right phrenic nerve injury. With the current set of catheters, real-time monitoring of PV-LA conduction is not possible. In the near future, a PV mapping catheter that can be passed via the central lumen into the PV during ongoing therapy will become available. This would enable a single transseptal procedure and for cryoenergy delivery to be stopped sooner once PVI is achieved early during a freeze. In turn, this could result in even shorter procedural times and lower rates of right phrenic nerve palsy.

Conclusions

In summary, PVI can be achieved in less than 2 hours by a simple cryoablation protocol. Excellent clinical outcomes, comparable to conventional RF ablation, can be achieved after a single intervention, particularly for paroxysmal AF. While the risk of complications arising from vascular and transseptal access is similar to conventional AF ablation, cryoablation is much less likely to cause PV stenosis or extracardiac fistulation. There remains a small (less than 2%) risk of transient right phrenic nerve palsy, and monitoring of right phrenic nerve function during cryoablation of the right-sided PVs is essential.

References

1. Bhargava M, Di Biase L, Mohanty P, et al. Impact of type of atrial fibrillation and repeat catheter ablation on long-term freedom from atrial fibrillation: results from a multicenter study. *Heart Rhythm.* 2009;6(10):1403–1412.
2. Jaïs P, Hocini M, Sanders P, et al. Long-term evaluation of atrial fibrillation ablation guided by noninducibility. *Heart Rhythm.* 2006;3:140–145.
3. O'Neill MD, Wright M, Knecht S, et al. Long-term follow-up of persistent atrial fibrillation ablation using termination as a procedural endpoint. *Eur Heart J.* 2009;30:1105–1112.
4. Marom EM, Herndon JE, Kim YH, et al. Variations in pulmonary venous drainage to the left atrium: implications for radiofrequency ablation. *Radiology* 2004;230:824–829.
5. Oral H, Scharf C, Chugh A, et al. Catheter ablation for paroxysmal atrial fibrillation: segmental pulmonary vein ostial ablation versus left atrial ablation. *Circulation.* 2003; 108:2355–2360.
6. Khairy P, Dubuc M. Transcatheter cryoablation part I: preclinical experience. *Pacing Clin Electrophysiol.* 2008; 31:112–120.

7. Packer DL. STOP-AF Trial. American College of Cardiology Annual Scientific Sessions, Atlanta, GA, 2010.
8. Moreira W, Manusama R, Timmermans C, et al. Long-term follow-up after cryothermic ostial pulmonary vein isolation in paroxysmal atrial fibrillation. *J Am Coll Cardiol*. 2008;51:850–855.
9. Tse HF, Reek S, Timmermans C, et al. Pulmonary vein isolation using transvenous catheter cryoablation for treatment of atrial fibrillation without risk of pulmonary vein stenosis. *J Am Coll Cardiol*. 2003;42:752–758.
10. Wong T, Markides V, Peters NS, et al. Percutaneous pulmonary vein cryoablation to treat atrial fibrillation. *J Interv Card Electrophysiol*. 2004;11:117–126.
11. Neumann T, Vogt J, Schumacher B, et al. Circumferential pulmonary vein isolation with the cryoballoon technique results from a prospective 3-center study. *J Am Coll Cardiol*. 2008;52:273–278.
12. Reddy VY, Neuzil P, d'Avila A, et al. Balloon catheter ablation to treat paroxysmal atrial fibrillation: what is the level of pulmonary venous isolation? *Heart Rhythm*. 2008;5:353–360.
13. Kojodjojo P, O'Neill MD, Lim PB, et al. Pulmonary venous isolation by antral ablation with a large cryo-balloon for treatment of paroxysmal and persistent atrial fibrillation: medium term outcomes and nonrandomised comparison with pulmonary venous isolation by radiofrequency ablation. *Heart*. 2010;96:1379–1384.
14. Van Belle Y, Janse P, Rivero-Ayerza MJ, et al. Pulmonary vein isolation using an occluding cryoballoon for circumferential ablation: feasibility, complications, and short-term outcome. *Eur Heart J*. 2007;28:2231–2237.
15. Van Belle Y, Janse P, Theuns D, et al. One year follow-up after cryoballoon isolation of the pulmonary veins in patients with paroxysmal atrial fibrillation. *Europace*. 2008;10:1271–1276.

Video Descriptions

Video 19.1 Double transseptal puncture guided by fluoroscopy and TEE.

Video 19.2 Left superior pulmonary venography via a 6-Fr NIH catheter.

Video 19.3 Left inferior pulmonary venography via a 6-Fr NIH catheter.

Video 19.4 Right superior pulmonary venography via a 6-Fr NIH catheter.

Video 19.5 Right inferior pulmonary venography via a 6-Fr NIH catheter.

Video 19.6 8-Fr SR0 transseptal sheath (St. Jude Medical, St. Paul, MN) exchanged over a wire in the left superior pulmonary vein to a 15-Fr deflectable FlexCath (Medtronic, Minneapolis, MN).

Video 19.7 Balloon cryoablation of the left superior pulmonary vein.

Video 19.8 Balloon cryoablation of the left inferior pulmonary vein.

Video 19.9 Balloon cryoablation of the right superior pulmonary vein.

Video 19.10 Balloon cryoablation of the right inferior pulmonary vein.

Video 19.11 Pullback technique to aid balloon cryoablation of the right inferior pulmonary vein.

Video 19.12 Capturing the right phrenic nerve by pacing in the SVC and monitoring right diaphragmatic contractions.

CHAPTER 20

HOW TO PERFORM PULMONARY VEIN ISOLATION USING LASER CATHETER ABLATION

Edward P. Gerstenfeld, MD

Background

Catheter-based PVI has advanced significantly since it was initially described in 1999.[1] However, the problem of PV reconnection after ablation[2] remains the Achilles heel of the procedure and is likely responsible for most late AF recurrences.[3,4] Use of a focal catheter for isolation of the PVs in a connect-the-dots approach is the major limitation of our current approach to PVI. Although use of irrigated catheters, electroanatomic mapping systems with image integration, and general anesthesia to promote greater catheter stability have improved the speed and safety of acute PVI, late recurrences continue to occur. Given the variable LA topology, thickness, variation in PV anatomy, and adjacent extracardiac structures such as the esophagus and lung, it is not surprising that contiguous full-thickness lesions over a wide area are difficult to achieve with consistency using a focal ablation catheter.

Balloon ablation technology offers a different approach to PVI. Rather than adapting catheters designed for focal ablation to wide-area encircling lesions, balloon catheters allow an approach adapted specifically to the PVs. This offers enhanced catheter stability and lesion delivery. Balloons typically use alternative energy sources that may be more suited to circumferential ablation compared to radiofrequency energy. Thus far, balloon energy sources have included ultrasound,[5-8] cryoablation,[9,10] and now laser ablation.[11,12]

The endoscopic laser balloon (Cardiofocus, Marlborough, MA) has gone through several design iterations (**Figure 20.1**). The original concept was to deliver a 360-circumferential beam that would allow complete PVI with one energy delivery. However, it was soon appreciated that the PVs are oval structures with variable branching and that no single circumferential pattern was suitable to PV anatomy. The second-generation balloon was a fixed-diameter balloon that came in 20-, 25-, and 30-mm diameter sizes. An endoscopic fiber allowed direct visualization of the LA endocardium in contact with the balloon, directing a 90° arc of laser energy around the PV periphery. It was felt that compared to the 360° laser, a 90° arc would allow a more directed delivery of energy in a pattern that could be "stitched" together to create complete isolation. While such an approach was successful in preclinical animal and initial human studies, the noncompliant balloon and 90° arc made the ablation procedures challenging.

The current-generation endoscopic laser ablation system has 3 components, an outer compliant balloon, a lesion generator, and the endoscope (**Figure 20.2**). The balloon is made of a compliant material that has an adjustable size depending on the inflation pressure, with diameter that varies from 25 to 32 mm, with internal inflation pressures varying from 1 to 5 PSI. The catheter shaft contains the lesion generator and endoscope. The laser is designed to ablate cardiac tissue using light energy in the infrared spectrum. The lesion generator produces a 30° arc of light

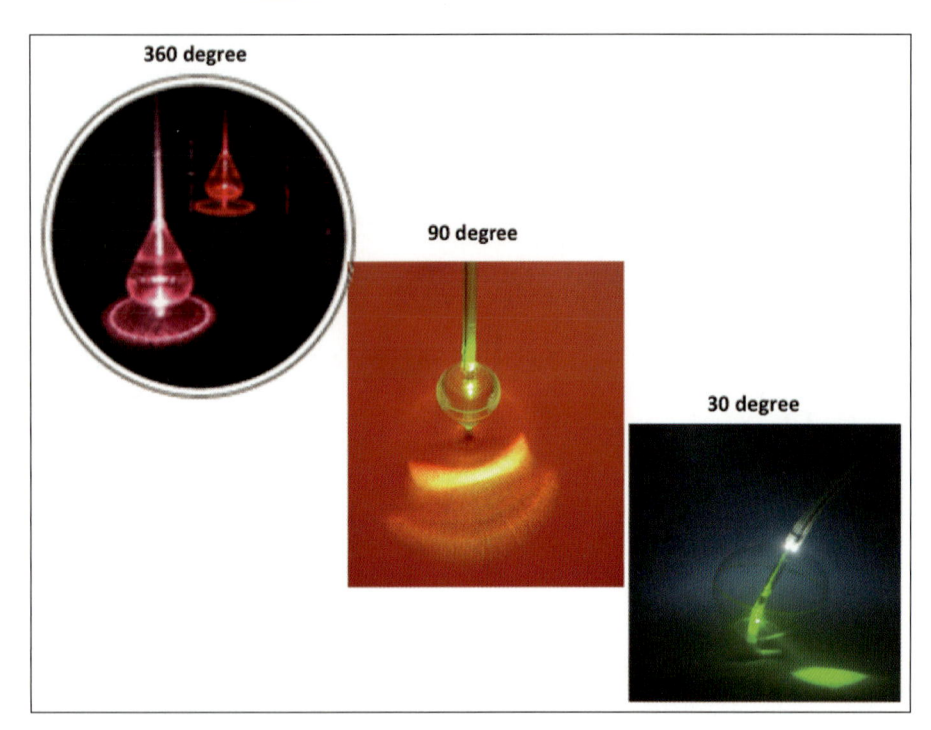

Figure 20.1 Evolution of the laser balloon concept from the original 360° circumferential design to the 90° noncompliant balloon to the current compliant balloon with 30° laser arc.

energy and is powered by a 980-nm diode laser. The 980-nm wavelength was chosen because it is optimal for absorption by H_2O, which allows tissue heating (**Figure 20.3**); it is poorly absorbed by deuterium oxide (D_2O, "heavy water"), which is an inert medium that can be used to inflate the balloon and provide a "loss-free" path for the projection of laser energy. The balloon is inflated with a mixture of sterile D_2O and sodium diatrizoate. The diode laser requires minimal power for energy generation (5.5–14 W). The endoscope has a 115° field of view and allows direct visualization of the area of the balloon in contact with the LA endocardium; tissue appears white and blood appears dark red; visualization cannot occur through moving blood. One must be careful not to ablate with the laser in areas of stagnant blood, or coagulum (thrombus) can occur. The catheter and lesion generator are disposable; the endoscope can be resterilized and reused during subsequent procedures.

Left Atrium Access and Balloon Deployment

One should perform some type of LA imaging to identify the PV anatomy, typically either computed tomography or magnetic resonance angiography, prior to the procedure. The maximum balloon diameter is 32 mm, so isolation cannot be performed on a single PV with an average of major and minor axes > 32 mm diameter. Most left common PVs can still be isolated more distally as individual PVs, but the

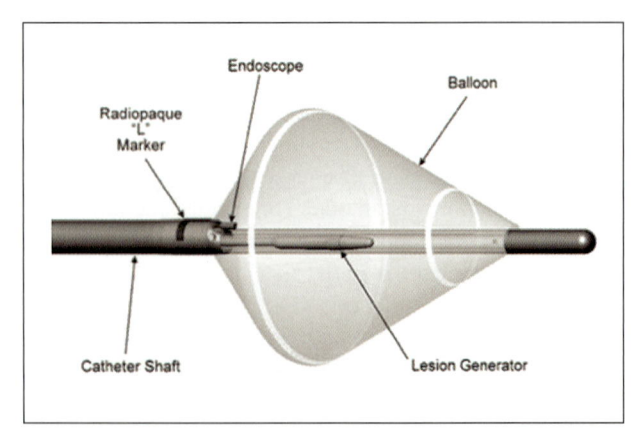

Figure 20.2 Schematic of the compliant laser balloon, which includes the central catheter shaft, compliant balloon, and catheter lumen that incorporates the lesion generator and endoscope. Courtesy of Cardiofocus.

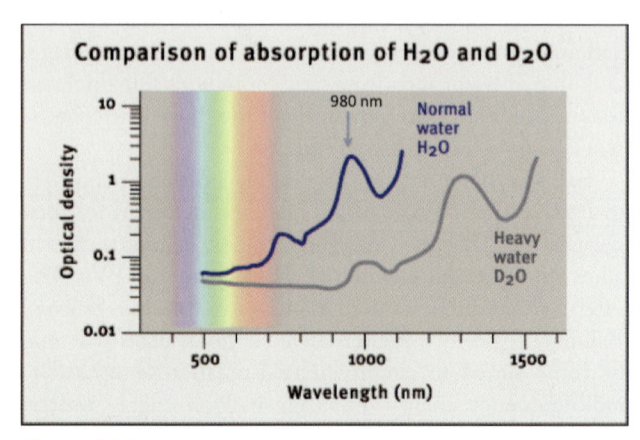

Figure 20.3 Absorption spectrum of water (H_2O) and deuterium oxide (D_2O) showing the difference in laser energy absorption at 980 nm for water compared to deuterium oxide. Used with permission.

trade-off of a more distal PVI should be considered. Finally, PVs with multiple proximal branches (**Figure 20.4**) may be difficult to isolate with balloon techniques, and a more standard catheter approach might be considered.

The laser ablation system is deployed using a custom 12-Fr-inner-diameter, 16-Fr-outer-diameter 180° deflectable sheath. The sheath comes with a soft-tipped dilator and has a distal fluoroscopic marker. The sheath should be flushed with heparinized saline under pressure throughout the procedure. If one is using ICE to guide transseptal access, full heparinization to an ACT > 300 secs can be performed prior to transseptal access. For those not comfortable with this approach, a heparin bolus should be given as soon as possible after LA access is obtained to prevent thrombus from forming on the transseptal sheath. LA access is first gained with a standard transseptal sheath; this sheath is then exchanged over a long wire for the custom laser ablation sheath. A low and anterior transseptal puncture (compared to the typical posterior punctures for catheter-based PVI) will facilitate balloon introduction into the RIPV, which often can be the most challenging approach for balloon catheters. A stiff long wire (Amplatz 240 cm extra stiff, 0.35" or smaller) is then introduced to the LA via the transseptal sheath and advanced out the left superior (or inferior) PVs. Securing the wire distally out one of the PVs before sheath exchange is important; the 16-Fr guiding sheath could otherwise injure the posterior LA wall during the exchange. The standard sheath is withdrawn over the wire and the 16-Fr laser sheath is advanced over the wire to the LA. One should be careful to withdraw blood and flush the 16-Fr sheath after any catheter exchange to avoid entraining air into the LA. We typically perform a second transseptal puncture to allow simultaneous LA access and PV mapping with a circular mapping catheter; however, others may perform a single transseptal puncture and exchange the balloon catheter for the mapping catheter sequentially.

Preparation of the balloon catheter can be performed simultaneously with LA access. The catheter tubing is connected to the console and the balloon and tubing are purged with D_2O. The console provides continuous circulation of fluid while the balloon is inflated to the desired pressure/size and maintains the catheter at a constant temperature. The endoscope needs to be advanced into place through the tubing and central catheter lumen to rest distally inside the balloon. The balloon is then deflated, immersed in saline, covered with the introducing tool, and advanced into the sheath. The sheath is typically kept in the mid-atrial cavity with the distal end oriented toward the PV of interest. Radio-opaque markers are present on the tip and distal end of the catheter to aid with fluoroscopic visualization. One should not advance the sheath out a PV as is often done for PV angiography. If one prefers to perform PV angiography, this should be done with a standard sheath before the exchange. Injecting contrast into the laser sheath should also be avoided. The deflated balloon is then advanced to the PV ostium under fluoroscopic and echocardiographic guidance and inflated. Although there is a soft tip on the balloon catheter, one should avoid advancing the balloon too far out of a PV. The sheath can then be withdrawn to the proximal "Z" marker on the balloon catheter to allow balloon inflation (**Figure 20.5**). The "Z" marker can be used to identify the balloon rotational orientation under fluoroscopy in order to ensure that the endoscopic image will be displayed in an anatomic view. We typically find phased-array intracardiac ultrasound extremely also helpful for guiding and confirming balloon position.

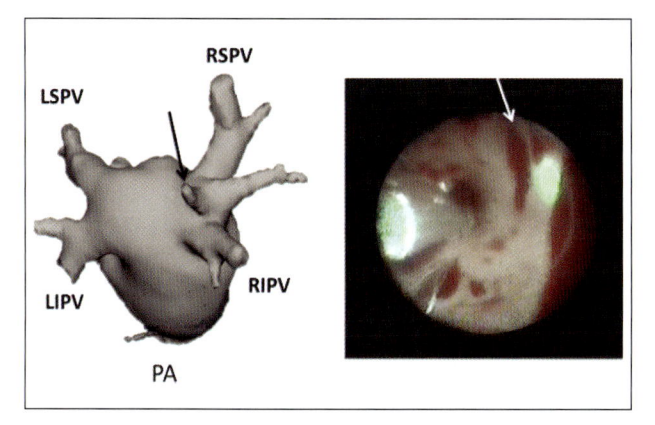

Figure 20.4 **Left panel**: CT angiogram of the LA demonstrating an early proximal posterior branch of the RSPV. **Right panel**: The endoscopic view through the laser balloon shows the posterior PV branch (arrow), which is compressed by the balloon with little clearance for ablation (aiming beam in green) on the posterior edge.

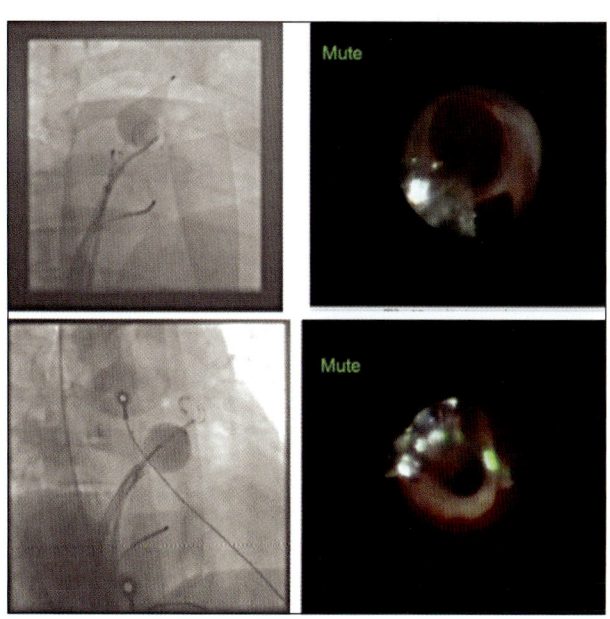

Figure 20.5 **Left panel**: fluoroscopic right anterior oblique views demonstrating the laser balloon in the LSPV (top) and LIPV (bottom) with the circular catheter in the other ipsilateral vein. **Right panel**: Endoscopic view of the LSPV (top) and LIPV (bottom). In the top panel, the LSPV, carina, and superior portion of the LIPV can be seen. In the bottom panel, the laser aiming beam (green) is shown on the anterior ridge between the LIPV and LAA.

PVI with the laser balloon is typically performed sequentially using a vein-by-vein approach. Stitching together lesions to isolate ipsilateral pairs of PVs as a unit is technically challenging and often not feasible[13]; tracking the level of lesion placement while moving the balloon from the superior to inferior PV is often difficult. Individual vein-by-vein isolation is the most efficient approach in our experience.

Once inflated, *every effort should be made to achieve optimal circumferential contact with the LA endocardium prior to beginning the ablation*. Ablation lesions on the pale atrial tissue are often not visible, and it is best to deliver contiguous lesions circumferentially around the PV with one balloon position rather than trying to stitch together lesions in multiple balloon orientations. Lesions delivered at different balloon inflations may be present at different depths into the PV, and gaps in the longitudinal direction may not be easily appreciated. The balloon has as many as 9 levels of expansion based on the inflation pressure, from low (1 PSI) to high (5 PSI) in 0.5 PSI increments. The balloon diameter varies from 25 mm at low pressure to 32 mm at highest inflation pressure. One should realize that at higher inflation pressures, the balloon is less compliant and therefore less able to mold to the PV anatomy. We typically have performed isolation at low to medium inflation pressures (1–3 PSI).

Laser Ablation

The available ablation energy is projected perpendicular to the catheter shaft and ranges from 5.5 to 14 W. Lesions delivered at the lowest power, 5.5 W, are delivered for 30 seconds; higher-power lesions are delivered for 20 seconds each and include 7 W, 8.5 W, 10 W, 12 W, and 14 W. Delivering laser energy into stagnant blood should always be avoided; thrombus will form that can (1) heat the balloon surface and melt the balloon and (2) cause char that can lead to a thromboembolic event. It should be noted that the D_2O in the balloon is inert and has no ill systemic effects if the balloon leaks; however, the balloon will need to be replaced, which can add significant time and cost to the procedure. Lesions can be delivered in moving blood only at 5.5 W, which has been shown in animal models not to lead to thrombus formation. One of the most technically demanding aspects of the laser ablation system is avoiding delivery of higher-power laser energy when the beam is in contact with blood. Therefore, in addition to maintaining "contact" with the endocardium, it is desirable to have a sufficient "width" of contact to allow delivery of higher power lesions at a safe distance from the blood pool. As with any ablation delivery system, nontransmural lesions can result in transient PVI that can lead to late PV reconnection and AF recurrence. Animal studies have demonstrated that 5.5-W lesions lead to more chronic PV reconnection than higher power lesions. Therefore, one should try to use at least the 8-W setting for energy delivery. As a general rule 7.5 to 8 W can be used on the posterior aspect of the PV, 8 to 10 W on the roof and inferior aspect, and 10 to 12 W on the anterior ridge between the left PVs and the LAA. It is important to be aware that with any method of PV ablation, acute isolation does not necessarily mean chronic isolation will be achieved. Therefore, obtaining adequate contact with the balloon in order to allow delivery of high-power lesions is of the utmost importance. We typically reserve use of the 5.5-W lesions for 3 circumstances: (1) posteriorly when delivery of laser energy leads to rapid esophageal temperature rises; (2) at the carina between upper and lower PV near the catheter shaft, where the beam intensity is highest and tissue thinnest; (3) when adequate contact cannot be obtained and some flowing blood can not be eliminated from the balloon tissue interface. One should realize that although the beam subtends a 30° arc, this 30° arc is larger the more proximally the beam is delivered and smaller distally near the catheter shaft. Therefore, lower powers may be sufficient when the catheter/PV orientation forces lesions to be delivered more distally. As with standard catheter ablation, one should try to deliver lesions as proximally as possible. Finally, in order to minimize patient movement, discomfort during phrenic nerve pacing, and pain during ablation, we have typically performed these procedures under general anesthesia.

Endoscopic View

The endoscopic view is projected on a monitor and allows a 270° view as seen down the shaft of the balloon (Figure 20.5). Approximately 90° of the view is obscured by the shaft of the lesion generator, and while it is in place, this represents a "blind spot" in the field of view. One should avoid delivering laser energy behind the blind spot, as one cannot be sure of contact with the endocardium or the presence of stagnant blood. The balloon must be inflated and in contact with the LA or PV surface for visualization. Blood appears red and areas of contact with the endocardium white. Using the "Z" marker on the catheter shaft to determine the catheter orientation, the endoscopic view can be rotated to orient the endoscopic orientation into an anatomic view (ie, superior aspect of the vein on top, inferior on bottom, etc.). We typically will rotate the balloon so the blind spot is oriented initially over the PV carina. Once ablation has been performed over the 270° visualized radius, the entire catheter shaft can be rotated to visualize the remaining carina region and complete the circumferential ablation.

Lesion Visualization Software

The placement of each lesion is determined by the operator using a green laser "aiming beam," which transmits no ablation energy but projects where the energy will be delivered. The user can rotate the 30° aiming beam anywhere in the 360° circumference around the PV and advance or withdraw the laser distally or proximally without moving the catheter itself. One should attempt to orient the lesions as proximally as possible, keeping in mind the goal of delivering a 360° arc of lesions at the same depth. Once the position of the aiming beam is satisfactory, the operator can then deliver an ablative lesion at this location. The green beam will turn red when in contact with blood, and delivering lesions above 5.5 W should be avoided. The green aiming beam will "flash" during energy delivery to allow visualization of the underlying endocardium. Since ablative lesions delivered with the laser can often not be visualized, the system comes with software to track delivery of lesions in order to avoid gaps in lesion delivery. Typically, about 30% overlap in lesion contiguity is recommended. The lesion visualization software (LightTrack; Cardiofocus, Marlborough, MA) stores each lesion and displays the last delivered lesion on the endoscopic viewscreen (**Figure 20.6**). The user then can rotate the aiming beam, allowing for 30% overlap, and deliver the next lesion (▶ **Video 20.1**). After the entire circumference of the PV has been ablated, the lesions can be reviewed to be sure there are no gaps. Keep in mind that when the catheter is rotated to complete delivery behind the 90° blind spot, the endoscopic view must be realigned in order to keep track of lesion delivery relative to the underlying anatomy.

Left PV Ablation

As mentioned above, the left PVs are typically ablated individually, with complete circumferential lesions around the LSPV and LIPV, overlapping at the carina. In order to obtain contact with the posterior wall, clockwise torque on the balloon and sheath, as well as a medium inflation pressure, may be required. Catheter manipulation may be required to eliminate blood "pockets," and typically forward pressure on the balloon catheter is required during ablation. Care should be taken when ablating near the esophagus, as rapid temperature rises may occur. A temperature probe should always be placed in the esophagus and manipulated opposite the nearest site of ablation. We typically limit esophageal temperature rises during an ablation to < 1°C. In the case of rapid, early temperature rises, one can decrease the delivered power or, on occasion, alter the path of lesion delivery more distally toward the PV.

On the anterior ridge, it is important to try and obtain a wide rim of contact in order to allow sufficient clearance from the blood pool. In our experience, powers of at least 10 W are often required on the anterior ridge between the left PVs and LAA in order to obtain chronic PVI. Adequate clearance from LA blood is required in order to deliver lesions at these powers. Paradoxically, lower inflation pressures may be required in order to obtain more contact with the anterior ridge (**Figure 20.7**). Often 1 to 2 PSI inflation pressure together with forward contact on the balloon is required for adequate contact. On the anterior carina, at the junction between the appendage, superior and inferior PVs, 12 to 14 W may be required for isolation. We typically ablate the PV carina last; lesions in this tissue near the center of the sheath may require only 5.5 to 7 W.

The LIPV can be isolated in a similar manner, with 8 to 10 W posteriorly and inferiorly, 10 to 12 W along the anterior ridge, and 5.5 to 7 W along the bottom of the carina overlapping with the LSPV lesions.

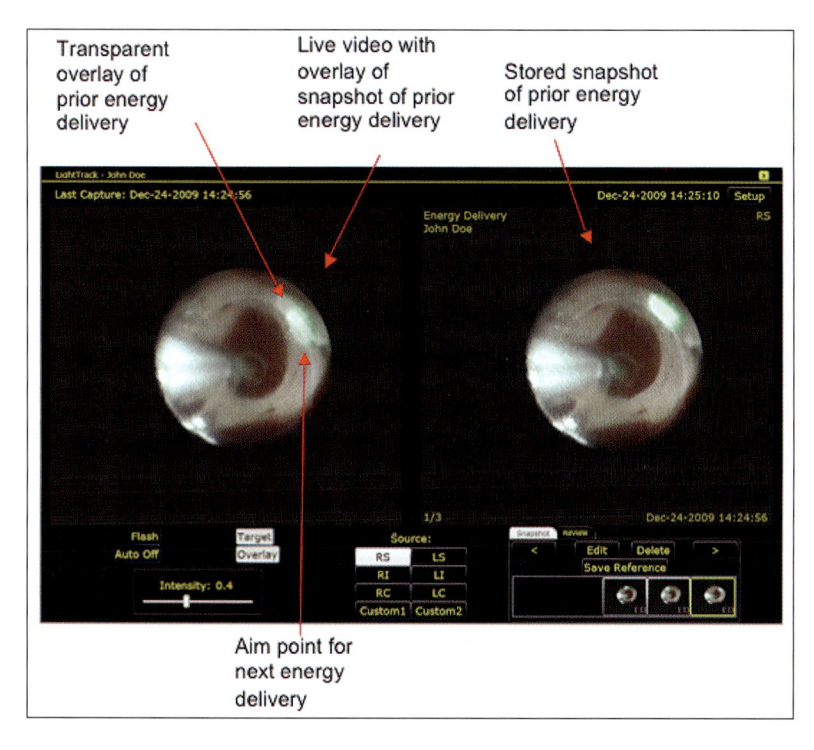

Figure 20.6 The view shown using the lesion visualization software that tracks lesion delivery during PVI. **Left panel**: The position of the lesion delivery at 2:00 on the PV circumference is saved. **Right panel**: The location of the prior lesion (light green) is shown overlapping with the current location of the aiming beam (bright green) to confirm 30% overlap before delivering the next lesion.

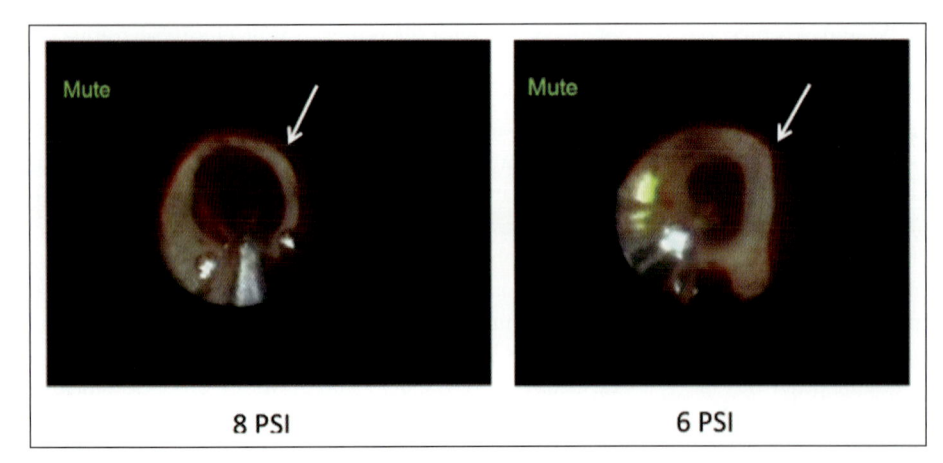

Figure 20.7 Endoscopic view with the laser balloon positioned in the LSPV. In the left panel, with the balloon inflated to 8 PSI, there is only a thin rim of contact on the anterior ridge (arrow) between the LSPV and LAA, limiting the maximum energy that can be delivered because of proximity to the blood pool. At lower balloon pressure (6 PSI), the right panel demonstrates a wider rim of contact (white), allowing higher energy delivery.

Right Pulmonary Veins

The RSPV is often the most suitable for balloon isolation. A larger balloon inflation pressure can often be used at moderate pressure, or about 3 to 4 PSI. Too small a balloon diameter may lead to too distal position and a higher likelihood of phrenic nerve damage. The phrenic nerve should be paced throughout septal (right) PV ablation. We typically place a multipolar catheter in the SVC and maneuver it while pacing at 10 mA, 2 ms pulse width, until consistent phrenic capture is obtained. Pacing is continued throughout ablation on the septal side of the right PVs and discontinued immediately if phrenic capture is lost. We typically use 10 W septally, 8 to 10 W posteriorly (unless limited by increasing esophageal temperature), and 5.5 to 7 W in the carina region between the superior and inferior PVs. The lower PV can be isolated similarly. As mentioned above, a low anterior transseptal access will facilitate balloon placement in the RIPV (**Figure 20.8**). During RIPV ablation, we typically use 10 W septally and inferiorly, 5.5 to 7 W at the carina, and 8 to 10 W posteriorly. Continuous pacing of the phrenic nerve should be continued during septal RIPV ablation. Occasionally a separate right middle PV is present. There are 2 options in this scenario: (1) trying to use a large balloon inflation size and include the right middle PV together with the superior or inferior PV, or (2) to perform a separate isolation of the right middle PV. We have typically used ICE to guide balloon placement balloon into the right middle PV to isolate its anterior and posterior aspect separately from the others.

Checking for PVI

After isolation, each PV is interrogated with a circular mapping catheter to confirm isolation (entry block). We also pace around the circular mapping catheter at 10 mA 2 ms pulse width to confirm exit block.[14] If isolation has not been achieved, we try to use the circular catheter to map the area of earliest entry into the PV and then move the laser balloon back into the PV to target this region. The presence of two transseptal punctures facilitates ease of moving the circular catheter into and out of the PV to check for isolation. Frequently, complete isolation of one PV may not occur until the other ipsilateral vein is isolated, so we will typically place the circular mapping catheter in the PV ipsilateral to the targeted PV to watch for isolation while ablation is being performed (Figure 20.5). The circular catheter can also be placed distally to the balloon to look for acute PVI during ablation. However, the shaft of the circular catheter often impairs contact of the balloon with the endocardial surface and makes isolation more difficult. We typically wait for 30 minutes after acute isolation to confirm persistent PVI. The balloon and sheath can then be withdrawn from the LA. We typically wait until the ACT is < 200 ms to pull the femoral sheath.

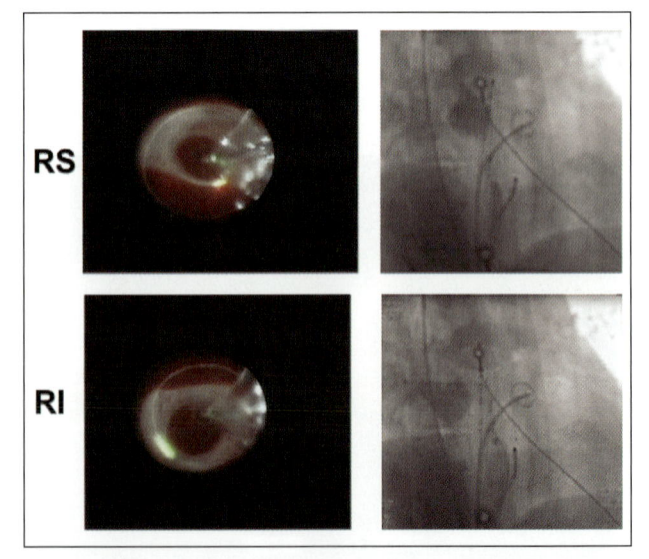

Figure 20.8 Endoscopic (**right panel**) and fluoroscopic (**left panel**) showing laser balloon position in the RSPV (**top**) and RIPV (**bottom**). An anterior and inferior transseptal puncture facilitates placing the balloon in the RIPV. A direct approach to the vein is preferable to looping the sheath in the LA.

Summary

The endoscopic laser balloon has several advantages over standard catheter ablation. These include (1) direct visualization of the endocardium and PV anatomy, (2) stability of catheter and energy source during lesion delivery, (3) minimal use of fluoroscopy and no need for complex electroanatomic mapping systems, and (4) transmural lesion delivery. Patients with very large veins (> 32 mm average diameter) or early proximal branching PVs may not be ideal for this approach. Results from a human feasibility trial and upcoming randomized trial against standard catheter ablation will determine whether this approach is safe, efficacious, and has a role in the armamentarium of AF ablation tools.

References

1. Haïssaguerre M, Jaïs P, Shah DC, et al. Spontaneous initiation of atrial fibrillation by ectopic beats originating in the pulmonary veins. *N Engl J Med.* 1998;339(10):659–666.
2. Gerstenfeld EP, Callans DJ, Dixit S, Zado E, Marchlinski FE. Incidence and location of focal atrial fibrillation triggers in patients undergoing repeat pulmonary vein isolation: implications for ablation strategies. *J Cardiovasc Electrophysiol.* 2003;14(7):685–690.
3. Tzou WS, Marchlinski FE, Zado ES, et al. Long-term outcome after successful catheter ablation of atrial fibrillation. *Circ Arrhythm Electrophysiol.* 2010;3(3):237–242.
4. Shah AN, Mittal S, Sichrovsky TC, Cotiga D, Arshad A, Maleki K, Pierce WJ, Steinberg JS. Long-term outcome following successful pulmonary vein isolation: pattern and prediction of very late recurrence. *J Cardiovasc Electrophysiol.* 2008;19(7):661–667.
5. Metzner A, Chun KR, Neven K, et al. Long-term clinical outcome following pulmonary vein isolation with high-intensity focused ultrasound balloon catheters in patients with paroxysmal atrial fibrillation. *Europace.* 2010;12(2):188–193.
6. Nakagawa H, Antz M, Wong T, et al. Initial experience using a forward directed, high-intensity focused ultrasound balloon catheter for pulmonary vein antrum isolation in patients with atrial fibrillation. *J Cardiovasc Electrophysiol.* 2007;18(2):136–144.
7. Schmidt B, Chun KR, Metzner A, Ouyang F, Kuck KH. Balloon catheters for pulmonary vein isolation. *Herz.* 2008;33(8):580–584.
8. Natale A, Pisano E, Shewchik J, et al. First human experience with pulmonary vein isolation using a through-the-balloon circumferential ultrasound ablation system for recurrent atrial fibrillation. *Circulation.* 2000;102(16):1879–1882.
9. Chun KR, Fürnkranz A, Metzner A, et al. Cryoballoon pulmonary vein isolation with real-time recordings from the pulmonary veins. *J Cardiovasc Electrophysiol.* 2009;20(11):1203–1210.
10. Neumann T, Vogt J, Schumacher B, et al. Circumferential pulmonary vein isolation with the cryoballoon technique results from a prospective 3-center study. *J Am Coll Cardiol.* 2008;52(4):273–278.
11. Reddy VY, Neuzil P, Themistoclakis S, et al. Visually-guided balloon catheter ablation of atrial fibrillation: experimental feasibility and first-in-human multicenter clinical outcome. *Circulation.* 2009;120(1):12–20.
12. Gerstenfeld EP, Michele J. Pulmonary vein isolation using a compliant endoscopic laser balloon ablation system in a swine model. *J Interv Card Electrophysiol.* 2010;29(1):1–9.
13. Schmidt B, Metzner A, Chun KR, et al. Feasibility of circumferential pulmonary vein isolation using a novel endoscopic ablation system. *Circ Arrhythm Electrophysiol.* 2010;3(5):481–488.
14. Gerstenfeld EP, Dixit S, Callans D, Rho R, Rajawat Y, Zado E, Marchlinski FE. Utility of exit block for identifying electrical isolation of the pulmonary veins. *J Cardiovasc Electrophysiol.* 2002;13(10):971–979.

Video Descriptions

Video 20.1 An example of laser ablation lesions delivered to the right inferior pulmonary vein (RIPV). The leftmost panel shows the live endoscopic view of the RIPV—white represents endocardial contact and red contact with blood. At 12:00 is the blindspot created by the laser generator. The green 30-degree arc is the laser aiming beam that guides lesion delivery; the aiming beam flashes during ablation. The duplicate image of the RIPV to the right saves the location of the lesion delivery so the next lesion can be aligned with approximately 30% overlap. The upper right panel is a fluoroscopic view of the balloon in the RIPV. The lower right panel shows intracardiac electrograms during ablation. Note the pacing stimulus that is delivered continuously to the phrenic nerve from a catheter in the superior vena cava during RIPV ablation.

CHAPTER 21

The Combined Surgical/Endocardial Ablation Procedure for Atrial Fibrillation

Rodney P. Horton, MD; Luigi Di Biase, MD, PhD; Andrew T. Hume, MD; James R. Edgerton, MD; Javier E. Sánchez, MD; Andrea Natale, MD[1]

Catheter-based ablation of AF has become a common treatment for patients who fail initial suppression with antiarrhythmic agents.[1] In the paroxysmal population, the acute and chronic efficacy is good, and the procedure is widely recognized as effective in this select group of patients. However, in the persistent AF and long-standing persistent AF populations, the efficacy is quite variable among high-volume centers and generally much lower than in their paroxysmal counterparts.[2] Two demographic variables that particularly predict lower success rates are duration of persistent AF[3,4] and enlargement in the LA.[5] Patients with more than 7 years of AF and those with LA dimensions over 5.0 cm on TTE have particularly low success rates from a single catheter ablation procedure.[6,7]

Surgical literature has offered the possibility of improving success rate in controlling AF from an open-chest approach since the first Cox MAZE procedure was first described.[8,9] While the initial procedure involved a sternotomy and was often performed concomitantly with other surgical procedures, less invasive, stand-alone approaches have been reported involving thoracoscopic ports on both sides of the chest and showing promising results.[10,11] Limitations to this approach appear to be postoperative pain, limited electrical confirmation of lesion integrity, and identification of nonvenous AF triggers. A combined or "hybrid" approach could offer the benefit of robust epicardial lesions with the detail and precision of an endocardial catheter ablation. The convergent approach involves combining an epicardial RF ablation device to deliver ablation lesions from the inferior, transdiaphragmatic approach followed by endocardial, voltage-guided catheter ablation of residual regions of PV conduction. This procedure offers the benefit of less postoperative pain but requires endocardial ablation, as the superior aspects of the LA cannot be easily accessed or visualized from the inferior approach. The following sections will outline and contrast the thoracoscopic and transdiaphragmatic approaches to the epicardial ablation lesion sets. The endocardial ablation section is virtually identical in both procedure types.

The Thoracoscopic Surgical Procedure

The patient is placed under general anesthesia with a double-lumen endotracheal tube and positioned according to the surgeon's preference and the available equipment. Two methods are available for proper positioning. In one method, the patient is placed at a 30° angle with the arm of the access site elevated toward the head (with repositioning of the thorax and the arms when working on the other side; see **Figure 21.1**). An alternative approach, developed in Dallas by Dr. Edgerton, is to place the patient

---

1. Dr. Di Biase is a consultant for Hansen Medical and Biosense Webster. Dr. Natale is a consultant for Biosense Webster and has also received a research grant from St. Jude Medical and received speaker honoraria from St. Jude Medical, Medtronic, Boston Scientific, Biotronik, and Biosense Webster.

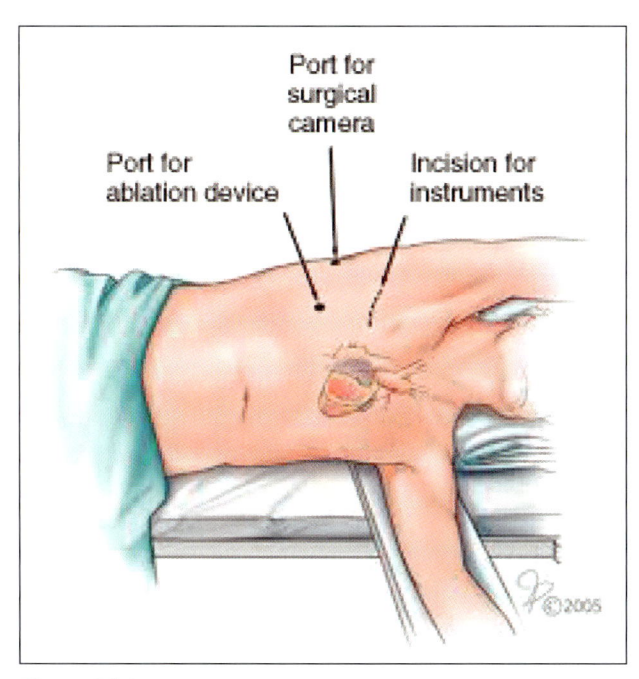

Figure 21.1 Positioning at a 30° angle with the arm of the access site elevated toward the head in a patient undergoing a thoracoscopic surgical procedure. (With permission from Atricure.)

in the supine position over a narrow deflated mattress, which upon inflation of the mattress elevates the patient and allows both arms to be securely placed below the level of the access port sites. Prophylactic systemic antibiotics are then administered and the entire chest and thorax is sterilely prepped.

An 8-level intercostal block is administered to the right hemithorax using 0.25% Marcaine with epinephrine. A 5-mm horizontal incision is placed in the third intercostal space at the midaxillary line and carbon dioxide gas is insufflated into the thoracic cavity while ventilation is maintained via the left lumen of the endotracheal tube. Two additional 10-mm incisions are placed in the right thorax. The first is horizontal in the second intercostal space and the midclavicular line. The second is placed horizontally in the sixth intercostal space and the midaxillary line.

After dissecting any adhesions, the right phrenic nerve is identified and nerve manipulation is minimized to avoid injury. The pericardium is opened 2 cm anterior to the phrenic nerve and the anterior portion of the pericardium is retracted via sutures from the posterolateral chest port. The SVC is approached from within the pericardium and dissected from the neighboring fat pad. The oblique sinus is opened and high-frequency stimulation is performed to map the ganglionated plexi.

With the assistance of the Lumitip™ Dissector to avoid posterior injury, the Isolator Synergy™ clamp is placed around the right PVs at the antral level and RF energy is delivered. Either electrical sensing or pacing in the vein is used to confirm entrance or exit block from the vein, respectively. This process is repeated to isolate the SVC and the IVC. Using a combination of the Coolrail™ linear pen and the Isolator® Multifunctional pen, a line is placed on the posterior aspect of the right atrium connecting the SVC and IVC lesion sets. Using the same linear lesion tools, a line is placed from the RSPV through the transverse sinus to the LSPV. A parallel line is placed from the RIPV through the oblique sinus to the LIPV. The right pericardial opening is then closed with interrupted suture. A 10-inch pain catheter is tunneled subpleural from caudad to cephalad, a 24 Blake drain is introduced, the lung is reinflated, and the skin incisions are closed.

The patient is repositioned with the left thorax raised, and identical skin incisions are placed in the left chest. Access to the left pericardium is similar except that the pericardial entry is posterior to the left phrenic nerve. Also, care is observed to avoid injury to the recurrent laryngeal nerve. The left PVs are ablated with isolation confirmation using the same technique as was used on the right PVs. Linear lesions are placed from the left PVs to the base of the LAA and to the mitral annulus, stopping at the CS. The AtriClip® is placed over the LAA and positioned at the base of the structure. The pericardium is closed with interrupted suture and a pain catheter and Blake drain are placed in the chest. The lung is reinflated and skin incisions are closed.

The Transdiaphragmatic Surgical Procedure

The patient is placed in the supine position and undergoes general anesthesia with a single endotracheal tube. After an appropriate prepping, the patient has a 2.0- to 2.5-cm incision approximately 2.0 to 4.0 cm below the xiphoid process in the midline of the epigastrium of the abdomen. The peritoneal cavity is entered under direct vision and a digital exploration is performed to ensure no abdominal adhesions that can interfere with additional port access. One or two additional 5- to 7-mm ports can be made in the left and right upper quadrants. Insufflation is instituted at 10 to 12 mmHg to expose the diaphragm and other anatomic structures within the abdomen. Reverse Trendelenburg may help demonstrate the tendinous portion of the diaphragm that is needed for access. The laparoscopic camera is placed in the center port and the following anatomic structures are identified: falciform ligament, liver, and the central tendon of the diaphragm. The location of the diaphragm opening should be as posterior as can be visualized and an adequate distance away from the falciform ligament. An oblique incision is performed with an adequate opening for the cannula to pass. This can be done with scissors or a hook electrocoagulation device. Each small vessel on the diaphragm should be cauterized, and the incision should not be too close, as stated above, to the falciform ligament or to the IVC. The diaphragm is grasped with an endoscopic instrument and opened obliquely through the tendinous portion of the diaphragm;

the pericardium is opened cautiously to protect the underlying cardiac structure. The pressure on the abdomen can cause hypotension, which is usually transient and may occasionally require decompression of the abdomen to restore normotensive pressures.

The cannula is inserted through the mid-epigastric incision with the endoscope in position inside the cannula to access the pericardial space under direct vision (**Figure 21.2**). Insufflation is maintained to access the diaphragmatic and pericardial opening. The suction is not attached to the cannula to prevent fat and omentum from occluding the suction ports. The tip of the cannula is placed in the opening and the cannula is gently rotated and advanced posteriorly into the pericardial space. Once in the pericardial space, insufflation is discontinued in the abdomen and the laparoscopic port removed to prevent injury to the abdominal contents. Suction is applied to the cannula inside the pericardial space and the pericardial fluid is removed. Exploration of the pericardium is performed to identify the left pulmonary veins, right pulmonary veins, coronary sinus, and IVC. Esophageal temperature is monitored continuously with a temperature probe placed by anesthesia and its positioned confirmed with fluoroscopy. When an increase in esophageal temperature is seen during the ablation greater than 0.5°C or greater than 38°C, ablation should be stopped and the ablation device repositioned as the temperature returns to baseline prior to any further ablation. The cannula requires small amounts of movement to explore the posterior aspect of the left atrium and should never be forced in any direction. The rotation of the cannula to expose the anatomic structures should be done to understand the different positions in which the device can be placed to achieve the desired ablation lesions. The ablation device is primarily placed on the fixed guide wire and the cannula oriented with the endoscope so that the epicardial lesion can be created according to the attached diagram as outlined.

The surgeon should confirm proper device position and irrigation before ablating the tissue. Additionally, the surgeon must confirm that the cannula and device are positioned such that energy is directed toward the myocardium. During the ablation, impedance is monitored as radiofrequency energy is delivered. The ablation lines are performed on the posterior surface of the heart and, once completed, the cannula is repositioned over the IVC for the anterior right and the right anterior intra-atrial groove lesions (**Figure 21.3**). The movement over the IVC must be done carefully so the tip of the cannula avoids any force into the IVC or atrium to avoid injury to these structures. The tip of the cannula is maintained in the lateral position into the pericardium to create space for the ablation device as well. This also ensures avoiding injury to the cardiac structures and the phrenic nerve. Also, some of the lesions may require the device to be removed off the guide wire to facilitate proper placement of the device. The final area to be ablated is the anterior left pulmonary veins up to the base of the LAA and ligament of Marshall (**Figure 21.4**). The patient can experience some hypotension from lifting the LV required to expose the LSPV. Upon completion of the epicardial ablation, a 19-Fr Blake is inserted and shortened to keep the fluted portion inside the pericardium. Intrapericardial steroids can now be instilled and left 30 minutes prior to connecting the drainage to suction to help alleviate postoperative pericarditis. The diaphragmatic opening is not closed. The cannula is removed from the pericardium, and the position of the drain is again confirmed to have not been accidentally dislodged and is remaining inside the pericardium. The abdominal wall wound is closed in layers and the drain brought out through one of the lateral port incisions.

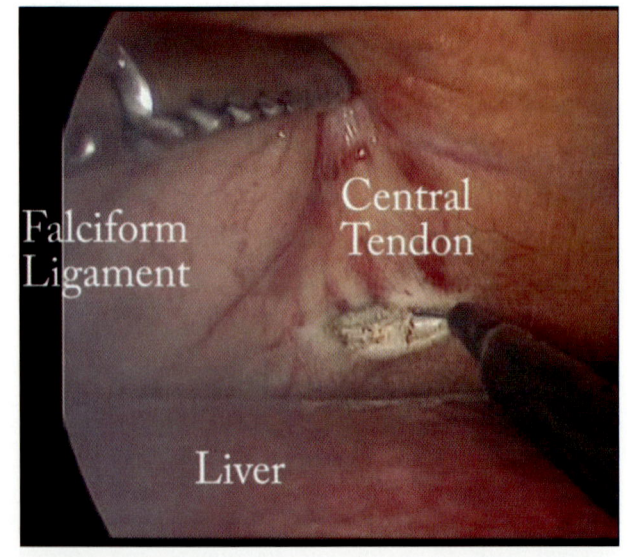

Figure 21.2 Cannula accessing the pericardial space. The liver, the central tendon, and the falciform ligament are shown.

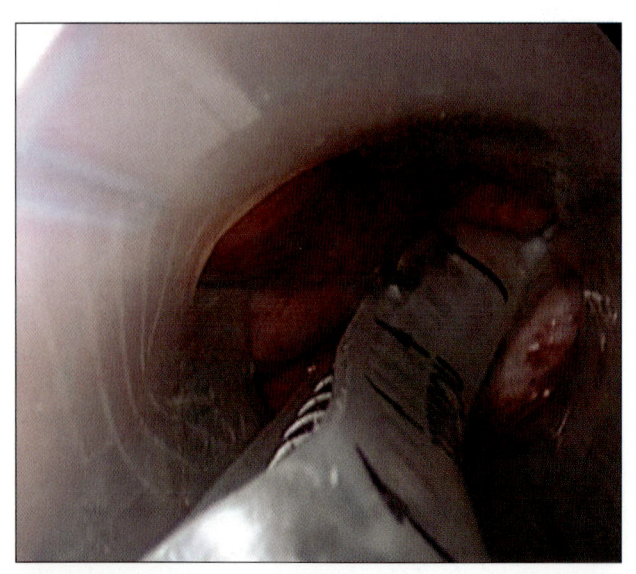

Figure 21.3 Arrows on the ablation cannula indicate the orientation for lesions delivery.

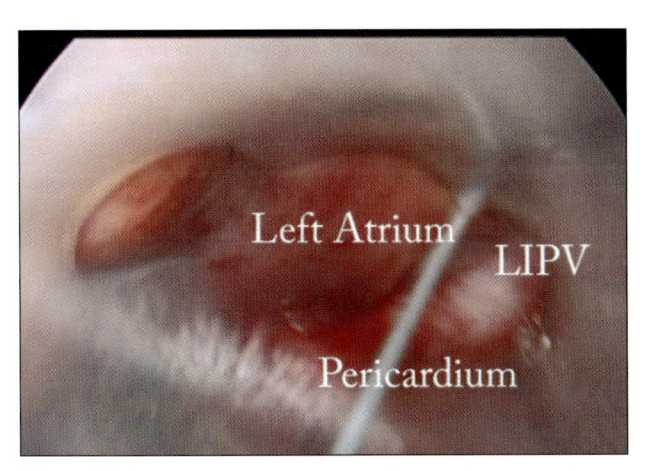

Figure 21.4 Ablation along the left inferior pulmonary vein.

The Endocardial Procedure

Regardless of which surgical approach is implemented, the endocardial approach is essentially the same. Either prior to or after the surgical portion of the procedure, bilateral femoral and right internal jugular venous access is obtained. A 20-pole catheter is placed from the jugular access and is placed in the CS. The proximal portion rests on the RA crista terminalis to provide real-time electrical insight into the AF characteristics from both the right and left atria as the procedure progresses. An ICE probe (Acuson, Acunav) is placed from the left femoral venous access into the RA. This is used to obtain real-time echocardiographic imaging of the septum, LA, PVs, and the pericardial space for the duration of the remaining procedure. The patient is then given heparin intravenously for full anticoagulation (target ACT > 350 seconds). Two transseptal sheaths replace the standard sheaths in the RFVs and these are used for transseptal access. This is achieved with ICE imaging of the septum, a transseptal needle (Brockenbrough, SJM). The transseptal access is then used to place a circular catheter and a mapping/ablation catheter into the LA. A 3-dimensional geometry is then obtained of the LA with particular attention to the PV/LA transition. Endocardial voltage mapping is then performed, identifying regions of successful epicardial transmural ablation as well as location of areas with residual conduction. RF ablation is then performed endocardially on the PV antra, concentrating on these areas. While much of the PV antra and posterior wall usually show little voltage, certain locations of conduction gaps are commonly seen. These tend to be located on the posterior and superior regions of both superior PVs, the inferoseptal region of the RIPV, and the ridge between the LSPV and the LAA. **Figure 21.5** demonstrates a voltage map during AF of the LA following the epicardial ablation procedure (CARTO, Biosense Webster). The arrows highlight the areas of common conduction gaps at this stage of the procedure. These gaps correlate with conduction along the IAS and the posterior pericardial reflection. While these areas require significant ablation energy to complete the isolation lesion set, complete circumferential ablation of these PVs is usually not required.

After complete isolation of the PV antra, mapping and ablation of complex fractionated atrial EGMs is performed as the atrial signals dictate. This usually involves ablation of the LA septum (not accessible from the epicardial surface), the anterior, superior LA and LAA (not directly visualized using the transdiaphragmatic epicardial approach), and the CS (epicardial access limited due to epicardial fat and proximity to the circumflex coronary artery). Upon completion of these ablation targets, the patient is cardioverted if sinus rhythm has not been restored spontaneously.

High-dose isoproterenol is then infused (20–30 mcg/min) to unmask early reconnection of isolated areas and nonvenous triggers for AF. Regions commonly observed to demonstrate triggering activity include the anterior, superior LA, the LA septum, the CS, and the LAA. After final confirmation of entrance and exit block from the PVs as well all other areas outlined above, the catheters are removed, heparin is reversed with protamine (ACT < 180 sec), suction is applied to the pericardial drain and the patient is transported to the ICU for extubation and sheath removal.

Postoperatively, the patients are admitted to the ICU and monitored carefully for drainage output, rhythm issues, and blood pressure control. The drain is left in place until the output is less than 50 to 75 cm^3 for a 24-hour period. Typically, a TTE is performed on postoperative day one to ensure no pericardial effusion.

Contraindications for the candidates for the convergent ablation procedure are those that have had previous cardiac surgery, extensive upper abdominal incisions, any significant structural or valvular abnormalities with the heart that would require an open procedure, or any other obvious comorbid conditions that would prevent the procedure from being performed safely. The hospital stay is usually 3 to 5 days, depending on drainage output and any rhythm issues. The patients have INR levels of 1.8 to 2.4 on the procedure day and postoperatively have their Coumadin continued on postoperative day zero.

Discussion

Interruption of the electrical conduction between the muscle sleeve of the PV and the LA (PV isolation) is widely considered to be an important goal of any surgical or catheter-based treatment of AF. However, this strategy alone is less effective in eliminating AF in the long-standing persistent AF population. In this group, several possible variables appear to be impacting the AF. First is the fact that the PVs appear to play a smaller role in the initiation and maintenance of AF in these patients. In this group, abnormal electrical tissue activity can be routinely seen in

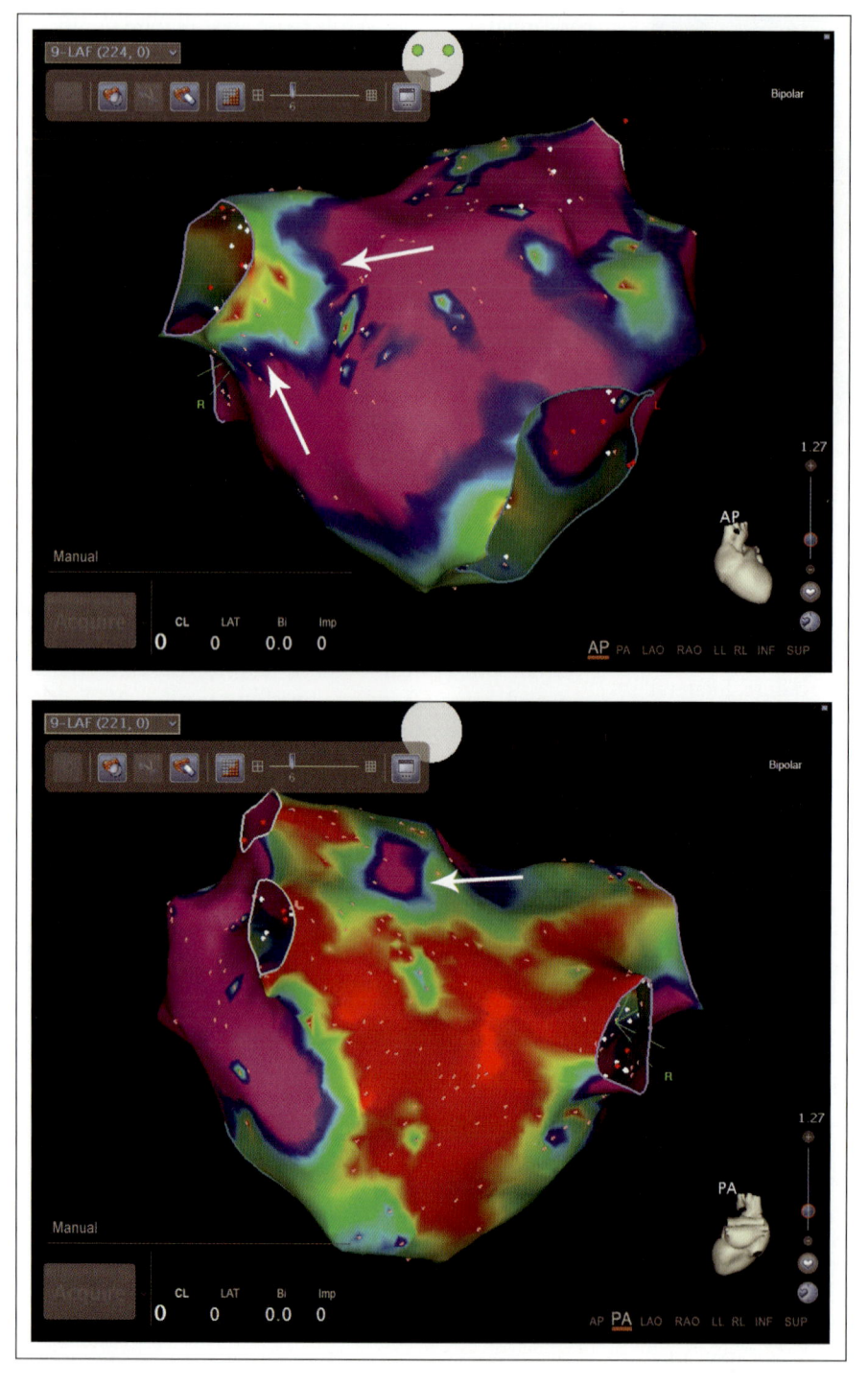

Figure 21.5 A voltage 3D Carto map reconstruction of the left atrium following epicardial ablation in two different views: AP upper panel and PA lower panel. The white arrows show the most common area of conduction gap at the level of the interatrial septum.

the LA regions surrounding the PVs (the PV antra). As such, isolating the PVs at the ostium may fail to fully eliminate the abnormal tissue activity.[12] Additionally, firing and abnormal electrical activity can be found in tissues remote from the PVs (nonvenous triggers). These tissues tend to occur in predictable locations such as the LA septum, anterior-superior LA, CS, RA septum, crista terminalis in the RA, and LAA.[13,14]

As a result, isolation of the PVs without addressing these other areas may account for lower success. As the duration of AF lengthens, the nature and histology of the atrial tissue changes.[15] Over extended time, the atrial myocardium thickens and becomes infiltrated with fibrous tissue. On gross inspection, this tissue is whiter in appearance as compared to normal atrial muscle.[16] Because of the fibrous infiltration and thickness, resistive heating as one achieves with RF ablation may be less likely to produce a transmural lesion as compared to similar lesions on normal atrial tissue. Published reports in the surgical literature suggest improved clinical results when the epicardial fat pads in which the GP reside are dissected or ablated.[17,18] However, consensus about the added value of GP ablation is still lacking[19] (especially when fairly antral ablation is performed[20]).

The principal advantage of surgical ablation of AF is the ability to apply larger lesions than can be applied with a catheter. This provides a debulking effect that may be effective, particularly with long-standing persistent AF. While direct visualization of ablation targets is possible with surgical ablation, the convergent access is at the level of the central tendon of the diaphragm. As a result, lesions on the inferior and posterior aspects of the LA can be well visualized. For the more anterior and superior lesions, direct visualization is not possible. In these locations, the lesions are applied without direct vision and rely on device angle/orientation and confirmation of tight suction against the tissue for device position. However, during the surgical approach, mapping and electrical confirmation of lesion set integrity is difficult and, in some locations, not possible with present technology.

In contrast, the principal advantage of endocardial catheter-based ablation of AF is the ability to perform point-by-point mapping along lesion sets, which allows identification and ablation of sites where electrical activity is present along previously ablated sites. The main disadvantages are smaller catheter size, less effective catheter–tissue contact, increased concern about energy delivery to collateral structures (particularly along the posterior LA wall), and the possibility of tissue overheating, resulting in steam pops. All of these limitations result in decreased energy delivery, thereby limiting lesion size. Late reconnection of PVs after confirmed acute isolation is more common with this approach.

From a morbidity standpoint, several points should be mentioned. While epicardial visualization offers an advantage, there remains the potential for collateral damage. If the device is angled toward the RA while ablating anterior to the right PVs (Waterston's groove), phrenic nerve injury is possible. While this complication is usually transient when observed during catheter ablation, the nature of the convergent lesion size may result in permanent injury in this situation. Similarly, when ablating the posterior LA, it remains possible to injure the esophagus, resulting in an atrioesophageal fistula. This is most likely to occur if the device is angled superiorly with suction applied to the posterior pericardial reflection. In this situation, energy could be delivered to both the LA and the mediastinum in direct contact to the esophagus. Finally, postoperative pericarditis and pericardial effusion remains the most common determinant of hospital length of stay. While a pericardial drain is left in place at the end of the procedure, drain obstruction from either clotting or kinking can lead to acute tamponade. Furthermore, late effusions and tamponade have been observed as late as 1 week after discharge. As a result, close monitoring for possible complications in house and detailed instructions of warning signs on discharge are crucial. In general, the pericardial drain is removed on days 2 to 4, allowing for discharge the following day. Although most centers perform both the epicardial and endocardial portions of the procedure in the same room in sequential fashion, some centers choose to perform the two components in separate rooms or on separate days.

Developing a combined endocardial/epicardial ablation strategy has been a focus of several studies. Intuitively, this offers the best of both approaches, as the strengths of one approach are the weaknesses of the other. However, most combined or hybrid approaches involve thoracoscopy from one or both hemi thoraces. As a result, postoperative pain is significant. Moreover, patient perception of procedure invasiveness is heightened with any thoracoscopic approach. This perception is not mitigated by euphemisms like "minimally invasive surgery."

The Atricure surgical component offers excellent exposure of the left and right atria via the respective thoraces. As such, the lesion set often results in complete isolation of the PVs as well as significant debulking of the LA. The notable disadvantage remains the relative invasiveness of the access with resultant postoperative pain.

The surgical component used for the convergent approach involves a midline upper-abdominal incision, peritoneal access, and entry into the pericardium from the central tendon of the diaphragm. By avoiding entry into the thorax, the postoperative pain perception is minimal. The primary disadvantage of this approach is the limited access to the superior aspects of the LA. The posterior wall is easily accessed and visualized; however, the posterior pericardial reflections limit access to the superior-most aspects of the SPVs from this window. Similarly, the inferior entry allows only indirect access to the anterior, superior LA as well as the ridge between the LAA and the LSPV.

It is because of these limitations that this approach in particular requires skilled endocardial ablation at the locations not accessible from the inferior epicardial access point. Once catheters are placed within the LA, mapping can be easily performed. This typically shows gaps in the epicardial lesion set at the location of the posterior pericardial reflection (posterior to both superior PVs), anterior and septal to the RIPV and the septal-most aspect of the ridge between the LAA and the LSPV. While endocardial ablation is required to complete this lesion set, large regions of the LA have already been ablated and debulked. As a result, this ablation is more focused on completing the lesion. As is the case with all long-standing persistent AF patients, nonvenous AF triggers can be a source of AF generation. As a result, during combined approaches, these are also mapped and ablated endocardially after completion of the PV isolation.

In conclusion, the convergent approach for the treatment of AF is a hybrid procedure involving a surgeon as well as an electrophysiologist. It is less invasive than other surgical techniques utilizing thoracic access ports and it allows for many of the advantages of surgical epicardial ablation. Further research and experience are needed to further elucidate its clinical role in the management of this complex arrhythmia.

References

1. Fuster V, Rydén LE, Cannom DS, et al. ACC/AHA/ESC 2006 guidelines for the management of patients with atrial fibrillation: full text: a report of the American College of Cardiology/American Heart Association Task Force on practice guidelines and the European Society of Cardiology Committee for Practice Guidelines (Writing Committee to Revise the 2001 guidelines for the management of patients with atrial fibrillation) developed in collaboration with the European Heart Rhythm Association and the Heart Rhythm Society. *Europace.* 2006;8:651–745.
2. Brooks AG, Stiles MK, Laborderie J, et al. Outcomes of long-standing persistent atrial fibrillation ablation: A systematic review. *Heart Rhythm.* 2010;7:835–846.
3. Sauer WH, McKernan ML, Lin D, Gerstenfeld EP, Callans DJ, Marchlinski FE. Clinical predictors and outcomes associated with acute return of pulmonary vein conduction during pulmonary vein isolation for treatment of atrial fibrillation. *Heart Rhythm.* 2006;3:1024–1028.
4. Bhargava M, Di Biase L, Mohanty P, et al. Impact of type of atrial fibrillation and repeat catheter ablation on long-term freedom from atrial fibrillation: results from a multicenter study. *Heart Rhythm.* 2009;6:1403–1412.
5. Lee SH, Tai CT, Hsieh MH, et al. Predictors of early and late recurrence of atrial fibrillation after catheter ablation of paroxysmal atrial fibrillation. *J Interv Card Electrophysiol.* 2004;10:221–226.
6. Berruezo A, Tamborero D, Mont L, Benito B, Tolosana JM, Sitges M, et al. Preprocedural predictors of atrial fibrillation recurrence after circumferential pulmonary vein ablation. *Eur Heart J.* 2007;28:836–41.
7. Matsuo S, Lellouche N, Wright M, et al. Clinical predictors of termination and clinical outcome of catheter ablation for persistent atrial fibrillation. *J Am Coll Cardiol.* 2009;54:788–795.
8. Cox J, Schuessler R, D'Agostino H, Stone C, Chang B, Cain M, Corr P, Boineau J. The surgical treatment of atrial fibrillation. III. Development of a definitive surgical procedure. *J Thorac Cardiovasc Surg.* 1991;101(4):569–83.
9. Prasad S, Maniar H, Camillo C, Schuessler R, Boineau J, Sundt T, Cox J, Damiano R. The Cox maze III procedure for atrial fibrillation: long-term efficacy in patients undergoing lone versus concomitant procedures. *J Thorac Cardiovasc Surg.* 2003;126(6):1822–8.
10. Wolf RK, Schneeberger EW, Osterday R, et al. Video-assisted bilateral pulmonary vein isolation and left atrial appendage exclusion for atrial fibrillation, *J Thorac Cardiovasc Surg.* 2005;130:797–802.
11. Edgerton JR, Edgerton ZJ, Weaver T, Reed K, Prince S and Herbert MA et al. Minimally invasive pulmonary vein isolation and partial autonomic denervation for surgical treatment of atrial fibrillation, *Ann Thorac Surg.* 2008;86:35–38
12. Rostock T, Steven D, Hoffman B, et al. Chronic atrial fibrillation is a biatrial arrhythmia. Data from catheter ablation of chronic atrial fibrillation aiming arrhythmia termination using a sequential ablation approach. *Circ Arrhythm Electrophysiol.* 2008;1:344–353.
13. Haïssaguerre M, Hocini M, Sanders P, et al. Catheter ablation of long-lasting persistent atrial fibrillation: clinical outcome and mechanisms of subsequent arrhythmias. *J Cardiovasc Electrophysiol.* 2005;16:1138–1147.
14. Elayi CS, Verma A, Di Biase L, et al. Ablation for longstanding permanent atrial fibrillation: results from a randomized study comparing three different strategies. *Heart Rhythm.* 2008;5:1658–1664.
15. Frustaci A, Chimenti C, Bellocci F, Morgante E, Russo MA, Maseri A. Histological substrate of atrial biopsies in patients with lone atrial fibrillation. *Circulation.* 1997;96:1180–1184.
16. Shirani J, Alaeddini J. Structural remodeling of the LAA in patients with chronic nonvalvular atrial fibrillation: implications for thrombus formation, systemic embolism, and assessment by transesophageal echocardiography. *Cardiovasc Pathol.* 2000;9(2):95–101.
17. Melo J, Voigt P, Sonmez B, et al. Ventral cardiac denervation reduces the incidence of atrial fibrillation after coronary artery bypass grafting. *J Thorac Cardiovasc Surg.* 2004;127:511–516.
18. Edgerton JR, Brinkman WT, Weaver T, Prince SL, Culica D, Herbert MA, Mack MJ. Pulmonary vein isolation and autonomic denervation for the management of paroxysmal atrial fibrillation by a minimally invasive surgical approach. *J Thorac Cardiovasc Surg.* 2010;140(4):823–828.
19. Cummings JE, Gill I, Akhrass R, Dery M, Biblo LA, Quan KJ. Preservation of the anterior fat pad paradoxically decreases the incidence of postoperative atrial fibrillation in humans. *J Am Coll Cardiol.* 2004;43:994–1000.
20. Verma A, Saliba WI, Lakkireddy D, et al. Vagal responses induced by endocardial left atrial autonomic ganglion stimulation before and after pulmonary vein antrum isolation for atrial fibrillation. *Heart Rhythm.* 2007;4:1177–1182.

CHAPTER 22

How to Perform a Hybrid Surgical Epicardial and Catheter Endocardial Ablation for Atrial Fibrillation

Srijoy Mahapatra, MD; Gorav Ailawadi, MD[1]

Introduction

Although catheter-based PV isolation is often successful in patients with paroxysmal AF, it has only a 40 to 70% single-procedure success rate in persistent and long-standing persistent AF.[1] Reasons for this poor success rate include inability to isolate the pulmonary antrum, the LAA, and the SVC.[2]

Many of these limitations can be addressed by a minimally invasive surgical approach via port access. In particular, animal studies suggest that the antrum is best isolated using bipolar clamps placed epicardially and providing energy on both sides of atrial tissue.[3]

However, surgical ablation can lead to multiple flutters caused by gaps in linear epicardial lines, which are typically made with spot burns or linear unipolar tools. Thus, most recurrent arrhythmias after minimally invasive surgery are due to gaps in lines.[4] However, these gaps can be touched up with endocardial catheter ablation.

In 2007, La Meir, Ailawadi, Mahapatra, Pison (LAMP) developed a hybrid epicardial-endocardial AF ablation that attempted to combine the advantages of minimally invasive surgery and catheter techniques. Although there are multiple variations of this hybrid procedure, here we describe our techniques using a bipolar clamp, LAA clip, unipolar pen for lines, and catheters for endocardial lines.

Procedure Goal and Summary

The goals of the procedure are:

1. Antral PV isolation with confirmed entrance and exit block, created with bipolar clamps.

2. Posterior wall isolation, created with linear surgical ablation tools; this always has required endocardial "touch-up" ablation.

3. Creation of a line of block from left IPV to mitral isthmus. This line is created partially epicardially but requires catheter ablation in both the LA and CS.

4. SVC isolation with bipolar clamp. This is done surgically.

5. Ganglia ablation done surgically.

6. Creation of CTI line done exclusively with catheters.

---

[1]. Disclosures: Drs. Mahapatra and Ailawadi have served as consultants to Atricure and, through the University of Virginia, have intellectual property related to epicardial access and ablation. Dr. Mahapatra is a shareholder of St. Jude Medical and EpiEP and was a consultant to Johnson and Johnson during the creation of this article. After submission, he became a consultant to and is currently a full-time employee of St. Jude Medical.

7. Ligament of Marshall ablation performed surgically/epicardially.

8. LAA exclusion performed epicardially by the surgeon.

9. Ablation of all inducible flutters. This is done endocardially by the electrophysiologist.

Figure 22.1 illustrates the lesion set.

Patient Selection

We initially selected only patients with symptomatic, persistent AF that had failed at least one antiarrhythmic drug and one catheter ablation. However, as our experience has grown, we have considered treating patients with paroxysmal AF that has failed one ablation or persistent AF that has not failed an ablation.

Preprocedural Planning

Imaging

All patients undergo cardiac imaging, including TEE, to assess LA dimensions, LVEF, and look for a thickened or aneurysmal atrial septum. This imaging is used for pre-procedure planning and for prediction of success.

All patients undergo coronary artery gated computed tomography (coronary CT) to define PV anatomy and rule out CAD. High-risk patients (smokers, known CAD, EF < 50, patients with diabetes, or any history of typical chest pain) undergo angiogram to evaluate coronary arteries. All patients receive a TEE just prior to the procedure in the operating room to rule out LAA clot.

Performing the LAMP Hybrid AF Procedure

The LAMP procedure can be divided into two portions: surgical and then catheter ablation. **Figure 22.2** is a flow chart delineating the procedure.

Surgical Procedure with EP Checking for Epicardial Block

Patient Positioning

Under general anesthesia, a double lumen endotracheal tube and Foley catheter are inserted. The patient is placed in a supine position, with arms placed at the sides. The left arm is positioned below the cushion of the operating table to allow access to the posterior portion of the left chest. An inflatable IV pressure bag is placed under each scapula and is inflated while the chest, abdomen, and groins are prepped widely.

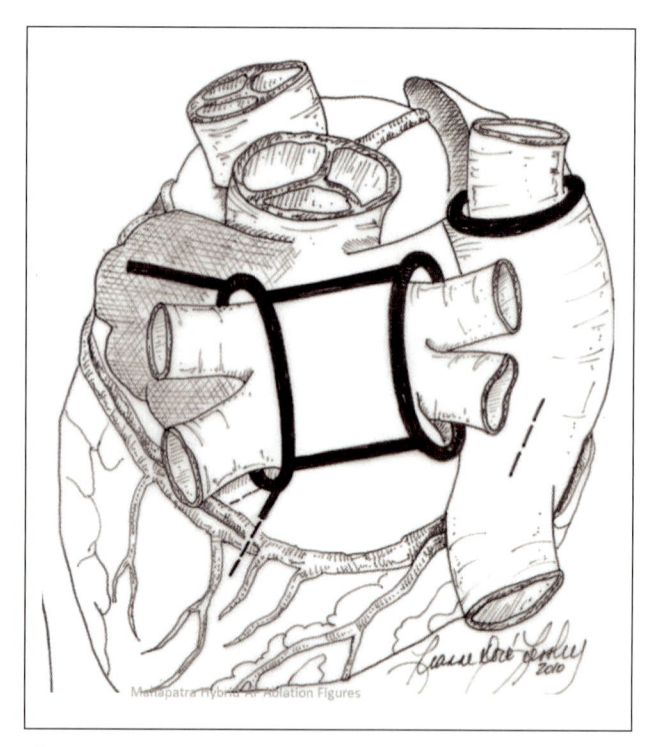

Figure 22.1 LAMP lesion set. Solid lines are surgical epicardial lesions. Dashed lines are catheter endocardial lesions. LAA is clipped or excluded. (With permission from reference 7.)

Right-Sided Entry and Setup

The left IV pressure bag is deflated. Single-lung ventilation of the left lung is begun. A 10-mm port is placed at the third or fourth interspace in the anterior axillary line and is used for the video thoracoscope. A second 10-mm port is placed in the inframammary crease in the midclavicular line and is used as the primary utility port. This incision should not be below the xiphoid, as the diaphragm will limit the utility of this incision. A third 5-mm port is placed in the second intercostal space in the midclavicular line (**Figure 22.3**).

We prefer to use a 10-mm 0° laparoscope. CO_2 insufflation is used at a pressure of 6 to 8 mmHg to help maintain working space in the right chest. The pericardium is opened 2 to 3 cm anterior to the phrenic nerve. Two 0-Ethibond stay sutures are placed in the lower edge of the pericardium and retracted through the chest wall with a suture passer. The oblique and transverse sinuses are opened bluntly. The SVC is mobilized off the pulmonary artery. The space between the RPA and RSPV is created bluntly. The interatrial groove is developed using low electrocautery. A lighted dissector (Atricure, West Chester, OH) is carefully placed under the right PVs and gently passed to see the lighted tip between the RPA and RSPV. A red rubber catheter is passed around the posterior veins and brought through to the 5-mm port. At this point, the inferior 10-mm trocar is removed and a 0-prolene purse-string suture is placed around the inferior working port to maintain CO_2 insufflation in the chest (▶ **Video 22.1**).

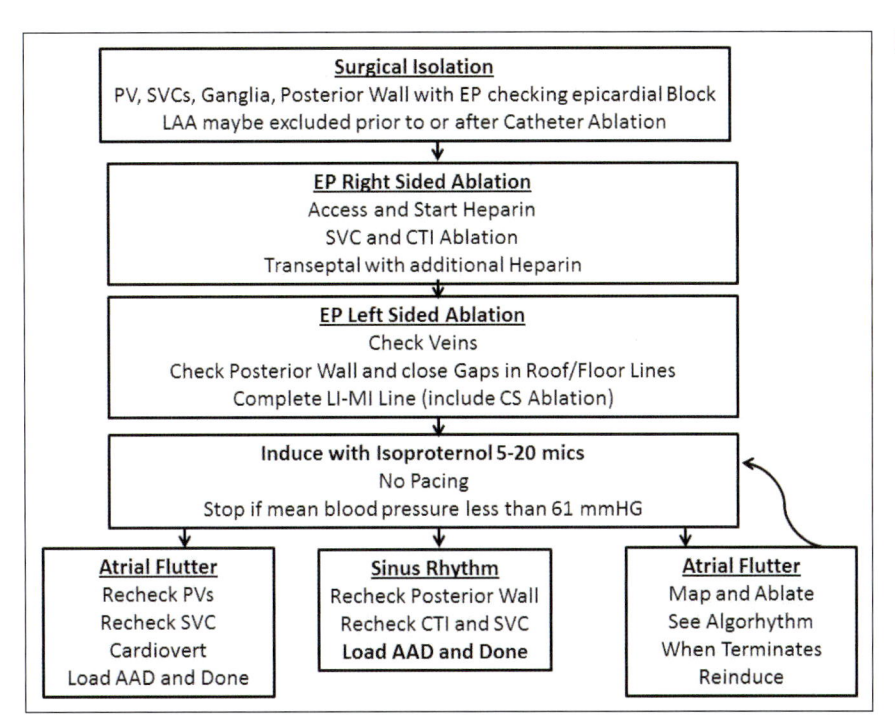

Figure 22.2 Workflow.

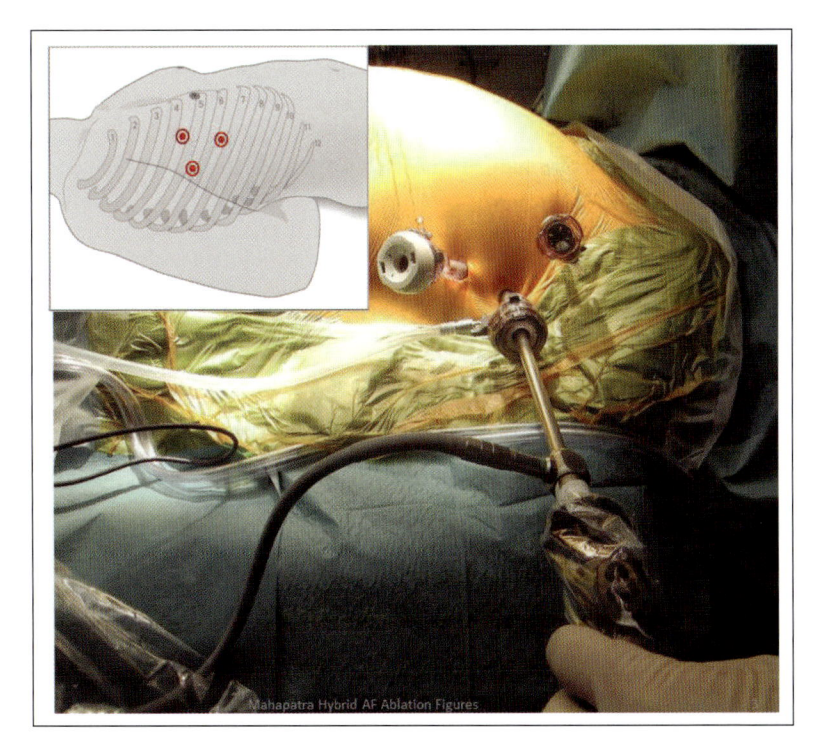

Figure 22.3 Left ports placed. (Photo courtesy of Mark La Meir, University Hospital Maastrich.)

Testing for Ganglia/Ganglia Ablation

The bipolar pen (Atricure) is placed through the inferior port. Next, autonomic ganglionic plexi are tested. Active ganglionic plexi are identified by prolongation of the ventricular cycle length by ≥ 50% during high-frequency stimulation. These are tested in 10 standardized locations. Active ganglionic plexi are ablated using the bipolar pen and are restested and reablated as necessary. Typically the R10 (as well as R11) region behind the IVC is commonly very active ganglionic plexi with profound asystole during high-frequency stimulation in this region (**Figure 22.4**; ▶ **Video 22.2**).

Right PV and Antral Isolation

Entrance block is tested with the bipolar pen sensing the RA and RSPV and IPV, as well as the carina. Exit block can be tested if the patient is in sinus rhythm by pacing the RSPV and right IPV at 10A using the bipolar pen. Generally, the veins are not completely isolated; even if they are, the antrum is not. Thus, a bipolar, bidirectional clamp (Synergy, Atricure) is then attached to the red rubber catheter and placed into the inferior port. It is carefully passed around the right PVs. Four to five successive bipolar lesions are made high on the antrum of the LA. This requires significant dissection of Waterson's groove (**Figure 22.5**; Video 22.3). The endpoint for PV ablation is complete entrance block (and exit block if in sinus rhythm) as described above. Up to 4 or 5 additional lesions are created if PV isolation and antral isolation are not obtained after the initial lesions.

Atrial Roof Line

Next, the Coolrail (Atricure) device is placed through the inferior port and placed across the atrial roof. Care must be taken to ensure the ablation is posterior to the LAA as the left main coronary artery/circumflex artery lies anterior to the LAA (**Figure 22.6**). Successive lesions are made with the Coolrail device until the power curve drops. This typically requires 60 to 80 seconds of ablation at 30 W. We have found that deeper lesions are created by putting gentle pressure on the ablating head of the Coolrail device during ablation. The atrial roof line lesion is then created and brought toward the right PVI lesion with generous overlap between lesions to minimize the risk of gaps in the roof line ablation (Video 22.4).

Atrial Floor Line

Similar to the roof line, the atrial floor line is created using the Coolrail device and is extended as far to the patient's left as visible. Often the CS may be visualized. The floor lesion is brought as close to the CS as feasible without ablating on the vein itself and brought toward and overlaps the right PVI lesion (Video 22.5).

Right Atrial Lesions

Two ablation lines are created on the RA. First, the SVC is isolated circumferentially with a single application of the bipolar clamp at least 2 cm superior to the RA/SVC junction. If central lines are present, they should be pulled back to ensure they are not within the ablated area. Using the bipolar pen, a line on the lateral RA from the SVC line to the IVC is created. Again, care is taken to ensure there is generous overlap of lesions to minimize the risk of incomplete line/flutter.

At the conclusion of these lesions, the pericardium is closed with a single suture. The phrenic nerve is carefully

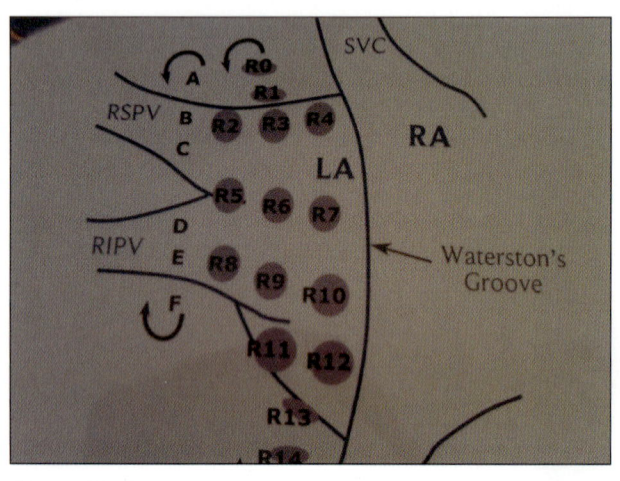

Figure 22.4 Right-sided ganglia map. (Courtesy of K Frazier, Atricure.)

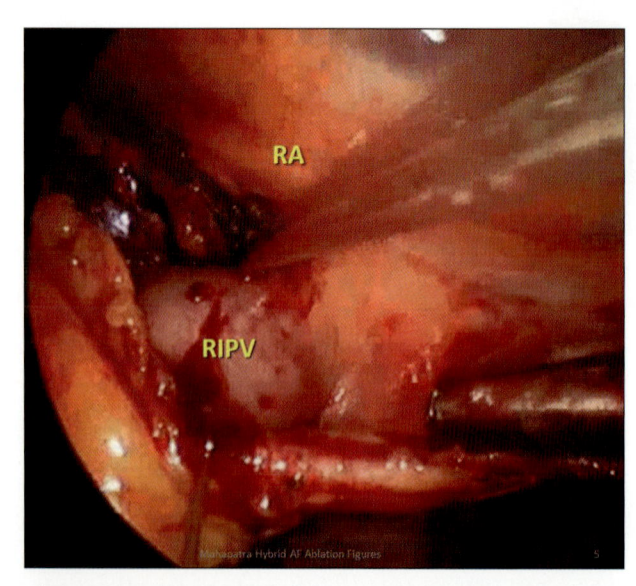

Figure 22.5 Image of RPV dissected prior to antral ablation.

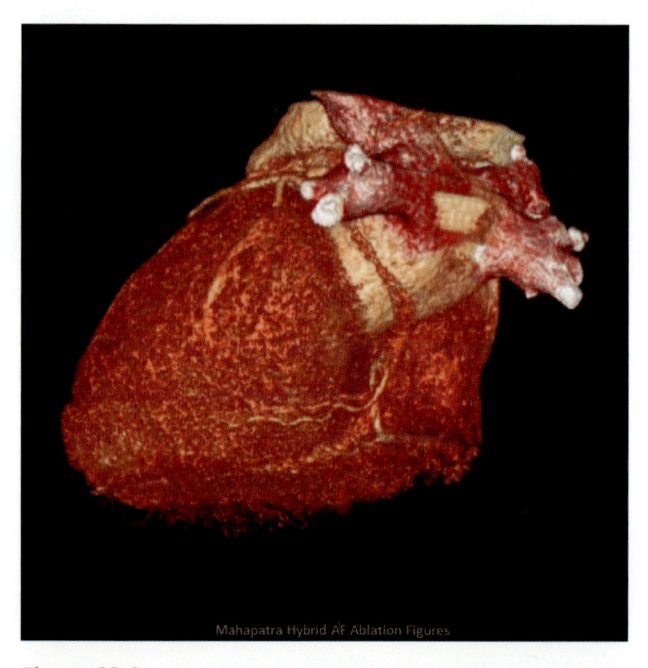

Figure 22.6 Preop CT scan with circumflex artery.

avoided. A single 19F Blake chest tube is inserted and brought through the right inferior working port. The tube is placed to waterseal.

Left-Sided Entry and Setup

The right lung is reinflated and the left lung deflated. The pressure bag under the right scapula is deflated and the pressure bag on the left is inflated to allow optimal exposure of the lateral chest wall. Three ports (2 10-mm and 1 5-mm) are placed in a similar fashion as on the right side (▶ Video 22.6). Typically, these are placed more posteriorly on the left chest wall than on the right. If the working port is placed too anteriorly, the LV apex lies in the way. CO_2 insufflation is used as on the right side. The phrenic nerve is identified and the pericardium is opened posterior to the phrenic nerve. The nerve can lie just above the left main pulmonary artery, so care must be taken to mobilize the nerve anteriorly to create enough working space to open the pericardium safely. Two 0-Ethibond stay sutures are placed in the inferior pericardium and retracted out of the chest wall laterally using an Endostitch (Ethicon).

Ligament of Marshall Ablation

The LSPV and LPA are identified. The Ligament of Marshall lies just between these two vessels and is divided with a hook cautery. An 0-prolene pursestring suture is placed around the inferior working port and the trocar removed.

Left Ganglia Ablation

The left-sided ganglionic plexi are tested as described above and ablated as necessary. Typically there are few active left-sided ganglionic plexi.

Left PV Isolation

Similar to the right side, the left PVs are assessed for evidence of entrance and exit block prior to any ablation. The lighted dissector (Atricure) is then placed through the inferior port and is carefully placed below the left PVs. The dissector is carefully reticulated and aimed toward the right scapula. The light is then visualized between the LSPV and LPA. This is often more medial than anticipated. A red rubber catheter is then passed from the inferior port, behind the veins, and through the superior 5-mm port. The bipolar Synergy clamp is then carefully placed around the left veins. Four to five successive ablations are created with the clamp. The veins are then tested for block with the bipolar pen as with the right-sided PVs. Up to four or five additional lesions may be required to obtain bidirectional block. We check block epicardially (**Figure 22.7**).

Completion of Roof and Floor Lines

The Coolrail device is then placed through the inferior port and the roof line is completed from the left side. Typically, the roof line ablation is evident by visualization and is completed toward the patient's left side. Thorough overlap with the left PVI line should be ensured. Similarly, the floor line ablation is completed from the floor ablation, which may be visualized to the left PVI line.

Once complete, the atrial posterior wall can be tested for evidence of bidirectional block using the bipolar pen to sense and pace within the posterior atrial box, although access to this area can be challenging.

Mitral Isthmus Line

The mitral isthmus line is then started epicardially using the bipolar pen from the left IPV toward the CS. For this particular lesion, it is important to understand the patient's coronary anatomy. The preoperative coronary CT scan can be extremely useful in understanding the size and dominance of the circumflex artery (Figure 22.6). It is important not to ablate over this artery. Thus, the mitral isthmus line is almost never completed, and a gap is left near the mitral valve that will need to be ablated from the LA and inside the CS by the EP.

LA Appendage Lesion and Exclusion

An additional line from the left PVI line to the tip of the LAA is created using the bipolar pen. As the LAA is often thin, 10-second burns are typically sufficient for each lesion; however, careful overlap of successive lesions is required (▶ Video 22.7).

The LAA is then removed either now or typically after the EP procedure. Our preference has been to use a no-knife 45-mm green-load EZ stapler (Ethicon, Blue Ash, OH). More recently, the Atriclip (Atricure) has been

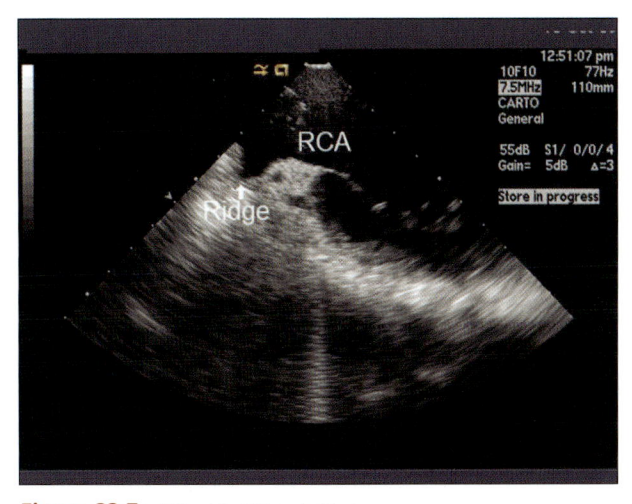

Figure 22.7 ICE with CTI and ridge.

approved by the FDA for exclusion of the LAA. The appendage can be safely excluded using this device. Although experience with this device is limited, the potential for bleeding complications is likely to be less than with a stapling device.

Depending on the comfort of the surgeon and electrophysiologist, the LAA can be excluded before or after the EP portion, although we typically remove the LAA after the EP portion. The EP portion of the LAMP procedure does require heparinization; thus, any potential bleeding from stapling the appendage may become more significant. However, in our experience, bleeding seems to be less of an issue with the new clip. One advantage of LAA exclusion prior to the EP procedure is LAA triggers are eliminated prior to EP testing. Since the LAA is the source of AF in a proportion of AF patients, this may shorten the EP procedure.

EP Procedure

Access

We place an 8.5-Fr, 8-Fr, and 6-Fr right femoral sheath for right-sided ablation, first transseptal and RV catheter respectively. We place 11-Fr and 6-Fr left femoral vein sheaths for ICE (SoundStar) and a decapolar catheter for CS. We typically do not place catheters from the internal jugular or subclavian veins (▶ **Video 22.8**).

Catheters

The TEE probe and Swan-Ganz used during surgery are pulled back. A quadrapolar catheter is placed in RV, a decapolar in CS. ICE (Soundstar, Biosense Webster, Diamond Bar, CA) is placed in RA and ablation (Thermacool, D/F curve irrigated tip, Biosense Webster) is placed in RA.

Heparin

After catheter insertion, we give 5000 U heparin. After first transseptal, we give an additional 5000 to 10,000 U for a total of 120 U/kg. A drip is started at 18 U/kg/h. The goal ACT is 350 seconds.

Right-Sided Lesion (CTI and SVC)

Typical AFL can complicate minimally invasive surgery for AF in up to 12% of patients.[5] Thus, we begin by burning on the isthmus using ICE and 3D mapping guidance using up to 50 W of power and 30 cm^3/min of irrigation (**Figure 22.8**). We then place a 20-pole Halo and check for block using standard pacing maneuvers from the RA, LA, and RV. In patients with prior CTI, we check for bidirectional block and ablate as needed. We then replace the Halo with a 20-mm spiral catheter (Biosense Webster) and place it into the SVC and check for block.

Transseptal Puncture

We do RA lesions first in order to maximize time from LA epicardial lesion creation to LA endocardial lesion check. In essence, we are working in the RA while allowing time for PV reconnection.

We perform a single transseptal puncture with a steerable sheath (Agillis, St. Jude Medical, Minnetonka, MN) using primarily ICE guidance (**Figure 22.9**). Successful transseptal puncture is confirmed with visualization of bubbles in the LA on ICE and pressure tracing. After the first transseptal puncture, we place the lasso catheter in the LA and pull the Agillis sheath back. We then attempt to place an ablation catheter into LA using the same transseptal puncture site. If it does not enter the LA easily, we perform a second transseptal with an SL-1 sheath.

Selection of Mapping and Ablation Catheter

We typically use a Thermacool F/J curve bidirectional steerable ablation catheter but use the D/F curve in atrium smaller than 45 mm (Biosense Webster). For mapping we

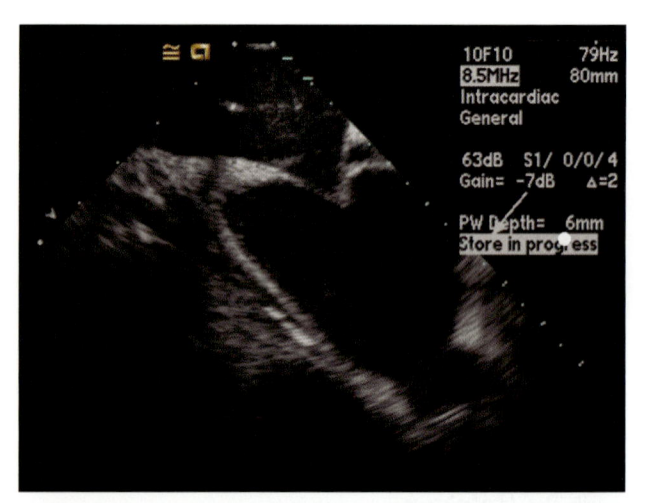

Figure 22.8 ICE of transseptal with needle tenting.

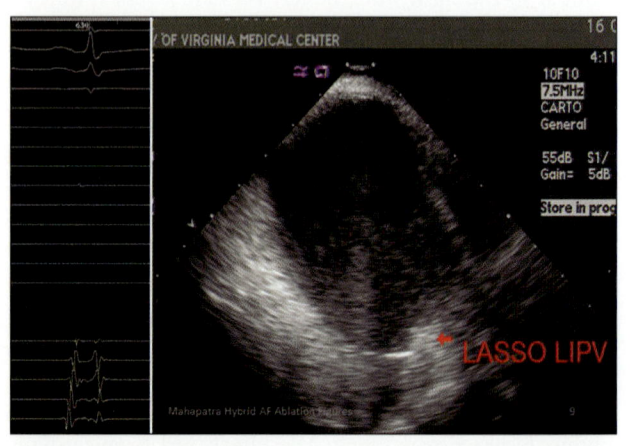

Figure 22.9 ICE image of lasso in left superior vein and no signal in vein (entrance block).

use a 15- or 20-mm 10-pole lasso catheter (Biosense Webster).

3D Mapping

3D mapping is used for catheter manipulation and to track flutters. We typically use a magnetic-based mapping system (CARTO XP, Biosense Webster) for two reasons. First, magnetic-based systems are not affected by injecting fluid, air, and moving tools around the heart, which we do especially while touching up the posterior wall and mitral line. A second issue is that impedance-based systems require multiple adhesive patches on the chest, which can interfere with the surgical field. Other groups have used impedance systems.

Phased-Array Intracardiac Echocardiography (ICE)

We use a 10-Fr phased-array ICE that integrates with 3D mapping (SoundStar, Biosense Webster). Phased-array ICE (either Biosense Webseter or ViewFlex, St. Jude, St. Paul, MN) may help in making a 3D map prior to insertion of transseptal guide catheters and ensure good contact. Later, it can be used to confirm appendage removal with Doppler. Rotational ICE (Galaxy, Boston Scientific, Natick, MA) is less helpful for lines and CS ablation and for confirming LAA removal since it does not have Doppler.

Left-Side Mapping and Ablation

If the patient is in AF, we cardiovert in order to ensure block on lines and PVs. If the patient is in AFL (defined as less than 10% variation in CL with fixed activation sequence), we skip to mapping the AFL as described below.

Antral Isolation

We first place the lasso into each PV to confirm entrance block. Next, we place the ablation catheter and lasso in each PV. By pacing off the catheter, we confirm exit block. The lasso is used to confirm local capture. In our experience, entrance and exit block are always achieved acutely after bipolar clamp use (**Figure 22.10**).

Posterior Wall Block and Isolation

We place the lasso on the posterior wall and use ICE to ensure contact (**Figure 22.11**). We then pace on lasso and ensure local capture on other poles. If there is local capture, but the atrial rate is not accelerated, the posterior wall has exit block. If there is atrial acceleration, then a gap exists in either the roof line or floor line. In our experience, the posterior wall has never been isolated prior to catheter touch-up.

If there are local gaps, we typically find them by going over the roof and floor line evaluating for any significant signals. We then ablate for 40 seconds using 25 to 30 W of power with 17 cm^3/min of irrigation and increase as needed to eliminate local signal. One difficulty of this technique is that the patients have multiple prior lines, so finding the correct line can be difficult. In general, prior catheter-based lines are posterior (toward the spine) to the surgical epicardial line. To help find the epicardial line, we can have the surgeon push on the roof line and position our ablation catheter with ICE. We repeat the same technique with the floor line. An alternative is to place radiographic clips on the roof and floor. Regardless, at the end of each ablation, we pace from lasso. If we cannot get block by simply ablating on the line, we create an activation map while pacing. Voltage maps can be difficult to interpret due to prior ablation. **Figures 22.12** and **22.13** illustrate an example of block after ablation. The posterior wall often shows significant signal even when isolated, but careful examination will show dissociation (Figure 22.12).

Line Check

Most of our patients have multiple linear lesions often crossing each other. This makes checking block across the roof and floor line using pacing techniques difficult. Instead, we rely on exit block from the posterior wall as the indicator of block across the floor and roof lines. We do use pacing maneuvers on the mitral isthmus and CTI line.

Mitral Line and CS Ablation

To find the location of the surgical epicardial partial mitral line, we have the surgeon push on the epicardial line. We then use ICE to place the ablation catheter on the endocardial side of this line. We perform ablation from the left IPV to the mitral isthmus and try to be directly on the endocardial side of the surgical line. We focus our attention

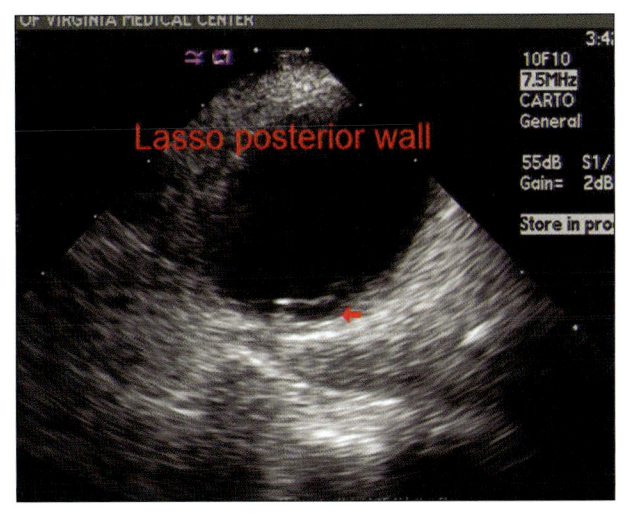

Figure 22.10 ICE image of lasso on posterior wall.

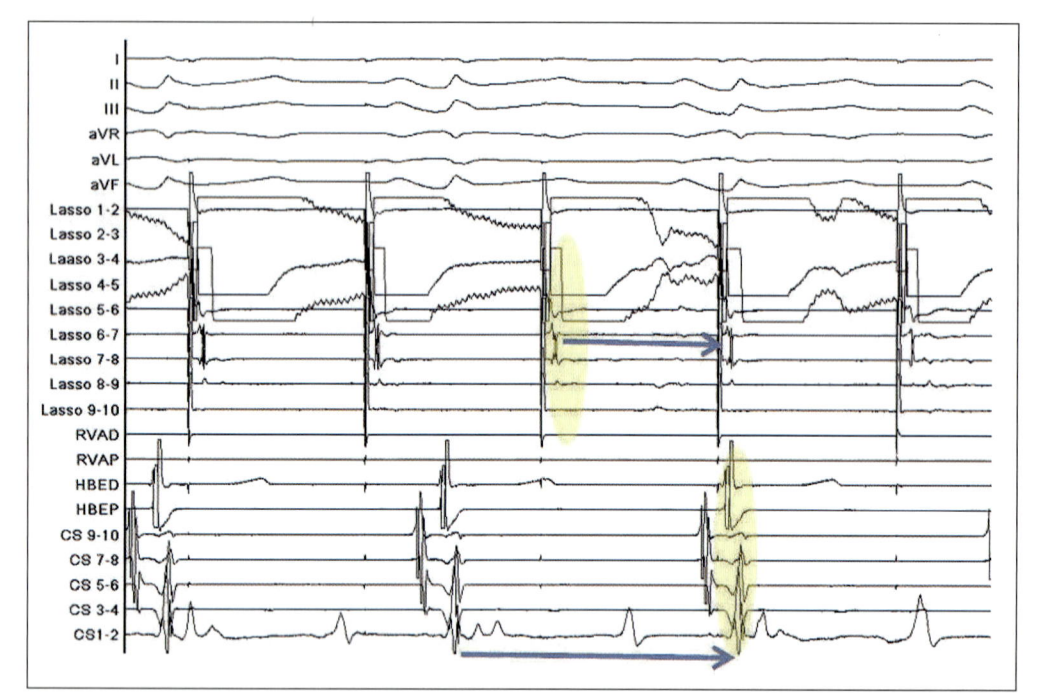

Figure 22.11 Pacing of posterior wall captures wall but does not accelerate CS. (Photo courtesy of Mark La Meir, University Hospital Maastrich.)

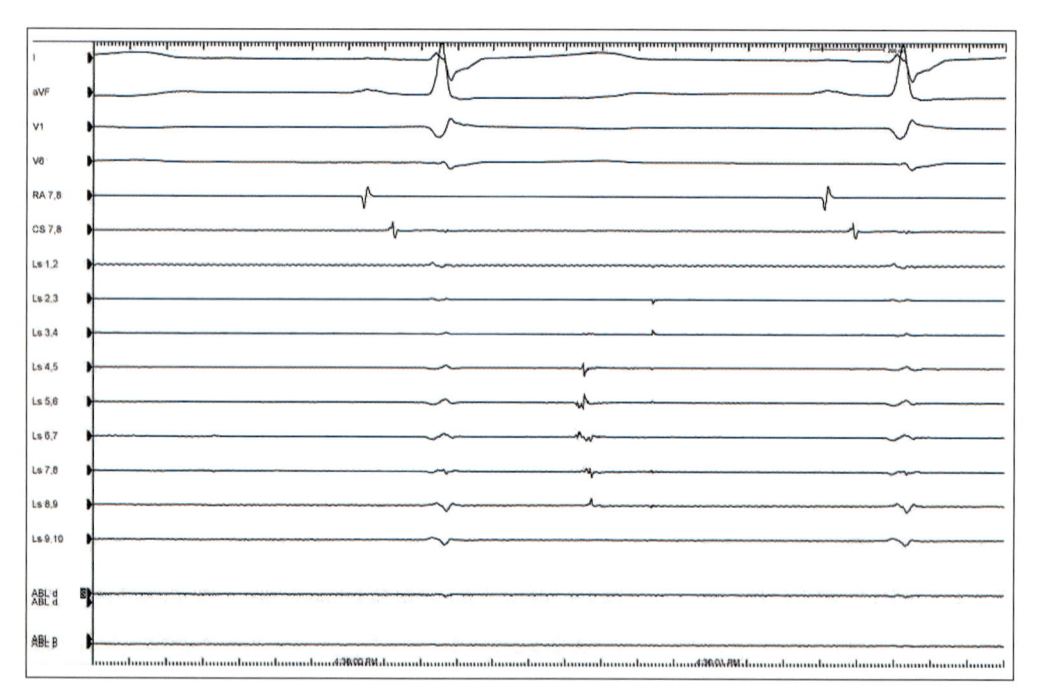

Figure 22.12 Isolated signal on posterior wall.

on the area near the mitral valve since the surgeon does not ablate here (because of the circumflex). Patients generally also require CS ablation in order to achieve block in both the CS and LA. On the mitral line, we typically use 40 W but sometimes use 50 W to achieve block. Inside the CS, we start with 15 W and titrate to 30 W with 17 cm³/min of irrigation, using ICE to stay on the atrial side of the CS. Our goal is demonstration of bidirectional block in the CS and in the LA (**Figure 22.14**).

Induction of Atrial Flutter

We then attempt to induce AFL or AF using isoproterenol. We begin with 5 mcg/kg/min and increase every 2 minutes by 5 mcg/kg/min increments to 20 mcg/kg/min as blood pressure tolerates. If we induce AFL (defined as a stable activation sequence with a less than 15% variation in CL), we map and attempt to ablate the flutter. If AF is induced, we recheck PV, SVC, and posterior wall isolation,

Figure 22.13 No block and block in LA and CS after surgical mitral isthmus line. (Photo courtesy of Mark La Meir, University Hospital Maastrich.)

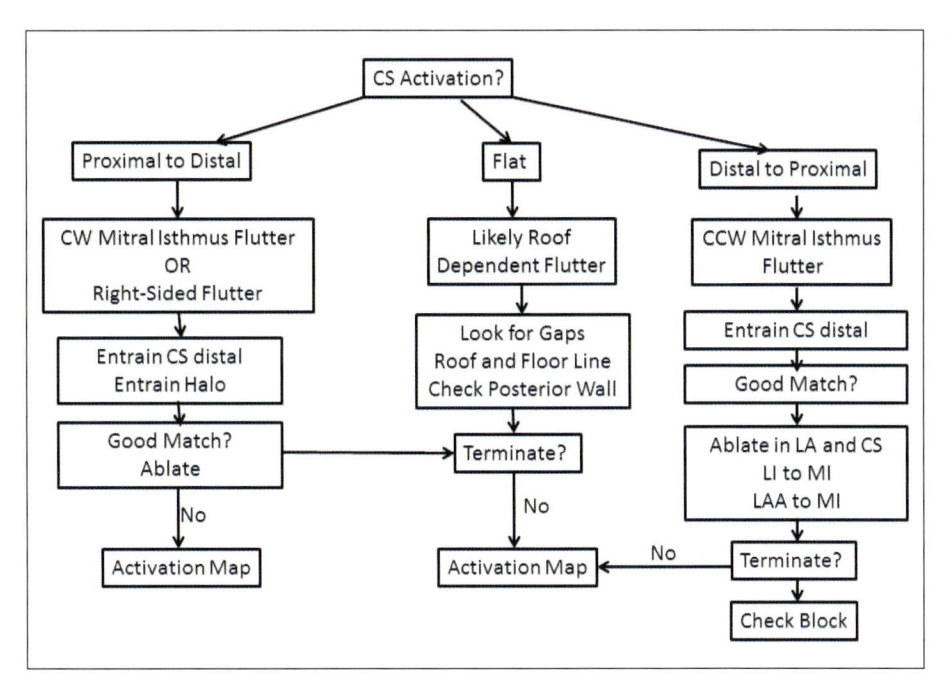

Figure 22.14 Algorithm for tracking flutter.

and then cardioversion. We do not pace the atrium to induce.

Tracking Flutters

Typically we do not use 3D activation mapping to track flutters. Instead we use a Halo and CS decapolar catheter to guide ablation as described by the Bordeaux group. The key to this strategy is that there are 3 common flutters, each with typical patterns (**Figure 22.15**): CTI flutter, mitral isthmus flutter, and roof flutter.

If the flutter occurs in CS distal to proximal, then it must be mitral isthmus flutter. We entrain from CS, and if PPI = TCL, we perform ablation along the LI-MI line and

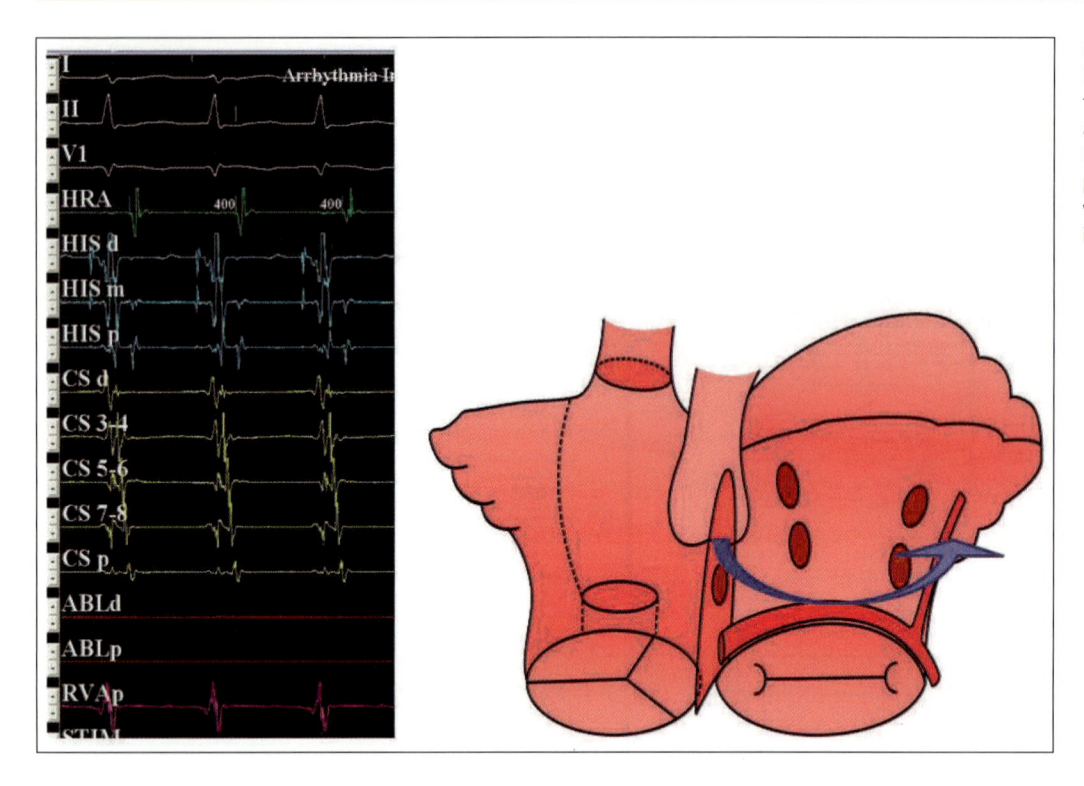

Figure 22.15 Example of clockwise flutter on mitral isthmus after surgical ablation. Note CS distal to proximal activation, which is typically mitral isthmus flutter.

in the CS. If the flutter is in CS proximal to distal, then we entrain from CS distal. If entrainment is good here and poor in RA, we presume it is a mitral isthmus counterclockwise flutter and perform ablation along this line. If CS activation is flat, then we presume a roof flutter and look for gaps on the roof line, usually near the LSPV. We only create an activation map if these techniques fail to resolve the flutter. **Figure 22.16** shows examples of flutters after surgery.

Ablation Technique

Using an irrigated-tip catheter, we begin with 15 to 30 W of power and titrate to a maximum of 40 W, with a maximum temperature of 42°C. Occasionally, a higher wattage is needed, especially at the junction of the LSPV and roof and on the line from MI to LI. Our approach is to deliver energy in a continuous manner, maneuvering the ablation catheter to different sites every 20 seconds or until the electrical signals is reduced by 75%. Contact can be seen with ICE **(Figure 22.17)** supplemented with 3D imaging. Our primary imaging modality is ICE.

In areas near the esophagus, we typically do not deliver energy at all and instead either move our catheter to a location away from the esophagus or have the surgeon separate the LA from the esophagus by lifting the atria slightly. Generally, we have not had issues with esophageal heating since we rarely need to ablate on the posterior wall. This is because the veins are usually isolated already and the roof line made during the LAMP procedure is more anterior (at the transverse sinus) than traditional catheter-based roof lines. The only time we have needed to ablate near the esophagus is on a floor-line touch-up.

Complex Fractionated Atrial Electrograms

Although there is evidence that ablation of complex fractionated electrograms may improve procedure success rates, we have not typically performed CFAE in every patient. CFAE ablation can add to procedural time, which can be potentially significant in an already long procedure. The ongoing FDA-approved DEEP-AF trial encourages the use of CFAEs if patients are still in AF after all other lesions are completed.

End of EP Procedure

We first load patients with amiodarone 300 mg IV over 10 minutes. Heparin is reversed with protamine until ACT is below 180 seconds. At this point, all catheters except ICE are removed; the LAA is typically excluded as guided by ICE (**Figure 22.18**).

Postprocedure Care

Recovery

Following ablation, the guiding sheaths are pulled out of the LA and heparin is stopped. Protamine can be given to help reverse the heparin, and access sheaths can be pulled once the ACT is less than 180 seconds. Unfractionated

Chapter 22: Hybrid Surgical Epicardial & Catheter Endocardial Ablation for AF • 199

Figure 22.16 ICE image showing ablation contact with wall.

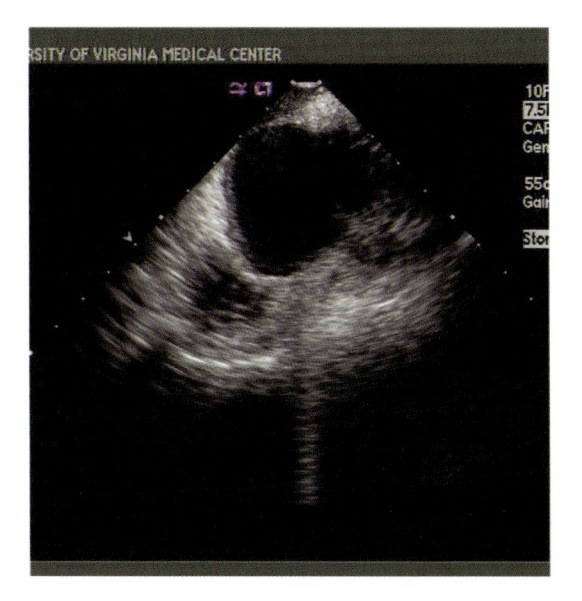

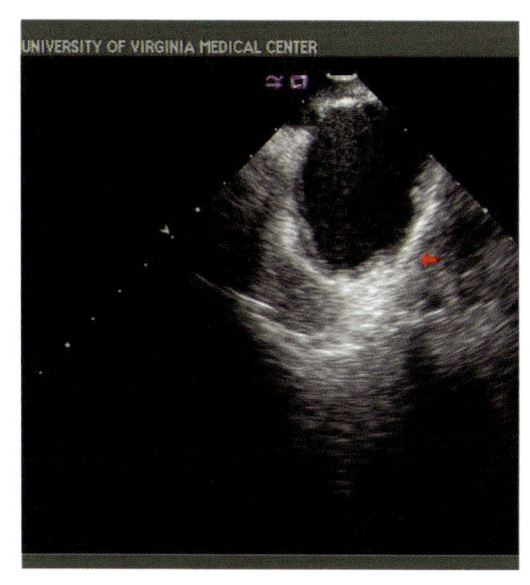

Figure 22.17 ICE image showing LAA before and after stapling.

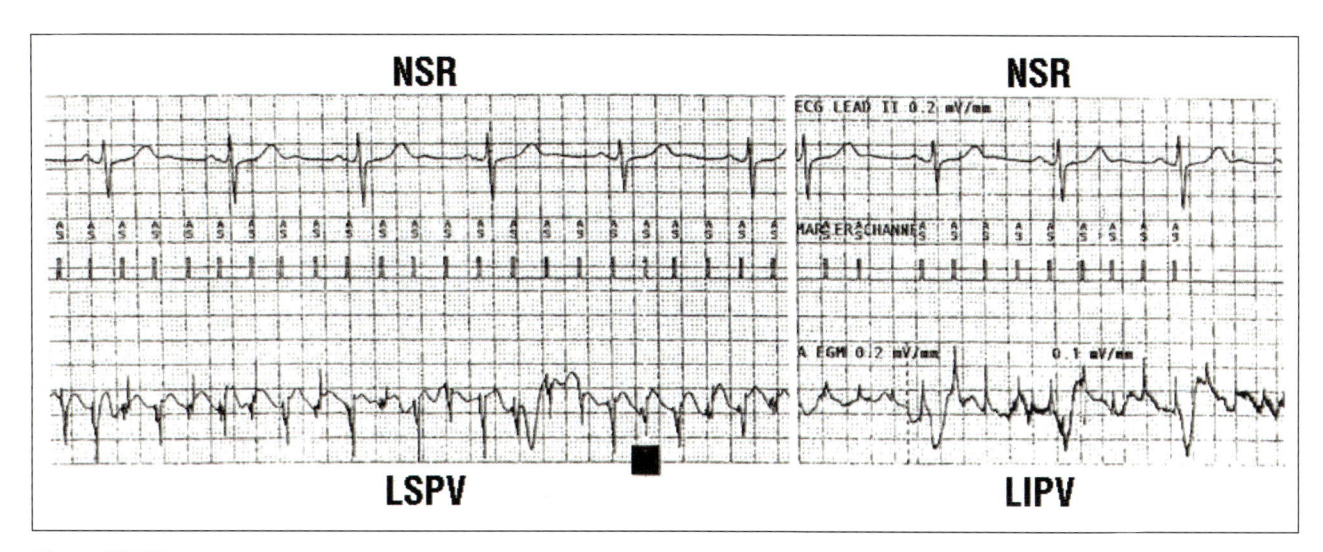

Figure 22.18 Exit block after antral isolation.

heparin is given approximately 18 to 24 hours after the procedure, and warfarin is started on postoperative day 1. Patients are discharged with INR > 2.

Patients are typically given 1000 mg of amiodarone during the 24 hours after the procedure and then given 1200 mg/day orally for 3 days, 400 mg/day until day 30, and then given 200 mg/day until day 90. In patients intolerant to amiodarone, we load dofetilide as appropriate for renal function.

Follow-Up

Patients are followed closely for the year following a hybrid ablation procedure. We typically ask our patients to be seen in an EP clinic at 1, 3, 6, 9, 12, 18, and 24 months afterward and annually thereafter. At each visit, we require at least a 24-hour monitor (either at our center or the referring center) and prefer a 7-day monitor.

Anticoagulation and Antiarrhythmic Drugs

Patients are left on antiarrhythmic drugs for 90 days, and then they are stopped. If AF recurs, we restart an antiarrhythmic drug. All patients, regardless of stroke risk, are anticoagulated with warfarin for the first 3 months. Patients with a CHA_2DS_2VAS score of 1 or less are taken off warfarin and switched to aspirin at day 90.

Procedural Complications

The complications of a hybrid ablation include all the potential complications of surgical ablation plus all the potential complications of catheter ablation. The most dramatic surgical complication is cardiac perforation requiring sternotomy, occurring in approximately 3% of procedures. This typically occurs while removing appendage or dissecting adhesions around the atrium that likely form after prior catheter ablation. Other surgical complications include phrenic nerve injury, wound infection, and lung injury due to deflation and reinflation.

Catheter complications include stroke or TIA related to LA ablation, cardiac perforation, vascular injury, heart block, PV stenosis, and esophageal injury. Overall, we feel that the complications from the catheter portion of the LAMP procedure is less than from a full catheter ablation of persistent AF because our LA times and ablation times are shorter.

Alternatives

Sequential Procedure (Surgery on Day # 0, Catheter Day #4)

Initially, starting in August 2007, we performed the surgical epicardial ablation on one day, followed approximately 4 days later by an endocardial catheter ablation as clinically indicated, especially in patients with flutter. The advantages of this included simpler logistics, since we did not need to coordinate the surgical and EP staff. In addition, by waiting 4 days, we felt we were giving more time for PV reconnection and to watch for clinical flutters. However, the requirement for 2 separate procedures can be less attractive to patients who desire a single procedure with a high success rate. Thus, in October 2009 we switched to the hybrid procedure (LAMP). Another approach that has been proposed is to perform a surgical procedure on day 0 and then bring patients back at day 90 only if they have recurrence. In this case, no line from the mitral to left inferior should be performed, since it frequently has gaps. This approach should be used carefully in patients with typical flutter, since no CTI line can be performed on day 0. It has the disadvantage of a 40% failure rate, which is not desirable in some patients.

Subxiphoid Approach

Although the VATS procedure is well tolerated by most patients, we have some concern that single-lung ventilation is poorly tolerated by some patients. Kiser reported AF-freedom in 80% of 65 patients at 1 year with a subxiphoid-delivered epicardial ablation device (Visatrax, NContact Surgical, Morrisville, NC) combined with an irrigated-tip catheter (Biosense Webster). A disadvantage of this approach is that there is no anterior ablation epicardially, because the Visatrax cannot go anterior from the subxiphoid approach. Thus, the catheter portion may be longer. In addition, the LAA cannot be removed from a subxiphoid approach using current tools. This may not only be important for stroke risk but also Di Biase et al.[6] have reported than the LAA is major trigger for AF. Tools that can perform a complete box lesion and remove the LAA from a minimally invasive or nonsurgical subxiphoid access point are being contemplated.

Initial Data

Initial data from US and European centers suggest that hybrid ablation with LAA removal is associated with at 84% success rate at one year. Comparisons to matched controls undergoing catheter ablation suggest that sequential ablation has higher success rates but may be associated with higher complication rates and longer hospital stays.[7,8]

Location of Gaps in Surgical Lesions

In our experience, the most common location of gaps are at the roof next to the LSPV. All patients have a gap at mitral valve to left IPV line with surgical lesions alone, since the surgeon cannot ablate close to the coronary artery.[9]

Conclusions

Persistent AF is a growing problem. Current drug therapy, catheter ablation techniques, and surgery therapies have suboptimal results. By combining the advantages of surgical and catheter ablations in a hybrid procedure, the LAMP procedure may increase AF-free rates. However, coordination is required between the surgical and EP teams in patient selection, preprocedure planning, during the procedure, and during follow-up. Overall, the surgical team's goal is to isolate veins, begin to isolate the posterior wall, begin lines, and remove the LAA. The EP teams goal is ensure isolation, touch up lines to ensure bidirectional block, and create a CTI line. Future experience will help improve this novel procedure.

Acknowledgments

We thank Drs. La Meir and Pison of University Hospital Maastrich for their assistance with figures and in the development of this procedure.

References

1. Crawford T, Oral H. Current status and outcomes of catheter ablation for atrial fibrillation. *Heart Rhythm.* 2009;6: S12–S27.
2. Haisaguerre M, Sanders P, Hocini M, et al. Catheter ablation of long-lasting persistent atrial fibrillation: critical structures for termination. *J Cardiovasc Electrophysiol.* 2005;16:1125–1137.
3. Schuessler RB, Lee AM, Melby SJ, et al. Animal studies of epicardial atrial ablation. *Heart Rhythm.* 2009;6:S41–S45.
4. Han FT, Kasirajan V, Kowalski M, et al. Results of a minimally invasive surgical pulmonary vein isolation and ganglionic plexi ablation for atrial fibrillation: single-center experience with 12-month follow-up. *Circ Arrhythm Electrophysiol.* 2009;2:370–377.
5. Chan D, Van Hare G, Makall J, Carlson M, Waldo A. Importance of atrial flutter isthmus in postoperative intra-atrial rentrant tachycardia. *Circulation.* 2000;102: 1283–1289.
6. Di Biase L, Burkhardt JD, Mohanty P, et al. Left atrial appendage: an underrecognized trigger site of atrial fibrillation. *Circulation.* 2010;122:109–118.
7. Mahapatra S, LaPar D, Kamath S, et al. Initial experience of sequential surgical epicardial-catheter endocardial ablation for persistent and long-standing persistent atrial fibrillation with long-term follow-up. *Ann Thorac Surg.* 2011;91: 1890–1898.
8. Mahapatra S, La Meir M, Pison L, Ailawadi G. One year follow-up of hybrid surgical-catheter ablation for AF at two centers. *Heart Rhythm* (Poster). 2011:PO4-79.
9. Mahapatra S, La Meir M, Pison L, Ailawadi G. Location of endocardial gaps after minimally invasive surgical AF ablation. *Heart Rhythm* (Poster). 2011:PO4-80.

Video Descriptions

Video 22.1 Right dissection.

Video 22.2 Ganglia.

Video 22.3 Right clamp.

Video 22.4 Roof line.

Video 22.5 Floor line.

Video 22.6 Left veins.

Video 22.7 Clip of LAA.

Video 22.8 EP portion.

CHAPTER 23

HOW TO ABLATE THE VEIN OF MARSHALL

SEONGWOOK HAN, MD, PHD; PENG-SHENG CHEN, MD; CHUN HWANG, MD

Introduction

The ligament of Marshall (LOM) is an epicardial vestigial fold that contains the oblique vein of Marshall (VOM), autonomic nerves, and myocardial sleeve, ie, the Marshall bundle (MB),[1] that serves as a terminal portion of the inferior interatrial pathway.[2] The left lateral ridge, an endocardial structure located in between the LAA and left PVs, is known to be important to AF ablation.[3] The LOM is located in the epicardial aspect of the left lateral ridge. The MB can develop automatic rhythm during isoproterenol infusion,[4] can serve as a source of paroxysmal AF,[5,6] and is known to activate rapidly during sustained AF.[7] A worldwide survey in 2005 showed that 22.8% of the clinical EP laboratories target LOM in their AF ablation sessions.[8] The LOM is a frequent source of paroxysmal AF in a young man with a history compatible with adrenergic AF,[9] ie, AF induced by exercise or a high catecholaminergic state. In the EP laboratory, a high dose (10 to 20 mcg/min) of isoproterenol is used to trigger AF in these patients. Ectopic beats from the MB often show biphasic or negative P waves in surface ECG lead II. The intracardiac recordings from the mid-CS may show double potentials. If the earliest activation of ectopic beats or AF is in the mid- or distal CS, and double potentials are present at those sites, the MB mapping should be considered. In addition, if the earliest endocardial activation is located inside the left PVs but the PV potential during triggered beat precedes the LA potential by < 45 msec, the LOM mapping should be considered. Finally, if EP study after complete PV isolations shows that a left PV site-premature complex seems to have triggered AF, but no left PV trigger can be found despite careful mapping, LOM mapping may be needed to identify the focus.

The Anatomy of Ligament of Marshall

The LOM can be divided anatomically into proximal, mid, and distal portions. The proximal portion directly connects to the muscle sleeve of the CS. The mid portion of the MB connects to the LA or the left PVs. The distal portion, which is often fibrotic and shows no electrical activity, extends beyond the left PVs. There are significant variations of the morphologies of the LOM on the epicardium. The postmortem histopathological studies of the proximal and the mid portions of the MB demonstrated multiple connections with the LA.[10,11] The major connections between the MB and the LA are located in the CS juncture, LA–left PV junction, and LA in between CS and PVs with wide multiple connections. At the CS junction, the MB completely encircles the VOM and inserts directly into the CS musculature or more distally into the posterior wall of the LA. At the middle or distal portions of the LOM, the MB gradually changes into multiple muscle fibers and then disappears or inserts into the epicardium of the anterior wall of the LA and left PVs, dominantly in the LIPV. There are three distinct groups of anatomical connections between MB and LA: single connection in the juncture of the CS, double connections in CS and LA–PVs, multiple connections in between CS and PVs. Typical examples of the LOM in human hearts are shown in **Figure 23.1**.[12] In addition to MBs, immunohistochemical studies of the LOM confirmed the presence of sympathetic nerve fibers and ganglion cells.[4,11] A more recent study by Ulphani et al[13] documented that, in addition to sympathetic nerves, the LOM is abundantly innervated by the parasympathetic nerves as well. These nerve structures may be responsible for the vagal responses observed during MB ablation and may contribute to the initiation and perpetuation of AF.

Electrophysiological Characteristics of the MB

Scherlag et al[2] first characterized the electrical activities of the LOM. The investigators reported that the MB was part of the inferior interatrial pathway that connects the left and right atria. A recent study showed three different EP characteristics of the MB in humans based on anatomical connections.[13]

Single Connection

This type of connection was documented in the beginning of the MB research.[5] In patients with a single connection, the activation from the sinus node crosses to the LA via Bachmann's bundle and the inferior interatrial pathway and activates the MB from a proximal-to-distal direction. Because there is no other connection between the MB and LA, the MB is not preexcited by the sinus wavefront from the Bachmann's bundle. The EGM recording during sinus rhythm shows a typical proximal-to-distal activation sequence (**Figure 23.2A**) and the same sequence of activation occurs during AF (**Figure 23.2, B and C**). Note that these activations are relatively regular as compared with the activations within the LA. This electrical activity of the MB during AF is much slower and more organized than in the other 2 types of connections. Because the MB only connects to CS muscle sleeves, the communication between the LA and MB is indirect. It is possible that delayed conduction with the CS muscle sleeves has prevented some of the AF wavefronts from reaching the MB. Therefore, the MB activation is slow. Some of this type of patients show additional ectopic activity from the distal MB during AF. Those activities (downward arrows in **Figure 23.2, B and C**) activate the MB in a distal-to-proximal direction with slower rate than passive activation of the MB. Although MB of this type may initiate AF through ectopic activity,[5] the slow activation during persistent AF suggests that it may not be a major contributor to AF maintenance.

Double Connections

If the MB has connections with both the CS and the LA (or PVs), the wavefronts from the CS and LA (or PVs) compete for MB activation.[14] As a result, the MB EGMs might not be clearly visible. **Figure 23.3A** shows the recordings during sinus rhythm. Note that the MB EGM and the local LA EGM are very close to each other at the distal MB and most of the MB EGMs are indistinguishable from the local LA EGM in sinus rhythm. However, by the premature complex from the LSPV (dashed arrow, **Figure 23.3B**), multiple MB potentials are revealed. The activation in the MB is distal to proximal, consistent with

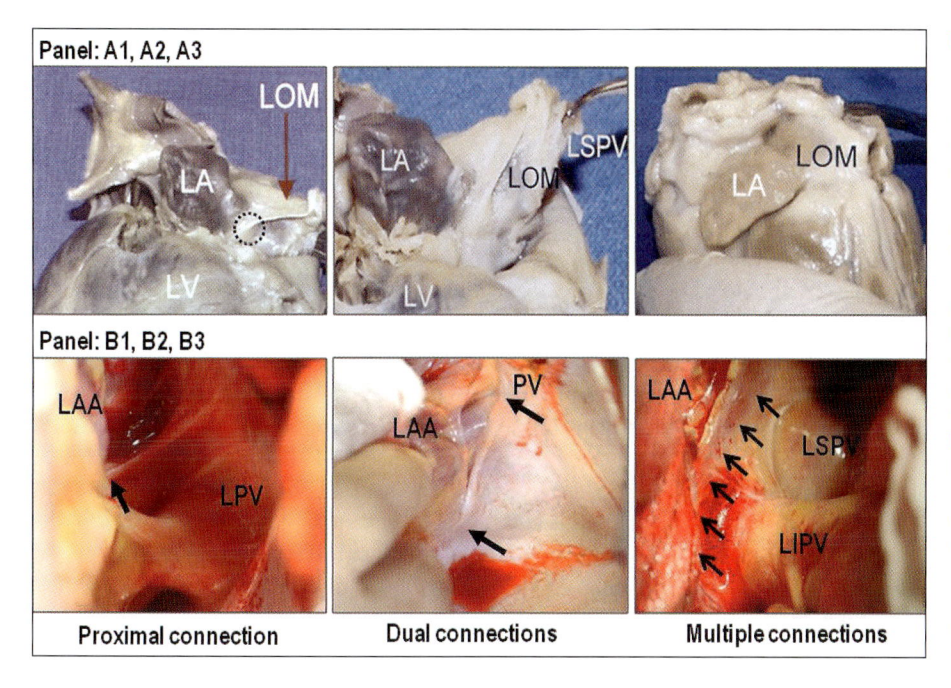

Figure 23.1 Variations of LOM anatomy. **A.** Pictures from autopsy specimens. **B.** Pictures taken during surgery. A black circle in **A1** indicates the proximal connection of the LOM to the CS. **A2.** A different view of the same heart. The distal end of the LOM inserts into the LSPV. **A3.** A second heart in which LOM was completely attached to the epicardium. A discrete ligament was not identified. **B1.** Proximal connection (arrow) between the LOM and the CS. **B2.** Both the proximal and distal connections of the LOM (2 arrows) in a second heart. **B3.** A third heart, which seems to have multiple muscle fibers (arrows) connecting the LOM and the LA. LIPV = left inferior pulmonary vein; LSPV = left superior pulmonary vein; LV = left ventricle; other abbreviations are as in the text. (Used with permission from reference 12.)

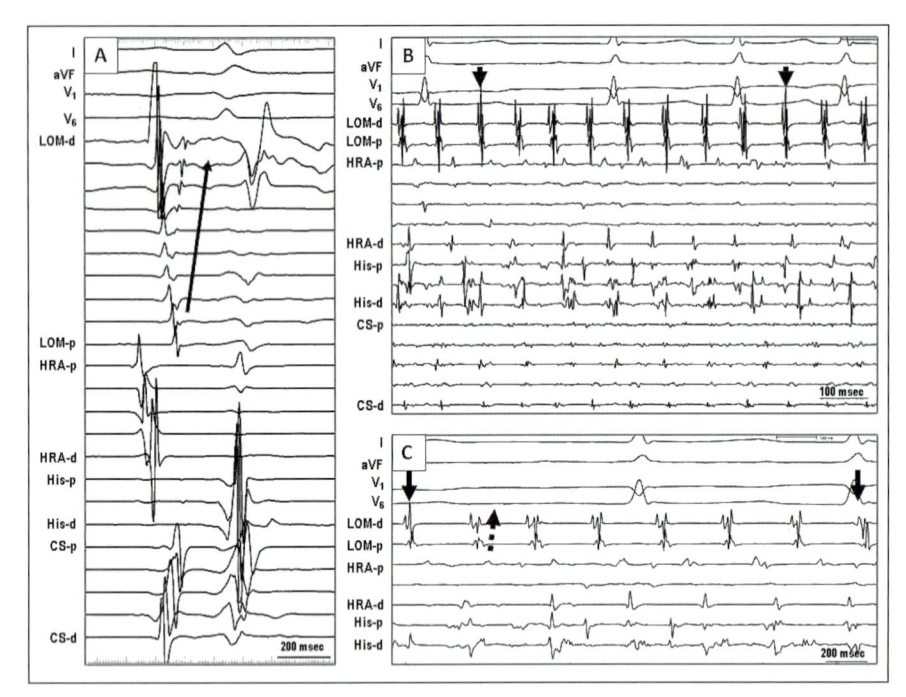

Figure 23.2 EGM characteristics of single MB-CS connection. **A.** Sinus rhythm. The second potentials in LOM channel, which were recorded by a duodecapolar catheter placed epicardially on the LOM, were MB potentials. The earliest activation site was the proximal site near the coronary sinus. The activation propagated to the distal MB (arrow). **B.** MB recordings of a single connection type during AF. The electrical activities of the MB (marked as LOM) were regular and organized without chaotic fibrillatory activities. Independent of passive activities of MB, ectopic beats (arrow) from the distal MB were observed. **C.** The MB is activated from proximal to distal (dashed arrow) during persistent AF, but the MB ectopy activated in a distal-to-proximal direction (arrow). AF = atrial fibrillation; other abbreviations are as in the text and previous figure. (Used with permission from reference 13.)

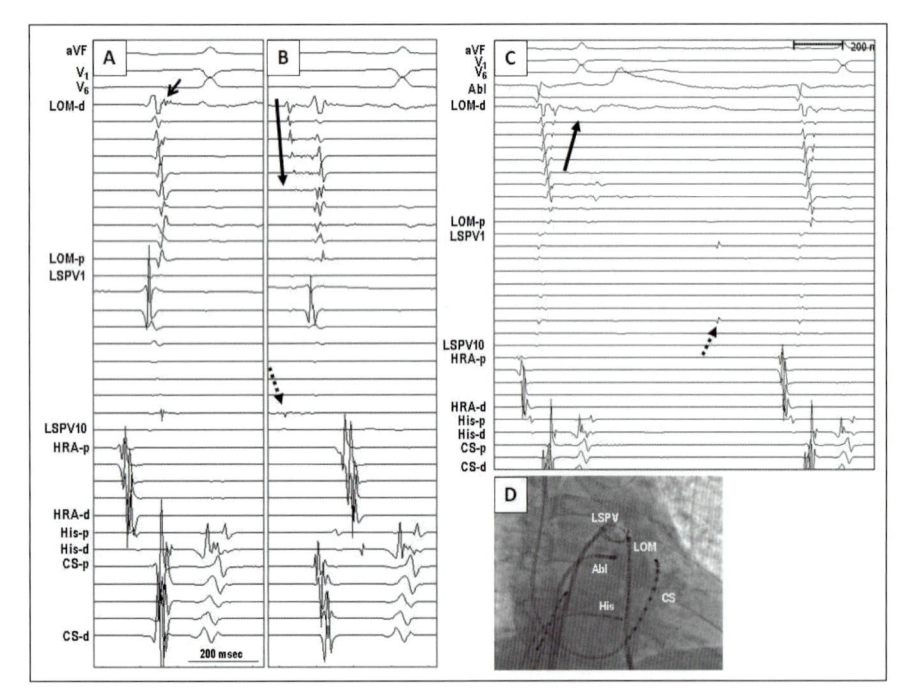

Figure 23.3 EGM characteristics of double-MB connections (to CS and to LA–PVs). **A.** Sinus rhythm. The MB EGM (arrow) and the local LA EGM were close to each other. Therefore, distinct MB potentials were not seen in most recordings. **B.** A premature beat from the LSPV (dashed arrow) propagated first into the distal MB and then activated the MB in a distal-to-proximal direction (solid arrow). **C.** A recording from a double-connection type after the ablation of the distal connection between the MB and LSPV. During sinus rhythm, the MB activation was consistent with a single-connection type (proximal-to-distal activation pattern, solid arrow). Note that there was dissociated PV potential (dashed arrow). **D.** Fluoroscopic image in the left anterior oblique projection. A circular mapping catheter was located in the LSPV, and a duodecapolar catheter was placed epicardially on the LOM. All abbreviations are in the text and previous figures. (Used with permission from reference 13.)

the existence of a distal connection within the LSPV. After successful RF catheter ablation of the distal MB–LA (PV) connection, only one connection (MB–CS) is left conducting. The MB activity should then be visible in sinus rhythm. In this situation, the propagation is proximal to distal (solid arrows, **Figure 23.3C**), simulating the activation patterns of a single connection. In this type, the MB may serve as a bypass tract that connects the CS to the left PVs without any LA involvement. This connection might provide a substrate for macroreentry. The rapid electrical interaction between the left PVs and the MB has been shown to participate in reentry during electrically induced AF in canine models.[15] An important clinical implication of this finding is that the PV–MB connection provides an epicardial conduit between PV and LA through the CS muscle sleeves. If this epicardial conduit (accessory pathway) is not eliminated, electrical stimulation within the PV would be followed by LA activation and vice versa. A clinical electrophysiologist performing AF ablation might interpret these findings as failed PV isolation. In half of the patients of this type, the MB is directly connected to the muscle sleeves of the left PVs. Direct ablation inside the PVs is needed to eliminate these distal connections and to achieve complete antral isolation. The sites of successful ablation within the PV may be either at the origin of MB ectopy or at the site of earliest activation during MB pacing.

Multiple Connections

In case of multiple MB–LA connections, the electrical activation patterns depend on the earliest MB–LA breakthrough sites and the number of MB–LA connections. In these patients, the electrical potentials from the MB are generally small due to thin muscle bundle, and they do not propagate in a uniform proximal-to-distal activation pattern as in a single connection or distal-to-proximal activation pattern during premature complex in double connections. Rather, both central and peripheral sites could serve as an independent early site, and the earliest MB activation is not at either end of the MB (**Figure 23.4, A and B**). Due to the presence of these additional connections, the interval between the local atrial EGMs and the MB may be either short or nonexistent. Therefore, distinct MB potentials are often difficult to identify during sinus rhythm. In patients with multiple connections, we might observe a premature MB activity breakthrough into the middle of the LA earlier than into either end of the LA. An example of the latter phenomenon is shown in **Figure 23.4C**, where the bold arrow points to the earliest LA activation. Due to conduction delay, there is a clear separation between MB and LA.

During AF, rapid and complex fractionated activations of the MB are noted in all patients with multiple connections (**Figure 23.5A**). After isolation of the MB, some of this type of patient shows dissociated MB potentials and MB tachycardia under isoproterenol infusion (**Figure 23.5B**). Experimental studies showed that the dominant source of AF maintenance might be the rotors that generate high-frequency spiraling waves and create spatially distributed frequency gradients.[16-18] Clinical studies demonstrated the existence of a hierarchical distribution of the rate of activation in the different regions during AF.[19,20] Ablation of the highest-frequency site was associated with slowing and termination of AF.[20] Thus, a very rapid focus producing fibrillatory conduction may be a driver of AF, and these drivers are often the targets of the catheter ablation.[21,22] Animal and human studies have shown that the MB had the highest dominant frequency during sustained AF.[7,23] The complex pattern of the electroanatomical connections between the MB and the LA can provide a substrate for reentry, leading to complex and fragmented MB activities. After isolating the MB from LA, localized MB tachycardia could be induced by sympathetic stimulation while the atria remain in sinus rhythm. These findings document that MB is capable of independent rapid activation and is not always activated passively by the neighboring AF wavefronts.

Methods of Marshall Bundle Mapping

The arrhythmia from the MB can be mapped via either epicardial or endocardial approaches.[5,7] The endocardial

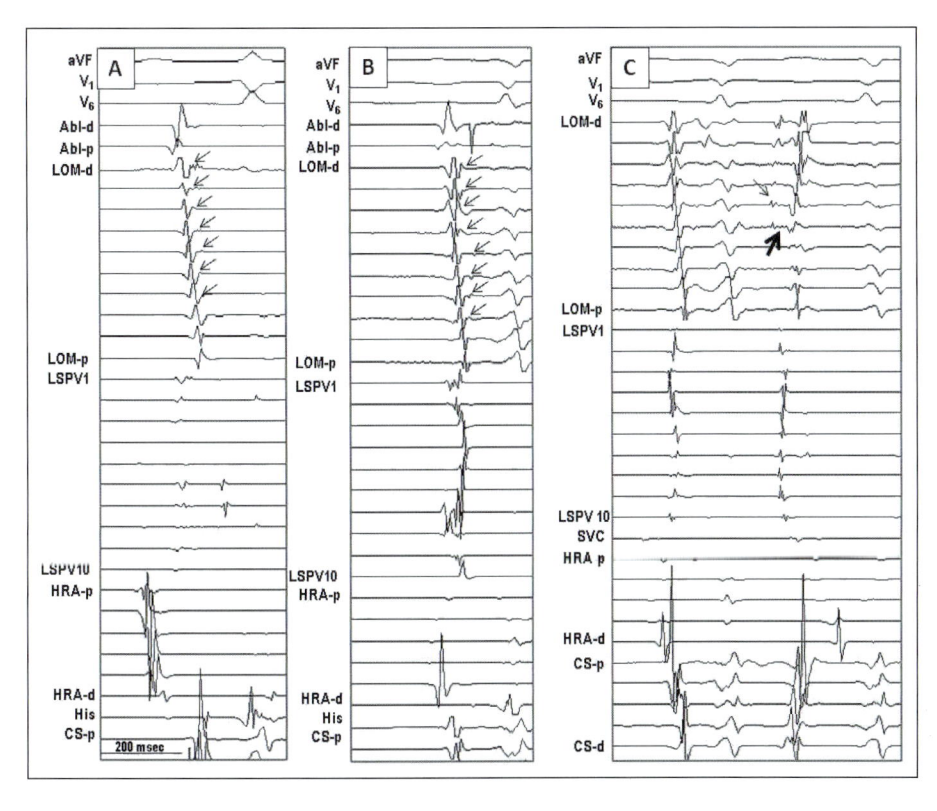

Figure 23.4 EGM characteristics of multiple connections. **A, B.** MB recordings during sinus rhythm. The earliest breakthrough was in the middle of the MB. The MB potentials were typically small (arrows), and the activation sequence of the MB was irregular and did not show either a distal or a proximal activation pattern. **C.** During premature complex from the MB (thin arrow), the earliest atrial breakthrough site (thick arrow) was not at either end but was in the middle. SVC = superior vena cava; other abbreviations as in the text. (Used with permission from reference 13.)

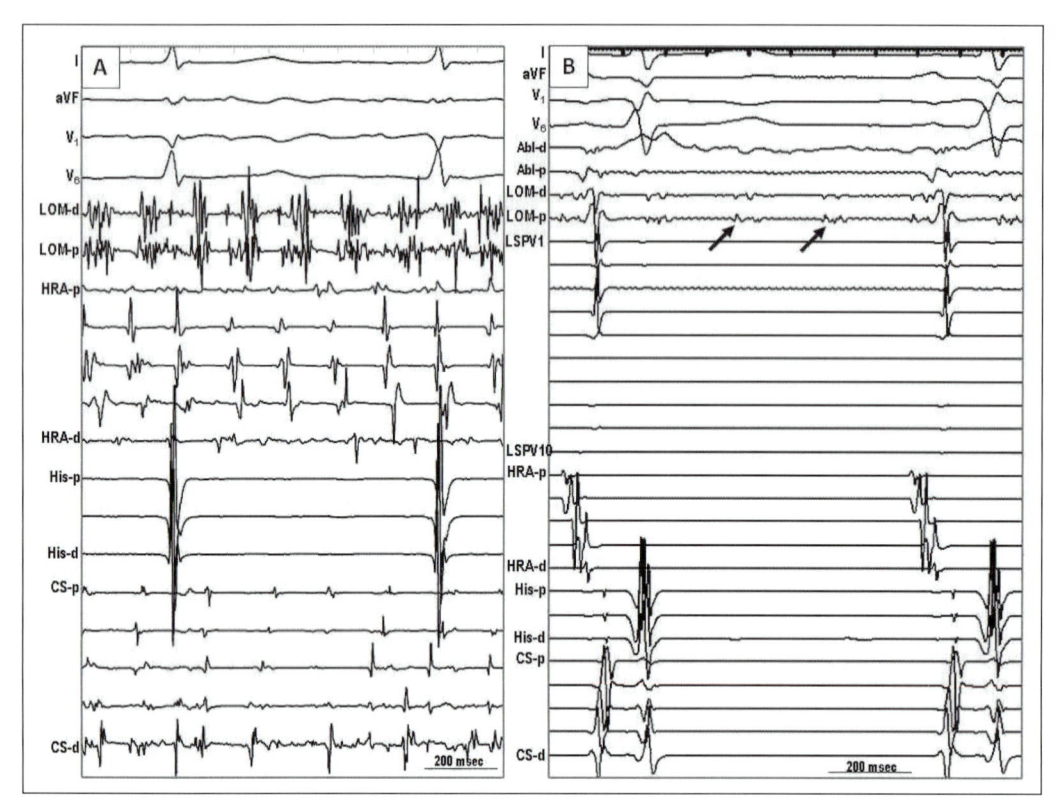

Figure 23.5 MB potentials before and after RF catheter ablation in a patient with multiple MB connections. **A.** Recording during AF. The MB activity demonstrated sustained complex fractionated activations. **B.** Recording after isolation and during infusion of 1 μg/min isoproterenol. The MB recording showed fast but organized tachycardia (arrows), which was dissociated with the rest of the LA. Abbreviations are as in the text. (Used with permission from reference 13.)

mapping was possible in approximately 45% of patients who underwent attempted VOM cannulation. It can be done by using a direct cannulation of CS with a 7-Fr luminal decapolar catheter. The right jugular vein is generally selected with an 8-Fr locking venous sheath. An occlusive CS venogram (**Figure 23.6A**) is obtained in both left and right anterior oblique view to visualize the VOM inside the CS. A 7-Fr luminal CS catheter is then engaged into the ostium of the VOM. The distal 10 mm of the CS catheter must be shaped so that the tip points upward to facilitate the engagement into the ostium of VOM. A 1.5-Fr quadripolar catheter (Cardima, Cardima Inc, Fremont, CA, USA) is inserted into the inner lumen of the CS catheter and advanced toward the VOM. Once the VOM is cannulated, the mapping catheter is advanced gradually in the direction of the left lateral ridge and the left PVs. A rare complication of this approach is the dissection of the VOM or CS. However, it does not result in major bleeding or other complications. The dissection usually resolves within 30 minutes. In patients whose VOM is not visible on CS angiogram or in whom it could not be cannulated, MB mapping can be performed by the epicardial approach, which had the advantage of free catheter movement and is not limited by the size of the VOM.[24,25] The epicardial

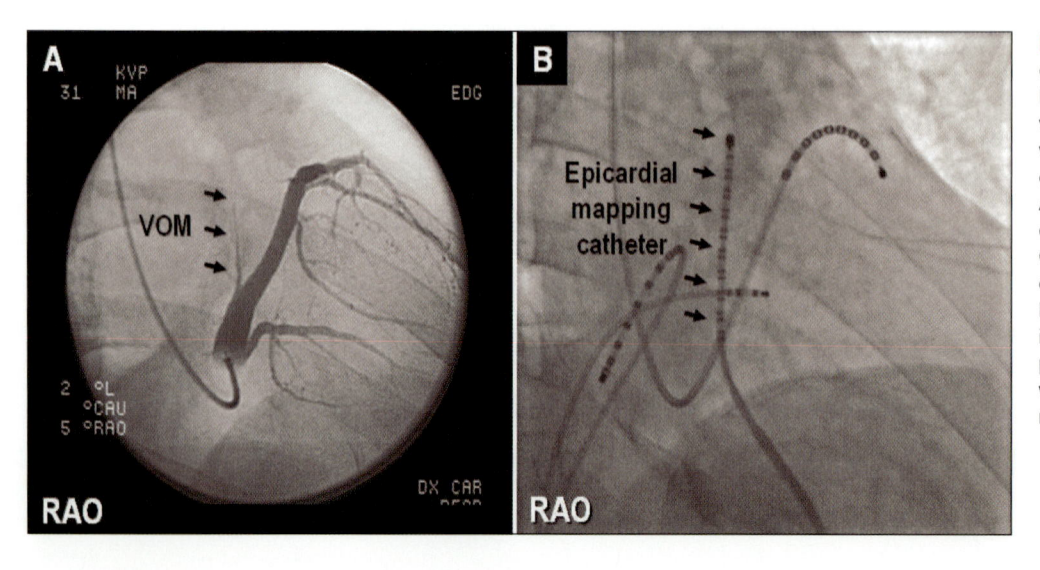

Figure 23.6 Two different approaches to MB mapping in the RAO view. **A.** Vein of Marshall is well visualized by balloon occlusion CS angiogram. A 1.5-Fr mapping catheter can be advanced via the CS into this VOM for endocardial mapping. **B.** Epicardial mapping catheter inserted via a subxiphoid pericardial puncture. (Used with permission from reference 24.)

mapping, also, can be done in patients who have already undergone AF ablation but have residual potentials inside the left PVs that are refractory to the complete antral or ostial PV isolations. The epicardial approach was performed via a subxyphoid pericardial puncture[26] followed by mapping with a deflectable duodecapolar catheter and 8-Fr SL 1 transseptal sheath (Fast-Cath guiding introducer, St. Jude Medical, Inc, St. Paul, MN) to stabilize the MB recordings (**Figure 23.6B**). The epicardial mapping catheter can be placed over the visible VOM by CS angiogram, or in cases in which the VOM was not visualized, the epicardial catheter can be located between left PVs and LAA. If VOM is not visualized, the ostium of VOM can be identified by a superior notch at the valve of Vieussens in the CS angiograms.[27] If there was a premature ectopic beat from the MB, small-amplitude potentials followed by large-amplitude (atrial) potentials could be verified as MB potentials (**Figures 23.2** and **23.3**). Otherwise, MB potentials can be verified by differential pacing from by CS, left PV, or appendage (**Figure 23.7**). The pacing from each site could separate the second small-amplitude potentials from the first large-amplitude (atrial) potentials, which allows us to verify that the second potentials are not from other parts of the LA.

Marshall Bundle Ablation

The multielectrode mapping catheter can also be used as the anatomical target to guide endocardial ablation and to confirm the successful ablation of the MB. Typically, successful ablation of the MB is associated with the elimination of MB potentials along the entire length of the ligament.[5] In addition, selective MB pacing from multiple sites within the VOM or from the epicardial mapping catheter can help determine whether there is exit block between the MB and the LA. Both of the elimination of MB EGMs and the presence of exit block during pacing are suggestive

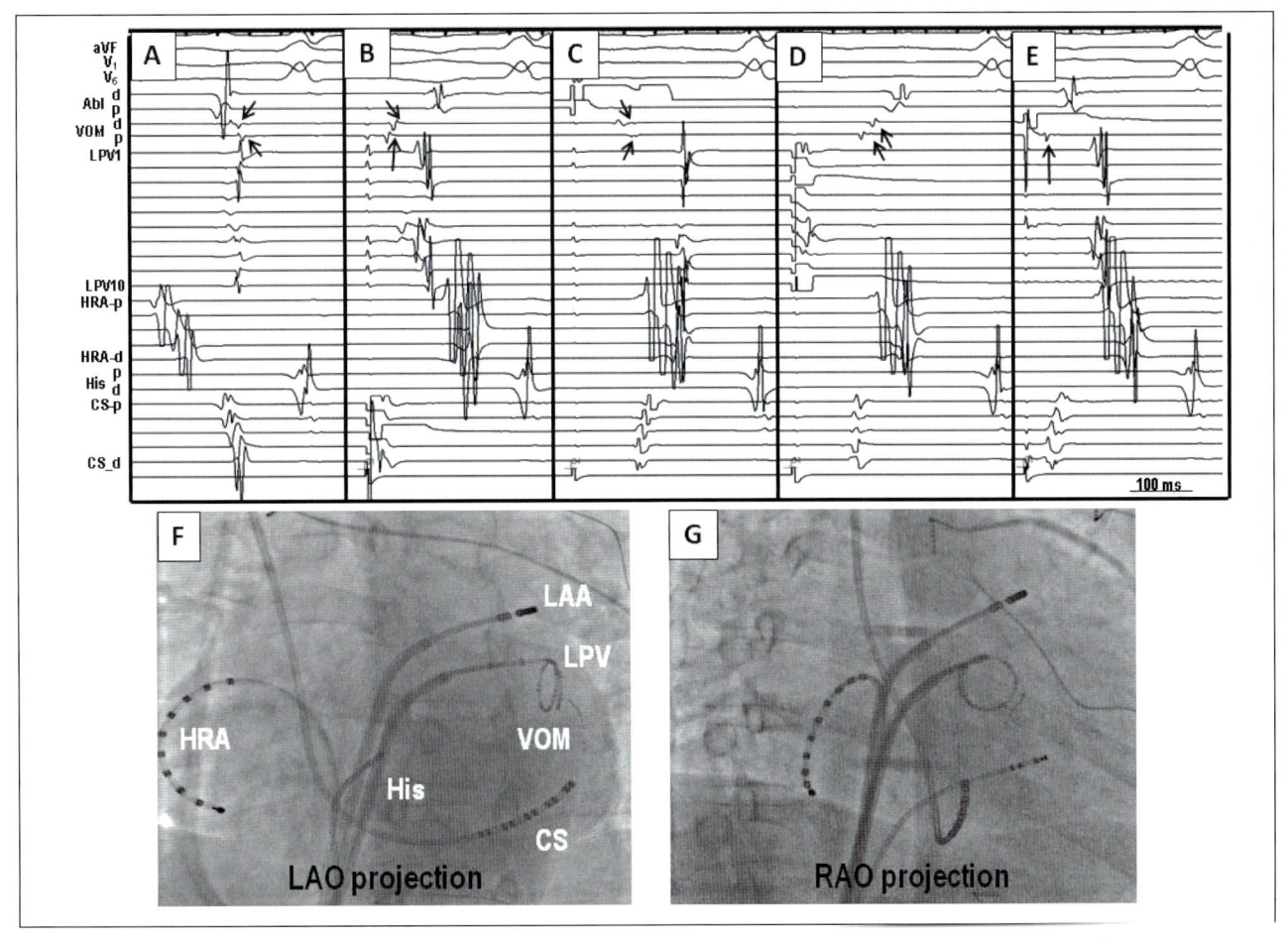

Figure 23.7 Example of differential pacing to map the MB potentials. **A.** Intracardiac recordings during sinus rhythm. **B.** Activation during CS pacing. The earliest activation was in CS, followed by proximal-to-distal propagation within the VOM. These VOM potentials *(arrows)* clearly preceded the onset of PV and HRA potentials. **C.** Pacing from distal pole of the ablation catheter located within the LAA. The potentials recorded by the VOM catheter *(arrows)* are completely separated from atrial and PV potentials. **D.** Pacing from left PV separated the VOM potentials *(arrows)* from the PV potentials. **E.** Pacing from the distal VOM showed that the proximal VOM potential *(arrow)* preceded the PV potential, indicating that these potentials are not from the PVs. **F.** and **G.** Fluoroscopic images during differential pacing. Abl = ablation; HRA = high right atrium; LAA = left atrial appendage; other abbreviations are as in the text. (Used with permission from reference 13.)

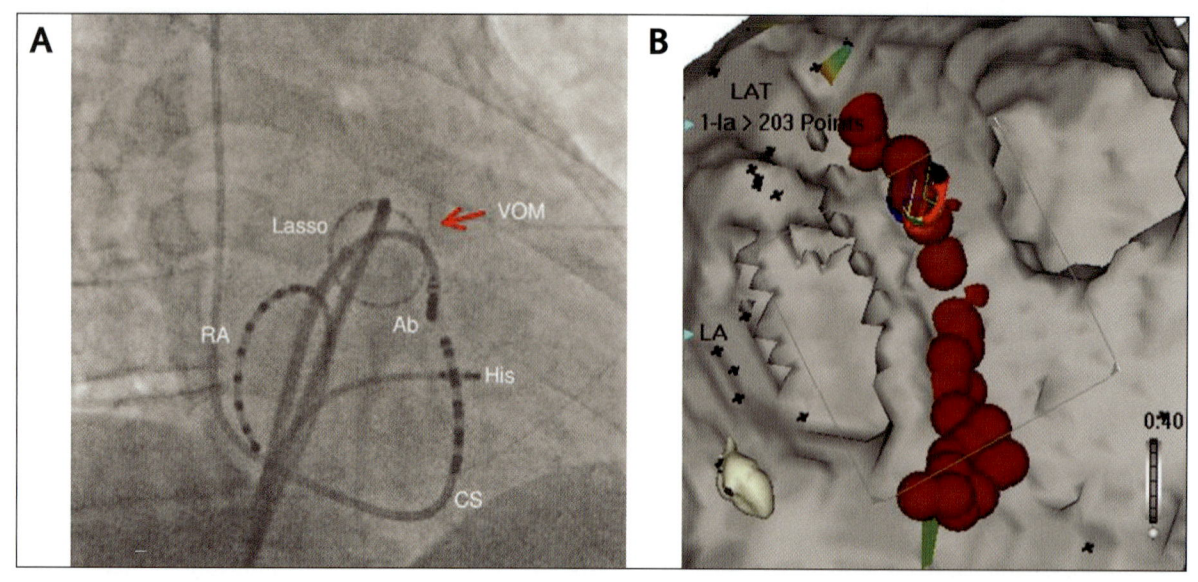

Figure 23.8 Ablation of MB connections. **A.** Catheter location. Arrow points to a 1.4 -F ablation catheter inside the VOM. RF energy application through the ablation catheter (Ab) placed in the proximal VOM may successfully ablate the CS–MB connection. **B.** A magnetic resonance imaging used in 3-dimensional mapping. Red dots on the left lateral ridge show ablation lesions. We found that 3-dimensional mapping-guided ablation of left lateral ridge is useful in ablating the connecting fibers in patients with the multiple MB-LA connections. All abbreviations are as in the text. (Used with permission from reference 12.)

of successful MB ablation. The electroanatomical mapping using the CARTO system (Biosense Webster, Diamond Bar, CA) indicates that the site having the shortest distance from LA endocardium to the MB is located at the inferior region of the left antrum, just under the left inferior pulmonary vein ostium,[24] and the mid portion of MB can be ablated from the inferoanterior aspect of the left lateral ridge under the LIPV ostium (**Figure 23.8A**). The RF energy applied with an open irrigation catheter (flow of 30 ml/min, 30 W) at that region eliminates the MB potentials in more than 90% of the patients. However, in rare cases, it is necessary to use higher power (35 W or more) over the left lateral ridges and the septoatrial bundle, near the orifice of the left pulmonary veins, and in the LAA to eliminate all MB connections (**Figure 23.8B**). The endocardial ablation can completely eliminate all MB potentials in the majority of patients. However, in < 4% of the patients, endocardial ablation alone could not eliminate all connecting fibers, as evidenced by the ability to still record ligament of Marshall potentials.[24] The epicardial approach may be needed to completely eliminate all connecting fibers in the remaining patients.

Additional Implications for Commonly Performed AF Ablation Procedures

The commonly practiced methods for persistent AF ablation include empiric all PVI or biantral ablation without trigger mapping. The biantral ablation is usually performed with linear ablation lines placed on the roof and the lateral isthmus of left atrium. A lateral isthmus ablation line is placed between the LIPV to the lateral or posterolateral mitral valve annulus. However, because of the absence of an anatomical landmark, there is no consensus on where to place the mitral isthmus ablation line. We proposed that the ablation lines can be placed with the guidance of a VOM catheter.[24] The benefits of this approach include the presence of a reliable anatomical target to guide the lateral isthmus ablation. In addition, this approach allows the operator to eliminate the proximal portion of the MB, which is connected to the CS myocardium, and to eliminate autonomic innervations around the LOM.

References

1. Marshall J. On the development of the great anterior veins in man and mammalia; including an account of certain remnants of foetal structure found in the adult, a comparative view of these great veins in the different mammalia, and an analysis of their occasional peculiarities in the human subject. *Philos Trans R Soc Lond B Biol Sci.* 1850;140:133–170.
2. Scherlag BJ, Yeh BK, Robinson MJ. Inferior interatrial pathway in the dog. *Circ Res.* 1972;31(1):18–35.
3. Cabrera JA, Ho SY, Climent V, Sanchez-Quintana D. The architecture of the left lateral atrial wall: a particular anatomic region with implications for ablation of atrial fibrillation. *Eur Heart J.* 2008;29(3):356–362.
4. Doshi RN, Wu TJ, Yashima M, et al. Relation between ligament of Marshall and adrenergic atrial tachyarrhythmia. *Circulation.* 1999;100(8):876–883.
5. Hwang C, Wu T-J, Doshi RN, Peter CT, Chen P-S. Vein of Marshall cannulation for the analysis of electrical activity in patients with focal atrial fibrillation. *Circulation.* 2000;101(13):1503–1505.

6. Katritsis D, Ioannidis JPA, Anagnostopoulos CE, et al. Identification and catheter ablation of extracardiac and intracardiac components of ligament of Marshall tissue for treatment of paroxysmal atrial fibrillation. *J Cardiovasc Electrophysiol.* 2001;12(7):750–758.
7. Kamanu S, Tan AY, Peter CT, Hwang C, Chen P-S. Vein of Marshall activity during sustained atrial fibrillation. *J Cardiovasc Electrophysiol.* 2006;17(8):839-846.
8. Cappato R, Calkins H, Chen SA, et al. Worldwide survey on the methods, efficacy, and safety of catheter ablation for human atrial fibrillation. *Circulation.* Mar 8 2005;111(9): 1100-1105.
9. Coumel P. Autonomic influences in atrial tachyarrhythmias. *J Cardiovasc Electrophysiol.* 1996;7(10):999–1007.
10. Kim DT, Lai AC, Hwang C, et al. The ligament of Marshall: a structural analysis in human hearts with implications for atrial arrhythmias. *J Am Coll Cardiol.* 2000;36(4): 1324–1327.
11. Makino M, Inoue S, Matsuyama TA, et al. Diverse myocardial extension and autonomic innervation on ligament of Marshall in humans. *J Cardiovasc Electrophysiol.* 2006;17(6):594–599.
12. Hwang C, Chen P-S. Ligament of Marshall: why it is important for atrial fibrillation ablation. *Heart Rhythm.* 2009;6(12, Supplement 1):S35–S40.
13. Han S, Joung B, Scanavacca M, Sosa E, Chen PS, Hwang C. Electrophysiological characteristics of the Marshall bundle in humans. *Heart Rhythm.* 2010;7(6):786-793.
14. Omichi CCC, Lee MH, Chang CM, Lai A, Chen PS. Demonstration of electrical and anatomic connections between marshall bundles and left atrium in dogs: implications on the generation of p waves on surface electrocardiogram. *J Cardiovasc Electrophysiol.* 2002;13(12): 1283–1291.
15. Tan AY, Chou C-C, Zhou S, et al. Electrical connections between left superior pulmonary vein, left atrium, and ligament of Marshall: implications for mechanisms of atrial fibrillation. *Am J Physiol Heart Circ Physiol.* 2006;290(1): H312–H322.
16. Jalife J, Berenfeld O, Mansour M. Mother rotors and fibrillatory conduction: a mechanism of atrial fibrillation. *Cardiovasc Res.* 2002;54(2):204–216.
17. Mandapati R, Skanes A, Chen J, Berenfeld O, Jalife J. Stable microreentrant sources as a mechanism of atrial fibrillation in the isolated sheep heart. *Circulation.* 2000;101(2): 194–199.
18. Skanes AC, Mandapati R, Berenfeld O, Davidenko JM, Jalife J. Spatiotemporal periodicity during atrial fibrillation in the isolated sheep heart. *Circulation.* 1998;98(12): 1236–1248.
19. Sahadevan J, Ryu K, Peltz L, et al. Epicardial mapping of chronic atrial fibrillation in patients: preliminary observations. *Circulation.* 2004;110(21):3293–3299.
20. Sanders P, Berenfeld O, Hocini M, et al. Spectral analysis identifies sites of high-frequency activity maintaining atrial fibrillation in humans. *Circulation.* 2005;112(6): 789–797.
21. Oral H, Chugh A, Good E, et al. A tailored approach to catheter ablation of paroxysmal atrial fibrillation. *Circulation.* 2006;113(15):1824–1831.
22. Waldo AL. Mechanisms of atrial fibrillation. *J Cardiovasc Electrophysiol.* 2003;14(12 Suppl):S267–S274.
23. Wu TJ, Ong JJ, Chang CM, et al. Pulmonary veins and ligament of Marshall as sources of rapid activations in a canine model of sustained atrial fibrillation. *Circulation.* 2001;103(8):1157–1163.
24. Hwang C, Fishbein MC, Chen PS. How and when to ablate the ligament of Marshall. *Heart Rhythm.* 2006;3(12):1505–1507.
25. Pak HN, Hwang C, Lim HE, Kim JS, Kim YH. Hybrid epicardial and endocardial ablation of persistent or permanent atrial fibrillation: a new approach for difficult cases. *J Cardiovasc Electrophysiol.* 2007;18(9):917–923.
26. Sosa E, Scanavacca M, d'Avila A, Oliveira F, Ramires JAF. Nonsurgical transthoracic epicardial catheter ablation to treat recurrent ventricular tachycardia occurring late after myocardial infarction. *J Am Coll Cardiol.* 2000;35(6): 1442–1449.
27. Chou CC, Kim DT, Fishbein MC, Chen PS. Marshall bundle and the valve of Vieussens. *J Cardiovasc Electrophysiol.* 2003;14(11):1254–1254.

CHAPTER 24

Diagnosis and Ablation of Atrial Tachycardias Arising in the Context of Atrial Fibrillation Ablation

Amir S. Jadidi, MD; Ashok J. Shah, MD; Mélèze Hocini, MD; Michel Haïssaguerre, MD; Pierre Jaïs, MD

Introduction

RF ablation of AF was developed in 1997. The discovery of the PVs as the main driving sources of paroxysmal AF[1] led to the global development of current ablation strategies that aim the electrical isolation of the PVs at their antral portion (proximal PV-LA junction).[2] Ablation strategies depend on clinical types of AF, but especially in persistent and long-standing persistent AF, the volume of atrial tissue ablated to treat AF is high (including PVI, ablation of rapid fractionated atrial sites, and linear lesions in both LA and RA). Paroxysmal AF can be treated by catheter ablation with a limited amount of atrial tissue destruction, because electrical isolation of PVs is sufficient for curing this type of AF.[2] Persistent and long-standing persistent (patients remaining for more than one year in AF) forms of AF may necessitate more extensive ablation to restore sinus rhythm.[3-7] These include, in addition to PVI, EGM-guided ablation at sites with continuous EGM fractionation/activity during AF until local "regularization" of EGMs has been achieved. Additional linear lesions at the LA roof (between LSPV and RSPV) and at the lateral mitral isthmus (linear ablation between LIPV or LSPV and the mitral annulus) may be necessary to restore sinus rhythm in patients with persisting AF.

The incidence of ATs occurring after PVI is low in young patients with paroxysmal AF. ATs occur frequently in the presence of structural heart disease and also when extensive ablation is undertaken. Therefore, their global incidence varies from 5% to 75% in patients undergoing AF ablation. In persistent AF, and more so in the long-standing persistent AF, atrial tachycardias are almost always observed during AF ablation as an intermediate rhythm prior to the restoration of sinus rhythm.

Incidence of Atrial Tachycardia after AF Ablation

Presence of structural heart disease, the LA size, the baseline AF CL, the type of AF (longer-lasting AF episodes), the type of AF-ablation procedure, and its endpoint impact the incidence of AT. Incidence of AT after PVI has been variably reported from 2.9% to 10%.[10-14] As the number and extent of ablative lesions are higher in the circumferential PVI technique, it may lead to a higher incidence of AT than segmental PVI.[12,13] In patients undergoing circumferential PVI and linear ablation, incidence of AT has been reported to be as high as >10% to 30%.[15-18] Though < 20% of patients develop AT after isolated ablation of complex fractionated signals, the incidence rises to 40% to 57% in patients wherein EGM-based atrial ablation accompanies PVI and linear ablation.[3,7,19] In a multicenter study on the effectiveness of ablation of complex fractionated signals without PVI and linear ablation in persistent AF, up to 40% patients were found to develop intraprocedural AT (unpublished European data from Bad Krozingen, Munich, and Bordeaux).

Classification of Atrial Tachycardia

AFL/AT are classified by the working group into the clinically relevant macroreentrant and focal categories.[20] Macroreentrant ATs are due to large reentrant circuits (> 3 cm diameter), but the EP mechanism of focal AT could be automaticity, triggered activity, or localized reentry.[22] Importantly, in the era of AF ablation, the majority of focal ATs seem to be due to localized reentry with the circuit comprising < 2 cm in diameter (see also **Figure 24.1**).[22] Among all forms of ATs, 46 to 70% represent the macroreentrant ATs and 30 to 53% represent the focal forms. Among the focal ATs, 26 to 50% are due to discrete focal source and 50 to 74% represent the localized reentrant variety.[21,22]

Mechanisms of Atrial Tachycardia

To simplify and facilitate the diagnostic approach, we consider atrial tachycardia as being due either to a macroreentrant circuit or a focal source. The latter forms are characterized by centrifugal atrial activation and are due to localized reentrant circuit (diameter < 2 cm) in most of the cases; however, a true focal origin may also be the underlying origin.

Drug Therapy

Usually, AF ablation is undertaken in patients who fail to respond to drug therapy. Patients with AF recurrence may show improved responsiveness to antiarrhythmic drug therapy after AF ablation. But ATs are less responsive to drugs than AF. In addition, ventricular rate is usually faster during AT than during AF, reducing the patient's level of arrhythmia tolerance. Hence, the risk of developing congestive heart failure due to tachymyopathy is higher under AT than AF. Both recurrence of AF or AT may be transient and limited to the blanking period, but in our experience, they tend to recur in most of the patients over a period of several months postblanking. As a consequence, our strategy is to ablate these ATs if they persist or recur after the first month following AF ablation. ATs are always targeted for ablation when they occur during an AF ablation procedure.

ATs Occurring During AF Ablation

Using the stepwise approach toward the ablation of longstanding AF, PVI is followed by EGM-based ablation of continuous activity/complex fractionated EGMs and sites with activation gradient. The final step involves linear lesions at the LA roof and at the left mitral isthmus. If AF is converted to sinus rhythm, no further lesion is delivered. If the intermediate rhythm is AT, it is mapped and ablated. Additional lesions, if required, are applied and complete isolation of the PVs and bidirectional block across prior linear lesions are ensured. Most of the time, AF ablation is associated with a progressive increase in AF CL until about 200 ms, when AF gets converted into AT. Thus, AT is often observed as a transitional rhythm from AF to sinus rhythm.[19] Such intraprocedural AT is suggestive of hidden organization in the disorganized-appearing AF. When AF organizes into slow, sustained AT, it is a sign of impending restoration of sinus rhythm, which can be achieved following accurate diagnosis and ablation of the critical isthmus/source maintaining the AT. In other words, the AT could be due to a mechanism that was present and active during AF and participated in the maintenance of the latter. Spectral analysis of AF CL in animals and humans has shown a relationship between the AF dominant frequency and the CL of the subsequently occurring AT.[23,24]

AT Occurring After AF Ablation

After AF ablation, a variable degree of inflammatory state exists in the atria. The tissue takes about 6 to 12 weeks to organize and form a fibrous scar at the sites of ablation. After AF ablation, this period is usually observed as a blanking period, marked by transient but recurrent and possibly nonclinical atrial arrhythmias. As inflammation heals, inhomogeneous areas of nonuniform scar interspersed with healthy and/or partially damaged atrial tissue remain.[25] Thus, the atrium gets transformed into an electrophysiologically heterogeneous chamber with unevenly distributed scar tissue. Areas of low voltage and slow conduction properties coexist as gaps amid the nonconducting scar tissue, generating a substrate highly favorable for reentrant arrhythmias. The likelihood of gaps (slowly conducting, incompletely scarred tissue) increases with increase in the extent of ablation. Arrhythmias observed beyond the blanking period may be attributed to a proarrhythmic effect of ablation. Alternatively, they may also be the consequence of the arrhythmia revealed by AF ablation (see above).[22]

Locations of Atrial Tachycardia Circuits

In paroxysmal AF, PVI is enough to treat AF in the vast majority of patients. Very few ATs are observed in this context. They consist of the localized reentry circuits at the PV ostia associated with the formation of gap in the previous PVI lesion. In the era of circumferential PVI involving higher volume of ablated tissue, few patients also develop roof-dependent and/or perimitral circuits.

In persistent AF, wherein more extensive ablation is required to terminate AF, all types of AT may be observed. Notably, patients with AT after previous linear ablations (roof and mitral isthmus lines) for AF/AT show most frequently macroreentrant circuits involving the LA. Perimitral flutters are the most common, followed by roof-dependent ATs. CTI-dependent AT is another likely macroreentrant RA tachycardia, although it is the least common type. These are the only macroreentrant circuits observed post–AF ablation. Importantly, the typical flutter wave morphology is not commonly observed on 12-lead ECG of CTI-dependent flutter in the context of extensive atrial ablation and spontaneous scarring. Although ablation of macroreentrant AT circuits could be challenging, it takes less than 10 minutes to rule them in or out.

Localized ATs with centrifugal activation of the atria may be due either to a localized reentrant circuit or a true focal mechanism. Localized reentry gets established in small areas most commonly at the venous ostia (PV ostia, ostium of SVC, and CS), the left septum, the base of the LAA, the junction of the LAA and the roof, the posterior LA, and the posterolateral mitral isthmus. Such localized, small circuits give rise to centrifugal atrial activation from these sites (Figure 24.1). Most of the time, but not necessarily always, they are located at LA sites with regional slow conduction at areas of prior ablation. However, the anterior wall of the LA can host them spontaneously, and they may have participated in AF maintenance, suggesting that this arrhythmia mechanism is not exclusively created by ablation.[32,21,22] Unlike the point sources of typical focal AT, these sites involve small regions of slowly conducting tissue harboring the entire or almost the entire tachycardia circuit locally within a diameter of 2 cm (Figure 24.1).

Diagnosis

Atrial Tachycardia Diagnosis on Surface ECG

Clinically, the diagnostic and localizing value of surface ECG is debatable in atrial tachycardias arising after extensive ablation, especially when linear lesions have been applied previously. Since the magnitude and direction of

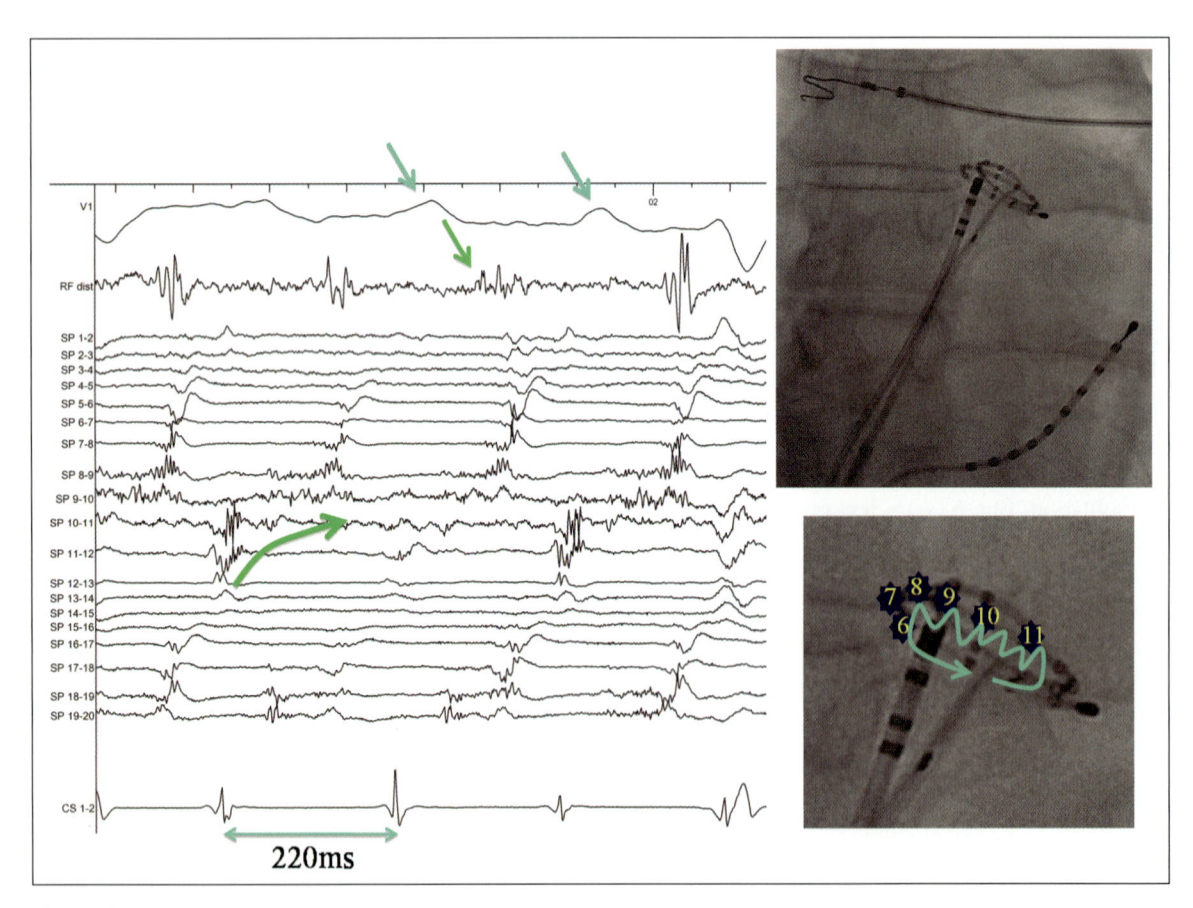

Figure 24.1 Cardiac fluoroscopy in postero-anterior view shows a multipolar spiral-like catheter (AFocus II, St. Jude Medical; 20 mm diameter) and a decapolar catheter within the CS. The spiral catheter is mapping LA roof. Within a small area of ~5 cm², electrical activity taking almost the entire CL (220 ms) of tachycardia is recorded from dipoles 11 to 12 to 6 to 7 on the spiral catheter (green curved arrows). The EGMs 11 to 7 to 8 display long, fractionated, diastolic potentials. These potentials represent the slow-conducting isthmus of the AT circuit and are targeted by the ablation catheter. Note the fractionated diastolic potentials on the RF catheter that precede the P wave on surface ECG (V₁, green straight arrows). The EGMs display low voltage with maximum amplitude of up to 0.2 mV. This is characteristic of localized reentrant forms of focal atrial tachycardia. Instead of a point source, a small area harbors a tiny circuit that sustains > 70% of the CL of reentrant tachycardia. The remainder of the atrium is activated centrifugally, which is consistent with focal tachycardia.

vector of atrial activation are tremendously influenced by the differential conduction velocity and voltage of extensively ablated or remodeled atria, surface P waves do not provide consistent information on the mechanism of AT and the location of focal ATs. Therefore, regular ECG clues cannot be applied effectively to patients subjected to extensive ablation of the atria.

However, when the AT occurs after lone (segmental or wide circumferential) PVI (without previous linear ablation of the LA), the 12-lead ECG can provide more guidance into the mechanism of AT. Under these circumstances, the presence of an isoelectric interval > 90 to 100 ms occurring simultaneously on all of the 12 ECG leads is a diagnostic marker of a localized reentry circuit.[28] This probably applies to all centrifugal arrhythmias.

The 12-lead ECG has also been used to predict perimitral circuits, but again, this has been validated in the context of lone PVI[30] and doesn't apply, in our experience, to more extensive AF ablation procedures.

Atrial Tachycardia Diagnosis in the EP Laboratory

In the EP laboratory, it is important to diagnose the mechanism underlying AT to achieve clinical success. As a preliminary step, it is important to acquire the information on previously ablated sites and determine if clear endpoint (bidirectional block at previous linear lesions) had been achieved.

If the patient is in sinus rhythm at the beginning of the repeat procedure, the evaluation for completeness of previously performed PVI should be the first step. If there is any evidence of PV reconnection, PVI should be completed before targeting other areas. This is important, as PVs are not just associated with AF but can also host AT, particularly in cases of incomplete isolation or reconduction. If linear ablation involving CTI, roof line, or mitral isthmus line was performed previously, bidirectional block should be reconfirmed. Reablation should be performed, wherever needed, to establish complete bidirectional block.

During ongoing tachycardia, we apply a 3-step approach **(Figure 24.2)** to diagnose the type of AT based on the classification (macroreentrant vs. focal) cited above.[22] We use a quadripolar irrigated-tip mapping/ablation catheter in the atrial chamber and a decapolar catheter in the CS and implement the diagnostic approach during ongoing AT as follows.

Step 1: Determination of Stability of AT

Using the EGMs recorded from the LAA and the CS for up to 1 minute, the mean CL and the range of variation in CL over 1 minute are assessed. If the variation is > 15% of the mean CL, focal mechanism is the most likely diagnosis. If the arrhythmia is stable (< 15% variation), the next step is to diagnose or rule out macroreentrant AT.[21]

Step 2: Determination of Left Atrial Activation Pattern and Entrainment of AT for Macroreentry

Consider that macroreentrant AT would usually represent one of the following three patterns: (1) mitral isthmus-dependent flutter (perimitral AT); (2) roof-dependent flutter; or (3) CTI-dependent flutter. Therefore, we

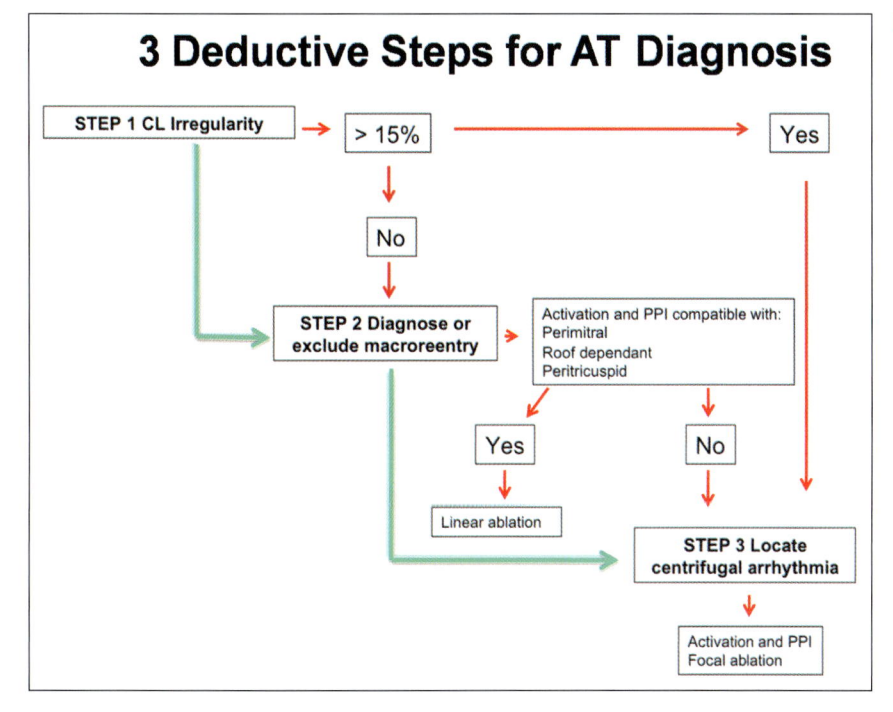

Figure 24.2 Atrial tachycardia diagnostic algorithm: A three-step approach for diagnosing atrial tachycardia during or after AF ablation. PPI = postpacing interval (measured during entrainment mapping). (Modified from Jaïs P, et al. *J Cardiovasc Electrophysiol.* 2009;20(5):480–491.)

deductively evaluate each of these possibilities based on LA and CS activation patterns.

The CS activation must be noted in particular because it is representative of the posteroinferior LA activation. A "chevron" activation (neither proximal to distal nor distal to proximal) is not in favor of a perimitral circuit. It is compatible with a roof-dependant circuit. Proximal-to-distal CS activation may be seen in both cavotricuspid and counterclockwise perimitral flutters while the distal-to-proximal CS activation favors a clockwise perimitral flutter more than a peritricuspid circuit. All 3 types of CS activation are equally observed with roof-dependent circuits.[22]

For tachycardias compatible with macroreentry, it is necessary to demonstrate opposite activation fronts in opposite segments of the circuit: a septal-to-lateral activation of the inferior LA (CS prox to dist) and lateral to septal anteriorly is compatible with a counterclockwise perimitral circuit. The reverse would work for a clockwise perimitral circuit (**Figure 24.3**).

To diagnose a roof-dependent flutter, the same concept applies to the analyses of the anterior and posterior segments of the LA. If the anterior and posterior walls activate high to low and low to high, respectively (or vice versa), roof-dependent AT rotating counterclockwise (or clockwise) around the antrum of right PVs is the most likely possibility. From a therapeutic standpoint, we do not need to categorize roof-dependent circuit as right or left, as the linear roof ablation will treat both of them uniformly (**Figure 24.4**).

The RA activation front in typical counterclockwise CTI-dependent flutter would be low to high on the right septum and high to low on the lateral RA. The LA is activated from the septum to the lateral wall and the CS activation occurs in the proximal-to-distal direction in the vast majority.

Entrainment of AT is very useful to demonstrate that the circuit depicted by the activation mapping is truly the one responsible for the arrhythmia. It is crucial to note that good return cycle in 2 opposite segments qualifies for macroreentry and excludes other possible mechanisms. In other words, a good return cycle from both the septum and the lateral LA implies a perimitral circuit. On the contrary, if the return cycle is good only in the lateral LA (PPI < 30 ms) and longer in the septum (usually > 50 ms), a centrifugal arrhythmia from the lateral LA cannot be excluded.

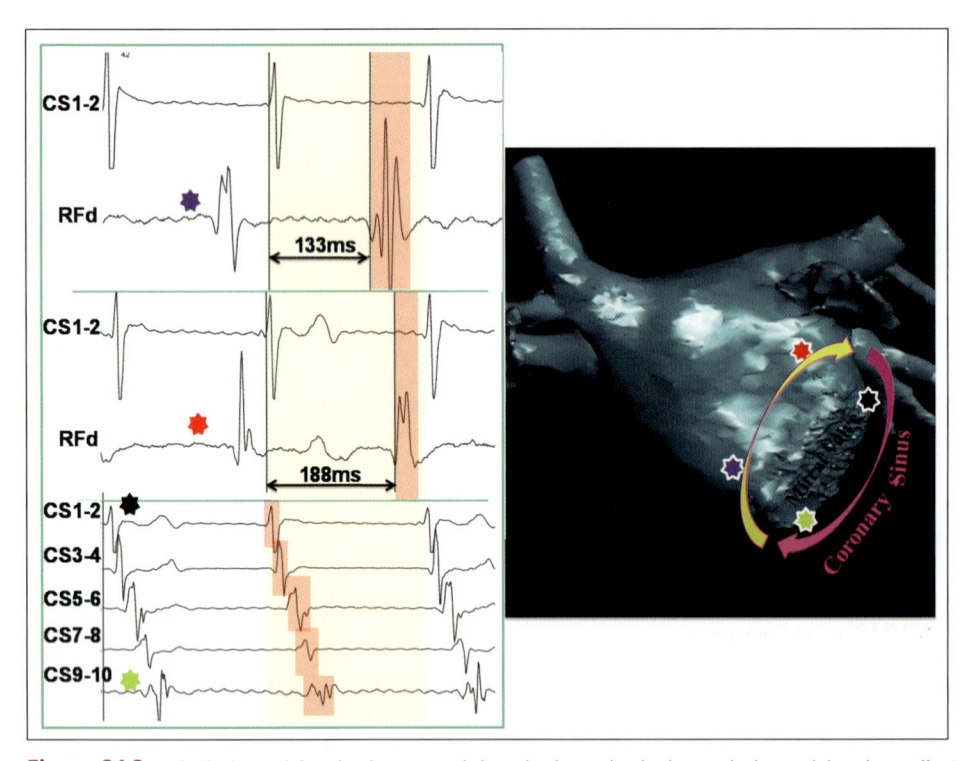

Figure 24.3 Clockwise atrial activation around the mitral annulus is shown during atrial tachycardia. Lateral- (black marker) to-septal (green marker) atrial activation pattern on decapolar CS catheter is shown. Electrical activity recorded on mapping catheter (RF) in reference to distal CS dipole 1 to 2 is demonstrated from two different sites (red and blue markers). Mapping catheter positioned at anterolateral mitral annulus (red marker) is activated 188 ms after distal CS. Mapping catheter positioned at anteroseptal mitral annulus (blue marker) is activated 133 ms after distal CS. Thus, during tachycardia, atrial activation proceeds septally from lateral in the posterior left atrium and laterally from the septal aspect of anterior LA. This pattern conforms to that of clockwise perimitral flutter. Activation pattern around the mitral annulus comprises the entire CL of this flutter. Prior to the linear ablation of mitral isthmus, the mechanism of perimitral flutter was confirmed by 2 just PPI values at opposite sites of the mitral annulus (lateral and septal side).

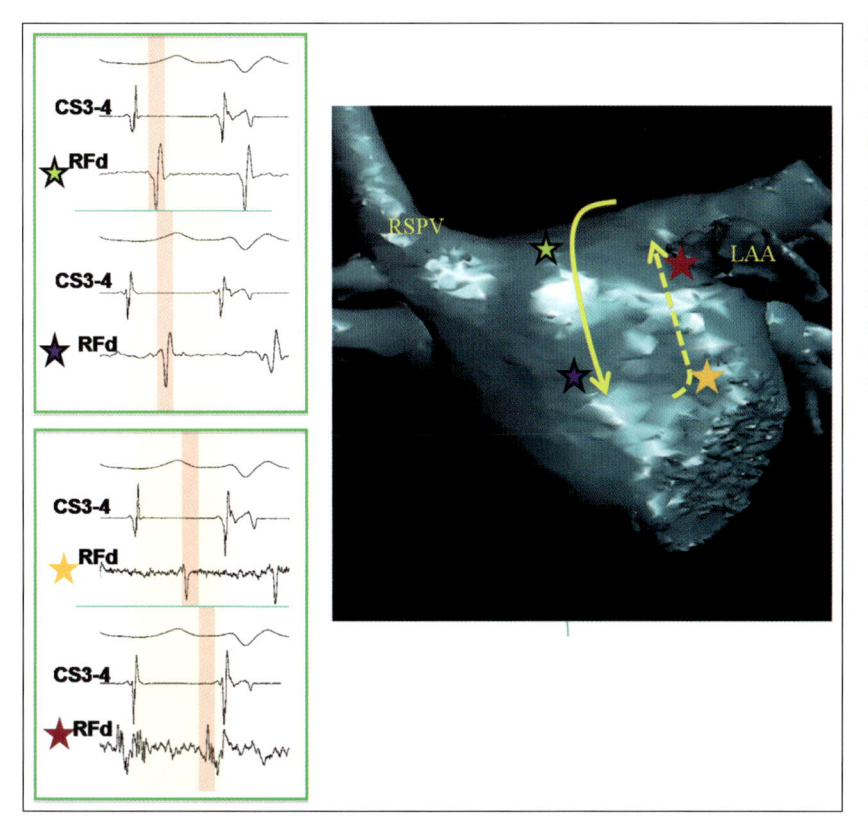

Figure 24.4 The EGM recordings from four sites (green, blue, yellow, and maroon stars) on anterior and posterior LA are timed with CS dipole (CS 3-4) as reference. Local EGMs recorded from the high (green star) and low (blue star) anterior sites are 168 ms and 214 ms, respectively, from the reference suggestive of high-to-low anterior LA activation pattern. Local EGMs recorded from high (maroon star) and low (yellow star) posterior sites are 274 ms and 262 ms, respectively, from the reference, suggestive of low-to-high posterior LA activation pattern. This pattern is consistent with roof-dependent flutter.

Step 3: Localization of Centrifugal Atrial Tachycardia: Focal and Localized Reentry

The atrial activation pattern reflects the direction of centrifugal propagation of AT from the source. In a single tachycardia cycle, the activation pattern of CS (proximal to distal or distal to proximal) and the LA activation pattern (based on local activation time of the anterior and posterior LA) that do not conform to macroreentrant mechanism provide a useful guide for mapping the source. Recording fragmented EGM spanning 50 to 75% of TCL is suggestive of localized reentry (small circuit) (Figure 24.1).

The entrainment response for centrifugal AT is characteristically distinct from macroreentry. In contrast to macroreentrant circuit, which is spread over 3 to 4 (all) atrial segments, centrifugal arrhythmia is localized to one atrial segment only. A crucial property to be understood is that the return CL increases with increasing distance from the source. In other words, the PPI continues to get shorter as the pacing site gets closer to the source. This phenomenon provides an important guide to segmental localization of the source of centrifugally spreading AT.[26] PPI < 30ms suggests that the pacing site is located near the source (**Figure 24.5**). Sometimes, it is difficult to establish capture at the site of interest even with the highest pacing output. The fractionation of the local EGM may also pose challenge to the measurement of the return CL. In such a situation, pacing from a relatively healthy area in proximity to the site of interest would yield PPI in the range of 30 ms to 50 ms, which is acceptable. If the segment of interest cannot be localized to the LA based on the AT activation pattern and entrainment criteria, RA mapping is performed similarly. Centrifugal arrhythmias are more difficult to localize when compared to macroreentrant forms, but they are much easier to ablate.

Focal AT demonstrating automatic mechanism of initiation and maintenance of tachycardia is less commonly encountered in post–AF ablation patients. High variability in atrial TCL is characteristically described for automatic tachycardia with spontaneous onset and offset and gradual warmup and decline. The centrifugal atrial activation pattern can be helpful in mapping the source of the focus. Instead of continuous low-voltage, fragmented local activity on EGMs, a sharp and high-frequency presystolic potential with high negative dV/dt monophasic (QS shaped) unipolar EGM can be obtained at the site of origin of AT. Overdrive pacing of automatic tachycardias usually demonstrates a variable response from the same site of pacing since the postoverdrive recovery time of automatic focus is highly variable.

Three-dimensional Mapping Tools

Three-dimensional electroanatomical mapping systems can be of significant help but are not indispensable for

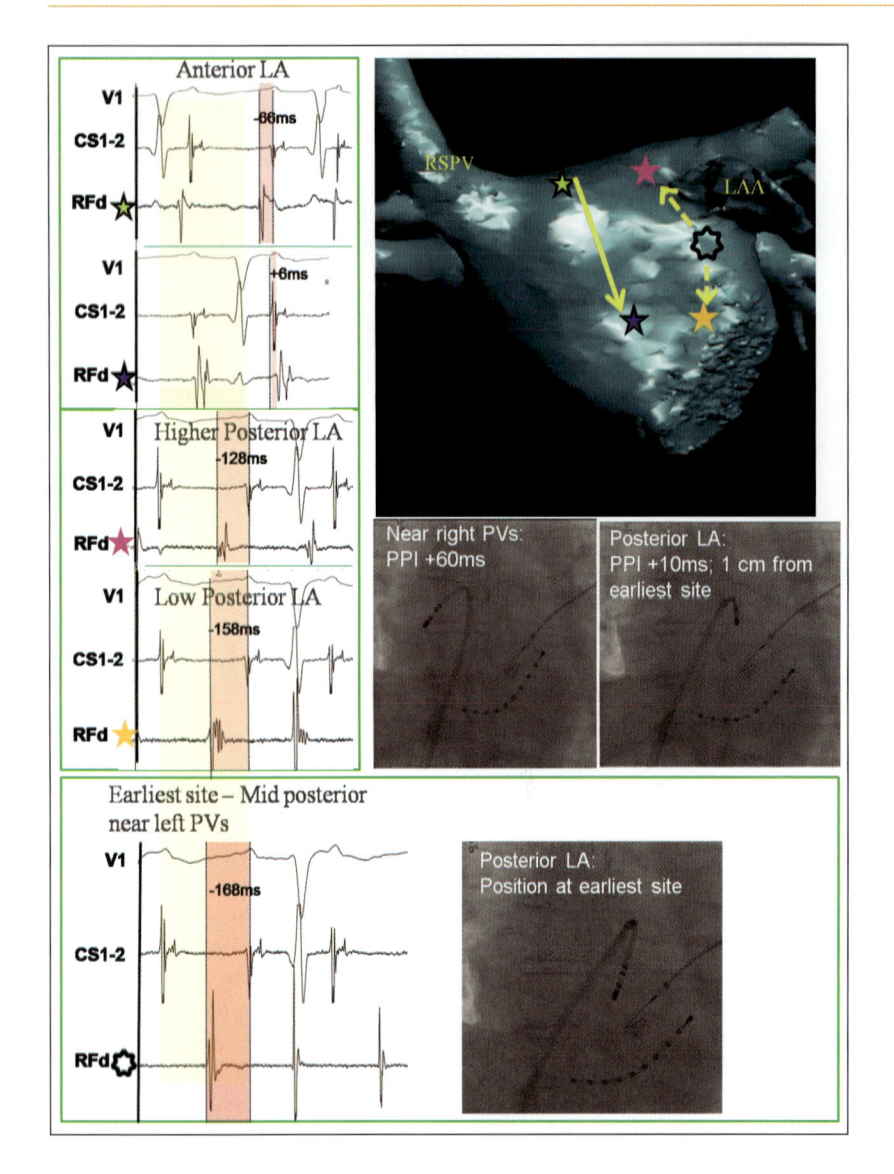

Figure 24.5 Top: The EGM recordings from four sites (green, blue, yellow, and pink stars) on anterior and posterior left atriums are timed with CS bipole (CS 1-2) as reference. Local EGMs recorded from high (green star) and low (blue star) anterior sites are −66 ms and +6 ms, respectively, from the reference, suggestive of high-to-low anterior LA activation sequence. Local EGMs recorded from the high (pink star) and low (yellow star) posterior sites are −128 ms and −158 ms from the reference. The earliest activation site during AT (−168 ms from reference CS 1-2 that preceded the surface P wave in V_1) was found next to the left PV ostia between the high and the low posterior mapping sites. This pattern is compatible with a focal tachycardia arising from a focus next to previously ablated pulmonary vein ostia. Notably, entertainment mapping showed good PPI values (PPI-TCL < 30 ms) around the mid posterior LA wall with longer values near right PVs (+60 ms) and at LA roof (+70 ms, not shown). Very long PPI values were measurable at the anterior LA wall (+200 ms, not shown). Scheme: The atrial tachycardia focus is shown in the mid posterior wall as "✡". The arrows display centrifugal activation of the atria. RF application targeting the site of earliest activation terminated this atrial tachycardia.

diagnosis and ablation of AT. Very often, more than one AT occurs sequentially before restoration of the sinus rhythm during ablation. Conversion of target tachycardia to another tachycardia will entail reconstruction of activation maps every time it happens. Moreover, areas of low-amplitude signals, which are frequently critical to the understanding of the tachycardia mechanism, may be below the system's noise level. None of the available systems automatically assign activation time to such EGMs, and manual adjustment of the local activation time is required on several adjacent points to have the system display slow conduction or localized reentrant source. This can cause disparity between clinical tachycardia and reconstructed electroanatomical map, especially for localized reentrant AT. However, especially for reentrant AT circuits, the use of 3-dimensional electroanatomical mapping systems allows the visualization of the critical AT isthmus and its spatial width. Multielectrode catheters may be used in combination with mapping systems such as the NavX System. They have the advantage of building atrial activation maps of high density within 8 to 10 minutes.[31] This can also be achieved noninvasively with body surface mapping systems such as the one developed by CardioInsight, Inc (Cleveland, OH). Nonsustained arrhythmias are amenable to this technology as long as few uncontaminated (not within the QRS or T waves) beats of arrhythmia occur during the mapping procedure. Such a technology could provide preprocedural diagnosis of the mechanism and localization of AT, but this area will require clinical validation.[29]

Catheter Ablation

Ablation of focal-source AT is accomplished more easily than its diagnosis. The reverse holds true for macroreentrant AT. Successful termination of target tachycardia is the common endpoint for both the types of AT, but the achievement of complete block is the final endpoint for macroreentry. Conversion of target tachycardia to another tachycardia with same/different CL and/or atrial activation pattern and/or surface P-wave morphology is frequently encountered before eventual restoration of sinus rhythm. Therefore, close monitoring of invasive and body-surface EGMs during tachycardia ablation is very important. Finer changes in activation pattern and CL may be the only subtle clues toward repeating diagnostic maneuvers, including the entrainment response. After significant RF delivery with no apparent effect, it is important to rediagnose the tachycardia, which may have changed even in the absence of any detectable change in CL or CS activation pattern.

Focal Atrial Tachycardia

Focal ATs are ablated at the site of origin. Using a saline irrigated-tip catheter (up to 60 ml/min) and a target temperature up to 42°C, RF energy with power of up to 30 W can be delivered for 30 to 60 seconds at each point with continuous monitoring of EGMs. Transient acceleration of tachycardia following the beginning of energy delivery may occur when ablation is localized at the right spot. If tachycardia fails to terminate or convert to another tachycardia after at least 60 seconds of energy delivery, further mapping is performed to localize a better target site for ablation.

Macroreentrant Atrial Tachycardia

Macroreentrant ATs are targeted by performing linear ablation at the site of critical isthmus. CTI ablation is performed conventionally for CTI-dependent flutters. Linear ablation of the LA roof is performed by joining the ostia of two superior PVs at the most cranial aspect of LA (in order to avoid esophageal injury, the posterior roof line is not recommended). It terminates both the types of roof-dependent flutters: the ATs around right and the left PVs that use the LA roof as a common isthmus.

Perimitral Flutter

Perimitral flutter is targeted by performing linear ablation at the posterolateral mitral isthmus. Ablation of mitral isthmus is performed by withdrawing the catheter from the ventricular side of the mitral isthmus (where the atrial to ventricular EGM ratio is 1:1 or 2:1) either to the LIPV (posterior mitral isthmus line) or to the anterior portion of the LSPV just behind the LAA (lateral mitral isthmus line). Ablation within the CS on the epicardial side of the mitral isthmus is frequently needed (60%). Power of up to 35 W endocardially (near the mitral annulus) and up to 25 W epicardially (distally within the CS) is required to achieve transmural lesion in most cases. The endpoint is the creation of a line of complete block. Confirmation of bidirectional block is undertaken following restoration of sinus rhythm. Mitral isthmus ablation can be facilitated by the use of a steerable sheath (Agilis, St. Jude Medical, St. Paul, MN).[33]

Block across the mitral isthmus linear ablation is demonstrated by differential pacing from distal and proximal CS bipoles sequentially and recording the time of activation in LAA. If LAA activation is earlier with proximal CS pacing than more distal CS pacing, it is suggestive of complete block in one direction. If subsequent pacing from the LAA shows that the activation in the CS proceeds from proximal bipole distally, it is conclusive of bidirectional block (**Figure 24.6**).

Estimation of block across the roof linear ablation is undertaken in sinus rhythm and/or LAA pacing. If the activation of posterior LA occurs low to high during sinus rhythm or pacing from the anterior LA, it suggests complete roof block. Subsequently, differential pacing of the posterior LA and recording the time of activation in LAA can be done to confirm bidirectional block. LAA activation

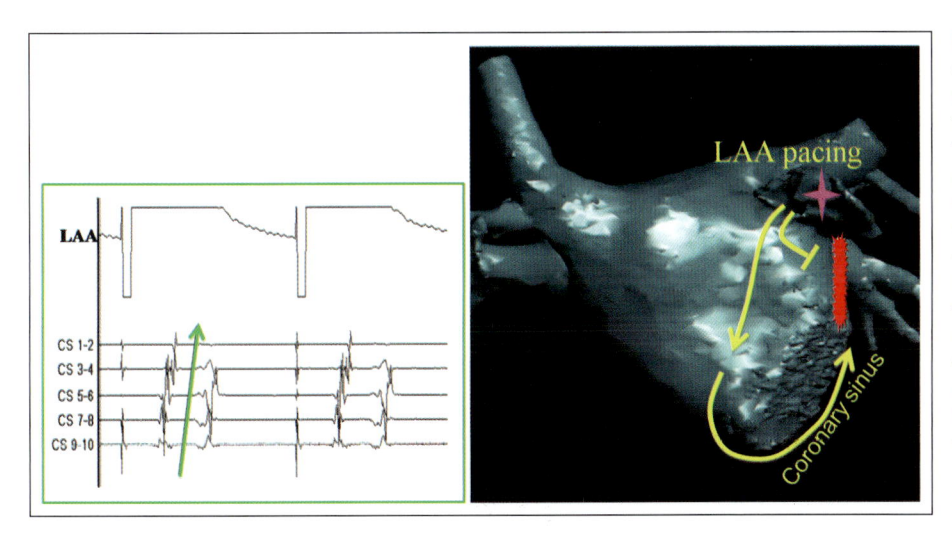

Figure 24.6 Pacing maneuver for confirmation of mitral isthmus block: LAA pacing (✚) results in proximal-to-distal activation (arrow) of CS. This is suggestive of blocked (✳) posterolateral mitral isthmus, at least unidirectionally. CS 9-10 – proximal CS, CS 1-2 – distal CS. In order to check for bidirectional mitral isthmus block, we compare activation delay to LAA when pacing posterior to the mitral isthmus line from CS 3-4 and CS 5-6. If the mitral isthmus is blocked, delay to LAA activation is longer when pacing from CS 3-4 than from CS 5-6.

with infero-posterior LA pacing should occur earlier than superoposterior LA pacing to conclude that the roof linear ablation is bidirectionally blocked. Since previous posterior LA ablation often disables local capture at supranormal pacing outputs, differential pacing from the posterior LA is not routinely undertaken in the clinical practice. Presence of widely split double potentials across the line of block reinforces the completeness of linear ablation.[7,27]

Procedural Outcome and Prognosis

Using the algorithm mentioned above, 97% of ATs were diagnosed in a mean time of < 11 minutes of mapping duration in a recently published report from our center. Incoherent mapping due to widespread areas of very low-voltage EGMs/scars and noninducibility after inadvertent termination of tachycardia caused difficulty in diagnosis. It should be noted that this limitation is much more frequent during the index AF procedure where edema obscures mapping. All the diagnosed cases were treated successfully. Complete line of block at mitral isthmus, LA roof, and CTI was achieved in 95%, 97%, and 100% of cases, respectively. At follow-up of 21 ± 10 months, recurrence of sustained AT was observed in 5%. After repeat ablation procedure, sinus rhythm was maintained in 95% of patients.[22]

Prevention of AT

Atrial tachycardia is partly an iatrogenic proarrhythmia that shows rising incidence since LA ablations are performed more widely. Since the volume of ablation drives the probability of occurrence of AT, limiting the ablation within the atrium may help reduce the incidence of certain forms of AT. Judicious use of ablative energy can help minimize the incidence of reentrant and focal AT. Macroreentrant AT develops frequently in patients with incompletely blocked previous linear ablation. Ensuring the achievement and documentation of bidirectional block after linear ablation is mandatory to prevent recurrent macroreentry. An important lesson learned from AF ablation procedures is that application of energy unscrupulously and indiscriminately is not helping cure AF. Therefore, limiting ablation to achieve isolation of PVs in paroxysmal AF and PVI plus necessary defragmentation and linear ablation with bidirectional block in persistent and long-lasting forms of AF can reduce development of AT following AF ablation. A more focused persistent AF strategy targeting precise areas hosting active sources maintaining AF would be desirable but remains to be discovered. But we also have to consider that if more ATs are observed in the context of AF ablation, it is also due to the efficacy of the procedure, which organizes AF and reveals underlying mechanisms.

Conclusion

In the era of AF ablation, there is an increase in the incidence of both macroreentrant and centrifugally spreading ATs. Extensive substrate modification generates focal areas of slow conduction and low voltage capable of sustaining localized reentry, a novel mechanism of reentrant atrial arrhythmias post–AF ablation. AT is also the final common pathway towards restoration of sinus rhythm in catheter ablation of long-lasting AF. Ascertaining bidirectional block after linear ablation and identifying key targets for successful AF termination by limited use of RF energy can help reduce the incidence of AT. Using conventional tools and EGM guidance for catheter ablation, the deductive algorithm presented here can help diagnose and cure AT.

References

1. Haïssaguerre M, Jaïs P, Shah DC, et al. Spontaneous initiation of atrial fibrillation by ectopic beats originating in the pulmonary veins. *N Engl J Med.* 1998; 339:659–666.
2. Ouyang F, Bansch D, Ernst S, et al. Complete isolation of left atrium surrounding the pulmonary veins: New insights from the double-Lasso technique in paroxysmal atrial fibrillation. *Circulation.* 2004; 110:2090–2096.
3. Nademanee K, McKenzie J, Kosar E, Schwab M, Sunsaneewitayakul B, Vasavakul T, Khunnawat C, Ngarmukos T. A new approach for catheter ablation of atrial fibrillation: mapping of the electrophysiologic substrate. *J Am Coll Cardiol.* 2004;43:2044–2053.
4. Haïssaguerre M, Sanders P, Hocini M, et al. Catheter ablation of long-lasting persistent atrial fibrillation: Critical structures for termination. *J Cardiovasc Electrophysiol.* 2005; 16:1125–1137.
5. Willems S, Klemm H, Rostock T, et al. Substrate modification combined with pulmonary vein isolation improves outcome of catheter ablation in patients with persistent atrial fibrillation: a prospective randomized comparison. *Eur Heart J.* 2006; 27:2871–2878.
6. Oral H, Chugh A, Good E, et al. Radiofrequency catheter ablation of chronic atrial fibrillation guided by complex electrograms. *Circulation.* 2007; 115:2606–2612.
7. Jaïs P, Hocini M, Hsu LF, et al. Technique and results of linear ablation at the mitral isthmus. *Circulation.* 2004; 110:2996–3002.
8. Gillinov AM. Ablation of atrial fibrillation with mitral valve surgery. *Curr Opin Cardiol.* 2005;20:107–114.
9. Mason PK, Dimarco JP. Atrial tachycardias after surgical ablations of atrial fibrillation: an incoming tide. *J Cardiovasc Electrophysiol.* 2007;18:356-357.
10. Gerstenfeld EP, Callans DJ, Dixit S, Russo AM, Nayak H, Lin D, Pulliam W, et al. Mechanisms of organized left atrial tachycardias occurring after pulmonary vein isolation. *Circulation.* 2004; 110:1351–1357.
11. Essebag V, Wylie JV Jr, Reynolds MR, et al. Bi-directional electrical pulmonary vein isolation as an endpoint for ablation of paroxysmal atrial fibrillation. *J Interv Card Electrophysiol.* 2006;17:111–117.

12. Karch MR, Zrenner B, Deisenhofer I, et al. Freedom from atrial tachyarrhythmias after catheter ablation of atrial fibrillation: a randomized comparison between 2 current ablation strategies. *Circulation*. 2005;111:2875–2880.
13. Shah D, Sunthorn H, Burri H, Gentil-Baron P, Pruvot E, Schlaepfer J, Fromer M. Narrow, slow-conducting isthmus-dependent left atrial reentry developing after ablation for atrial fibrillation: ECG characterization and elimination by focal RF ablation. *J Cardiovasc Electrophysiol*. 2006;17:508–515.
14. Cummings JE, Schweikert R, Saliba W, et al. Left atrial flutter following pulmonary vein antrum isolation with radiofrequency energy: linear lesions or repeat isolation. *J Cardiovasc Electrophysiol*. 2005;16:293–297.
15. Deisenhofer I, Estner H, Zrenner B, et al. Left atrial tachycardia after circumferential pulmonary vein ablation for atrial fibrillation: incidence, electrophysiological characteristics, and results of radiofrequency ablation. *Europace*. 2006;8:573–582.
16. Daoud EG, Weiss R, Augostini R, et al. Proarrhythmia of circumferential left atrial lesions for management of atrial fibrillation. *J Cardiovasc Electrophysiol*. 2006;17:157–165.
17. Mesas CEE, Pappone C, Lang CCE, et al. Left atrial tachycardia after circumferential pulmonary vein ablation for atrial fibrillation: electroanatomic characterization and treatment. *J Am Coll Cardiol*. 2004;44:1071–1079.
18. Chae S, Oral H, Good E, et al. Atrial tachycardia after circumferential pulmonary vein ablation of atrial fibrillation: mechanistic insights, results of catheter ablation, and risk factors for recurrence. *J Am Coll Cardiol*. 2007;50:1781–1787.
19. Matsuo S, Lim KT, Haïssaguerre M. Ablation of chronic atrial fibrillation. *Heart Rhythm*. 2007;4(11):1461–1463.
20. Saoudi N, Cosio F, Waldo A, et al. Classification of atrial flutter and regular atrial tachycardia according to electrophysiologic mechanism and anatomic bases: a statement from a joint expert group from the Working Group of Arrhythmias of the European Society of Cardiology and the North American Society of Pacing and Electrophysiology. *J Cardiovasc Electrophysiol*. 2001;12:852–866.
21. Morady F, Oral H, Chugh A. Diagnosis and ablation of atypical atrial tachycardia and flutter complicating atrial fibrillation ablation. *Heart Rhythm*. 2009;6:S29–S32.
22. Jaïs P, Matsuo S, Knecht S, et al. A deductive mapping strategy for atrial tachycardia following atrial fibrillation ablation: importance of localized reentry. *J Cardiovasc Electrophysiol*. 2009;20(5):480–491.
23. Berenfeld O, Mandapati R, Dixit S, et al. Spatially distributed dominant excitation frequencies reveal hidden organization in atrial fibrillation in the langendorff-perfused sheep heart. *J Cardiovasc Electrophysiol*. 2000;11:869–879.
24. Yoshida K, Chugh A, Ulfarsson M, et al. Relationship between the spectral characteristics of atrial fibrillation and atrial tachycardias that occur after catheter ablation of atrial fibrillation. *Heart Rhythm*. 2009;6:11–17.
25. Takahashi Y, O'Neill MD, Hocini M, et al. Effects of stepwise ablation of chronic atrial fibrillation on atrial electrical and mechanical properties. *J Am Coll Cardiol*. 2007;49:1306–1314.
26. Mohamed U, Skanes AC, Gula LJ, Leong-Sit P, Krahn AD, Yee R, Subbiah R, Klein GJ. A novel pacing maneuver to localize focal atrial tachycardia. *J Cardiovasc Electrophysiol*. 2007;18:1–6.
27. Hocini M, Jaïs P, Sanders P, et al. Techniques, evaluation, and consequences of linear block at the left atrial roof in paroxysmal atrial fibrillation: A prospective randomized study. *Circulation*. 2005;112:3688–3696.
28. Shah D, Sunthorn H, Gentil-Baron P, Pruvot E, Schlaepfer J, Fromer M. Narrow, slow-conducting isthmus dependent left atrial reentry developing after ablation of atrial fibrillation: ECG characterization and elimination by focal radiofrequency ablation. *J Cardiovasc Electrophysiol*. 2006;17:508–515.
29. Cuculich P, Wang Y, Lindsay B, Faddis M, Schuessler R, Damiano R, Li L, Rudy Y. Noninvasive characterization of epicardial activation in humans with diverse atrial fibrillation patterns. *Circulation*. 2010;122:1364–1372.
30. Gerstenfeld EP, Dixit S, Bala R, Callans DJ, Lin D, Sauer W, Garcia F, Cooper J, Russo AM, Marchlinski FE. Surface electrocardiogram characteristics of atrial tachycardias occurring after pulmonary vein isolation. *Heart Rhythm*. 2007;4(9):1136–1143.
31. Patel AM, d'Avila A, Neuzil P, Kim SJ, Mela T, Singh JP, Ruskin JN, Reddy VY. Atrial tachycardia after ablation of persistent atrial fibrillation: identification of the critical isthmus with a combination of multielectrode activation mapping and targeted entrainment mapping. *Circ Arrhythm Electrophysiol*. 2008;1(1):14–22.
32. Jaïs P, Sanders P, Hsu LF, et al. Flutter localized to the anterior left atrium after catheter ablation of atrial fibrillation. *J Cardiovasc Electrophysiol*. 2006 Mar;17(3):279–285.
33. Arya A, Hindricks G, Sommer P, Huo Y, Bollmann A, Gaspar T, Bode K, Husser D, Kottkamp H, Piorkowski C. Long-term results and the predictors of outcome of catheter ablation of atrial fibrillation using steerable sheath catheter navigation after single procedure in 674 patients. *Europace*. 2010;12(2):149–150.

CHAPTER 25

How to Perform 3-Dimensional Entrainment Mapping to Treat Post–AF Ablation Atrial Tachycardia/AFL

Philipp Sommer, MD; Christopher Piorkowski, MD; Gerhard Hindricks, MD, PhD

Introduction

In the past decade, ablation of AF has become standard procedure in the treatment of AF patients. Wide atrial circumferential ablation lines are drawn around the ipsilateral PVs in order to isolate this region in almost all patients as the cornerstone of ablation procedures. During the development of today's techniques, noncontinuous ablation lines with gaps due to bad tip-to-tissue contact caused post–AF ablation atrial tachycardias and atypical AFL in up to 20% of patients (**Figure 25.1**). With improved mapping and catheter navigation technologies, the rate of these iatrogenic tachycardias has decreased to approximately 5%. Understanding of the tachycardia mechanism is crucial for a successful treatment of these arrhythmias.

Preprocedural Planning

Imaging

Before their initial AF ablation procedure, all patients undergo cardiac imaging, mostly with a 128-slice CT or an MRI (especially in very young patients). For all post–AF arrhythmia ablations, the initial imaging is being used for the reablation as well. Nevertheless, it can be very helpful to redo the 3-dimensional reconstruction of the DICOM data because not only the LA but also the RA may play a role in this form of arrhythmias. Otherwise, a combination of electroanatomical reconstruction and registered (superimposed) 3-dimensional CT model is necessary (**Figure 25.2**).

Echo Before Ablation

In all patients, regardless of their rhythm and individual thromboembolic risk, atrial thrombus formation is ruled out the day before the ablation procedure by TEE. Furthermore, LVEF is measured in all patients with TTE to identify patients who developed a tachycardiomyopathy with impaired LVEF under their atrial tachycardia and fast conduction over the AV node. This might have implications on the periprocedural planning and sedation regimens (eg, negative inotropic effects of propofol in patients with impaired LVEF) as well as follow-up.

Procedure

Patient Preparation

All patients undergo their PVI as well as their post–PVI AT ablation under deep analgosedation. Before puncture of the femoral veins, midazolam and fentanyl are administered in low doses. Then a bolus of propofol is delivered followed by continuous application. The

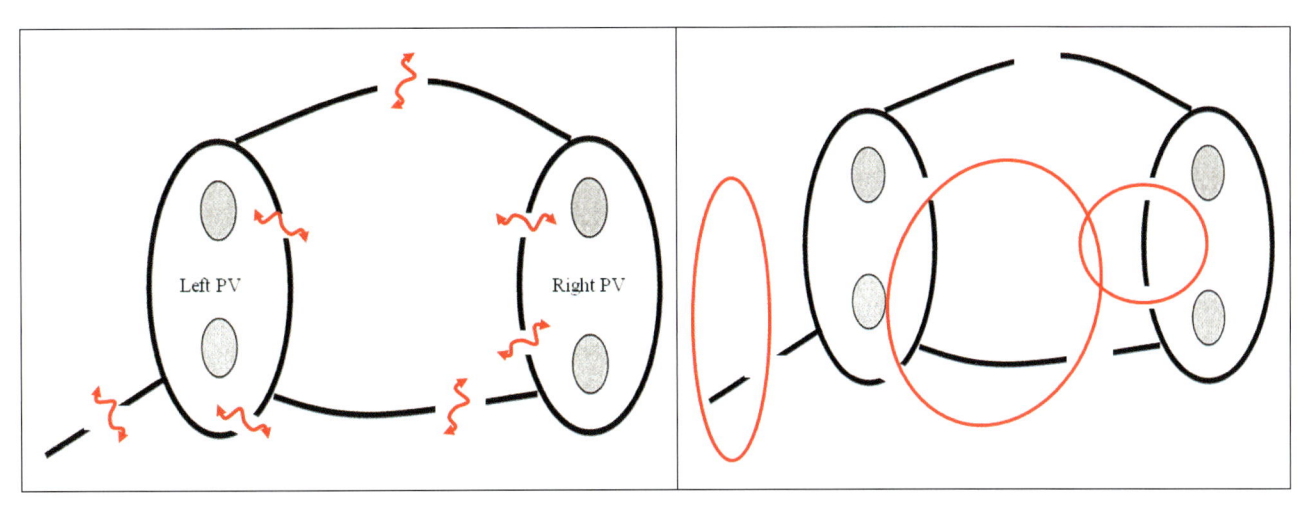

Figure 25.1 Schematic picture of the 4 PVs and an ablation pattern for persistent AF patients with circumferential lesions, posterior box lesions, and mitral isthmus line. The red flashes indicate possible locations for gaps in the ablation lines (left panel). Based on these gaps, several LA MRTs can occur (red circles, right panel).

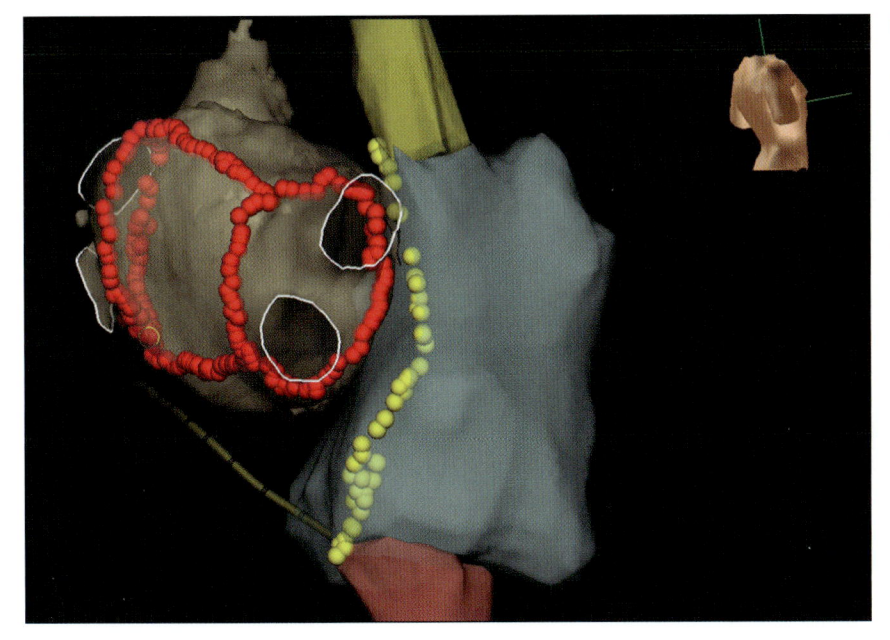

Figure 25.2 Combination of 3-dimensional mapping modalities: CT-reconstructed and registered 3-dimensional model of a LA (grey shell), electroanatomically mapped SVC (yellow shell), RA (blue shell), decapolar diagnostic catheter in coronary sinus (yellow), LA ablation with PVI and linear lesions (red points), and RA linear lesion between SVC and IVC (yellow points).

LFV accommodates a 5-Fr (RVA) and 6-Fr (CS) sheath for the standard diagnostic catheters. We routinely use deflectable decapolar CS catheters that can be inserted via a femoral access. On the right side, a short 12-Fr sheath is placed for insertion of the transseptal sheath. Additionally, an arterial line (4-Fr) is punctured for invasive blood pressure measurement. Finally, a temperature probe is inserted in the esophagus to monitor temperature increase during ablation.

Transseptal Puncture

Single transseptal puncture for LA access is typically performed after initial entrainments within CS and HRA have suggested a LA origin of the arrhythmia. The puncture is guided by contrast dye injection and fluoroscopy mainly. Another tool is pressure recording at the needle tip with the RR measurement line. Successful puncture is confirmed by contrast dye injection and fluoroscopical control. TEE guided transseptal punctures are only rarely necessary (< 1%). After the transseptal puncture, an initial bolus of 100 U/kg is given and the ACT controlled every 20 minutes in order to maintain target ACT values between 250 and 350s. If necessary, repeated heparin boluses are delivered during the ablation.

Selection of Guiding Sheaths and Catheters

The guiding sheath for the spiral and the ablation catheter is a deflectable sheath that allows bidirectional movement during the ablation procedure (Agilis®, St. Jude Medical, St. Paul, MN). In patients with normal or moderately enlarged LA diameter (< 45 mm), we use the small curve; in enlarged left atria, "med" curve is preferred. The sheath is constantly flushed with a heparinized saline drip at a flow rate of 2 ml/h. In clinical routine, we use RF as the energy source exclusively. An open irrigated-tip catheter (Cool Path duo, M-Curve, IBI, Irvine, CA) is the standard ablation catheter, irrigation rate is 30 ml/min, and the preferred spiral catheter is an adjustable (15–25 mm) Optima (IBI, Irvine, CA).

Mapping

3-Dimensional Mapping System

For ablation of AF, but especially for AT/AFL procedures, the use of 3-dimensional mapping systems has increased efficacy significantly. When combined with image integration, 3-dimensional mapping systems allow reproducible identification and visualization of reentrant circuits. For AT/AFL ablations, we routinely use the EnSite NavX Navigation & Visualization Technology (St. Jude Medical, St. Paul, MN).

Registration of 3-Dimensional CT Model

After the transseptal puncture, the spiral diagnostic catheter is inserted into all PVs and separate geometries are acquired over all 10 poles. The 3-dimensional CT model is superimposed visually (**Figure 25.3**; ▶ **Video 25.1**) and registration is completed with additional 10 to 15 characteristic points acquired manually with the ablation catheter (eg, mitral annulus 3, 6, 9, 12 o'clock, roof).[2] Once the CT model is registered, the electroanatomical information can be displayed on this shell without acquiring any further geometries.

PPI Mapping

The main problem in AT/AFL procedures is understanding the mechanisms of tachycardias. Initially, conventional activation mapping within 3-dimensional mapping

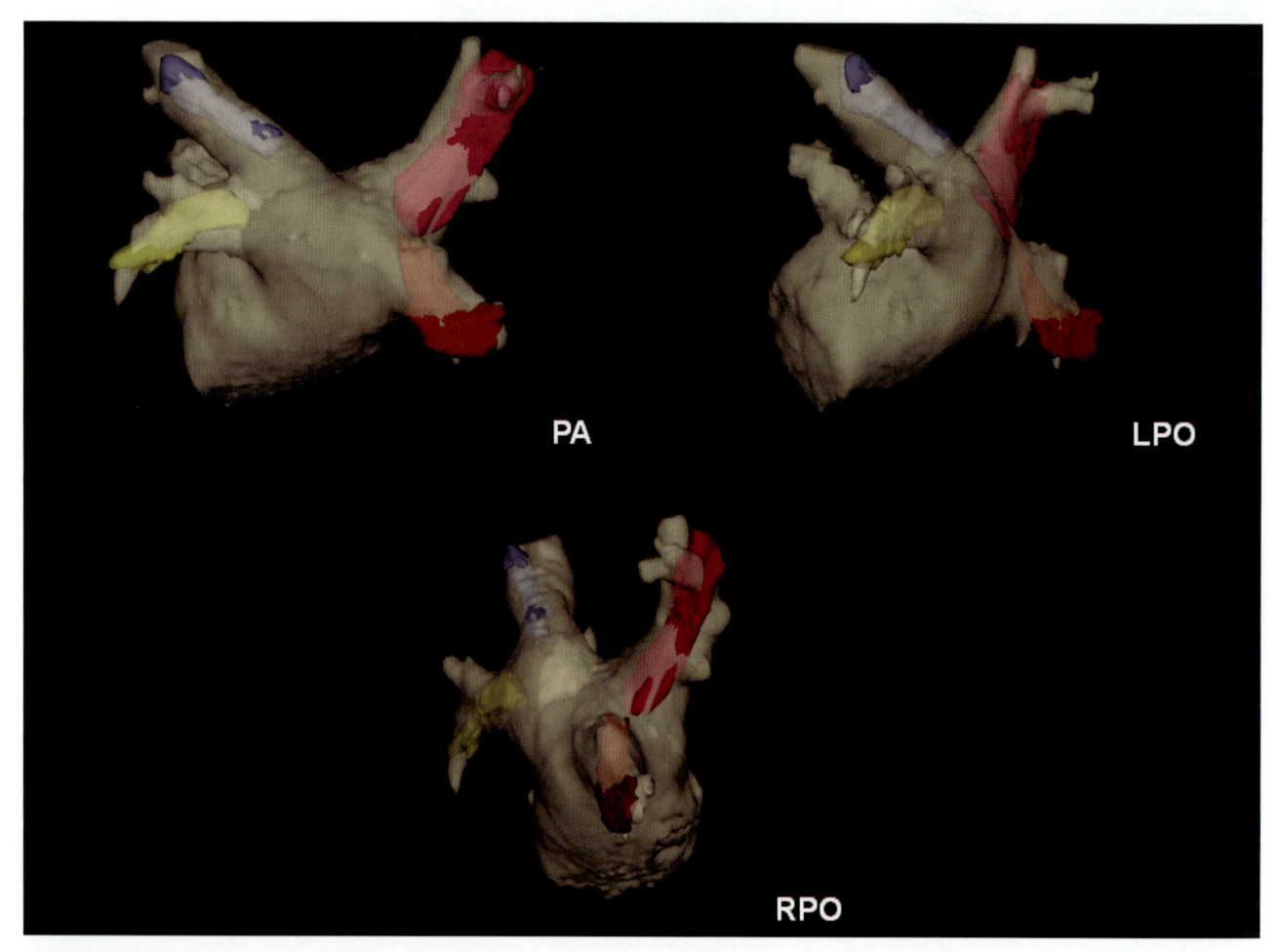

Figure 25.3 Registration of 3-dimensional reconstructed CT model with geometries acquired by 3-dimensional mapping system: LSPV (blue), LIPV (yellow), RSPV (pink), and RIPV (brown) were reconstructed electroanatomically and fused with the CT-derived model (grey shell) in posteroanterior (PA), left posterior oblique (LPO), and right posterior oblique (RPO) views. (Used with permission from Piorkowski C, Kircher S, Arya A, et al. Computed tomography model-based treatment of atrial fibrillation and atrial macro-re-entrant tachycardia. *Europace*. 2008;10(8):939–948.)

systems was the standard approach to understanding atrial MRT. Besides the uncertainty of assigning early and late activation within a continuously running reentrant circuit, slow conduction outside the circuit can further confuse correct allocation of local activation times. To separate out late local activation resulting from bystander zones of slow conduction (not involved into the critical circuit), entrainment was occasionally used to determine the anatomical distance of the stimulation site from the reentrant circuit. Entrainment stimulation is typically being performed 30 ms slower than the TCL. Too-fast stimulation may terminate or change the activation pattern. Too-slow stimulation may fail to capture the tachycardia. The difference between the entrainment return cycle (PPI) and the TCL has been shown to be an indicator for the anatomical distance from the critical reentrant circuit.[1] When PPI equals TCL, stimulation is being performed from within the circuit (**Figure 25.4A**). The bigger the difference, the further apart the stimulation site is located (**Figure 25.4B**). Use of entrainment within fluoroscopical environment is limited with respect to spatial orientation. In order to fully understand the 3-dimensional path of the reentrant circuit, we have introduced a method of 3-dimensional color-coded display of entrainment information. The entrainment information obtained from the EP recording system is being transferred to the 3-dimensional mapping system using the activation map interface. Annotation, however, is only based on the numeric PPI value, disregarding any EGM timing on the mapping system. Calibrating the annotation bar, a PPI-TCL of 0 ms should be visualized in red, and a PPI-TCL of 150 ms in purple. Using a registered CT image, this information can directly be projected on the surface. With sequential entrainment in different anatomical locations point by point, a map of the tachycardia is being developed that no longer shows the relative precocity of local activation toward a reference signal but

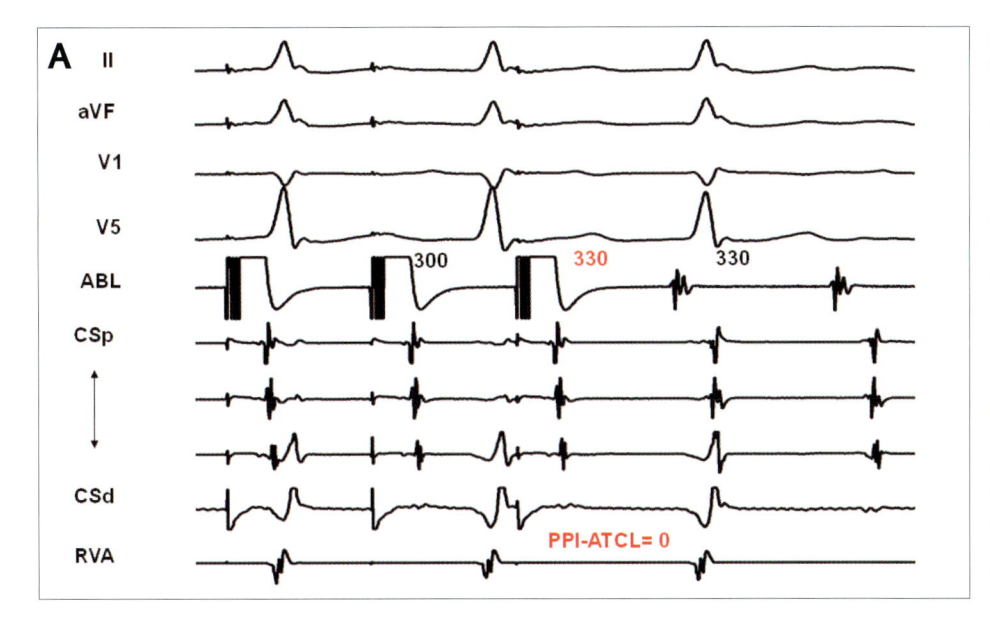

Figure 25.4 A. Recordings from the EP system: four surface ECG leads, signals from the ablation catheter (ABL) with stimulation artifacts; intracardiac EGM from proximal (CSp) to distal (CSd) coronary sinus and right ventricular apex (RVA). TCL is 330 ms, tachycardia is entrained from the ablation catheter at a CL of 300 ms; the PPI is 330 ms, the difference between PPI and TCL is 0 ms. The spot of the ablation catheter must be part of the reentrant circuit. **B.** Same recordings as in panel **A**; here, the PPI is 485 ms, and the difference between PPI and TCL is 155 ms. The spot of the ablation catheter must be quite distant from the reentrant circuit.

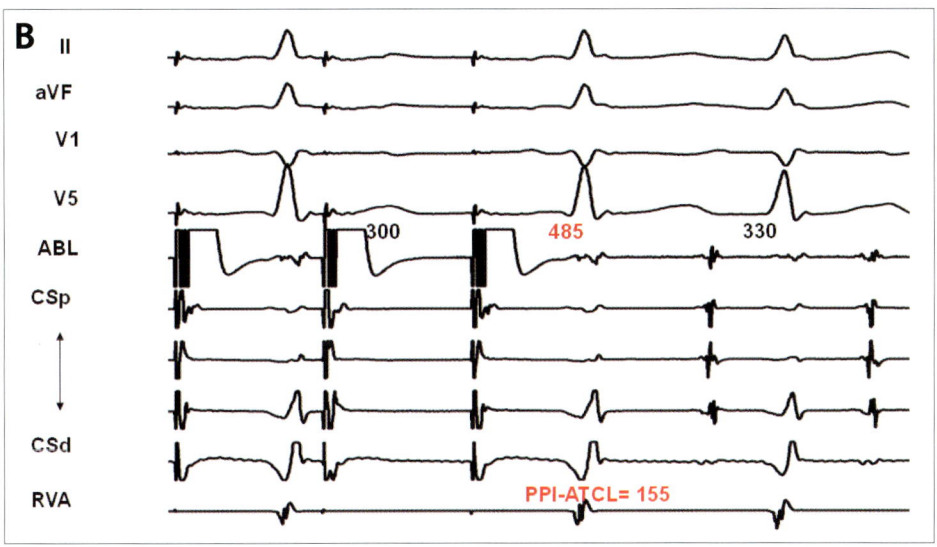

the anatomical proximity towards the reentrant circuit (**Figure 25.5**).[3]

Ablation

Once the reentrant circuit is visualized, the ablation line can be performed. There are typical reentrant mechanisms appearing after PVI as the initial procedure: MRT around the mitral annulus (**Figure 25.6A**; ▶ **Video 25.2**), roof-dependent (**Figure 25.6B**), around the septal or lateral PVs due to gaps in the circumferential line (**Figure 25.6C**; ▶ **Video 25.3**) or tachycardias originating from the LAA (**Figure 25.6D**) or the posterior wall (**Figure 25.6E**). For example, in the frequent case of perimitral tachycardia, a mitral isthmus line must be performed. During ablation, the TCL typically increases, and the tachycardia terminates. Alternatively, the MRT can change its reentrant circuit when a line of block is created; therefore, increase of TCL or change of activation pattern in the CS are often indicators that a different tachycardia appeared. In this case, a remap of the new reentrant circuit must be performed. Usually ablation is started using 40 W of energy with a maximum temperature of 48°C. If the esophageal probe reveals temperature rises of > 41°C, the power settings and/or the location of the ablation line are adapted. Once the tachycardia is converted to sinus rhythm, the isolation of the PVs is controlled using the spiral catheter and completed if necessary. At the end of the procedure, burst pacing is performed to evaluate inducibility. Noninducibility of any regular atrial tachycardia is the procedural endpoint.

Postprocedure Care

Recovery

At the end of the procedure, the steerable sheath is removed, protamin is delivered in order to antagonize the heparin effect, and finally, the sheaths are pulled. When stopping the propofol drip, it usually takes 10 to 15 minutes for the patient to awaken. The patients must lie flat for 6 hours after the procedure and are carefully monitored during that time under intermediate care conditions (blood pressure, oxygen saturation, heart rate). On day 0 (ablation), no more heparin is given; on day 1, we administer low-molecular-weight heparin 1 mg/kg of body weight once daily, and at day 2, 1 mg/kg twice daily. All patients are treated with vitamin K antagonists regardless of their individual thromboembolic risk for at least 3 months postprocedure. Patients usually are discharged on day 1 or day 2.

Follow-Up

Patients are followed with sequential 7-day Holter immediately after the ablation procedure, and again after 3, 6, and 12 months. In general, preexisting antiarrhythmic drug therapy is discontinued with the ablation, and the patients are discharged under beta blockers. The decision to discontinue oral anticoagulation after 3 months mainly is driven by the individual risk for thromboembolic events (CHA_2DS_2-VASc-Score). All patients with a score ≥ 2 will, in general, have to continue anticoagulation; exceptions are individually based decisions in patients with no

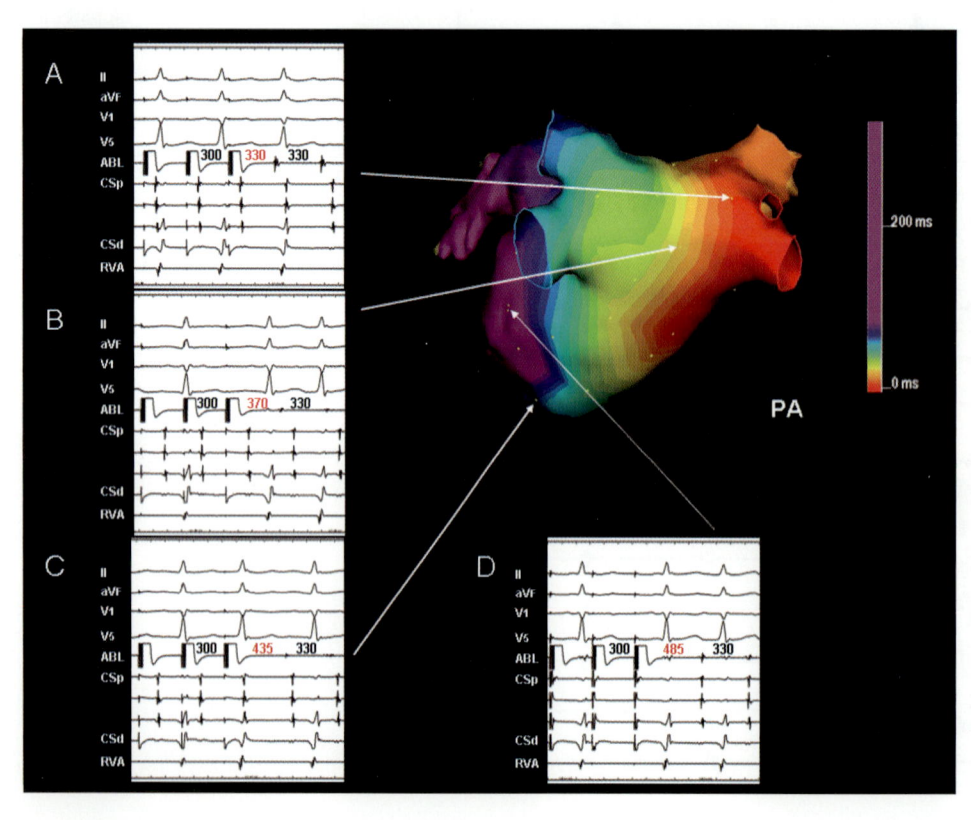

Figure 25.5 Concept of color-coded 3-dimensional entrainment mapping. At each 3-dimensional mapping point (small yellow points within the 3-dimensional image), entrainment stimulation was performed from the tip of the ablation catheter. Examples are given at four distinct 3-dimensional locations, **A–D**). The time difference between return cycle and TCL was displayed for each 3-dimensional mapping point in color-coded fashion. Color bar displays encoding of the entrainment information. Red represents short return cycles with stimulation close to the reentrant circuit. Blue and purple represent long return cycles with stimulation distant from the reentrant circuit. (Used with permission from Esato M, Hindricks G, Sommer P, et al. Color-coded three-dimensional entrainment mapping for analysis and treatment of atrial macroreentrant tachycardia. *Heart Rhythm.* 2009;6(3):349–358.)

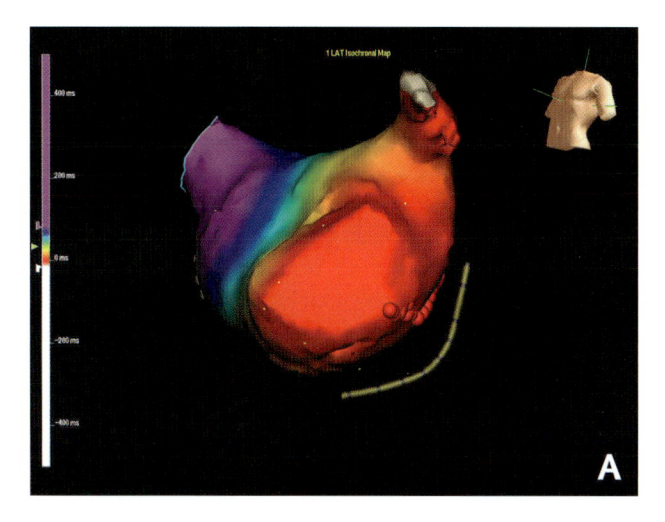

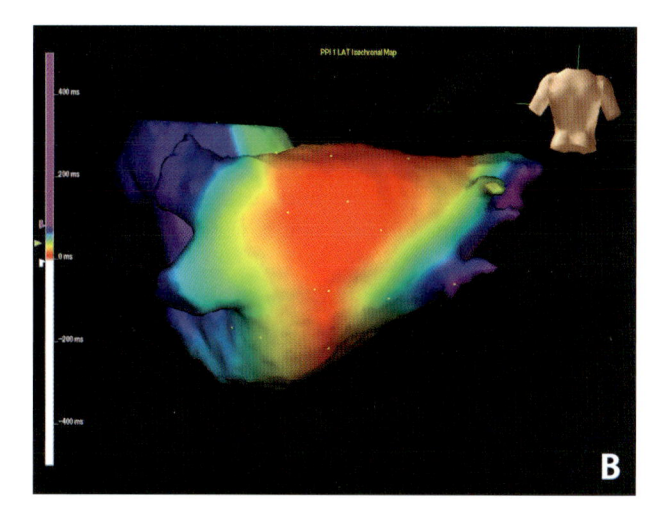

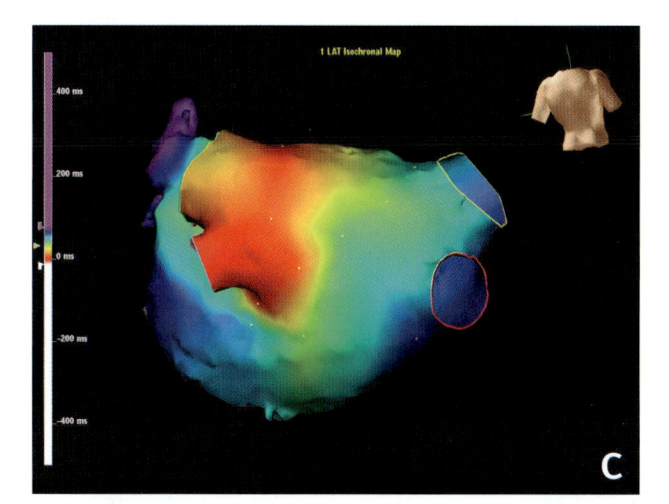

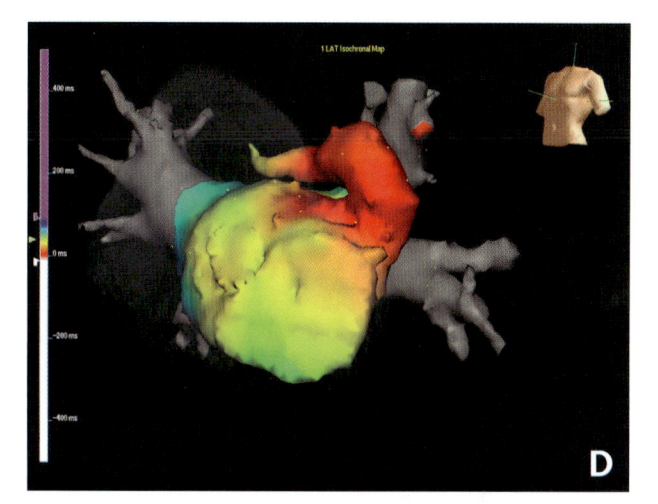

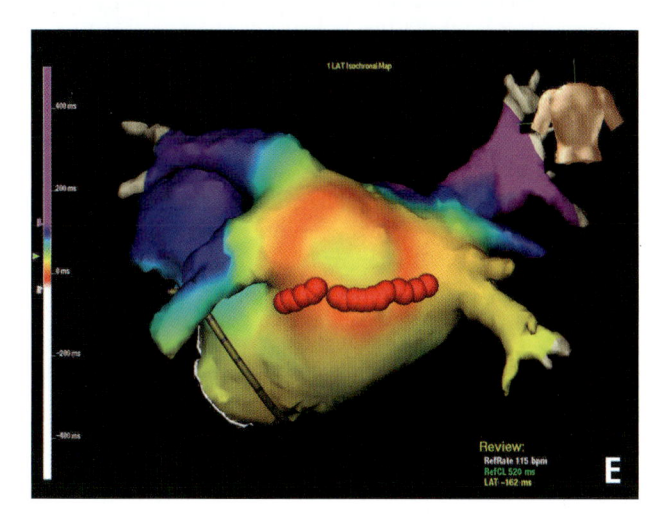

Figure 25.6 Example of typical reentrant mechanisms following PVI procedure in color-coded entrainment maps: LAMRT around the mitral annulus (**A**), roof-dependent (**B**), around the left PVs (**C**), around the LAA (**D**), and a macroreentry at the posterior wall (**E**).

recurrences on Holter or an implantable device (pacemaker or implantable loop recorder).

Success Rates

With the achievement of the procedural endpoints such as tachycardia termination and noninducibility, the success rates are typically high (~90%). Disease progression with newly developed fibrosis serving as arrhythmia substrate, however, may be one reason for further tachycardia occurrence after long and very long follow-up periods.

Procedural Complications

Hemodynamic monitoring with continuous, invasive blood pressure measurement is helpful in early detection of complications such as pericardial effusion with tamponade. In experienced centers, pericardial effusion should not exceed 1% of the patients. Most frequent is vascular complications with 1 to 2%; PV stenosis after ablation of atrial tachycardia is rare since the substrate is mostly in the LA, no longer in the PV. Thromboembolic events are very rare, as are phrenic nerve paralysis or esophagoatrial fistulas (0.4 and 0.2%).[4] A specific complication that maybe associated with MRTs involving the IAS is the risk of damage to the compact AV node. In any such circumstances, AV nodal conduction must be carefully monitored during ablation line placement.

Advantages and Limitations

In contrast to standard activation mapping, entrainment-based mapping of post–PVI tachycardias is easily reproducible and allows fast understanding of the underlying mechanisms, especially in combination with integration of 3-dimensional imaging. As a limitation, 3-dimensional PPI mapping requires stable tachycardias at an entrainable TCL. Therefore, the method cannot be used for arrhythmia description in patients with continuously changing tachycardia pathways, unstable arrhythmias, or repetitive degeneration into AF. Entrainment stimulation performed from within an area of slow conduction carries the risk of paradoxically long PPIs, tachycardia termination, and tachycardia degeneration. Our published experience with this method still is monocentric; a comparison of our approach with the established method of activation mapping with respect to procedural and efficacy data clearly requires a larger comparative study.

Conclusion

Color-coded 3-dimensional entrainment ("PPI") mapping is a new method for direct visualization of the entire reentrant circuit and the selection of a strategic ablation line not necessarily targeting the area of slow conduction of the arrhythmia. The approach is feasible, provides detailed information on the location of the reentrant circuit, and results in an excellent rate of tachycardia termination with satisfying long-term clinical efficacy.

References

1. Waldo AL. AFL: entrainment characteristics. *J Cardiovasc Electrophysiol.* 1997;8:337–352.
2. Piorkowski C, Kircher S, Arya A, et al. Computed tomography model-based treatment of atrial fibrillation and atrial macro-re-entrant tachycardia. *Europace.* 2008;10(8): 939–948.
3. Esato M, Hindricks G, Sommer P, et al. Color-coded three-dimensional entrainment mapping for analysis and treatment of atrial macroreentrant tachycardia. *Heart Rhythm.* 2009;6(3):349–358.
4. Dagres N, Hindricks G, Kottkamp H, et al. Complications of atrial fibrillation ablation in a high-volume center in 1,000 procedures: still cause for concern? *J Cardiovasc Electrophysiol.* 2009;20(9):1014–1019.

Video Descriptions

Video 25.1 Four PV geometries acquired by the spiral catheter (grey) are fused with the 3-dimensional reconstructed CT data (dark red shell). The decapolar diagnostic catheter is placed in the CS (yellow). The roving ablation catheter is displayed with a green tip and is used for approval of the registration.

Video 25.2 Rotation of 3-dimensional CT in NavX after successful ablation of perimitral flutter. PPI map shows reentrant circuit around mitral valve. Ablations (red points) were performed in the mitral isthmus (2 lines endocardially) and from the CS (epicardially, yellow points) with site termination of the tachycardia (green point). Finally, the PVI was completed.

Video 25.3 Rotation of 3-dimensional CT in NavX after successful ablation of roof-dependent AFL around the right PVs. The patient has undergone mitral valve repair with cryoablation previously. The mitral ring can be seen in LAO projection. Ablations (red points) were performed at the roof of LA with site termination of the tachycardia (yellow points). Finally, the PVI was completed.

CHAPTER 26

Catheter Ablation of Autonomic Ganglionated Plexi in Patients with Atrial Fibrillation

Hiroshi Nakagawa, MD, PhD; Benjamin J. Scherlag, PhD; Warren M. Jackman, MD[1]

Introduction

Multiple different approaches have been used for catheter ablation of AF.[1-8] These involve PV ostial isolation, extending the PV-encircling lesions in the posterior LA to include much of the PV antrum (antrum isolation), adding linear LA lesions (roof line and/or mitral isthmus line), isolation of the SVC, and ablating sites exhibiting fractionated APs in the RA, LA, and CS[9-11] during AF (CFAE[7]). Recent experimental and clinical studies on AF suggest that activation of the intrinsic cardiac autonomic nervous system may plays a significant role in the generation of fractionated AP and the initiation and maintenance of AF.[9-21]

Autonomic influences on the heart are generated by both the extrinsic (central) and intrinsic cardiac autonomic nervous systems. The extrinsic cardiac autonomic nervous system is comprised of the vagosympathetic system from the brain and spinal cord to the heart. The intrinsic cardiac autonomic nervous system includes autonomic ganglionated plexi (GP) on the epicardial surface of the left and right atria.[22,23] The intrinsic system receives the input from the extrinsic system but acts independently to modulate cardiac functions, including automaticity, contractility, and conduction.[12,15]

The intrinsic cardiac autonomic nervous system contains clusters of autonomic GP located in epicardial fat pads on the left and right atria and in the ligament of Marshall.[22,23] The GP contain afferent neurons from the atrial myocardium and from the central autonomic nervous system (extrinsic system), efferent cholinergic and adrenergic neurons (with heavy innervation of the PV myocardium and the atrial myocardium surrounding the GP), and an extensive array of interconnecting neurons.[22,23]

It has been postulated that AF induced by increased GP activity is produced by triggered firing resulting from early after-depolarizations (EADs).[16,17] GP activation includes both parasympathetic and sympathetic stimulation of the atrium surrounding the GP and the PV. Parasympathetic stimulation markedly shortens action potential duration, especially in the PV myocardium (**Figures 26.1** and **26.2**). Sympathetic stimulation increases calcium loading and calcium release from the sarcoplasmic reticulum (enhancing calcium transient). The combination of short action potential duration (early repolarization) and enhanced calcium release results in high intracellular calcium concentrations during and immediately after repolarization. The high calcium concentration during and immediately after repolarization drives Na^+/Ca^{++} exchange, with 3 Na^+

---

1. Disclosures: H. Nakagawa and W. M. Jackman are consultants for Biosense Webster, Inc.

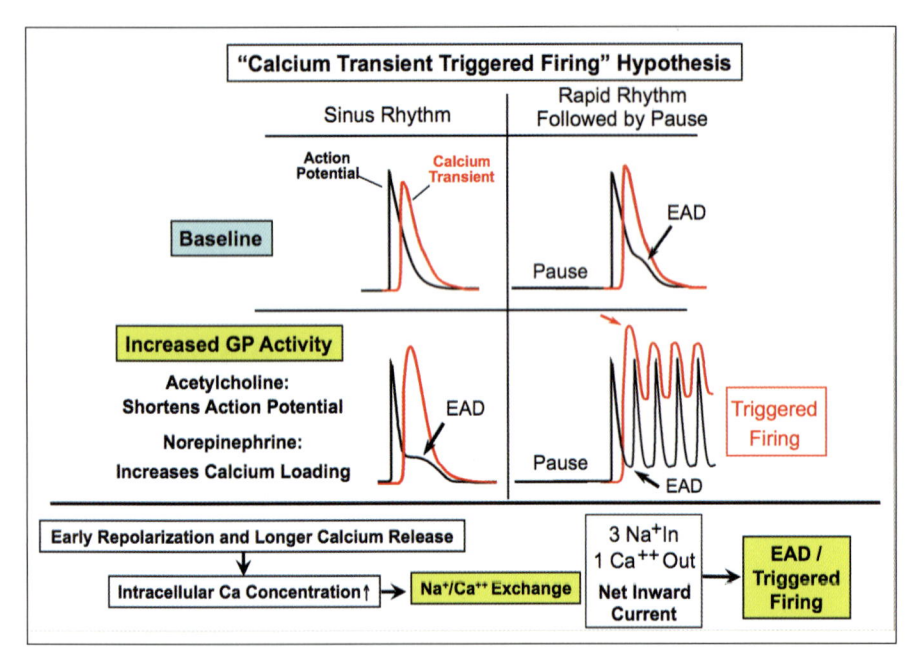

Figure 26.1 "Calcium Transient Triggered Firing" hypothesis for the mechanism of short episodes of very rapid irregular firing in the pulmonary vein (PV) initiating atrial fibrillation (AF). Action potential is drawn in black and the calcium transient is drawn in red. Ganglionated plexi (GP) activation results in both sympathetic and parasympathetic stimulation. Acetylcholine shortens the action potential duration and norepinephrine enhances the calcium transient. The disparity between the short action potential duration and the enhanced calcium transient can produce early after-depolarization (EAD) with inward sodium–calcium exchange current. Further enhancement of the calcium transient is observed after rapid rhythm followed by pause, initiating triggered firing. (Modified with permission from reference 17.)

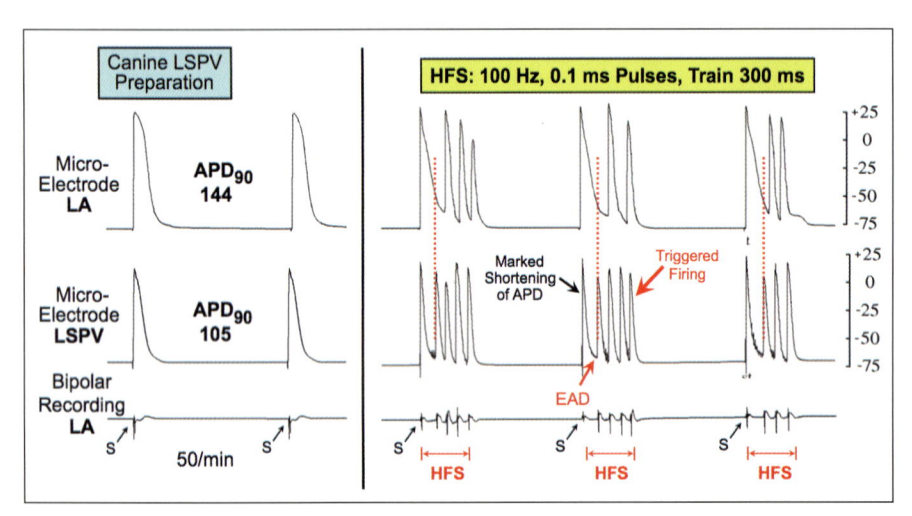

Figure 26.2 Pulmonary vein triggered firing during high-frequency stimulation (HFS) of the ganglionated plexi (GP) in a canine model. Microelectrode recordings from the left atrium (LA) and left superior pulmonary vein (LSPV) in the isolated canine PV preparation. **Left panel:** During LA pacing at 50/min without HFS, the action potential duration at 90% of repolarization (APD_{90}) was markedly shorter in the PV myocyte (105 ms) than the LA myocyte (144 ms). **Right panel:** Short trains of high-frequency stimulation (HFS, CL 10 ms, 0.1 ms pulse width, train duration 300 ms, 100 volts) were delivered to the LA pacing site, immediately after each pacing stimulus (without capture of the LA). HFS produced significant shortening of action potential duration in both the LA and LSPV myocytes, EADs, and triggered firing. At the first triggered beat of each episode, activation of the LSPV precedes the LA activation, indicating the occurrence of triggered firing from the LSPV. The greater APD_{90} shortening and occurrence of triggered firing in the PV myocyte suggests the PV has greater sensitivity to autonomic stimulation than the LA. (Modified with permission from reference 16.)

atoms entering the cell for each Ca^{++} atom exiting the cell, creating a net inward current and producing EADs and triggered firing ("Calcium Transient-Triggered Firing Hypothesis," **Figure 26.1**).[17] Myocardial contractility, EADs, and triggered firing are enhanced by a pause, especially when the pause follows rapid rate. The rapid rate increases Ca^{++} loading in the cells (shorter diastolic periods prevent extrusion of all of the Ca^{++} that enter the cell during systole). The increased Ca^{++} accumulates in the sarcoplasmic reticulum during the pause. Activation of the cell at the end of the pause results in an exaggerated release of Ca^{++} from the sarcoplasmic reticulum (increased calcium transient), producing triggered firing (**Figure 26.1**).[17]

In a canine isolated LSPV preparation with a rim of adjacent LA, selective electrical stimulation (high-frequency stimulation, HFS: CL 10 ms, 0.1 ms pulse width, train duration 300 ms) of axons originating from the GP produced a striking shortening of action potential duration with EAD and triggered firing in the PV myocardium (**Figure 26.2**).[16,17] The response to HFS was completely blocked by superfusion with tetrodotoxin in low concentration, which blocks neurons without affecting the action potential of the LA or PV myocardium, confirming that HFS produces its effects by stimulating autonomic axons (ie, GP activity), and not by direct electrical stimulation of the myocardial cells. In this model, atropine prevents the shortening of action potential duration by HFS and prevents triggered firing.[17] Atenolol allows the shortening of action potential duration by HFS but prevents the triggered firing. Ryanodine, which prevents the release of Ca^{++} from the sarcoplasmic reticulum, allows some shortening of the action potential duration, but totally prevents EAD formation and triggered firing.[17] The response to ryanodine supports the role of the primary Ca^{++} release from the sarcoplasmic reticulum in the generation of EADs and triggered firing. The EADs and triggered firing in this preparation are increased by a pause following rapid pacing, similar to the pause-dependant pattern of PV firing seen clinically (**Figure 26.3**).[17]

The magnitude of action potential shortening, EAD formation, and triggered firing produced by HFS is greater in the PV myocardium than in the adjacent LA myocardium (**Figure 26.2**).[16] The increased sensitivity of the PV myocardium may explain the clinical observation, in patients with paroxysmal AF, that the focal firing which triggers AF is often located in the PV myocardial sleeves.

We have shown that, in an in vivo canine model, epicardial HFS of a fat pad containing GP produces: (1) a vagal response (sinus bradycardia or AV block); (2) marked shortening of the atrial refractory period close to the activated GP; and (3) initiation of sustained AF either spontaneously or by a single atrial extrastimulus delivered close to the GP.[10,11,14,15] Testing in the LA distant from the stimulated GP shows little or no decrease in atrial refractory period and sustained AF can not be induced by a single atrial extrastimulus.[10,11,15] During AF produced by HFS of GP, rapid and fractionated atrial potentials are consistently located in the adjacent PV and LA surrounding the stimulated GP (**Figure 26.4**). Intracardiac EGMs recorded at sites distant from the stimulated GP exhibit more organized atrial potentials and longer CLs. These experimental data suggest a relationship between fractionated AP and autonomic activity from GP (Figure 26.4).

In the canine model, the GP can be localized from the endocardium using HFS.[10,14] When close to a GP, an endocardial application of HFS through a mapping catheter produces a vagal response manifested by a marked lengthening of the R-R interval during AF (transient AV block). Endocardial RF ablation at those sites eliminated the vagal response to repeat endocardial HFS. The RF ablation often decreased or eliminated the fractionated AP close to the stimulated GP.[19,23] The above animal studies suggest that the GP may play a significant role in clinical AF, especially in patients with paroxysmal AF.

Localization of LA Ganglionated Plexi by Endocardial High-Frequency Stimulation

GP can be identified and localized using endocardial HFS in patients undergoing catheter ablation of AF.[10,11] We begin with a high-density bipolar electroanatomical map (CARTO-XP, Biosense Webster, Inc, Diamond Bar, CA) of the LA and each of the 4 PVs, obtained during AF to provide both an anatomical shell of the LA and PVs and the location of fractionated AP areas in the LA. We found that the LA fractionated APs were located primarily in 4 areas: (1) LAA ridge fractionated AP area (between LAA and left PVs); (2) superior left fractionated AP area; (3) infero-posterior fractionated AP area; and (4) anterior right fractionated AP area (**Figure 26.5A**). Endocardial high-frequency stimulation (HFS, CL 50 ms, 12–15 volt actual output, 10 ms pulse width, using a Grass stimulator

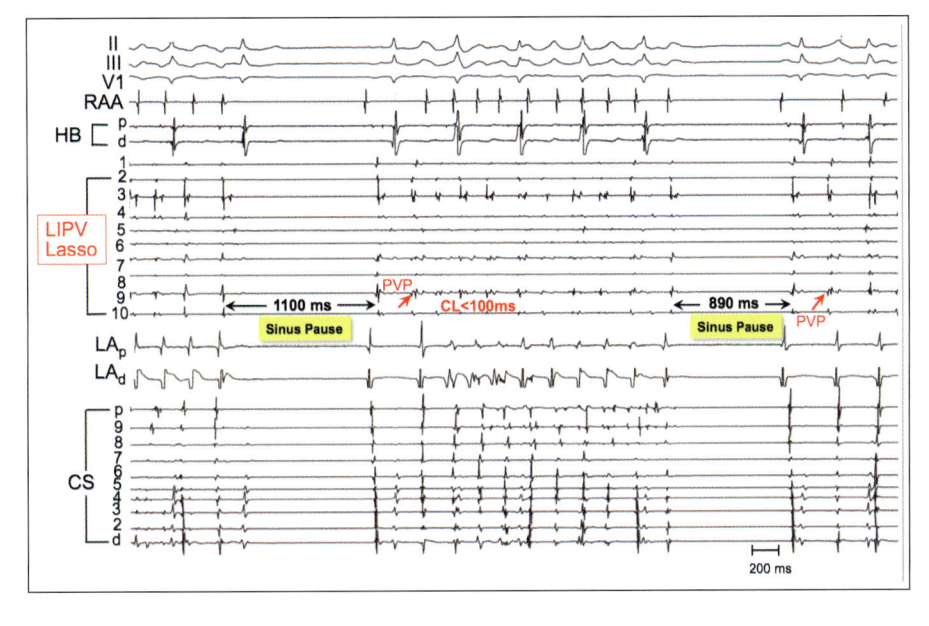

Figure 26.3 Spontaneous pause-dependent PV firing from the LIPV in a patient with paroxysmal AF. Tracings from the top are surface ECG leads II, III, V_1, and intracardiac EGMs from RAA, HB region, the LIPV, the LA, and the CS. A spontaneous termination of brief AF episode resulted in a sinus pause (1100 ms), followed by very rapid (mean CL < 100 ms), irregular firing in the LIPV, initiating AF. The AF episode terminated again, resulting in another sinus pause (890 ms) and PV firing. PVP: pulmonary vein potential (red arrows).

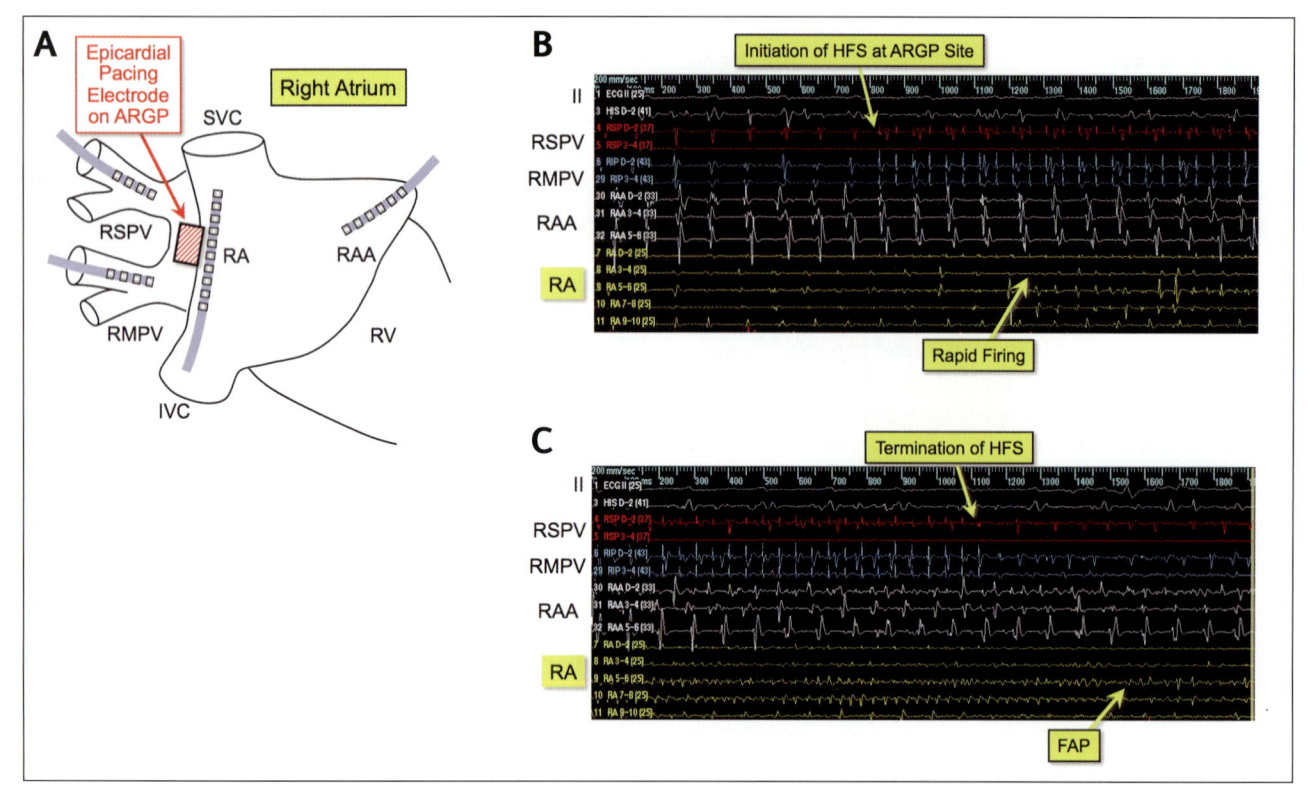

Figure 26.4 Effects of anterior right GP stimulation on intracardiac EGMs during AF in a canine model. **A.** Schematic representation of the RA showing position of epicardial recording electrodes (blue electrode catheters) and epicardial pacing electrodes (red cross-hatched areas) over the fat pads containing the anterior right GP. The epicardial pacing electrode was used to deliver HFS to the anterior right GP. RSPV: right superior pulmonary vein; RMPV: right middle pulmonary vein; RA: right atrium close to the anterior right GP; RAA: right atrial appendage; RV: right ventricle. **B.** Rapid RA stimulation initiated only nonsustained episodes of relatively organized AF (beginning of the tracing). HFS at the anterior right GP region (without capture of the atrial myocardium) was initiated during organized AF (top yellow arrow). The HFS resulted in rapid firing, recorded initially in the RA EGMs (RA3-4, bottom yellow arrow) located close to the stimulated anterior right GP, accelerating AF. **C.** With the continuation of HFS for 30 seconds, AF became sustained and continued to accelerate in EGMs close to the anterior right GP (RA EGMs), exhibiting fractionated APs with very short CLs (< 30–40 ms) even after the termination of HFS. (Modified with permission from reference 16.)

coupled to an isolation unit) was delivered through the distal pair of the electrodes on a mapping/ablation catheter to sites in the LA and within the 4 PVs.[14-17] The sites with a positive vagal response to HFS were localized in 5 major areas (**Figure 26.5B**). We refer to these areas as the Marshall tract GP, superior left GP, anterior right GP, inferior left GP, and inferior right GP (**Figures 26.5A** and **26.6**). The sites of vagal response to HFS were generally located outside of the PVs, except for the Marshall tract GP along the LAA ridge. The superior left GP, inferior left GP and inferior right GP are usually located > 1.0 to 2.0 cm from the adjacent PVs. The anterior right GP is usually located < 1 cm from the RSPV ostium. Importantly, each of the 5 LA GP are generally located within a large 4 fractionated AP area (**Figures 26.5A** and **26.6**). In addition, HFS of a GP often produced increased fractionation in both the adjacent PV and distant PVs.[10] These findings suggest a relationship between GP activation and the occurrence of fractionated AP and communication between GP (activation of one GP may lead to activation of other GP).

Catheter Ablation of LA Ganglionated Plexi

For endocardial catheter ablation of the GP, RF energy is applied to each site exhibiting a positive vagal response to HFS.[10,11] HFS is repeated after each RF application. If a vagal response is still present, RF energy is reapplied until the vagal response is eliminated. Elimination of the vagal response to HFS at each GP generally requires 2 to 12 (median 6) RF applications (usually 30–40 Watts for 30–40 seconds, but the RF power is reduced when close to the esophagus).

The vagal response (transient AV block) to HFS may not identify the entire GP area. HFS-induced transient AV block is driven by activation of the crux GP in the crux fat pad, which is located between the inferior vena cava and CS ostium. Therefore, activating the superior left GP, inferior left GP, Marshall tract GP, or anterior right GP by HFS is followed by activation of other GP, including the inferior right GP, which then results in activation of the

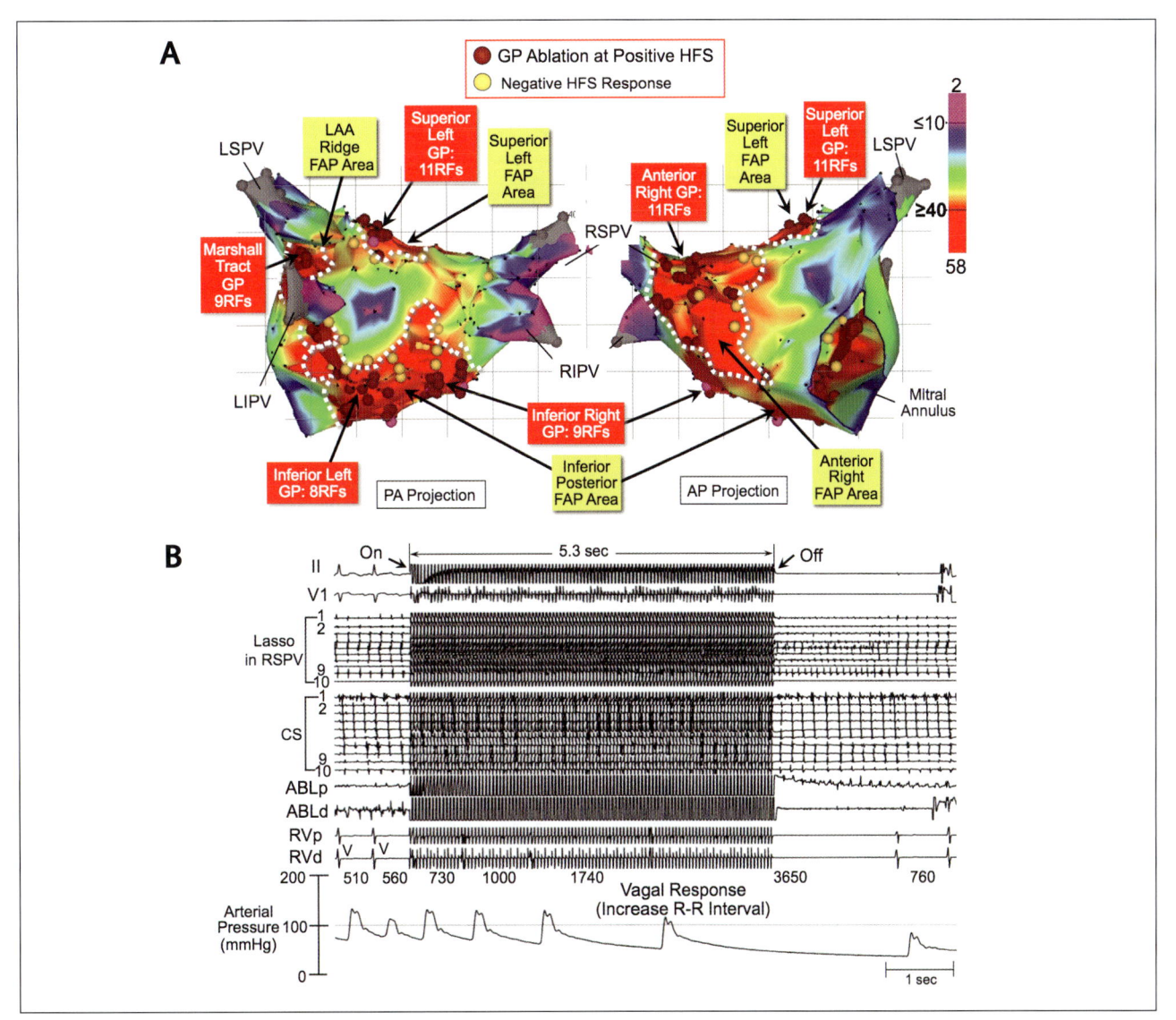

Figure 26.5 Relationship between locations of fractionated APs and GP in a 59-year-old man undergoing catheter ablation of paroxysmal AF. **A.** An electroanatomical map of fractionated APs in a patient with paroxysmal AF. Intracardiac EGMs were recorded for 2.5 seconds at each site in the LA and all 4 PVs. Sites exhibiting continuous or transient fractionated AP were and colored red (fractionated AP segments ≥ 40 per 2.5 seconds). Sites exhibiting periods of irregular amplitude, polarity, and CL, but not rapid were classified as intermediate, fractionated AP and colored green-light blue. Sites exhibiting large amplitude, discrete APs with average CL ≥ 180 ms were classified as slow, organized APs and colored purple (fractionated AP segments ≤ 10 per 2.5 sec). Four fractionated AP areas were identified (LAA ridge fractionated AP area, superior left fractionated AP area, inferior posterior fractionated AP area, and anterior right fractionated AP area). Sites where endocardial HFS produced a vagal response (shown in Figure 26.5B) are marked by brown tags, corresponding to the 5 major GP areas; (1) Marshall tract GP; (2) superior left GP; (3) inferior left GP; (4) inferior right GP; and (5) anterior right GP. HFS failed to produce a vagal response at the sites marked by yellow tags. Note that all 5 GP are located within the 4 fractionated AP areas. PA: posterior-anterior, AP: anterior-posterior. **B.** The tracings from the top are ECG lead II, V$_1$, EGMs from the lasso catheter in the RSPV, CS, RV, and arterial pressure. During AF, endocardial HFS (CL 50 ms, pulse width 10 ms, 5.3 second stimulation) was delivered from the ablation catheter (ABL) positioned in the anterior right fractionated AP area (1.0 cm anterior to the ostium of the RSPV) results in transient complete AV block (R-R interval increased up to 3650 ms) and hypotension (vagal response), identifying the anterior right GP.

crux GP, which innervates the AV node. The vagal response to HFS (transient AV block) may not occur due to ablation of one of the intermediate GP along the line to the crux GP. In order to minimize the loss of the vagal response, we perform ablation of the GP in the following order: Marshall tract GP, superior left GP, anterior right GP, inferior left GP, and finally, inferior right GP. Other signs of GP activation (such as the onset of PV firing other than the PV adjacent to the stimulated GP)[10,24] are occasionally observed during HFS, which does not produce a vagal response.

In 70 patients with paroxysmal AF undergoing ablation of the LA via GP ablation followed by PV antrum isolation, GP ablation alone (prior to PV antrum isolation)

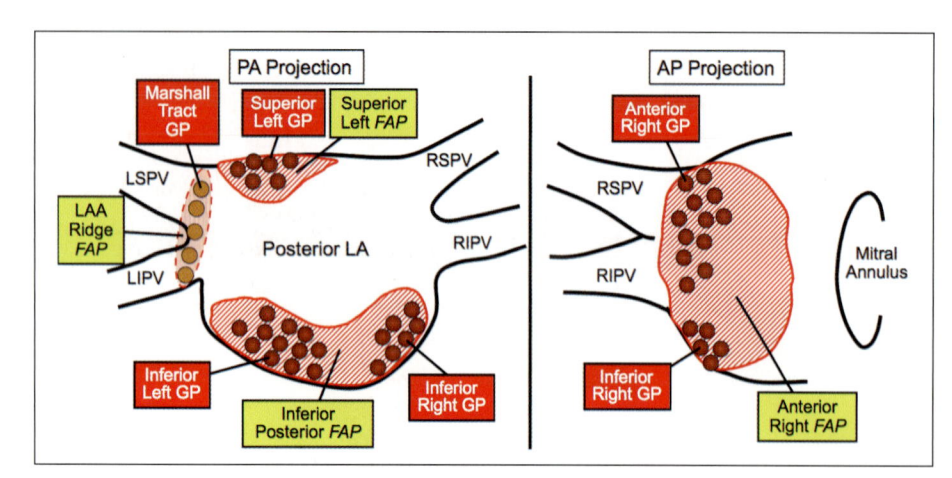

Figure 26.6 Schematic representation of the relationship between the fractionated AP (FAP) areas and GP locations. Brown tags indicate sites with a positive HFS response (GP location). Red cross-hatched areas indicate fractionated AP areas. LAA ridge fractionated AP area and Marshall tract GP are located anterior to the left PVs along the appendage ridge. All 5 GP are located within one of the 4 fractionated AP areas. PA Projection: posterior-anterior, AP Projection: anterior-posterior. (Modified with permission from reference 10.)

decreased the occurrence of PV firing from 53 (76%) of 70 patients before GP ablation to only 11 (16%) of the 70 patients ($p < 0.01$) after GP ablation. PV antrum isolation was then performed, which eliminated PV firing in the remaining 11 patients (0/70 patients), suggesting that additional PV antrum isolation interrupted axons extending from GP which were not ablated by the GP ablation alone. The description in earlier studies of the elimination of PV firing by PVI without targeting the PV firing sites,[10,25] may be explained by the interruption of the axons extending from the GP to the PV myocardium. PV myocardium may require sympathetic and parasympathetic stimulation to produce focal firing. Since axons may regenerate after PV antrum isolation, and PV antrum isolation may not be permanent, axon regeneration may account for recurrence of PV firing and AF in some patients. GP ablation (targeting the GP cell bodies) may be more permanent, complementing PV antrum isolation. GP ablation alone usually eliminates the majority of CFAE, despite ablating a significantly smaller area than the CFAE area. CFAE ablation may eliminate much of the fractionation by ablating the axons without ablation of the GP cell bodies, which may be less likely to be permanent.

GP ablation also decreased the inducibility of sustained AF (> 3 minutes duration) from 48 (69%) of 70 patients to 25 (36%) of 70 patients ($P < 0.01$). The addition of PV antrum isolation further decreased the inducibility of sustained AF to 12 (17%) of 70 patients ($P < 0.01$).[9,10] Fractionated AP mapping of the LA and 4 PVs was obtained before and after GP ablation (prior to PV antrum isolation) in 8 patients in whom sustained AF continued after GP ablation. Although ablation sites were limited to sites of positive vagal response to HRS, GP ablation markedly reduced the area of fractionated AP (median 27.9 cm^2 to 2.8 cm^2, $P < 0.01$) in all 8 patients. These findings are consistent with animal studies showing progressive decrease in fractionated AP with serial ablation of 4 GP.[26] The clinical and experimental studies suggest that fractionated AP may result from GP activation and GP ablation reduces or eliminates the large areas of fractionated AP produced by the extension of axons. Targeting the GP (cell bodies) directly may have advantages over targeting the more peripheral fractionated AP areas, since fractionated AP may be eliminated transiently by ablation of the axons peripherally. The axons may regenerate, whereas ablation of the cell bodies in the GP is likely permanent (no regeneration).

References

1. Haïssaguerre M, Jaïs P, Shah DC, et al. Spontaneous initiation of atrial fibrillation by ectopic beats originating in the pulmonary veins. *N Engl J Med.* 1998;339:659–666.
2. Chen SA, Hsieh MH, Tai CT, et al. Initiation of atrial fibrillation by ectopic beats originating from the pulmonary veins: electrophysiological characteristics, pharmacological responses, and effects of radiofrequency ablation. *Circulation.* 1999;100:1879–1886.
3. Haïssaguerre M, Shah DC, Jaïs P, et al. Electrophysiological breakthrough from the left atrium to the pulmonary veins. *Circulation.* 2000;102;2463–2465.
4. Pappone C, Oreto G, Rosanio S, et al. Atrial electroanatomic remodeling after circumferential radiofrequency pulmonary vein ablation: efficacy of an anatomical approach in a large cohort of patients with atrial fibrillation. *Circulation.* 2001;104:2539–2544.
5. Harken O, Scharf C, Chugh A, et al. Catheter ablation for paroxysmal atrial fibrillation: segmental pulmonary vein ostial ablation versus left atrial ablation. *Circulation.* 2003;108:2355–2360.
6. Marrouche NF, Martin DO, Wazni O, et al. Phased-array intracardiac echocardiography monitoring during pulmonary vein isolation in patients with atrial fibrillation: impact on outcome and complications. *Circulation.* 2003;107:2710–2716.
7. Nademanee K, McKenzie J, Kosar E, et al. A new approach for catheter ablation of atrial fibrillation: mapping of the electrophysiologic substrate. *J Am Coll Cardiol.* 2004;43:2044–2053.
8. O'Neill MD, Jaïs P, Takahashi Y, et al. The stepwise ablation approach for chronic atrial fibrillation-evidence for a cumulative effect. *J Interv Card Electrophysiol.* 2006; 16:153–167.
9. Nakagawa H, Jackman WM, Scherlag BJ, et al. Relationship of complex fractionated atrial electrograms during atrial

fibrillation to the location of cardiac autonomic ganglionated plexi in patients with atrial fibrillation. *Circulation.* 2005; 112:II–746. Abstract
10. Nakagawa H, Scherlag BJ, Patterson E, et al. Pathophysiologic basis of autonomic ganglionated pelxus ablation in patients with atrial fibrillation. *Heart Rhythm.* 2009;6:S26–S34.
11. Nakagawa H, Yokoyama K, Scherlag BJ, et al. Ablation of autonomic ganglia. Pp. 218–230 in Calkins H, Jaïs P, Steinberg JS, eds. *A Practical Approach to Catheter Ablation of Atrial Fibrillation.* Philadelphia, PA: Wolters Kluwer/Lippincott Williams & Wilkins, 2008.
12. Armour JA, Hageman GR, Randall WC. Arrhythmias induced by local cardiac nerve stimulation. *Am J Physiol.* 1972;223:1068–1075.
13. Sharifov OF, Fedorov VV, Beloshajeko GG, et al. Roles of adrenergic and cholinergic stimulation in spontaneous atrial fibrillation in dogs. *J Am Coll Cardiol.* 2004;43:483–490.
14. Scherlag BJ, Yamanashi WS, Patel U, et al. Autonomically induced conversion of pulmonary vein focal firing into atrial fibrillation. *J Am Coll Cardiol.* 2005;45:1575–1880.
15. Scherlag BJ, Nakagawa H, Jackman WM, et al. Electrical stimulation to identify neural elements on the heart: their role in atrial fibrillation. *J Interv Electrophysiol.* 2005;13:37–42.
16. Patterson E, Po SS, Scherlag BJ, et al. Triggered firing in pulmonary veins initiated by in vitro autonomic nerve stimulation. *Heart Rhythm.* 2005;2:624–631.
17. Patterson E, Lazzara R, Szabo B, et al. Sodium-calcium exchange initiated by the Ca2+ transient: an arrhythmia trigger within pulmonary veins. *J Am Coll Cardiol.* 2006;47:1196–1206
18. Po SS, Scherlag BJ, Yamanashi, et al. Experimental model for paroxysmal atrial fibrillation arising at the pulmonary vein-atrial junctions. *Heart Rhythm.* 2006;3:201–208.
19. Lin J, Scherlag BJ, Zhou J, et al. Autonomic mechanism to explain complex fractionated atrial electrograms (CFAE). *J Cardiovasc Electrophysiol.* 2007;18:1197–1205.
20. Lemola K, Chartier D, Yeh YH, et al. Pulmonary vein region ablation in experimental vagal atrial fibrillation: role of pulmonary veins versus autonomic ganglia. *Circulation.* 2008;117:470–477.
21. Lin J, Scherlag BJ, Lu Z, et al. Inducibility of atrial and ventricular arrhythmias along the ligament of Marshall: role of autonomic factors. *J Cardiovasc Electrophysiol.* 2008;9:955–962.
22. Armour JA, Yuan BX, Macdonald S, et al. Gross and microscopic anatomy of the human intrinsic cardiac nervous system. *Anat Rec.* 1997;247:289–298.
23. Pauza DH, Skripka V, Pauziene N, et al. Morphology, distribution, and variability of the epicardiac neural ganglionated subplexuses in the human heart. *Anat Rec.* 2000;259:353–382.
24. Hou YL, Scherlag BJ, Lin J, et al. Interactive atrial neural network: determining the connection between ganglionated plexi. *Heart Rhythm.* 2007;4:56–63.
25. Macle L, Jaïs P, Scavee C, et al. Electrophysiologically guided pulmonary vein isolation during sustained atrial fibrillation. *J Cardiovasc Electrophysiol.* 2003;14:255–260.
26. Niu G, Scherlag BJ, Lu Z, et al. An acute experimental model demonstrating 2 different forms of sustained atrial tachyarrhythmias. *Circ Arrhythm Electrophysiol.* 2009;2:384–392.

CHAPTER 27

How to Use Electroanatomic Mapping to Rapidly Diagnose and Treat Post–AF Ablation Atrial Tachycardia and Flutter

Aman Chugh, MD[1]

Introduction

Patients who undergo catheter ablation of AF may develop AT during follow-up, which may require a repeat ablation procedure. These tachycardias may arise from the LA, RA, and also the CS. Unlike CTI-dependent AFL, which can be readily recognized based on its stereotypical features and can be eliminated in virtually every patient without significant difficulty, mapping and ablation of postablation AT remains challenging. The reasons for this include lack of specific ECG clues, the diversity of mechanisms, and sites of origin. Nonetheless, these tachycardias can be eliminated in the vast majority of patients. This chapter will offer a practical approach to mapping these tachycardias using electroanatomic mapping.

Preprocedure Planning

The planning phase in some ways has its beginnings at the initial consultation for consideration of AF ablation. We discuss with patients, particularly those with persistent AF, that they may require a repeat ablation procedure for AT. The referring physicians are also included in this discussion, since they are part of the team that will be managing the patients even after the procedure. Approximately 50% of patients will require a repeat procedure after an ablation procedure for persistent AF. Not uncommonly, patients may develop AT shortly after LA ablation for persistent AF. However, these patients should not necessarily be committed to a repeat procedure since in some patients, the AT may be a transient finding. In our practice, all patients with a recurrence within the first few months after an ablation procedure undergo transthoracic cardioversion or are treated medically in case of paroxysmal AT. If the arrhythmia then recurs, then we consider a catheter ablation procedure. Most patients elect to undergo a repeat ablation procedure as opposed to taking antiarrhythmic therapy because many patients have either failed medical therapy for AF and/or wish to be arrhythmia free without the need for long-term rhythm-controlling medications and anticoagulation.

If patients were taking antiarrhythmic medications to suppress the arrhythmia while waiting for the procedure, these medications should be discontinued at least 5 half-lives before the procedure. Amiodarone should be discontinued at least 2 months before the procedure. In patients with paroxysmal AT, we typically discontinue the rhythm-controlling medications, except for amiodarone, about 4 to 6 weeks prior the procedure to increase the

---

1. Disclosures: Supported in part by the Leducq Transatlantic Network.

chance of arrhythmia recurrence. Ideally, the ablation procedure for AT should be performed during the arrhythmia. In some patients, AT may not be inducible in the EP laboratory despite isoproterenol infusion and an aggressive induction protocol. An empiric ablation strategy in such an instance may not eliminate the culprit arrhythmia, leading to recurrence.

Rate-controlling medications are usually discontinued a few days prior to the procedure. For patients with persistent AT, this may be associated with improvement in AV nodal conduction. In most patients, transient tachycardia is reasonably well tolerated. However, in others, abrupt discontinuation of rate-controlling medications may be associated with 1:1 AV nodal conduction during AT, leading to hemodynamic compromise. These patients may require urgent cardioversion, which of course helps alleviate the acute symptoms but also results in interruption of the tachycardia, which may not be inducible in the EP laboratory. To guard against this possibility, patients who are known to have very facile AV nodal conduction are admitted to the hospital on the day prior to the procedure for washout of cardiac medications. If they develop tachycardia, then intravenous rate-controlling medications can be used in a monitored setting. These medications can then be discontinued a few hours before the procedure.

Our preference is to perform LA ablation procedures on therapeutic oral anticoagulation with warfarin. This has been shown to be safe and is probably associated with not only a lower risk of thromboembolic complications but also decreased prevalence of access-site complications. The decision to perform TEE to rule out thrombus is individualized. In patients with therapeutic international normalized ratio, without significant structural heart disease and present in sinus rhythm, TEE may be deferred. Patients presenting in AT routinely undergo TEE prior to the procedure. Patients with significant structural heart disease (eg, severe left ventricular dysfunction or severe LA enlargement (> 5.5 cm) or atrial myopathy or delayed activation of the LAA noted during a prior procedure) should probably undergo TEE irrespective of their presenting rhythm or anticoagulation status.

CT or MRI may have a role in the management of a patient presenting for an AT procedure. In most instances, preprocedure imaging is obtained to evaluate for variant PV anatomy. However, this information is unlikely to alter the approach to the patient with AT. The course of the circumflex or the sinus nodal artery may influence the operator's decision to perform prophylactic linear ablation at the mitral isthmus and the LA roof, respectively (see below). The anatomy of the coronary branches may be difficult to interpret on imaging studies for most electrophysiologists and consultation with a cardiothoracic radiologist may be needed.

Mapping and Ablation of Postablation AT

Venous and LA Access

A minimum of two catheters is required for a repeat procedure for postablation ATs. Occasionally, patients presenting for a repeat procedure may have significant soft tissue resistance or scarring over the femoral vessels, making it challenging to utilize 3 sheaths within an ipsilateral femoral vein. In this circumstance, the operator has the option to simply use 2 sheaths or obtain venous access on the contralateral side. Our practice is to use 2 sheaths, especially in female patients or those with small stature, to minimize the risk of vascular complications. LA access may also be challenging owing to a thickened interatrial septum secondary to repeat transseptal punctures. In such an instance, the transseptal puncture may be performed using RF energy applied at the tip of the needle.

P-Wave Morphology

Prior to performing detailed mapping, it is helpful to review the P-wave morphology during AT on the ECG. Although the majority of postablation ATs arise from the LA, AFL from the CTI is frequently encountered. Negative flutter waves any of the precordial leads are consistent with a RA source (**Figure 27.1**).[1] Negative flutter waves in the inferior leads are also suggestive but less specific for a RA origin. The flutter waves may not be readily apparent during 2:1 AV nodal conduction. Ventricular pacing can help unmask the atrial activity. Adenosine can also help visualize the flutter waves but the fact it may result in AF or alter the tachycardia makes it less attractive. Identifying a RA origin probably does not preempt transseptal catheterization since documenting PVI after elimination of the tachycardia is critical in preventing recurrence. The ECG is also helpful in ruling out organized AF. During AT, the P-wave morphology should be consistent, owing to consistent atrial activation. During organized AF, the P-wave morphology should vary, even subtly, which should prompt mapping of AF.

Defining the Reference for Electroanatomic Mapping

A stable reference is required for both activation and entrainment mapping. Typically, a decapolar catheter is inserted into the CS for this purpose. During activation mapping, it is preferable to use the CS bipole with the largest atrial and smallest ventricular EGM. Rarely, the EGM amplitude of the CS EGM is extremely small or the catheter may not be stable within the CS. In this instance, the reference catheter can be placed in the RAA. Alternatively, a small-caliber electrode (Medtronic Model 6416) can be

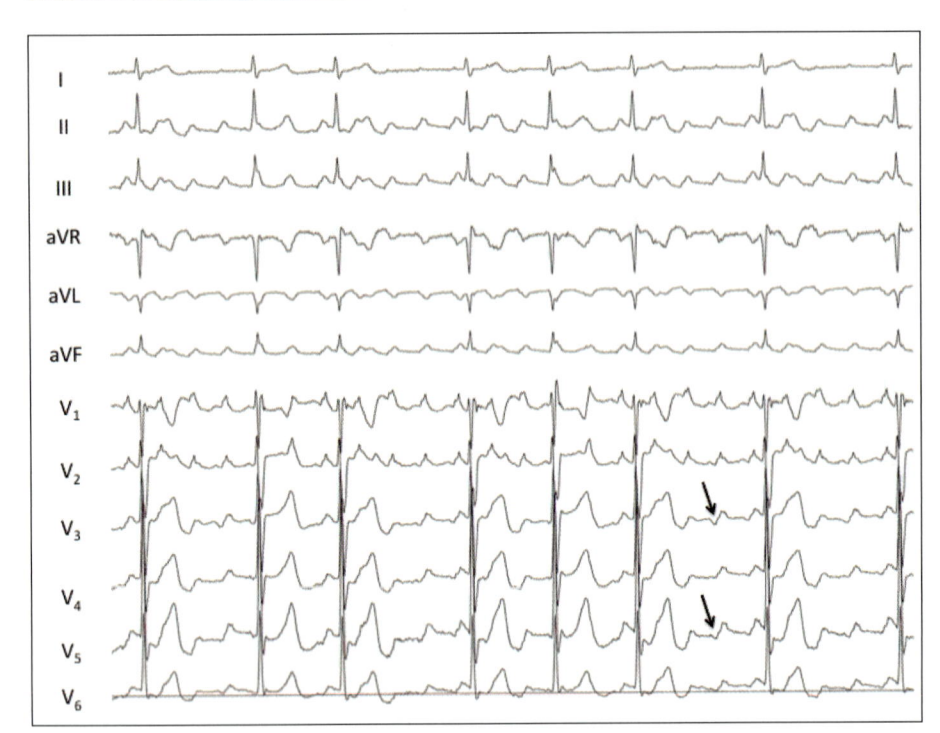

Figure 27.1 A 12-lead electrocardiogram (ECG) during counterclockwise, CTI-dependent AFL. The negative component of the flutter waves in the inferior leads is attenuated due to extensive LA ablation for atrial fibrillation. However, the initial negativitiy of the flutter waves in the precordial leads (arrows) is consistent with the diagnosis of typical flutter. Paper speed = 25 mm/s.

temporarily fixed in the RA, which may then serve as a reference. Either the CARTO (Biosense Webster, Diamond Grove, CA) or NAVX (St. Jude Medical, St. Paul, MN) system may be used for mapping of AT.

Creating the LA Shell

Unless the P-wave morphology is suggestive of an RA origin, we typically obtain LA access prior to RA mapping, since about 80% tachycardias are successfully ablated from the LA. Prior to creating an activation map, it is reasonable to obtain some geometry of the LA using a circular mapping catheter (Lasso, Biosense Webster) and a new-generation 3-dimensional mapping system (CARTO 3, Biosense Webster). This provides a much richer rendering of the PVs and the LA and can be achieved much more efficiently (< 1 minute) as compared with mapping with an ablation catheter (Thermocool, Biosense Webster).

Activation Mapping

It is important to document CL stability prior to constructing an activation map. Variability of more than 10% may be associated with a nonsensical activation pattern. The mechanism of these tachycardias is probably best explored by mapping the diastolic interval.

Prior to collecting activation data, the window of interest is defined on the 3-dimensional mapping system. There are a number of methods in defining the window of interest. A practical approach is to aim to cover approximately 90% of the TCL. For example, for an AT with a CL of 230 ms, the window is selected to span 210 ms. This interval is then divided in half, and values of −105 ms and 105 ms (before and after the reference, respectively) are entered to define the window of interest. One may also define the window based on the mechanism of the tachycardia, ie, focal versus macroreentrant. In the case of the former, the window of interest would be set to account for a fraction of the TCL. However, this presupposes the mechanism, which in itself may be problematic.

The window of interest may also be defined with respect to the P wave during tachycardia.[2] This helps to highlight the mid-diastolic isthmus. If the P wave is not apparent on the ECG (e.g., due to 2:1 AV block), ventricular pacing or adenosine is required to fully define the P wave. Although this method would not alter the ablation approach to macroreentrant tachycardias, it may be helpful in delineating the critical site in the setting of small reentrant circuits.

A point-by-point activation map is then constructed on the shell created by the circular mapping catheter. It is important to acquire each point during the end expiration, which avoids virtual anatomy created by catheter movement during the respiratory cycle. As the catheter is moved from point to point, additional geometry is acquired. The number of points that is needed to construct a map depends on several variables. Of course, larger atria require acquisition of more activation data in order to glean the mechanism of the tachycardia. A more detailed map may be required in patients with multiple areas of low-voltage/scar or conduction block. A higher-density map may also be required if the initial map does not yield an obvious diagnosis.

A critical step in constructing an activation map is properly assigning timing to each acquired point. Inconsistent annotation may lead to a nonsensical map and longer procedure times. The bipolar EGM recorded by the distal bipole of the mapping catheter is typically used to acquire activation data. Local activation is probably best defined by the peak of the bipolar EGM. When a point is selected, the mapping system automatically assigns timing by placing an annotation icon on the EGM within the window. However, the operator must verify the timing and may have to move the icon to the point on the EGM which best coincides with local activation.

With low-amplitude signals, it may difficult to identify true local activation. Differentiating far- from near-field signals may also be difficult. Pacing may help discern between near- and far-field potentials; however, it may alter or terminate the tachycardia. Adjudicating local activation timing to fractionated or split EGMs may also be challenging. In this case, it is best to be consistent and revisit these sites after completion of the map to ensure that the EGMs were correctly annotated. If EGMs consistently span beyond the window of interest, it is possible that the window was not defined appropriately or that there is significant CL variation. If a small part of the EGM does span beyond the window, it is reasonable to assign timing to the earliest or the latest portion of the EGM *within* the window of interest. It is important to be consistent in annotating EGMs; otherwise one will end up with a meaningless map.

While creating an activation map, it is helpful to accurately define anatomic obstacles, which will serve as anchors to linear lesions. Areas without appreciable electrical activity should be tagged as "scar." Sites of conduction block, defined as widely split potentials that are separated by an isoelectric interval, should be tagged as "double potentials." The mitral and tricuspid annuli should be accurately depicted. Not uncommonly, one may encounter fractionated, long-duration EGMs early during the mapping procedure, and it may be tempting to perform entrainment mapping at or even ablate such an "attractive" site. However, it is best to construct the map and understand the mechanism of the tachycardia prior to entrainment mapping and ablation.

Classically, an activation map during macroreentrant tachycardias should reveal an early-meets-late pattern (areas color coded as red (early) and purple (late) adjacent to each other). In addition, mapping should account for nearly the entire CL of the tachycardia. Otherwise one should suspect an origin from the contralateral chamber or the CS. It is important to bear in mind that in a large reentrant circuit, there are no absolute early or late areas, and are only deemed such with respect to an arbitrary reference. To target the "early" area on such a map with RF energy would be the wrong approach. One first confirms the mechanism with entrainment mapping and then identifies anatomical barriers to which the linear lesion is anchored. Other mechanisms include a small reentrant circuit, which is relegated to only one segment of the LA, eg, anterior or posterior walls, but not both (see below). An activation map during a small reentrant AT may demonstrate an early-meets-late pattern (see below). For focal tachycardias, one should observe a centrifugal activation from the point of origin (red followed by yellow, green, blue, and purple). Despite sampling the entire chamber of origin, only a fraction of the CL may be covered.

Prior to commencing with ablation, it is critical that one understand the mechanism of the tachycardia. It must be borne in mind that patients presenting for AT have previously undergone an extensive ablation procedure for persistent AF, including ablation of PV antra, complex, fractionated EGMs, and lines at the roof and/or mitral isthmus. Thus, one should expect to encounter areas of scar, slow conduction, and conduction block. These findings may obfuscate the activation patterns, leading to nonsensical maps. This is why it is good practice to confirm the findings of activation mapping with entrainment mapping.

LA Macroreentrant ATs

Mitral Isthmus–Dependent AFL

The most common macroreentrant AT after catheter ablation of AF is mitral isthmus–dependent AFL.[3] The mitral isthmus is defined as the region between the lateral mitral annulus and the left-sided PVs. Perimitral flutter is usually seen after prior linear ablation at the mitral isthmus, but it may also be encountered even without prior ablation in this region. In contradistinction to typical AFL, which is predominantly due to counterclockwise activation (around the tricuspid valve), mitral isthmus–dependent flutter is equally likely to be due to clockwise or counterclockwise activation around the mitral valve. The following criteria are required for the diagnosis of perimitral flutter: activation mapping accounts for entire CL of the tachycardia; the activation map shows an early-meets-late pattern around the mitral valve (**Figure 27.2**); and entrainment mapping at any point around the valve reveals a postpacing interval (PPI) within 20 to 30 ms of the TCL (**Figure 27.3**). (Note: If only entrainment mapping is utilized, PPIs within 20 to 30 ms of the TCL, from opposite, eg, lateral and septal aspects of the mitral annulus, confirm the diagnosis.)

Linear ablation is commenced from the lateral annulus and extended to the anterior aspect of the left-sided PVs. In about 20% of patients, a pouch is present at the lateral mitral isthmus, making it difficult to deliver RF energy to the region.[3] If the catheter consistently "skips" during catheter pullback from the lateral annulus, a pouch is likely present. The real-time impedance profile during ablation may also suggest the presence of a pouch. In such a case, it is reasonable to extend the line from the posterolateral or even anterolateral annulus. Typically, high power (35 W of irrigated RF energy) is required during endocardial ablation of the mitral isthmus.

Frequently, endocardial ablation fails to terminate the tachycardia. Epicardial ablation within the CS is required in about two-thirds of the cases to terminate perimitral flutter and/or achieve bidirectional block at the isthmus (**Figure 27.4**). The ablation catheter is advanced into the distal CS to the level of the endocardial line. Prior to commencing with RF energy, the catheter is torqued toward the atrial side to avoid power delivery within a ventricular branch, which is more likely to be associated with arterial injury. If a large ventricular EGM is present on the distal bipole of the ablation catheter, it is useful to perform high-out pacing to rule out ventricular capture.

During RF energy delivery within the CS, the power is reduced to 20 W, and the catheter is withdrawn slowly to the mid CS. If the tachycardia does not terminate, the process is repeated until the local atrial EGM is abolished. While ablating in the CS, it is critical to follow the impedance/temperature curves to monitor for overheating or catheter dislodgement into a ventricular branch. The latter will be associated with a sudden impedance rise. If after several attempts there is no slowing of the tachycardia or change in the activation sequence/P-wave morphology, it is useful to perform entrainment mapping to make sure one is still dealing with the same tachycardia (see "Multi-Loop ATs" below).

After tachycardia termination (**Figure 27.4**), the next step is to demonstrate linear block at the mitral isthmus. This may be accomplished either during pacing from the proximal CS (**Figure 27.5**) or the LAA (**Figure 27.6**). We typically place the ring catheter at the base of the LAA and observe for an abrupt change in activation during RF energy delivery. In the absence of conduction block, pacing from the LAA results in distal-to-proximal activation of the CS. When conduction block is achieved, there is a sudden change in the activation sequence to proximal-to-distal. Pacing from multiple bipoles of the CS catheter is helpful in ruling out slow conduction and confirming bidirectional block (**Figure 27.7**). Bidirectional block across the mitral isthmus can be achieved in up to 90% of patients, but it may be quite challenging in some. The most likely reason for the inability to create complete mitral isthmus block is the presence of the circumflex artery, interposed between the CS and the epicardial isthmus.[4] The artery likely acts as a heat sink, preventing adequate heating of the mitral isthmus. Herein lies the possibility of injury to the circumflex artery. If block cannot be achieved, the next step is to repeat RF energy delivery, perhaps using higher power. Since the interposition of the circumflex is the likely reason for lack of success, additional attempts, especially if using higher power, may not only fail to yield block but may also increase the risk of arterial injury.

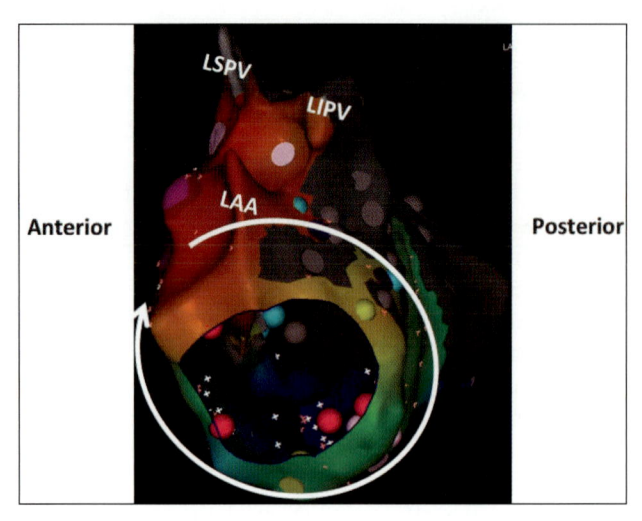

Figure 27.2 An activation map during clockwise mitral isthmus–dependent AFL in a left anterior oblique (LAO) view. The gold tags refer to sites that afforded perfect return cycles during entrainment mapping (see Figure 27.3). LSPV = left superior pulmonary vein. LIPV = left inferior pulmonary vein. LAA = left atrial appendage.

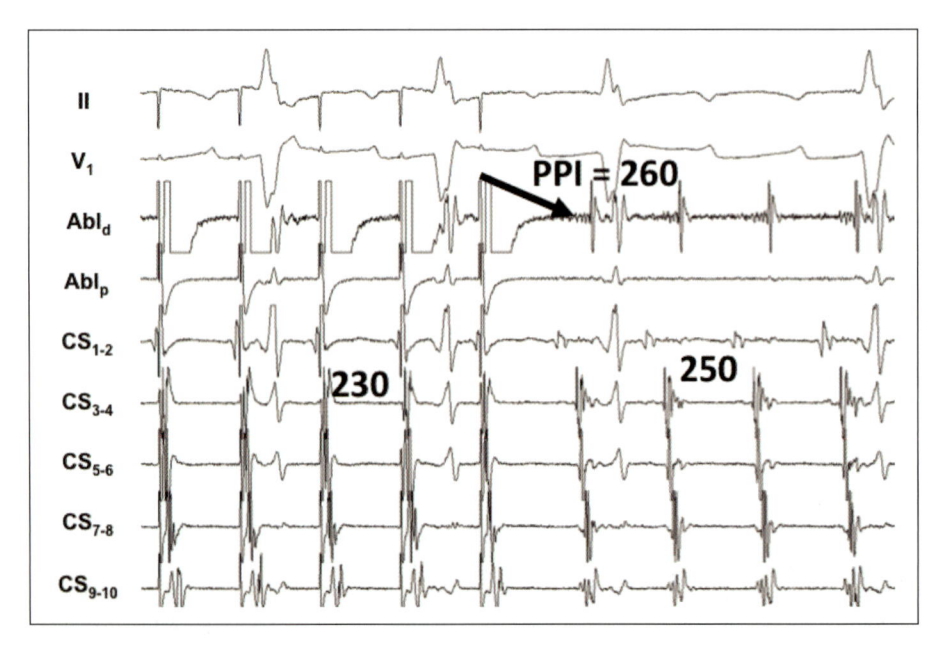

Figure 27.3 Entrainment mapping from the mitral isthmus from the same patients as shown in Figure 27.2. The tachycardia is accelerated to the pacing rate (230 ms). Upon cessation of pacing, the postpacing interval (PPI) approximates the TCL (250 ms), confirming the diagnosis of perimitral flutter. Note that the initial portion of the EGM recorded by the distal bipole of the ablation (Abl) catheter is very fractionated. CS = CS.

Figure 27.4 (Continuation of Figure 27.3.) Termination of perimitral flutter during RF (RF) energy delivery within the distal CS. LA = left atrial.

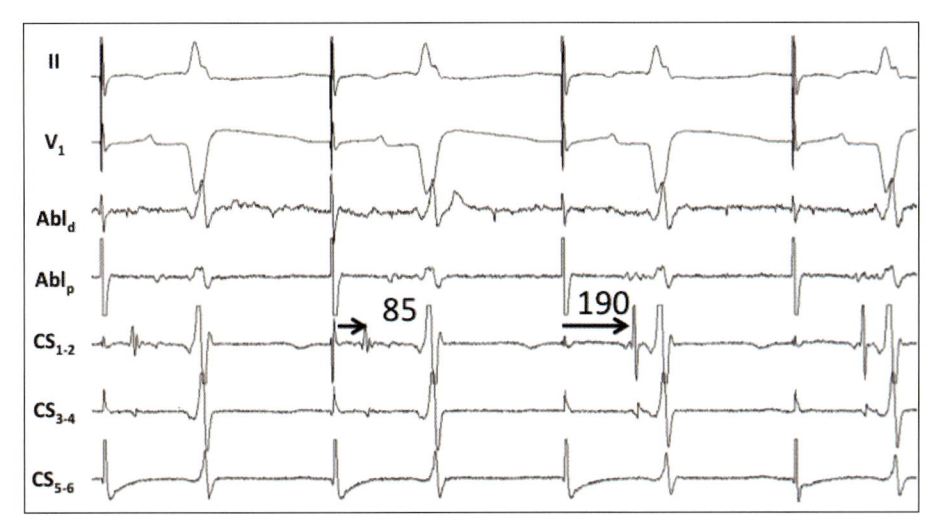

Figure 27.5 (Continuation of Figure 27.4.) Demonstration of linear block across the mitral isthmus during RF energy delivery within the distal CS and during proximal CS pacing. Note the sudden increase in the stimulus-atrial EGM interval from 85 ms to 190 ms. Pacing from the LAA showed proximal-to-distal activation of the CS, confirming linear block at the mitral isthmus (not shown).

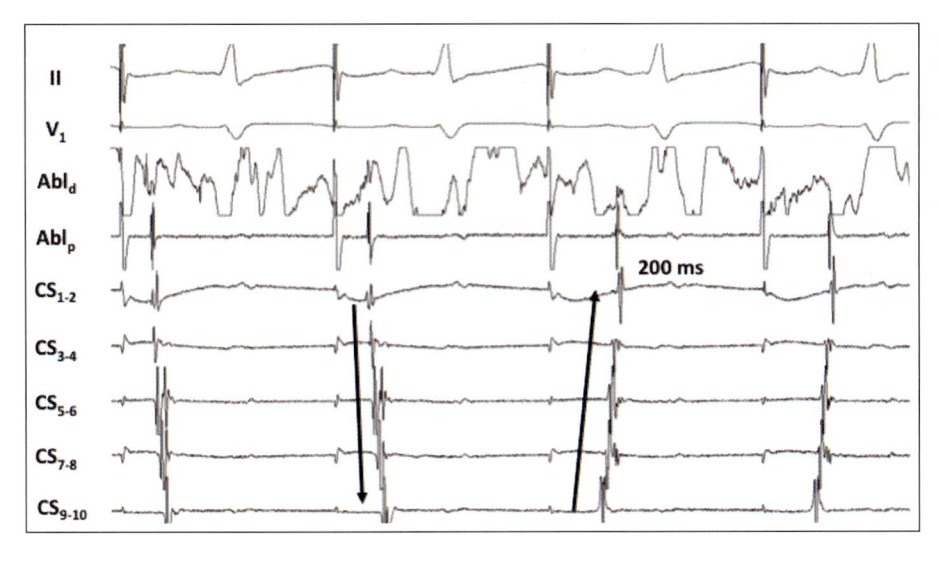

Figure 27.6 Demonstration of conduction block at the mitral isthmus during RF energy delivery in the distal CS and LAA pacing. Note the abrupt change in the sequence of CS activation, from distal to proximal to proximal to distal.

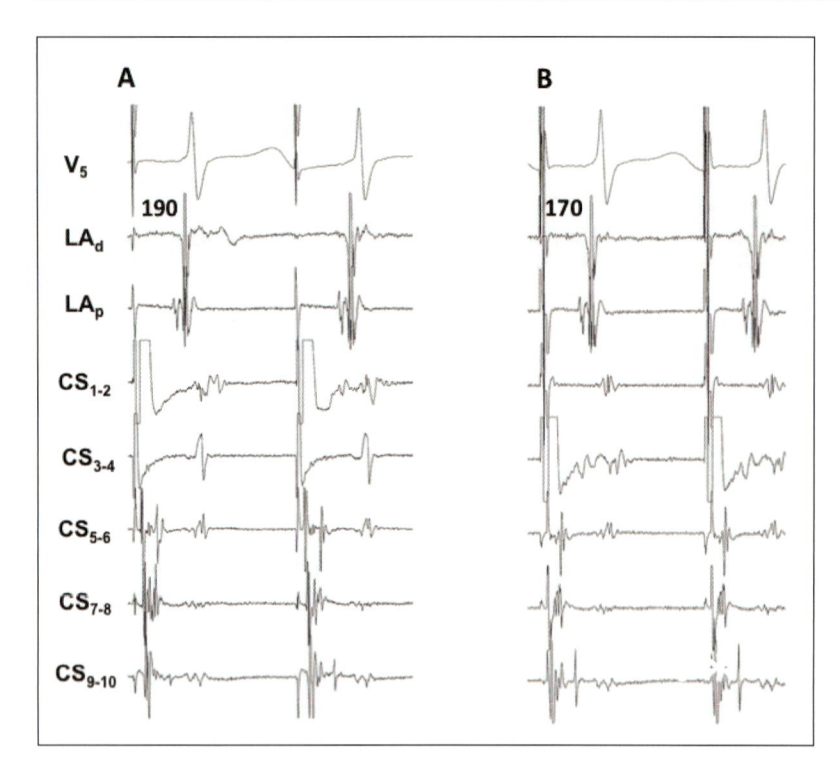

Figure 27.7 Differential pacing to confirm mitral isthmus block. Pacing from the distal bipole (CS_{1-2}) in panel A results in a longer stimulus-atrial EGM interval than pacing from a proximal bipole (CS_{3-4}), ruling out slow conduction and confirming bidirectional block at the isthmus. The numbers refer to activation delay (in milliseconds) from the CS to the LA mapping catheter placed anterior to the ablation line.

Three-dimensional mapping is advantageous in the mapping and ablation of perimitral AFL for a number of reasons. First, it helps reduce to exposure to ionizing radiation, since catheter navigation across the isthmus may be performed without continuous fluoroscopy. "Tagging" the line with ablation points helps insure lesion continuity and prevent gaps in the line. Second, one is able to readily identify the endocardial linear lesion, which helps to determine the starting point of epicardial ablation within the distal CS (**Figure 27.8**). During energy delivery in the CS, the ability to follow the temperature and impedance curves may also be helpful in prevent complications such as perforation and inadvertent energy delivery in a ventricular branch.

Roof-Dependent Macroreentry

After the mitral isthmus, the roof is the second most common site of LA macroreentry after catheter ablation of AF. The wavefront may revolve around either left- or right-sided PVs and in either direction (**Figures 27.9** and **27.10**). One may also encounter more uncommon activation patterns, such as a double-loop tachycardia (one around each of the upper PVs) during which the two loops intersect at the roof. CS activation may either be proximal to distal or distal to proximal, depending on the exit site. Entrainment mapping will show good return cycles along the entire circumference of the macroreentrant loop, ie, anterior and posterior LA, inferior LA/mid CS regions, and of course, the myocardium at the roof, between the upper PVs. RF energy (25 W) is delivered at the most cranial aspect of the roof, connecting the two upper PVs. If the initial attempt

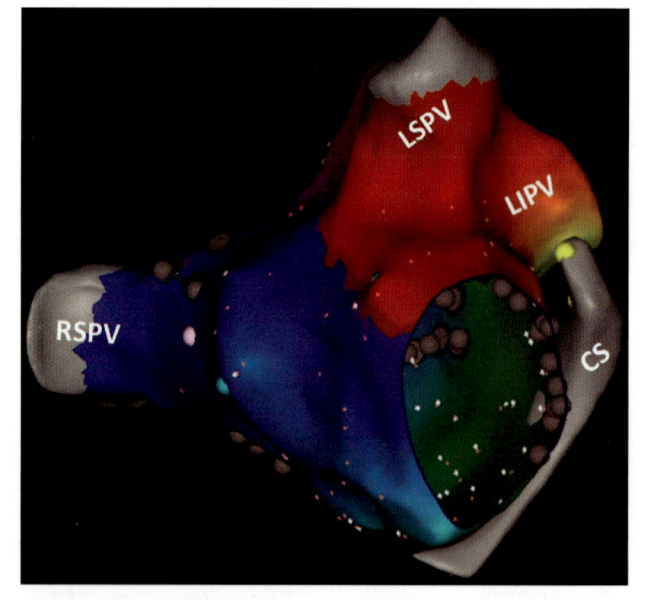

Figure 27.8 Relationship of the mitral isthmus and the CS shown in a shallow LAO view. In this patient, there were no appreciable EGMs on the endocardial aspect of the isthmus (gray tags), prompting RF energy delivery within the distal CS. The lower yellow tag in the CS, seen tangentially, represents the site at which RF energy terminated perimitral AT. The more superior tag denotes the site at which RF energy delivery resulted in complete bidirectional block. The appendage is not seen, as it had been oversewn at the time of arrhythmia surgery. The time required to construct this activation map utilizing more than 100 points was 20 minutes. RSPV = right superior pulmonary vein.

is unsuccessful, the next step is to try a bit more posterior or anterior to the initial line. If a more posterior line is chosen, the operator has to account for the esophagus.

Figure 27.9 An example of a macroreentrant AT utilizing the LA roof seen in a right lateral view. The gold tag represents the site which afforded an excellent return cycle during entrainment mapping (see Figure 27.10).

electrical silence at the roof, a corridor of double potentials during LAA pacing.

Linear block is easier to achieve at the LA roof than at the mitral isthmus and may be demonstrated in about 90% of patients. In some cases, however, linear block may be impossible to attain (or, perhaps, demonstrate) despite extensive ablation and voltage abatement at the roof and anterior and posterior to the line. A recent study suggests that the course of the left-sided sinus nodal artery may act as a heat sink as it courses at the roof or the high anterior LA and may hinder linear ablation at the roof.[5]

Using a 3-dimensional mapping system to guide linear ablation at the LA roof can be very helpful. First, it facilitates ideal lesion placement at the cranial aspect of the roof. One advantage of this approach as compared to a more anterior or posterior line is catheter stability. Further, this approach requires very little fluoroscopy. Utilizing 3-dimensional mapping can also guide the alternative anterior or posterior LA ablation in case of failure of the initial linear lesion. Fluoroscopy alone does not afford this level of resolution. Lastly, limited activation mapping using a 3-dimensional mapping can help discriminate between incomplete and complete roof ablation. Whether the posterior LA is activated in a descending or ascending fashion can be determined by collecting just a few activation points on the posterior LA during LAA pacing or sinus rhythm.

Catheter stability with a more anterior approach may be suboptimal and therefore calls for slightly higher power (30 W). After tachycardia termination (**Figure 27.11**), the completeness of the line is analyzed during LAA pacing or sinus rhythm. During RF energy delivery, one may observe a sudden appearance of a double potential (**Figure 27.12**), consistent with linear block at the roof. This may be confirmed with activation mapping. With intact conduction across the roof, there is descending activation of the posterior LA (**Figure 27.13**). After the roof line has been completed, the sinus rhythm or the paced (from the LAA) wavefront blocks at the roof, and the posterior LA must be activated in an ascending fashion (**Figure 27.14**). Additionally, one may be able to document, barring

Other Macroreentrant ATs

The mitral isthmus and the roof account for the majority of LA macroreentrant ATs after catheter ablation of AF. After elimination of these isthmi, one may encounter macroreentry from other sites such as the anterior LA and the LAA. In case of the former, linear ablation is commenced from the anterior mitral annulus toward the RSPV. Frequently, these tachycardias will terminate during RF

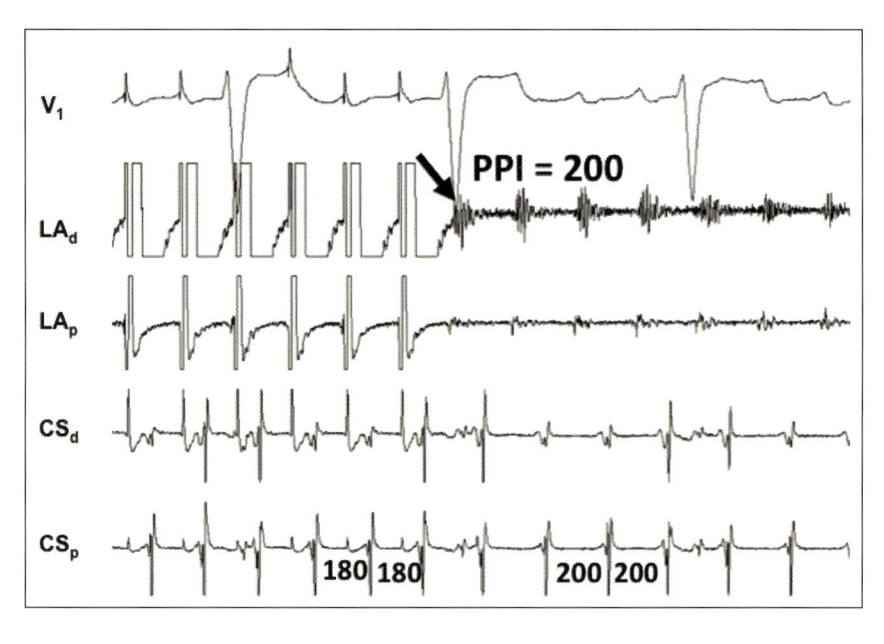

Figure 27.10 Entrainment mapping from the same patient as shown in Figure 27.9. The tachycardia is accelerated to the pacing rate (180 ms) and the PPI matches the TCL, confirming that the pacing site is a critical component of the reentry circuit.

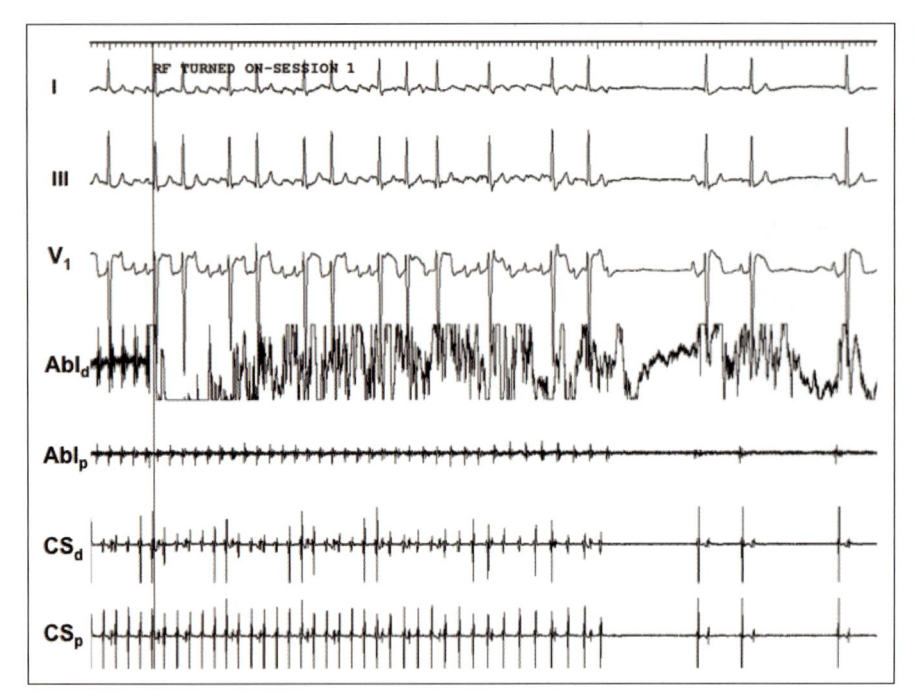

Figure 27.11 (Continuation of Figure 27.10.) A single RF lesion at the site shown in Figures 27.10 and 27.11 terminated the tachycardia to sinus rhythm.

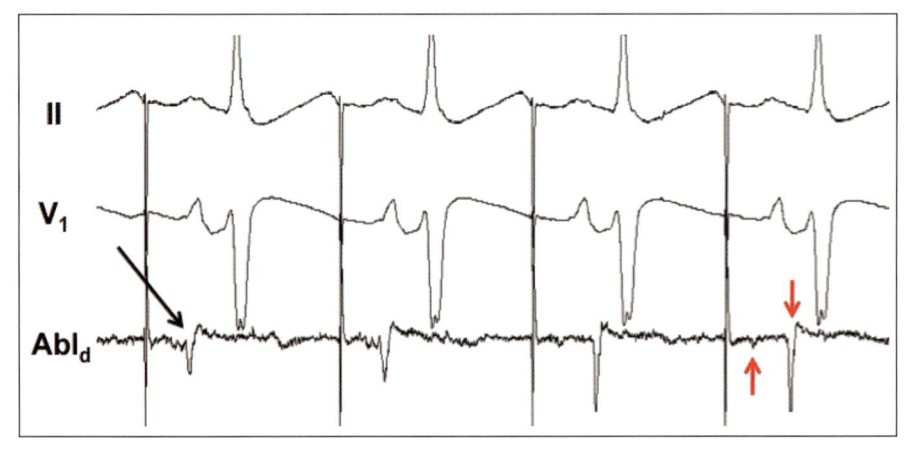

Figure 27.12 Achievement of linear block at the roof during RF energy delivery. During pacing from the LAA, a fractionated EGM (black arrow) was recorded at the mid roof. RF energy delivery at this site led to the sudden appearance of widely split double potentials (red arrows), consistent with linear block at the LA roof.

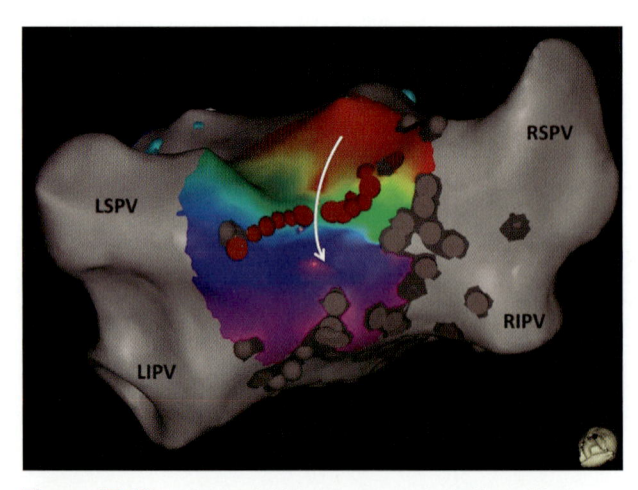

Figure 27.13 After an initial attempt to obtain linear block at the roof, there was evidence of descending activation of the posterior LA during sinus rhythm. This implies that there is conduction across the roof and the line is incomplete.

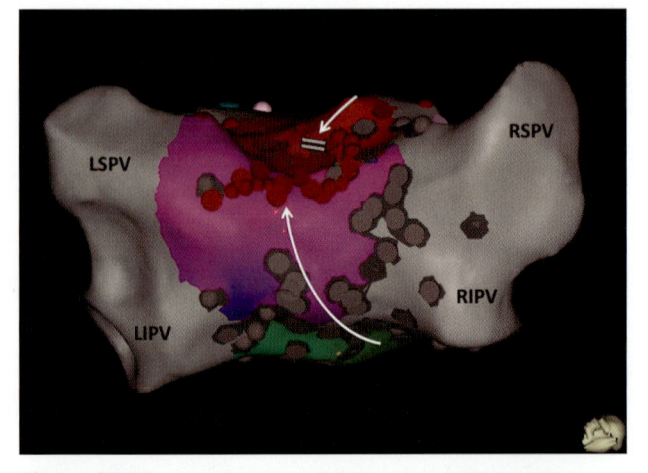

Figure 27.14 (Continuation of Figure 27.13.) After further ablation at the high anterior wall, the sinus rhythm wavefront now blocks at the roof, and as a result, the posterior LA is activated in an ascending fashion, confirming linear block at the roof.

energy delivery in the region of Bachmann's bundle (antero-superior LA, outside the RSPV). However, high power (35 W) may be required, which implies that the portion of the circuit may involve the epicardium. With high-power energy delivery, there is a risk of injury to the sinus nodal artery if it arises from the left circumflex. Occasionally, complete elimination of these tachycardia may require ablation at the septal aspect of the RAA. Recall that Bachmann's bundle in essence connects the right and left atrial appendages. Therefore, in some cases, RF energy delivery may be required over the entire course of this connection. Since a component of the macroreentrant ATs involving of the Bachmann's bundle tachycardias is likely to be epicardial, endocardial ablation may fail to terminate the tachycardia. Thus, complete elimination of these tachycardias may require a formal epicardial approach in some patients.

Ideally, the endpoint of ablation of macroreentrant ATs is demonstration of linear block and not just tachycardia termination. However, this may be difficult to achieve or show and may not be desirable with respect to ATs involving the anterior LA. Transecting the anterior LA has important implications with respect to the mechanical function of the LA. Since patients presenting for a repeat procedure for AT have already undergone extensive ablation of the posterior LA (for PVI), LA systolic function is critically dependent on the integrity of the anterior LA. Also, extensive ablation of the anterior wall often involves ablation in the region of Bachmann's bundle. Ablation of this structure, especially in the context of prior procedures or preexistent atrial myopathy, may lead to interatrial disconnection or even isolation of the LAA. Lastly, there is also a chance of injury to the AV node if ablation is also required at the low atrial septum, adjacent to the mitral annulus.

Multi-Loop ATs

A multi-loop tachycardia is defined as a tachycardia that requires ablation of multiple isthmi or target sites prior to termination. These tachycardias may be found in about 20% of patients presenting for a procedure for AT.[2] The multiple loops may be engaged simultaneously or may be encountered sequentially. Frequently, despite extensive ablation at the initial isthmus, there is no change in atrial activation, CL, or P-wave morphology. The only clue is a change in PPIs, that is, a long PPI from a site that afforded excellent return cycles prior to ablation. Because each isthmus (eg, mitral, LA roof, cavotricuspid isthmus) requires dedicated ablation and demonstration of linear block at each, these procedures can be quite long (**Figure 27.15**). Since resumption of conduction may occur any of the multiple lines, patients presenting with a multi-loop AT may be more likely to recur than those with a single isthmus.

Small-Reentrant ATs

After ruling out macroreentry, the operator should consider the possibility of small-reentrant ATs. In contradistinction to macroreentrant ATs, these tachycardias are confined to a discrete segment of the LA, eg, either anterior or posterior walls, but not both, which would be case during roof-dependent macroreentry. The diameter of these circuits is on the order of a few centimeters, which is much smaller than that of macro-reentrant circuits but larger than that of focal tachycardias (see below). With careful mapping, one should be able to account for the majority of the TCL. Frequently, activation mapping may account for nearly all of the TCL. This by itself should not be considered diagnostic of macroreentry, as the presence of areas with conduction block and slow conduction, which is requisite

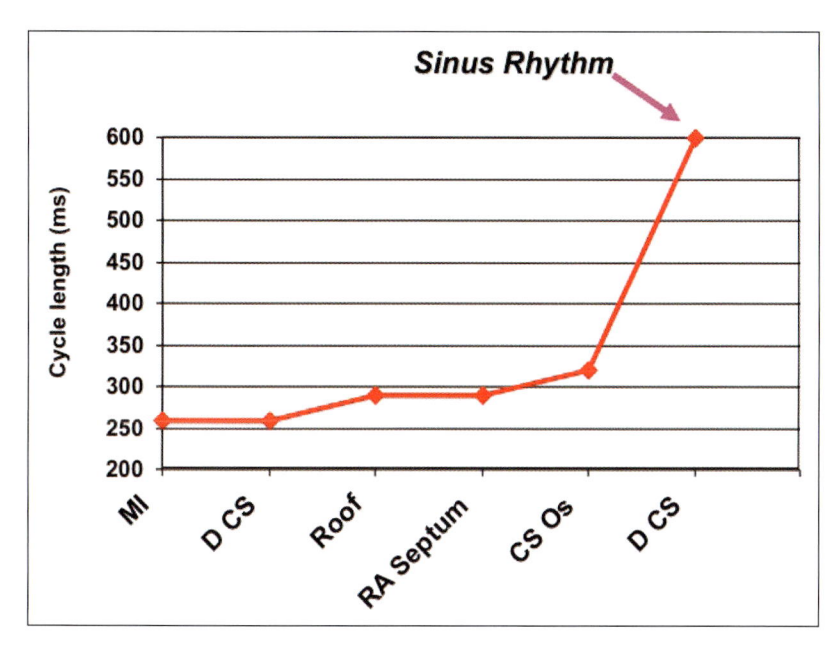

Figure 27.15 An example of target sites that required ablation prior to termination of a multi-loop AT to sinus rhythm. Note that prior to repeat ablation within the distal CS, there was little change in the CL of the tachycardia. Despite the existence of multiple isthmi, there was no change in the P-wave morphology or atrial activation throughout the procedure. RA = right atrial.

for the formation of small reentrant circuits, may be responsible for this finding. As a result of areas of conduction slowing or block, a classic early-meets-late pattern may or may not be observed and a nonsensical activation pattern may be the result.

An important diagnostic feature of small-reentrant circuits is the presence of fractionated EGMs at the critical site that account for a significant portion of the TCL. The long-duration EGMs are inscribed due to the extremely slow conduction at the culprit site (**Figure 27.16**). Entrainment mapping at the critical site will reveal excellent return cycle over the circumference of the circuit. The remaining atrial myocardium will be activated passively, and hence these tachycardias, along with focal tachycardias, are categorized as "centrifugal."[6] This centrifugal spread may not be obvious on the activation map in the presence of slow conduction/conduction block at adjacent sites. Entrainment mapping at sites even a short distance away from the circuit may reveal very long return cycles, which is another distinguishing feature of small reentrant circuits. Such behavior is not seen with macroreentrant ATs.

Occasionally entrainment mapping may slow or terminate small reentrant ATs owing to the presence of extremely slow conduction along the circuit. They are also vulnerable to mechanical termination during mapping. Tagging sites on the 3-dimensional map at which entrainment mapping or mechanical trauma changed or terminated tachycardia allows the operator to identify and ablate these sites despite alteration of the tachycardia. The endpoint of ablation of these small circuits is tachycardia termination during RF energy delivery and noninducibility.

Small-reentrant ATs may originate from numerous LA and RA sites. These include the base of the LAA, the anterior LA, septum, the perivenous atrial myocardium outside the PVs, the posterior and inferior LA, the CS, and the region bounded by the CS ostium and the eustachian ridge.

These tachycardias respond readily to RF energy delivery (25–30 W) owing to presence of atrial uncoupling and markedly slow conduction at the critical site (Figure 27.16).

Focal ATs

Focal ATs originate from a discrete site within the LA or RA. Focal ATs may be due to microreentry, triggered activity, or abnormal automaticity. Activation mapping using a 3-dimensional mapping system reveals centrifugal activation from a point source (**Figure 27.17**). In the case of a focal mechanism, mapping the entire chamber of origin will not be able to account for the entire CL. The reason is that the CL of the tachycardia is usually longer than the time required for complete activation of the chamber. It is important to note that in the presence slow conduction or conduction block, the time required to activate the chamber of origin may be significantly longer, which may falsely suggest the presence of macroreentry.

Simply noting centrifugal activation on the activation map is not enough to establish the mechanism and commence with RF energy delivery. In the case of a focal mechanism, the operator must first demonstrate that the local EGM at the "earliest" site on the activation map indeed precedes the P wave on the electrocardiogram, usually by at least 20 ms. Recall that the activation map is typically constructed with respect to an intracardiac reference and not the P wave on the electrocardiogram. Thus, the red area on the map simply identifies the site of earliest activation as compared to the reference and may not represent the actual site of origin. If the onset of the P wave is obscured by the QRS or the T wave, ventricular pacing may be employed to unmask the P wave. If the EGM at the "earliest" site is not presystolic, this site cannot be the site of origin of a focal tachycardia, and further mapping is required. This scenario is frequently encountered when the

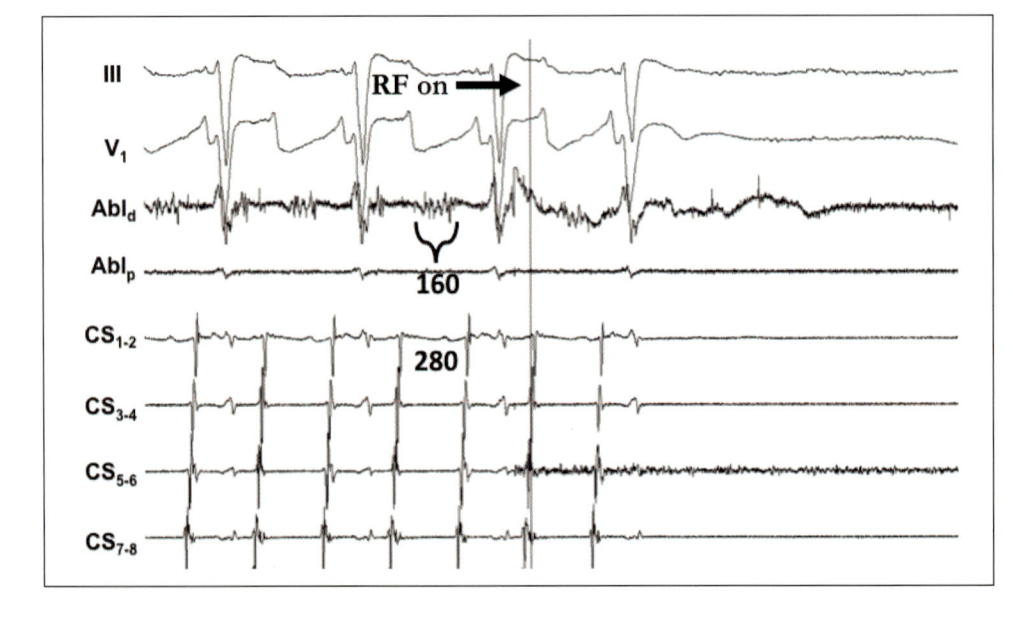

Figure 27.16 Effect of RF energy delivery at the LA septum. The AT was due to a small-reentrant circuit near the septal aspect of the mitral annulus. Note the mid-diastolic, fractionated EGM (160 ms) that accounts for > 50% of the TCL (280 ms). RF energy delivery at 25 W immediately terminates the tachycardia to sinus rhythm, after which it was no longer inducible.

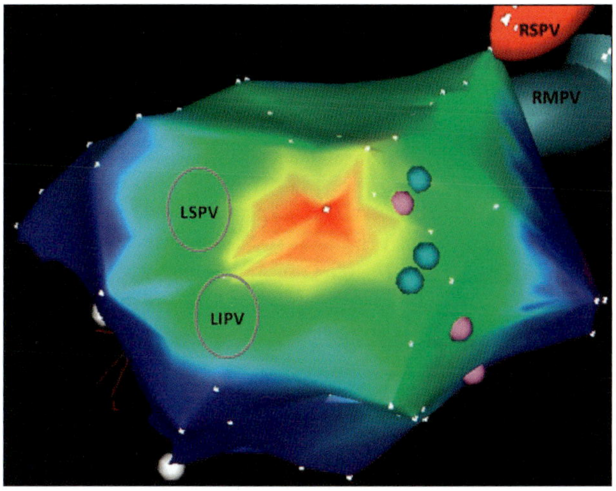

Figure 27.17 An example of a focal AT from the left PV antrum. Note the centrifugal spread of activation from the site of origin.

tachycardia originates from the chamber contralateral to the one being mapped. The focal spread simply represents the earliest breakthrough of the chamber being mapped and ablation at the site of "early" activation will be futile.

Focal ATs may originate from anywhere in the LA or RA or the CS. Possible target sites include reconnected PVs, the LAA, the posterior LA, atrial myocardium around the mitral or tricuspid valves, ligament of Marshall, septum, SVC, posterior RA/crista terminalis, ostium of the CS, and the base of the RAA. The endpoint of ablation of focal ATs is tachycardia termination and noninducibility during isoproterenol infusion.

Procedural Endpoints

After elimination of the clinical AT, the operator should document complete PVI to prevent arrhythmia recurrence. If linear ablation was performed at the mitral isthmus or the LA roof during the prior or current procedure, our endpoint is demonstration of linear block by strict EP criteria. We no longer perform prophylactic ablation of the mitral isthmus, that is, in patients without perimitral flutter, for a number of reasons. First, it may be challenging to achieve linear block. Since RF energy delivery is required within the CS in most patients, there is also a risk of arterial injury. Resumption of conduction across previously complete lines is frequent and may result in pro-arrhythmia. Lastly, long linear lesions, even when complete, may act as lateral barriers and promote the formation of small reentrant circuits. In patients who have previously undergone arrhythmia surgery, empiric ablation should be based on the operative report. If the mitral isthmus was targeted during surgery, it may be reasonable to ensure complete block at the mitral isthmus, even in the absence of perimitral flutter.

In patients with a history of persistent AF presenting for an AT procedure, we routinely perform ablation of the CTI, even if the arrhythmia was not inducible. The rationale is that these patients may develop typical flutter during follow-up and that ablation of this isthmus is usually straightforward and unlikely to be met with complications or pro-arrhythmia.

We also perform programmed atrial stimulation during isoproterenol infusion (10–20 mcg/min). If the patient is inducible for another AT, it is important to target it despite the length of the procedure up to that point. If the arrhythmia is deemed "nonclinical" and not eliminated, there is very good chance of recurrence requiring yet another procedure or antiarrhythmic medications. Another reason to perform programmed atrial stimulation is that occasionally one may find AV nodal reentrant tachycardia or even orthodromic reciprocating tachycardia, the elimination of which will likely prevent arrhythmia recurrence.

Postprocedure Care

After the ablation procedure, patients are observed in a telemetry unit. Occasionally, a patient may develop recurrent AT, most often after a procedure during which complete elimination of all tachycardias was not possible. The acute management depends on hemodynamic stability, symptoms, and the ventricular rate of the tachycardia. A 12-lead ECG should be obtained immediately after the procedure and prior to discharge to evaluate for ischemia, especially if RF energy was delivered within the CS, and pericarditis. Mild pericarditis is relatively common and typically abates within a few days of the procedure. Short-term administration of oral nonsteroidal analgesics is effective for ongoing symptoms. Patients with severe pain or hemodynamic instability should undergo urgent echocardiography to evaluate for a pericardial effusion.

An often-overlooked aspect of performing ablation procedures using open-irrigation catheters is the saline load that patients receive. To counteract this, we infuse intravenous furosemide during and after the procedure, aiming for an even fluid balance. In some patients it may not be possible to administer diuretics during or shortly after the procedure due to relative hypotension related to anesthetic medications. In this case, it is advisable to prescribe oral diuretics for a few days after the procedure. This practice has led to a significant decrease in the number of patients presenting to the emergency department after discharge for dyspnea related to volume overload.

If the clinical AT was eliminated and the patient was rendered noninducible at the end of the procedure, antiarrhythmic medications are not prescribed. Patients are asked to continue taking the same rate-controlling medications until they are seen in follow-up. If all of the ATs could not be eliminated, then rhythm- and rate-controlling medications are prescribed.

Anticoagulation should be continued for at least 3 months. In most instances, the decision to discontinue oral anticoagulation should be based on the patients' underlying risk of thromboembolism. We perform long-term (4 weeks) monitoring, with an autotrigger monitor, at 6 to 9 months after the ablation procedure. We discontinue oral anticoagulation in patients with no objective evidence of recurrence in the absence of antiarrhythmic medications and without a history of thromboembolism or another indication for oral anticoagulation.

Procedural Outcomes

The endpoint of elimination of the clinical AT and noninducibility may be achieved in approximately 90% of patients. However, about 25% of patients require yet another procedure for recurrent tachycardia. About half of the recurrences are due to resumption of conduction across previously complete lines, and the other half to small-reentrant tachycardias that were not present or inducible during the prior session. During long-term follow-up, about 80% of patients are arrhythmia free in the absence of antiarrhythmic therapy.

In a consecutive series of 173 patients undergoing 226 ablation procedures for AT at the University of Michigan, serious complications occurred during 2 procedures (1%). One patient developed pericardial tamponade immediately after the procedure and responded to percutaneous drainage. In another patient, occlusion of the distal circumflex was discovered several months after the ablation procedure, during which complete mitral isthmus block could not be achieved.

In addition, permanent intra-atrial or inter-atrial conduction block or LAA isolation occurred in 5 (2%) patients. One of these patients required a permanent pacemaker as a result of intra-atrial dissociation. Extensive biatrial scarring was present in all of these patients prior to the ablation procedure.

Advantages and Limitations of Activation Mapping

Postablation AT may be mapped with either activation mapping using a 3-dimensional mapping system or exclusively by entrainment mapping. One advantage of activation mapping is that it allows the operator to appreciate the full extent of the reentrant circuit. The operator can readily recognize the anatomic obstacles, which must be connected by the linear lesion. Also, utilization of a mapping system significantly reduces the exposure to ionizing radiation. Another advantage of activation mapping is that the operator can extract a tremendous amount of mechanistic information without perturbation of the tachycardia. The biggest disadvantage of the entrainment mapping is that it may alter or terminate the tachycardia, which may not be inducible thereafter. The operator can also tag "interesting" sites, eg, those harboring fractionation, on the 3-dimensional map. These sites may be critical to the clinical AT or perhaps to another tachycardia induced after elimination of the former.

The main criticism of activation mapping is that it may be time consuming since the map is constructed by point-by-point mapping. In the near future, multipolar catheters will allow the operator the obtain activation data over a significantly larger surface area and more efficiently as compared to the distal bipole of the ablation catheter. Still, it is currently possible to construct a high-density map within 15 to 20 minutes (Figure 27.8). Occasionally, even a high-density map may fail to provide an accurate diagnosis. This typically occurs in the setting of severely diseased myocardium or prior linear ablation. Hence, the diagnosis suggested by the activation map should always be corroborated by entrainment mapping.

The precise clinical setting may also be important in determining whether to employ activation or entrainment mapping. In patients presenting for an ablation procedure for AT, we perform an activation map at the outset for the reasons enumerated above. Not infrequently, patients may develop another tachycardia after elimination of the clinical AT. Constructing multiple activation maps for multiple tachycardias is not efficient. In this setting, it is best to use the 3-dimensional shell to tag sites that do and do not afford matching PPIs during entrainment mapping. This approach allows the operator to visualize the circuit and facilitates RF energy delivery and may also be associated with lower fluoroscopy times. In patients presenting for an ablation procedure for persistent AF, a stepwise ablation strategy may terminate AF and give way to an AT. This conversion usually requires several steps and at least a few hours and, therefore, activation mapping of the resultant AT will only prolong an already long procedure. This setting also calls for strategic entrainment mapping. In short, neither activation nor entrainment mapping is clearly superior to the other and, in fact, they are truly complementary.

Conclusions

Due to the multiplicity of mechanisms and sites of origin, mapping and ablation of post–AF ATs may be quite challenging. Even when the diagnosis is straightforward, eg, perimitral AFL, elimination of the tachycardia and demonstration of linear block may prove to be very difficult in some patients. Given these limitations, it stands to reason that we should do our utmost in preventing these tachycardias in the first place. There is no question that extensive ablation strategies are responsible for generating or, in some cases, unmasking these tachycardias. In an effort to decrease the prevalence of AT, we no longer perform prophylactic LA linear ablation in patients with persistent AF. In an effort to decrease the prevalence of post-ablation AT, we no longer perform empiric linear ablation in all patients with persistent AF.

No matter the strategy, the electrophysiologist who performs catheter ablation of AF is sure to encounter AT in his/her practice. Whether one employs activation or entrainment mapping, it is critical to establish the mechanism prior to ablation. If linear ablation is performed, then the line must be shown to be complete by objective criteria. After elimination of the AT, the procedural endpoint should also include PVI and noninducibility.

Although our understanding of the various mechanisms of postablation AT has improved significantly over the last several years, the tools at our disposal in dealing with these tachycardias have not kept pace. Point-by-point ablation in creating linear lesions is time consuming. A linear ablation catheter that can safely deliver RF energy over the entire isthmus simultaneously would simplify matters. The ability to rapidly diagnose the mechanism of the tachycardia, perhaps with the combination of the ECG and mapping system, would also be helpful. Supplementing an endocardial with an epicardial approach may also help improve outcomes in patients with challenging tachycardias. Hopefully, these advances and others will lead to an improvement in efficacy and efficiency and a reduction in the prevalence of repeat procedures in patients with postablation ATs.

References

1. Chugh A, Latchamsetty R, Oral H, et al. Characteristics of cavotricuspid isthmus–dependent atrial flutter after left atrial ablation of atrial fibrillation. *Circulation*. 2006;113: 609–615.
2. De Ponti R, Verlato R, Bertaglia E, et al. Treatment of macro-re-entrant atrial tachycardia based on electroanatomic mapping: identification and ablation of the mid-diastolic isthmus. *Europace*. 2007;9:449–457.
3. Chae S, Oral H, Good E, et al. Atrial tachycardia after circumferential pulmonary vein ablation of atrial fibrillation: mechanistic insights, results of catheter ablation, and risk factors for recurrence. *J Am Coll Cardiol*. 2007;50: 1781–1787.
4. Yokokawa M, Sundaram B, Garg A, Stojanovska J, Oral H, Morady F, Chugh A. Impact of mitral isthmus anatomy on the likelihood of achieving linear block in patients undergoing catheter ablation of persistent atrial fibrillation. *Heart Rhythm*. 2011;8(9):1404–1410.
5. Yokokawa M, Sundaram B, Oral H, Morady F, Chugh A. The course of the sinus node artery and its impact on achieving linear block at the left atrial roof in patients with persistent atrial fibrillation. *Heart Rhythm*. 2012, Apr 16. [Epub ahead of print]
6. Jaïs P, Matsuo S, Knecht S, et al. A deductive mapping strategy for atrial tachycardia following atrial fibrillation ablation: importance of localized reentry. *J Cardiovasc Electrophysiol*. 2009;20:480–491.

CHAPTER 28

How to Utilize Frequency Analysis to Aid in Atrial Fibrillation Ablation

Yenn-Jiang Lin, MD, PhD; Li-Wei Lo, MD; Shih-Ann Chen, MD

Introduction

Atrial fibrillation (AF) is the most common cardiac arrhythmia in clinical practice. It is well known that AF depends on the interaction between the triggers and substrate.[1] It is also well known that the elimination or isolation of the PVs and non-PV triggers can cure AF.[1-3] Some patients with paroxysmal AF and nearly all patients with nonparoxysmal AF may require additional substrate modification to improve the clinical outcome. In recent years, growing knowledge of atrial substrate mapping has helped us to learn more about the maintenance of AF and to identify the critical atrial substrate for catheter ablation in spite of the elimination of all triggers initiating AF. However, how to identify the critical arrhythmogenic atrial substrate remained unclear.

It is well known that AF is characterized by a spatiotemporal organized activation with a variable frequency and spectral morphology throughout the atria. Therefore, mapping of the atrial substrate would be difficult during a complex rhythm such as AF. The complex activation patterns of AF can result in fractionated signals separated by short and variable intervals that prohibit a reliable identification of the precise local activation rate or CL. Furthermore, it is difficult to represent sustained episodes of AF by only a small sample of fibrillatory EGMs within a limited period of time, and it is technically difficult to link and compare the regional distribution of the AF from time-domain signals alone.[4,5] One reasonable method for a transformation is to transform the time-domain EGM signal into a frequency-domain EGM signal, that is, to elucidate the data beyond the time-domain EGM. Frequency-domain signals provide a feasible method to analyze the temporal and spatial distribution of fibrillatory waves during AF.[4,5] The regional frequency analysis can identify local sources of AF with rapid repetitive activation and reveal their mechanism. From animal studies to the clinical setting, dominant-frequency (DF) mapping is emerging as a technique for guiding EGM-based approaches to substrate modification.

Preprocedural Planning: Technological Considerations

A Fourier transform is based on the concept that the signals can be approximated by the sum of the sinusoidal waveforms with different frequencies. Therefore, the resultant power spectrum is a graph of the DFs that are present within the period of the duration they were collected. The DF of the EGM represents the frequency of the highest power in the spectrum. Assuming an

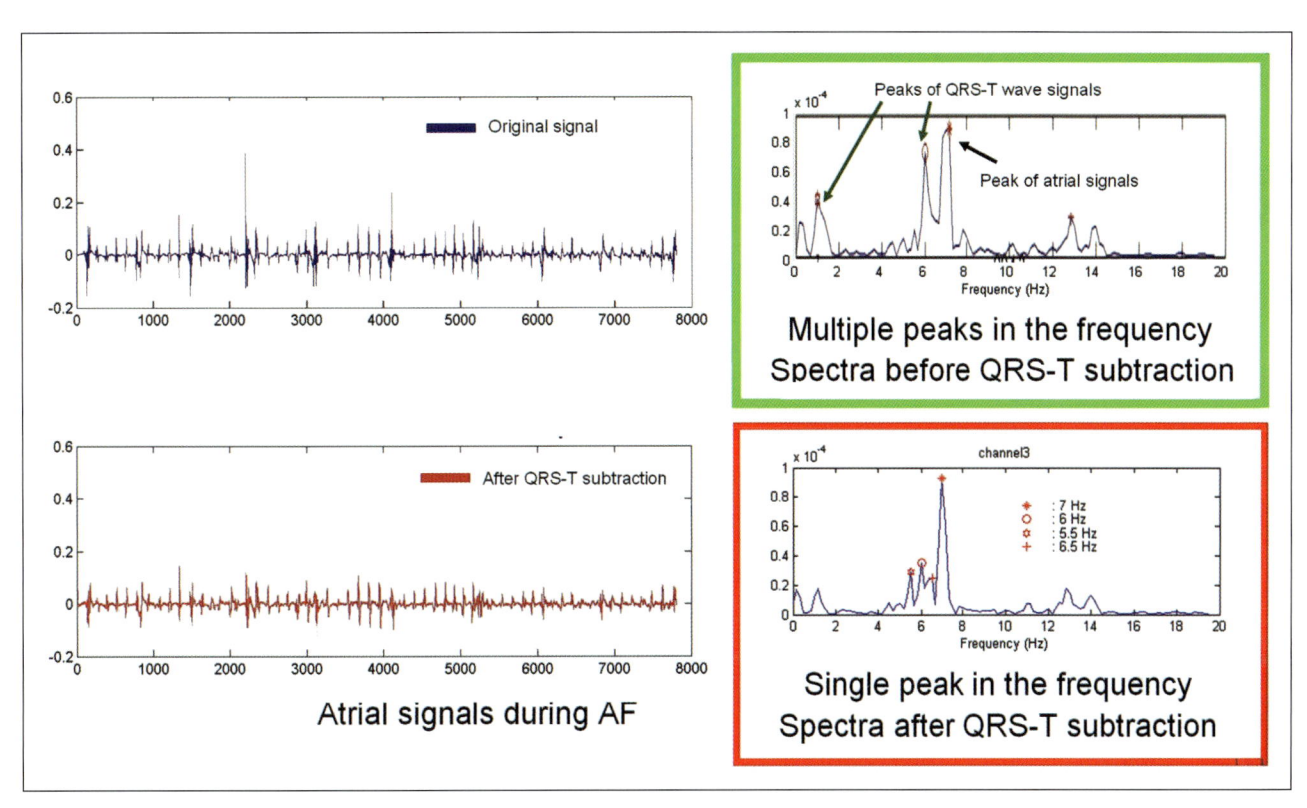

Figure 28.1 Schematic presentation of frequency analysis from time-domain signals.

appropriate pretreatment of filtering is applied, the DF is related to the inverse of the average CL. Therefore, the purpose of a frequency analysis is to map the mean activation rate of seemly chaotic signals during AF. The sites with the highest DFs were considered to be the drivers of AF by analyzing the intracardiac fibrillatory signals throughout the RA and LA.

Requirement of QRS-T Subtractions

The DF calculation is not a flawless process due to the nature of the fibrillatory activities during AF. Various factors, such as preprocessing filtering, QRS-T far field, and the duration of the recording may affect the DF analysis.[6] For example, the identification of DF values within the spectra of the physiologically relevant range from 3 to 15 Hz. However, the harmonic peaks of the low frequency range due to the QRS-T complexes may interfere with the atrial DF peaks of interest. The determination of the atrial DF peaks may be inaccurate. This is especially frequently observed with unipolar recording (**Figure 28.1**).[6] Our laboratory routinely applied QRS-T subtraction as signal preprocessing before spectral analysis (**Figure 28.2**). In our experience, QRS subtraction is required for frequency analysis of fibrillation signals if the recording sites show low atrial voltage or prominent far-field ventricular potentials. The QRS subtraction techniques improve the reliability of the frequency spectra obtained from intracardiac AF signals.

Reliability and Stability of DF Value

Reliability of the DF sites, spatially and temporally, is an important issue for the application of clinical DF mapping. The reproducibility of DF values over time remains a controversial issue. Recently, Habel et al used a stationary 64-electrode basket catheter in the LA to record the atrial activity over 5 minutes. They reported that inaccuracy occurred during repeated measurements of the DF value. These data raised more questions about the accuracy of DF mapping by the sequential site-by-site approach. However, the investigation from other laboratories showed the opposite results.[7,8] Sander et al showed the temporal stability of the DF values in patients with AF presenting for ablation, and the stability of the DF improved after a recording duration of > 5 seconds.[7,8] Verma et al examined the stability of fractionated EGMs in 24 patients with AF. There was no significance of a mean interval of < 120 ms (> 8.3 Hz), as compared to sites with a mean interval of > 120 ms.[9] Lin et al further demonstrated that only the sites with the shortest fractionated interval harbored the least temporal variation.[10] These data suggest the temporal stability in the highest DF region, and a temporal variation of the DF may be observed in the rest of the atrium. Thus, DF mapping with simultaneous multiple electrode catheters or Ensite-array DF mapping may be alternatives to improve the accuracy of the DF (**Figures 28.3** and **28.4**, ▶ **Video 28.1**). However, these limitations do not preclude the application of sequential DF mapping, because only the high-DF regions are of interest during AF in the electrophysiologic mapping and ablation procedure.

Spectral Analysis During Sinus Rhythm: AF Nest Identification

In most of the laboratories, DF value was calculated during AF. An alternative approach is to use the spectral analysis to characterize the sinus EGMs based on the consistency of the sinus EGMs over time. Previous studies showed that abnormal atrial sites were characterized by fractionated EGMs as shown in the time-domain EGMs and high-frequency peaks in the frequency domain analysis during sinus rhythm.[11-15] According to Pachon's study,[11] the high-DF sites (or AF nest) were identified by visual inspection of the frequency spectra, especially in the high-frequency range of > 80 Hz. This laboratory[12] applied a 30-Hz

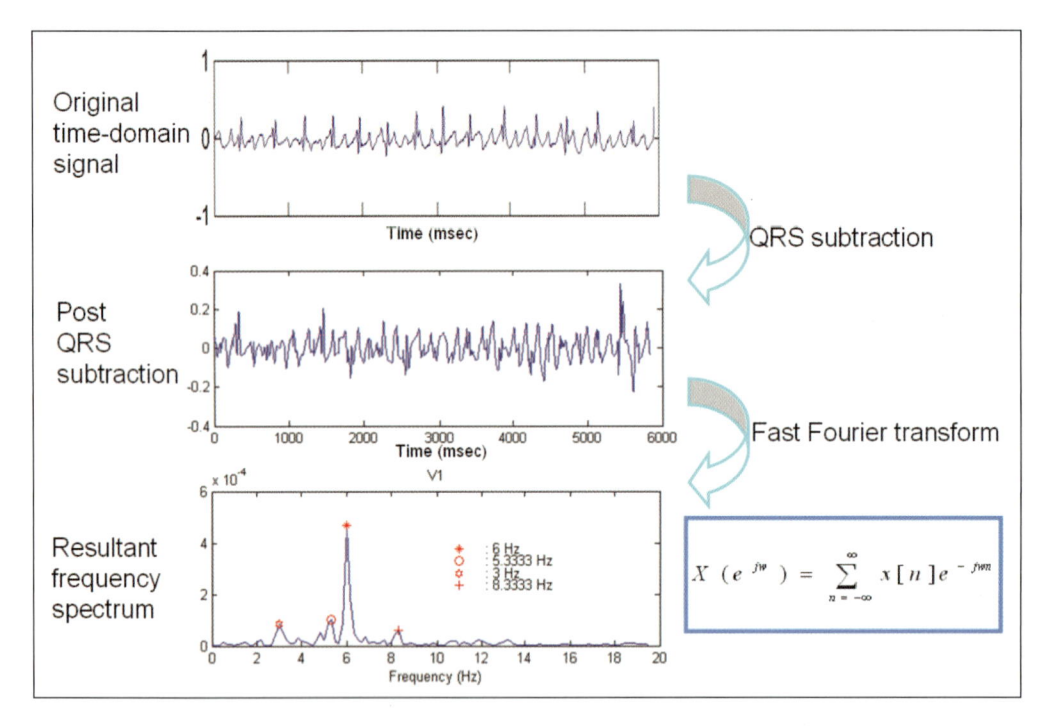

Figure 28.2 An example of frequency analysis before and after QRS subtraction. The frequency peaks (right upper) obtained from frequency analysis without QRS subtraction are difficult to analyze because of multiple harmonic peaks of QRS-T wave signals. On the other hand, the frequency analysis showed single and dominant peak if the signals were processed after QRS subtraction. These results indicate that QRS subtraction before frequency analysis is mandatory in this ventricular far-field dominant atrial signals.

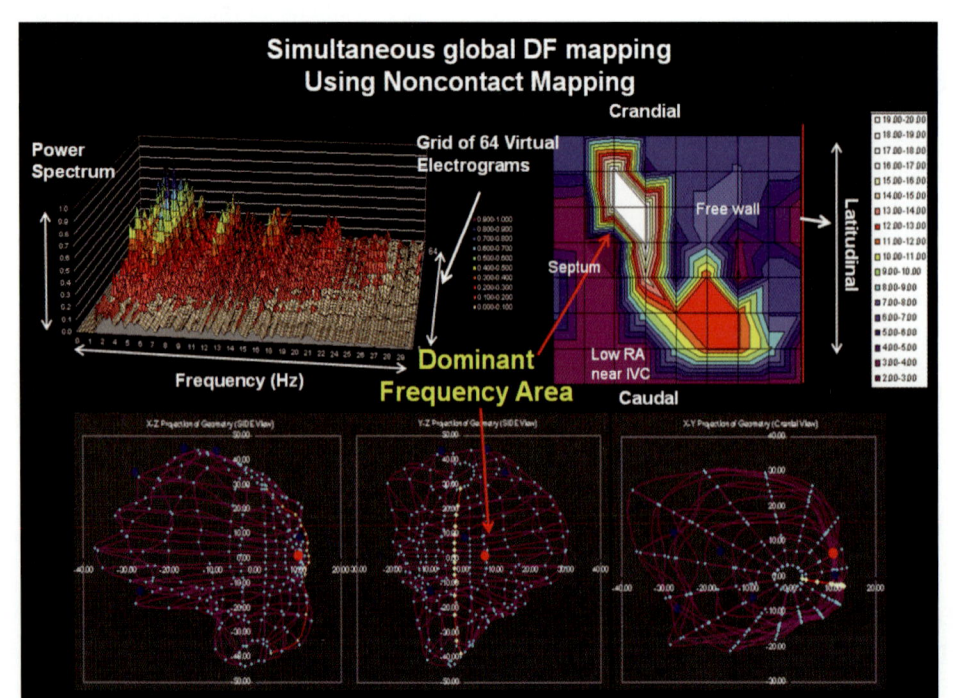

$$X(e^{j\omega}) = \sum_{n=-\infty}^{\infty} x[n] e^{-j\omega n}$$

Figure 28.3 A schematic example demonstrating the global frequency analysis in the atrial chamber, the overall power spectrum, and the 2-dimensional display of the DF value distribution. The 256 noncontact unipolar EGMs of each chamber were exported for a dominant frequency analysis (6.8 seconds, 1200 Hz, using surface ECG lead V_1 as the template to subtract the QRS-T far-field signal, and the 2-dimensional DF map was performed using SPSS software version 11.0).

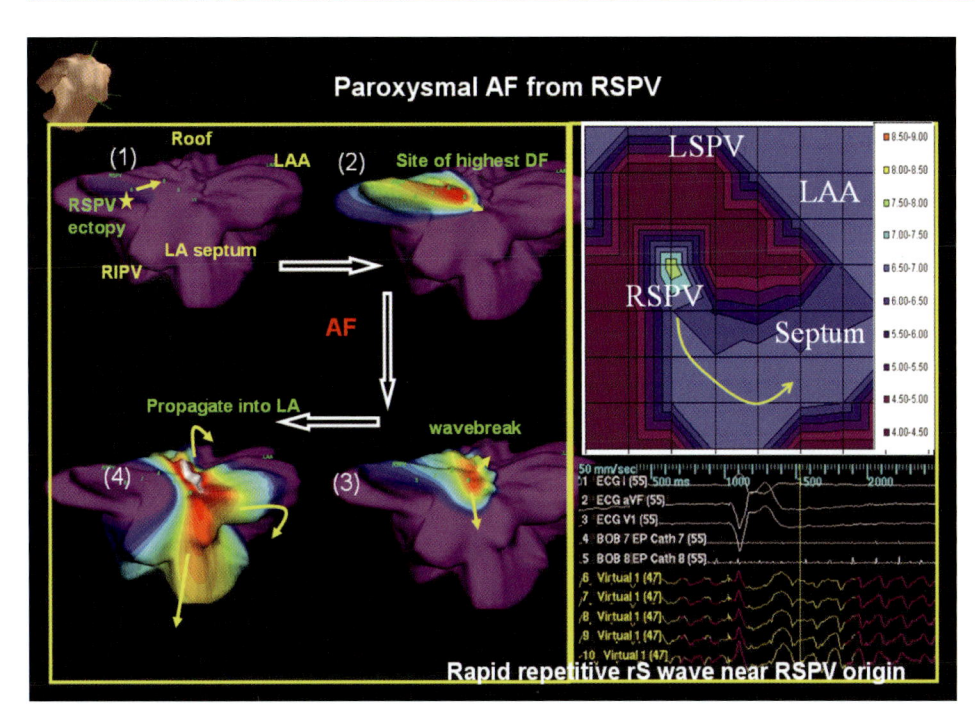

Figure 28.4 Activation map, frequency map of the LA, and the unipolar EGMs in a patient with paroxysmal AF from RSPV. The high-DF site was near the RSPV ostium, where repetitive rS unipolar EGMs were observed near the origin of RSPV triggers.

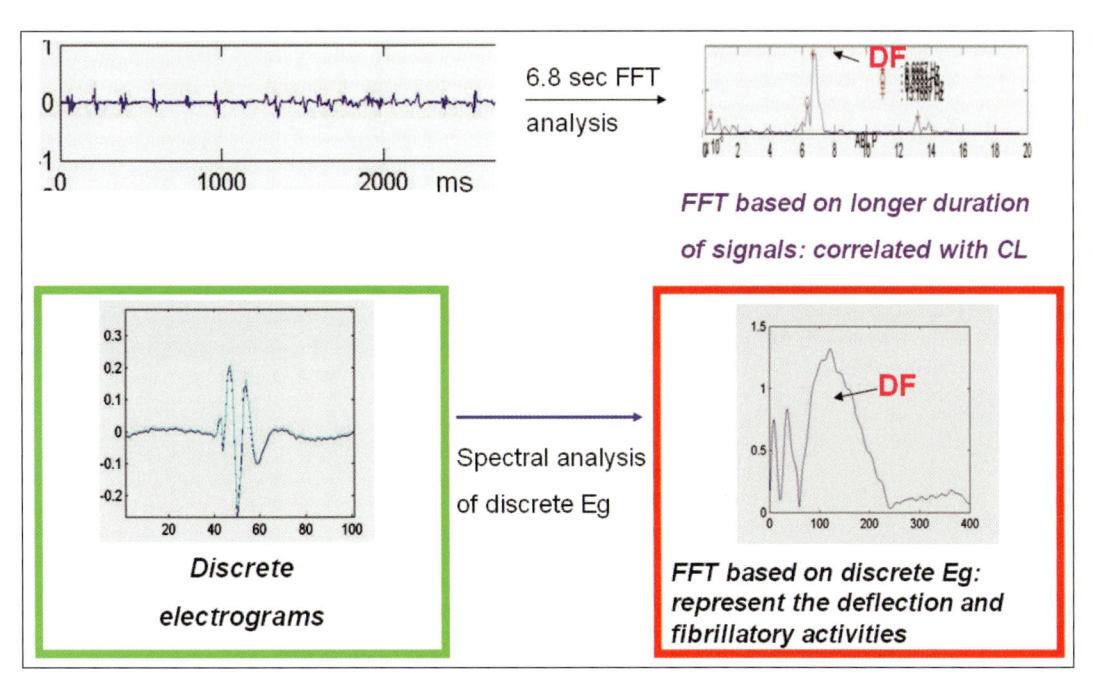

Figure 28.5 Illustration of the frequency analysis during AF and spectral analysis during sinus rhythm (AF nest). The data were reproduced from reference 12, with the permission of the publisher.

high-pass filtering to exclude the fundamental peaks to highlight the corresponding high DF sites of the abnormal atrial substrate in Pachon's study. Technically, the spectral analysis of sinus EGMs was based on bipolar EGMs (**Figure 28.5**). A low-frequency resolution (> 0.5 Hz) owing to a short recording duration of the sinus EGMs makes a sophisticated quantitative analysis of the DF value of a single site less likely. The advantage of AF nest analysis is the reliability and consistency of the EGM during sinus rhythm.

Procedure

The application of DF mapping in the substrate mapping and ablation is summarized in **Table 28.1**. Current evidence has demonstrated that DF mapping could be used to (1) classify the atrial substrate, (2) locate the abnormal arrhythmogenic regions, and (3) as an endpoint for substrate modification. Prospective DF-guided ablation was mostly performed in paroxysmal AF patients.[11,13,14] The

Table 28.1 Summary of the role of DF-guided mapping and ablation in atrial fibrillation

	PAF/CAF (No.)	Rhythm for FFT	Data acquisition for the signal analysis	Location of the high-DF sites	Application of DF analysis during procedure	Ablation strategy	DF-guided mapping ablation (Yes/No)	PV isolation (Yes/No)
Pachon et al *Europace* 2004[11]	34/0	Sinus rhythm	Sequential bipolar recording	Outside PV	Guide ablation	AF nest ablation	Yes	No
Lin et al *Circulation* 2005[13]	13/0	Atrial fibrillation	Simultaneous unipolar recording of each intracardiac region	Right atrium*	Identify the arrhythmogenic region in the RA*	Target the high-DF region	Yes	No
Atienza et al *Heart Rhythm* 2009[14]	32/18	Atrial fibrillation	Sequential bipolar recording	Left atrium/PV	Guide ablation	DF ablation with PVI	Yes	Yes
Sander et al *Circulation* 2005[17]	19/13	Atrial fibrillation	Sequential bipolar recording	Left atrium/PV	Nil+	PVI with CFAE ablation	No	Yes
Yokoyama et al *JCE* 2009[18]	61/0	Atrial fibrillation	Sequential bipolar recording	Left atrium/PV	Nil+	PVI	No	Yes
Yoshida et al *Heart Rhythm*, 2010[22]	0/100	Atrial fibrillation	Continuous recording from surface ECG and CS	Nil**	Decrease of DF as endpoint of substrate modification	PVI with CFAE ablation	No	Yes
Lin et al *Heart Rhythm*, 2010[19]	0/50	Atrial fibrillation	Sequential bipolar recording	Left atrium	Identify the culprit CFAEs in the LA	PVI with CFAE ablation	Yes	Yes

ABBREVIATION: CFAE: complex fractionated atrial EGMs, DF = dominant frequency, LA = left atrium, PVI = pulmonary vein isolation.
* PV-AF patients were excluded from the baseline electrophysiological study.
** FFT was only performed on the surface ECG and CS rather than the intracardiac recordings.
+ These studies were based on retrospective study.

application of a DF-guided ablation in nonparoxysmal AF patients remains limited in the literature.

DF Mapping in Paroxysmal AF Patients

In the majority of patients with paroxysmal AF, there is an LA-to-RA DF gradient; this is compatible with the animal model of acute AF, in which AF waves emanating from the high-frequency sources of the LAPV resulted in an LA-to-RA DF gradient, suggesting that the LAPV area is important for maintaining sustained AF. However, in patients with AF originating from SVC,[15] the highest-DF sites were located inside the arrhythmogenic SVC to the SVC-ostium, and no LA-to-RA DF gradient was observed (**Figures 28.6** and **28.7**). Recently, Suenari et al used 3-dimensional high-density DF mapping for paroxysmal AF prior to the PV isolation. High DFs (> 8 Hz) were identified in 1.5 ± 0.9 regions per patient and were mostly located within 15 mm of the PV ostia. Of those, 75% of the high DF regions were related to arrhythmogenic veins. There was a significant steep DF gradient from the arrhythmogenic PV ostium to the left atrium. Therefore, the DF valve could be used to identify the potential thoracic vein triggers during AF.

In patients with reentrant dominant AF (3% of all paroxysmal and persistent AF), initiation ectopies could be identified and the mean CL obtained from the right atrial catheter was significantly shorter than the LA/CS catheters. Electroanatomic mapping during AF demonstrated that there was a reentrant driver for the AF maintenance. High-DF regions were recorded around a stationary reentrant circuit in part of the right atrium with an aperiodic pattern with fibrillatory conduction to the rest of the atrium (**Figure 28.8**, ▶ **Video 28.2**). In these patients, selectively ablating the conduction channels successfully eliminated AF in these patients. Taken together, in paroxysmal AF, the highest-DF drivers were located within the arrhythmogenic thoracic veins and to the nearby atrial substrate.[10,20] A frequency analysis can demonstrate a regional distribution throughout the atria and detect the location of the rapid firing of triggers or reentrant sources during AF.

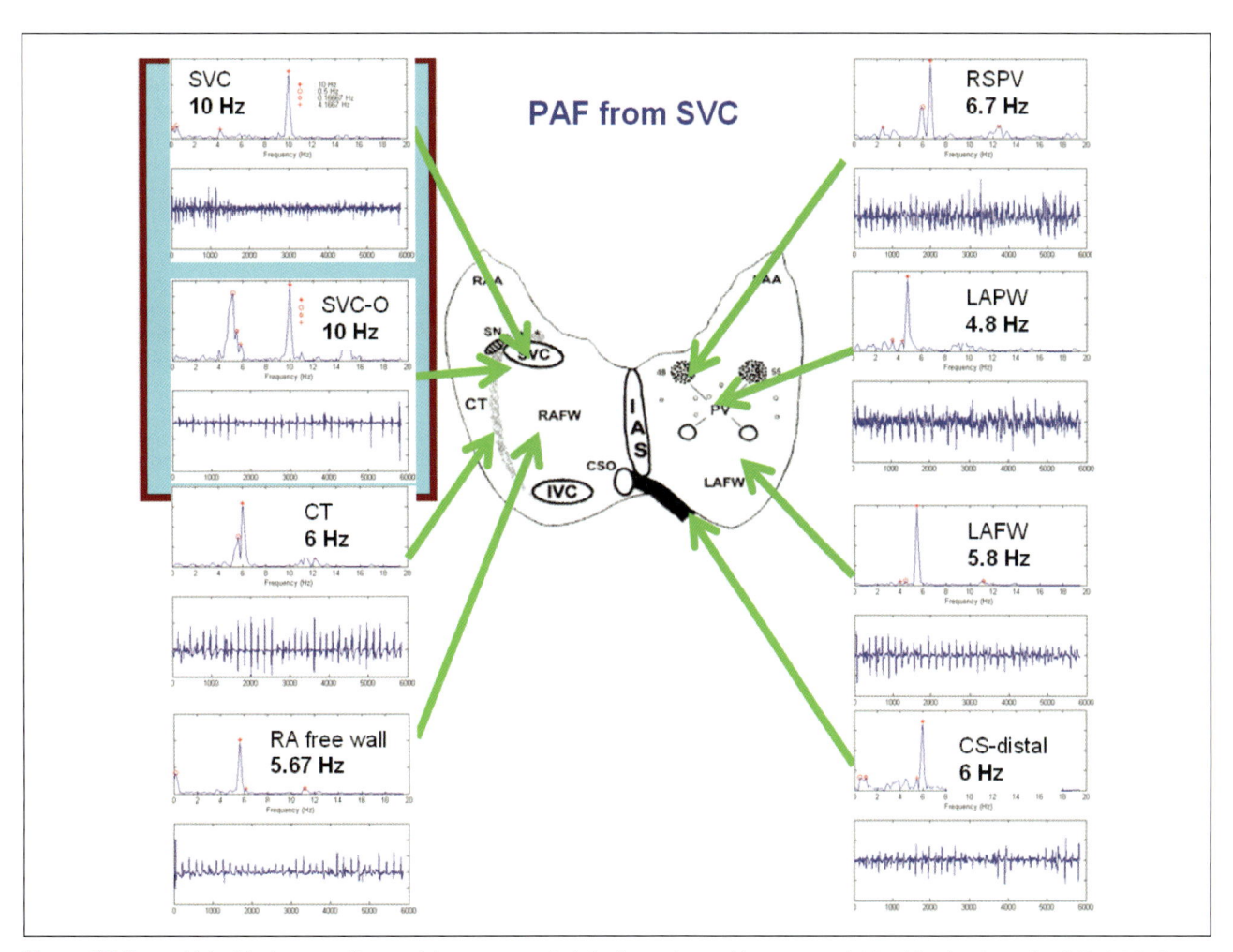

Figure 28.6 Multisite bipolar recordings and frequency analysis in the patients with paroxysmal AF originating from the SVC. A DF of 10 Hz was found inside the SVC. The DFs of the RA sites were lower, ranging from 5.67 to 6.1 Hz. There was a frequency gradient from the arrhythmogenic SVC to the rest of the atria and other thoracic veins. The frequency gradient of LA to RA was not evident in this patient. The data were reproduced from reference 15, with the permission of the publisher.

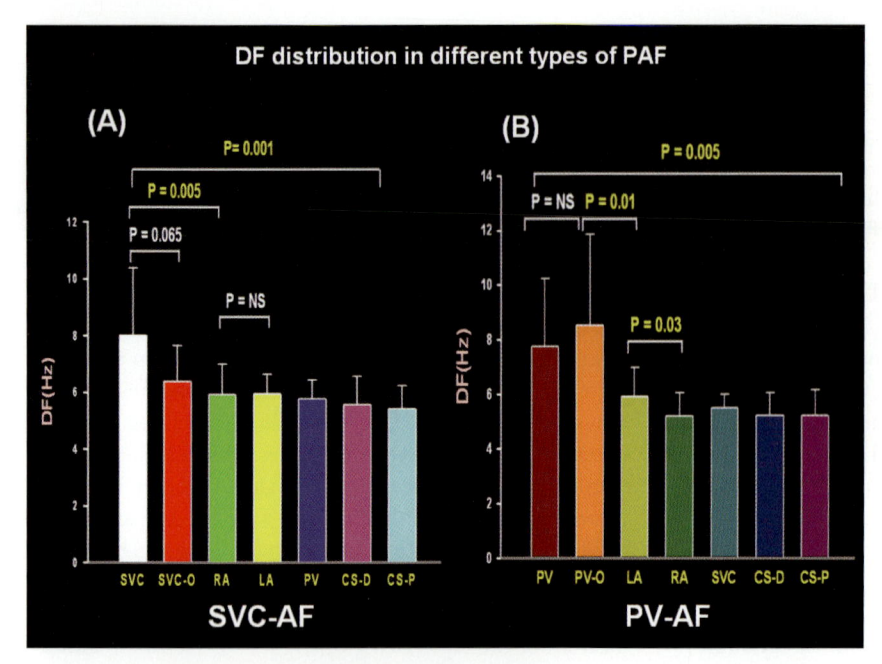

Figure 28.7 **A.** In the patients with SVC-AF, the DF was the highest inside the SVC or SVC ostium, with a significant frequency gradient to the RA, LA, PV, and CS. **B.** In the PV-AF patients, the DF of the PV ostium was higher than the DF of the LA (near the PV ostium), and the DF of the LA was significantly higher than that of the RA. The lowest DFs were located in the CS, RA, and SVC, which were far away from the highest DF and site of the ectopy initiating AF. The data were reproduced from reference 15, with the permission of the publisher.

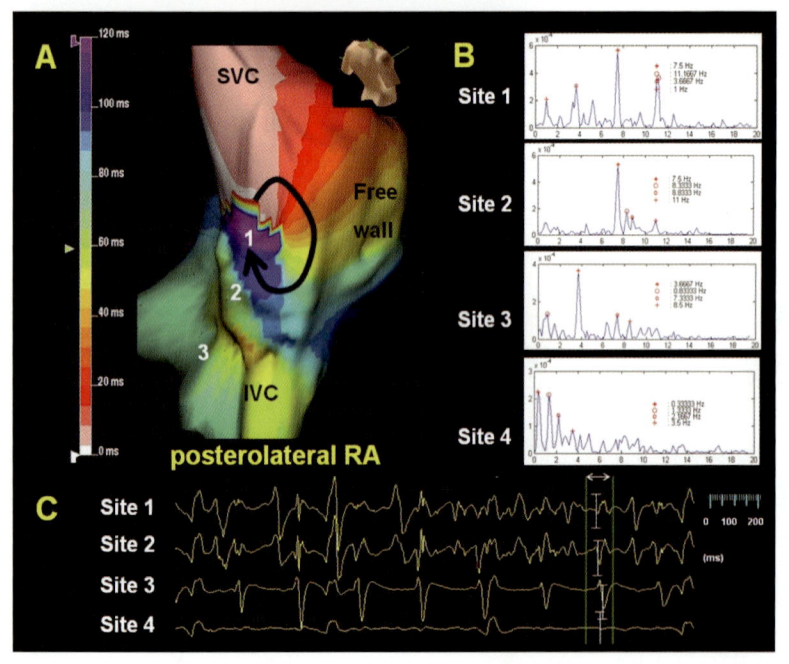

Figure 28.8 Activation map (**A**), frequency-domain analysis (**B**), and intracardiac unipolar EGMs (**C**) in a patient with right atrial AF. **A.** Isochronal activation maps with the high-DF region demonstrating a vortex-like reentrant circuit propagating around the crista terminalis with a mean cycle length of 120 ms. **B.** Frequency analysis around the reentrant circuit showing fast and organized activity with the highest-DF peak (7.3 Hz, site 1). The margin of the reentrant circuit exhibited a variable activation (site 2). The rest of the RA exhibited a slow and disorganized activity. Frequency analysis revealed multiple frequency peaks with a low DF value (3.8 Hz, site 3). The data were modified and reproduced from reference 13.

AF Nest Analysis in Paroxysmal AF Patients

In our experience, spectral analysis (AF nest) can detect an abnormal atrial substrate in paroxysmal AF. The high-frequency sites were associated with multiple rapid deflections, prolonged EGM, and low bipolar voltage of EGM morphology. The regional distribution of the high-DF sites (higher than 70 Hz) in the LA predicted the efficacy of PV isolation and the requirement for substrate modification (**Figure 28.9**). Approximately 75 to 80% of the AF nests were observed near the PV ostium, and the presence of the high-frequency site in the LA predicted positive AF inducibility test and the requirement of substrate medication.

DF Mapping in Nonparoxysmal AF

In persistent AF, the mean DF was higher than that in paroxysmal AF and the LA-to-RA DF gradient became less evident.[8,16,17] The absence of an intra-LA DF gradient (PV to LA) correlated with a positive AF inducibility after PVI.[18] In the patients with a lesser intra-LA DF gradient, the PVI was less likely to terminate the AF and subsequent substrate modification would be necessary.[18,19] Those patients were characterized by a larger LA, longer activation time, more non-PV ectopy, and widely distributed fractionated EGMs. Thus, these patients contain a greater abnormal atrial substrate and may facilitate numerous

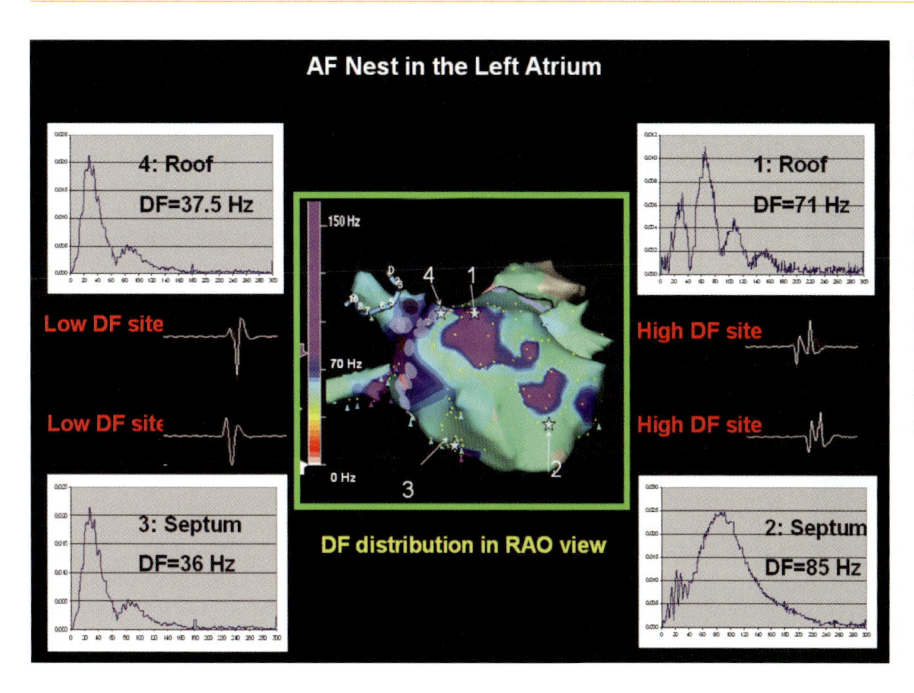

Figure 28.9 The regional distribution of the high-frequency sites in a patient with paroxysmal AF and positive AF inducibility of PVI. The high-frequency sites were in the PV and LA. The intracardiac bipolar EGMs and the corresponding frequency spectra of the high-DF sites and the low-DF sites were shown. The spectral morphology is the AF termination site in the LA anterior off (site) showed a high DF peak of 71 Hz during sinus rhythm. EGM morphology showed multiple and rapid deflections. The data were reproduced from reference 12, with the permission of the publisher.

high-DF sites, and the DF value could decrease the spatial heterogeneity of the DF distribution.[19]

DF-Guided Catheter Ablation in Nonparoxysmal AF Patients

An ablation strategy guided by frequency analysis may be a better way for finding the critical substrate involved in the maintenance of AF.[13] Retrospective analysis showed that the DF sites corresponded to the successful ablation sites.[16,17] Prospective studies using real-time DF mapping-guided ablation have remained limited in the literature. The Jalife group prospectively applied real-time DF mapping for catheter ablation in 32 patients with paroxysmal AF and 18 with persistent AF (Table 28.1).[14] DF-guided substrate modification followed by PV isolation leads to the elimination of LA-to-RA frequency gradients with an optimal long-term clinical outcome. In that study, after a mean follow-up of 9.3 ± 5.4 months, 88% of the paroxysmal and 56% of the persistent AF patients were free of AF. In that study, the presence of an inter-atrial DF gradient indicated a better response to this procedure, and the endpoint of the substrate modification was the elimination of the DF gradients between the LA and RA. Those studies emphasized the importance of extensive mapping of the DFs and the elimination of those foci was important for the long-term maintenance of sinus rhythm.

As Adjunctive Tool for Substrate Mapping in Nonparoxysmal AF

In our laboratory, the substrate modification was guided by a continuous CFAE ablation postpulmonary vein isolation. We found that the variation of the frequency and fractionation were partly related to the PV activities. After PV isolation, regional DF and degree of fractionation decreased. DF mapping was an adjunctive treatment to identify the critical CFAEs for procedural AF termination (**Figure 28.10**). The fractionated sites in the vicinity of the highest DF were frequently associated with AF procedural termination compared to the other CFAE sites.[20] This finding indicated that a combined analysis of both the fractionation and frequency analysis may allow for a more specific approach to identify the critical atrial substrate that remains after PVI.

AF procedural termination was related to the long-term success during chronic AF ablation. However, procedural AF termination may be difficult to achieve in patients with long-lasting AF. Furthermore, the favorable effect of AF termination decreased when the LA diameter was > 45 mm.[21] Michigan's laboratory used a reduction in the DF value in surface ECG lead V_1 and CS of more than 11% as the endpoint of the substrate modification with an optimal long-term sinus rhythm maintenance rate.[22] Therefore, a DF analysis could also be applied to serve as the endpoint of the substrate modification in patients with nonparoxysmal AF.

Clinical Perspective

Before performing PVI, the spectral analysis and frequency analysis results provide valuable information with respect to the ablation strategy. In patients with paroxysmal AF, the spectral analysis data of the LA during sinus rhythm provide important information about the degree of atrial remodeling in the LA, especially in the area of the PV ostia. In our experience, we determined the optimal isolating lines of the right PVs and left PVs based on the spectral analysis results before the PV ablation. The

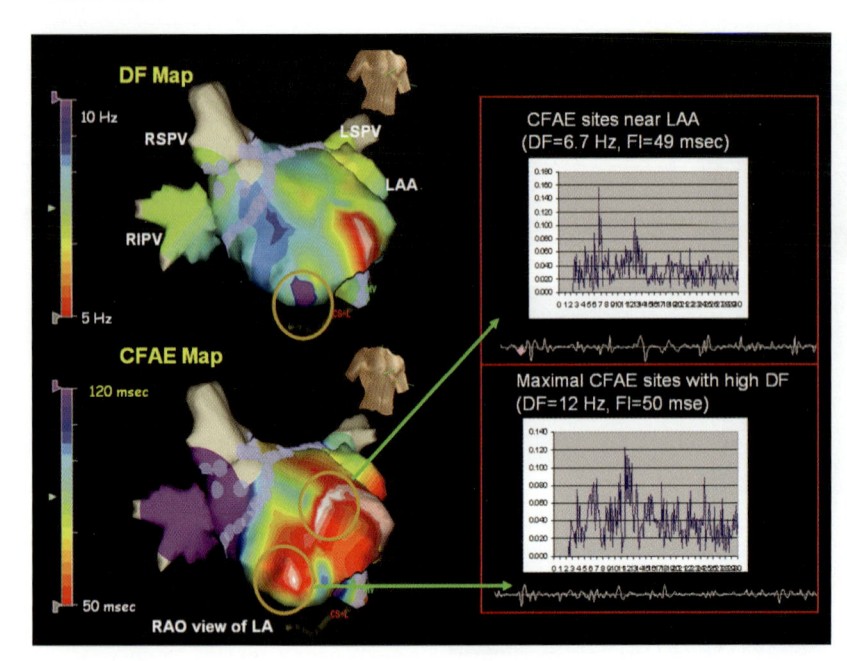

Figure 28.10 Comparison of the regional distribution of the fractionation interval (degree of fractionation) and DF (left panels) in a patient with nonparoxysmal AF. The CFAE map and DF map were obtained after complete PVI. The local intracardiac bipolar EGM and its corresponding frequency spectra during AF are shown in the right panels. Continuous CFAE sites in the low LA septum were compatible with the highest-DF sites and with the location where the radiofrequency ablation successfully terminated the AF. The data were reproduced from reference 20.

optimal ablation lines were positioned 1.0 to 1.5 cm from the angiographically determined PV ostium encircling the AF nests. Around 70 to 80% of the AF nests were within 1.0 to 1.5 cm from the ostia, especially near the arrhythmogenic veins.[23] In a randomized controlled trial, the single-ablation procedure efficacy of this new approach was better when compared with the conventional technique (84.2% vs. 65.6 %, with a mean follow-up duration of 11 months).[24] The time required to isolate the PVs was similar in both groups. The next question is whether it is necessary to treat the AF nests in the LA away from the PV isolating lines. Currently, we do not routinely target them or do a linear ablation unless there is the presence of a mappable, organized LA tachycardia. In these patients, a more aggressive identification of the nonpulmonary vein triggers initiating AF would be applied.

In patients with persistent AF and nearly persistent AF patients with incessant AF at the beginning of the procedure, the substrate modification was guided by a continuous CFAE ablation post–PVI. DF mapping during AF would be helpful to identify the high-frequency AF drivers and arrhythmogenic veins when sinus rhythm is difficult to restore before the catheter ablation.

Limitations

Frequency mapping could be an accessible tool to identify the AF source regardless of the mechanism of AF. First, sequential mapping of the intracardiac EGMs is a widely used tool. Simultaneous mapping from multiple sites may provide more accurate information. The filter setting, pronounced harmonic peaks, low signal-to-noise ratio, and study duration may affect the quality of the frequency spectra.[6]

The signal analysis based on the DF gradients provides limited value when the regional DF gradient was limited in patients with long-lasting persistent AF. Real-time DF mapping and catheter ablation are difficult in these patients. In these patients, an atrial substrate with continuous complex fractionated EGMs was considered to be a maintainer of AF. Investigators may apply the organization index or harmonic index to quantify the degree of fractionation.[25] The organization and harmonic index (the area of the DF peaks with the harmonic peaks over the total spectra) represented the irregularity of the DF value over time and provided some information about the consistency of the DF (**Figure 28.11**). However, the spectral morphology index (DF and harmonic index) may be overcome by the presence of chaotic signals in the background of the power spectra. In fact, in seemly chaotic fibrillatory signals, identification of a DF may be ambiguous and would be technically challenging. In the future, a nonlinear processing for the highly disorganized fractionated activity on the intracardiac recordings may allow for a more targeted approach to identify the critical atrial substrate in the patients with long-lasting AF.

Conclusions

DF mapping is emerging as a technique for guiding EGM-based approaches in the catheter ablation of AF. Although much data indicated that the high-DF sites play a role in the maintenance AF, only a few studies have demonstrated that DF-site ablation independently predicts clinical success. Current clinical evidence has demonstrated that intra-atrial DF mapping could be used to classify the atrial substrate, facilitate the identification of PV or extra-PV foci, and serve as an endpoint for substrate

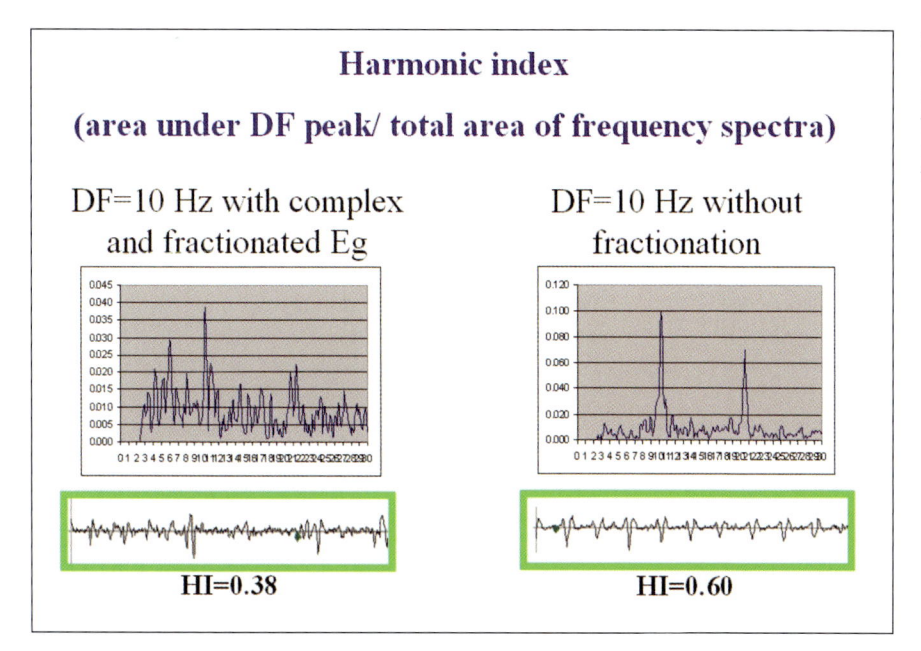

Figure 28.11 A schematic example of a harmonic index analysis in sites harboring similar DF values but different levels of fractionation. The lower harmonic index indicated more fractionation based on the time-domain EGM analysis.

modification with or without PV isolation in patients with paroxysmal AF. In patients with long-lasting AF, the regional DF distribution could be homogeneous. These may cause difficulty for the identification of the high-DF sites. A sophisticated reevaluation of the frequency spectra, high-density mapping of the high-DF sites, and simultaneous DF mapping are still required to enhance the high-DF site determination. Currently, most observational and ablation studies using DF analyses have been primarily based on paroxysmal AF patients; the data based on prospective studies and nonparoxysmal AF patients remain limited. Whether the ablation strategy will evolve as a sole guide to ablation or as a hybrid together with other approaches remains to be seen.

References

1. Haïssaguerre M, Jaïs P, Shah DC, et al. Spontaneous initiation of atrial fibrillation by ectopic beats originating in the pulmonary veins. *N Engl J Med*. 1998;339(10):659–666.
2. Chen SA, Hsieh MH, Tai CT, et al. Initiation of atrial fibrillation by ectopic beats originating from the pulmonary veins: electrophysiological characteristics, pharmacological responses, and effects of radiofrequency ablation. *Circulation*. 1999;100(18):1879–1886.
3. Lin WS, Tai CT, Hsieh MH, et al. Catheter ablation of paroxysmal atrial fibrillation initiated by non-pulmonary vein ectopy. *Circulation*. 2003;107(25):3176–3183.
4. Konings KT, Kirchhof CJ, Smeets JR, Wellens HJ, Penn OC, Allessie MA. High-density mapping of electrically induced atrial fibrillation in humans. *Circulation*. 1994;89(4):1665–1680.
5. Ropella KM, Sahakian AV, Baerman JM, Swiryn S. The coherence spectrum. A quantitative discriminator of fibrillatory and nonfibrillatory cardiac rhythms. *Circulation*. 1989;80(1):112–119.
6. Ng J, Kadish AH, Goldberger JJ. Technical considerations for dominant frequency analysis. *J Cardiovasc Electrophysiol*. 2007;18(7):757–764.
7. Stiles MK, Brooks AG, John B, et al. The effect of electrogram duration on quantification of complex fractionated atrial electrograms and dominant frequency. *J Cardiovasc Electrophysiol*. 2008;19(3):252–258.
8. Sanders P, Berenfeld O, Hocini M, et al. Spectral analysis identifies sites of high-frequency activity maintaining atrial fibrillation in humans. *Circulation*. 2005;112(6):789–797.
9. Verma A, Wulffhart Z, Beardsall M, Whaley B, Hill C, Khaykin Y. Spatial and temporal stability of complex fractionated electrograms in patients with persistent atrial fibrillation over longer time periods: relationship to local electrogram cycle length. *Heart Rhythm*. 2008;5(8):1127–1133.
10. Lin YJ, Tai CT, Kao T, et al. Consistency of complex fractionated atrial electrograms during atrial fibrillation. *Heart Rhythm*. 2008;5(3):406–412.
11. Pachon MJ, Pachon ME, Pachon MJ, et al. A new treatment for atrial fibrillation based on spectral analysis to guide the catheter radiofrequency ablation. *Europace*. 2004;6(6):590–601.
12. Lin YJ, Kao T, Tai CT, et al. Spectral analysis during sinus rhythm predicts an abnormal atrial substrate in patients with paroxysmal atrial fibrillation. *Heart Rhythm*. 2008;5(7):968–974.
13. Lin YJ, Tai CT, Kao T, et al. Electrophysiological characteristics and catheter ablation in patients with paroxysmal right atrial fibrillation. *Circulation*. 2005;112(12):1692–1700.
14. Atienza F, Almendral J, Jalife J, et al Real-time dominant frequency mapping and ablation of dominant frequency sites in atrial fibrillation with left-to-right frequency gradients predicts long-term maintenance of sinus rhythm. *Heart Rhythm*. 2009;6(1):33–40.
15. Lin YJ, Tai CT, Kao T, et al. Frequency analysis in different types of atrial fibrillation. *J Am Coll Cardiol*. 2006;47(7):1401-1407.

16. Lazar S, Dixit S, Marchlinski FE, Callans DJ, Gerstenfeld EP. Presence of left-to-right atrial frequency gradient in paroxysmal but not persistent atrial fibrillation in humans. *Circulation.* 2004;110(20):3181–3186.
17. Sanders P, Nalliah CJ, Dubois R, et al. Frequency mapping of the pulmonary veins in paroxysmal versus permanent atrial fibrillation. *J Cardiovasc Electrophysiol.* 2006;17(9):965–972.
18. Yokoyama E, Osaka T, Takemoto Y, Suzuki T, Ito A, Kamiya K, Kodama I. Paroxysmal atrial fibrillation maintained by nonpulmonary vein sources can be predicted by dominant frequency analysis of atriopulmonary electrograms. *J Cardiovasc Electrophysiol.* 2009;20(6):630–636.
19. Lin YJ, Tsao HM, Chang SL, et al. Role of high dominant frequency sites in non-paroxysmal AF patients: Insights from high-density frequency and fractionation mapping. *Heart Rhythm.* 2010;7(9):1255–1262.
20. Lin YJ, Tai CT, Kao T, et al. Spatiotemporal organization of the left atrial substrate after circumferential pulmonary vein isolation of atrial fibrillation. *Circulation Arrhythm Electrophysiol.* 2009;2:233–241.
21. Lo LW, Lin YJ, Tsao HM, et al. The impact of left atrial size on long-term outcome of catheter ablation of chronic atrial fibrillation. *J Cardiovasc Electrophysiol.* 2009;20(11):1211–1216.
22. Yoshida K, Chugh A, Good E, et al. A critical decrease in dominant frequency and clinical outcome after catheter ablation of persistent atrial fibrillation. *Heart Rhythm.* 2010;7(3):295–302.
23. Huang SY, Lin YJ, Tsao HM, et al. The biatrial substrate properties in different types of paroxysmal atrial fibrillation. *Heart Rhythm.* 2011;8(7):961–967.
24. Lin YJ, Chang SL, Lo LW, et al. A prospective, randomized comparison of modified pulmonary vein isolation versus conventional pulmonary vein isolation in patients with paroxysmal atrial fibrillation. *J Cardiovasc Electrophysiol.* 2012 (in press).
25. Everett TH, Kok LC, Vaughn RH, Moorman JR, Haines DE. Frequency domain algorithm for quantifying atrial fibrillation organization to increase defibrillation efficacy. *IEEE Trans Biomed Eng.* 2001;48(9):969–978.

Video Descriptions

Video 28.1 Wavefront dynamics during atrial fibrillation from simultaneous bi-atrial Ensite array in paroxysmal AF patient originating from RSPV, shown in Figure 28.4. Rapid and repetitive activities were observed in the RSPV ostium.

Video 28.2 Wavefront dynamics during atrial fibrillation from simultaneous right atrial Ensite array in paroxysmal AF. The high-DF region was compatible with small-radius reentry in the right atrial posterior wall, and linear ablation connecting the conduction channels successfully eliminated and prevented further induction of AF.

CHAPTER 29

Utilization of the Hansen Robotic Catheter Navigation System: The Austin Approach

G. Joseph Gallinghouse, MD; Luigi Di Biase, MD, PhD; Andrea Natale, MD[1]

Introduction

Ablation has become a common method of treating AF, as antiarrhythmic drug therapy is relatively ineffective and fraught with side effects. While there have been significant advances in technology that facilitate safe and effective application of ablation lesions, manual catheter navigation remains essentially unchanged since the mid-1990s. Recently, remote catheter navigation systems have emerged that may result in refined catheter positioning and contact titration relative to manual navigation. There are also advantages to the operator, allowing ablation from an ergonomically favorable seated position, removed from the radiation field. Our group at the Texas Cardiac Arrhythmia Institute at St. David's Medical Center (Austin, TX) has amassed the world's largest experience in robotic catheter navigation. This chapter describes our approach.

Background

For those of us in cardiac EP training programs during the mid-1990s, the concept of taming AF with ablation seemed to be the proverbial "Holy Grail." We fondly recall the excitement of eliminating accessory pathway-mediated tachycardias and AV nodal reentry. The typical flutter circuit had just been defined, and lesions at the tricuspid isthmus would terminate the arrhythmia—to our delight. However, AF was our nemesis. Then, Haïssaguerre and colleagues[1] published the seminal observation in 1998 that the great majority of AF triggers resided in the PVs, finding that the arrhythmia could be suppressed by targeting these sites with ablation. This led to intensive investigation of the optimal approach to elimination of these triggers, ultimately evolving to the current "PV isolation" procedure—of which there are several variations.[2-8]

The past decade has seen tremendous strides in the development of technology to facilitate safe and effective ablation of the AF substrate. The medical device industry, driven by market opportunity and competition, has quickly provided tools that allow the modern electrophysiologist to approach even the most complex arrhythmias. Advanced 3-dimensional electroanatomical mapping systems allow the operator to reconstruct the anatomy of the chamber of interest in real time and to track electrical activation on a beat-by-beat basis.[9] Availability of voltage mapping with

---

All the authors contributed equally to the drafting and editing of this chapter.

1. Disclosure/Conflict of Interest: Dr. Gallinghouse has consulting agreements with Hansen Medical and St. Jude Medical. Dr. Di Biase is a consultant for Hansen Medical and Biosense Webster. Dr. Natale is a consultant for Biosense Webster and has also received a research grant from St. Jude Medical and received speaker honoraria from St. Jude Medical, Medtronic, Boston Scientific, Biotronik, and Biosense Webster.

these systems has facilitated ventricular tachycardia ablation and assessment of PV isolation. The development of ICE provides continuous visualization of catheter location relative to important structures, facilitates transseptal catheterization, and allows early detection of ablation-related complications such as pericardial tamponade.[10,11] However, lagging behind has been improvement of the navigational capabilities of the primary therapeutic tool—the ablation catheter itself.

Ablation catheters have been enhanced with tip irrigation for cooling, which has advantages in lesion formation and avoidance of char.[12] Contact sensors are in clinical trials, given that tactile feedback and visual cues are a poor gauge for the operator of proximity to tissue targets. Remarkable, however, is the fact that the steering mechanisms of modern ablation catheters are little different than those found in catheters from the mid-1990s.[13-16] Even though we are now required to create much more complex lesion sets covering large geometric areas, the manual ablation catheter is still limited to uni- or bidirectional movement using pull wires.

Recently, remote navigation systems have emerged that allow movement of the ablation catheter with computer-guided precision not attainable manually. Navigation may be linked to a 3-dimensional mapping system that provides intuitive catheter "driving" based on the real-time anatomy generated during the case. Very fine contact titration can be performed during ablation, which may allow delivery of more effective RF energy to tissue with reduced power requirements.

There are two current commercially available remote navigation systems. One utilizes application of magnetic field vectors to a proprietary catheter (Stereotaxis, St. Louis, MO), and the other maneuvers standard ablation catheters robotically (Hansen Medical, Mountain View, CA).[17-30] This review will describe our experience with the robotic system for ablation of AF, which is the most extensive in the world to date.

As with any new medical technology applied to a challenging clinical problem, there are individual and collective learning curves that must be overcome to achieve optimal utilization—both from safety and efficacy standpoints. The manufacturer may make recommendations as to the intended operation of the system, but ultimately it is the responsibility of the operator to determine "best practices" with regard to the care of patients. Robotic catheter navigation is no different.

After clinical trials in Europe, the first installation of a Hansen system in the U.S. occurred at the Cleveland Clinic in May 2007, followed by St. David's Medical Center in Austin, TX, in September of that year. Our group endeavored to learn the system quickly and began to perform AF ablation procedures in high volume immediately. We accepted the concept that our early experience would be relatively time consuming, but the hope was that repetitive use would lead to rapid mastering of the technology. This in fact was the case, and within the first 30 cases, our ablation times to achieve clinical endpoints were equivalent to those cases performed manually.

In an attempt to accelerate "ascent of the learning curve" through the shared experience of many operators, several users' group meetings were held in 2008 and 2009. This allowed us to quickly determine the most successful approaches to various technical aspects of the robotic ablation procedure. While the methods have thus become fairly standardized, there are slight variations from center to center.

The "Austin approach" will be detailed below.

Description of the Hansen System

The Hansen robotic catheter navigation system allows remote manipulation of an ablation catheter utilizing computer-driven input to a bedside robotic arm. After placement of the robotically driven catheter in the chamber of interest, the operator sits at a console with controls that input commands to the catheter via the robotic arm (**Figure 29.1**).

The system consists of two primary components, the Sensei Robotic Catheter System and the Artisan Guide Catheter, a remotely controlled steerable sheath (**Figure 29.2**). The physician remotely directs the movement of the Artisan Guide Catheter through the Sensei Robotic Catheter System—an electronically controlled mechanical system for remotely controlling the Artisan. The Sensei is comprised of a physician workstation, an electronics rack, and a patient-side Remote Catheter Manipulator (RCM) (**Figures 29.1** and **29.2**).

The system allows the clinician to direct the catheter tip to a desired intracardiac location based on visual feedback from 3-dimensional electroanatomic maps, fluoroscopic images, and ICE images while seated at the workstation. The RCM electromechanically manipulates the steerable guide catheter in response to commands received from the physician through a special 3-D joystick (Intuitive Motion Controller, or IMC) at the physician workstation. A basic principle of the system is that operator input is "intuitive" relative to an image in the "navigation window" monitor, which is in the center of the monitor console. For example, if the navigation window is an LAO fluoroscopic image of the LA, movement to the right with the IMC will direct the Artisan toward the lateral wall, and pushing the IMC away from the operator (or "into the monitor") will direct it toward the posterior wall.

The Artisan Guide Catheter is a pull-wire-actuated open-lumen guide catheter. The inner lumen is 8-Fr diameter and the guide catheter fits through a standard 14-Fr hemostatic introducer. The Artisan attaches to the RCM through a sterile drape barrier and the RCM in turn actuates the catheter pull-wires in response to commands from the physician. The Artisan is a guide catheter and is not capable of therapy or diagnostics on its own. Rather,

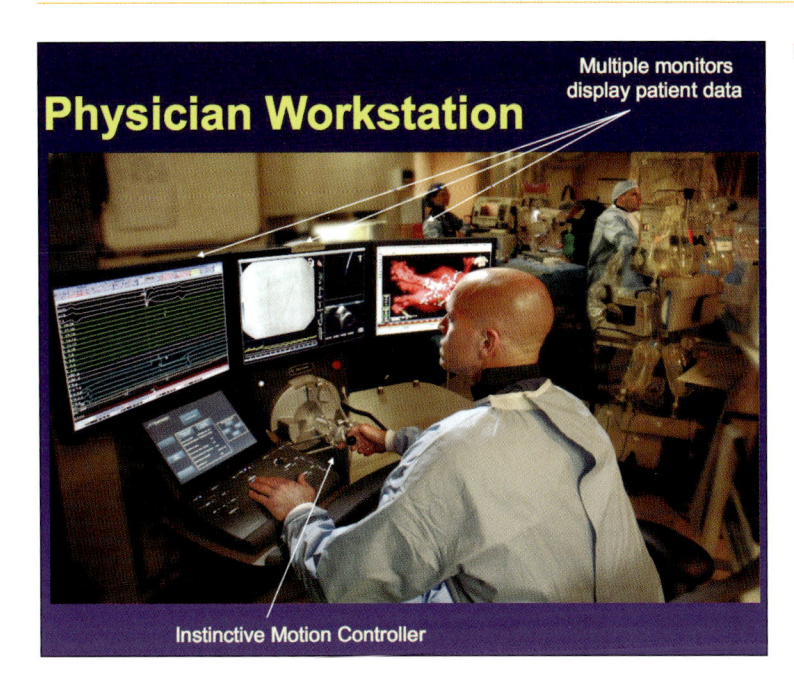

Figure 29.1 Physician workstation.

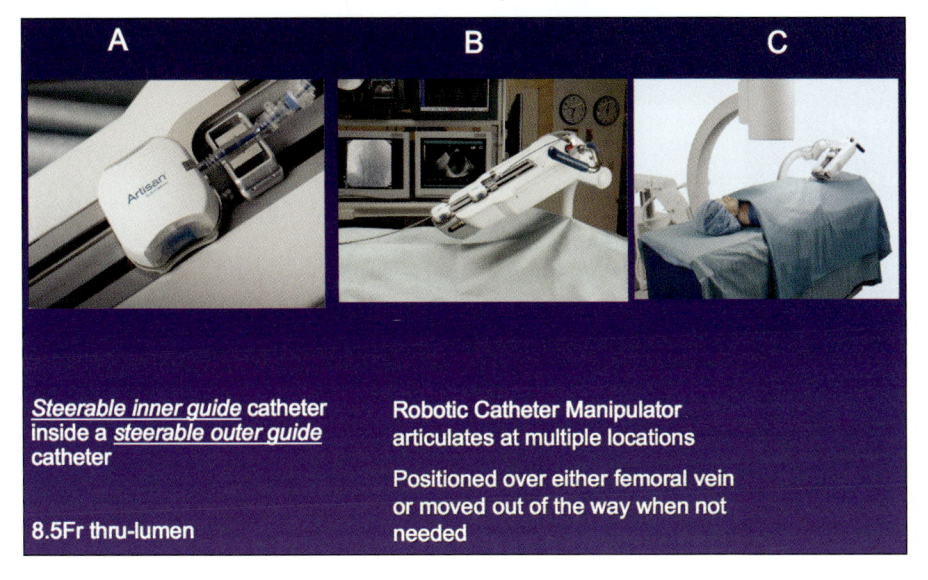

Figure 29.2 The Sensei Robotic Catheter System and the Artisan Guide Catheter.

commercially available ablation catheters are placed into the Artisan, with just the distal two electrodes extending beyond the Artisan tip.

The Artisan can articulate in any direction to 270 degrees, with a minimal working curve diameter of 30 mm (**Figure 29.3** and ▶ **Video 29.1**)

Introduction of the Artisan Catheter

In the majority of laboratories, the robotic arm is positioned on the patient's left side, and therefore the Artisan catheter is inserted via the left femoral vein. This leaves the right side unobstructed for the operator when manipulation of a second mapping catheter or ICE catheter is required. Early-experience placement of the Artisan from the left was occasionally problematic, particularly in a tortuous iliac vein, given the size and stiffness of the catheter relative to typical EP equipment. There were reports of retroperitoneal bleeding complications attributed to iliac tears.[22]

The solution was to insert a long (30 cm) sheath under fluoroscopic guidance extending into the IVC. The Artisan was then placed through the long sheath, with the relatively soft ablation catheter approximately 5 cm beyond the tip of the inner guide. Once safely in the IVC, the Artisan could be manually advanced to the RA under fluoroscopic guidance, leading with the steerable ablation catheter. The Artisan could then be advanced over the fixed ablation catheter into position in the low RA (▶ **Video 29.2**).

Occasionally, we find that insertion of the long introducer sheath to the IVC is difficult depending on the left iliac anatomy. Shaping the tip of the sheath/dilator with a

30-degree bend and use of a stiff wire (Amplatz) will usually facilitate this step. However, we are occasionally required to remove the dilator and insert our 10-Fr steerable ICE catheter into the sheath in the distal iliac vein (**Figure 29.4** and ▶ **Video 29.3**).

The ICE catheter is then directed into the IVC and used as a "rail" for the long sheath. We have yet to encounter a case where the left-sided Artisan access site had to be abandoned, but ultimately the access site could be shifted to the right if necessary. To demonstrate the course of the left iliac vein, we always insert a CS catheter from the left before inserting the long sheath.

Transseptal Access

Robotic LA ablation requires placement of the Artisan catheter through a transseptal puncture site, as with any other such procedure. Even if a PFO is present, transseptal access obtained via puncture as the ideal crossing is at the antero-inferior aspect of the fossa. This provides an ideal angle of attack for ablation near the right PVs.

Our practice is to utilize an SL1 (St. Jude Medical, St. Paul, MN) or similar sheath, along with a Brockenbrough needle, to access the LA with ICE guidance. We then place a circular mapping catheter (Lasso, Biosense Webster, Diamond Bar, CA) into the LA via the sheath and carefully build the geometric reconstruction of the chamber using the Endocardial Solutions NavX 3-dimensional electroanatomical mapping system (St. Jude Medical, USA) or with the Carto 3D mapping system (Biosense Webster, Diamond Bar, CA). After the geometric map has been obtained, the Lasso is removed and a guidewire placed through the transseptal sheath into a left PV for support. The sheath is then withdrawn into the RA, which leaves its transseptal access site available for passage of the Artisan.

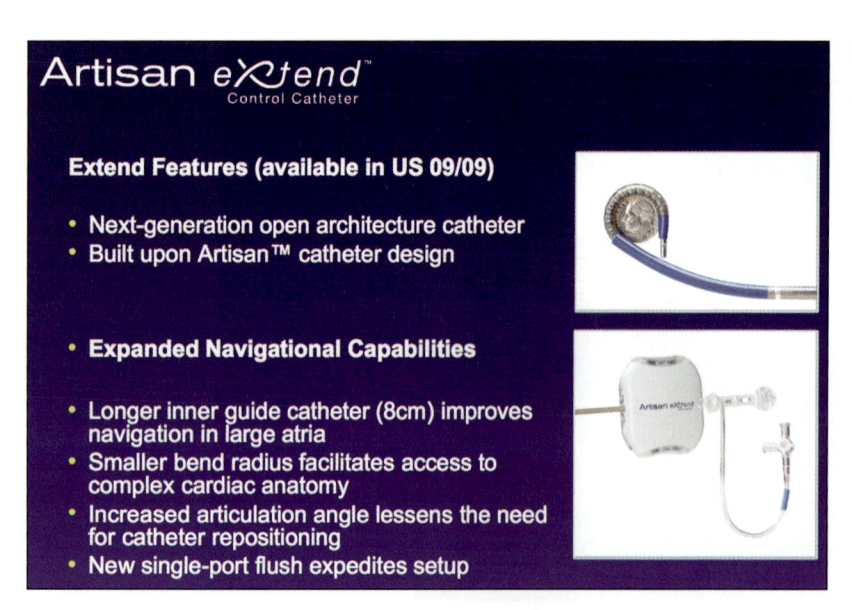

Figure 29.3 The Artisan catheter max degree of articulation (270 degrees), with a minimal working curve diameter of 30 mm.

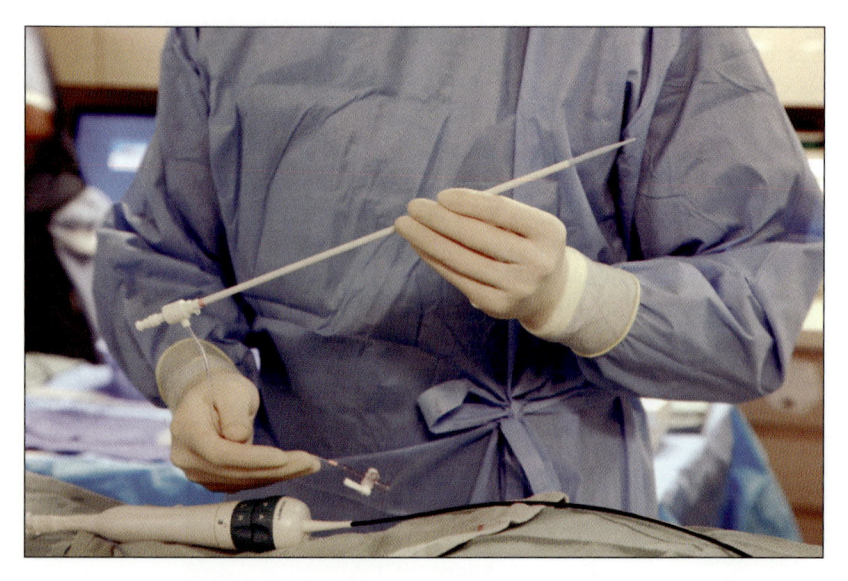

Figure 29.4 14-Fr sheath introducer.

With a guidewire marking the location of the fossa ovalis puncture site, along with the trajectory from RA to LA, safe transseptal placement of the Artisan is relatively simple. We robotically position the Artisan-ablation tip near the fossa using both fluoroscopy and ICE guidance. Using orthogonal fluoroscopic views, the ablation tip is robotically aligned to the guidewire and then carefully "driven" through the puncture site until saline echo contrast is seen in the LA (▶ Videos 29.4 and 29.5). The outer guide can be advanced for support if there is any difficulty passing the inner guide into the LA, as for example in the case of a thickened fossa.

An alternative transseptal approach used by some operators is to manually maneuver the ablation catheter through the puncture site in the fossa and then advance the Artisan over the ablation catheter—similar to the technique used for RA positioning. In our lab, we have occasionally utilized this technique if there was difficulty driving the Artisan into the LA due to a scarred or thick fossa. In over 650 cases, we have never failed to successfully achieve transseptal placement of the catheter and typically require no longer than 1 to 2 minutes for this aspect of the procedure.

Titration of Contact and Catheter Stability

In our view, a clear advantage of the Hansen robotic catheter system over manual or magnetic navigation is the ability to control contact force. Ablation lesion formation results from a complex interplay of catheter contact with tissue, power settings, catheter stability, and duration of RF delivery. Until ablation catheters become available with contact sensors, operator assessment of pressure at the catheter tip–tissue interface will remain a "guesstimate." This is dramatically illustrated with the recent Toccata preliminary study findings,[15] which showed that experienced ablationists grossly over- and underestimated contact in positions that they felt were optimal for RF delivery when they were blinded to pressure data.

The stable platform provided by the inner guide of the Artisan sheath prevents "rebound" of the ablation tip when placed against tissue, as occurs with relatively soft manual ablation catheters. As a result, the power required to achieve effective RF lesions is typically in the range of 15 to 25 W, as opposed to 35 to 45 W with manual ablation. Further, very small adjustments of the catheter tip contact can be made by utilizing both the IMC ("joystick") and the auto-retract button, which withdraws the catheter at a programmable rate—typically set at 1 cm/sec. This capability allows refinement of the catheter tip location and pressure on a millimeter-by-millimeter basis.[13,24]

The support provided by the inner guide has generated concern among some operators that there may be an increased risk of cardiac or vascular perforation with the Artisan. This has not been our experience. While the sheath is clearly "stiffer" than a manual ablation catheter, use of the long introducer sheath from the left femoral vein allows safe passage through tortuous iliac anatomy. A novel pressure-sensing mechanism is also built into the system, termed "Intellesense" (**Figure 29.5**). This feature involves automated dithering of the ablation catheter and normalizing to 0 grams of pressure with a baseline measurement in the heart. A load sensor on the robotic arm then calculates the contact force with tissue and displays this graphically in real time for the operator. Haptic feedback is available, wherein the IMC may be programmed to vibrate above a set cut-point, for example 40 grams. Intellesense has been demonstrated to be highly accurate when the catheter is perpendicular to tissue but becomes less so as the ablation tip orientation nears parallel.

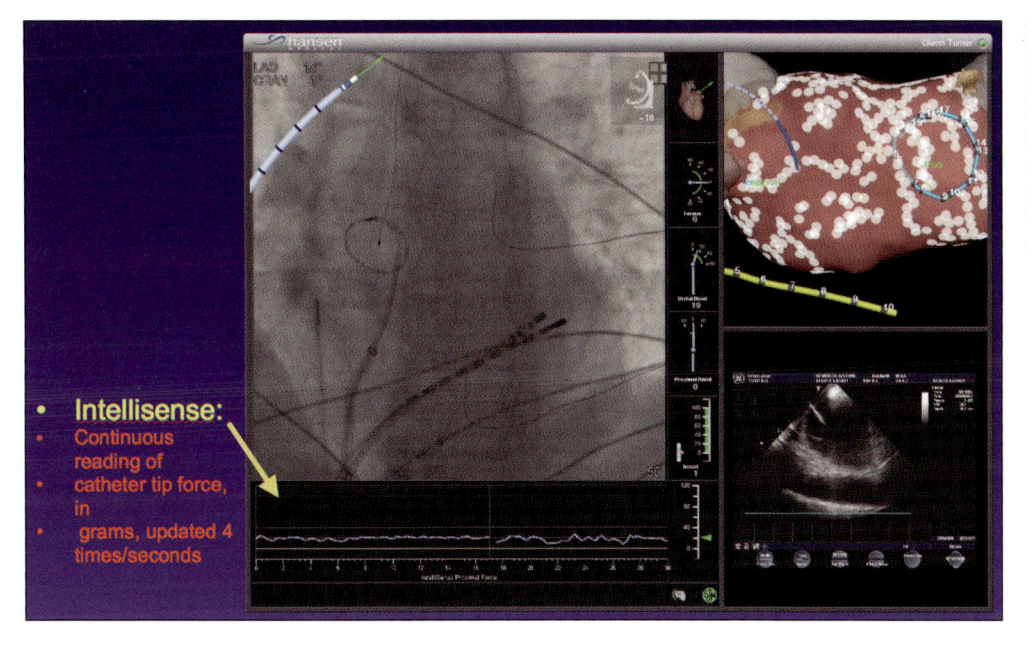

Figure 29.5 Screen shot obtained from the physician workstation showing fluoroscopy, ICE, 3-dimensional mapping, and the Intellisense, a continuous reading of the catheter tip force in grams, updated 4×/sec.

Therefore, while less than perfect, Intellesense provides a safety mechanism where catheter forces on the myocardium are greatest: perpendicular.[13]

We have found that the ability to navigate the Artisan utilizing a 3-dimensional electroanatomical map (NavX, St. Jude Medical) provides further contact titration advantages. A software module available in the Sensei system, termed "Cohesion," allows the operator to place the 3-dimensional map of the LA in the navigation window and to move the catheter intuitively based on the map orientation. The operator can continuously reorient the 3-dimensional map display with a trackball on the Sensei pendant, allowing for point-by-point adjustments during the course of the ablation procedure (▶ Video 29.6). In our practice, we find this feature invaluable for fine manipulation of the Artisan to ablation sites on the 3-dimensional map, giving complete control of both catheter movement and map orientation to the operator for optimal ablation target acquisition.

Finally, the 270-degree out-of-plane maneuverability of the Artisan allows for contact titration adjustments not possible with uni-/bidirectional manual catheters. As an example, the LAA ridge can be a very challenging location to maintain stable ablation tip contact with a manually directed catheter, requiring rotation and torque together with pull and release of curve to optimize lesion formation. The catheter frequently slips out of position on a narrow ridge, requiring reorientation of the tip. In contrast, the Artisan can be directed to the center of the vein at its antrum, then simply maneuvered out of plane in the third dimension to achieve contact on the ridge. Reliably stable contact is then achieved even with drag lesions along the ridge using the interplay of the IMC and Cohesion adjustments. This degree of catheter tip control has also been found to be of great value in other relatively difficult manual catheter locations, such as at the LA roof near the right SPV, the inferior aspect of the right IPV, and within the CS.

Ablation Lesion Sets

As for most groups around the world, our first priority in ablation of AF is antral PV isolation. However, our approach to achieving this endpoint is somewhat different. We manipulate a circular mapping catheter (Biosense Webster "Lasso") in the antra of the veins and ablate electrograms recorded on the lasso bipoles until isolation is complete (▶ Video 29.7). These lesions are extended across the posterior wall with the intent of eliminating all atrial electrograms, roughly from a line extending from the upper aspect of the superior veins to the lower aspect of the inferior veins (**Figure 29.6**). During the course of ablation, a pediatric temperature probe in the esophagus is continually moved to the location of the ablation catheter tip, and ablation is terminated in that location if a temperature rise exceeding 39°C is observed. ICE is utilized to ensure appropriate ablation catheter contact and to periodically view the potential pericardial space for effusion.

When utilizing the robotic catheter ablation system, power requirements to achieve effective lesion formation are significantly lower than with manual ablation—likely because of improved and constant catheter contact without rebound. This is a critically important point, as excessive power delivery can result in steam pops and pericardial effusion/tamponade. Our practice is to limit power on the posterior wall to 15 to 20 W and anterior to the veins 25 to 30 W. We have never been required to up-titrate power beyond 35 W to achieve PV isolation, and have used 35 W on rare occasions. This is consistent with what Di Biase et al reported in animal models.[13]

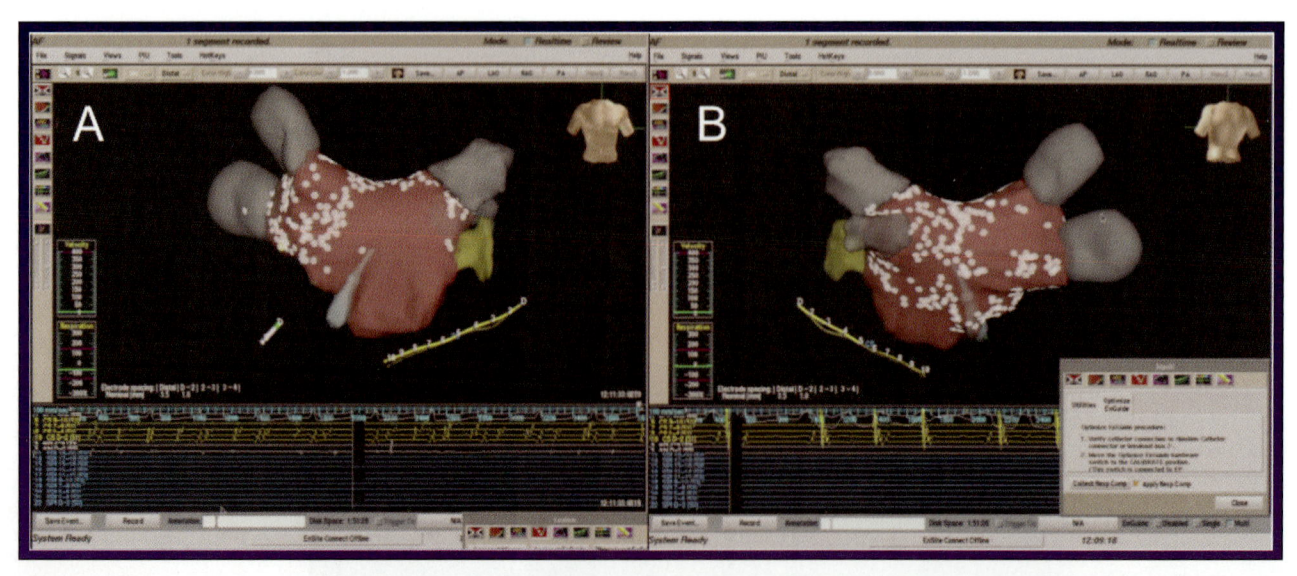

Figure 29.6 NavX™ map with the ablation lesion set (white dots) in AP and PA view at the level of the PV antrum and the posterior wall utilizing the Hansen robotic system.

In patients who have long-standing persistent AF, ablation is performed in a stepwise fashion. Antral PV isolation is performed first, in the same manner as in paroxysmal patients. However, a larger area of posterior wall in the LA is isolated with lesions extending from the roof to the floor of the CS. Ablation is continued with the goal of organizing and terminating the arrhythmia, typically targeting CFAE on the IAS and at the base of the LAA. If required, the CS is then isolated (▶ Video 29.8), followed by targeting of CFAE in the RA (crista terminalis/septum) and isolation of the SVC. Should typical RA flutter be seen or induced, the subeustachian isthmus is ablated with documentation of bidirectional isthmus block. Finally, the LAA is isolated if tachycardia appears to be driven by that structure.[8]

In both paroxysmal and persistent AF patients, isoproterenol (20 mcg/min × 20 minutes) is infused after ablation has been completed. During this period, PV isolation is confirmed and additional focal atrial tachycardias ablated if induced.[8]

Our experience with the Hansen robotic catheter navigation system suggests that it may offer significant advantages over manual navigation for ablation of the AF substrate. The benefits to the operator are inarguable; one is able to perform the procedure in a comfortable seated position, without a lead apron and removed from the fluoroscopy field. Robotic navigation may offer improved procedural outcomes for patients as well, although randomized data are currently unavailable. We have published a nonrandomized series comparing almost 400 consecutive patients undergoing robotic and manual ablation.[24] This demonstrated a trend, albeit not statistically significant, toward improved efficacy outcomes in both paroxysmal and persistent AF patients. Complication rates were similarly low in both groups.

A multicenter randomized clinical trial is now underway to better assess the value of robotic navigation in patients with paroxysmal AF. Efficacy and safety will be compared in two groups of patients who have failed antiarrhythmic drug therapy, with a 2:1 randomization schedule of robotic vs. manual ablation. The availability of new pressure sensors ablation catheters, when combined with robotic navigation, may be an ideal combination for RF lesion formation, due to stability of the ablation platform, and for precise titration of contact force.

References

1. Haïssaguerre M, Jaïs P, Shah DC, et al. Spontaneous initiation of AF by ectopic beats originating in the PVs. *N Engl J Med.* 1998;339:659–666.
2. Oral H, Scharf C, Chugh A, et al. Catheter ablation for paroxysmal AF: segmental PV ostial ablation versus LA ablation. *Circulation.* 2003;108:2355–2360.
3. Nakagawa H, Scherlag BJ, Lockwood DJ, et al. Localization of LA autonomic ganglionated plexuses using endocardial and epicardial high frequency stimulation in patients with AF. *Heart Rhythm.* 2005;2005:S10.
4. Pappone C, Santinelli V, Manguso F, et al. PV denervation enhances long-term benefit after circumferential ablation for paroxysmal AF. *Circulation.* 2004;109:327–334.
5. Bhargava M, Di Biase L, Mohanty P, et al. Impact of type of AF and repeat catheter ablation on long-term freedom from AF: results from a multicenter study. *Heart Rhythm.* 2009;6:1403–412.
6. Pachon MJ, Pachon ME, Lobo TJ, et al. A new treatment for AF based on spectral analysis to guide the catheter RF-ablation. *Europace.* 2004;6:590–601.
7. Nademanee K, McKenzie J, Kosar E, et al. A new approach for catheter ablation of AF: mapping of the EP substrate. *J Am Coll Cardiol.* 2004;43:2044–2053.
8. Di Biase L, Burkhardt JD, Mohanty P, et al. LAA: an under-recognized trigger site of AF. *Circulation.* 2010;122:109–118.
9. Karch MR, Zrenner B, Deisenhofer I, et al. Freedom from atrial tachyarrhythmias after catheter ablation of AF: a randomized comparison between 2 current ablation strategies. *Circulation.* 2005;111:2875–2880.
10. Verma A, Marrouche NF, Natale A: PV antrum isolation: intracardiac echocardiography-guided technique. *J Cardiovasc Electrophysiol.* 2004;15:1335–1340.
11. Di Biase L, Burkhardt JD, Mohanty P, et al. Periprocedural stroke and management of major bleeding complications in patients undergoing catheter ablation of AF: the impact of periprocedural therapeutic international normalized ratio. *Circulation.* 2010;121:2550–2556.
12. Wilber DJ, Pappone C, Neuzil P, et al. Comparison of antiarrhythmic drug therapy and radiofrequency catheter ablation in patients with paroxysmal AF: a randomized controlled trial. *JAMA.* 2010;303:333–340.
13. Di Biase L, Natale A, Barrett C, et al. Relationship between catheter forces, lesion characteristics, "popping," and char formation: experience with robotic navigation system. *J Cardiovasc Electrophysiol.* 2009;20:436–440.
14. Nakagawa H, Kautzner J, Natale A, et al. Electrogram amplitude and impedance are poor predictors of electrode-tissue contact force in ablation of AF. *Heart Rhythm.* 2010;7:S65.
15. Kuck KH. TOCCATA European Clinical Study—First multi-clinical study using irrigated ablation catheters with an integrated contact force sensor, presented at Boston Atrial Fibrillation Symposium, 2010.
16. Neuzil P, Shah D, Herrera C, et al. Does catheter contact force during RF ablation relate to AF recurrence rate? 17th World Congress Cardiostim 2010, Nice Acropolis, France, 16–19 June 2010. *Europace.* 2010;12(Suppl 1), 176P/7, i107.
17. Pappone C, Vicedomini G, Manguso F, et al. Robotic magnetic navigation for AF ablation. *J Am Coll Cardiol.* 2006;47:1390–1400.
18. Di Biase L, Fahmy TS, Patel D, et al. Remote magnetic navigation: human experience in PV ablation. *J Am Coll Cardiol.* 2007;50:868–874.
19. Miyazaki S, Shah AJ, Xhaet O, et al. Remote magnetic navigation with irrigated tip catheter for ablation of paroxysmal AF. *Circ Arrhythm Electrophysiol.* 2010;3:585–589.

20. Chun KR, Wissner E, Koektuerk B, et al. Remote-controlled magnetic PV isolation using a new irrigated-tip catheter in patients with AF. *Circ Arrhythm Electrophysiol.* 2010;3:458–464.
21. Pappone C, Vicedomini G, Frigoli E, et al. Irrigated-tip magnetic catheter ablation of AF: a long-term prospective study in 130 patients. *Heart Rhythm.* 2011;8:8–15.
22. Wazni OM, Barrett C, Martin DO, et al. Experience with the Hansen robotic system for AF ablation—lessons learned and techniques modified: Hansen in the real world. *J Cardiovasc Electrophysiol.* 2009;20:1193–1196.
23. Saliba W, Reddy VY, Wazni O, et al. AF ablation using a robotic catheter remote control system: initial human experience and long-term follow-up results. *J Am Coll Cardiol.* 2008;51:2407–2411.
24. Di Biase L, Wang Y, Horton R, et al. Ablation of AF utilizing robotic catheter navigation in comparison to manual navigation and ablation: single-center experience. *J Cardiovasc Electrophysiol.* 2009;20:1328–1335.
25. Schmidt B, Tilz RR, Neven K, et al. Remote robotic navigation and electroanatomical mapping for ablation of AF: considerations for navigation and impact on procedural outcome. *Circ Arrhythm Electrophysiol.* 2009;2:120–128.
26. Hlivák P, Mlãochová H, Peichl P, Cihák R, Wichterle D, Kautzner J. Robotic navigation in catheter ablation for paroxysmal atrial fibrillation: midterm efficacy and predictors of postablation arrhythmia recurrences. *J Cardiovasc Electrophysiol.* 2011;22(5):534–540.
27. Di Biase L, Davies W, Horton R, et al. Acute complication rate with the robotic navigation for catheter of atrial fibrillation: the worldwide experience. *Circulation.* 2008;118:S978–S979.
28. Arya A, Zaker-Shahrak R, Sommer P, et al. Catheter ablation of AF using remote magnetic catheter navigation: a case-control study. *Europace.* 2011;13:45–50.
29. Kautzner J, Peichl P, Cihák R, Wichterle D, Mlãochová H. Early experience with robotic navigation for catheter ablation of paroxysmal AF. *Pacing Clin Electrophysiol.* 2009;32 Suppl 1:S163–S166.
30. Willems S, Steven D, Servatius H, et al. Persistence of PV isolation after robotic remote-navigated ablation for AF and its relation to clinical outcome. *J Cardiovasc Electrophysiol.* 2010;21:1079–1084.

Video Descriptions

Video 29.1 The video shows the articulation and rotations up to 270 degrees of the Artisan catheter, which is composed of two sheaths. The guide catheter is an 8-Fr sheath that navigates in the LA. This is the same size as a regular transseptal sheath. The outer sheath (more proximal) sits in the RA and gives support with some forward bend as needed.

Videos 29.2 and 29.3 After the insertion of a 14-Fr long sheath (30 cm) over a guidewire (Video 29.2), the Artisan catheter is advanced into the RA using the open irrigated ablation catheter as a guidewire (Video 29.3). Once safely in the IVC, the Artisan could be manually advanced to the RA under fluoroscopic guidance, leading with the steerable ablation catheter.

Video 29.4 After a manual transseptal access is obtained and a guidewire is placed into the tip of the left SPV, the guidewire is used as a marker of the fossa ovalis, along with the trajectory from right to LA. This video shows a safe transseptal placement of the Artisan. Robotically, the Artisan-ablation tip is positioned near the fossa, using both fluoroscopy and ICE guidance. Using orthogonal fluoroscopic views, the ablation tip is robotically aligned to the guidewire and then carefully "driven" through the puncture site until saline echo contrast is seen in the LA.

Video 29.5 Following the initial positioning shown in Video 29.4, the outer guide can be advanced for support and the ablation catheter is able to map and ablate into the LA.

Video 29.6 Using the trackball on the Sensei pendant, the operator is orienting the 3-dimensional map with the ablation catheter to target the circular mapping catheter at the level of the electrodes 5 and 6. This feature, only available with the NavX system, is invaluable for fine manipulation of the Artisan to ablation sites on the 3-D map, giving complete control of both catheter movement and map orientation to the operator for optimal ablation target acquisition.

Video 29.7 PA and AP rotational 3-dimensional view of a PV antrum isolation extended to the posterior wall and to CS in a patient with persistent AF. Note the circular mapping catheter at the antrum of the left PVs.

Video 29.8 The video shows the artisan catheter advanced robotically into the CS to obtain CS isolation guided by a mapping decapolar catheter positioned manually into the CS in patients with long-standing persistent AF. The circular mapping catheter is positioned into the LA.

CHAPTER 30

How to Perform Atrial Fibrillation Ablation Using Remote Magnetic Navigation

J. David Burkhardt, MD; Matthew Dare, CEPS; Luigi Di Biase, MD, PhD;
Pasquale Santangeli, MD; Andrea Natale, MD

Introduction

AF ablation requires the electrical isolation of all PVs. In addition, the posterior wall, septum, CS, mitral valve annulus, SVC, and occasionally the LAA require significant ablation or isolation.[1,2] This very complex ablation requires significant skill, manual dexterity, and experience. Remote magnetic navigation is the manipulation of specially designed ablation catheters within a magnetic field inside the patient's chest. This field is the composite magnetic field created by two large rare earth magnets that are present on the sides of a patient. These magnets tilt, rotate, and move in and out, changing the direction of the magnetic field and allowing a catheter to be directed anywhere in the x, y, or z axes. Remote magnetic navigation has been shown to be useful in AF ablation and may allow less experienced operators to perform the complex maneuvers required in this complex ablation.[3-5]

Preprocedural Planning

Patients are interviewed prior to the planned procedure. During this interview, the procedure is described in detail, including the risks and benefits. Preprocedure testing includes documentation of AF, echocardiography, and stress testing (if any risk factors are present). The echocardiogram is carefully reviewed for valvular heart disease, LA size, and any potential congenital anomalies that may impact the ablation procedure. If the echocardiogram or cardiac catheterization suggest the need for an open-chest procedure such as coronary artery bypass grafting or valvular repair, then the patient is referred to a cardiac surgeon for concomitant surgery and a "cut and sew" MAZE procedure. If the patient has had a previous LA ablation procedure, a contrast-enhanced cardiac CT is performed to evaluate for the presence of PV stenosis or other anomaly (**Figure 30.1**). If the patient has an implantable cardiac device such as a pacemaker or ICD, appropriate plans are made for reprogramming the device at the time of the procedure due to the fact that the magnetic field can impact the device's function. A pacemaker may act in magnet or DOO mode, and an ICD may not charge the capacitors appropriately in the magnetic field.

Patients should be anticoagulated prior to the procedure with warfarin if possible. In general, patients should have therapeutic INRs for at least a month prior to the procedure. Coumadin is not withdrawn prior to the procedure.

If the patient arrives for the procedure in AF without documented therapeutic INRs, then a TEE is performed to evaluate for the presence of LAA thrombus. If thrombus is present, the procedure is cancelled for 2 months, and a repeat TEE is performed prior to the procedure.

Procedure

The patient arrives in the fasting state and is intubated for general anesthesia. At the same time, an esophageal temperature probe is placed for monitoring during the ablation. After sterilely prepping and draping the patient, two 8-Fr introducers are placed in the right femoral vein, one 10.5-Fr introducer is placed in the left femoral vein, and one 7-Fr introducer is placed in the right internal jugular vein. All venous access is guided by ultrasound. The artery appears to pulsate on ultrasound and does not compress with pressure. The vein does not have as robust pulsation and collapses with compression. The use of ultrasound guidance appears to reduce vascular injury events and complications in patients that are anticoagulated.

After introducers are placed, a heparin bolus is given to the patient to achieve a goal ACT of about 400 seconds. A duodecapolar recording catheter is placed in the CS from the right internal jugular introducer. The distal 10 poles are placed in the CS for recording and pacing of the LA, and the proximal 10 poles lie along the lateral RA for pacing and recording of this location (**Figure 30.2**).

A phased-array sideways-looking intracardiac ultrasound catheter is placed into the RA. This is used to visualize the atrial septum, PVs, and to monitor for complications such as pericardial effusion. Careful attention is paid to the septum to see if it is thick or floppy or if an atrial septal defect is present. The PVs are evaluated for general direction in relation to the LA, the presence of common ostia, and size. The depth of ultrasound is usually set to 90 to 100 mm for the LA. To evaluate the presence of pericardial effusion or to evaluate LV function, the ultrasound depth is increased to 160 mm and the catheter is retroflexed across the tricuspid valve with the array facing the ventricular septum. This provides an excellent view of the cardiac border and LV structures.

A 180-cm wire is placed from the lower right femoral introducer into the SVC or subclavian system. The introducer is exchanged for a long LAMP90 transseptal sheath. The sheath is placed into the high SVC over the wire, and the wire is withdrawn. A syringe with heparinized saline is attached to the sheath and suction is performed until blood is withdrawn. After this, the sheath is flushed with the saline. The syringe is removed and a transseptal needle (BRK) is shaped according to the patient's distance from IVC to septum seen on ultrasound. The needle is placed into the sheath and advanced to within a centimeter of the tip of the introducer tip. A contrast syringe on the hub of the transseptal needle is flushed. The arrow of the needle is pointed to the 5 o'clock position, and the entire system is withdrawn to the upper septum. The ICE catheter is rotated to show the septum and the left PVs. A puncture

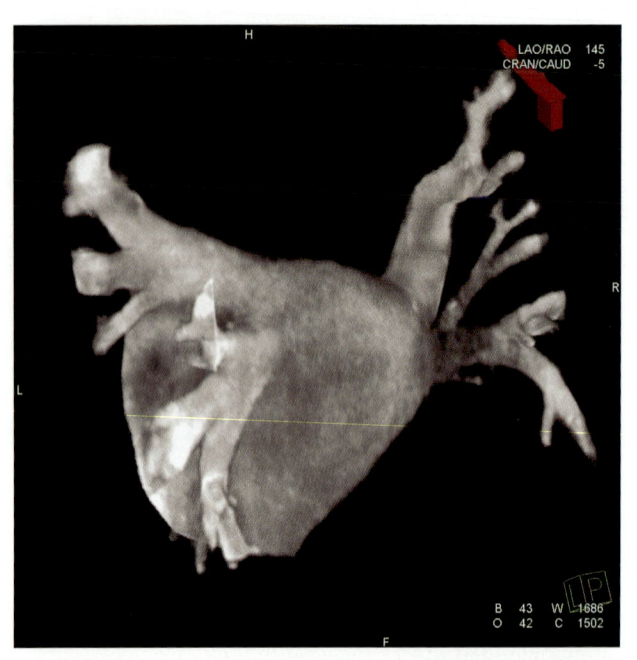

Figure 30.1 A CT-type image of the LA acquired by rotational angiography with 3-dimensional reconstruction.

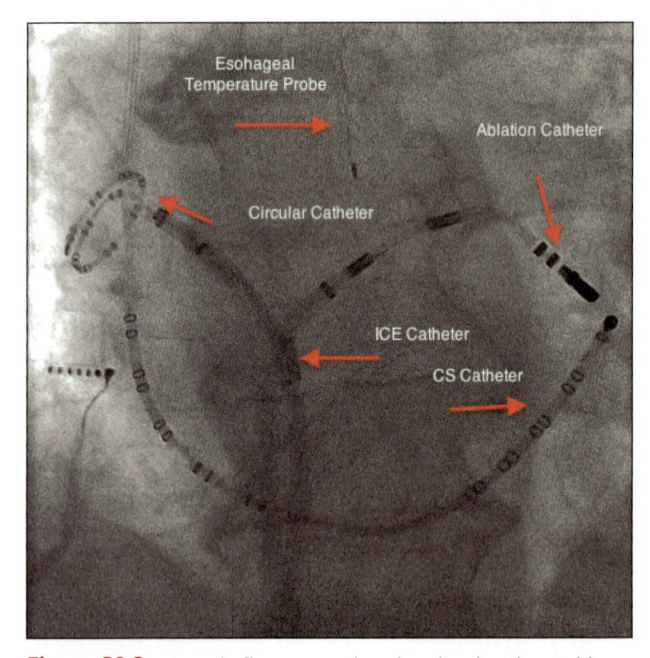

Figure 30.2 A static fluoroscopy imaging showing the positions of the equipment.

in this location allows optimal movement of the circular catheter. The needle and sheath are further withdrawn until the needle is seen tenting the septum. The sheath is rotated until the tenting and needle tip are seen in the view with the left PVs in sight (**Figure 30.3**). At this point, the needle is advanced until the septum is punctured. Once punctured, contrast is injected through the needle. (**Figure 30.4** and ▶ **Videos 30.1** and **30.2**) This is viewed on fluoroscopy as well as ICE to confirm position in the LA. Once confirmed, the introducer is

Chapter 30: AF Ablation by Remote Magnetic Navigation • 269

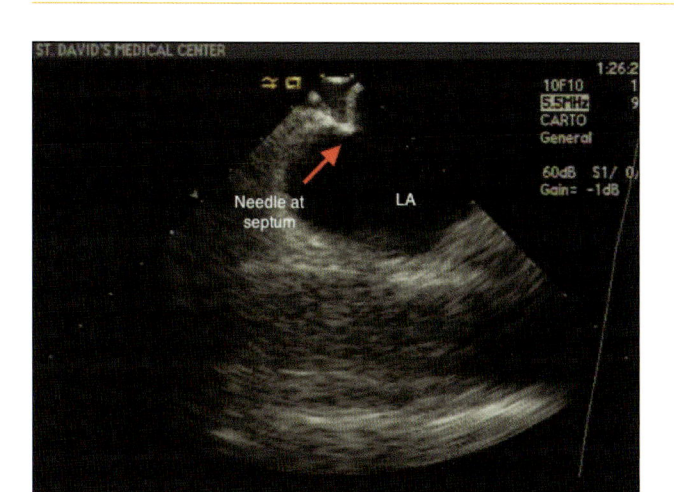

Figure 30.3 ICE image showing tenting of the septum.

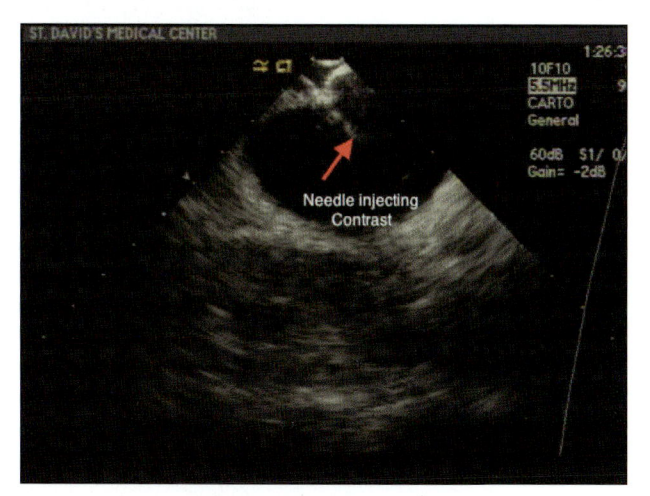

Figure 30.4 ICE image showing contrast injected into the LA.

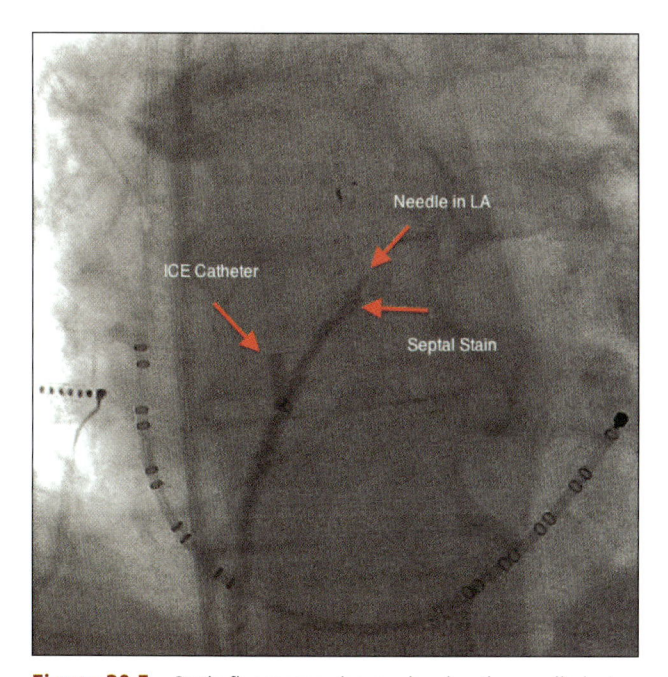

Figure 30.5 Static fluoroscopy image showing the needle just after puncturing the septum.

advanced through the septum and over the needle tip. Once the introducer is past the needle tip, the outer sheath is advanced over the introducer (**Figure 30.5**). Once past the needle tip, the introducer and needle are withdrawn as a single unit. The sheath is aspirated until blood is withdrawn, and hooked up to pressure tubing. A LA pressure is recorded. Once fully flushed, a 20-pole adjustable-diameter circular catheter is inserted. This is placed into the LSPV. Recordings are confirmed from this catheter.

The second transseptal puncture is performed identically to the first, except an SL0 transseptal sheath is used, and the puncture site should be slightly anterior to the previous puncture to allow all of the magnets of the magnetic navigation catheter to be out of the sheath when approaching the right-sided veins.

After the second transseptal sheath and ablation catheter are flushed, the magnetically enabled ablation catheter is inserted into the LA. The sheath is withdrawn to the right side of the septum, which allows the optimal movement of the ablation catheter.

At this point, mapping may begin. It is critical to create a high-quality and high-density map to accurately depict the position of the magnetic catheter, since the tactile feedback from using the manual catheter is not present. The mapping system is set to collect geometry from the circular catheter. The circular catheter is initially positioned in the central LA. Once data collection is started, it is moved into the LSPV. The catheter is moved deep into the vein and rotated and pulled back until it is at the antral position. The ICE catheter determines the optimal position of the catheter in the antrum. The left veins are best viewed with the ICE catheter in an unflexed position in the RA. A slightly posterior rotation shows the left veins in a long axis view. To achieve a long axis view of the right veins, the ICE catheter is retroflexed just below the IAS. The circular catheter is similarly placed into all PVs, and the antrum is identified on the map. The catheter is rotated into the superior, inferior, posterior, and anterior positions in each antrum to fully appreciate the anatomy. The catheter is then moved along the posterior wall, roof, anterior wall, septum, and valvular area. A separate map is created for the LAA to fully visualize the carina between the LSPV and the LAA (▶ **Videos 30.3** and **30.4**). Regional scaling is applied to the map to optimize the anatomy of the veins (**Figure 30.6**).

The next step is to prepare for registration and setting the fluoroscopic window. The fluoroscopy table is positioned to show the entirety of the LA in the x-ray field, making sure the CS catheter, septum, and lateral LA are visible with minimal lung in view. The table is left locked into place and must not be moved until after the magnets are in position and registration is complete.

The location pad of the mapping system is put into position, with the six dots being clearly seen in the x-ray

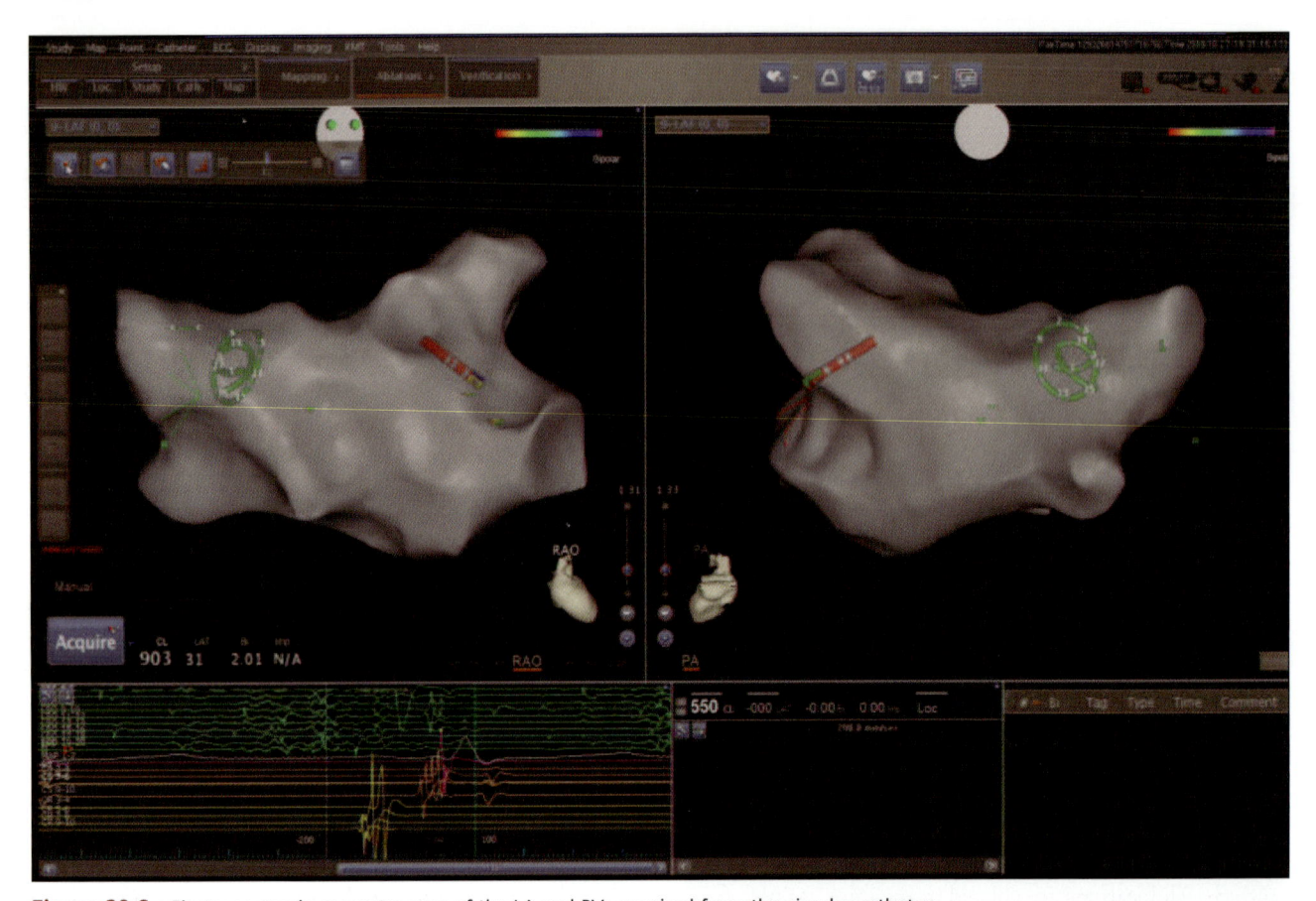

Figure 30.6 Electroanatomic geometry map of the LA and PVs acquired from the circular catheter.

field. A short cine shot is made to serve as the registration image (**Figure 30.7**).

All obstacles within the tracks of the magnets are removed, and the patient's arms are positioned to allow the magnets to come close to the body of the patient without tripping the force sensor alarm of the magnet covers. The two appropriate buttons are depressed, allowing the magnets to automatically move into navigation position, as indicated by an audible beep and display message on the computer control system for the magnets.

The physician takes the position in front of the consolidated display monitor allowing control over the magnetic system, mapping system, and recording system and displays the ICE image, fluoroscopy, and anesthesia monitor. The physician selects the magnetic catheter from the menu and registers the previously acquired cine image. This is done by making sure that the 6 dots of the location pad are correctly located as identified by green X marks that should be on top of each black dot in the image. The physician sets the controls to display an anatomic model to aide in navigation (▶ **Video 30.5**).

The first step is to complete any gaps in the anatomic map or more clearly define any anatomy that appears suboptimal. Once the map appears to be adequate, the physician moves the circular catheter into the antrum of the left superior vein; it is fully opened into its largest

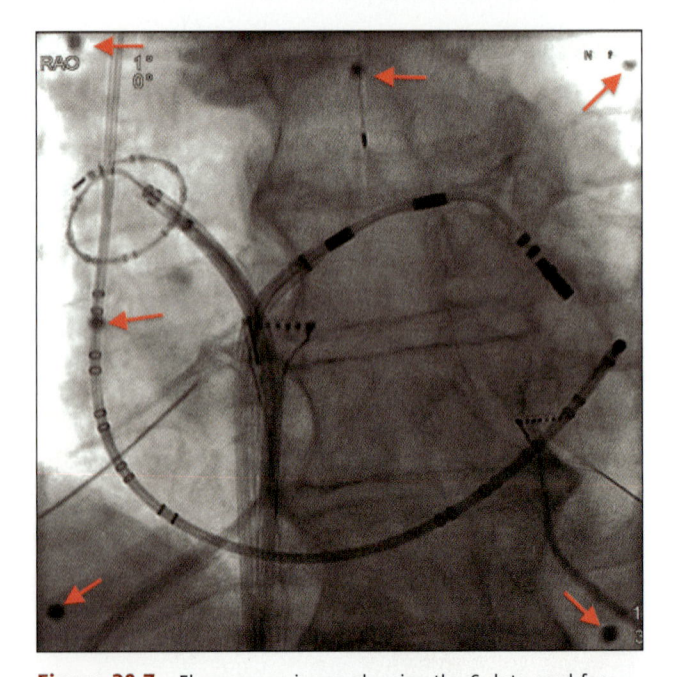

Figure 30.7 Fluoroscopy image showing the 6 dots used for registration. The dots are shown by arrows.

diameter and rotated so that it lies against the anterior segment of the antrum.

With the circular catheter in this position, the magnetic catheter is directed to the circular catheter. This is done by moving the vector on the anatomic model toward the LSPV posteriorly and then moving the vector more anteriorly and advancing the catheter with the catheter-advancing joystick. Once in position, ablation is started (▶ **Video 30.6**). The RF generator is set to manual ablation at 40 W. Ablation throughout the LA is performed at this power unless tip temperatures rise above 40°C. If this occurs, the power is decreased until the temperature drops below 40°C. Ablation is performed at a single site for up to 20 seconds, and the catheter is moved to the next position with ablation remaining on. Careful attention is paid to catheter impedances and changes. If the EGMs are not disappearing with standard settings, the power may be increased as necessary. All EGM determinations are made by observing the circular catheter. The anterior segment of the left superior antrum is first ablated, the circular catheter is moved to the posterior segment, and ablation is performed, then the sequence is repeated with the inferior and superior segments. At this point the vein should be isolated. The circular catheter is moved slightly into the vein to confirm this (**Figures 30.8** and **30.9**). If any gaps exist, they are ablated. The circular catheter is moved to the left inferior antrum, right superior antrum, and finally the right inferior antrum. All locations are ablated in the same fashion.

Magnetic navigation around the left PVs, roof, and posterior wall is relatively straightforward. The catheter can be advanced nearly directly, with the navigation vector facing the point of interest. Small vector movements superiorly and inferiorly allow movement around the circular catheter. To achieve optimal contact force, the catheter is advanced just until a slight buckling is seen on fluoroscopy. This is also seen by contact with the map surface and a high level on the contact meter.

Navigation along the right PVs and septum may be more difficult. Small atria are the most challenging due to the difficulty in having all of the magnets outside the transseptal sheath. In cases where the right side cannot be reached directly, a looping maneuver is performed. The catheter is advanced posteriorly toward the left superior veins, and then the vector is directed inferiorly, then toward the right veins, while advancing the catheter. This forms a loop, with the major portion fixed against the left veins. This allows the catheter tip to be manipulated with good support from the lateral LA. The tip alone can be manipulated with small vector movements. Slight movements can still be performed by advancing and retracting the catheter. All areas of the right side can be accessed with this maneuver. Also, minimizing the active length of the catheter increases the contact force (**Figure 30.10** and ▶ **Video 30.7**).

Once all of the veins are isolated, the circular catheter is moved to the posterior wall. Ablation is performed here with careful monitoring of the esophageal temperature probe. The probe is advanced or retracted to be in the location nearest the ablation catheter. Ablation is terminated in that location if the esophageal temperature rises above 38°C or is rapidly rising. After the posterior wall, the roof and septum are ablated (**Figure 30.11**). If the patient is in sinus rhythm, ablation is terminated at this point, and an isoproterenol infusion is started at 20 mcg/kg/min to

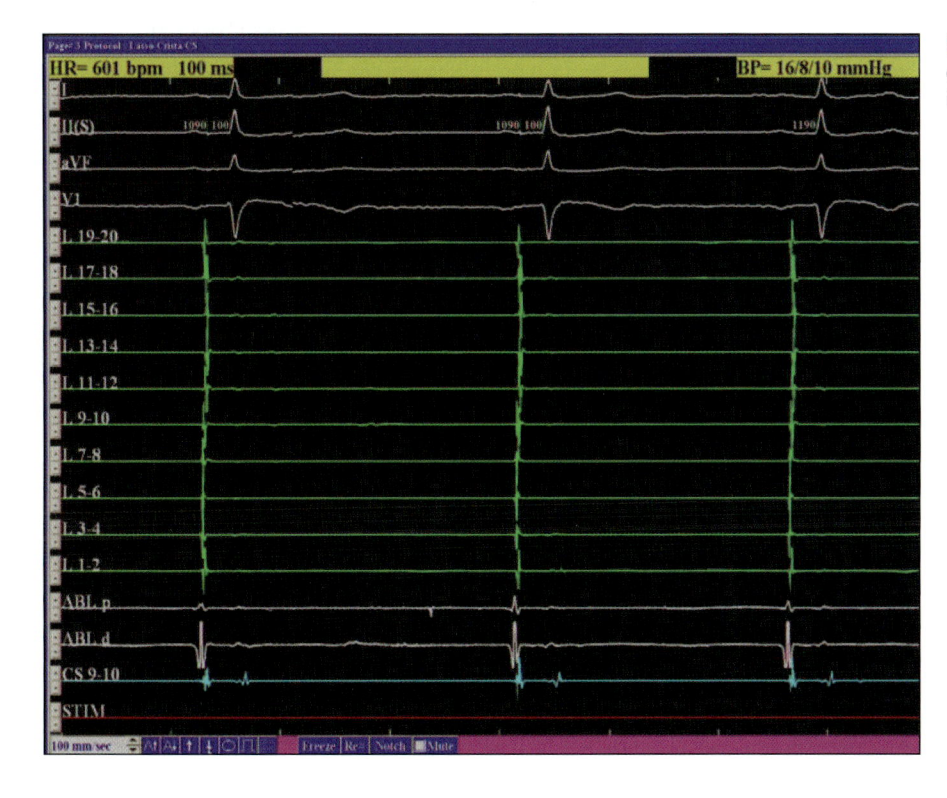

Figure 30.8 EGMs on the circular catheter (green signal) before venous isolation.

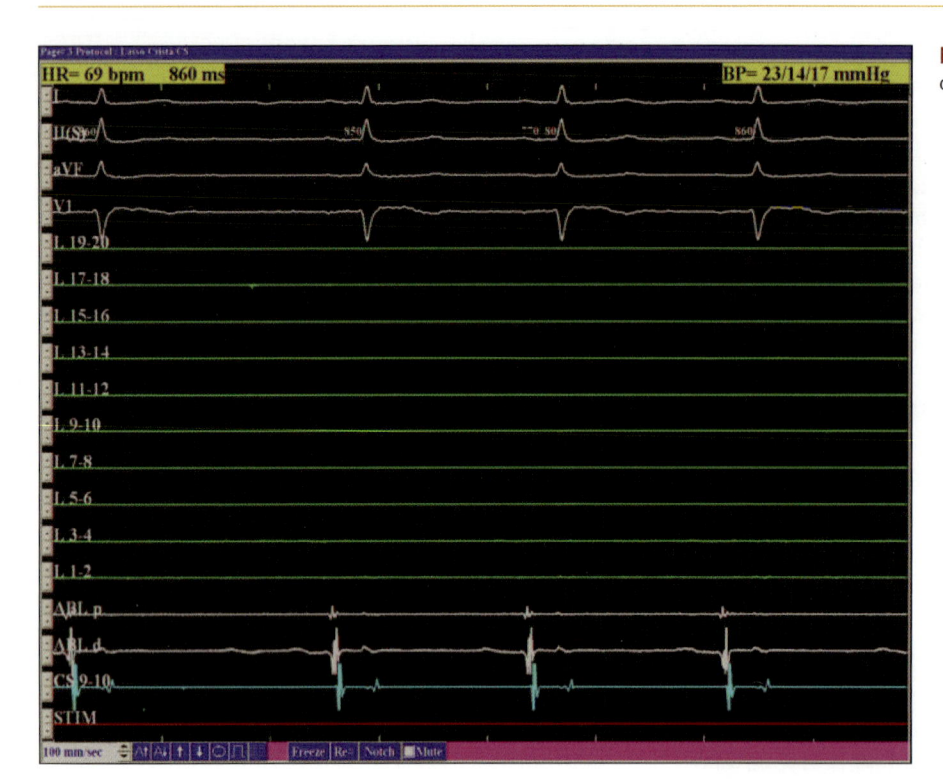

Figure 30.9 EGMs on the circular catheter (green signal) after isolation.

uncover any potential triggers of AF. If the heart rate response is inadequate, this in increased to 30 mcg/kg/min. If any triggers are seen, they are ablated. Typically these may come from the CS, LAA (which may require complete isolation), or crista terminalis. After trigger ablation is completed, the circular catheter is moved back to all veins to confirm isolation. Further ablation is performed as needed.

If the patient remains in AF or organizes into an AT, steps are performed to terminate these rhythms. Ablation is performed in areas of complex fractionated EGMs in the case of AF, or the LAA is isolated. In the case of stable ATs, these are mapped by activation mapping and entrainment mapping techniques. If termination is achieved, the isoproterenol protocol is performed as above to uncover potential trigger sites.

Once left-sided ablation is completed, the circular catheter is moved to the SVC. Optimal position is confirmed by advancing the ICE catheter superiorly and rotated until the pulmonary artery is seen. The circular catheter should be placed at the inferior portion of the pulmonary artery on ICE. Ablation is performed around the circular catheter until the SVC is isolated. High-output pacing is performed near areas of the phrenic nerve. If stimulation is present, ablation is avoided at those sites (▶ **Video 30.8**).

Postprocedure Care

After the procedure, protamine is given for partial heparin reversal. Sheaths are pulled when the ACT is less than 250 seconds. The patient is advised to lie flat for 4 hours. In

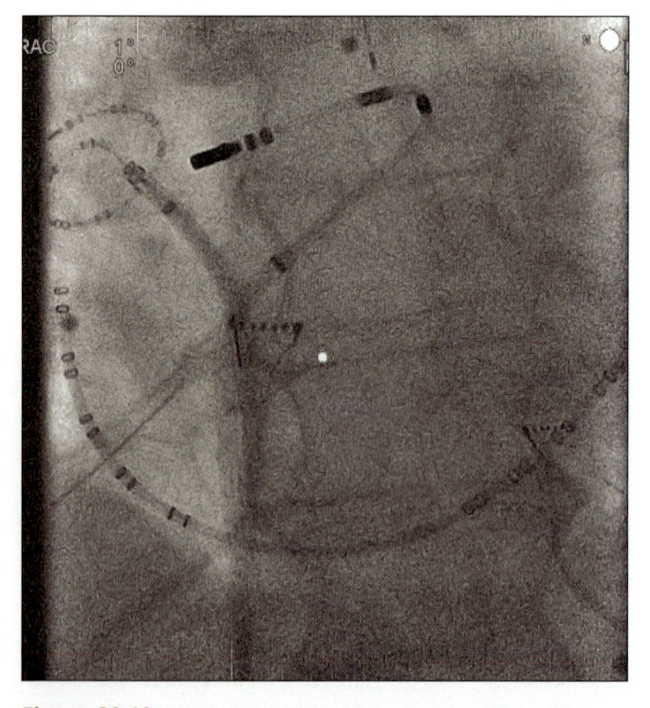

Figure 30.10 Static fluoroscopy image showing the looping technique.

general, furosemide is given at the end of the procedure to counteract the saline load and effect of volume retention seen with atrial ablation. The patient remains in the hospital overnight unless complications are seen. Postprocedure education is given prior to discharge. The patient is given an arrhythmia transmitter and contact for specialized AF nurses. The patient is advised to discontinue antiarrhythmic

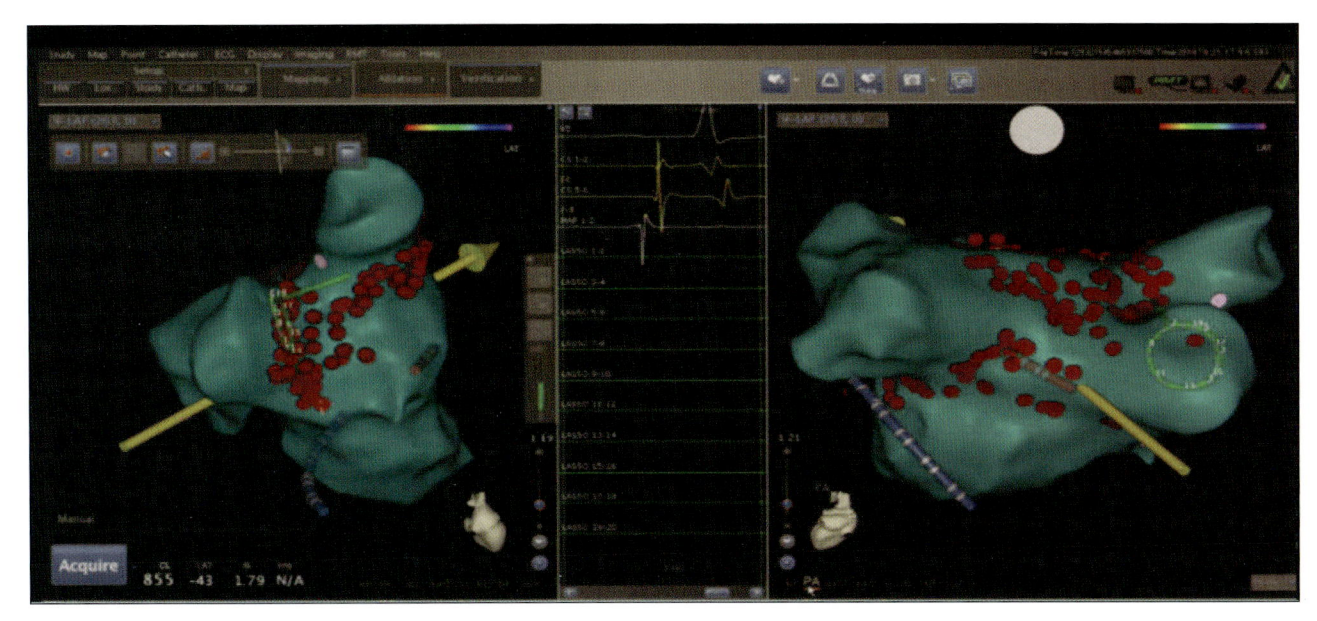

Figure 30.11 Electroanatomic map after ablation is completed.

medications in 8 weeks and counseled on symptoms of potential complications. All patients are advised to remain on warfarin until follow-up.

Follow-Up

Patients are seen in every 3 months for a year. Event monitor transmissions are reviewed on the first 2 visits, and 7-day Holter monitors are performed at 3-, 6-, and 12-month visits. If the patient experiences recurrence outside of the early period, repeat ablation procedures are discussed. Any suspicions of PV stenosis require the ordering of a cardiac CT. Echocardiograms are ordered for any patients in which LV dysfunction was previously seen. If after extensive monitoring, no recurrence is seen, then anticoagulation may be discontinued based on a discussion of stroke risk, guidelines, and available data.

Procedural Complications

Procedural complications associated with magnetic navigation seem similar to manual navigation, except they occur less frequently.[6] Pressure appears to be a significant contributor to cardiac tamponade and possibly atrial esophageal fistula. These may occur less frequently with magnetic navigation, since the contact force is lower than with manual ablation.[7] Vascular complications may be minimized by the use of ultrasound-guided venous access.

Phrenic nerve paralysis occurs less frequently with antral ablation and careful monitoring around the lateral SVC.[8] Rarely, some patients experience esophageal or gastric motility problems, this is usually treated conservatively and resolves.[9]

Advantages and Limitations

Remote magnetic navigation appears to have similar efficacy compared to manual navigation in AF ablation. Safety appears to favor magnetic navigation, but procedure times and ablation times are usually longer. Fluoroscopy times are usually shorter.[6]

The main advantages appear to be safety, fluoroscopy reduction, and operator comfort. These should not be underestimated. Safety, certainly, is the most important. It makes sense that the lower contact force may reduce the complications associated with high pressure. This clearly benefits patients and is usually not included when looking at efficiency. Fluoroscopy reduction should be viewed as a safety factor, and it generalizes to all people involved, patient and staff. The improvement in operator comfort is also important. The reduction in orthopedic burden may improve the longevity of the operator and could reduce fatigue.

The main limitations appear to be in increased procedure and ablation time. In expert ablation hands, this may be more pronounced than in less expert centers.[4,5] In some cases of less expert centers, the procedure time may be shorter. The majority of increase in the time is the time between movements and longer ablation time. Improvement in contact force and magnet speed may decrease these times further.

Conclusion

Remote magnetic navigation is a valuable tool in AF ablation. It allows the operator to perform this procedure in a location that is not at the bedside. This allows the operator to avoid the burden of heavy lead and fatigue. The system appears to offer an excellent safety profile and, with improvements, could make procedure times similar to manual if not better. Techniques such as looping are invaluable when encountering obstacles such as difficult right-sided veins. With further enhancement of automation features and magnetic movement, remote magnetic navigation could become a preferred technology for AF ablation.

References

1. Di Biase L, Burkhardt JD, Mohanty P, et al. Left atrial appendage: an underrecognized trigger site of atrial fibrillation. *Circulation.* 2010;122:109–118.
2. Elayi CS, Di Biase L, Barrett C, et al. Atrial fibrillation termination as a procedural endpoint during ablation in long-standing persistent atrial fibrillation. *Heart Rhythm.* 2010;7:1216–1223.
3. Arya A, Kottkamp H, Piorkowski C, Bollmann A, Gerdes-Li JH, Riahi S, Esato M, Hindricks G. Initial clinical experience with a remote magnetic catheter navigation system for ablation of cavotricuspid isthmus-dependent right atrial flutter. *Pacing Clin Electrophysiol.* 2008;31:597–603.
4. Chun KR, Wissner E, Koektuerk B, et al. Remote-controlled magnetic pulmonary vein isolation utilizing a new irrigated tip catheter in patients with atrial fibrillation. *Circ Arrhythm Electrophysiol.* 2010.
5. Di Biase L, Fahmy TS, Patel D, et al. Remote magnetic navigation: Human experience in pulmonary vein ablation. *J Am Coll Cardiol.* 2007;50:868–874.
6. Katsiyiannis WT, Melby DP, Matelski JL, Ervin VL, Laverence KL, Gornick CC. Feasibility and safety of remote-controlled magnetic navigation for ablation of atrial fibrillation. *Am J Cardiol.* 2008;102:1674–1676.
7. Yokoyama K, Nakagawa H, Shah DC, Lambert H, Leo G, Aeby N, Ikeda A, Pitha JV, Sharma T, Lazzara R, Jackman WM. Novel contact force sensor incorporated in irrigated radiofrequency ablation catheter predicts lesion size and incidence of steam pop and thrombus. *Circ Arrhythm Electrophysiol.* 2008;1:354–362.
8. Bai R, Patel D, Di Biase L, et al. Phrenic nerve injury after catheter ablation: should we worry about this complication? *J Cardiovasc Electrophysiol.* 2006;17:944–948.
9. Di Biase L, Dodig M, Saliba W, Siu A, Santisi J, Poe S, Sanaka M, Upchurch B, Vargo J, Natale A. Capsule endoscopy in examination of esophagus for lesions after radiofrequency catheter ablation: a potential tool to select patients with increased risk of complications. *J Cardiovasc Electrophysiol.* 2010;21:839–844.

Video Descriptions

Video 30.1 Transseptal puncture on fluoroscopy.

Video 30.2 Transseptal puncture in ICE.

Video 30.3 Map generation as seen on the electroanatomic mapping system.

Video 30.4 Map generation using the circular catheter as seen on fluoroscopy.

Video 30.5 Operator at consolidated console. The vector and catheter advancing movements can be seen in the lower left.

Video 30.6 View of entire consolidated console screen during ablation.

Video 30.7 Looping of the catheter and directing the tip toward the right side.

Video 30.8 Phrenic nerve stimulation seen on fluoroscopy from high output pacing at the lateral SVC.

CHAPTER 31

How to Perform Accurate Image Registration with Electroanatomic Mapping Systems

Francesco Perna, MD, PhD; Moussa Mansour, MD

Introduction

Catheter ablation for cardiac arrhythmias, including AF, has been facilitated in recent years by the development of new technologies allowing precise localization of mapping and ablation catheters in relation to the relevant cardiac anatomy. Electroanatomical mapping, in which 3-dimensional anatomical information is combined with local electrical information during real-time catheter mapping, can create 3-dimensional representations of cardiac structures and associated electrical function. However, even with extensive and high-density mapping, the anatomic information provided by this technique remains inferior to that provided by imaging modalities such as cardiac MRI and CT. This is due in part to the complex anatomy of the PV and the LA. There are thin ridges separating the PVs from each other and from structures such as the LAA. As a result, navigating the catheter in the LA can sometimes be challenging and the availability of a detailed representation of the LA anatomy at the time of the procedure is important to ensure a safe and effective outcome.

Image integration has been developed with the aim of incorporating the detailed anatomy of the LA into the operative field. By allowing the fusion of CT and MRI acquired prior to the procedure with a catheter localization tool, this technology provides the operator with a 3-dimensional view of the heart with the catheter position superimposed in an anatomically accurate manner.[1] Currently, the available image integration algorithms can be used with magnetic and impedance-based electroanatomic mapping systems. In addition to CT and MRI, anatomy of the LA can also be acquired using 3-dimensional rotational angiography, which in turn can be integrated with a catheter-localization tool.

Image integration allows better visualization of the location of the ablation catheter in relation to critical LA structures such as the PV ostia and the LAA ridge. Observational and prospective randomized studies have demonstrated that image integration improves the procedural outcome by reducing fluoroscopy time and improving the success rate.[2-6] However, in order to fulfill these promises, image integration must be accurate. One major limitation of this approach is that is that the CT and MRI are not obtained in real time coincident with the catheter mapping, and any error in integration will translate into error in identification of catheter position in relation to the superimposed images. Accurate integration is therefore necessary for precise catheter localization relative to the imported MRI and CT images in order to ensure maximum safety and efficacy during ablation. In this chapter, some techniques that may improve the accuracy of image integration are discussed.

Preprocedural Planning

Patient Preparation

Before performing imaging studies, the patient's medical history should be investigated in order to rule out the presence of contrast medium allergies or devices which are not compatible with MRI (ie, cardiac devices or metallic implants). It is advisable to test blood hCG levels in all premenopausal women undergoing CT scan. Renal function must be assessed because of the risk of iodine contrast medium-induced nephropathy or gadolinium-induced nephrogenic systemic fibrosis. Claustrophobia may also be an issue, especially in patients undergoing MRI study.

Imaging

Both cardiac CT and MRI are used to obtain images to be integrated with electroanatomical maps, and they seem to provide comparable image quality and information, thus making the choice largely determined by an institution's expertise and availability. MRI avoids ionizing radiation exposure and the use of iodine-based contrast media, which may carry harmful effects for the patients. However, it has been suggested that serious clinical consequences in patients with significantly impaired renal function may be caused by gadolinium as well, even though evidence in this matter is not conclusive. Furthermore, MRI equipment is not as widely available as CT equipment is. Finally, patients' tolerance to MRI is poor, primarily due to the duration and confinement associated with the exam.

Changes in hemodynamic status between the time of imaging and catheter ablation have the potential to influence registration accuracy. In order to minimize differences between the geometry at the time of image acquisition and the ablation procedure, the intervening period should be reduced as much as possible.

CT Scan

The helical scanning of multidetector tomographs enables acquisition of images within a breath hold. In more evolved tomographs, more series of detectors are present, which further reduces procedural time. This allows acquiring simultaneously data relative to large volumes. For cardiac studies, equipment must be furnished with at least 16 series of detectors. Recently, the introduction of wide-area detectors or dynamic volume scanners, such as the 320-row multidetector CT scanner (Aquilion One, Toshiba, Otawara, Japan) provides full cardiac coverage enabling whole-heart imaging without helical scanning. This new technology may reduce not only radiation dose to less than one-fourth of that for a typical multidetector CT scan but also the total amount of contrast material needed for ECG-gated scanning. The "ECG-pulsing technique," in which the tube current is modulated between 40% and 80% of the R-to-R interval, has the potential to reduce by 80% the effective radiation dose. A bolus of iodinated contrast is injected intravenously, followed by a saline chaser.

MRI

The LA and PVs anatomy can also be studied using gadolinium-enhanced MRI. Such studies are performed on 1.5- to 3-Tesla MRI systems during a breath-hold in the postabsorptive state. Angio-MRI is usually obtained with a 3-dimensional fast-field Spoiled Gradient Echo imaging sequence. Slices with a thickness of about 1.5 mm are acquired. The acquisition is performed after the injection of paramagnetic contrast medium. Revelation systems which can synchronize the acquisition of the image at the exact time when the bolus passes the LA are used in order to reduce the exposure time.

Rotational Angiography

Intraprocedural acquisition of LA volumes using rotational angiography has recently been introduced.[7,8] After contrast medium injection in the right heart chambers, the fluoroscopy c-arm is rapidly rotated around the patient, and images are acquired throughout the rotation to generate 3-dimensional volumetric anatomical rendering of the LA-PVs. Such images can be superimposed to the fluoroscopic projections of the heart or integrated into an electoanatomical mapping system. This innovative technique might overcome the limitation of acquiring the images in a different time with respect to the ablation procedure, but the consistent iodinated contrast agent load and radiation dose are important limiting factors.

Once the image is acquired, it is stored in a proprietary format. The data can then be exported from the scanner. A medical image standard known as DICOM (Digital Information and Communications in Medicine) has been devised and is widely used. This allows data to be exchanged between different scanners and viewing consoles.

Procedure

Image Segmentation

After performing the CT/MRI studies, the images are imported into the electroanatomic mapping system using customized softwares (CartoMerge, Biosense Webster, Inc., Diamond Bar, CA; or NavX Fusion/Verismo, St. Jude Medical, St. Paul, MN). The process of isolating the structures of interest from the remainder of the radiological image is called segmentation. First, the intensity threshold is set by selecting a transverse slice at the level of the LA, which is the chamber of interest where contrast density should be maximized. Pixels with intensities below a threshold value are assigned one class and the remaining pixels a different class. Regions are then formed by connecting adjacent pixels of the same class. After that, labels or "seeds" are placed in the center of each anatomical structure to optimize separation of the chamber of interest. When any structures are not adequately separated by the semi-automatic software, the image can be manually edited using the "slice and punch" tools to differentiate the structures. The PVs are often cut at a more proximal level, where an excessive branching does not create problems in distinguishing vascular structures from each other. Since ablation deep inside the PVs must be avoided, excluding their distal portion does not negatively affect the ablation procedure. Once the 3-dimensional reconstruction of the LA-PVs block has been separated from the surrounding structures, it can be exported into the real-time mapping system for registration.

Three-Dimensional Geometry Creation

Before performing image integration itself, the 3-dimensional anatomic shell of the LA must be created using an electroanatomical system. Two such systems are currently available: the magnetic-based Carto system (Biosense Webster Inc, Diamond Bar, CA), and the impedance-based EnSite NavX system (St. Jude Medical, St. Paul, MN). The latest versions of both systems use contact mapping for chamber geometry reconstruction by sweeping the catheter tip along the endocardial surface of the chamber of interest, which allows for quicker acquisition of a large number of points and a better definition of anatomy, especially when using multielectrode catheters.

Adequate catheter contact while acquiring surface points is determined by fluoroscopic visualization of catheter mobility in relation to cardiac motion, a discrete atrial EGM, and the catheter icon on the 3-dimensional navigation system. Uniform point sampling is essential to avoid geometry distortion. Regions of the LA susceptible to deformation (roof, anterior wall, appendage) should be approached carefully (**Figure 31.1**).

Algorithms aimed at balancing heart shift during the breathing cycle (respiratory compensation) and manual elimination of "false spaces" (ie, geometry with sparse points) and erroneous structure definition are also important to the purpose of better reproducing the true cardiac anatomy. The field-scaling algorithm available with the NavX system compensates for variations in impedance between the heart chambers and vascular structures, hence rendering a final geometry that is more physiological and more closely resembles the 3-dimensional radiological image.

Registration

Registration describes the process of aligning the segmented 3-dimensional LA image with the real-time

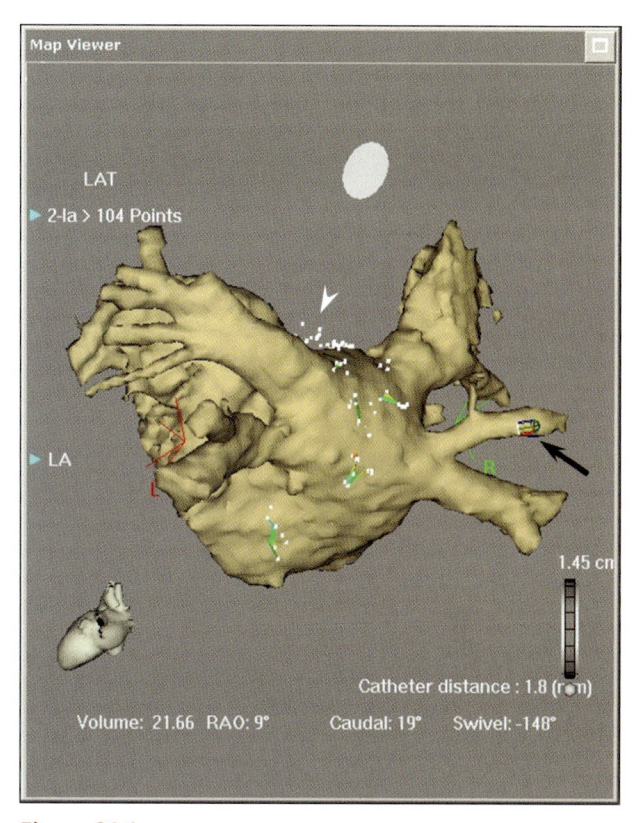

Figure 31.1 Accurate image registration. Posterior view of the LA showing an integrated MRI image. The ablation catheter (black arrow) is advanced into a small branch of the right inferior pulmonary vein without protruding outside the MRI shell. The white points along the roof (white arrowhead) protrude outside the shell which is the result of distention of the roof during map acquisition.

electoanatomical map in an anatomically accurate manner.

CartoMerge

Two strategies have been developed to accomplish this step: landmark registration and surface registration. A combination of these two approaches is mostly used to perform image registration with the CartoMerge software.

Landmark registration is an approach in which fiducial points are selected at different anatomic structures that can be easily recognized on both fluoroscopy and the 3-dimensional CT/MRI image. The LA posterior wall and PV ostia are largely anchored by pericardial attachments so that they are ideal as landmark points for registration. The catheter tip is positioned to the chosen location and a point is acquired on the electoanatomical map. The corresponding point on the radiological image is selected and paired to the point on the electoanatomical map. At least three corresponding points are used to perform landmark registration. Following this, the 3-dimensional left LA image from the CT or MRI is superimposed upon the electoanatomical map created by the mapping system by anchoring each fiducial point to the corresponding one.

When mapping a left-sided cardiac chamber, it has been shown that using a left-sided structure (LA, PV branches, aorta) for surface registration significantly improves registration accuracy.

Surface registration aims to refine the orientation of the integrated image by minimizing the distance between the electoanatomical map and the 3-dimensional radiological image surfaces. When sufficient points (typically at least 20 points spanning the body of the LA) have been acquired on the electoanatomical mapping system, surface registration is performed, which serves to further adjust the radiological image, thus providing a satisfying fit to the atrial geometry. The more accurate the landmark registration, the smaller the number of points required for surface registration. Different strategies may also focus on surface registration with single landmark points. Theoretically, at least one landmark pair is required to complete image registration, but this approach lacks accuracy and should be discouraged.

NavX Fusion

With this technology, the process of fusion dynamically molds the created geometry to the CT/MRI image. The electoanatomical map is "fused" to the radiological image in two stages, called primary fusion and secondary fusion.

Primary fusion uses three fiducial points on the geometry and the radiological image of the LA to superimpose these images. Just like with the CartoMerge software, posterior wall points are preferred for image registration due to their relative fixity to surrounding structures.

For *secondary fusion*, more fiducial points are applied at sites of local mismatch between the two geometries superimposed during the primary fusion. In this phase, the created geometry is molded to the CT/MRI surface while also "bending" the 3-dimensional navigation space within the geometry. After disabling the geometry display at the end of the fusion, all lesions, labels, and catheters should be projected on the 3-dimensional CT/MRI image.[2]

Registration is a critical step in the image integration process, since it is liable for error, which can invalidate the entire image integration process. It is sometimes difficult to achieve perfect registration. A very close correspondence is crucial at the sites which can potentially affect the efficacy and safety of the ablation procedure, that is, the PV-LA junctions and the ridges between adjacent structures, such as PVs and LAA. The CartoMerge software module provides an estimate of the registration error by determining the smallest average distance between the electoanatomical map points and the CT/MRI image points ("surface-to-point distance"). A mean registration error smaller than 3 mm is desirable for good registration. However, this surrogate tool for accuracy should be considered in combination with clinical information provided by EP data (EGM, impedance) and fluoroscopic and ultrasound visualization of catheter location.

Intracardiac Ultrasound-Based Image Integration (CartoSound)

One limitation associated with image integration is chamber deformation during catheter manipulation, which can result in suboptimal image integration. Also, chamber status changes occurring in the time interval between CT/MRI image acquisition and intervention, including changes in volume, rhythm, cardiac cycle, or respiration, may play a role in limiting the reliability of radiological images that have been acquired in a different moment with respect to the ablation procedure. A new technology, CartoSound (Biosense Webster, Diamond Bar, CA), enables rapid collection of a large quantity of spatial data derived from LA endocardial surfaces, which is apparent on ICE. A 3-dimensional reconstruction of the LA can be obtained using a phased-array transducer–catheter incorporating a position sensor (SoundStar, Biosense Webster, Diamond Bar, CA), which records individual 90° sector image planes, including their location and orientation, to the Carto workspace. This catheter renders real-time images while positioned within the RA or even the LA through a transseptal puncture.[9] Once ECG-gated echocardiographic images of the LA have been obtained, its endocardial surfaces may be identified, delineated, and collated to create a 3-dimensional volume-rendered image of the LA. This technique of recreating LA anatomy is advantageous, as it minimizes chamber deformity with contact mapping, permits detailed visualization of the LA and the surrounding structures, and has the potential to minimize radiation exposure. Moreover, 3-dimensional ultrasound image volumes have the advantage of real-time confirmation by combined 2-dimensional ICE imaging and electoanatomical measurements. Other electoanatomical points can also be acquired by using a separate mapping catheter and registered to the reconstructed 3-dimensional ultrasound volume, within the same coordinate system as the ICE images. This technology can be employed either as a stand-alone tool or as a facilitator of integration of preoperatively obtained CT/MRI using the CartoMerge software.

Factors Affecting Integration Error

There are technique- and patient-related factors that can affect the accuracy of the image integration process.

Respiratory Cycle During Image Acquisition

It is advisable that MRI, CT, or rotational angiography imaging is acquired at end expiration, when the patient is instructed to maintain a breath hold. This has been demonstrated to allow more accurate image integration with the electoanatomical maps also acquired during end expiration.[10]

Cardiac Chamber Volume

It has been demonstrated that the LA size affects the accuracy of image integration.[11] An LA volume larger than 110 ml has been associated with increased integration error.[11] This may be due to greater difficulty in obtaining similar precision when defining a relatively large structure. It is possible that a large LA is more difficult to map accurately than a small LA. A dilated LA may be more deformable by the pressure applied by a manually deflected catheter, producing a less accurate electroanatomic map.

Other factors have been studied and were found to have no effect on the accuracy of image integration. These include left ventricular ejection fraction, type of AF (persistent vs. paroxysmal), imaging modality (CT vs. MRI), and presenting rhythm (AF vs. sinus rhythm).[11,12]

Postprocedure Care

Image integration does not usually entail any adjunctive postprocedure care with respect to the ablation procedure. For patients undergoing CT who are at high risk to develop contrast-induced nephropathy, intravenous hydration should be continued after the imaging procedure and renal function should be assessed for at least 48 hours. Postprocedural complications including pleural or pericardial effusions and PV stenosis can be evaluated by CT or MRI.

Procedural Complications

Since image integration only requires imaging procedures in addition to the standard procedure, it does not carry a significant increase of procedural complications as compared to the conventional fluoroscopic approach.

Contrast-induced nephropathy can occur in patients undergoing CT with the administration of iodinated contrast medium. Although transient in the majority of cases, serum creatinine elevation—and the underlying renal impairment this reflects—can lead to increased morbidity and even death in some patients with contrast-induced nephropathy. To date, periprocedural plasma volume expansion is the only measure with an established role in reducing the risk of contrast-induced nephropathy.

Nephrogenic systemic fibrosis is a recently described, debilitating systemic disease most commonly seen in patients with renal insufficiency. Exposure to gadolinium-based contrast agents has been associated with skin lesions, fibrosis of skeletal muscle, joints, liver, lung, and heart, with possible fatal outcomes. There is no consistently effective therapy for this disease. Improving renal dysfunction appears to slow or arrest the progression of nephrogenic systemic fibrosis.

Suboptimal image quality or registration with poor accuracy can reduce procedure efficacy by targeting ablation lesions to inappropriate sites. It can also potentially increase the risk of complications during AF ablation, such as PV stenosis or atrio-esophageal fistula, by giving an inaccurate assessment of the distance from the ablation catheter to vulnerable cardiac structures.

Advantages and Limitations

The major advantage of this strategy is the precise representation of anatomical variations and structures that are critical for safe and successful catheter ablation, such as PV ostia and LA ridges. Radiological imaging using CT or MRI provides a detailed representation of the cardiac anatomy with an average accuracy of 1 to 3 mm. In addition, catheter-related myocardial wall stretch occurring during electroanatomical mapping does not affect LA wall reconstruction obtained from radiological images. Localization of surrounding structures, such as the esophagus, can also improve the safety profile of the ablation procedure by helping avoid high-output energies while ablating in close proximity of these structures.[13] Moreover, CT and MRI also have the potential to detect postprocedural complications such as PV stenosis.

A number of studies have investigated the effect of image integration on the outcome of the procedure and found a beneficial effect. This ranges from reduced fluoroscopy time to improved rate of AF elimination.[2-6]

Patient's movement after image registration can significantly reduce the accuracy of the image integration. Performing AF ablation under general anesthesia has the advantage of preventing patient movement and is thus preferred by some operators. If the radiological image of the LA is of insufficient quality or is not accurately registered, image integration may be deleterious to guiding catheter manipulation.

The main limitation of this approach is that the CT/MRI are not obtained at the same time catheter mapping is done, and any error in integration will translate into error in identification of catheter position in relation to the superimposed images. Accurate integration of images is therefore necessary for precise catheter localization relative to the imported images in order to ensure maximum safety and efficacy during ablation. In the future, preacquired image integration may be replaced by real-time MRI.

Conclusions

Understanding the anatomical substrate is essential for safe and successful catheter ablation. Novel imaging technologies have been implemented to improve the knowledge of the true anatomy, thus helping navigate the ablation catheter through the complex anatomy of the LA and the PVs and locating the lesion sets. One such technology is image integration, which has been developed to allow detailed information on complex LA anatomy derived from MRI and CT imaging to be applied directly to the mapping and ablation procedures. This technology is beneficial because it improves the visualization of cardiac structures such as the pulmonary vein ostia, which are difficult to render with precise anatomic detail by electroanatomic mapping alone. Ensuring accurate image registration is crucial. Registration with poor accuracy will not only reduce the procedure efficacy by targeting ablation lesions to inappropriate sites but will also increase the risk of complications by giving an inaccurate assessment of the distance from the ablation catheter to vulnerable cardiac structures.

Acknowledgment

This work has been partially supported by the Deane Institute for Integrative Research in Atrial Fibrillation and Stroke.

References

1. Reddy VY, Malchano ZJ, Holmvang G, Schmidt EJ, D'Avila A, Houghtaling C, Chan RC, Ruskin JN. Integration of cardiac magnetic resonance imaging with three-dimensional electroanatomic mapping to guide left ventricular catheter manipulation: feasibility in a porcine model of healed myocardial infarction. *J Am Coll Cardiol.* 2004;44: 2202–2213.
2. Brooks AG, Wilson L, Kuklik P, et al. Image integration using NavX Fusion: initial experience and validation. *Heart Rhythm.* 2008;5(4):526–535.
3. Della Bella P, Fassini G, Cireddu M, et al. Image integration-guided catheter ablation of atrial fibrillation: a prospective randomized study. *J Cardiovasc Electrophysiol.* 2009;20(3):258–265.
4. Caponi D, Corleto A, Scaglione M, et al. Ablation of atrial fibrillation: does the addition of three-dimensional magnetic resonance imaging of the left atrium to electroanatomic mapping improve the clinical outcome? a randomized comparison of Carto-Merge vs. Carto-XP three-dimensional mapping ablation in patients with paroxysmal and persistent atrial fibrillation. *Europace.* 2010;12(8):1098–1104.
5. Dewire J, Calkins H. State-of-the-art and emerging technologies for atrial fibrillation ablation. *Nat Rev Cardiol.* 2010;7(3):129–138.
6. Kistler PM, Earley MJ, Harris S, et al. Validation of three-dimensional cardiac image integration: use of integrated CT image into electroanatomic mapping system to perform catheter ablation of atrial fibrillation. *J Cardiovasc Electrophysiol.* 2006;17:341–348.
7. Thiagalingam A, Manzke R, D'Avila A, Ho I, Locke AH, Ruskin JN, Chan RC, Reddy VY. Intraprocedural volume imaging of the left atrium and pulmonary veins with rotational X-ray angiography: implications for catheter ablation of atrial fibrillation. *J Cardiovasc Electrophysiol.* 2008;19(3): 293–300.
8. Al-Ahmad A, Wigström L, Sandner-Porkristl D, et al. Time-resolved three-dimensional imaging of the left atrium and pulmonary veins in the interventional suite—a comparison between multisweep gated rotational three-dimensional reconstructed fluoroscopy and multislice computed tomography. *Heart Rhythm.* 2008;5(4):513–519.
9. Singh SM, Heist EK, Donaldson DM, Collins RM, Chevalier J, Mela T, Ruskin JN, Mansour MC. Image integration using intracardiac ultrasound to guide catheter ablation of atrial fibrillation. *Heart Rhythm.* 2008;5 (11): 1548–1555.
10. Noseworthy PA, Malchano ZJ, Ahmed J, Holmvang G, Ruskin JN, Reddy VY. The impact of respiration on left atrial and pulmonary venous anatomy: implications for image-guided intervention. *Heart Rhythm.* 2005;2(11):1173–1178.
11. Heist K, Chevalier J, Holmvang G, Singh J, Ellinor P, Milan D, D'Avila A, Mela T, Ruskin J, Mansour M. Factors affecting error in integration of electroanatomic mapping with CT and MR imaging during catheter ablation of atrial fibrillation. *J Interv Card Electrophysiol.* 2006;17(1):21–27.
12. Patel AM, Heist EK, Chevalier J, Holmvang G, D'Avila A, Mela T, Ruskin JN, Mansour M. Effect of presenting rhythm on image integration to direct catheter ablation of atrial fibrillation. *J Interv Card Electrophysiol.* 2008;22(3): 205–210.
13. Aleong R, Heist EK, Ruskin JN, Mansour M. Integration of intracardiac echocardiography with magnetic resonance imaging allows visualization of the esophagus during catheter ablation of atrial fibrillation. *Heart Rhythm.* 2008; 5(7):1088.

SECTION III

ABLATION OF VENTRICULAR TACHYCARDIA

CHAPTER 32

How to Localize Ventricular Tachycardia Using a 12-Lead ECG

Hicham El Masry, MD; John M. Miller, MD

Introduction

Over the past decade, the use of catheter procedures to identify and ablate sustained VT has increased dramatically. The success of these ablation procedures is dependent on the localization and destruction of the arrhythmogenic tissue, while minimizing unnecessary damage to more normal areas of myocardium. This critical step depends in turn on the identification of a small target area serving as the isthmus of slow conduction in reentrant rhythms or the repetitively firing focus in automatic and triggered rhythms. The target in most cases is microscopic; hence a precise method of localization is of paramount importance in ensuring success within an acceptable procedure time. The process of localization of the target site starts with the use of the ECG characteristics of the VT, which provides a simple, noninvasive method to define a general area of interest in which focused efforts of mapping and testing can subsequently lead to successful ablation. Because of this, every effort should be made to record any nonsustained or sustained episodes of the VT on a 12-lead ECG. This will serve not only in the regionalization of the target site, as we will discuss in this chapter, but also as a template for pace mapping (replication of the ECG appearance of VT by pacing at candidate sites). On the other hand, in most patients with structural heart disease, multiple VTs may be induced, and focusing ablation efforts on the clinically encountered VT ("clinical VT") is the primary objective, with elimination of other VTs a secondary goal.

It is important to use correct lead placement when an ECG is obtained: in many cases a slight change in the position of leads (especially precordial) can result in significant differences in the ECG of the same VT, confounding regionalization efforts. Occasionally, when VT cannot be readily induced in the lab, it is helpful to mark the ECG electrode positions at the time of obtaining the ECG during a subsequent spontaneous episode, or retaining those electrodes until the patient is brought to the lab.

In this chapter we will discuss the current knowledge of the ECG localization of VT based on the different clinical entities encountered, including coronary disease and NICM as well as VT originating from the RVOT, LVO, epicardial origin, and Purkinje-associated VT.

Bundle Branch Reentrant Ventricular Tachycardia

BBRVT occurs due to reentry within a well-defined circuit involving the right and left bundle, connected proximally by the His bundle and distally by the septal myocardium. BBRVT typically occurs in patients with structural heart disease, especially dilated cardiomyopathy, where a longer circuit and/or HPS disease provide sufficient delay to sustain reentry.[1] It is crucial to rule out this diagnosis by EP testing in any patient with cardiomyopathy presenting with VT, especially those demonstrating LBBB or a non-specific intraventricular conduction delay on baseline ECG. BBRVT is characterized by a typical BB pattern (similar to sinus rhythm) with rapid rates of 180 to 300/min, often causing hemodynamic instability. A LBBB pattern during VT is more common, and a normal or left axis can be encountered.[2] In contrast to most other VTs, a short intrinsicoid deflection is typical of BBRVT, consistent with the initial activation of the HPS and not myocardial cell-to-cell propagation.

Ventricular Tachycardia in Patients with Coronary Artery Disease

Post-infarct VT is typically based on a reentrant mechanism and relies on a circuit incorporating a region of slow conduction in or near the infarct (scar) zone; hence the resultant ECG represents the activation spreading from the exit site of the circuit. In general, the QRS patterns in these patients are less accurate in localizing the target zone compared to patients with focal VTs. This is related to altered conduction in areas damaged by prior infarct; nevertheless, the ECG offers the capacity to regionalize the exit site to an area of 10 to 15 cm^2.[3] Several algorithms have been proposed for noninvasive localization of the VT circuit's exit; however, starting with the following basic principles is invaluable:

1. Post-MI VTs almost always arise in the left ventricle or IVS. In this respect, knowledge of the location of the prior infarct facilitates the localization process: VTs associated with inferior MI arise from the inferobasal septum or free wall, and those associated with anterior MI arise from the antero-apical or infero-apical septum or free wall.
2. Overall, VTs arising from the IVS have narrower QRS durations compared to free wall VTs.
3. LBBB VTs almost always localize to the septum, while RBBB VTs can arise anywhere in the left ventricle, posing a greater challenge for localization.
4. The presence of positive or negative concordance in the precordial leads strongly suggests a basal or apical exit site, respectively.
5. A superior axis in general points to an IVT exit location (thus many inferior MI VTs have a superior axis) or apical locations (in anterior MI), while an inferior axis generally implies an antero-basal location.

Using these simple principles, an adequate localization of the VT exit site can be inferred in most cases encountered in daily practice. More sophisticated algorithms have been suggested by Miller et al.[3] and Kuchar et al.[4], and more recently by Segal et al.[5], and will be summarized in the following discussion.

In the algorithm described by Miller et al.[3], VTs were analyzed based on the location of the prior infarct, BBB pattern, QRS axis, and R-wave progression. Eight patterns of R-wave progression were described and are illustrated in **Figure 32.1**. In patients with prior inferior MI, large R waves were usually observed in leads V_2 to V_4. Decreasing or reversing R-wave amplitude is seen when the exit site moves more laterally or posteriorly. A left axis was usually seen in VTs arising near the septum; the more the VT moves laterally, the more "right" or superior the axis will become. In patients with anterior MI, the accuracy of the ECG localization is lower than in patients with inferior MI, probably due to the more extensive myocardial damage. In these patients, most LBBB VTs arise from the apical septum, and an anterior vs. inferior location is dependent on the axis (inferior vs. superior axis, respectively). Most RBBB VTs in these patients have a right-superior axis and arise from the antero-apical septum but are usually the most difficult to localize, probably due to variation in extent of infarction and residual myocardium that contributes to the ECG.

An algorithm proposed by Kuchar et al.[4] (**Figure 32.2**) was based on results of pace mapping in patients with prior infarction. The left ventricle in this study was divided into 3 parts in each of 3 axes (apical/middle/basal; septal/central/lateral; and anterior/middle/inferior zones); this is of somewhat limited utility because of the variability of propagation from scarred regions (nonspecific results).

In the algorithm of Segal et al.[5], VTs were studied based on the BBB pattern and polarity in the limb leads (**Figure 32.3**). The studied population was not limited to patients with anterior or inferior infarcts but included any MI location. Although R-wave progression was studied, it had no specific bearing on the localization of the VT exit site representing an important variation compared to the Miller et al.[3] algorithm. The left ventricle was divided similarly to the study by Kuchar et al.[4] All LBBB VTs studied were mapped to the septum; a superior axis correlated with basal- and mid-septal locations. LBBB VTs with an inferior axis were mostly localized to the mid-septum. All RBBB VTs were mapped away from the septum: a positive lead I polarity and superior axis pointed to a mid- or basal-posterior location, while a negative lead I and superior axis mapped to an apical-posterior location. Inferior axis RBBB VTs were mapped to the anterior wall, with localization to the mid-anterior wall if lead I is negative vs. basal location if it is positive. This algorithm had an overall ≥ 70% positive predictive value when validated prospectively.[5]

Note that in these studies, 15% to 20% of all VTs couldn't be localized using these algorithms. For this reason, they should be used as regionalizing tools to help guide mapping. It is our practice to construct a comprehensive activation map of the whole ventricle with dense mapping

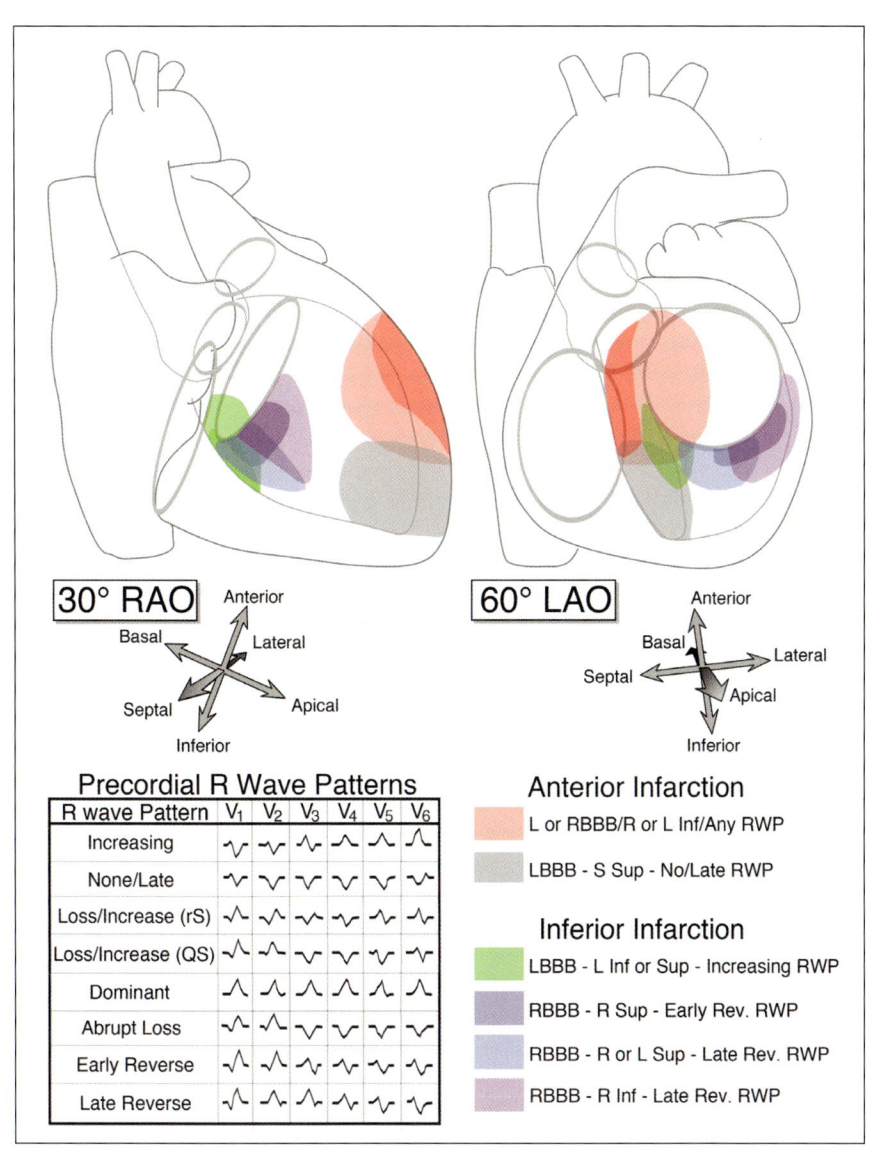

Figure 32.1 Correlation of ventricular tachycardia exit sites in patients with prior MI according to Miller et al.[3] RAO and LAO outlines of the heart are shown at top. ventricular tachycardias were characterized by infarct location, BBB pattern, quadrant of frontal plane axis (right [R] or left [L], superior [Sup] or inferior [Inf]), and precordial R-wave progression (RWP) pattern (examples at lower left). Combinations of these features having > 70% PPV for an endocardial region are listed at lower right with color shading at the corresponding left ventricular regions in the 2 common fluoroscopic views above.

focused on the suspected culprit area of the exit, especially in patients with sustained, hemodynamically stable VTs.

Less information is available regarding ECG regionalization of VT in patients with various forms of NICM, except that in most cases, circuits and their respective exit sites are more likely to be in the basal third of either left or right ventricles.[6,7] In addition, epicardial circuits and exits are more common in myopathies than in post-MI substrates,[7] and BBRVT is far more common in these cases.

In ARVC, right ventricular basal sites (peritricuspid annulus, outflow tract) predominate and epicardial ablation is often necessary for complete effect.[8] Sarcoidosis-related VT tends to affect the RV more than the LV, but in most cardiomyopathic hearts, the LV is the source of VT.[9] VTs uniformly have an LBBB pattern, generally with gradually increasing R-wave amplitude from right to left in precordial leads; frontal plane axis is typically a reliable indicator of exit region (ie, leftward superior axis suggests exit on the inferolateral RV free wall, strongly inferior axis suggests outflow tract exit, etc).

Of note, these algorithms for scar-based VT regionalize the exit site of the VT, rather than the more optimal ablation site (within a mid-diastolic corridor). Most evidence suggests that the exit site and diastolic corridor are within 2 cm of each other, however. In addition, many patients with VT episodes in the setting of structural heart disease already have an ICD, which generally treats VT episodes quickly and precludes obtaining a 12-lead ECG in order to use its features to plan mapping and ablation studies.

Idiopathic Ventricular Tachycardias

Idiopathic VTs constitute around 10% of clinically encountered VTs and occur, by definition, without identifiable associated structural heart disease. Several classifications have been proposed for these VTs including their site of origin as well as their response to pharmacologic intervention: 2 categories have been widely recognized including verapamil-sensitive VTs and adenosine-sensitive VTs.

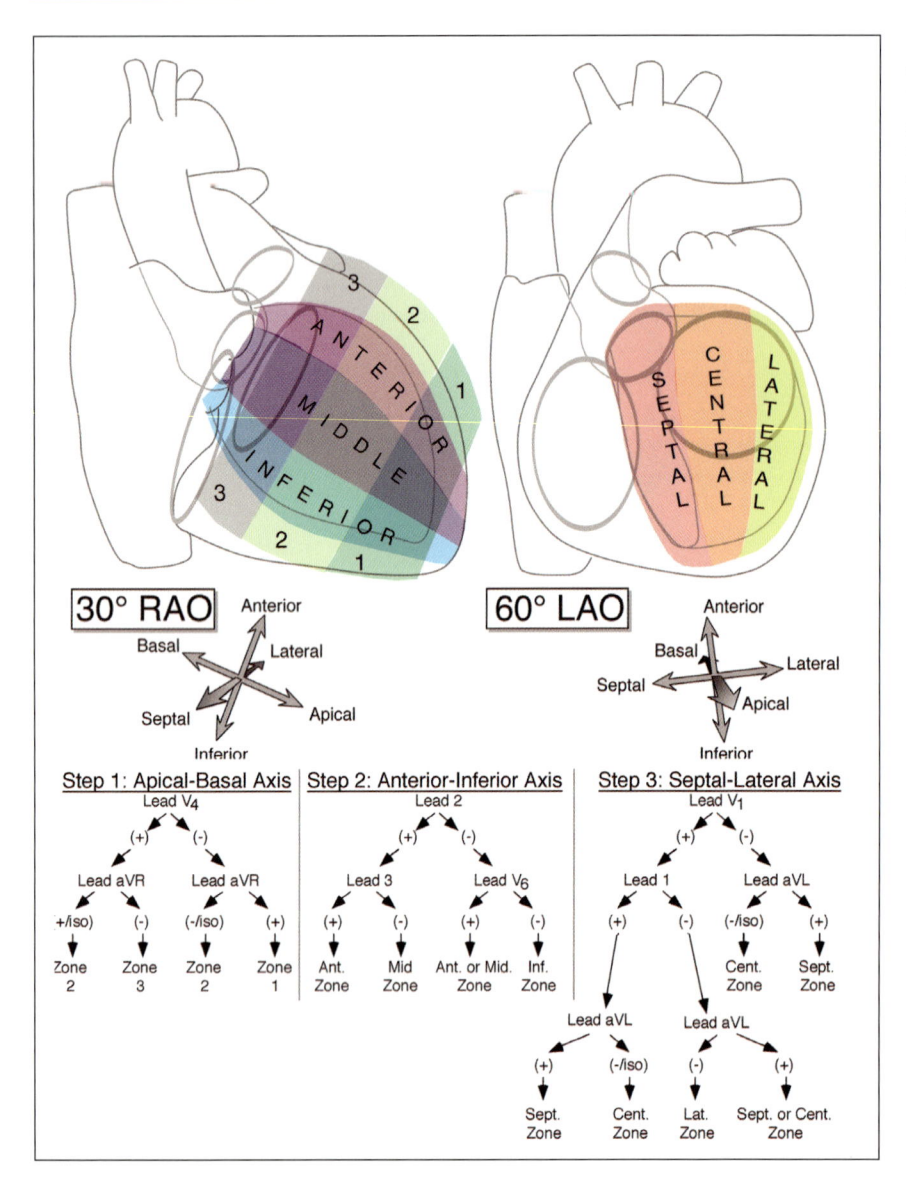

Figure 32.2 Correlation of ventricular tachycardia exit sites in patients with prior MI according to Kuchar et al.[4] Format similar to Figure 32.1. A 3-step algorithm was used as indicated at bottom. Specific ventricular tachycardia patterns having > 70% PPV for an endocardial region are represented in the algorithm. The left ventricle was divided into 3 zones in each of 3 planes as shown.

Verapamil-Sensitive, Purkinje-Associated Ventricular Tachycardias

These VTs—previously known as fascicular VTs—are now identified as Purkinje-associated VTs pertaining to their inclusion of Purkinje fibers in a moderately large circuit on the left ventricular aspect of the septum. These are the major type of idiopathic VTs based on reentry (others being focal in origin); the exit site (a sharp Purkinje potential) had served as the target for ablation, but more recent evidence suggests targeting sites with smaller diastolic potentials on the septum.[10] These VTs have a classical ECG appearance of RBBB and left-anterior or less commonly left-posterior fascicular block pattern (**Figure 32.4**). A relatively narrow QRS (140 ms) is the rule corresponding to a septal exit site of the VT. A left superior axis is usually associated with more posterior exit site along the septum (towards the posteromedial papillary muscle) while a more apical exit site has a right-superior axis. Often, there is a "shelf" or "step" in the upstroke of the inferior leads. Because these VTs have a relatively narrow QRS, occur in younger patients, are usually hemodynamically stable, and terminate in response to verapamil (but not adenosine), they are often mistaken for SVT.

Adenosine-Sensitive, Outflow Tract, and Basal Ventricular Tachycardias

This group of VTs has a focal origin rather than being based in reentry, and since slow conduction and scar-related disruption of propagation of wave fronts are not present, the exit site of the VT and its actual source (the target for ablation) are fundamentally the same site. These terminate in response to a variety of physical maneuvers and drugs, most particularly adenosine. Most idiopathic VTs originate from the outflow tract regions of either ventricle. These VTs have a variety of clinical manifestations, ranging from frequent monomorphic ectopy to long

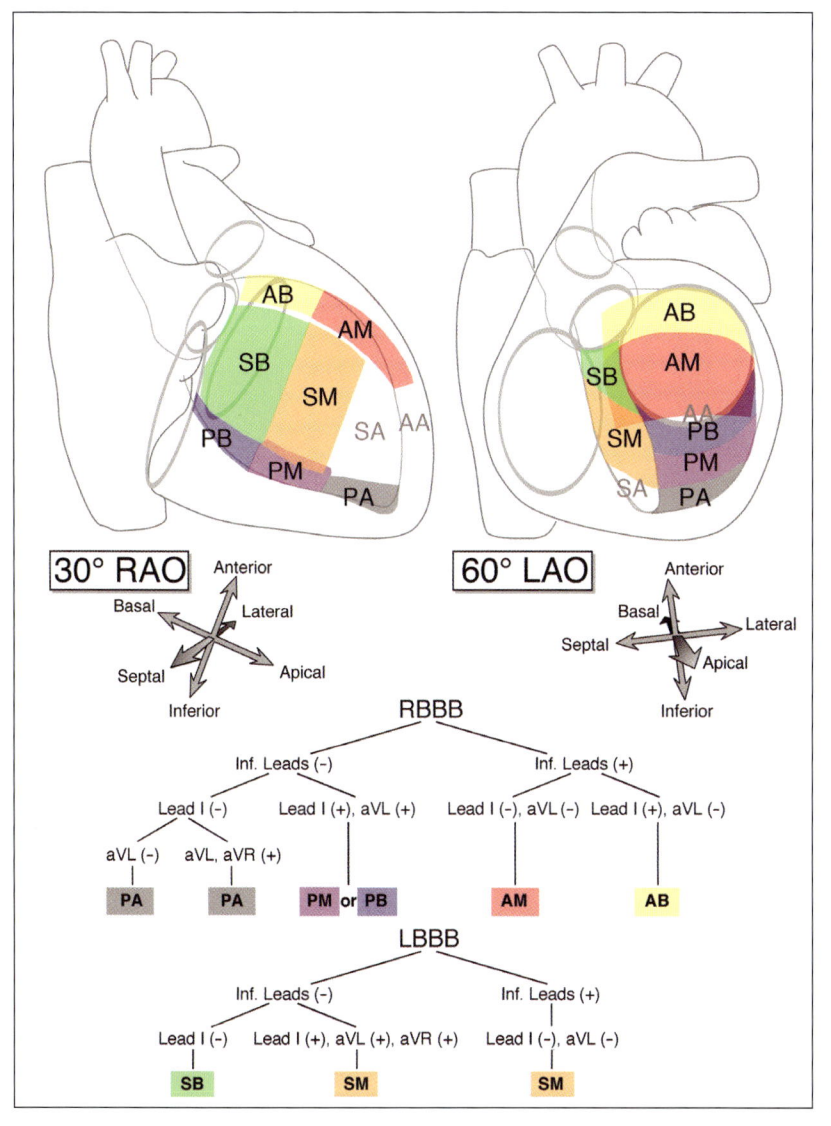

Chapter 32: Localizing Ventricular Tachycardia by 12-Lead ECG • 287

Figure 32.3 Correlation of ventricular tachycardia exit sites in patients with prior MI according to Segal et al.[5] Format similar to Figure 32.1. Separate algorithms were developed for RBBB and LBBB ventricular tachycardias irrespective of infarct location. Specific ventricular tachycardia patterns having > 70% PPV for an endocardial region are represented in the algorithm. The left ventricle was divided into 9 zones, combinations of apical, mid, and basal and septal, anterior, and posterior regions (ie, PA, postero-apical; PM, postero-mid; PB, postero-basal; AM, antero-mid; AB, antero-basal; SB, septal-basal; SM, septal-mid). Color-shaded regions on the diagrams at top correspond to results of the algorithm below.

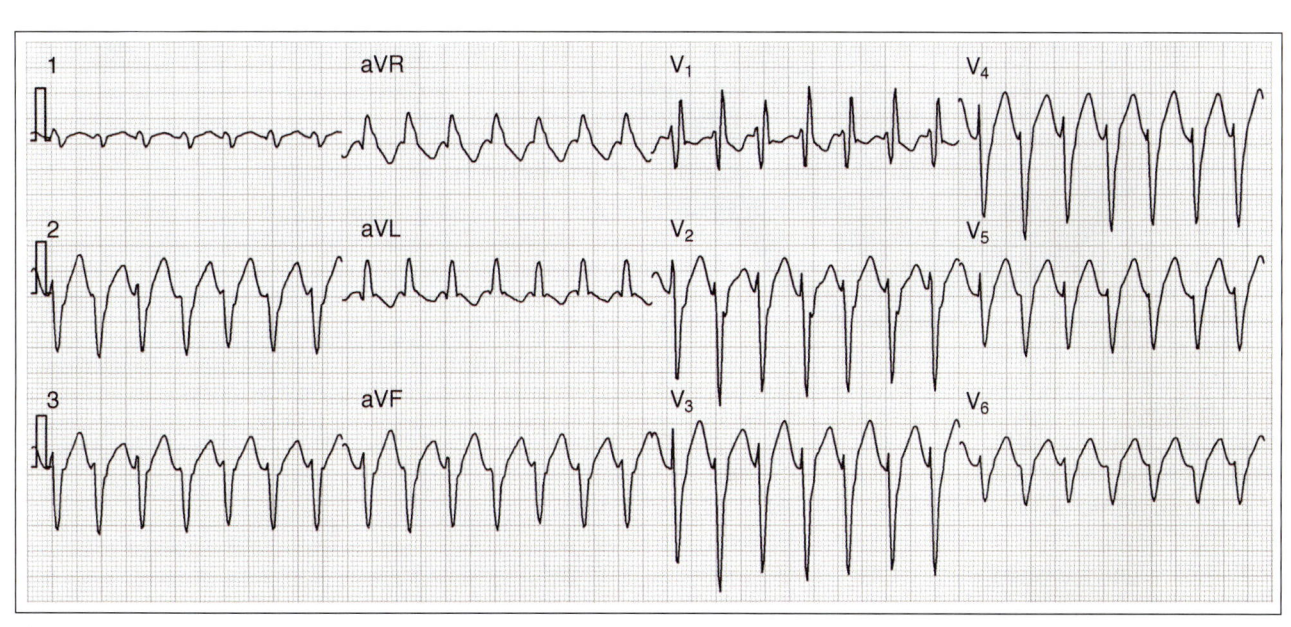

Figure 32.4 RBBB, left-superior-axis ventricular tachycardia (verapamil-sensitive, Purkinje-related). Note the relatively narrow QRS complex and superior axis, and a slurring in the upstroke of the inferior lead as it returns to the baseline.

episodes of VT interrupted by short interludes of sinus rhythm. Their clinical occurrence is tightly related to autonomic modulation, with special sensitivity to exercise. Irrespective of their clinical presentation and behavior, all these VTs have an inferior-axis morphology (usually with LBBB), and their exact localization is challenging due to the complex anatomy and the close proximity of the aortic cusps, RVOT, LVO, and the epicardial surface (**Figure 32.5**). On the other hand, localization of the VTs noninvasively is particularly rewarding since it affords the opportunity of planning for the procedure including the possible use of a deep-seated CS catheter in the anterior interventricular vein (epicardial surface of the basal LV), reliance on ICE as well as fluoroscopy to define the aortic cusps region and the RVOT border/pulmonic valve area, and the possible need for coronary arteriography to ascertain safety of ablation in certain locations. Moreover, although we advocate mapping both outflow tract areas in most patients with suspected outflow tract VTs to define the earliest endocardial site, the ECG features of the tachycardia are key in targeting electroanatomical mapping and reducing procedure time and radiation exposure. In this respect, it is important to remember the anatomical relation of both outflow tracts, especially the leftward direction of the RVOT and the pulmonary artery vs. a rightward direction of the LVO and the aortic root (important in evaluating lead I and V_5, V_6 for the presence of S waves). Moreover, examining lead V_1 for the presence of an initial R wave is critical since it correlates with the anteroposterior distribution of the outflow tracts.[11]

RVOT Ventricular Tachycardias

Most of these VTs originate from the so-called septal RVOT (actually free wall but on the leftward aspect, below the pulmonic valve) and exhibit a characteristic ECG pattern of LBBB, inferior axis with large positive QRS in the inferior leads, and large negative complexes in aVR and aVL. The QRS complex in lead I is multiphasic with near zero or slightly positive net voltage. For most other foci in the RVOT, an exact localization can be predicted with reasonable accuracy by analysis of the complexity and duration of the QRS complex in the inferior leads as well as the axis and precordial transition (**Figure 32.5**).

A "septal" vs. free wall location of these VTs determines the QRS duration in leads II and III, where a duration of < 140 ms correlates with a leftward outflow tract location (close access to the conduction system) while a longer, notched, and smaller R wave is associated with a rightward free wall focus. Moreover, an earlier precordial R-wave

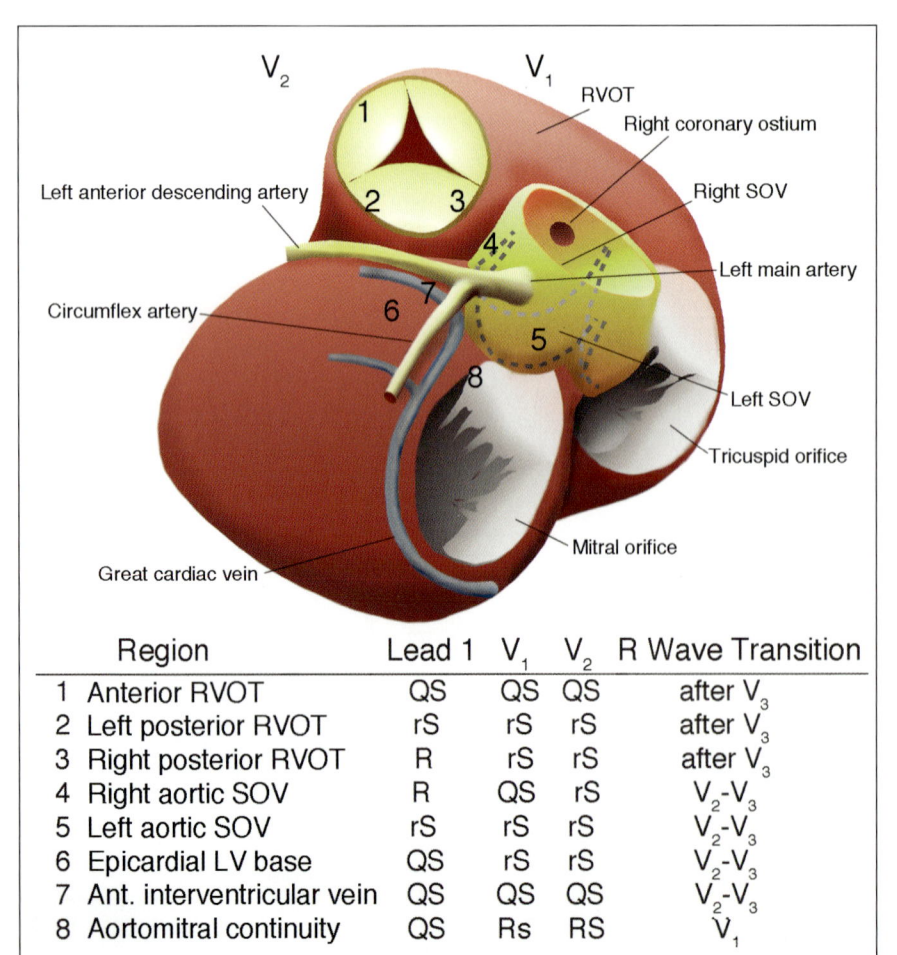

Figure 32.5 Outflow tract regions corresponding to idiopathic ventricular tachycardia exit sites. The heart is viewed from approximately the left shoulder, looking down on the outflow tract regions of both ventricles. Anatomic regions are labeled; dashed lines indicate attachments of aortic valve cusps. Approximate relative locations of ECG leads V_1 and V_2 are shown. ECG features associated with numbered regions on the diagram are shown below. RVOT, right ventricular outflow tract; SVO, sinus of Valsalva; LV, left ventricle.

Region	Lead 1	V_1	V_2	R Wave Transition
1 Anterior RVOT	QS	QS	QS	after V_3
2 Left posterior RVOT	rS	rS	rS	after V_3
3 Right posterior RVOT	R	rS	rS	after V_3
4 Right aortic SOV	R	QS	rS	V_2-V_3
5 Left aortic SOV	rS	rS	rS	V_2-V_3
6 Epicardial LV base	QS	rS	rS	V_2-V_3
7 Ant. interventricular vein	QS	QS	QS	V_2-V_3
8 Aortomitral continuity	QS	Rs	RS	V_1

transition is usually due to a more basal source or even aortic root/sinus of Valsalva.[12] Due to the slanted direction of the RVOT, as the focus moves posteriorly it also moves in a lateral direction; hence the R wave in lead I becomes positive.[12] Similarly, as the focus moves inferiorly it also moves rightward and posteriorly; hence, the precordial transition shifts to the left, and a more positive/taller R wave in lead I occurs as well as positive QRS in aVL.[13] The amplitude of the initial R wave in V_1 and V_2 has also been suggested as a distinguishing ECG feature, where > 0.2 mV suggests a superior origin.[12,14]

Foci above the pulmonary valve level are associated with taller R wave in the inferior leads and earlier precordial transition than RVOT VTs. A QS or rS wave is typically seen in lead I corresponding to the leftward location of the focus.[15,16]

LVO Ventricular Tachycardias

Less commonly, outflow tract tachycardias originate from the LV outflow region (there is no tubular muscular "tract"), and these share many of the ECG characteristics of the RVOT VTs due to the anatomical proximity of these two structures. However, an early precordial transition in leads V_1 or V_2 (R wave in lead V_1 and V_2) as well as an S wave or QS complex in lead I, distinguishes an LVO origin.[17-19]

A supravalvular location of an LVO VT has similar features but specifically lacks S waves in V_5 or V_6 and has taller R waves in V_1 and V_2 (R/QRS duration more than 50% and R/S amplitude more than 30%).[20] Among these VTs, a right SOV origin is the most common and is characterized by a taller R wave in lead I vs. a QS or rS complex in lead I for a left SOV origin. Left SOV VTs typically have an "M" or "W" pattern in V_1 giving either a possible RBBB or LBBB classification. The noncoronary SOV is rarely the origin of VT due to paucity of muscle fibers extending from it to the LV.[18,20] Note that localization of VTs in the region of the aortic cusps remains challenging due to the variation of the ECG characteristics with the position of the heart (a vertical heart results in more posterior location and more negative lead I characteristics) and the derivation of the above ECG characteristics from pace mapping protocols.[20] In addition, there have been several reports of the same focus producing very different QRS configurations of VT or premature ventricular complexes, as proven by elimination of more than one configuration by a single ablation lesion.[21,22]

ECG Characteristics of Epicardial Ventricular Tachycardias

An epicardial origin of VT has been more commonly identified in recent years. The frequency of an epicardial focus or reentrant circuit is variable depending on the underlying substrate: it is rare in post-MI VT (ranging from 1% to 2%), while it accounts for 5% to 10% of VTs in ARVC, 25% to 45% of VTs in NICM, and up to 30% to 40% of VTs in Chagas disease. Careful consideration should be given to ECG features of the clinical VT, especially in the setting of NICM, where it is reasonable to obtain pericardial access at the beginning of the procedure to avoid having to do so after initiation of anticoagulation necessary for endocardial LV mapping.

Many ECG criteria have been identified for localizing epicardial VTs, including:

1. Pseudo–delta wave (measured from the earliest ventricular activation to the earliest fast deflection in any precordial lead) of 34 ms or more[23]

2. Intrinsicoid deflection time in V_2 (measured from the earliest ventricular activation to the peak of the R wave in V_2) of more than 85 ms[23]

3. Shortest RS complex duration (measured from the earliest ventricular activation to the nadir of the first S wave in any precordial lead) of 121 ms or more[23]

4. Maximal deflection index (MDI), measured by dividing the earliest time to maximum deflection in any precordial lead by total QRS duration, of 0.55 or more[24]

5. QRS duration of more than 200 ms[25]

Most of these criteria, however, are site-specific and, except for MDI, apply to patients with structural heart disease. These are illustrated in **Figure 32.6**.

Morphologic criteria have been suggested that strongly correlate with an epicardial VT origin in the absence of scar (structural heart disease) and are site-specific. These criteria include the presence of a Q wave in lead I for basal and apical SVTs; the absence of a Q wave in any of the inferior leads for basal SVTs; and the presence of a Q wave in the inferior leads for basal IVTs and apical IVTs (**Figure 32.7**).[25] For VTs originating from the RV, the presence of an initial Q wave in lead I and QS in lead V_2 for anterior sites in the RV strongly predicts an epicardial origin while an initial Q wave in leads II, III, and aVF predicts an inferior epicardial location of the RV.[26]

Screening the ECG for many of these morphologic and quantitative criteria is helpful in increasing the sensitivity and specificity of detecting an epicardial VT origin. This was elegantly demonstrated in a study by Vallès et al.[27] in which a stepwise approach yielded a 96% sensitivity and 93% specificity in detecting an epicardial location in the setting of NICM.

Conclusion

The ECG during VT provides many clues as to the site of myocardial breakthrough, after which the remainder of ventricular myocardium is activated. A number of

290 • Ablation of VT

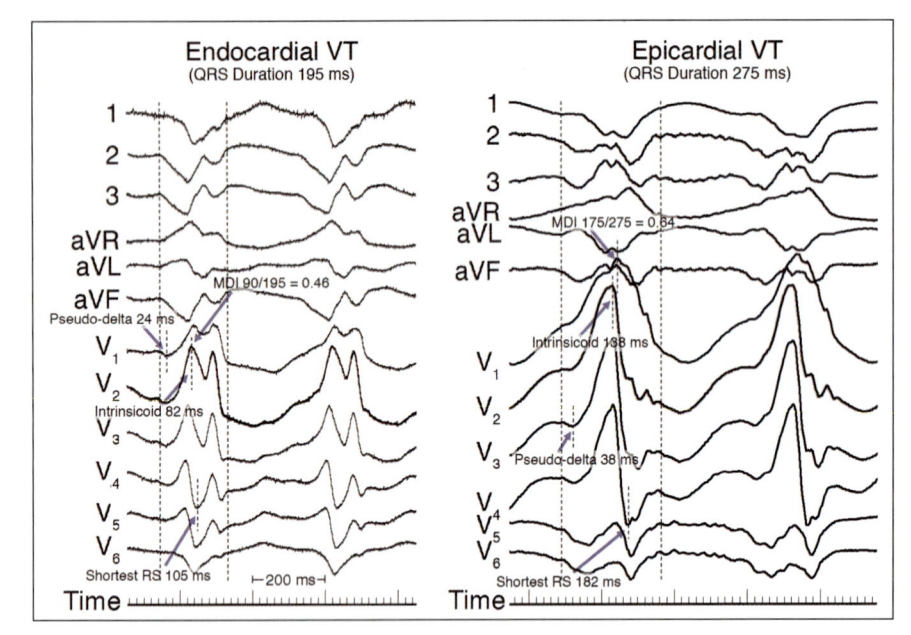

Figure 32.6 ECG features of epicardial ventricular tachycardia exit sites. 12-lead ECGs of 2 ventricular tachycardias are shown with measurements corresponding to several criteria for epicardial exit sites. At left, all indices correctly suggest an endocardial exit site, whereas at right, a ventricular tachycardia with a wider QRS complex has indices that suggest epicardial exit.

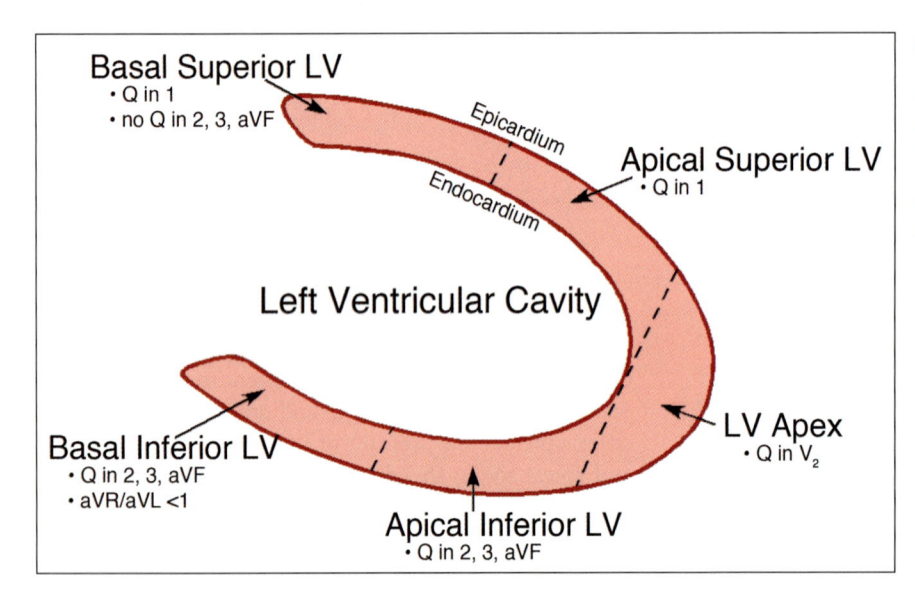

Figure 32.7 ECG features of epicardial ventricular tachycardia origins in left ventricular idiopathic ventricular tachycardia. The left ventricle is viewed from a right anterior oblique perspective. Specific features of individual ECG leads that correlate with epicardial ventricular tachycardia origins are shown.

algorithms have been developed that have moderately high accuracy (> 70% positive predictive value) for designating a 2 to 5 cm² region that is the earliest activated during VT. In the absence of structural heart disease, ECG algorithms denote the site of actual impulse origin (since most VTs in this group are focal in origin). However, in the presence of structural heart disease (almost always accompanied by substantial scarring), algorithms designate the site of exit from a reentrant circuit, during most of which activation is "silent" in the ECG (diastole). Since sites activated during diastole are generally the most attractive ablation sites, the algorithm-designated region is almost never the ideal site for ablation. Whether or not heart disease is present, ECG clues to VT breakthrough sites are very useful as a guide to focus initial mapping efforts toward regions most likely to contain appropriate ablation sites. As experience grows with different varieties of focal VT as well as epicardial mapping and ablation, it is likely that existing algorithms will be further refined and new ones developed to enhance the ability of the ECG during VT to guide mapping and ablation.

References

1. Blanck Z, Dhala A, Deshpande S, Sra J, Jazayeri M, Akhtar M. Bundle branch reentrant ventricular tachycardia: cumulative experience in 48 patients. *J Cardiovasc Electrophysiol.* 1993;4(3):253–262.
2. Daoud E. Bundle branch reentry. In: Zipes DP, Jalife J, eds. *Cardiac Electrophysiology: From Cell to Bedside.* Philadelphia: WB Saunders, 2004:683–688.

3. Miller JM, Marchlinski FE, Buxton AE, Josephson ME. Relationship between the 12-lead ECG during ventricular tachycardia and endocardial site of origin in patients with coronary artery disease. *Circulation.* 1988;77:759–766.
4. Kuchar DL, Ruskin JN, Garan H. ECG localization of the site of origin of ventricular tachycardia in patients with prior myocardial infarction. *J Am Coll Cardiol.* 1989;13:893–903.
5. Segal OR, Chow AW, Wong T, et al. A novel algorithm for determining endocardial ventricular tachycardia exit site from 12-lead surface ECG characteristics in human, infarct-related ventricular tachycardia. *J Cardiovasc Electrophysiol.* 2007;18(2):161–168.
6. Hsia HH, Callans DJ, Marchlinski FE. Characterization of endocardial electrophysiological substrate in patients with NICM and monomorphic ventricular tachycardia. *Circulation.* 2003;108:704–710.
7. Soejima K., Stevenson WG, Sapp JL, Selwyn AP, Couper G, Epstein LM. Endocardial and epicardial radiofrequency ablation of ventricular tachycardia associated with dilated cardiomyopathy: the importance of low-voltage scars. *J Am Coll Cardiol.* 2004;43:1834–1842.
8. Marchlinski FE, Zado E, Dixit S, et al. Electroanatomic substrate and outcome of catheter ablative therapy for ventricular tachycardia in setting of right ventricular cardiomyopathy. *Circulation.* 2004;110:2293–2298.
9. Jefic D, Joel B, Good E, Morady F, Rosman H, Knight B, Bogun F. Role of radiofrequency catheter ablation of ventricular tachycardia in cardiac sarcoidosis: report from a multicenter registry. *Heart Rhythm.* 2009;6:189–195.
10. Nogami A, Naito S, Tada H, et al. Demonstration of diastolic and presystolic Purkinje potentials as critical potentials in a macroreentry circuit of verapamil-sensitive idiopathic left ventricular tachycardia. *J Am Coll Cardiol.* 2000;36:811–823.
11. Bala R, Marchlinski FE. ECG recognition and ablation of outflow tract ventricular tachycardia. *Heart Rhythm.* 2007;4;366–370.
12. Dixit S, Gerstenfeld EP, Callans DJ, Marchlinski FE. ECG patterns of superior right ventricular outflow tract tachycardias: distinguishing septal and free-wall sites of origin. *J Cardiovasc Electrophysiol.* 2003;14:1–7.
13. Tada H, Tadokoro K, Ito S, et al. Idiopathic ventricular arrhythmias originating from the tricuspid annulus: Prevalence, ECG characteristics, and results of radiofrequency catheter ablation. *Heart Rhythm.* 2007;4:7–16.
14. Tada H, Ito S, Naito S, et al. Prevalence and ECG characteristics of idiopathic ventricular arrhythmia originating in the free wall of the right ventricular outflow tract. *Circ J.* 2004;68:909–914.
15. Timmermans C, Rodriguez LM, Medeiros A, Crijns HJ, Wellens HJ. Radiofrequency catheter ablation of idiopathic ventricular tachycardia originating in the main stem of the pulmonary artery. *J Cardiovasc Electrophysiol.* 2002;13:281–284.
16. Sekiguchi Y, Aonuma K, Takahashi A, et al. ECG and electrophysiologic characteristics of ventricular tachycardia originating within the pulmonary artery. *J Am Coll Cardiol.* 2005;45:887–895.
17. Kamakura S, Shimizu W, Matsuo K, et al. Localization of optimal ablation site of idiopathic ventricular tachycardia from right and left ventricular outflow tract by body surface ECG. *Circulation.* 1998;98:1525–1533.
18. Hachiya H, Aonuma K, Yamauchi Y, et al. ECG characteristics of left ventricular outflow tract tachycardia. *Pacing Clin Electrophysiol.* 2000;23:1930–1934.
19. Ito S, Tada H, Naito S, et al. Development and validation of an ECG algorithm for identifying the optimal ablation site for idiopathic ventricular outflow tract tachycardia. *J Cardiovasc Electrophysiol.* 2003;14:1280–1286.
20. Lin D, Ilkhanoff L, Gerstenfeld E, et al. Twelve-lead ECG characteristics of the aortic cusp region guided by ICE and electroanatomic mapping. *Heart Rhythm.* 2008;5:663–669.
21. Yamada T, Platonov M, McElderry HT, Kay GN. Left ventricular outflow tract tachycardia with preferential conduction and multiple exits. *Circ Arrhythm Electrophysiol.* 2008;1:140–142.
22. Yamada T, Murakami Y, Yoshida N, et al. Preferential conduction across the ventricular outflow septum in ventricular arrhythmias originating from the aortic sinus cusp. *J Am Coll Cardiol.* 2007 Aug 28;50(9):884–891.
23. Berruezo A, Mont L, Nava S, Chueca E, Bartholomay E, Brugada J. ECG recognition of the epicardial origin of ventricular tachycardias. *Circulation.* 2004;109:1842–1847.
24. Daniels DV, Lu YY, Morton JB, Santucci PA, Akar JG, Green A, Wilber DJ. Idiopathic epicardial left ventricular tachycardia originating remote from the sinus of Valsalva: electrophysiological characteristics, catheter ablation, and identification from the 12-lead ECG. *Circulation.* 2006;113(13):1659–1666.
25. Bazan V, Gerstenfeld EP, Garcia FC, et al. Site-specific twelve-lead ECG features to identify an epicardial origin for left ventricular tachycardia in the absence of myocardial infarction. *Heart Rhythm.* 2007;4:1403–1410.
26. Bazan V, Bala R, Garcia FC, et al. Twelve-lead ECG features to identify ventricular tachycardia arising from the epicardial right ventricle. *Heart Rhythm.* 2006;3:1132–1139.
27. Valles E, Bazan V, Marchlinski FE. ECG criteria to identify epicardial ventricular tachycardia in NICM. *Circ Arrhythm Electrophysiol.* 2010;3:63–71.

CHAPTER 33

How to Diagnose and Ablate Ventricular Tachycardia from the Outflow Tract and Aortic Cusps

Takumi Yamada, MD, PhD; G. Neal Kay, MD

Introduction

The ventricular outflow tracts and ASCs are major sites of origin of ventricular arrhythmias with or without structural heart diseases.[1-11] The ventricular arrhythmias arising from these regions are being increasingly recognized as targets for catheter ablation.[2-12] Although the ECG and EP characteristics of these ventricular arrhythmias may be helpful for identifying the site of origin, it is well known that the complex anatomy of this region may limit the reliability of algorithms based on those characteristics.[9-14] In these ventricular arrhythmias, endocardial catheter ablation is usually successful, but an epicardial catheter approach to ablation via the cardiac vein and subxiphoidal pericardial approach may sometimes be required.[2-17] In this chapter, we discuss our approach to catheter ablation of outflow tract and ASC ventricular arrhythmias.

Preprocedural Planning

Although the RVOT, LVOT, and ASCs are located anatomically close to each other,[18,19] the techniques and equipment used for mapping and catheter ablation may differ among these regions. Therefore, a preprocedural planning of the mapping and catheter ablation approach is important to save procedural time and to reduce costs and complications. The preprocedural planning is usually based on the ECG characteristics and several other considerations.

ECG Diagnosis

ECG characteristics are helpful for predicting the site of origin of ventricular arrhythmias originating from these regions.[5,8-11,20] The most important diagnosis to make by an ECG may be whether the ventricular arrhythmias originate from the right or left side. The BBB pattern, the precordial transition zone, and the magnitude and width of the R wave or QRS complex in leads V_1 and V_2 may be helpful for localizing the site of origin. An RBBB QRS morphology clearly suggests the ventricular arrhythmia originates on the left side. When an LBBB QRS morphology is observed, the precordial transition pattern, the magnitude and width of R wave or QRS complex in leads V_1 and V_2 (R/S wave amplitude and duration indexes), should be evaluated next (**Figure 33.1**). The R/S wave amplitude ratio in leads V_1 and V_2 is calculated using the amplitude of the QRS complex peak or nadir to the isoelectric line. The R/S wave amplitude index, which is a greater value of the R/S wave amplitude ratio in lead V_1 or V_2, is considered more useful than the R/S wave amplitude ratio alone in lead V_1 or V_2. The R-wave duration index is calculated by dividing the longer R-wave duration in lead V_1 or V_2 by the QRS-complex duration. A precordial transition later than lead V_4 or R/S amplitude index of < 0.3

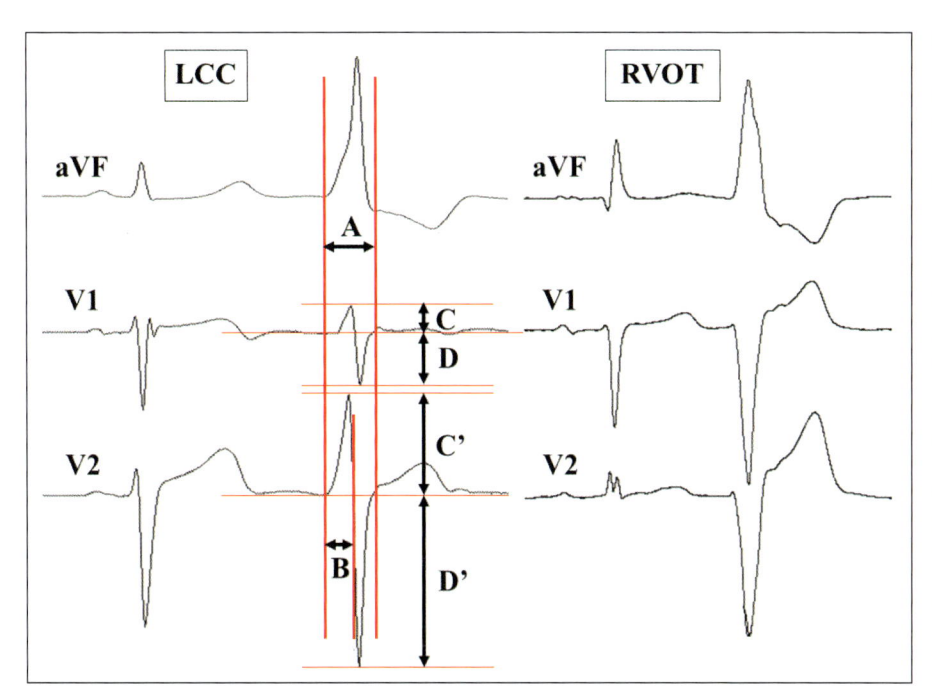

Figure 33.1 Examples of an ECG analysis of ventricular arrhythmias. The first beats are sinus and the second beats are ventricular arrhythmias originating from the LCC and RVOT. **A** indicates the total QRS duration, **B** the longer R-wave duration in lead V_1 or V_2, determined in lead V_2 from the QRS onset to the R-wave intersection point where the R wave crosses the isoelectric line, **C** the R-wave amplitude, measured from the peak to the isoelectric line, and **D** the S-wave amplitude measured from the QRS nadir to the isoelectric line. The R/S wave amplitude ratio in lead V_2 (C'/D') is greater than that in lead V_1 (C/D) and C'/D' is determined as the R/S wave amplitude index. The R/S amplitude index is less than 0.3 and R wave duration index less than 0.5 during RVOT ventricular arrhythmias whereas they are not during LCC ventricular arrhythmias.

and R-wave duration index of < 0.5 may strongly suggest a ventricular arrhythmia origin on the right side (**Figure 33.1**).[8] Otherwise, a ventricular arrhythmia origin on the left side may be suggested (**Figure 33.1**). The presence of S waves in lead I may also be helpful for differentiating ventricular arrhythmia origins in the ASCs or RVOT.[5,8] The presence of "notching" in the middle of the QRS complex strongly suggests a ventricular arrhythmia origin in the free wall of the RVOT.[21] The presence of S waves in lead V_6 may suggest a ventricular arrhythmia origin in the endocardial LV, which indicates the area below the aortic valve.[5] A qrS pattern in the right precordial leads may be highly specific for a ventricular arrhythmia origin at the junction between the left and right ASCs.[9]

The ECG features as to whether ventricular arrhythmias can be successfully ablated from the endocardial or epicardial side are also important to recognize. The maximum deflection index (MDI), which is calculated by dividing the shortest time to the maximum deflection in any precordial lead by the QRS duration and the ratio of the Q-wave amplitude in leads aVL to aVR (aVL/aVR ratio), may be helpful for making such a diagnosis.[20,22] An MDI of > 0.55 and aVL/aVR ratio of > 1.4 suggest that ventricular arrhythmias may be ablated epicardially, although these algorithms are reliable for ventricular arrhythmias arising from the endocardial LVOT and less reliable for those arising from the ASCs and epicardial LVOT.

Because of their anatomical close proximity, ventricular arrhythmias originating from the RVOT, LVOT, and ASCs may exhibit similar ECG features. In addition, the complex anatomy of these regions may limit the reliability of these ECG algorithms. In the preprocedural planning, these limitations should be kept in mind, and all possibilities should be considered.

Other Considerations

RVOT ventricular arrhythmias occur more frequently in women than in men while males consistently predominate with LVOT ventricular arrhythmias.[10,23] The RVOT ventricular arrhythmias are usually caused by abnormal automaticity. They can be induced by exercise or intravenous isoproterenol and may be suppressed by beta-blockers. The LVOT ventricular arrhythmias are likely to occur based on a mechanism of triggered activity and can be induced by ventricular stimulation.

Procedure

Patient Preparation

All patients are brought to the EP laboratory in a fasting state. EP study and catheter ablation are performed under deep sedation with intravenous midazolam, fentanyl, and propofol. In patients with PVCs, the 12-lead surface ECGs of clinical PVCs should be recorded before sedation is initiated, because sedation may sometimes suppress PVCs.

A total of 3 sheaths are inserted in the right femoral vein for catheter placement with an 8-Fr sheath for an ablation catheter. Access in the right femoral artery is obtained with an 8-Fr sheath for LV mapping. A heparin bolus of 100 to 150 units/kg is typically given immediately thereafter, and intravenous heparin is administered to maintain an ACT > 250 seconds during LV mapping and ablation procedure. It is also important to prepare for possible arterial access in the left femoral artery with a 6-Fr sheath for coronary angiography.

EP Study

For mapping and pacing, a quadripolar catheter is positioned at the HB region via the right femoral vein and a 6- or 7-Fr deflectable decapolar catheter in the CS. The CS catheter is advanced into the GCV as far as possible, even into the AIVV until the proximal electrode pair records an earlier ventricular activation than the most distal electrode pair during the ventricular arrhythmias (**Figures 33.2** and **33.3**). When this is impossible, a 2.3-Fr multielectrode catheter (PATHFINDER™, CARDIMA, Fremont, CA, USA) is advanced through a 7-Fr Amplatz angiographic catheter via the right femoral vein for mapping within these veins (**Figure 33.4**). Endocardial mapping and pacing in the ventricular outflow tracts are usually performed using a 7-Fr, 4- or 5-mm-tip ablation catheter via the right femoral vein or artery. When few PVCs are observed at the beginning of the EP study, induction of ventricular tachycardia or PVCs is attempted by burst pacing from the RVOT or right ventricular apex with the addition of an isoproterenol infusion.

Mapping

Because preprocedural ECG diagnosis is imperfect, mapping in the RV should be first performed in all patients with an LBBB QRS morphology. Activation mapping seeking the earliest bipolar activity and/or a local unipolar QS pattern during ventricular arrhythmias is most reliable for identifying a site of origin of the ventricular arrhythmia. In some patients, when the VT or PVCs are frequent, electro-anatomic mapping can facilitate the procedure and improve procedural outcomes.[24] Pace mapping may be helpful when ventricular arrhythmias are infrequent and can roughly localize a site of origin. Pace mapping is especially helpful for RVOT ventricular arrhythmias[3,12], but may be less helpful for ASC ventricular arrhythmias because pacing in the ASCs may not exactly reproduce the QRS morphology of the ventricular arrhythmias because of preferential conduction (**Figure 33.5**)[13] or the inability to obtain myocardial capture despite the use of high pacing current. A comparison of the pace maps from the right and left side may be helpful to predict whether a ventricular arrhythmia can be ablated from the right or left ventricle (**Figure 33.6**). When an earlier precordial transition during ventricular arrhythmias cannot be reproduced by pace mapping from the right ventricle, a site of origin may be considered to be located in the left ventricle. A comparison of the pace maps from the ASCs, endocardial LVOT, and GCV may be helpful to predict whether a ventricular arrhythmia can be ablated from the endocardial or epicardial side (Figure 33.6). In this comparison, the MDI as well as the pace map score should be evaluated. When the MDI during ventricular arrhythmias is closer to that during pace mapping from the GCV than that during pace mapping from the ASCs and LVOT, the epicardial surface may be considered to be the source of the ventricular arrhythmia. Pace mapping is performed using the distal bipolar electrodes at a pacing cycle length of 500 ms and at a minimum stimulus amplitude required for consistent capture (up to a maximum output of 20 mA and pulse width of 2.0 ms). The score for the pace mapping is determined as the number of leads with an identical height of the R wave/depth of the S wave (R/S) ratio match (12 represents a perfect R/S ratio match in all 12 leads), as well as the number of leads with a fine notching match in the 12-lead ECG as previously reported (perfect pace mapping

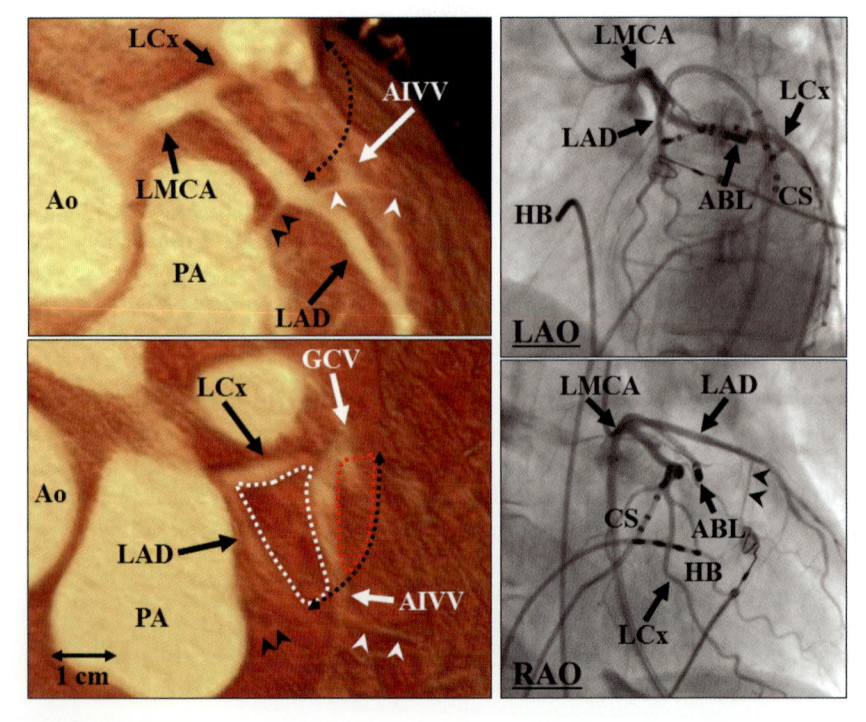

Figure 33.2 Computed tomographic (left panels) and fluoroscopic (right panels) images exhibiting the LV summit. The LV summit was defined based on the fluoroscopy and coronary angiography as the region on the epicardial surface of the LV near the bifurcation of the left main coronary artery that is bounded by an arc (black dotted line) from the LAD, superior to the first septal perforating branch (black arrowheads), anteriorly to the LCx, and then laterally along the LCx. The GCV bisects the LV summit into a superior portion surrounded by the white dotted line (the *inaccessible area*) and an inferior portion surrounded by the red dotted line (the *accessible area*). The white arrowheads indicate the first diagonal branch of the LAD. The ablation catheter is positioned in the accessible area and a decapolar catheter in the GCV. ABL = ablation catheter; AIVV = anterior inter-ventricular cardiac vein; Ao = aorta; CS = coronary sinus; HB = His bundle; LAO = left anterior oblique; LMCA = left main coronary artery; PA = pulmonary artery; RAO = right anterior oblique. (Used with permission from reference 17.)

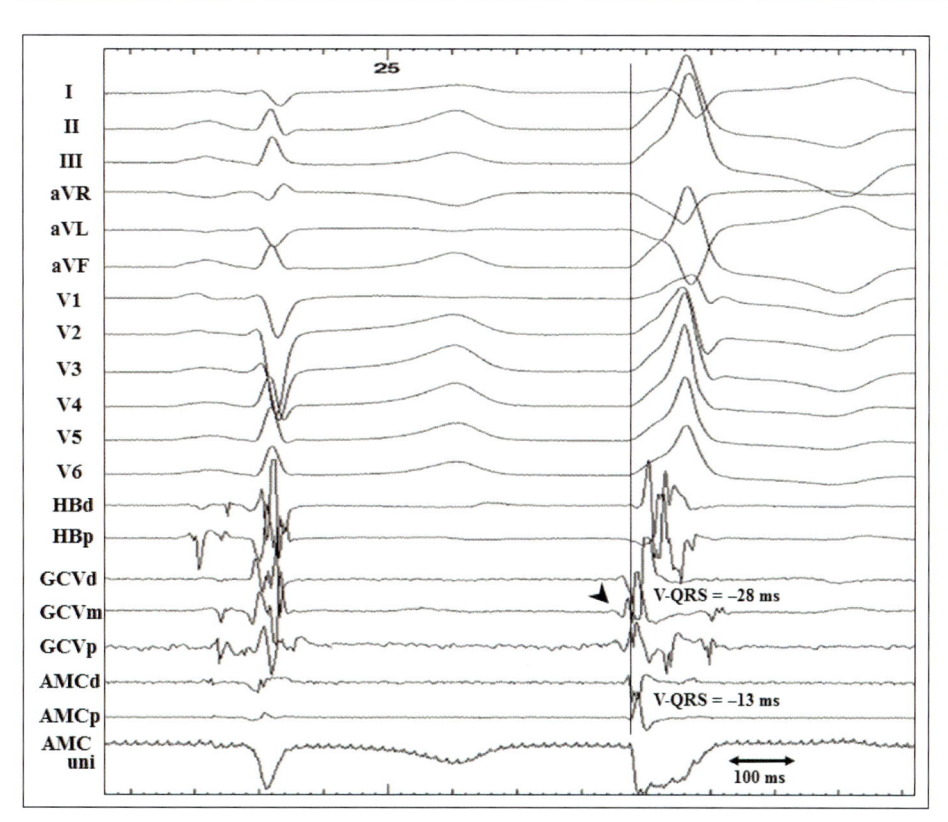

Figure 33.3 Cardiac tracings recorded from a micro multielectrode catheter positioned in the GCV. During ventricular arrhythmias, the ventricular activation recorded from the middle electrode pair of the micro multielectrode catheter (arrowhead) was earlier than that recorded from the distal electrode pair and that recorded from the AMC. AMC uni = the distal unipolar electrode of the mapping catheter positioned at the AMC; V-QRS = the local ventricular activation time relative to the QRS onset; d (m, p) = the distal (middle, proximal) electrode pairs of the relevant catheter. The other abbreviations are as in Figure 33.2.

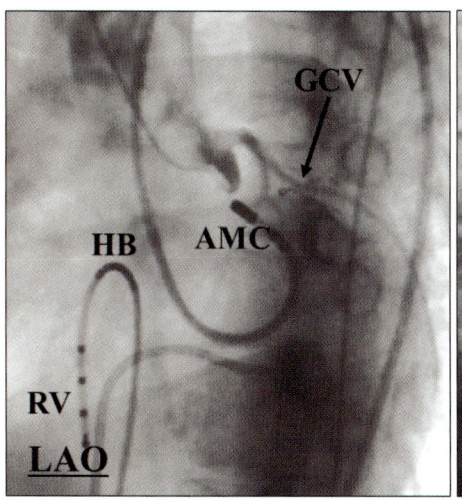

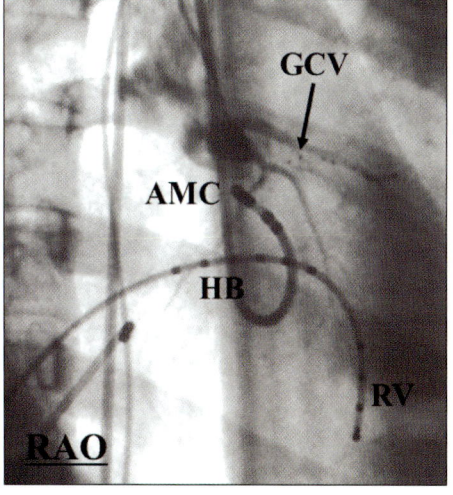

Figure 33.4 Fluoroscopic images exhibiting a micro multielectrode catheter positioned in the GCV through an Amplatz angiographic catheter via the right femoral vein. The ablation catheter is positioned in the AMC underneath the left coronary cusp. RV = right ventricle. The other abbreviations are as in Figure 33.1.

is equal to 24 points).[3] An excellent pace map is defined as a pace map that obtains a score of > 20. The pace map score can also be automatically calculated with computer software by comparing the paced QRS complex with a template of the spontaneous PVC or VT morphology.

When the earliest ventricular activation in the RV precedes the QRS onset by more than 20 ms and is earlier than that recorded in the GCV, RF catheter ablation may be performed at that site when there is confirmation of an excellent pace map match to the QRS complex of the clinical ventricular arrhythmias. When there are no sites with early activation in the RV, or when RV catheter ablation is unsuccessful, mapping in the ASCs and LVOT should follow. Because the posterior portion of the RVOT is in close apposition to the LV near the aortic root, when catheter ablation has not been successful in the LVOT, the RV should be carefully mapped before determining that an epicardial approach is required.

Before mapping and catheter ablation above the aortic valve, selective angiography of the coronary artery and aorta should be performed to carefully determine the coronary artery ostium in the ASCs, to precisely define the location of the ablation catheter, and to avoid arterial injury (**Figure 33.7**).[10,11] The 3 ASCs can be readily identified during biplane aortography or coronary angiography. The LCC is most easily identified in the LAO projection

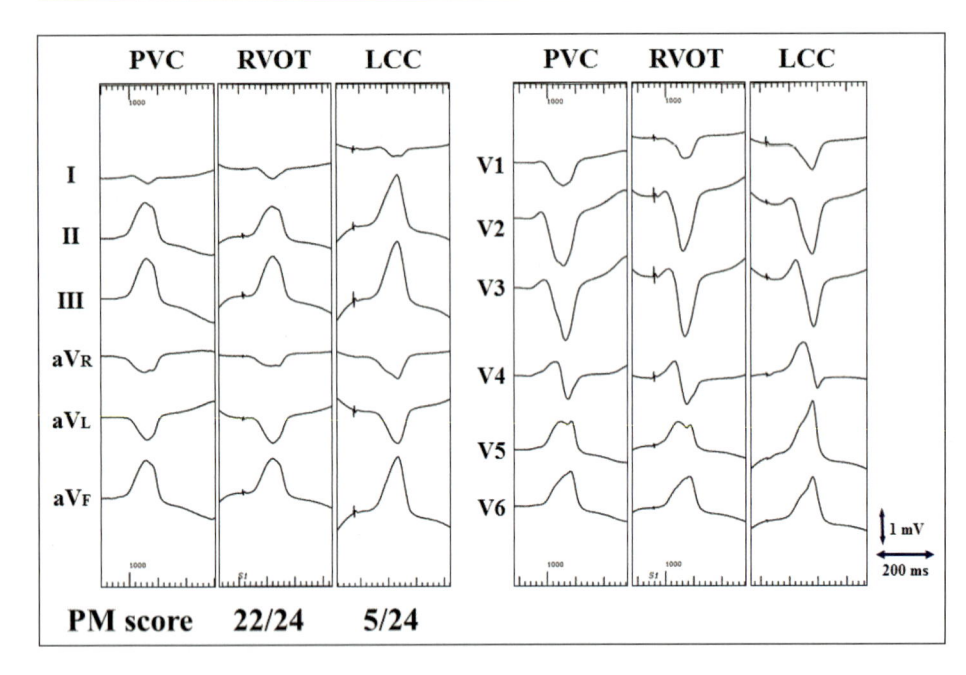

Figure 33.5 Premature ventricular contractions (PVCs) with an LCC origin showing a left bundle branch block and inferior QRS axis morphology with a precordial transition between V_4 and V_5. An excellent pace map was obtained at the site of the earliest ventricular activation in the RVOT (pace map [PM] score 22/24). However, a poor PM was obtained at the successful ablation site in the LCC (PM score 5/24). The pacing stimulus to QRS interval was 0 ms and 50 ms during pace mapping from the RVOT and LCC, respectively. The other abbreviations are as in Figure 33.1. (Used with permission from reference 13.)

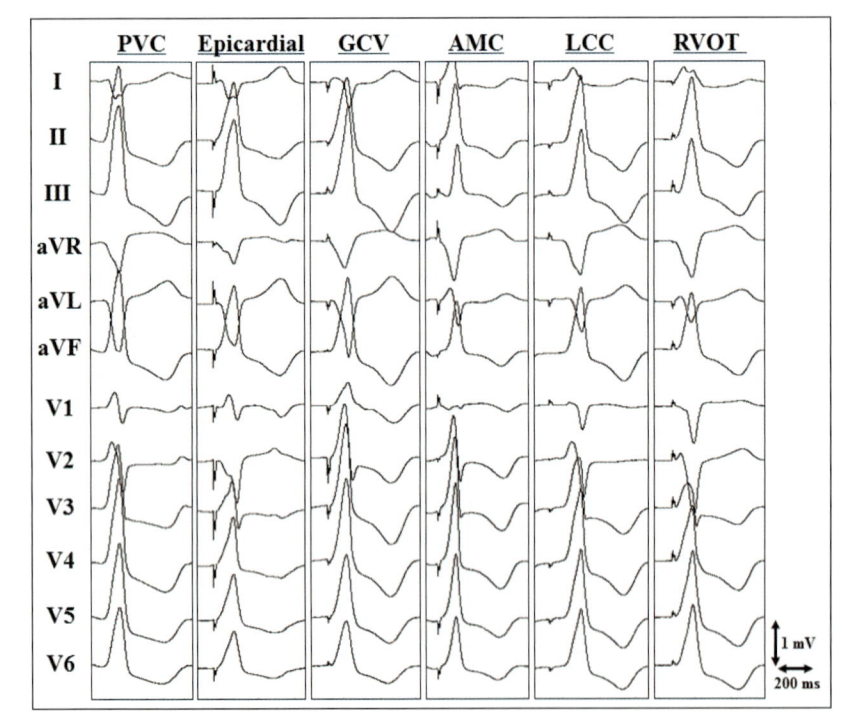

Figure 33.6 Comparison of the 12-lead ECGs between the PVCs arising from the inaccessible area and pace maps from various right and left ventricular outflow tract locations. Note that pacing from any endocardial or epicardial sites never produced an excellent pace map especially with higher amplitudes of the R waves in the inferior leads. The abbreviations are as in the previous figures. (Used with permission from reference 17.)

where this cusp is on the far lateral aspect of the aortic root, leftward and superior to the HB catheter (**Figure 33.7A**). The RCC usually requires coronary angiography in both the RAO and LAO projections for accurate identification of the cusp relative to the RCA ostium (**Figure 33.7B**). In the RAO projection, the ablation catheter is typically located anterior and inferior to the RCA ostium. In the LAO projection, the typical ablation site is more leftward in the cusp than the RCA ostium. The NCC is readily identified as the most inferior of the three cusps and by its close relation to the HB catheter. In the RAO projection (**Figure 33.7C**), a catheter in the NCC is posterior and inferior to the RCA ostium, just above the HB catheter. In the LAO projection (Figure 33.7C), the NCC is just superior to the HB catheter, well posterior to the RCA ostium. ICE may also be useful for identifying the site of the ablation catheter. Because the NCC overlies the atrial septum, amplitude of an atrial electrogram is usually larger than that of a ventricular electrogram within the NCC.

When ventricular arrhythmias exhibit an R wave in lead I and a local ventricular activation recorded from the HB catheter precedes the QRS onset, mapping in the RCC,

Figure 33.7 Coronary angiograms and the catheter positions. **A.** The left coronary angiograms. **B.** The right coronary angiograms. **C.** The right coronary angiograms with the ablation catheter within the NCC. Note that the typical site of the catheter ablation for ventricular arrhythmias arising from the LCC and RCC is at the nadir of those cusps. RCA = right coronary artery. The other abbreviations are as in the previous figures. (Used with permission from reference 11.)

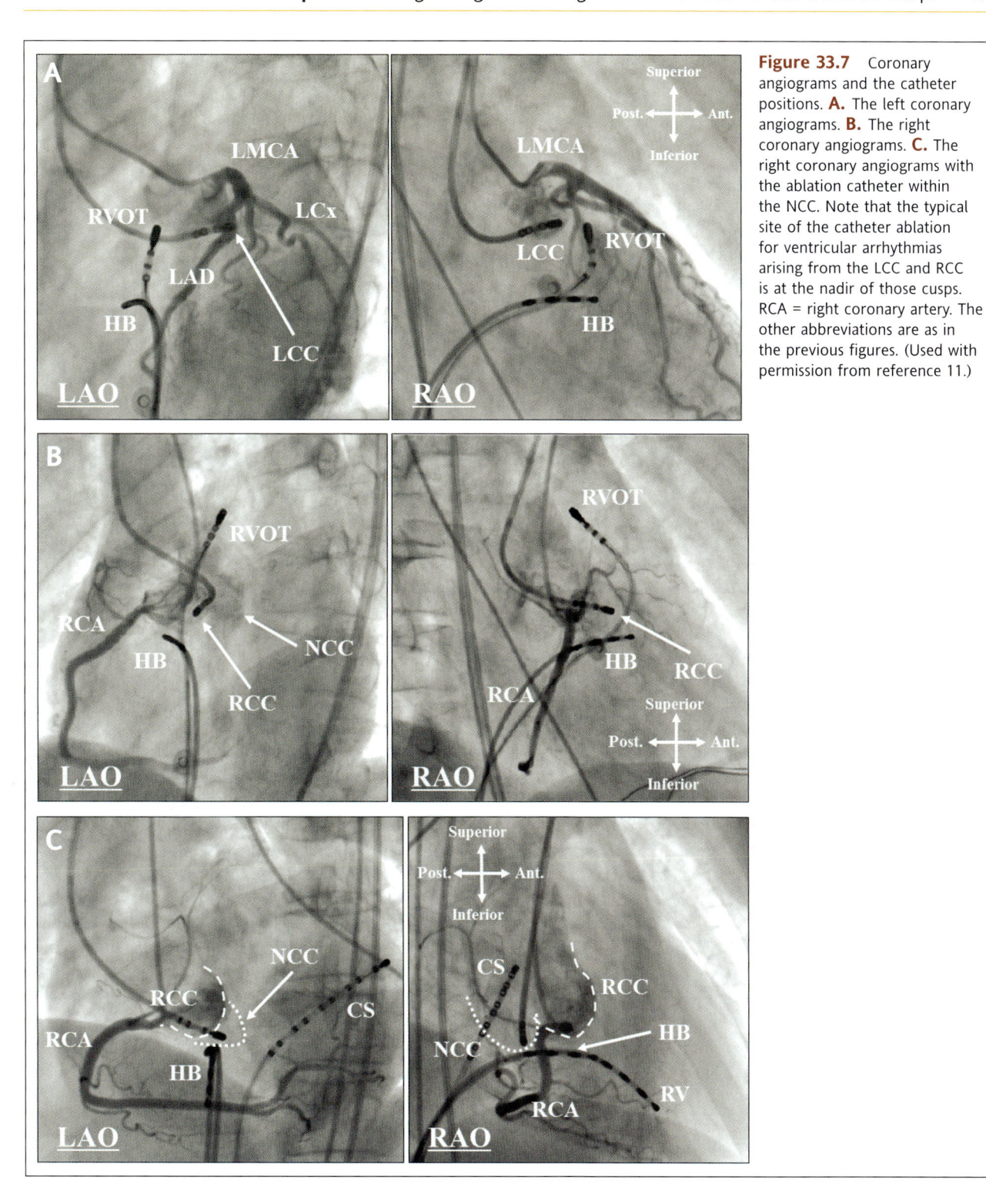

NCC, and sites underneath those cusps should be considered first. Otherwise, mapping in the LCC and AMC should be first performed because ventricular arrhythmias are more likely to arise from these sites. A ventricular prepotential preceding the QRS onset is often recorded within the ASCs during ventricular arrhythmias, and it may suggest a successful ablation site (**Figure 33.8**). Pacing within the ASCs often exhibits a long stimulus to QRS interval (more likely in the LCC than the RCC) whereas that below the aortic valves does not (Figures 33.5 and 33.6).

When the earliest ventricular activation in the ASCs and endocardial LVOT precedes the QRS onset by more than 20 ms and is earlier than that within the GCV, RF catheter ablation may be performed at that site. When endocardial catheter ablation is unsuccessful or the local

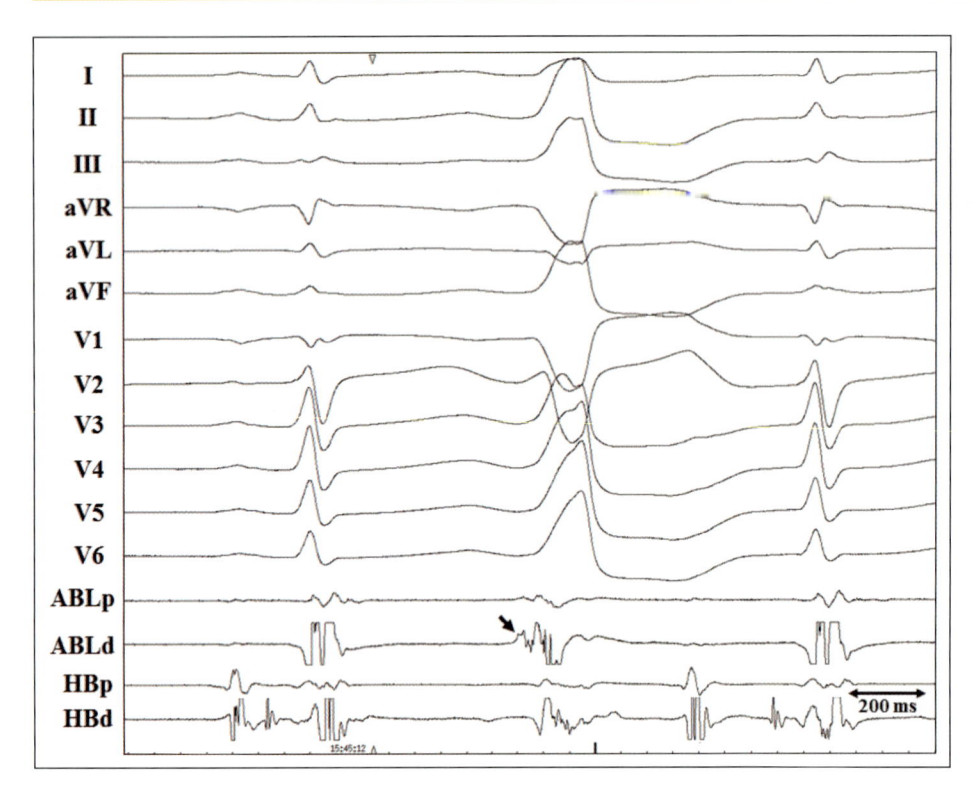

Figure 33.8 Cardiac tracings recorded at the site of the successful ablation of PVCs originating from the RCC. The arrow indicates a prepotential preceding the QRS onset. The abbreviations are as in the previous figures.

ventricular activation during the ventricular arrhythmias is earlier in the GCV than at any endocardial site, epicardial catheter ablation using transvenous or transpericardial approaches should be considered.

A region of the LV epicardial surface bounded by the LAD and LCx that lies superior to the aortic portion of the LV ostium occupies the most superior portion of the LV and has been termed the LV summit by McAlpine (**Figures 33.2** and **33.9**).[18] This region near where the GCV ends and the AIVV begins is one of the major sources of epicardial idiopathic ventricular arrhythmias. The LV summit is bisected by the GCV into an area lateral to this structure that is accessible to epicardial catheter ablation (the *accessible area*) and a superior area that is inaccessible to catheter ablation due to the close proximity of the coronary arteries and the thick layer of epicardial fat that overlies the proximal portion of these vessels (the *inaccessible area*). The LAA may sometimes override the accessible area (Figure 33.2), and cause a problem during mapping in this area. When a mapping catheter is placed on the LAA, a large atrial electrogram should be recorded at the mapping site, and catheter-induced premature atrial contractions may be observed. When the local ventricular activation within the GCV or AIVV precedes the QRS onset by more than 20 ms and pacing from the site of the earliest ventricular activation within the GCV or AIVV produces an excellent match to the QRS complex of the ventricular arrhythmias, RF catheter ablation within the GCV or AIVV is attempted. Otherwise, or when the RF ablation within the GCV or AIVV fails to eliminate the ventricular arrhythmias, epicardial mapping and ablation via a subxiphoid approach are performed. During this epicardial mapping, the mapping catheter within the GCV is helpful as a landmark, and epicardial mapping is performed around the site with the earliest ventricular activation within the GCV. Because the inaccessible area of the LV summit is covered with a thick fat pad, far-field electrograms are usually recorded, the local impedance is high, and pacing even with a maximal output may not capture the ventricular myocardium in this area. When the earliest ventricular activation is recorded in the inaccessible area, catheter ablation is usually abandoned because of the close proximity to the left coronary arteries. When the earliest ventricular activation is recorded in the accessible area, catheter ablation should be attempted if the site is located more than 5 mm away from the coronary arteries. In the accessible area with lesser fat pads, catheter ablation may be effective even at the site with far-field electrograms.

Catheter Ablation

For catheter ablation in the RVOT, ASCs, and endocardial LVOT, a nonirrigated ablation catheter is usually used for several reasons. First, the cooling effect by much blood flow through the ventricular outflow tract is enough to deliver desirable RF energy. Second, irrigated RF current application may cause perforation of the free wall of the RVOT and destroy the aortic valves. Nonirrigated RF current is delivered with a target temperature of 55°C to 60°C and maximum power output of 50 W. In the ASCs, RF ablation is applied under continuous fluoroscopic observation with an angiographic catheter positioned within the

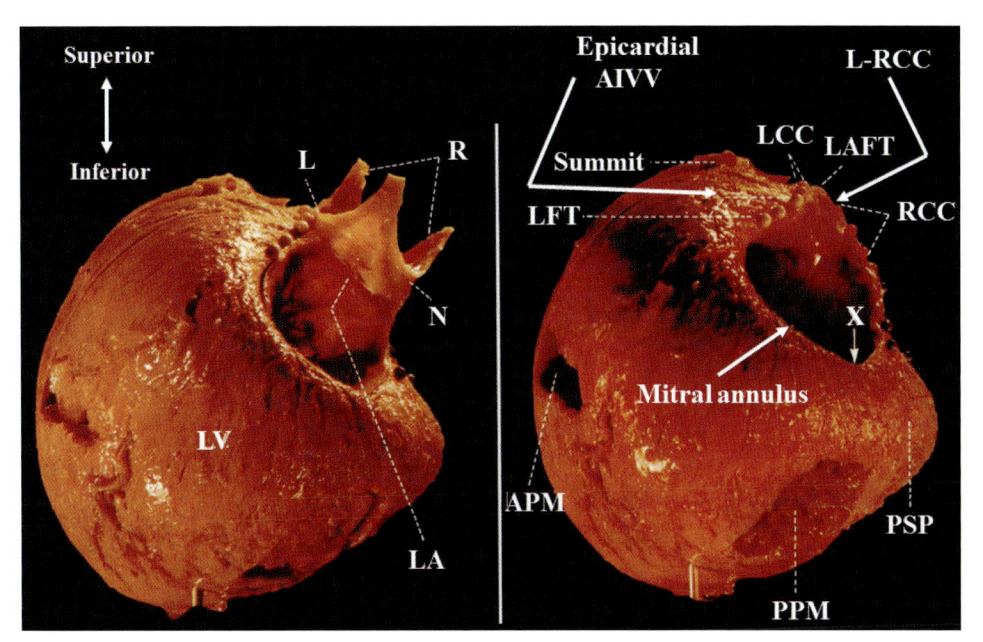

Figure 33.9 An autopsy heart exhibiting the LV summit (postero-cranial view). Reproduced with permission from reference 18. The left panel includes the aortic root with the right coronary sinus (R), left coronary sinus (L), and noncoronary sinus (N). In the right panel, the root of the aorta has been removed to demonstrate the elliptical ostium of the LV with the junction of the RCC, LCC, and LV summit demonstrated. APM = anterior papillary muscle; LA = left atrium; LAFT = left anterior fibrous trigone; LFT = left fibrous trigone; L-RCC = the junction between the LCC and RCC; PPM = posterior papillary muscle; PSP = posterosuperior process of the LV; X = attachment of the LA to the AV membrane. The other abbreviations are as in the previous figures. (From reference 18. Used with kind permission from Springer Science + Business Media.)

ostium of the coronary artery (Figure 33.7). The outline of the ASCs and flow in the coronary artery are observed by hand injections of contrast every 15 seconds. An RF application should never be delivered within 5 mm of the coronary artery.

In an epicardial catheter ablation using transvenous or percutaneous subxiphoid approaches, an externally irrigated ablation catheter is usually used. When an intramural ventricular arrhythmia origin is suggested, irrigated RF current may be delivered from the endocardial side. Irrigated RF current is delivered in the power-control mode starting at 20 W in the GCV and AIVV and 30 W on the epicardial surface with an irrigation flow rate of 30 ml/min. The RF power is titrated to as high as 30 W and 50 W, respectively, with the goal being to achieve a decrease in the impedance of 8 to 10 Ω and with care taken to limit the temperature to < 41°C. During the epicardial catheter ablation using transvenous and transpericardial approaches, simultaneous left coronary angiography should be performed every 15 seconds to ensure the location of the ablation catheter relative to the left coronary arteries and to minimize the risk of thermal injury to these vessels (Figure 33.2). An RF application is never delivered within 5 mm of the coronary artery.

When an acceleration or reduction in the frequency of the VT or PVCs is observed during the first 10 seconds of the application, the RF delivery is continued for 30 to 60 seconds. Otherwise, the RF delivery is terminated, and the catheter is repositioned. The endpoint of the catheter ablation is the elimination and noninducibility of VT or PVCs during an isoproterenol infusion (2 to 4 mg/min) and burst pacing from the RV (to a cycle length as short as 240 ms). After epicardial catheter ablation, left coronary angiography is repeated to ensure that there is no evidence of injury to the coronary arteries.

In either endocardial or epicardial approach via the cardiac veins or subxiphoid access, efficacy of RF energy delivery may be limited because of the inaccessibility, high impedance within the venous system, intramural ventricular arrhythmia origins, close proximity to the coronary artery, or epicardial position underneath a fat pad. Cryothermal ablation may be a viable alternative to RF ablation in cases with high impedance within the venous system or when the origin is located close to a coronary artery.[16]

Postprocedural Care

Recovery

Following ablation, the groin sheaths are pulled out after a bedside echocardiogram demonstrates no evidence of pericardial effusion. If patients are anticoagulated, protamine can be given to help reverse the effects of heparin, and the groin sheaths can be pulled once the ACT is less than 170 seconds. Patients will typically lie flat for 6 hours after the sheaths are removed. In patients with a pericardial approach, all pericardial sheaths are removed at the end of the procedure unless there is continued bleeding. Intrapericardial injection of 0.5 to 1 mg/kg of methylprednisolone or 2 mg/kg of intermediate-acting corticosteroid (triamcinolone) are given to prevent postprocedural pericarditis or inflammatory adhesion formation. As long as the pericardial drain is in place because of continued bleeding, an intravenous cephalosporin antibiotic should be administered. We administer 81 mg of aspirin for 6 weeks after the catheter ablation in the LVOT and ASCs to prevent any clot formation at the ablation site. Patients are usually monitored overnight.

Follow-up

Patients are usually followed without any antiarrhythmic drugs after a successful catheter ablation. Patients are seen in clinic with 12-lead ECGs and 24-hour ambulatory (Holter) monitoring. An exercise stress test is especially useful for a patient with exercise-induced ventricular arrhythmias. Recurrence of ventricular arrhythmias in this region usually occurs early after the catheter ablation (within the first 3 months), and late recurrence is rare.

Procedural Complications

Catheter ablation in this region is in close proximity to several important anatomical structures, raising concern for potential complications. The most serious complication is coronary artery injury with an inadvertent application of RF current over the coronary arteries being potentially lethal.[25] Because of this possibility, it is essential that some form of imaging be used to ensure that the ablation catheter is not near or directly overlying a coronary artery. Aortic regurgitation may occur as a result of mechanical trauma or RF current applied directly to valvular tissue. In addition, inadvertent damage to the AV conduction system may occur during catheter ablation within the RCC and NCC and underneath these cusps, because the HB runs through the central fibrous body, which is located underneath these cusps. Though previous studies have reported very low complication rates,[1-12,14-17] it should be emphasized that those reports generally have come from highly experienced centers with highly skilled personnel. VF induced during RF energy delivery in the RVOT has been reported.[26] Transient sinus bradycardia followed by transient complete AV conduction block has been observed during RF ablation within the RCC.[10] RF energy deliveries within the RCC may have a thermal effect on the anterior epicardial fat pad containing parasympathetic ganglia, resulting in vagal stimulation.[10,27] A pericardial effusion or cardiac tamponade may occur during catheter ablation in the RVOT with its relatively thin wall. Perforation of the free wall of the RVOT is almost always critical, leading to rapid hemodynamic collapse. In this situation, pericardiocentesis should be performed very quickly, but a surgical repair is often required since the injury is usually a linear tear. Complications associated with the pericardial procedure via a subxiphoid approach such as intra-abdominal bleeding or laceration of an epicardial coronary artery should also be considered with epicardial mapping and catheter ablation.[28]

Conclusions

The ventricular outflow tracts and ASCs are major sites of origin for ventricular arrhythmias, and catheter ablation can cure ventricular arrhythmias originating from this region safely. Because the anatomy of this region is complex and some ventricular arrhythmia origins are epicardial, it may sometimes be difficult to locate the site of the ventricular arrhythmia origin. Meticulous mapping of the ventricular outflow tracts, ASCs, GCV, and LV epicardial surface may be required to achieve successful catheter ablation of ventricular arrhythmias arising from this region. Catheter ablation in this region may cause critical damage to important anatomical structures such as the coronary arteries and AV conduction system because of their close proximity. Accurate recognition of the anatomy of this region is essential for the prevention of complications associated with catheter ablation.

References

1. Buxton AE, Waxman HL, Marchlinski FE, Simson MB, Cassidy D, Josephson ME. Right ventricular tachycardia: clinical and electrophysiological characteristics. *Circulation.* 1983;68:917–927.
2. Morady F, Kadish AH, DiCarlo L, et al. Long-term results of catheter ablation of idiopathic right ventricular tachycardia. *Circulation.* 1990;82:2093–2099.
3. Coggins DL, Lee RJ, Sweeney J, et al. Radiofrequency catheter ablation as a cure for idiopathic tachycardia of both left and right ventricular origin. *J Am Coll Cardiol.* 1994;23:1333–1341.
4. Dixit S, Gerstenfeld EP, Callans DJ, Marchlinski FE. Electrocardiographic patterns of superior right ventricular outflow tract tachycardias: distinguishing septal and free-wall sites of origin. *J Cardiovasc Electrophysiol.* 2003;14:1–7.
5. Ito S, Tada H, Naito S, et al. Development and validation of an electrocardiographic algorithm for identifying the optimal ablation site for idiopathic ventricular outflow tract tachycardia. *J Cardiovasc Electrophysiol.* 2003;14:1280–1286.
6. Callans DJ, Menz V, Schwartzman D, Gottlieb CD, Marchlinski FE. Repetitive monomorphic tachycardia from the left ventricular outflow tract: electrocardiographic patterns consistent with a left ventricular site of origin. *J Am Coll Cardiol.* 1997;29:1023–1027.
7. Kanagaratnam L, Tomassoni G, Schweikert R, et al. Ventricular tachycardias arising from the aortic sinus of valsalva: an under-recognized variant of left outflow tract ventricular tachycardia. *J Am Coll Cardiol.* 2001;37:1408–1414.

8. Ouyang F, Fotuhi P, Ho SY, et al. Repetitive monomorphic ventricular tachycardia originating from the aortic sinus cusp: electrocardiographic characterization for guiding catheter ablation. *J Am Coll Cardiol.* 2002;39:500–508.
9. Yamada T, Yoshida N, Murakami Y, Okada T, Muto M, Murohara T, McElderry HT, Kay GN. Electrocardiographic characteristics of ventricular arrhythmias originating from the junction of the left and right coronary sinuses of Valsalva in the aorta: the activation pattern as a rationale for the electrocardiographic characteristics. *Heart Rhythm.* 2008;5:184–192.
10. Yamada T, McElderry HT, Doppalapudi H, et al. Idiopathic ventricular arrhythmias originating from the aortic root: prevalence, electrocardiographic and electrophysiological characteristics, and results of the radiofrequency catheter ablation. *J Am Coll Cardiol.* 2008;52:139–147.
11. Yamada T, Litovsky SH, Kay GN. The left ventricular ostium: an anatomic concept relevant to idiopathic ventricular arrhythmias. *Circ Arrhythmia Electrophysiol.* 2008;1:396–404.
12. Stevenson WG, Soejima K. Catheter ablation for ventricular tachycardia. *Circulation.* 2007;115:2750–2760.
13. Yamada T, Murakami Y, Yoshida N, et al. Preferential conduction across the ventricular outflow septum in ventricular arrhythmias originating from the aortic sinus cusp. *J Am Coll Cardiol.* 2007;50:884–891.
14. Yamada T, McElderry HT, Doppalapudi H, Kay GN. Catheter ablation of ventricular arrhythmias originating from the vicinity of the His bundle: significance of mapping of the aortic sinus cusp. *Heart Rhythm.* 2008;5:37–42.
15. Chun KR, Satomi K, Kuck KH, Ouyang F, Antz M. Left ventricular outflow tract tachycardia including ventricular tachycardia from the aortic cusps and epicardial ventricular tachycardia. *Herz.* 2007;32:226–232.
16. Obel OA, d'Avila A, Neuzil P, Saad EB, Ruskin JN, Reddy VY. Ablation of left ventricular epicardial outflow tract tachycardia from the distal great cardiac vein. *J Am Coll Cardiol.* 2006;48:1813–1817.
17. Yamada T, McElderry HT, Doppalapudi H, et al. Idiopathic ventricular arrhythmias originating from the left ventricular summit: anatomic concepts relevant to ablation. *Circ Arrhythm Electrophysiol.* 2010;3:616–623.
18. McAlpine WA. *Heart and Coronary Arteries.* New York: Springer-Verlag; 1975.
19. Anderson RH. Clinical anatomy of the aortic root. *Heart.* 2000;84:670–673.
20. Daniels DV, Lu YY, Morton JB, Santucci PA, Akar JG, Green A, Wilber DJ. Idiopathic epicardial left ventricular tachycardia originating remote from the sinus of Valsalva: Electrophysiological characteristics, catheter ablation, and identification from the 12-lead electrocardiogram. *Circulation.* 2006;113:1659–1666.
21. Yoshida Y, Hirai M, Murakami Y, et al. Localization of precise origin of idiopathic ventricular tachycardia from the right ventricular outflow tract by a 12-lead ECG: a study of pace mapping using a multielectrode "basket" catheter. *Pacing Clin Electrophysiol.* 1999;22:1760–1768.
22. Yamada T, McElderry HT, Okada T, Murakami Y, Doppalapudi H, Yoshida N, Yoshida Y, Inden Y, Murohara T, Epstein AE, Plumb VJ, Kay GN. Idiopathic left ventricular arrhythmias originating adjacent to the left aortic sinus of valsalva: electrophysiological rationale for the surface electrocardiogram. *J Cardiovasc Electrophysiol.* 2010;21:170–176.
23. Nakagawa M, Ooie T, Ou B, Ichinose M, Takahashi N, Hara M, Yonemochi H, Saikawa T. Gender differences in autonomic modulation of ventricular repolarization in humans. *J Cardiovasc Electrophysiol.* 2005;16:278–284.
24. Yamada T, Murakami Y, Yoshida N, et al. Efficacy of electroanatomic mapping in the catheter ablation of premature ventricular contractions originating from the right ventricular outflow tract. *J Interv Card Electrophysiol.* 2007;19:187–194.
25. Pons M, Beck L, Leclercq F, Ferriere M, Albat B, Davy JM. Chronic left main coronary artery occlusion: a complication of radiofrequency ablation of idiopathic left ventricular tachycardia. *Pacing Clin Electrophysiol.* 1997;20:1874–1876.
26. Ito S, Tada H, Lee JD, Miyamori I. Ventricular fibrillation induced by a radiofrequency energy delivery for idiopathic right ventricular outflow tachycardia. *Int J Cardiol.* 2008;128:e65–67.
27. Cummings JE, Gill I, Akhrass R, Dery M, Biblo LA, Quan KJ. Preservation of the anterior fat pad paradoxically decreases the incidence of postoperative atrial fibrillation in humans. *J Am Coll Cardiol.* 2004;43:994–1000.
28. Yamada T, Kay GN. Recognition and prevention of complications during epicardial ablation. In: Shivkumar K, Boyle NG, Thakur RK, Natale A, eds. *Cardiac Electrophysiology Clinics: Epicardial Interventions in Electrophysiology*. Elsevier Inc., 2010;2:127–134.

CHAPTER 34

How to Diagnose and Ablate Fascicular Ventricular Tachycardia

Frederick T. Han, MD; Nitish Badhwar, MBBS

Introduction

Fascicular VT represents a subset of the idiopathic LV tachycardias. Fascicular VT is an uncommon, but well-studied, ventricular arrhythmia that has several characteristic features: (1) a verapamil-sensitive mechanism; (2) induction with atrial pacing; and (3) occurrence in patients without structural heart disease.[1] These tachycardias also have an excellent prognosis and, thus, do not require an ICD after a successful ablation.[2] Given its origin in the fascicles of the LV, each subtype of VT has a characteristic ECG morphology[1] and can be classified as:

1. Left posterior fascicular VT (LPF VT)—RBBB with left-axis deviation (common form)
2. Left anterior fascicular VT (LAF VT)—RBBB with right-axis deviation (uncommon form)
3. Left upper septal fascicular VT (septal VT)—narrow QRS and normal frontal-plane axis (rare form)

Although a number of studies have demonstrated the presence of mid- and late-diastolic potentials (DPs) during VT, the presence of a slow conduction zone during entrainment, and the presence of constant and progressive fusion,[3-8] not all fascicular tachycardias demonstrate features of a reentrant mechanism.[9,10] As a result, one should not assume that a fascicular tachycardia is purely dependent upon a microreentrant and/or macroreentrant circuit involving the Purkinje network. Recently, multiform fascicular tachycardias with an interfascicular reentrant mechanism have also been described.[11] Fortunately, the ECG morphology of these multiform VTs is based on the fascicular circuit(s) involved and can be elucidated with a combination of fascicular potential mapping and entrainment pacing. Defining the mechanisms and circuits of fascicular tachycardias has led to an improved understanding of the ideal ablation targets and a long-term success rate of > 95% with a single ablation.[12]

Preprocedural Planning

Since by definition fascicular VTs occur in patients without structural heart disease, standard preprocedural planning involves screening with a history and physical, imaging, and work-up to exclude structural or ischemic heart disease. Since a retrograde aortic approach is commonly taken to access the LV for mapping and ablation, the presence of significant peripheral vascular or aortic disease should be identified as well. If anatomic considerations or coexistent medical conditions preclude retrograde aortic access, an antegrade transseptal approach can be pursued. If possible, all antiarrhythmic medications are stopped at least 5 half-lives prior to the procedure.

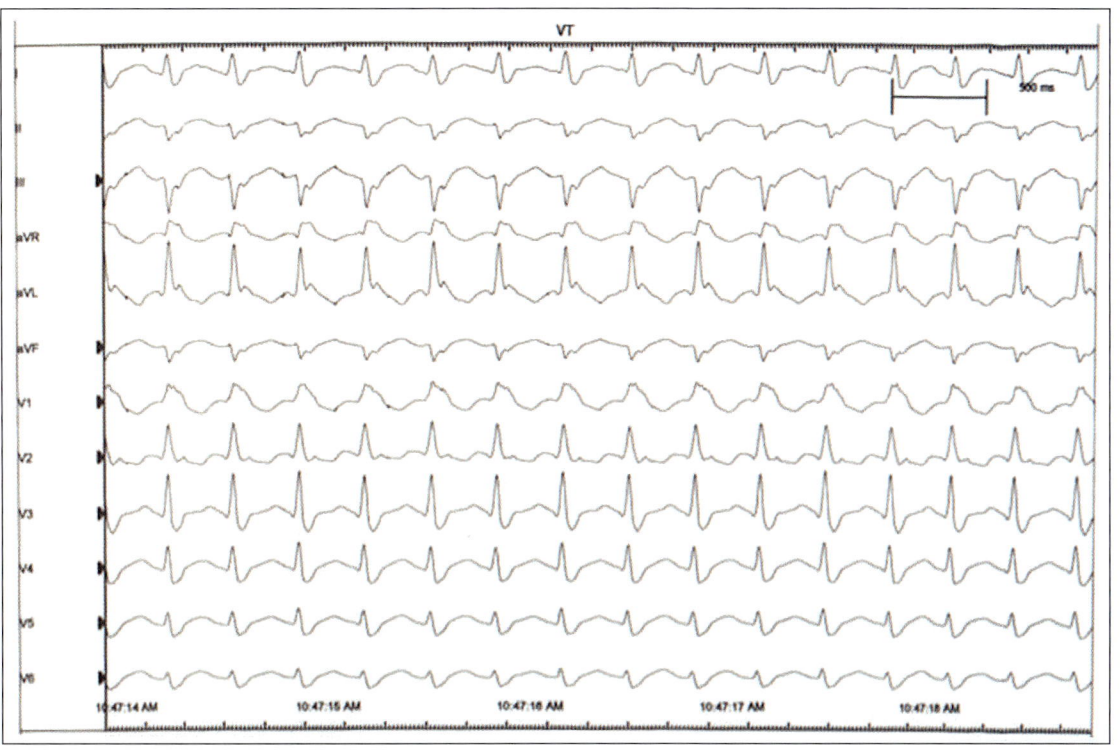

Figure 34.1 Surface ECG of verapamil-sensitive left posterior fascicular ventricular tachycardia (LPF VT) demonstrating an RBBB left-axis morphology.

Reviewing the ECG morphology of the VT serves to confirm the diagnosis as well as to plan on the approaches of endocardial mapping and ablation. **Figure 34.1** shows a 12-lead ECG of LPF VT. Both LPF and LAF VTs have proximal and distal subtypes corresponding to the exit site of the VT along the proximal or distal aspect of the respective fascicle. Nogami and colleagues have shown that the LAF proximal subtype (midseptal exit site) is characterized by an "RS" or "Rs" morphology in leads 1, V_5, and V_6, whereas the LAF distal subtype (anterolateral wall exit site) manifests a "QS" or "rS" morphology in those leads (**Figure 34.2**).[6] Unfortunately, the proximal and distal subtypes of LPF VT cannot be distinguished by QRS morphology variations, so they are distinguished by the location of the late DPs during LV endocardial mapping. The LPF proximal subtype is characterized by late DPs in the basal to mid inferior septum, whereas the LPF distal subtype has late DPs found in the apical inferior septum. **Figure 34.3** shows a 12-lead ECG of a left upper septal VT. Due to their high septal exit sites, these VTs can have a narrow QRS and may not satisfy criteria based on QRS morphology.

Procedure

Patient Preparation

Most patients presenting for EP study and ablation of fascicular VTs are generally healthy without significant comorbid illnesses, and unless otherwise indicated, conscious sedation and monitored anesthesia care are preferred methods of analgesia. In addition, some fascicular VTs occur in the setting of exercise or heightened sympathetic tone, which may be inhibited with the use of general anesthesia.

For vascular access, we place a decapolar CS catheter from the right internal jugular vein, a quadripolar catheter to the HRA, a quadripolar catheter to the HB, and a quadripolar catheter to the RVA through the femoral vein. The HRA catheter can be moved to the RVOT after atrial programmed stimulation has been completed. The right femoral artery is used for placement of an 8-Fr sheath through which a bidirectional 7-Fr, 4-mm quadripolar ablation catheter with 2-mm distal electrode spacing is navigated to the LV via retrograde aortic access. Given that patients with fascicular VTs lack significant pathologic LV dilatation, an ablation catheter that has a medium-size curve is usually sufficient for LV mapping/ablation. Once arterial access is obtained, an intravenous bolus of unfractionated heparin at a dose of 70 U/kg is given, and an infusion at 1000 U/hour is started. Additional heparin boluses and adjustment of the heparin infusion are titrated for a goal ACT of 250 to 350 seconds measured every 15 minutes.

Diagnosis

Baseline EP measurements are obtained. Then, burst pacing and programmed electrical stimulation with up to

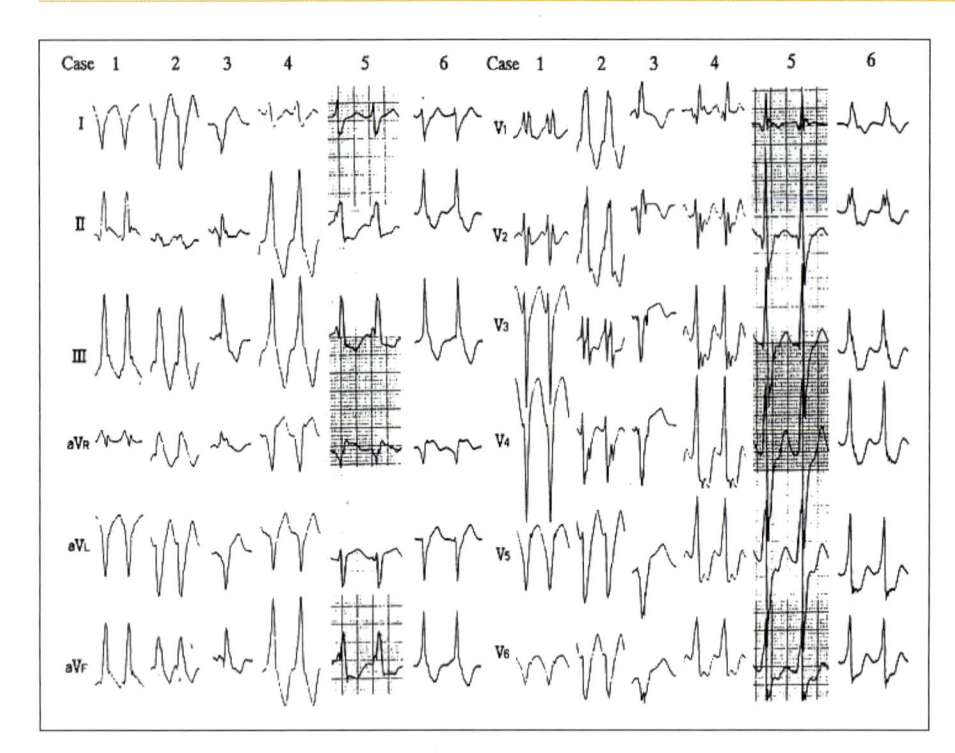

Figure 34.2 Surface ECG morphology of verapamil-sensitive left anterior fascicular VT (LAF VT) demonstrating an RBBB right-axis morphology. The first 3 patients have an exit site in the distal left anterior fascicle, whereas patients 4-6 have a proximal left anterior fascicle exit site. (Reprinted from Nogami A, et al. *J Cardiovasc Electrophysiol.* 1998;9:1269–1278, with permission from John Wiley and Sons, Inc.)

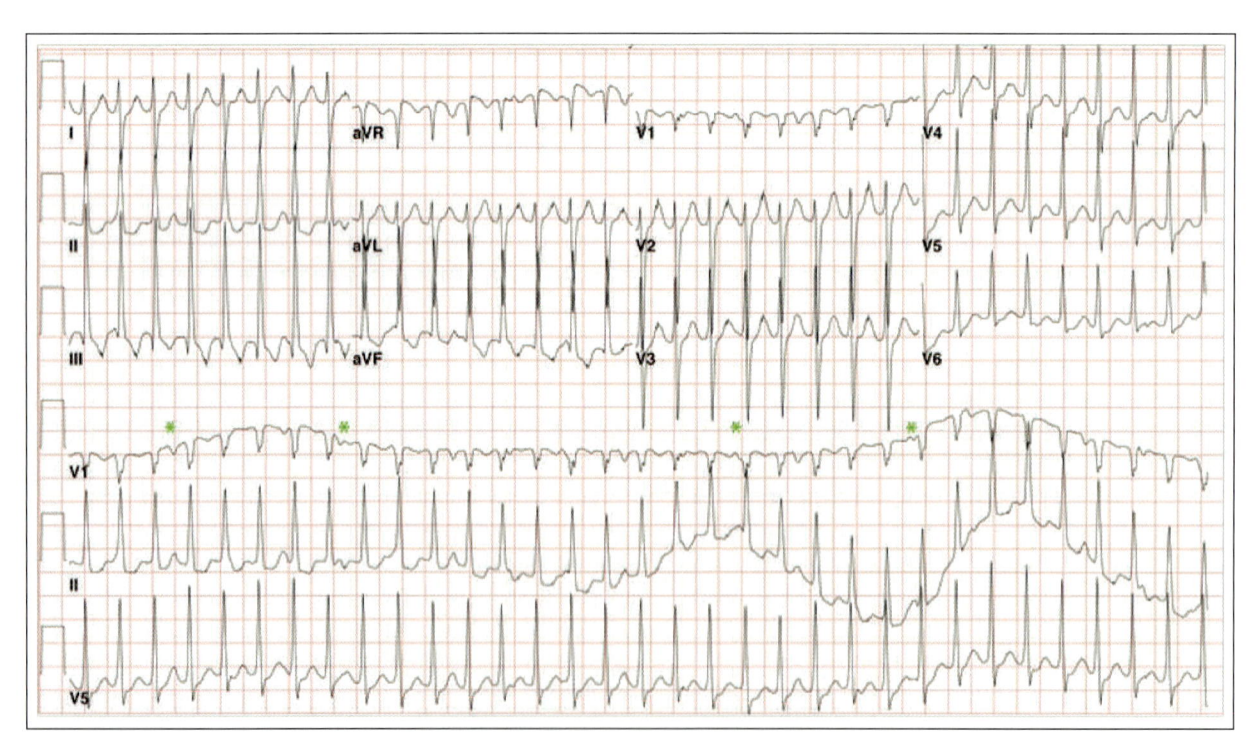

Figure 34.3 Surface ECG of verapamil-sensitive left upper septal fascicular VT demonstrating a LBBB right-axis morphology. The QRS morphology does not satisfy traditional VT precordial lead criteria; however, the presence of atrioventricular dissociation with discrete P waves (*) identified in the rhythm strip of V_1 proves the diagnosis of VT.

3 extrastimuli at twice the diastolic threshold and a 2-ms pulse width are initiated from the HRA, RVA, and LV (**Figure 34.4**). Burst pacing is usually pursued up to a minimum cycle length of 200 ms. The HRA catheter can be moved to the RVOT if VT cannot be initiated from the RVA and LV. If VT is still not induced, an isoproterenol infusion is started, and the same protocol is repeated. The isoproterenol infusion is titrated up to (10 mcg/min) in order to achieve a goal of 20% increase in heart rate.

The reentrant circuit of fascicular VT was elegantly described by Nogami and colleagues (**Figure 34.5**).[4] The orthodromic limb is hypothesized to be an accessory Purkinje fiber or a branch of the Purkinje network demonstrating decremental conduction and verapamil sensitivity.

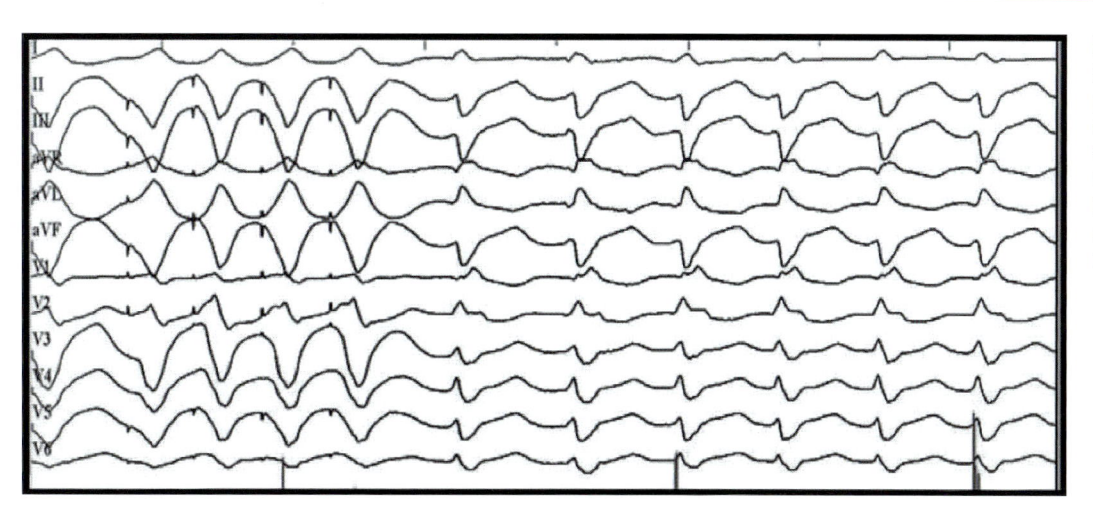

Figure 34.4 Surface ECG showing programmed electrical stimulation from the right ventricular apex leading to induction of left posterior fascicular VT.

This limb of the VT circuit is oriented parallel to the fascicle, with or without an intervening myocardial bridge to the antidromic limb of the circuit, with the antidromic limb being the fascicle itself. Thus, during sinus rhythm, Purkinje potentials (PP) are noted to proceed in a basal-to-apical activation pattern, with the distal PP demonstrating fusion with the earliest ventricular activation (VT exit site). Conversely, during VT, late DPs can be visualized to proceed in a basal to apical activation pattern with PPs demonstrating a distal to proximal activation pattern.

Once ventricular tachycardia is induced, several diagnostic maneuvers are employed to confirm the diagnosis of fascicular VT and to define the location of the circuit. First, PPs and DPs preceding ventricular activation (V) are mapped. Second, changes in the PP-PP and DP-DP intervals should precede changes in the V-V intervals. Third, in the case of LPF and LAF tachycardias, His activation should follow the QRS onset. In left upper septal fascicular VT, a short HV interval is present. This short HV interval during VT will be shorter than the HV interval during sinus rhythm. Careful mapping can also reveal the presence of an LBB potential prior to the His potential during VT (**Figure 34.6**). Finally, the tachycardia should demonstrate entrainment with ventricular and/or atrial pacing.

Entrainment from the HRA or the RVOT is favored for the demonstration of constant and progressive fusion (**Figure 34.7**). In addition, as the pacing rate is increased, a prolongation of the stimulus-DP interval should be identified. During entrainment, we seek to identify constant and progressive fusion as well as changes in the stimulus-DP interval or DP-PP interval in order to prove that the diastolic potential is in a zone of slow conduction critical to maintenance of the tachycardia.

If a suitable DP cannot be mapped, pacing from the VT exit site can be used to demonstrate concealed entrainment. In addition, a PPI–TCL of < 20 ms confirms that the VT entrainment site is within the circuit of the tachycardia (**Figure 34.8**). As pacing rates are progressively increased, there is an increase in the stimulus to DP interval, thus demonstrating decremental conduction of the VT slow conduction zone (Figure 34.7). With continued decremental pacing, eventually the tachycardia should terminate upon cessation of pacing, thus providing evidence for the upper limit of the excitable gap.

Usually several diastolic potential sites can be mapped, and they are subsequently tagged as candidate sites for ablation. However, if these sites cannot be identified, the

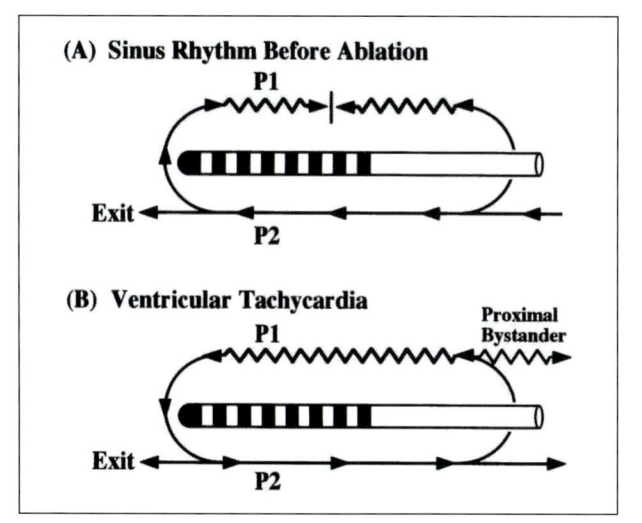

Figure 34.5 Schematic diagram of the reentrant circuit of left posterior fascicular VT. P2 represents activation of the left posterior fascicle or Purkinje fiber near the left posterior fascicle and forms the retrograde limb of the VT circuit. P1 represents an accessory limb of the left posterior fascicle composed of Purkinje fibers or ventricular myocardium forming the antegrade limb of the VT circuit. The undulating line indicates the portion of the circuit with decremental properties and verapamil sensitivity. **A.** Activation of the circuit during sinus rhythm. Since activation of P1 occurs in a retrograde fashion during sinus rhythm, the DP is obscured by the QRS complex. **B.** During VT, P1 is activated orthodromically and is manifested as a DP, whereas P2 is activated antidromically. P1 = diastolic potential, P2 = Purkinje potential. (Reprinted from Nogami A, et al. *J Am Coll Cardiol.* 2000;36: 811–823, with permission from Elsevier Science, Inc.)

306 • Ablation of VT

earliest PPs and the VT exit site are tagged as potential targets for ablation as well.

Electroanatomic Mapping

Three-dimensional electroanatomic mapping systems, while not required, enable activation mapping; if VT cannot be induced, electroanatomic mapping facilitates a linear ablation strategy. An initial strategy of activation mapping also helps to identify the minority of fascicular tachycardias that are due to an automatic fascicular focus. Once an automatic focus has been excluded, maneuvers to identify a reentrant focus can be pursued. In addition, for cases in which anatomical variations or other medical conditions preclude retrograde aortic access, we find that remote magnetic catheter navigation (Stereotaxis, St. Louis, MO) provides a useful alternative via a transseptal antegrade approach. This approach may also be less susceptible to inadvertent termination of VT associated with catheter contact.

If VT is induced and is hemodynamically tolerated, 3-dimensional electroanatomic activation mapping is performed using either the St. Jude NavX (St. Jude Medical, St, Paul, MN) or CARTO (Biosense-Webster, Diamond Bar, CA) systems. During activation mapping, the LV is mapped with the ablation catheter from an apical to basal position along the LV inferior septum (for a LPF VT) or along the anterolateral LV (LAF VT). The same approach is taken with a left upper septal VT with detailed mapping concentrated on the basal septum of the LV. During activation mapping, care is taken to identify 3 potential targets of ablation during VT, in order of preference: (1) diastolic potentials or sites of continuous or fractionated diastolic activity, (2) PPs with the earliest PPs being favored, and (3) sites of earliest ventricular activation with a fused presystolic Purkinje-ventricular potential identifying the VT

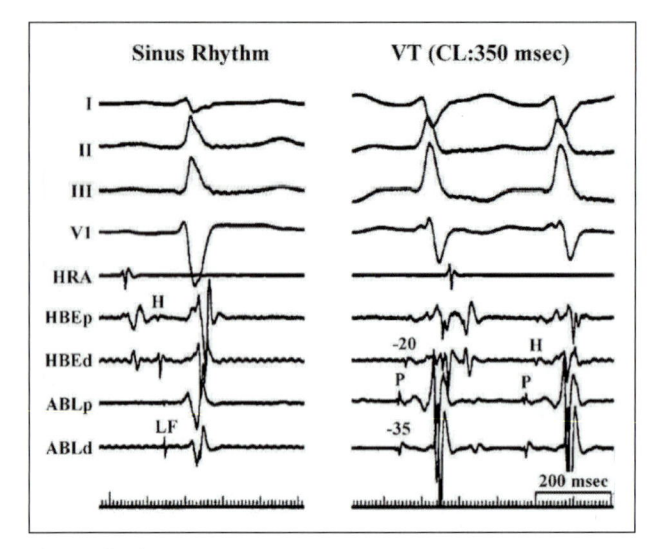

Figure 34.6 Intracardiac EGM at the successful ablation site of a left upper septal fascicular VT. This site demonstrated the presence of an LBB potential during VT. During VT, the LBB potential preceded the His potential. ABLd = distal electrode of ablation catheter, ABLp = proximal electrode of ablation catheter, CL = cycle length, H = His potential, HBEd = distal electrode at His bundle, HBEp = proximal electrode at His bundle, HRA = high right atrium, LF = LBB potential during sinus rhythm, P = LBB potential during VT. (Reprinted from Nogami A, et al. *Card Electrophysiol Rev.* 2002;6:448-457, with permission from Kluwer Academic Publishers.)

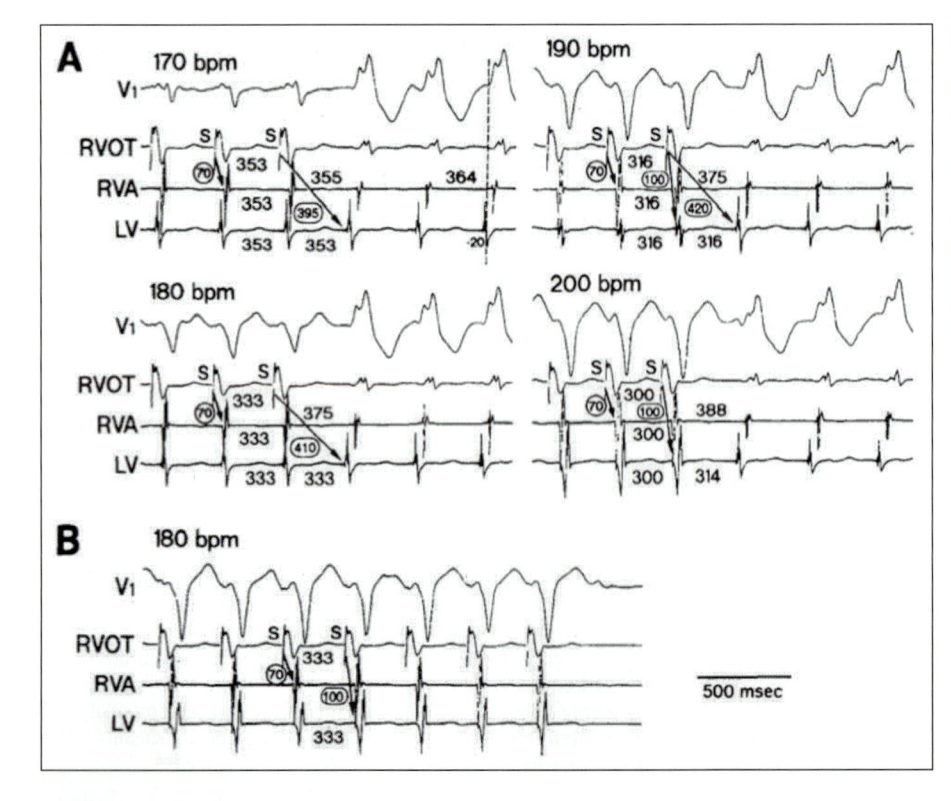

Figure 34.7 Surface ECG lead V_1 and intracardiac EGMs recorded at the right ventricular outflow tract (RVOT), right ventricular apex (RVA), and left ventricle (LV). **A.** Ventricular pacing at rates of 170, 180, 190, and 200 beats per minute (bpm) from the RVOT demonstrates progressive fusion during VT entrainment. **B.** RVOT pacing at 180 bpm during sinus rhythm. (Reprinted from Okumura K, et al. *Am J Cardiol.* 1996;77:379–383, with permission from Elsevier Inc.)

exit site. Pace mapping can be performed in order to confirm the ideal VT exit site for ablation. However, since activation mapping is often based on diastolic potentials (from the antegrade slow conduction zone) or the fascicular potentials (retrograde limb of the circuit), pace mapping more often than not fails to produce perfect concealed entrainment (**Figure 34.8**) because the antegrade slow conduction zone and the retrograde fascicular sites are not equivalent to the precise exit site. In addition, pace mapping is often plagued by variations in current strength with resulting QRS morphology variations, and variability in the amount of myocardium captured at each pacing site (**Figure 34.9**).

Unfortunately, in some cases VT cannot be induced or is terminated and rendered noninducible by catheter contact during contact mapping. If the electroanatomic activation map is insufficient for localizing the ideal target for ablation, one of 2 approaches can be employed: (1) mapping/ablation of a retrograde PP (retrograde PP, representing antidromic activation of the slow conduction zone of the VT circuit during sinus rhythm) or (2) linear ablation strategy in mid to mid-apical portion of the fascicle. Both approaches entail constructing a detailed 3-dimensional electroanatomic map of the LV during sinus rhythm, during which the HB, the LBB, and the anterior and posterior fascicles are mapped and tagged.

The retrograde PPs have been localized to sites within the posterior and anterior fascicles in patients presenting with fascicular VT. The ideal retrograde PP is the earliest fascicular retrograde potential that can be mapped during sinus rhythm (**Figure 34.10**). Ouyang and colleagues demonstrated that these potentials represent a slow conduction zone of the circuit, as evidenced by the presence of decremental conduction (gradual prolongation of the stimulus-retrograde PP) during pacing. These sites were also shown to correlate with the presence of diastolic potentials at the same sites during fascicular VT (**Figure 34.11**).[7]

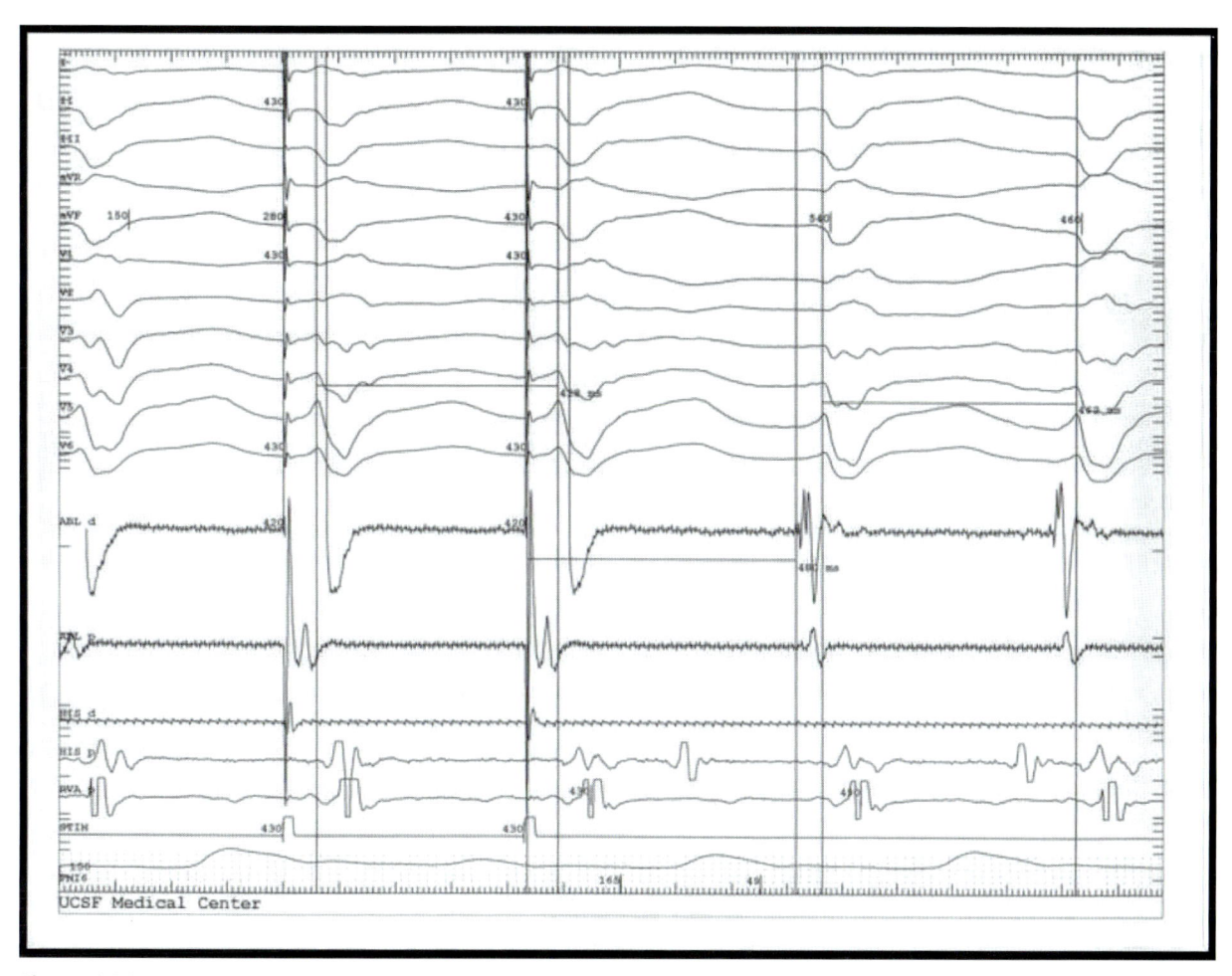

Figure 34.8 Manifest entrainment with pacing from the VT exit site. Surface ECG leads I, II, III, aVR, aVR, V_1, V_2, V_3, V_4, V_5, V_6 with intracardiac EGMs from the ABLd = distal ablator, ABLp = proximal ablator, HISd = distal His, HISp = proximal His, RVAp = proximal RVA. Pacing at the distal ablator from the VT exit site entrained the tachycardia at a cycle length of 420 ms and produced a QRS morphology similar to the left posterior fascicular VT. The post pacing interval (PPI = 480 ms) minus the tachycardia cycle length (TCL = 462 ms) was < 20 ms, indicating that the pacing site is within the VT circuit. (Figure provided courtesy of Dr Melvin M. Scheinman at the University of California, San Francisco Medical Center)

If a retrograde PP cannot be mapped, then we pursue a linear ablation strategy. Based on the presence of PPs and pace mapping, a site in the distal half to the distal third of the LV is targeted for a linear lesion across the fascicular tract (**Figure 34.12**). While some investigators have used left posterior fascicular block (LPFB) as an endpoint for this strategy, LPFB is not critical to a successful linear ablation.[13,14]

Ablation

Ideally, ablation is undertaken during VT in order to document termination of VT with successful ablation. RF energy is delivered to the mid-LV septal (for LPF VT) or the mid-anterior LV septal (for LAF VT) sites demonstrating a DP within the slow conduction zone. For LPF and LAF VT, RF energy is titrated for a maximum power of 40 W and a maximum electrode temperature of 60°C to 65°C for 60 seconds and a goal impedance drop of 8 to 10 ohms. The earliest DPs do not necessarily need to be targeted for successful ablation. However, if ablation fails to terminate or slow the VT within 20 seconds, then the catheter can be withdrawn to target an earlier DP. For left upper septal fascicular VT, the DP and fused PP sites are located in the basal septum. After identifying the HB and LBB sites, RF energy is delivered during sinus rhythm while monitoring for junctional rhythm and AV block. Ablation is started at 10 W and uptitrated gradually until goal temperature and/or an impedance drop is achieved. Reinduction of VT is then attempted to assess for ablation success.

Alternatively, if a DP cannot be mapped along the ventricular septum, then the presystolic fused PP at the VT exit site can be targeted using the same ablation parameters as above.

If a DP cannot be found and/or a suitable VT exit site cannot be mapped, then the retrograde PP along the posterior or anterior fascicle is targeted. After confirming that the target site is the earliest retrograde PP along the fascicle and that the site demonstrates decremental conduction with pacing, RF lesions are delivered.

If a retrograde PP cannot be mapped, we pursue a linear ablation strategy with a series of lesions placed perpendicular to the long-axis of the LV approximately midway between the base and the apex. For LPF VT, these lesions extend from the mid-ventricle to the junction of the septum and the inferior wall, and for LAF VT, these lesions extend from the mid-ventricle to the junction of the septum and anterior wall (Figure 34.12). This ablation is guided by the presence of presystolic PPs (**Figure 34.13**), and occasionally by pace mapping.

The endpoint of ablation (assuming VT could be induced prior to ablation) is the noninducibility of VT 30 minutes after the last ablation. Atrial and ventricular pacing protocols are repeated with and without isoproterenol infusion.

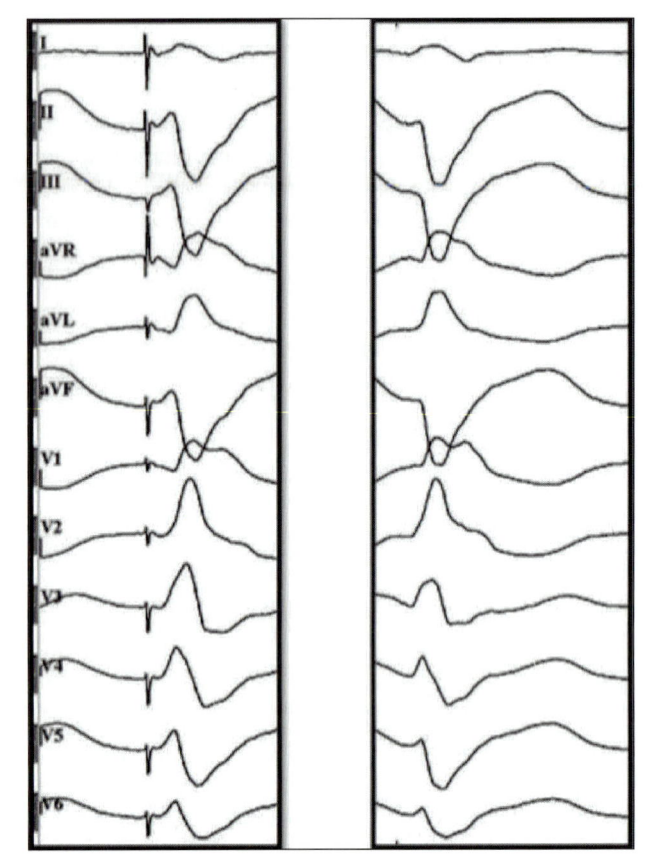

Figure 34.9 Surface ECG showing attempts at pace mapping to identify the exit site of left posterior fascicular VT. Despite pacing at minimal output, a 12/12 pace map match could not be obtained due to capture of surrounding myocardium. Ablation at this site terminated the VT.

Postprocedure Care

Recovery

After the postablation monitoring period has been completed, the ablation catheter is removed from the LV. Protamine is given to reverse the heparin, and the venous and arterial access sheaths are removed once the ACT < 180 seconds. Patients are monitored for a 6-hour bed rest interval. Aspirin (325 mg orally daily) is administered for 8 to 12 weeks, after which time it may be discontinued. If transseptal access is performed, patients are monitored overnight in a telemetry bed. Patients are discharged home without any antiarrhythmic medications.

Follow-up

Patients are seen within 4 to 6 weeks after their procedure as an outpatient, then followed yearly thereafter for recurrent arrhythmias. Depending upon the frequency of their symptoms prior to ablation, a Holter or event monitor is obtained 3 months after ablation and as needed thereafter for recurrent symptoms.

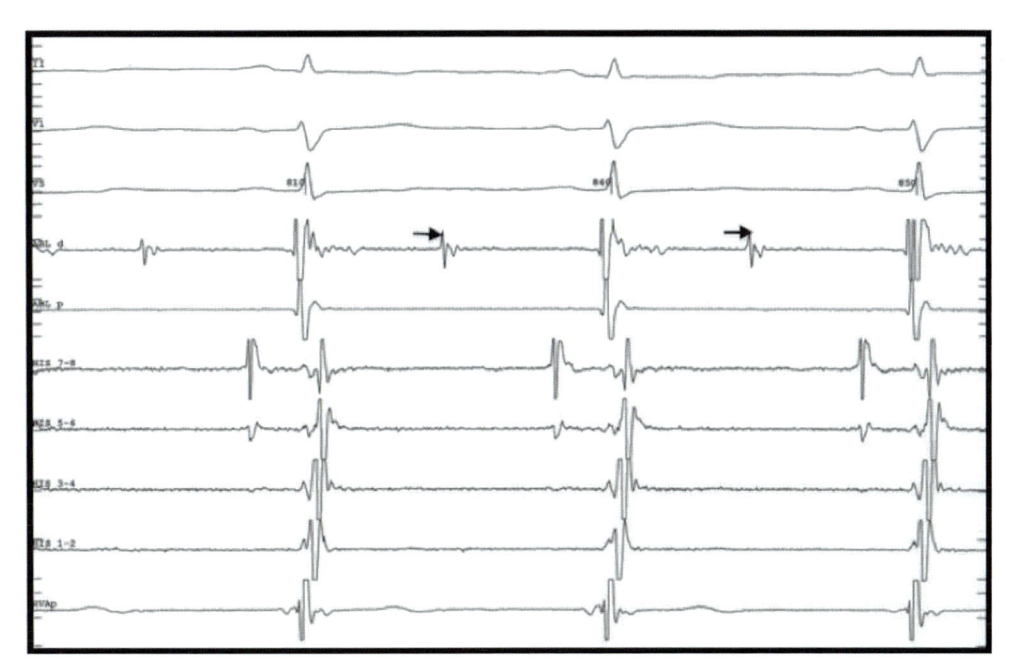

Figure 34.10 Surface ECG and intracardiac EGMs demonstrating retrograde PP (arrow) during sinus rhythm that was recorded on the ablator (Abl) in the left posterior fascicular region. Surface ECG leads II, V_1, V_5. Intracardiac EGMs: ABLd = distal ablator, ABLp = proximal ablator, HIS7, 8 = proximal His, HIS3, 4 and HIS5, 6 = mid-His, HIS1, 2 = distal His, and RVAp = proximal RVA. Ouyang and colleagues have shown that the earliest retrograde PP correlates with DP during VT and can be a target for ablation in patients with noninducible VT.

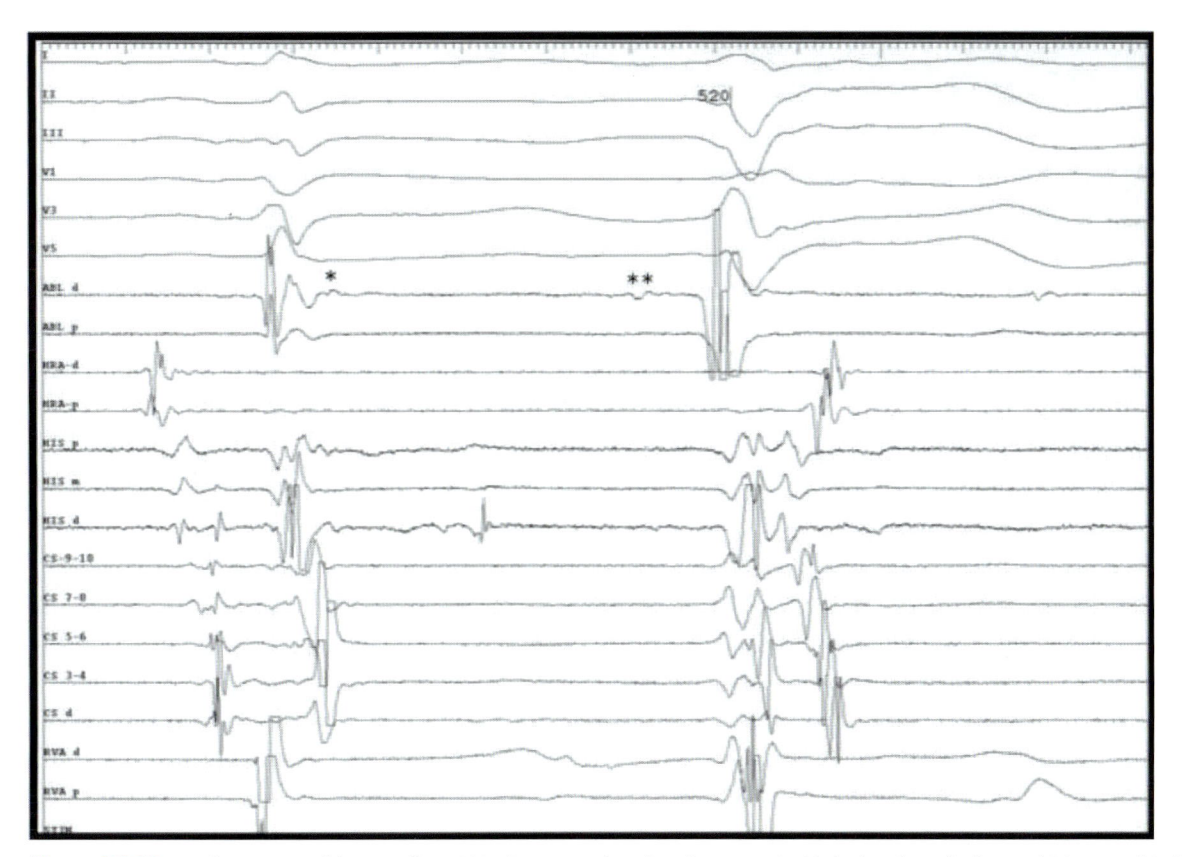

Figure 34.11 Surface ECG and intracardiac EGMs demonstrating site of retrograde PP during sinus rhythm and DP preceding left posterior fascicular PVC. Surface ECG leads I, II, III, V_1, V_3, V_5. Intracardiac EGMs: ABLd = distal ablator, ABLp = proximal ablator, HRAd = distal high right atrium, HRAp = proximal high right atrium, HISp = proximal His, HISm = mid-His, HISd = distal His, CS9-10 = proximal CS (CS), CS7-8 = CS bipole 7-8, CS5-6 = CS bipole 5-6, CS3-4 = CS bipole 3-4, CSd = distal CS, RVAd = distal right ventricular apex (RVA), RVAp = proximal RVA. The site of successful ablation of left posterior fascicular PVC demonstrating a retrograde PP (*) during sinus rhythm and a DP (**) preceding a left posterior fascicular premature ventricular contraction. The retrograde PP occurred 75 ms after the local EGM on the distal ablator. The DP occurred 85 ms prior to the onset of the QRS and the local EGM on the distal ablator.

310 • Ablation of VT

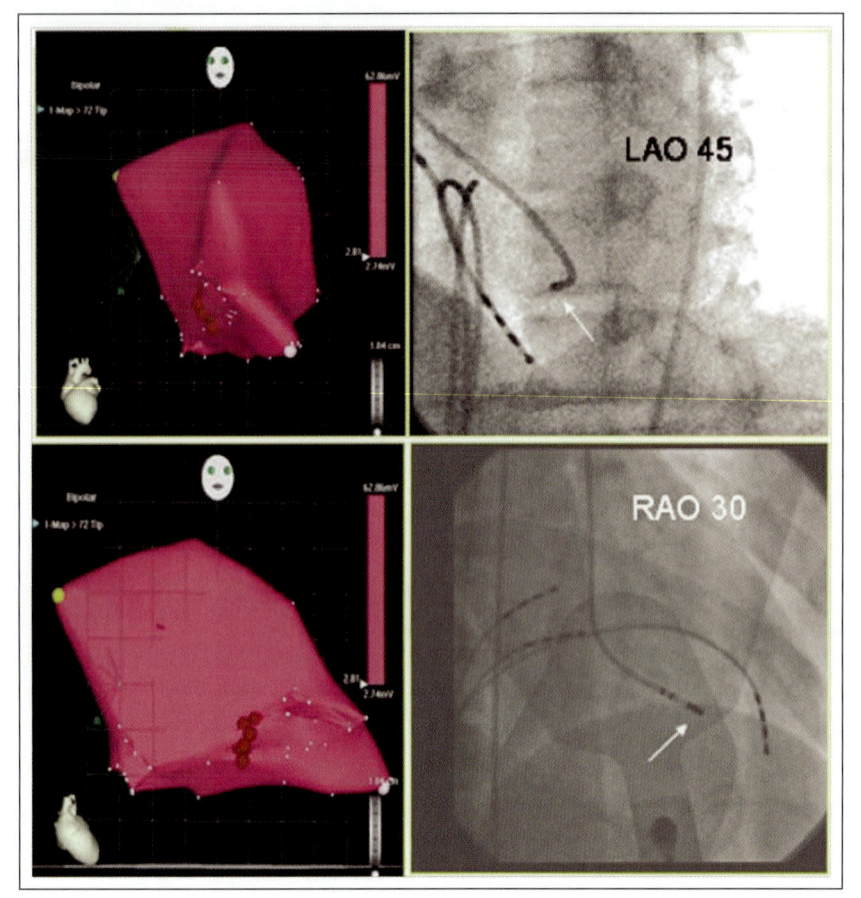

Figure 34.12 Three-dimensional electroanatomic map of the LV from the LAO and RAO projections with their corresponding fluoroscopic images at 45° LAO and 30° RAO. The line of small red circles represents the location of radiofrequency ablation lesions delivered in a linear fashion. (Reprinted from Lin D, et al. *Heart Rhythm.* 2005;2:934–939, with permission from Elsevier Science, Inc.)

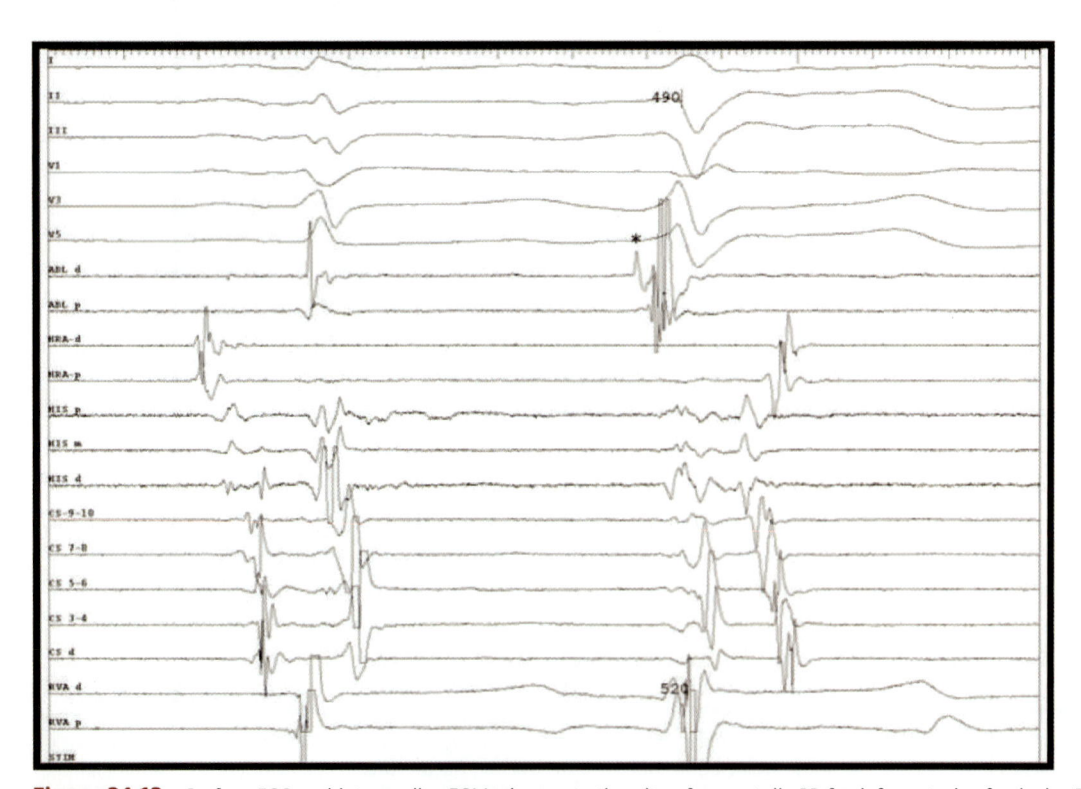

Figure 34.13 Surface ECG and intracardiac EGMs demonstrating site of presystolic PP for left posterior fascicular PVC. Surface ECG leads I, II, III, V$_1$, V$_3$, V$_5$. Intracardiac EGMs: ABLd = distal ablator, ABLp = proximal ablator, HRAd = distal high right atrium, HRAp = proximal high right atrium, HISp = proximal His, HISm = mid-His, HISd = distal His, CS9-10 = proximal coronary sinus (CS), CS7-8 = CS bipole 7-8, CS5-6 = CS bipole 5-6, CS3-4 = CS bipole 3-4, CSd = distal CS, RVAd = distal right ventricular apex (RVA), RVAp = proximal RVA. Mapping of the left posterior fascicle identified a presystolic PP (*) preceding the local intracardiac EGM at the distal ablator.

Repeat Ablations

If patients develop recurrent VT and they choose to undergo repeat ablation, we again map DPs and fused Purkinje-ventricular potentials during VT. These potentials are targeted with ablation for the goal of noninducible VT. If VT cannot be induced, then retrograde PP potentials are mapped along the left bundle and left fascicles. These potentials are targeted for ablation. However, the endpoint of noninducibility cannot be used in these cases, and the ablation endpoint becomes the abolition of these retrograde PP potentials. If VT cannot be induced and retrograde PP potentials cannot be mapped, then an ablation strategy of a linear ablation through the fascicle is performed. These ablation lines are guided by the presence of PPs and pace mapping. We do not pursue an endpoint of fascicular block, but other groups have pursued this as an endpoint with high success rates.

Procedural Complications

As with any procedure that entails intravascular access, LV access, and ablation, potential complications including bleeding, arteriovenous fistula, pseudoaneurysm, cardiac perforation, stroke, and thromboembolism are always possible. Complications specific to fascicular VT ablation include LBBB and AV block, especially with targeting the left basal septum. Transient LBBB and AV block have also been reported during mapping with catheter-induced block or after ablation in the mid-septum. Another reported complication in 1 patient undergoing fascicular VT ablation was a torn chordae tendinae of the mitral valve associated with mild mitral regurgitation.

Advantages and Limitations

Given the low incidence of fascicular VTs, especially the rare form of left upper septal VT, randomized approaches to the ablation of the fascicular VTs do not exist. When fascicular VT can be induced and mapped, demonstrating entrainment of the VT, identifying DPs and VT exit sites, and mapping the slow conduction zone of the VT have the advantages of proving the reentrant VT mechanism and localizing an ablation target. Mapping and ablation of retrograde PPs during sinus rhythm and linear ablation perpendicular to the fascicle have a high success rate, despite the absence of inducible tachycardia. Whether or not left posterior or left anterior fascicular block created during ablation leads to an increased risk of advanced conduction system disease over long-term follow-up is unknown.

Conclusions

Fascicular VT has characteristic ECG features, which can be used to identify those patients who may benefit from a curative ablation. Diagnosing and ablating fascicular VT can be definitively accomplished with the induction of VT and entrainment mapping for the critical limb of the VT circuit. The critical limb of the VT circuit manifests DPs that lie in a zone of slow conduction with decremental properties and verapamil sensitivity. Ablation at the critical limb of the circuit has a high rate of success.

Since not all fascicular VTs can be induced at the time of EP study, sinus rhythm mapping of the left bundle branch and the left anterior and posterior fascicles can be performed to facilitate mapping of retrograde PPs and to identify sites for linear ablation of the fascicles along the mid-distal ventricular septum. These approaches also have a high rate of success. Mapping and ablation during VT and/or sinus rhythm are facilitated by the use of electroanatomic mapping systems, which can help to reduce the use of fluoroscopy and radiation exposure.

References

1. Nogami A. Idiopathic left ventricular tachycardia: assessment and treatment. *Card Electrophysiol Rev.* 2002; 6:448–457.
2. Ohe T, Aihara N, Kamakura S, Kurita T, Shimizu W, Shimomura K. Long-term outcome of verapamil-sensitive sustained left ventricular tachycardia in patients without structural heart disease. *J Am Coll Cardiol.* 1995;25:54–58.
3. Okumura K, Yamabe H, Tsuchiya T, Tabuchi T, Iwasa A, Yasue H. Characteristics of slow conduction zone demonstrated during entrainment of idiopathic ventricular tachycardia of left ventricular origin. *Am J Cardiol.* 1996; 77:379–383.
4. Nogami A, Naito S, Tada H, Taniguchi K, Okamoto Y, Nishimura S, Yamauchi Y, Aonuma K, Goya M, Iesaka Y, Hiroe M. Demonstration of diastolic and presystolic Purkinje potentials as critical potentials in a macroreentry circuit of verapamil-sensitive idiopathic left ventricular tachycardia. *J Am Coll Cardiol.* 2000;36:811–823.
5. Tsuchiya T, Okumura K, Honda T, Iwasa A, Yasue H, Tabuchi T. Significance of late diastolic potential preceding Purkinje potential in verapamil-sensitive idiopathic left ventricular tachycardia. *Circulation.* 1999;99:2408–2413.
6. Nogami A, Naito S, Tada H, Oshima S, Taniguchi K, Aonuma K, Iesaka Y. Verapamil-sensitive left anterior fascicular ventricular tachycardia: results of radiofrequency ablation in six patients. *J Cardiovasc Electrophysiol.* 1998; 9:1269–1278.
7. Ouyang F, Cappato R, Ernst S, Goya M, Volkmer M, Hebe J, Antz M, Vogtmann T, Schaumann A, Fotuhi P, Hoffmann-Riem M, Kuck KH. Electroanatomic substrate of idiopathic

left ventricular tachycardia: unidirectional block and macro-reentry within the purkinje network. *Circulation.* 2002; 105:462–469.
8. Okumura K, Matsuyama K, Miyagi H, Tsuchiya T, Yasue H. Entrainment of idiopathic ventricular tachycardia of left ventricular origin with evidence for reentry with an area of slow conduction and effect of verapamil. *Am J Cardiol.* 1988;62:727–732.
9. Gonzalez RP, Scheinman MM, Lesh MD, Helmy I, Torres V, Van Hare GF. Clinical and electrophysiologic spectrum of fascicular tachycardias. *Am Heart J.* 1994;128:147–156.
10. Zipes DP, Foster PR, Troup PJ, Pedersen DH. Atrial induction of ventricular tachycardia: reentry versus triggered automaticity. *Am J Cardiol.* 1979;44:1–8.
11. Kim AM, Tseng ZH, Viswanathan MN, et al. Diagnosis and ablation of multiform fascicular tachycardia. *Heart Rhythm.* 2009;6:S176.
12. Aliot EM, Stevenson WG, Almendral-Garrote JM, et al. EHRA/HRS expert consensus on catheter ablation of ventricular arrhythmias: developed in a partnership with the European Heart Rhythm Association (EHRA), a Registered Branch of the European Society of Cardiology (ESC), and the Heart Rhythm Society (HRS); in collaboration with the American College of Cardiology (ACC) and the American Heart Association (AHA). *Heart Rhythm.* 2009;6:886–933.
13. Ma FS, Ma J, Tang K, Han H, Jia YH, Fang PH, Chu JM, Pu JL, Zhang S. Left posterior fascicular block: a new endpoint of ablation for verapamil-sensitive idiopathic ventricular tachycardia. *Chin Med J* (Engl). 2006;119: 367–372.
14. Lin D, Hsia HH, Gerstenfeld EP, Dixit S, Callans DJ, Nayak H, Russo A, Marchlinski FE. Idiopathic fascicular left ventricular tachycardia: linear ablation lesion strategy for noninducible or nonsustained tachycardia. *Heart Rhythm.* 2005;2:934–939.
15. Tada H, Nogami A, Naito S, Tomita T, Oshima S, Taniguchi K, Aonuma K, Iesaka Y. Retrograde Purkinje potential activation during sinus rhythm following catheter ablation of idiopathic left ventricular tachycardia. *J Cardiovasc Electrophysiol.* 1998;9:1218–1224.

CHAPTER 35

HOW TO MAP AND ABLATE HEMODYNAMICALLY TOLERATED VENTRICULAR TACHYCARDIAS

Kojiro Tanimoto, MD; Henry H. Hsia, MD

Introduction

Sustained VT is an important cause of morbidity and mortality in patients with structural heart disease. Although ICDs are effective in terminating VTs and reducing mortality, defibrillators do not prevent arrhythmia recurrences. ICD shocks, particularly when recurrent, cause significant decreases in patients' quality of life.[1] Furthermore, multiple shocks during an arrhythmia "storm" have been associated with an increased risk of death.[2] Additional intervention is needed when VT becomes recurrent or incessant. Antiarrhythmic drugs are sometimes useful but are associated with cardiac and noncardiac toxicities, and the long-term efficacy is limited.[3] Catheter ablation offers an alternative therapy for controlling ventricular arrhythmia recurrences, especially in patients with hemodynamically tolerated VTs. Although catheter ablation of VT remains a challenging procedure, VT ablation can be performed safely and successfully with careful procedural planning and detailed mapping.

Preprocedure Planning

History and Data Review

Patients for VT ablation should undergo a careful cardiovascular evaluation prior to the procedure. Tachycardia mechanisms and origins usually depend on patients' underlying heart diseases, which should be carefully characterized. In patients with ischemic heart disease, the reentrant VT circuits are often located at the subendocardial surface near the infarct region.[4] However, in patients with NICMs, such predilections for endocardial VT circuits do not exist. Limited LV endocardial low-amplitude EGM abnormalities were observed,[5] with larger epicardial low-voltage areas, usually located over the basal lateral LV near the valve annulus.[6-8] Furthermore, intramural scars have been demonstrated by cardiac MRI.[9,10] Substrate for ventricular arrhythmias in patients with NICMs may be endocardial, epicardial, or intramural.

In patients with ARVC/D, sizable low-voltage areas may involve the infundibulum, the free wall, and the basal perivalvular regions that constitute the endocardial VT substrate in this disease.[11,12] In addition, the presence of extensive epicardial scars has recently been identified,[13] with the reentrant VT circuits often located at the epicardial surface. In patients with congenital heart disease with prior surgical correction, the reentrant circuits are often related to the procedural incisions and surgical reconstructions.

Assessment of Coronary Artery Disease

In patients with structural heart disease, the presence of a monomorphic VT usually denotes a relatively "fixed" arrhythmia substrate, commonly related to scar-based reentry. However, it is important to qualify that patients with structural heart disease occasionally have idiopathic VTs.

Although myocardial ischemia and acute infarction alone are rare causes of monomorphic VTs, the potential of ischemia should always be assessed, especially in patients with coronary artery disease and prior myocardial infarction.

Evaluation of Cardiac Function and Wall Motion Abnormalities

The severity of cardiac dysfunction and the locations of wall motion abnormalities should be evaluated by a transthoracic echocardiogram before VT ablation. The presence of wall motion abnormalities or thinning suggests areas of scar and potential locations for the arrhythmogenic substrate. Furthermore, the presence of a mobile intracavitary thrombus is a contraindication for endocardial mapping procedures, particularly in patients with severe ventricular dysfunction or LV aneurysm.

Gadolinium-delayed enhancement on cardiac MRI may also help to define the locations of the scar in patients with ICM or NICM.[9,10] The scar locations (endocardial, epicardial, or intramural) on a preprocedure image facilitate procedural planning and approach.

The Electrocardiogram (ECG)

Careful review of the electrocardiogram (ECG) is a critical step of the preprocedure planning. Focusing on VT initiation, termination and cycle length oscillations, insights into the arrhythmia mechanisms (macroreentry or focal), and sites of origins of VT may be obtained. A "warm-up" phenomenon with significant cycle length oscillation ($\geq$ 20–30 ms) suggests a focal, automatic mechanism, whereas an abrupt initiation or termination with PVC implies reentry.

The presence of Q waves during sinus rhythm may reveal the locations of myocardial scars and the potential arrhythmia substrates. The presence of a bundle branch block suggests the presence of a diseased conduction system that may participate in a reentrant arrhythmia using the Purkinje fibers or bundle branch reentry. If the 12-lead ECG during VT is available for review, the QRS morphology of VT or PVC reflects the earliest site of ventricular activation, and the VT site of origin (reentry exit site or focal early activation) can be regionalized with a reasonable accuracy.

Some general rules can be applied to the ECG analysis.[14] We focus on (1) the "bundle branch block" configurations in lead V_1, (2) the frontal QRS axis in lead I, (3) the inferior lead (II, III, aVF) QRS axis, and (4) patterns of precordial R-wave transition. Left bundle branch block (LBBB with lead V_1 predominantly negative) configuration and positive R wave in lead I (leftward axis) suggest the ventricular arrhythmia originates at the interventricular septum or the right ventricle. Right bundle branch block (RBBB with lead V_1 predominantly positive) configuration and negative QRS in lead I (rightward axis) suggest an arrhythmia site of origin located near the free wall of the left ventricle. Positive QRS in the inferior leads (inferior axis) indicates an exit on the anterior/superior walls, whereas a negative QRS in the inferior leads (superior axis) indicates an exit on the inferior/posterior walls. An early R-wave transition in precordial leads (positive by lead V_3) suggests a basal site of origin, and a poor/late R-wave transition with dominant Q wave in V_4 to V_6 suggests an exit near the ventricular apex.

Other electrocardiographic characteristics help to distinguish endocardial versus epicardial site of origin. In general, ventricular arrhythmia originating near the epicardium tends to have a wider QRS duration with a slurred initial QRS upstroke, compared to arrhythmias arising from the endocardium. The presence of (1) a pseudo–delta wave of more than 34 ms in duration, (2) a delayed intrinsicoid deflection to the peak R wave in V_2 of more than 85 ms, or (3) the shortest RS complex, measured from the earliest ventricular activation to the nadir of the first S wave in any precordial lead, of greater than 121 ms, favors the diagnosis of epicardial arrhythmia.[15] In addition, a precordial maximum deflection index (MDI) of more than 0.55 suggests arrhythmias of epicardial origin.[16] MDI is calculated by dividing the earliest time to maximum deflection (MDT) in any of the precordial leads by the total QRS duration.

Since most patients have multiple induced VTs during the procedure, it is also useful to identify the clinical VT.[17] Since the 12-lead ECGs of the spontaneous arrhythmias are often not available, the stored EGM recordings from the ICD interrogation can provide useful data. By comparing the real-time ICD EGM morphologies and cycle lengths during intraoperative VT inductions with the stored EGM data from the spontaneous VT episodes (**Figure 35.1**), the clinical VT can often be identified.[18] In addition, analysis of the EGM recording during sinus rhythm is important. If the intracardiac EGMs during the spontaneous tachycardia recorded by the ICD are similar to those recorded during the sinus rhythm, the ventricular activation pattern during the tachycardia is thus similar to that during the sinus rhythm. This suggests the VT may utilize the native conduction system (**Figure 35.2**). Bundle branch reentry or a fascicular VT should be considered.

Procedure

Patient Preparation

Since the 12-lead ECG analysis is essential to regionalize the VT exit as well as for pace mapping, correct surface ECG electrode placement is critical. Erroneous ECG leads

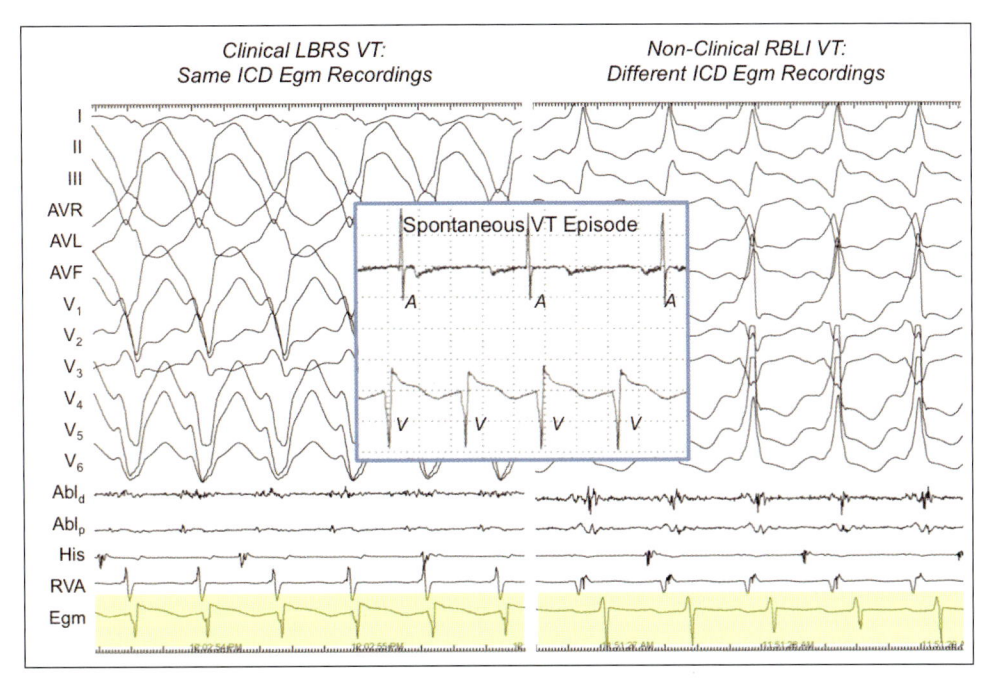

Chapter 35: Ablating Hemodynamically Tolerated VTs • 315

Figure 35.1 Utility of ICD EGM recordings in VT ablation. Two different morphologies of VTs were induced during the procedure. The 12-lead ECG and EGM of a LBRS QRS VT were shown (left panel). The ICD EGMs during the tachycardia matched the stored ICD EGM during the spontaneous VT episodes (inset). A RBLI VT was also induced with the ICD EGM during the tachycardia but did not match that recorded during a spontaneous VT episode (right panel). The LBRS VT was considered to be the "clinical" arrhythmia. Of note, the timing of the real-time ICD EGM was often different and "off-set" from the rest of the intracardiac recordings during the tachycardia due to variable delays between the ICD programmer outputs and the EP recording system.

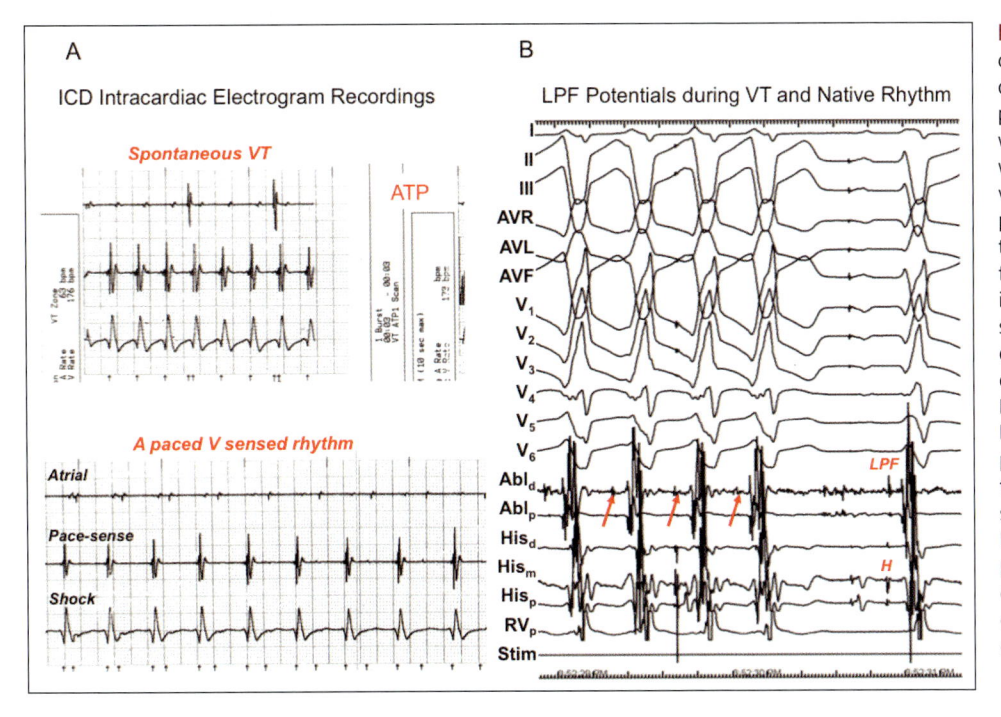

Figure 35.2 A. Comparison of the ICD EGM recordings during VT and during an atrial-paced rhythm. VA dissociation was evident during VT, which was terminated by ATP. The ventricular EGMs on both the pace-sense (near-field) and the shocking electrode (far-field) recordings demonstrated identical morphologies, suggesting identical activation during VT and during native conducted beats. **B.** The 12-lead ECG during VT showed an RBBB left anterior fascicular block pattern that was identical to the ECG during atrial pacing, suggesting conduction down the LPF during both rhythms. A LPF potential (arrow) was recorded during VT. The LPF potential occurred after the HB recording during atrial pacing.

positioning or ECG misinterpretations will result in confusion, procedural delay, and failed outcome.

Our protocol recommends the use of the electroanatomic system for VT mapping and ablation (CARTO, Biosense Webster, Diamond Bar, CA, USA). Care must be taken for placement of the reference patch to compensate for the dilated left ventricles that are often leftward rotated. The reference patch should be placed in the center of the ventricular silhouette in the anterior-posterior fluoroscopic projection to ensure proper registration of the navigational data. For the real-time ICD EGM recordings, a vendor-specific junction box may be obtained from the company that connects the programmer to the EP recording system in the analog channels for display.

The arterial access is obtained through the right femoral artery with an 8-Fr sheath for the retrograde aortic approach. A "long" sheath (≥ 30 cm) may be helpful, particularly in those with significant peripheral vascular disease or tortuosity of the aorto-iliac system. For accurate hemodynamic monitoring, a separate arterial line may be necessary in patients with advanced heart disease. In patients who have severe peripheral artery disease or aortic valve disease/prosthesis, a transseptal approach should be considered. Two right ventricular catheters are routinely placed at the right ventricular apex and near the HB. The RVA catheter marks the ventricular apex, and the His catheter marks the ventricular base, opposite of the aortic valve.

For the patient in whom an epicardial approach is anticipated, or in those who may have VTs originate near the mitral annulus, an additional CS catheter, inserted either from the right internal jugular vein or from the femoral vein, is used to outline the basal LV silhouette and mapping. For VTs that originate from near the LVOT, a 4-Fr catheter or a microcatheter (Pathfinder, Cardima, Fremont, CA) is useful to record epicardial EGMs from the "summit" of the left ventricle near the anterior coronary vein or great cardiac vein.

ICE imaging is also useful for creating the 3-dimensional anatomical shell of the ventricular chamber and for identifying the scar with wall motion abnormalities.[19] Moreover, the real-time monitoring using ICE to ensure contact between the catheter tip and tissue is useful, especially for VT originating near complex anatomical structures such as the LV outflow tract and papillary muscles. ICE is also helpful for early detection of the intracavitary thrombus or cardiac tamponade. The right femoral vein is usually accessed to accommodate an 11-Fr sheath for the placement of a 10-Fr phased-array ICE catheter.

Anesthesia

Most of patients who undergo catheter VT ablation in our laboratory are under general anesthesia. Multiple episodes of poorly tolerated arrhythmias are often induced during the procedure that require shock terminations. General anesthesia helps to control patients' discomfort, minimizes movement, and improves mapping accuracy. The disadvantages of general anesthesia include (1) VT induction may be more difficult and (2) lower blood pressure may occur during VTs due to the abolition of sympathetic tone for compensatory vasoconstriction. Close communication and collaboration between the anesthesiologists and the electrophysiologists are needed to perform VT ablation safely and successfully.

Anticoagulation

Placement of intravascular catheters, creation of ablation lesions, activation of coagulation factors, and potential disruption of atherosclerotic plaques all contribute to a risk of thromboembolism during and after the ablation procedures. The risk of stroke or thromboembolism for LV catheter VT ablation is at least as high as any left heart catheterization at ~1%. We recommend meticulous monitoring of the ACT every 20 to 30 minutes. The target ACT is maintained at ~300 seconds. A lower-level anticoagulation for prevention of venous thromboembolic complications is also recommended during right heart catheterization/ablation procedures as most patients have prolonged placement of multiple intravascular catheters.

If epicardial mapping/ablation is being considered, pericardial access should be obtained before anticoagulation is initiated. Otherwise, complete reversal of anticoagulation must be achieved before attempting the percutaneous subxyphoid pericardial puncture.[8,20]

General Principles

A systematic approach of VT ablation should be followed (**Figure 35.3**). A hybrid protocol with a combination of conventional and substrate-based mapping techniques is utilized to optimize the procedural efficiency and maximize success.

Induction of VT should be performed before ablation to confirm the diagnosis, to evaluate for bundle branch reentry, and to ascertain which arrhythmias are the clinical VTs. Programmed stimulation is usually performed from 2 ventricular sites (RV apex and RVOT) with up to 3 extra stimuli after basic drive cycle lengths of 600 and 400 ms.

Most patients have multiple inducible arrhythmias (mean 4 ± 3 VT morphologies), with hemodynamically and morphologically unstable VTs that do not allow extensive mapping during arrhythmias. Characterization of the electrophysiological substrate during sinus or paced rhythm should therefore be performed to minimize VT induction/episodes, especially in patients with advanced structural heart disease.

Substrate Mapping

Substrate characterization identifies areas of abnormal myocardium, particularly regions of slow conduction within the low-voltage scar that may constitute the potential reentry circuit. It allows more detailed mapping focusing on limited areas of interest and facilitates the design of the ablation lesion sets. Even for hemodynamically tolerated VTs, sustained arrhythmias of prolonged duration may induce ischemia or exacerbation of heart failure. Substrate mapping is therefore recommended even in patients with hemodynamically stable VTs. Integrating substrate mapping and conventional mapping techniques is essential for successful and efficient ablation procedures. Substrate mapping techniques include (1) analyzing the local EGM voltage, (2) defining the conducting channels, (3) identifying EGMs with isolated delayed components (E-IDC) or LPs, (4) pace mapping, and (5) detecting the EUS. Detailed descriptions of the substrate mapping techniques are beyond the scope of this chapter, and only a brief discussion is provided.

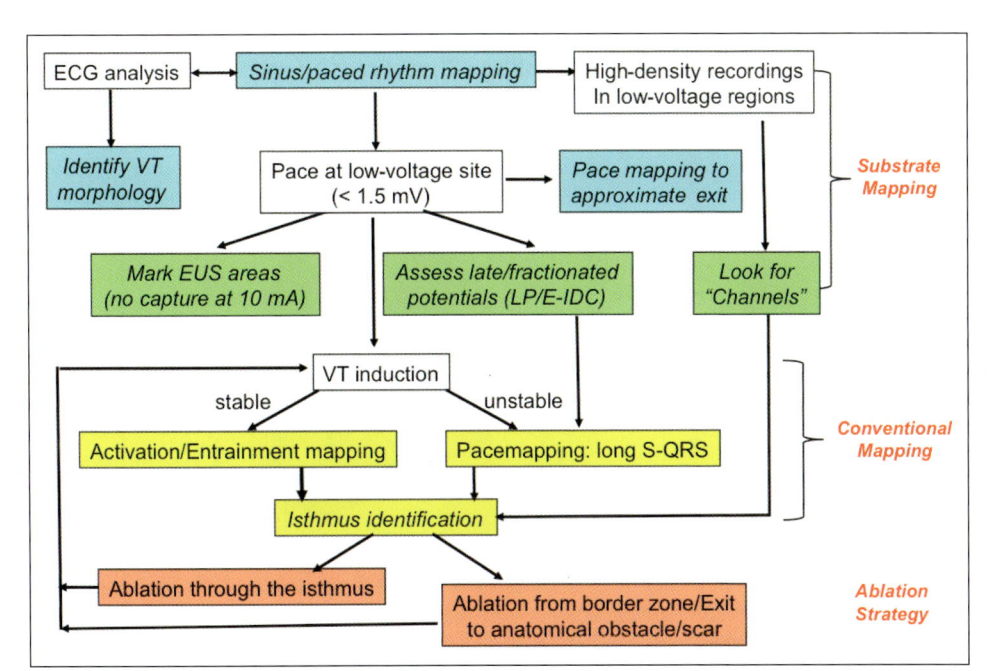

Figure 35.3 A flow diagram for the approach of catheter mapping and ablation of VT. A "hybrid" protocol with a combination of both "conventional" and "substrate-based" mapping techniques is utilized.

Voltage Mapping

The normal endocardium is defined as bipolar EGM voltage ≥ 1.5 mV. "Dense scar" is arbitrarily defined as areas with voltage less than 0.5 mV. The "border zone" is defined as the transition zone between dense scar and normal tissue (0.5–1.5 mV).[21] Most isthmus sites are located in areas of low-voltage scar (< 0.5 mV) while exits are often located in the border zone (0.5–1.5 mV).[22,23] Analysis of the voltage profiles identifies the approximate location of the VT circuit, and mapping efforts should then be directed toward the low-voltage scar (< 0.5 mV) for localizing the isthmus.

Conducting Channels

By careful voltage color adjustment, VT-related conducting channels may be identified as visible corridors with consecutive EGM recordings of relatively higher signal amplitude bordered by lower-voltage scars (**Figure 35.4**). The majority of channels can be identified when the voltage threshold is set between 0.2 and 0.3 mV.[23,24] The potential VT-related conducting channels should be confirmed by other collaborative methods such as activation mapping, pace mapping, and entrainment mapping.

Late Potentials

EGMs with isolated delayed components (E-IDC) or LPs recorded after the completion of the surface QRS reflect local conduction delay in the diseased myocardium and have been associated with the VT isthmus.[24-26] The majority of VT isthmus sites are associated with the presence of LPs, which are commonly found inside the dense scar. Furthermore, the degree of local conduction delay (QRS–LP interval) is significantly longer (≥ 200 ms) at sites near the entrance and mid-isthmus of a VT circuit compared to that of an exit site (**Table 35.1**; **Figure 35.5**). LPs may be better identified during RVA pacing or introduction of ventricular extrastimuli compared to sinus rhythm, suggesting that changes in wave front activation or decremental impulse propagation might unmask areas of block and slow conduction into the channels.[24]

Pace Mapping

The VT isthmus may also be identified by pace mapping.[27] Pacing near or at the exit of a VT should produce a QRS morphology similar to that of the VT. After defining the VT exit, pacing progressively away from the border zone into the dense scar (< 0.5 mV) should be performed to identify the potential isthmus site. Pace mapping in the VT isthmus should produce a QRS similar to that of the VT with a longer stimulus-to-QRS interval (S-QRS) due to slow conduction within the channel (**Figure 35.6**). A long S-QRS (> 40 ms) recorded deeper into the scar is a marker for abnormal conduction that is often associated with the VT isthmus.[27]

Electrically Unexcitable Scar (EUS)

Scar areas with noncapture at high-output unipolar pacing (> 10 mA at 2-ms pulse width) defines the EUS.[28] These areas often have bipolar EGM amplitudes of ≤ 0.2 mV and are located in proximity to the reentry circuit isthmuses and conduction channels.

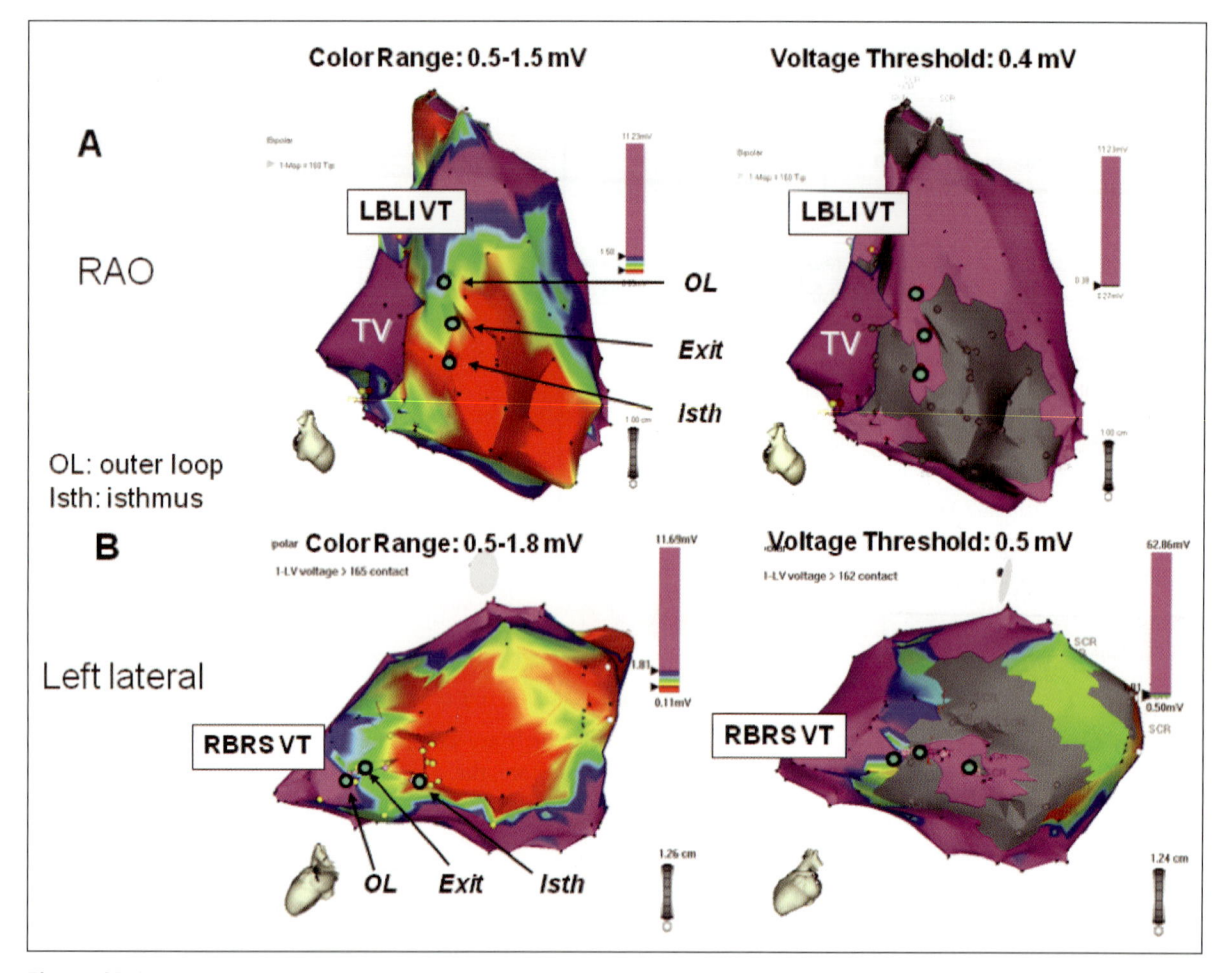

Figure 35.4 Identification of the conducting channels of VT reentrant circuits. Bipolar voltage maps in 2 patients with monomorphic VT were shown. Endocardial sites within the circuits were identified by entrainment mapping for the corresponding VTs. The standard color range for the voltage maps were depicted on the left panels, and the maps after voltage threshold adjustment were depicted on the right panels. **A.** Right ventricular maps in a patient with an ARVC and sustained LBBB-left inferior axis VT. At a voltage threshold of 0.4 mV (dense scar depicted by gray at 0.38 mV), a corridor characterized by a higher voltage that followed the path defined by orthodromically activated VT sites was visualized. **B.** Left ventricular maps in a patient with an ICM and prior infarction who presented with an RBRS axis VT. At a voltage threshold of 0.5 mV (dense scar depicted by gray at 0.4 mV), evidence of a conduit with a higher voltage that follows orthodromic activating sites during reentrant VT was identified. (Adapted with permission from Hsia H et al. *Heart Rhythm.* 2006;3:503–512.)

Table 35.1 Relationships of Late Potentials and the VT Circuit

	Entrance	Isthmus	Exit	Outer Loop
Number of sampled sites	13	86	101	11
VT circuits with LP	60%	90%**	36%	0%
% sampled sites with LP	53.8%	82.6%**	25.7%	0%
QRS-LP (msec)	203 ± 26*	201 ± 65*	115 ± 39	n/a

LP: late potentials

* $p < 0.05$ Exit vs. Isthmus and Entrance

** $p < 0.05$ Isthmus vs. Entrance and Exit

Adapted with permission from Hsia H. *J Interv Card Electrophysiol.* 2009;26:21–29.

Information obtained during substrate mapping should be classified and tagged on the voltage map for reference (potential VT-related conducting channel, EUS, LPs, good pace map sites). These data help to define the geometry of the circuit and its relationship to the underlying scar, identifying the VT isthmus and designing the ablation lesion set(s). After substrate mapping, the putative VT circuit must be confirmed by collaborative mapping methods. The mapping/ablation catheter should be placed at the presumed sites within the VT circuit for limited activation mapping and entrainment mapping during arrhythmias.

Mapping During Hemodynamically Stable VT

For hemodynamically stable VTs, mapping should be done during VT using conventional mapping techniques, guided

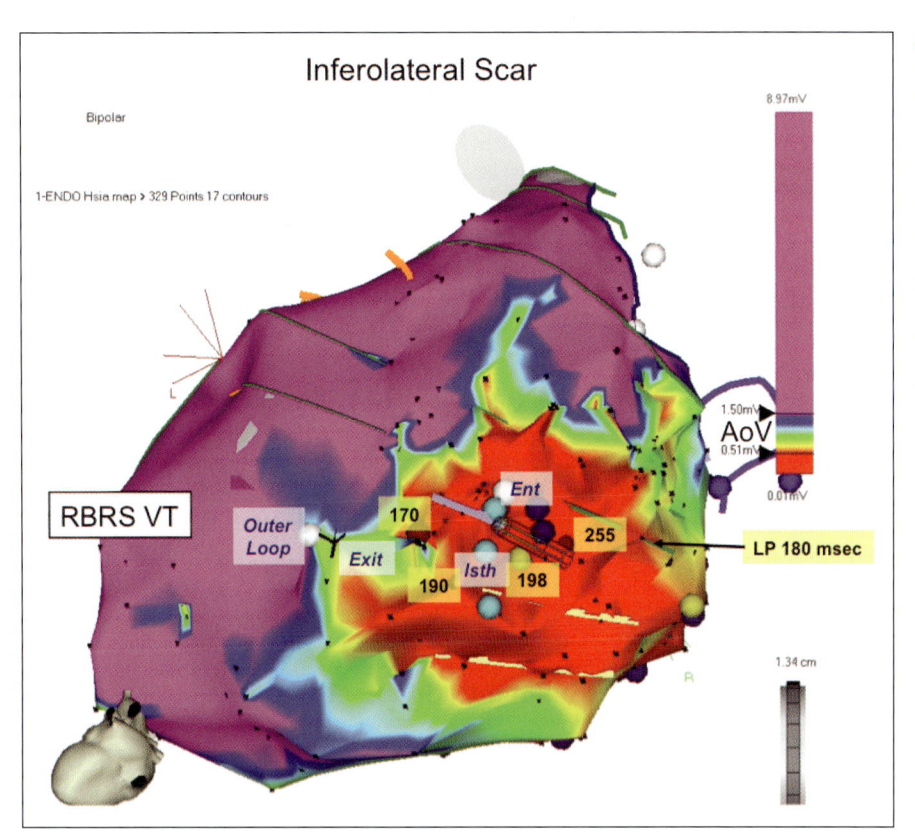

Chapter 35: Ablating Hemodynamically Tolerated VTs • 319

Figure 35.5 The relationship between LPs and the VT circuit. A left ventricular voltage map in a patient with a large inferolateral scar and RBRS VT was shown. The exit (Exit), isthmus (Isth), entrance (Ent), and outer loop were defined by entrainment. The locations of LPs were shown (yellow), and the QRS-LPs (in ms) were measured from the beginning of QRS to the latest LPs. The degree of local conduction delay (QRS–LP interval) was significantly longer at sites near the entrance and isthmus of the VT circuit.

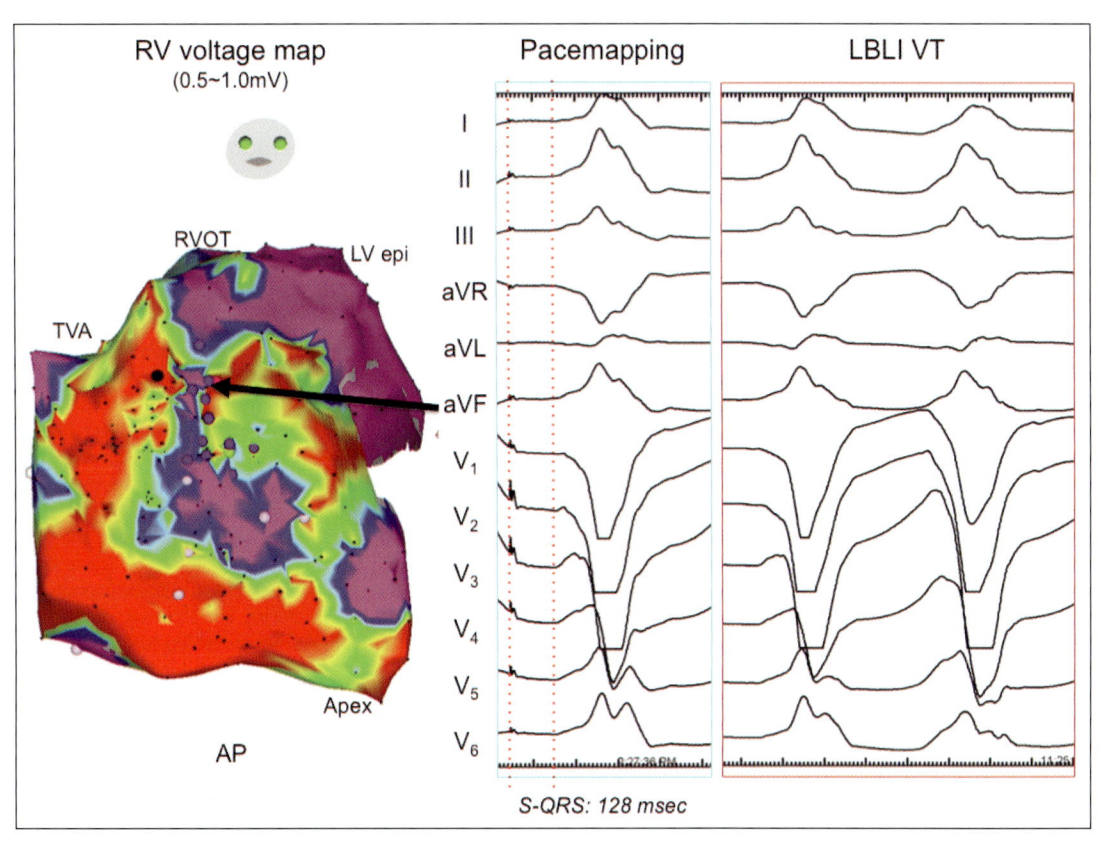

Figure 35.6 Pace mapping for identification of the VT isthmus. An epicardial voltage map in a patient with ARVC (left) was shown. Large low-voltage areas were found in the anterior aspect of the right ventricular epicardium. A potential "channel" was identified that corresponded to the VT isthmus. Pace mapping along the "channel" (blue dots) resulted in progressively longer stimulus-to-QRS (S-QRS) intervals. The pace map (arrow) showed a good match of RBRI VT with a long S-QRS interval of 128 ms, suggesting a VT isthmus site. RF ablation transecting the isthmus rendered the VT noninducible.

by prior substrate characterization. Such conventional mapping includes (1) ECG localization, (2) activation mapping, (3) entrainment mapping, and 4) pace mapping.

Activation Mapping

For monomorphic ventricular tachycardias, activation mapping measures the local activation time relative to the QRS onset. The beginning of the surface QRS during VT is usually used as the reference. Bipolar EGM recordings are utilized with the local activation time defined by the sharpest signal that crosses the baseline. For focal idiopathic VTs, the earliest site of depolarization is presumably the site of origin. Unipolar recordings at the site of origin often demonstrate a qS configuration. However, unipolar mapping may not be useful for nonidiopathic arrhythmias due to low signal amplitude and poor resolution commonly associated with scar-based reentry.

During sustained macroreentry VTs, the beginning of the QRS depicts when the activation wave front exits from the circuit. Mapping should be performed systematically, starting at the presumptive exit site. The location of the exit can be approximated by analysis of the QRS patterns from the ECG as well as the voltage maps. At the exit sites, presystolic potentials preceding the QRS (< 100 ms pre-QRS) are commonly recorded. Mapping should then proceed from the exit site located near the border zone (0.5-1.5 mV) toward the more proximal sites located in the dense scar (< 0.5 mV), with the majority of VT isthmuses located in areas of 0.2-0.3 mV[23,29,30] or near the EUS.[28] Inside the dense scar, low-amplitude MDPs should be sought, which may be recorded in up to 50% of the isthmus sites during VT (**Figure 35.7**).[31,32] However, not all MDPs are suitable targets for the ablation because they could be bystander signals, or dissociated potentials (**Figure 35.8**). To confirm whether the site is involved in the reentry circuit, overdrive pacing with entrainment must be performed.

In patients with extensive myocardial scar, the ECG QRS pattern may be an unreliable tool for rapid localization of the VT circuit during sustained monomorphic VT, particularly in those with prior anterior-apical infarctions who present with an RBBB pattern VT (R/S ratio > 1 in lead V_1). The QRS-RVA interval, measured from the beginning of the QRS to the right ventricular apical EGM recordings, can be helpful to quickly regionalize the VT circuit during activation mapping, identifying septal versus lateral site of origin of the RBBB VT. The QRS-RVA interval differs for different site of origin and is correlated with the exit locations (septal VT exit: < 100 ms versus lateral VT exit: > 125 ms).[33]

Entrainment and Resetting

Activation mapping alone is insufficient to define the VT circuit. Recorded potentials during sustained arrhythmia may be related to sites outside the zone of slow conduction, bystander locations, or remote sites unrelated to the VT circuit (**Figure 35.9**).

Most macroreentrant VT circuits have an excitable gap, such that an appropriately timed premature ventricular extrastimulus can reset the reentry. An early impulse enters the circuit and advances the subsequent wave front exiting the circuit. A flat, increasing, or mixed pattern of the

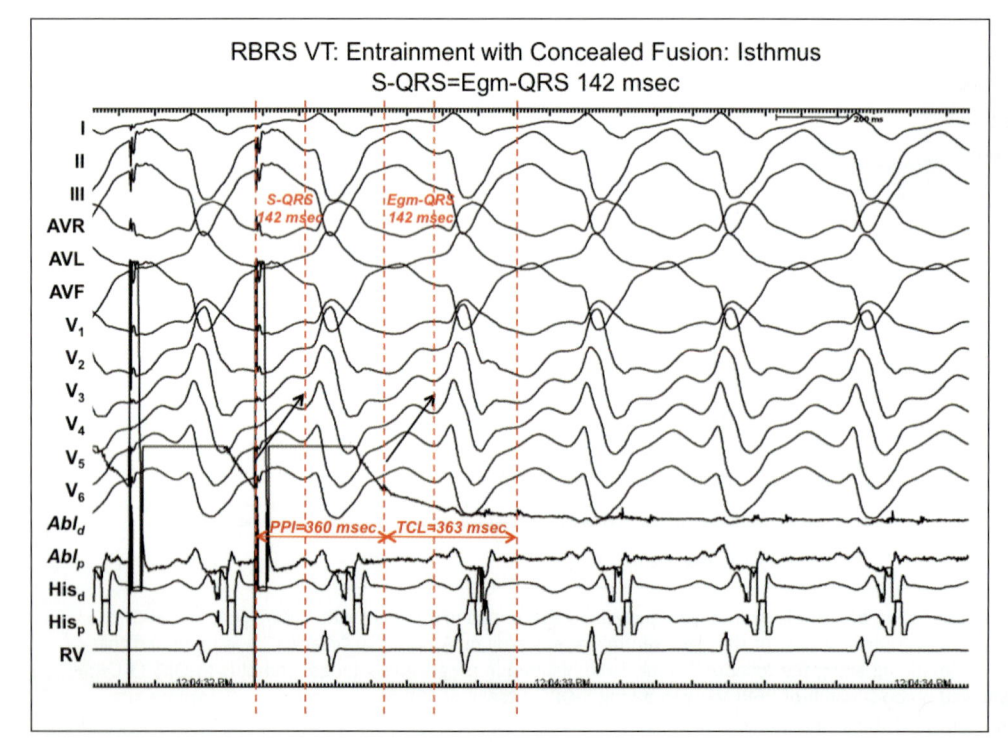

Figure 35.7 MDP recordings during sustained monomorphic VT. The ECG and intracardiac EGMs during overdrive pacing at central isthmus site were shown. Fractionated MDPs were recorded during sustained reentry. During entrainment, pacing accelerated all EGMs and QRS complexes to the pacing cycle length. There was no change in QRS morphology during entrainment, consistent with concealed fusion. The last pacing stimulus to the first noncaptured EGM after pacing, the PPI was 360 ms that matched the TCL. The S-QRS interval was 142 ms, which matched the EGM-to-QRS interval during VT. The S-QRS/EGM-QRS was ~39% of the VT cycle length consistent with pacing at the central isthmus of the circuit.

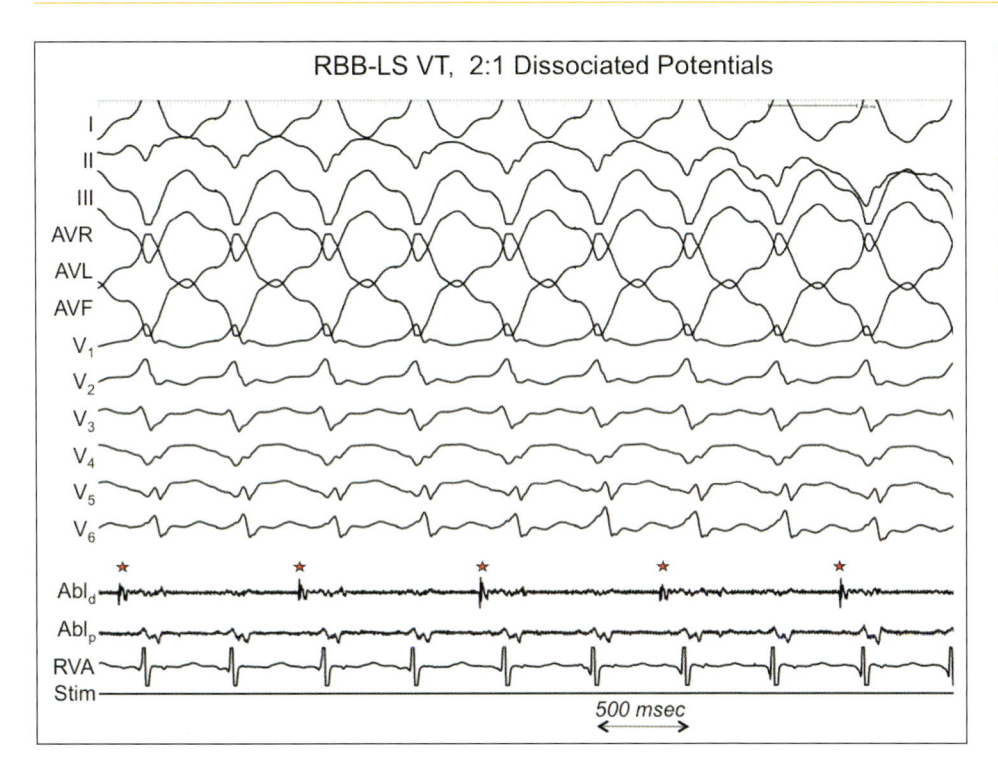

Figure 35.8 Two to one dissociated potential during a RBLS axis VT. The diastolic potentials with 2:1 conduction ratio were recorded at the distal ablation catheter electrodes. These diastolic potentials were dissociated and obviously not related to the VT reentrant circuit.

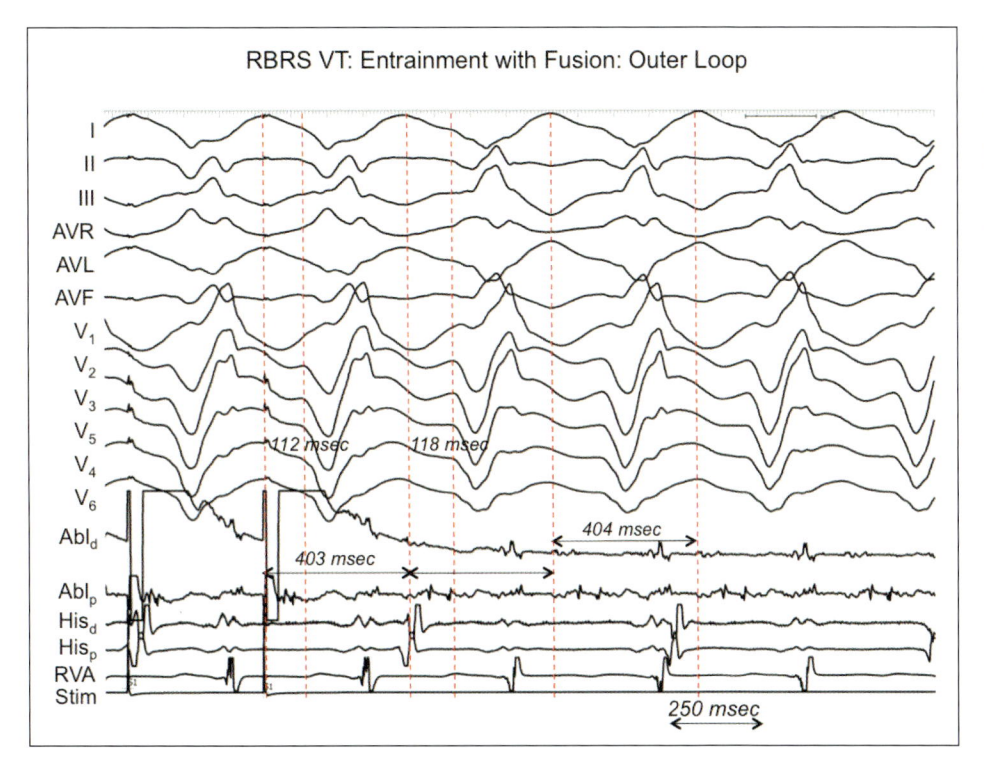

Figure 35.9 Overdrive pacing during VT with entrainment at the outer loop site was shown. Fractionated mid-diastolic potentials were recorded during VT. Pacing accelerated all intracardiac EGMs and the QRS complexes to the pacing cycle length. QRS fusion with changes in QRS morphology during overdrive pacing was shown. The PPI was 403 ms, which matched the VT cycle length (404 ms) and was consistent with pacing at a site in the reentry circuit. These findings suggested the site was at the outer loop site (EGM-QRS = S-QRS = 112 ms).

returned cycle (RC) slope can be defined. Such resetting response establishes the presence of an excitable gap and confirms the mechanism of reentry.[34-37]

Entrainment is the continuous resetting of the reentry by overdrive pacing during the tachycardia. Similar to the single beat resetting, pacing at a slightly faster rate than the tachycardia accelerates all QRS complexes and local ventricular EGMs to the pacing rate, and cessation of pacing is followed by resumption of the same tachycardia.[38] When pacing from sites outside the reentry circuit, entrainment can be confirmed by (1) the presence of constant QRS fusion during rapid pacing at a constant rate except for the last captured beat, which is entrained but not fused, (2) the presence of progressive QRS fusion during different pacing rates (**Figure 35.10**), or (3) evidence of local conduction block terminating the tachycardia.[39] Establishment of entrainment can distinguish reentry from other mechanisms (automaticity or triggered activity) (**Figure 35.11**).

The ventricular TCL should be measured immediately before overdrive stimulation, and entrainment pacing should be performed at 20 to 30 ms shorter than the VT cycle length. Excessively faster pacing rates (< 50 ms shorter cycle length) should be avoided as they may induce decremental conduction delay within the circuit with erroneous return cycle measurements or result in termination of reentry. Appropriate pacing rates and duration are required to ensure adequate capture of the tachycardia. If adequate capture and acceleration of the tachycardia circuit cannot be ascertained, a slightly faster (10 ms faster) or longer overdrive pacing duration should be attempted. Unipolar pacing is preferable although bipolar output is acceptable. Entrainment pacing should be performed at a minimum output just above the threshold for consistent local capture (with capture of the local EGMs). High-output pacing often results in anodal capture that depolarizes tissues outside the circuit (**Table 35.2**). Of note, inadequate outputs or poor catheter contact may result in intermittent loss of capture of the tachycardia and can easily be misinterpreted as entrainment without fusion.

In addition to distinguishing reentry from nonreentrant arrhythmia mechanisms, entrainment is an essential tool to identify the relationship of the pacing site to the reentry circuit (**Table 35.3**). Entrainment with overdrive pacing during VT can be quickly assessed by analyzing the (1) PPI, (2) surface QRS, (3) comparison of stimulus-QRS vs. EGM-QRS intervals, and (4) stimulus-QRS as a percentage of the TCL (S-QRS/TCL).

Postpacing Interval (PPI)

After cessation of overdrive pacing, the PPI is measured from the last pacing stimulus that accelerated the VT to the next noncaptured local potential at the pacing site (Figures 35.7 and 35.9). Similar to resetting response to a single extrastimulus, the PPI is equivalent to the returned cycle (RC), and three patterns of the PPI can also be observed. At relatively long paced cycle lengths that capture the VT, a constant return cycle (PPI) with a fully excitable gap can be demonstrated (Figure 35.10). At rapid paced cycle lengths, there is an increase in the return cycle with progressive prolongation in the PPI with each incremental paced beat until a longer equilibrium PPI is reached or the tachycardia terminates.[40]

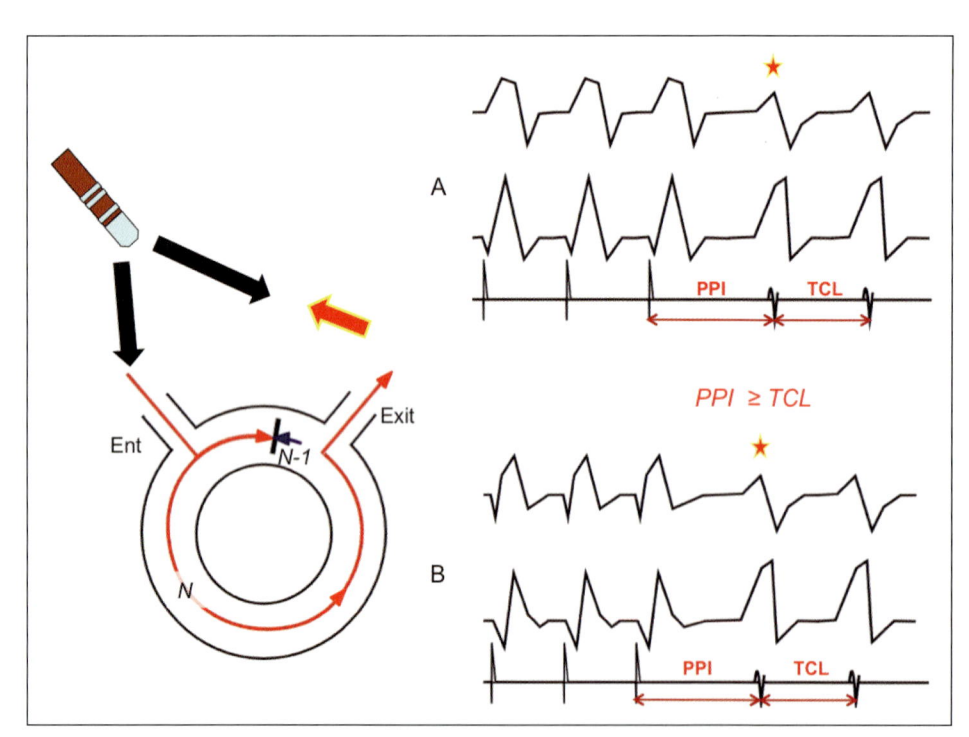

Figure 35.10 A schematic representation of entrainment. Pacing impulse from a site outside of the circuit propagates toward the reentry circuit, enters the circuit, and results in the both orthodromic and antidromic wave fronts (left panel). The orthodromic wave front (N, red arrow) resets tachycardia, whereas the antidromic wave front collides with the orthodromic wave front of the previous beat (N–1, blue arrow). **A.** Pacing from sites outside the reentry circuit results in QRS fusion with activation of myocardial tissues by both the paced wave fronts (large black arrow, N) and the previous wave front existing from the VT circuit (large red arrow, N–1). While entrainment pacing at a constant cycle length continues, the amount of fusion by both the pacing and VT exiting wave fronts is the same and results in "constant fusion." The last captured beat (star) is entrained but not fused. The PPI measures the conduction time from the pacing site to the reentry circuit, from entrance to exit, and back to the recording electrode. PPI is therefore longer than the conduction time around the reentry circuit (~TCL). **B.** At a faster pacing cycle length, more tissues are activated by the paced wave front than the VT circuit, and this results in a different activation pattern with "progressive fusion" and a different QRS morphology.

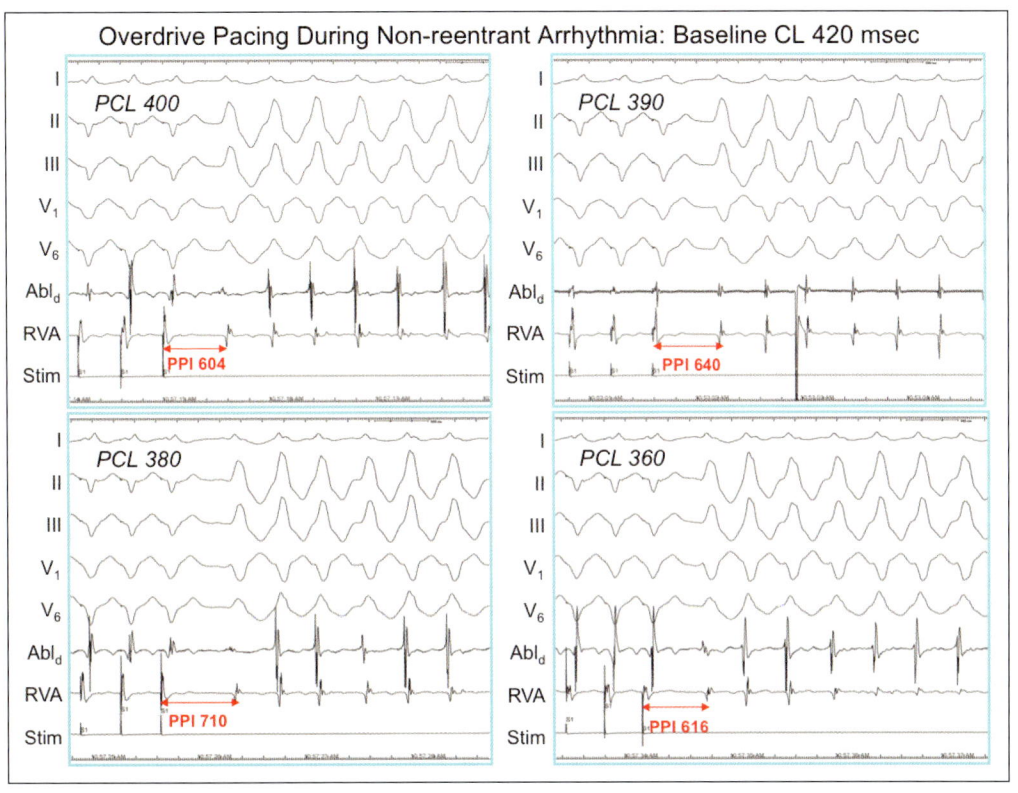

Figure 35.11 Overdrive pacing during a nonreentrant arrhythmia in a patient with an idiopathic VT originating from the right ventricular outflow tract (RVOT). The 12-lead ECG and the intracardiac EGMs during overdrive pacing at 400 ms, 390 ms, 380 ms, and 360 ms were shown. The PPIs at different overdrive pacing cycle length were not constant, suggesting the arrhythmia was not entrained and was not based on a reentrant mechanism.

The postpacing interval reflects the distance of the pacing site from the reentrant circuit. Pacing at sites remote from the circuit, PPI must be longer than the TCL as additional conduction time is required for impulse propagation from the pacing electrode to the circuit and back from the circuit to the pacing site (Figure 35.10). The PPI-TCL difference is therefore an indicator of the proximity of the pacing site to the reentrant circuit.

Pacing at sites within the circuit (entrance, isthmus, exit, or outer loop) during reentry produces two wave fronts of propagation. The paced orthodromic wave front (N) propagates through the circuit and resets the tachycardia. The antidromic wave front travels in the opposite direction in the circuit and collides with the orthodromic wave front of the previous beat (N–1). One revolution time around the reentry circuit (TCL) equals the postpacing interval, and the PPI-TCL difference should be less than 30 ms (**Figure 35.12**).[41]

Within the scar substrate, multicomponent, fractionated EGMs are often recorded during VTs, and the PPI should be measured to the local potential that is captured by pacing stimuli. It is important to distinguish near-field recordings of local tissue depolarization from the far-field

Table 35.2 Tips and Tricks of Entrainment Mapping

(1) Anodal capture of sites outside of the reentrant circuit: use minimal output to capture use unipolar pacing
(2) No local capture: not paced fast enough as VT rate changes not captured due to too low output
(3) Incorrect interpretations of entrainment results: PPI off due to too-fast pacing anodal capture with changing QRS catheter instability
(4) Use the proximal electrogram signals as surrogate recordings
(5) Use "N+1" method to assess entrainment if local EGM is not visible.

Table 35.3 Use of Entrainment to Delineate the Reentrant VT Circuits

(1) At sites within a circuit: PPI = TCL S-QRS = EGM-QRS (assumed equivalent latencies)
(2) At sites outside of a circuit: PPI > TCL S-QRS > EGM-QRS
(3) Use other intracardiac electrogram recordings as surrogates/references

PPI: post-pacing interval; TCL: tachycardia cycle length
S-QRS: stimulus to QRS intervals
EGM-QRS: local electrogram to QRS intervals

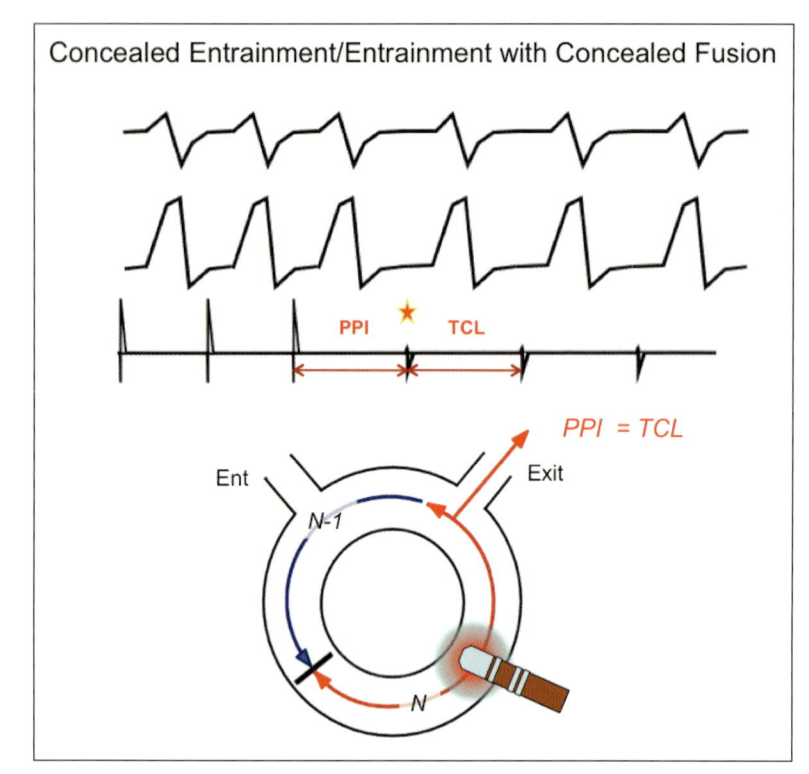

Figure 35.12 A schematic representation of entrainment with concealed fusion. Pacing at sites within the circuit during reentry produces 2 wave fronts of propagation. The orthodromic wave front (N, red arrow) propagates through the circuit and resets the tachycardia. The antidromic wave front collides with the previous reentry beat (N–1, blue arrow). The PPI is measured from the last paced stimulus to the first noncaptured local potential that is reset by pacing stimuli (star). The PPI equals to 1 revolution time around the reentry circuit that is approximated by the TCL, thus PPI = TCL. Since the overdrive pacing occurred within the "protected" corridor in the circuit, no surface QRS fusion is observed, and thus the entrainment is "concealed."

EGMs from depolarization of tissue adjacent or remote from the recording site. The largest potentials may not represent the local recordings, which may be of very low amplitude (Figure 35.7). Far-field potentials are not captured by pacing stimuli and can often be identified and separated from the stimulus artifact during pacing.

When the local EGM is obscured after the last pacing stimulus artifact, the PPI can be measured from the proximal electrode pair of the mapping catheter as a surrogate marker (**Table 35.2**). Alternatively, the PPI can be measured by the "N+1 method" using reliable references (QRS or other intracardiac recordings) of the second beat after the stimulus (**Figure 35.13**).[42]

QRS Fusion

The QRS morphology during entrainment indicates whether the pacing site is likely to be in a protected corridor (exit, isthmus, entrance, and bystander sites). Entrainment from a site outside the protected corridor produces manifested fusion that is the product of both paced wave front and the wave front that exits from the reentrant circuit (Figure 35.10). The degree of the fusion depends on the extent of the tissues activated by the 2 activation wave fronts. The morphology of a fused QRS can provide useful information on the location of the pacing site relative to the exit site. Pacing from the sites near the exit, minimal QRS fusion is observed compared to distinctly manifested QRS fusion with pacing from distant locations (Figure 35.10).

When pacing within the protected corridor of a reentrant circuit, tachycardia can be entrained without changing the QRS morphology because the paced orthodromic wave front (N) emerges from the circuit the same way as the spontaneous tachycardia. The paced antidromic wave front collides with the previous orthodromic wave front (N–1) within the circuit without recognizable QRS fusion on the ECG (concealed) (Figure 35.13). The presence of entrainment with concealed fusion indicates that the pacing site is located within a protected zone of slow conduction; however, adjacent bystander sites must be excluded.

Stimulus-to-QRS and EGM-to-QRS Intervals

With comparable wave front of propagation, the pacing stimulus to QRS onset (stimulus-to-QRS: S-QRS) interval indicates the conduction time from the pacing site to the circuit exit and should be the same as the interval from the EGMs recorded at that site to the QRS onset (exit) (EGM-QRS) interval. This holds true for sites along the reentry activation wave front (entrance, isthmus, exit and outer loop).[41] However, pacing at the adjacent bystander site off the main path of the reentry usually results in a longer S-QRS interval compared to the EGM-QRS despite "concealed" entrainment without QRS fusion (**Figure 35.14**).

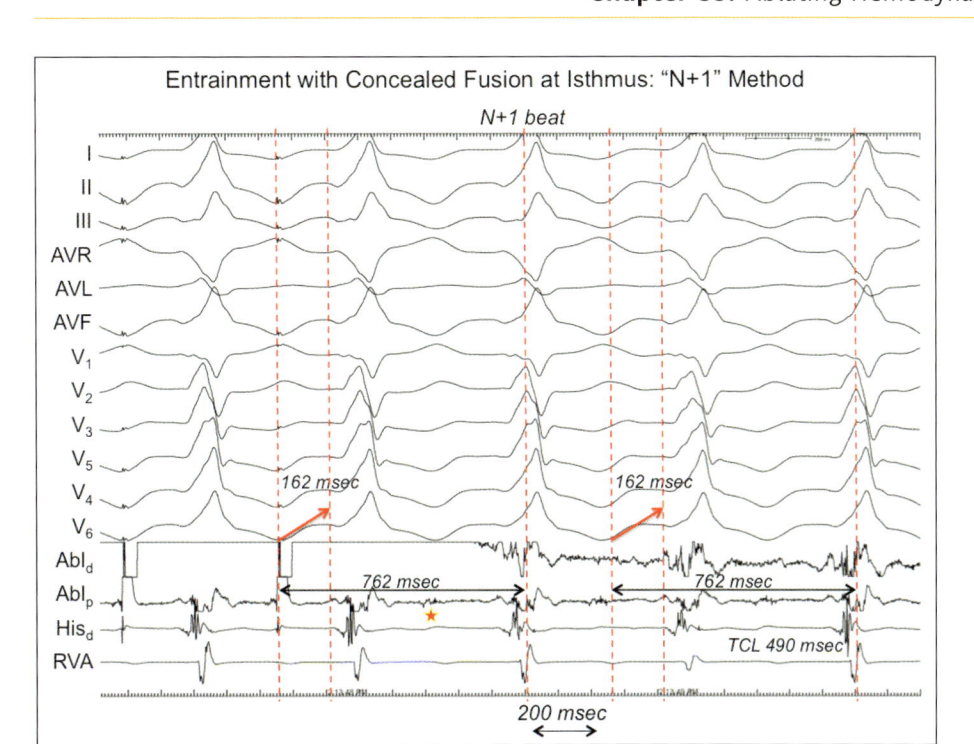

Figure 35.13 Entrainment with "N+1" method. The 12-lead ECG and the intracardiac recordings during a LBBB VT with a cycle length of 490 ms were shown. Overdrive pacing accelerated all EGMs and QRS complexes to the pacing cycle length. There was no change in QRS morphology during entrainment, consistent with entrainment with concealed fusion. However, the PPI was difficult to measure due to small signal amplitude at the distal electrode recording and pacing stimuli artifacts. The N+1 method for assessing the entrainment response was applied. The interval from the last pacing stimulus to the second postpacing right ventricular apical (RVA) EGM after stimulus was 762 ms. This measurement was compared to the interval from the local EGM at the stimulus site in any following beat to the second RVA EGM after this local EGM. The tachycardia was entrained since both intervals were the same (762 ms). A very low-amplitude signal was recorded on the proximal electrode (star). The S-QRS interval equaled the EGM-to-QRS interval at 162 ms. The S-QRS/TCL ratio was ~33%, consistent with an isthmus site. Ablation at this site resulted in immediate VT termination.

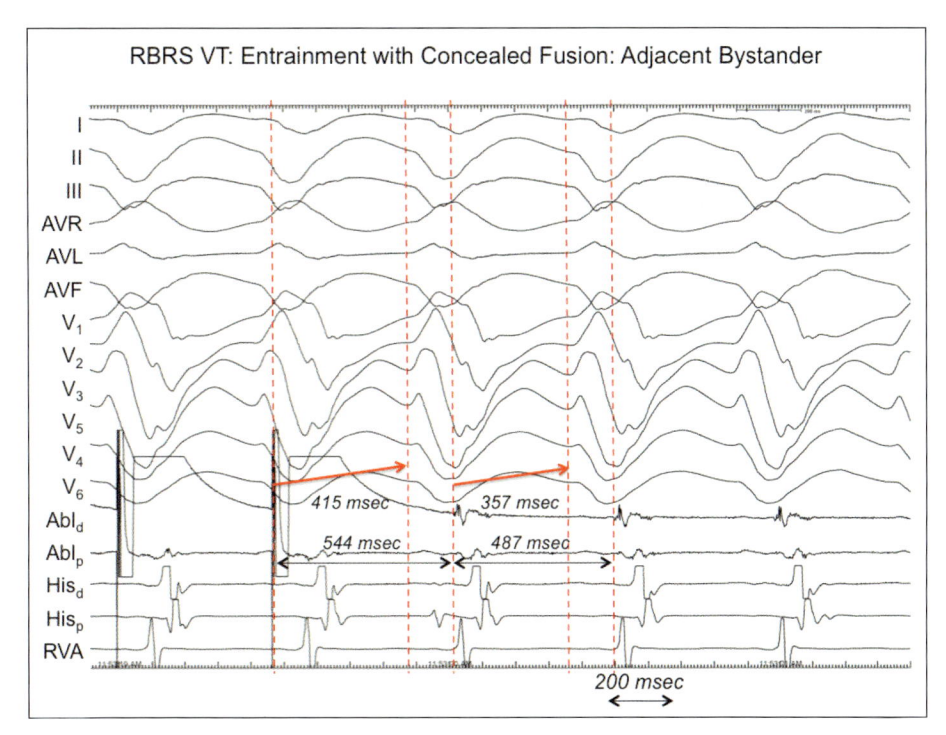

Figure 35.14 The 12-lead ECG and intracardiac recordings of entrainment pacing at an adjacent bystander site were shown. Pacing accelerated all EGMs and QRS complexes to the pacing cycle length. There was no change in QRS morphology during entrainment, consistent with entrainment with concealed fusion. The PPI was 544 ms, which was longer than the VT cycle length. The interval of the S-QRS was 415 ms, which was longer than the EGM-QRS interval. These findings suggested the pacing site was located at an adjacent bystander site.

S-QRS/TCL

The stimulus-to-QRS (S-QRS) intervals can also be interpreted as a percentage of the TCL. This identifies the relative locations within the reentrant circuit. The S-QRS interval gets progressively longer from the exit, to the isthmus, to the entrance sites. The exit is arbitrarily defined by an S-QRS/TCL ratio of < 30%, the central isthmus by a ratio of 30%-50%, the entrance site by an S-QRS/TCL ratio of 50%-70%, and the inner loop site by an S-QRS/TCL ratio of > 70% (**Figure 35.15**). Locations where ablation is most likely to interrupt reentry are those with features of isthmus sites with an S-QRS/TCL less than 70% of the VT cycle length and with an isolated potential.[32]

Pacing stimulation occasionally produces VT termination without global capture (**Figures 35.16 and 35.17**). Such finding of "noncapture termination" suggests local capture of the tissue within the protected isthmuses without depolarizing the surrounding myocardium and is generally a desirable surrogate target for ablation. Similarly, mechanical termination of VT due to catheter pressure can also be an indication that the catheter is located at the isthmus.

Ablation

The optimal target site for ablation is the central isthmus as it is most likely to interrupt reentry, although the exit site is also acceptable. For hemodynamically tolerated VT, ablation during sustained arrhythmia is desirable as termination of VT provides further evidence that the ablation site is in the tachycardia circuit. However, the isthmuses can be relatively broad and may require multiple radiofrequency energy applications to successfully transect the isthmus.[43]

After locations of the VT circuit (exit, isthmus, and entrance) have been identified, linear ablation lesions should be deployed extending from the exit site into the scar (< 0.5 mV), targeting the isthmuses (0.2–0.3 mV).

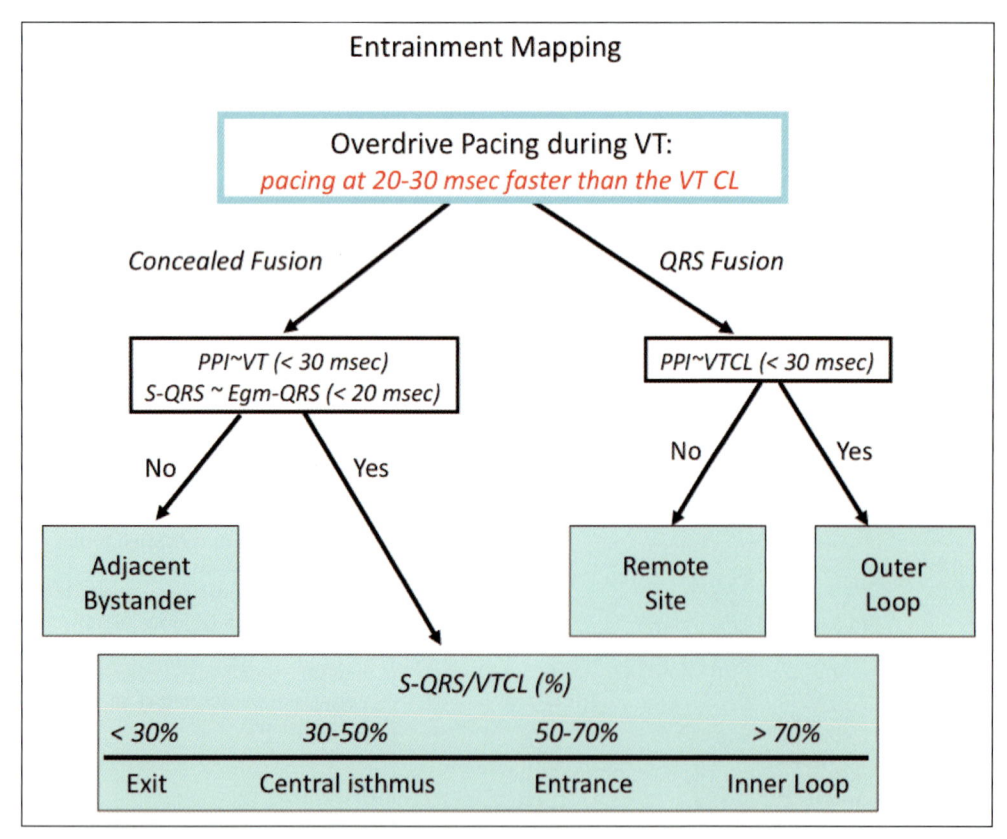

Figure 35.15 A flow diagram for the entrainment mapping. Overdrive pacing at 20–30 ms faster than the VT CL is performed. After adequate capture is confirmed by acceleration of the local signals and surface QRS to the pacing rate, changes of the surface QRS morphology during pacing are analyzed. When pacing within the "protected corridor" of the circuit (exit, isthmus, entrance, inner loop, and adjacent bystander sites), concealed fusion without changes of surface QRS is observed. The postpacing interval (PPI), the stimulus-to-QRS interval (S-QRS), and the local EGM-to-QRS (EGM-QRS) interval are then measured. When the PPI equals the VTCL, or the S-QRS is equal to the EGM-QRS intervals, the pacing site is located within the reentry circuit/wave front. The adjacent bystander site is defined by a PPI > TCL and/or a S-QRS > EGM-QRS. The S-QRS interval is expressed as a percentage of the TCL that describes the different locations within the circuit and relative to the reentry arrhythmia. If pacing entrains VT with QRS fusion and the PPI is consistent with a reentry circuit site (PPI = TCL), the site is classified as an outer loop site. Pacing at remote sites distant from the circuit results in QRS fusion and long PPIs that exceed the TCL.

Figure 35.16 Termination of VT without global capture. The 12-lead ECG and intracardiac recordings were shown. Stimulation from the ablation catheter was delivered at a site with diastolic potentials. Although the pacing stimuli did not capture the ventricle, VT was terminated (star). Such "sub-threshold" stimulation that terminated the reentry without global QRS activation suggested local tissue capture within the critical isthmus that interrupted the reentry.

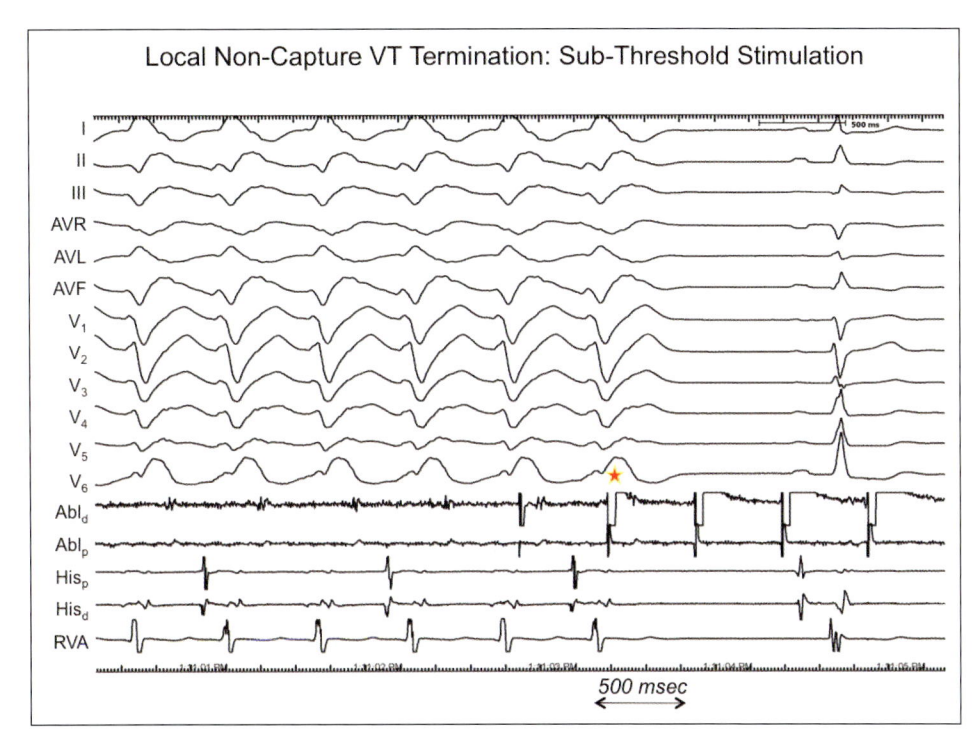

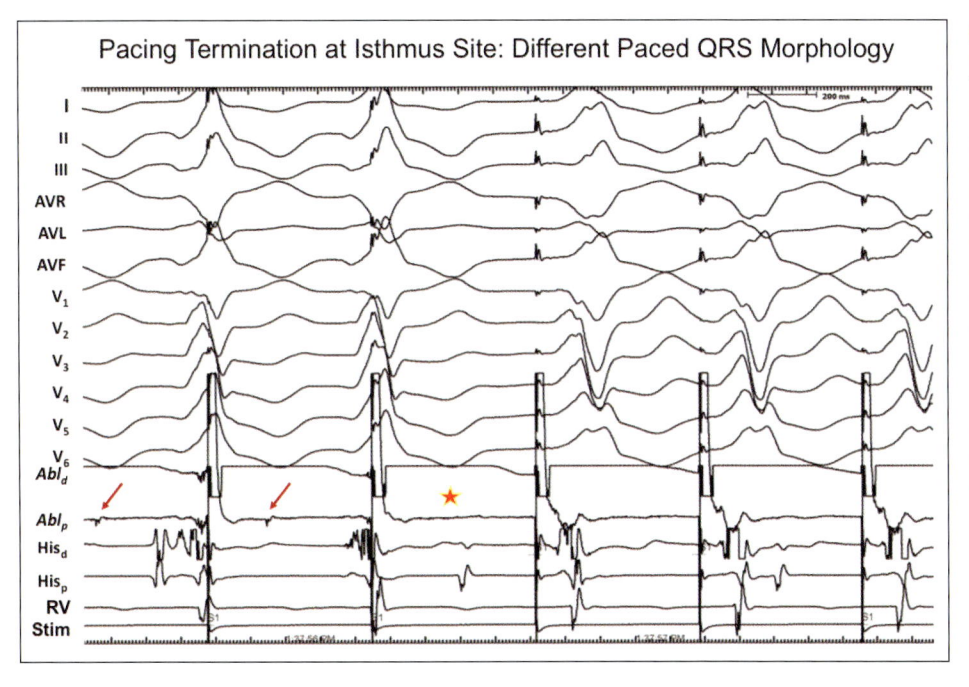

Figure 35.17 Termination of VT by a local capture at isthmus site. The 12-lead ECG and intracardiac recordings were shown. Overdrive pacing at a site with mid-diastolic potentials captured the local potential (star) and terminated the VT without QRS manifestation. Subsequent pacing showed different QRS morphologies from that of the VT. This indicated that local tissue capture interrupted the reentry within the protected corridor but pace mapping did not produce a perfect pace match, perhaps due to antidromic wave front emerging from the entrance or capturing adjacent tissues.

Multiple ablation lines, either parallel or perpendicular to the "exit" are often needed for successful substrate modification. Ablation energy delivery should be focused within areas of low EGM voltage to minimize damages to the normal myocardium. Ablation lines can be also deployed connecting between the dense scars (EUS) and/or connecting the scar to other anatomical obstacles such as a mitral valve annulus. Noncapture by high-output pacing (10 mA/2 ms) helps to confirm the effect of the ablation lesions.

Ablation Endpoint and Assessment

The acute effect of ablation is categorized into (1) noninducibility, (2) inducible but modified VTs with different morphologies and cycle lengths that are faster than the previously "targeted" VTs, and (3) persistently inducible, clinically sustained monomorphic VTs. After ablation, noninducibility of clinical VT is associated with a lower risk of VT recurrence, compared with persistent inducibility of the clinical VT.[44] The elimination of all VTs seems to be associated with a lower risk of recurrence but remains controversial.[45,46] The minimum ablation endpoint is termination and noninducibility of the "target" VT by programmed stimulation. Despite occasional arrhythmia recurrences, catheter VT ablation has been shown to be an effective therapy that markedly reduces the overall frequency/burden of recurrent VTs.[47]

Postprocedure Care

Standard postoperative care protocol is recommended. Protamine may be given to help reverse the heparin, and access sheaths can be pulled once the ACT is less than 180 seconds. A large net-positive fluid balance is expected when using irrigated-tip catheters for extensive endocardial ablations. Additional diuretics and heart failure assessment, including echocardiographic assessments, are often required in patients with advanced ventricular dysfunction.

Postoperative anticoagulation is recommended after endocardial VT ablation for a duration of ~1 month. Oral warfarin or dabigatran can be started the day of the procedure for stroke prevention and minimizing thromboembolic complication. Lovenox, or low-molecular-weight heparin, is generally not required to "bridge" these patients. In all other patients (right ventricular ablation, epicardial ablation, patients who are poor candidates for anticoagulation), aspirin (325 mg daily) is recommended.

In patients with pacemakers or ICDs, a postoperative device interrogation is essential to ensure stable lead parameters and device function. Catheter manipulations can cause lead dislodgement or lead damage, and radiofrequency energy delivery near the lead tip may result in elevation of pacing threshold and generator malfunction.[48] Based on the result of ablation procedure, ICD reprogramming may be needed to accommodate changes in lead thresholds/device function and to minimize underdetections of slower VTs.

Follow-up

Patients are followed closely after VT ablation, typically every 3 to 4 months. Antiarrhythmic drug therapy is often maintained for several months even after successful VT ablation. However, simplification of multiple antiarrhythmic drug regimen and/or reduction of amiodarone dosage should be considered. ICDs (or pacemakers) may need to be reprogrammed to ensure detection of "slower" VTs. The device should be interrogated to detect any arrhythmia recurrences. Serial device interrogation data can be very helpful for managing patients' antiarrhythmic drug regimen and assessment of the overall VT burden.

Of 55 consecutive patients with structural heart disease (38 ICM and 17 NICM patients) referred for VT ablation at our institution between 2009 and 2010, 11% had only mappable VTs, 64% had only unmappable VTs, and 25% had both mappable and unmappable VTs. During EP procedures, 160 VT morphologies were induced, consisting of 32 (20%) mappable VTs and 128 (80%) unmappable VTs. The ablation was successful in eliminating all but 1 mappable VT at the end of procedures. At the 3-month follow-up, 76% of patients who had mappable VTs are free of any VT recurrence, including 6 of 6 patients who had only mappable VTs.

Procedural Complications

In a multicenter trial of 226 patients with structural heart disease, VT ablation with open-irrigation catheters had a procedure-related mortality rate of 3%. Most death was due to uncontrollable VT (2.6%), and one patient died of tamponade.[47] Nonfatal significant complications rate was 7.3%, which included heart failure (2.6%) and mitral regurgitation exacerbation in 1 patient (0.4%). No patient had a thromboembolic complication or stroke.

In a multicenter trial of 146 patients with mappable VT, VT ablation with internal irrigation catheters had a procedure-related mortality of 2.7% that included 1 stroke, 1 tamponade, 1 valve injury, and 1 myocardial infarction due to coronary embolus.[45] Major procedure-related complications occurred in 8%, with stroke or transient ischemic attack occurring in 2.7%.

Conclusion

Catheter ablation is indicated in patients with recurrent episodes of VTs that are not controlled by antiarrhythmic drug therapy and required frequent ICD shocks. Although VT ablation for hemodynamically stable VT remains a challenging procedure, it can be performed safely and successfully with careful planning and using a hybrid strategy of both conventional mapping technique and substrate characterization. A thorough understanding and proficiency in entrainment are essential for detailed mapping of hemodynamically stable VTs.

References

1. Schron EB. Quality of life in the antiarrhythmics versus implantable defibrillators trial: impact of therapy and influence of adverse symptoms and defibrillator shocks. *Circulation*. 2002;105(5):589–594.
2. Moss AJ, Greenberg H, Case RB, et al. Long-term clinical course of patients after termination of ventricular tachyarrhythmia by an implanted defibrillator. *Circulation*. 2004;110(25):3760–3765.
3. Connolly SJ, Dorian P, Roberts RS, et al. Comparison of beta-blockers, amiodarone plus beta-blockers, or sotalol for prevention of shocks from implantable cardioverter defibril-

lators: the optic study: a randomized trial. *JAMA.* 2006; 295(2):165–171.
4. Horowitz LN, Josephson ME, Harken, AH. Epicardial and endocardial activation during sustained ventricular tachycardia in man. *Circulation.* 1980;61(6):1227–1238.
5. Hsia HH, Callans DJ, Marchlinski FE. Characterization of endocardial electrophysiological substrate in patients with NICM and monomorphic ventricular tachycardia. *Circulation.* 2003;108(6):704–710.
6. Soejima, K, Stevenson, WG, Sapp, JL, Selwyn, AP, Couper, G, and Epstein, LM, Endocardial and epicardial radiofrequency ablation of ventricular tachycardia associated with dilated cardiomyopathy: the importance of low-voltage scars. *J Am Coll Cardiol.* 2004;43(10):1834–1842.
7. Cano O, Hutchinson M, Lin D, et al. Electroanatomic substrate and ablation outcome for suspected epicardial ventricular tachycardia in left ventricular nonischemic cardiomyopathy. *J Am Coll Cardiol.* 2009;54(9):799–808.
8. Sacher F, Roberts-Thomson K, Maury P, et al. Epicardial ventricular tachycardia ablation a multicenter safety study. *J Am Coll Cardiol.* 2010;55(21):2366–2372.
9. Nazarian S, Bluemke DA, Lardo AC, et al. Magnetic resonance assessment of the substrate for inducible ventricular tachycardia in nonischemic cardiomyopathy. *Circulation.* 2005;112(18):2821–2825.
10. Bogun FM, Desjardins B, Good E, et al. Delayed-enhanced magnetic resonance imaging in nonischemic cardiomyopathy: utility for identifying the ventricular arrhythmia substrate. *J Am Coll Cardiol.* 2009;53(13):1138–1145.
11. Marchlinski FE, Zado E, Dixit S, et al. Electroanatomic substrate and outcome of catheter ablative therapy for ventricular tachycardia in setting of right ventricular cardiomyopathy. *Circulation.* 2004;110(16):2293–2298.
12. Verma A, Kilicaslan F, Schweikert RA, et al. Short- and long-term success of substrate-based mapping and ablation of ventricular tachycardia in arrhythmogenic right ventricular dysplasia. *Circulation.* 2005;111(24):3209–3216.
13. Garcia FC, Bazan V, Zado ES, Ren JF, Marchlinski FE. Epicardial substrate and outcome with epicardial ablation of ventricular tachycardia in arrhythmogenic right ventricular cardiomyopathy/dysplasia. *Circulation.* 2009;120(5):366–375.
14. Miller JM, Marchlinski FE, Buxton AE, Josephson ME. Relationship between the 12-lead electrocardiogram during ventricular tachycardia and endocardial site of origin in patients with coronary artery disease. *Circulation.* 1988;77(4):759–766.
15. Berruezo A, Mont L, Nava S, Chueca E, Bartholomay E, Brugada J. Electrocardiographic recognition of the epicardial origin of ventricular tachycardia. *Circulation.* 2004;109(15):1842–1847.
16. Daniels D, Lu Y, Morton J, Santucci P, Akar J, Green A, Wilber D. Idiopathic epicardial left ventricular tachycardia originating remote from the sinus of valsalva: electrophysiological characteristics, catheter ablation, and identification from the 12-lead electrogram. *Circulation.* 2006;113(13):1659–1666.
17. EHRS/HRS expert consensus on catheter ablation of ventricular arrhythmias. *Heart Rhythm.* 2009;6(6):886–933.
18. Yoshida K, Liu TY, Scott C, Hero A, Yokokawa M, Gupta S, Good E, Morady F, and Bogun F. The value of defibrillator electrograms for recognition of clinical ventricular tachycardias and for pace mapping of post-infarction ventricular tachycardia. *J Am Coll Cardiol.* 2010;56(12):969–979.
19. Khaykin Y, Skanes A, Whaley B, et al. Real-time integration of 2d intracardiac echocardiography and 3d electroanatomical mapping to guide ventricular tachycardia ablation. *Heart Rhythm.* 2008;5(10):1396–1402.
20. Hsia HH. Epicardial ventricular tachycardia ablation an evolution of needs. *J Am Coll Cardiol.* 2010;55(21):2373–2375.
21. Marchlinski FE, Callans DJ, Gottlieb CD, Zado E. Linear ablation lesions for control of unmappable ventricular tachycardia in patients with ischemic and NICM. *Circulation.* 2000;101(11):1288–1296.
22. Verma A, Marrouche N, Schweikert R, et al. Relationship between successful ablation sites and the scar border zone defined by substrate mapping for ventricular tachycardia post-myocardial infarction. *J Cardiovasc Electrophysiol.* 2005;16(5):465–471.
23. Hsia H, Lin D, Sauer W, Callans D, Marchlinski F. Anatomic characterization of endocardial substrate for hemodynamically stable reentrant ventricular tachycardia: identification of endocardial conducting channels. *Heart Rhythm.* 2006;3:503–512.
24. Arenal A, Glez-Torrecilla E, Ortiz M, et al. Ablation of electrograms with an isolated, delayed component as treatment of unmappable monomorphic ventricular tachycardias in patients with structural heart disease. *J Am Coll Cardiol.* 2003;41:81–92.
25. Bogun F, Good E, Reich S, et al. Isolated potentials during sinus rhythm and pace-mapping within scars as guides for ablation of post-infarction ventricular tachycardia. *J Am Coll Cardiol.* 2006;47(10):2013–2019.
26. Hsia H, Lin D, Sauer W, Callans D, Marchlinski F. Relationship of late potentials to the ventricular tachycardia circuit defined by entrainment. *J Interv Card Electrophysiol.* 2009;26:21–29.
27. Brunckhorst C, Delacretaz E, Soejima K, Maisel W, Friedman P, Stevenson W. Identification of the ventricular tachycardia isthmus after infarction by pace mapping. *Circulation.* 2004;110:652–659.
28. Soejima, K, Stevenson W, Maisel W, Sapp J, Epstein L, Electrically unexcitable scar mapping based on pacing threshold for identification of the reentry circuit isthmus: feasability for guiding ventricular tachycardia ablation. *Circulation.* 2002;106:1678–1683.
29. Soejima K, Suzuki M, Maisel WH, et al. Catheter ablation in patients with multiple and unstable ventricular tachycardias after myocardial infarction: short ablation lines guided by reentry circuit isthmuses and sinus rhythm mapping. *Circulation.* 2001;104(6):664–669.
30. Arenal A, del Castillo S, Gonzalez-Torrecilla E, et al. Tachycardia-related channel in the scar tissue in patients with sustained monomorphic ventricular tachycardias: influence of the voltage scar definition. *Circulation.* 2004;110(17):2568–2574.
31. Bogun F, Bahu M, Knight BP, et al. Comparison of effective and ineffective target sites that demonstrate concealed entrainment in patients with coronary artery disease undergoing radiofrequency ablation of ventricular tachycardia. *Circulation.* 1997;95(1):183–190.

32. Kocovic D, Harada T, Friedman P, Stevenson W. Characteristics of electrograms recorded at reentry circuit sites and bystanders during ventricular tachycardia after myocardial infarction. *J Am Coll Cardiol.* 1999;34:381–388.
33. Patel VV. Right bundle-branch block ventricular tachycardias: septal versus lateral ventricular origin based on activation time to the right ventricular apex. *Circulation.* 2004;110(17):2582–2587.
34. Almendral JM, Stamato NJ, Rosenthal ME, Marchlinski FE, Miller JM, Josephson ME. Resetting response patterns during sustained ventricular tachycardia: relationship to the excitable gap. *Circulation.* 1986;74(4):722–730.
35. Rosenthal ME, Stamato NJ, Almendral JM, Gottlieb CD, Josephson ME. Resetting of ventricular tachycardia with electrocardiographic fusion: incidence and significance. *Circulation.* 1988;77(3):581–588.
36. Stamato NJ, Frame LH, Rosenthal ME, Almendral JM, Gottlieb CD, Josephson ME. Procainamide-induced slowing of ventricular tachycardia with insights from analysis of resetting response patterns. *Am J Cardiol.* 1989:63(20):1455–1461.
37. Gottlieb CD, Rosenthal ME, Stamato NJ, Frame LH, Lesh MD, Miller JM, Josephson ME. A quantitative evaluation of refractoriness within a reentrant circuit during ventricular tachycardia: relation to termination. *Circulation.* 1990;82(4):1289–1295.
38. Waldo AL. From bedside to bench: entrainment and other stories. *Heart Rhythm.* 2004;1(1):94–106.
39. Waldo AL. Atrial flutter: entrainment characteristics. *J Cardiovasc Electrophysiol.* 1997;8(3):337–352.
40. Callans DJ, Hook BG, Josephson ME. Comparison of resetting and entrainment of uniform sustained ventricular tachycardia. Further insights into the characteristics of the excitable gap. *Circulation.* 1993;87(4):1229–1238.
41. Stevenson WG, Khan H, Sager P, Saxon LA, Middlekauff HR, Natterson PD, Wiener I. Identification of reentry circuit sites during catheter mapping and radiofrequency ablation of ventricular tachycardia late after myocardial infarction. *Circulation.* 1993;88(4 Pt 1):1647–1670.
42. Soejima K, Stevenson WG, Maisel WH, Delacretaz E, Brunckhorst CB, Ellison KE, Friedman PL. The n + 1 difference: a new measure for entrainment mapping. *J Am Coll Cardiol.* 2001;37(5):1386–1394.
43. Tanimoto K, Hsia H. Pace mapping for the confirmation of bidirectional block after mitral isthmus ablation in a patient with inferior myocardial infarction (abstr). *J Arrhythmia.* 2010;26(Suppl):17.
44. O'Donnell D, Bourke JP, Furniss SS. Standardized stimulation protocol to predict the long-term success of radiofrequency ablation of postinfarction ventricular tachycardia. *Pacing Clin Electrophysiol.* 2003;26(1 Pt 2):348–351.
45. Calkins H, Epstein A, Packer D, et al. Catheter ablation of ventricular tachycardia in patients with structural heart disease using cooled radiofrequency energy: results of a prospective multicenter study. Cooled RF Multicenter Investigators Group. *J Am Coll Cardiol.* 2000;35(7):1905–1914.
46. Della Bella P, De Ponti R, Uriarte JA, et al. Catheter ablation and antiarrhythmic drugs for haemodynamically tolerated post-infarction ventricular tachycardia; long-term outcome in relation to acute electrophysiological findings. *Eur Heart J.* 2002;23(5):414–424.
47. Stevenson WG, Wilber DJ, Natale A, et al. Irrigated radiofrequency catheter ablation guided by electroanatomic mapping for recurrent ventricular tachycardia after myocardial infarction: the Multicenter Thermocool Ventricular Tachycardia Ablation Trial. *Circulation.* 2008;118(25):2773–2782.
48. Lakkireddy D, Patel D, Ryschon K, et al. Safety and efficacy of radiofrequency energy catheter ablation of atrial fibrillation in patients with pacemakers and implantable cardiac defibrillators. *Heart Rhythm.* 2005;2(12):1309–1316.

CHAPTER 36

How to Map and Ablate Unstable Ventricular Tachycardia: The University of Pennsylvania Approach

Wendy S. Tzou, MD; Francis E. Marchlinski, MD

Introduction

Ventricular tachycardia most commonly occurs in the setting of structural heart disease, with patients with prior myocardial infarction and chronic coronary artery disease comprising the majority of cases.[1] However, individuals with nonischemic heart disease, including NICM and ARVC),[2-4] can have large areas of scar that lead to VT. In all of these patients, the predominant mechanism for VT is reentry. The presence of surviving myocardium intermixed within the scar provides the appropriate milieu for reentry to initiate and propagate in areas with (1) fixed or functional unidirectional block, and (2) slow conduction that permits recovery of previously depolarized tissue.

Due to limitations in antiarrhythmic drugs or ICDs,[5-8] percutaneous catheter mapping and ablation has evolved as an alternative and effective treatment strategy for the management of these often challenging cases.[9-11] Critical VT circuit elements can be identified and targeted successfully with ablation as long as the VT is inducible and hemodynamically tolerated. However, the vast majority of clinical VTs are "unmappable." This chapter will delineate the approach utilized by the EP Program at the Hospital of the University of Pennsylvania for ablation of unstable VT.

Preprocedural Planning

Surface ECG

We scrutinize available surface ECGs for clues about underlying disease substrate, scar burden, and, when possible, potential VT site(s) of origin. In sinus rhythm, the presence of Q waves in contiguous leads or ST elevations in absence of acute ischemia suggests the presence of prior myocardial infarction or aneurysm, and helps identify locations of potential VT substrates (described in detail in another chapter). The presence of a widened QRS at baseline, which may be a marker of His-Purkinje disease, suggests a predisposition for bundle-branch reentry or fascicular VT. A pronounced R wave in V_1 along with a pronounced S wave in V_6 in the absence of marked conduction disturbances suggests presence of basal-lateral scar in a patient with NICM.[12] Discovering epsilon waves or T-wave inversions in the right-sided precordial leads should heighten suspicion for ARVC, particularly in a younger person with multiple VT morphologies. In both of the latter situations, one should be prepared for possible epicardial in addition to endocardial ablation.[4,13] Further clues from an ECG in VT in a patient with NICM that may suggest the need for an epicardial approach include Q waves in lead I, along with an absence of Q waves in the inferior leads, a pseudo–delta wave of ≥ 75 ms, and a maximum-deflection index of ≥ 0.59, all of which are highly sensitive and specific for a basal and superior lateral epicardial focus.[14] Finally, an ECG acquired during VT not only assists in preprocedural planning but aids in the procedure itself (described below).

Noninvasive Cardiac Imaging

We obtain noninvasive cardiac imaging in all patients planning to undergo VT ablation. This is particularly helpful when no ECGs of VT exist. Information verifying extent of underlying disease, ventricular function and dimensions, scar or aneurysm location, and any significant valvular disease is important in procedural planning. Echocardiography has traditionally been the mainstay for acquiring all of this information; nuclear scintigraphy is often additionally helpful in verifying substrate information and to assess for active ischemia. We are increasingly performing cardiac MRI in patients presenting with VT, as it is a more sensitive tool for assessing for nontransmural scar in NICM.[15,16] Presence of an ICD or pacemaker has long been a contraindication for performing an MRI, but our center and several other centers have shown that it can be done safely in those who are not pacemaker dependent.[17,18] There are, however, limitations in image quality and interpretation due to artifact from the ICD pulse generator and right ventricular lead. The optimal approach, when possible, is to obtain the MRI prior to device implantation.

ICD Electrogram

In patients with ICDs, stored information during the VT episodes should be carefully reviewed. The number of events, both nonsustained and those resulting in therapy, can guide urgency with which subsequent medical care is executed. Additionally, device-recorded intracardiac EGMs may be especially helpful for (1) determining if there is potential utility of catheter ablative therapy, and (2) to help target ablation if a surface 12-lead ECG of the clinical VT is not available. Events predominated by polymorphic VT, for instance, may be less amenable to ablation unless a reproducible PVC trigger is evident that may be targeted. Depending on patient stability, one could consider NIPS testing through the device to see if any VT is induced whose intracardiac EGM resembles those stored from spontaneous clinical events in order to identify on 12-lead ECG the VT that has occurred clinically.

Additional Preparation

Before pursuing more invasive evaluation and treatment, a recent evaluation of the presence and status of coronary artery disease and determination of LV function and reserve, either noninvasively, as described above, or via cardiac catheterization, is important. Deaths related to the procedure are often due to underestimation of the importance of ischemic burden prior to and volume overload during the procedure. Documentation of anticoagulation status and exclusion of an unstable LV thrombus with echocardiography also are important. Identification of vascular access problems prior to the procedure facilitates its success and safety. Presence of severe arterial or aortic valvular disease, including mechanical prosthesis, will require a transseptal approach to the LV. Prior cardiac surgery and prior pericarditis may limit or preclude epicardial access and mapping/ablation. Details of present and past antiarrhythmic therapy are also important. Ideally, discontinuation of antiarrhythmic therapy for at least 5 half-lives should occur before the procedure, although this is often not possible because of the unstable nature of our patients. Furthermore, the EP effects of amiodarone often cannot be reversed due to its long half-life, even if the drug were stopped several days before the procedure. The results of programmed stimulation and subsequent mapping maneuvers should be interpreted with this knowledge.

Procedure

Patient Preparation

We initiate most VT ablations using conscious sedation or MAC, due to occasional difficulty in arrhythmia induction and the hypotension that can result from deeper levels of sedation. Occasionally, intubation and general anesthesia are necessary at the outset due to patient discomfort or ongoing or anticipated instability. In the setting of marginal hemodynamic stability and/or severe disease at baseline, additional mechanical support may also be initiated at the outset if not already present. This is usually accomplished by IABP insertion, as long as there is not severe peripheral arterial disease or aortic insufficiency. At our institution, this procedure has been increasingly performed in our EP laboratory, occasionally with the assistance of the interventional cardiologists. VT ablation can and is also performed in patients with surgically placed ventricular assist devices. Placement of temporary ventricular assist devices (eg, Impella, Abiomed Inc., Danvers, MA, or TandemHeart PTVA, CardiacAssist, Inc., Pittsburgh, PA) to provide support during ablation is now also an option; these may also be inserted percutaneously.

Foley urinary catheters are placed in all patients, given the long procedure lengths and significant volume administered with irrigated-tip ablation, and to accurately track urine output. The latter is particularly important in management of patients with severe ventricular dysfunction. Two sets of defibrillation pads, anterior-posterior and lateral, are often placed to prepare for shock-refractory VT/VF. The chest and upper abdomen are sterilely prepped if epicardial mapping and ablation are anticipated. If present, the patient's ICD is reprogrammed to disable tachycardia detection and therapies, after placement of ECG electrodes and external defibrillation pads. Baseline pacing mode is usually changed to maximize intrinsic ventricular conduction. However, presence of significant bradycardia, high-grade AV block, or ventricular ectopy may make continuous ventricular pacing preferable. Importantly, the ICD programmer remains in communication with the patient throughout the case, so that instantaneous intracardiac EGMs can be recorded during induced or spontaneously occurring VTs.

Vascular Access and Catheter Placement

The standard catheters used for ablation of LV VT include a quadripolar catheter for placement in the apical RV, an ICE catheter, and an ablation catheter. Occasionally, simultaneous recordings of His, RA, and/or CS signals are desired, in which case vascular access to accommodate additional quadripolar or decapolar catheters is obtained. We generally place sheaths that are at least 1-Fr caliber larger than the catheter that will be inserted within them to allow for continuous fluid and/or drug infusions via the sheath side ports. In general, each femoral vein can accommodate in the range of up to two 11.5-Fr or two 7-Fr and one 11-Fr sheaths.

Depending on whether retrograde aortic or transseptal approach to the left ventricle is planned, vascular access is obtained either via the RFA or the RFV, respectively. A short 8- or 9-Fr sheath is initially placed and exchanged later for a longer (transseptal or braided) sheath, if indicated. In the standard LV VT ablation, we also insert 7-Fr and 9-Fr sheaths in the LFV, for the RV quadripolar and standard ICE catheters, and up to 1 additional (eg, a 7-Fr catheter for a dynamic decapolar catheter) if necessary. Another 4-Fr catheter is often placed in the LFA in cases where IABP insertion is not performed at the outset, to facilitate urgent insertion during the case if needed. In the case of LV transseptal access, this also functions as a means to continuously monitor arterial blood pressure during the case. If RV mapping or ablation is anticipated, an 8-Fr sheath is placed in the RFV, which can later be exchanged for a longer sheath if necessary. Occasionally, either initial or continuous pulmonary artery pressure recordings are obtained using a balloon-tipped catheter, to assist in hemodynamic monitoring.

Once sheaths are in place, heparin is initiated (bolus of 100 to 120 U/kg and infusion of 12-15 U/kg/min). The ACT is checked every 15 to 30 minutes during the procedure, with additional heparin bolus and drip titrated as needed to maintain an ACT of 250 to 300 seconds (350–400 seconds for transseptal cases).

ICE imaging is performed at baseline to assess for anatomical features (eg, valvular disease, wall motion abnormalities, LV size and overall function, and presence of pericardial effusion) and throughout the case to monitor for acute complications, as well as to assist in mapping and ablation. ICE is particularly helpful in confirming adequate catheter contact when mapping or ablating in the proximity of the papillary muscles (**Figure 36.1**). Finally, ICE is also a valuable tool in assisting with transseptal puncture when required and can be used to actually track lesion formation.

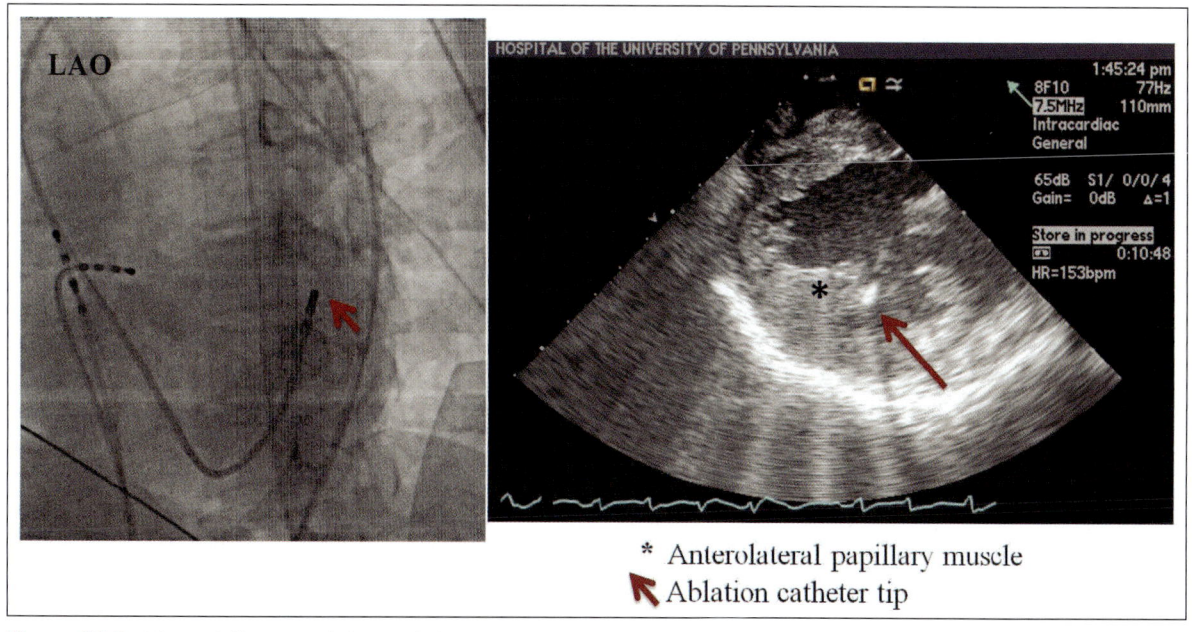

Figure 36.1 The LAO fluoroscopic image (left panel) depicts the ablation catheter at roughly the site of the anterolateral papillary muscle, although good contact is difficult to confirm. Only with simultaneous visualization of the catheter tip on ICE (right panel) is adequate contact with the papillary muscle confirmed.

Retrograde Aortic Versus Transseptal LV Access

The retrograde aortic approach is the preferred method for LV access, even when an IABP is present. Exceptions to this include presence of severe peripheral arterial, aortic, and/or severe aortic valvular disease. Also, in some cases, ablation of VT suspected to originate from the LV septum might be performed with greater contact and catheter stability using the transseptal method. In patients with CAD, known mild to moderate peripheral arterial disease, or elderly patients with tortuous vessels, we frequently exchange the short sheath placed in the RFA for a 45- to 65-cm-long, 8- or 9-Fr braided sheath (Arrow, Teleflex Medical, Research Triangle Park, NC), over a long, stiff, J-tipped wire (eg, Amplatz, Cook Medical, Bloomington, IN) under fluoroscopic guidance. Care is made to prevent the sheath or wire from crossing the aortic valve, to minimize the amount of hardware that can cross and potentially damage valve leaflets. This is usually only a consideration when using the 65-cm-long sheath. In the absence of these characteristics, mapping and ablation through the initially placed short sheath is preferable.

Transseptal puncture is performed under ICE and fluoroscopic guidance once heparin has been initiated, as above. For VT ablation, we often use a large-curve Agilis or LAMP90 Transseptal (St. Jude Medical, St. Paul, MN) sheath with a transseptal needle (BRK Transseptal, St. Jude Medical). LA access is obtained with manual pressure once the sheath and needle assembly are seen to tent the IAS with the LPVs and LAA in view. A somewhat more anterior approach than is used for pulmonary vein isolation is preferred, to better direct the sheath toward the left ventricle. Pressure transduced through the needle tip is additionally observed throughout this maneuver to confirm successful LA access.

We typically use a ThermoCool 3.5-mm-tip catheter (Biosense Webster, Inc., Diamond Bar, CA) for VT ablation. A standard F-curve radius is usually sufficient. However, if an LV outflow tract or cusp VT is suspected, a D curve may be more effective and allow for greater maneuverability in more confined spaces. Conversely, for maneuvering within a severely dilated ventricle, a J curve may provide greater reach. Increasingly, we have been using bidirectional catheters, because they often allow for greater maneuverability, especially when choosing a catheter with differing radius per direction (eg, F-J curve).

VT Induction

Particularly when no 12-lead ECGs of the clinical VT exist, we routinely attempt to induce VT. Depending on the clinical situation, this may be performed before, during, or after electroanatomic mapping is completed. If epicardial mapping is anticipated, we typically perform programmed stimulation after acquisition of the endocardial map. Similar to the goals of NIPS testing described above, we aim to see if there is a VT induced that matches the ICD EGM VT morphology. This may help to define our "clinical" or principally targeted VTs, and guide our mapping and ablation strategy. In addition, limited activation and entrainment mapping can sometimes be performed by positioning the mapping catheter at a suspected site of importance based on analysis of the 12-lead ECG of VT and regions of abnormal bipolar voltage just before VT induction. During VT and in the short interval before hemodynamic instability necessitates arrhythmia termination, mid-diastolic potentials at that or immediately adjacent sites often can be quickly characterized.

Methods for programmed electrical stimulation (PES) vary significantly. Pacing for 8 beats with basic drive cycle lengths of 600 and 400 ms followed by the introduction of 1 to 3 extrastimuli is generally the most accepted protocol. On occasion a short-long-short stimulation sequence may be advantageous. This stimulation has been described for the induction of bundle branch reentry but can be used for the induction of other VT associated with structural heart disease that is not induced with a more standard stimulation protocol. Burst pacing or sympathetic stimulation, for instance with isoproterenol infusion or stress testing, is often more useful for inducing arrhythmias based on triggered activity. Specific VT morphologies may require unique VT sites of stimulation. We have found that VTs with an RBBB morphology may frequently require stimulation from the lateral left ventricle.

Endocardial Mapping

A detailed, endocardial, electroanatomical voltage map is created, typically using CARTO (Biosense Webster, Diamond Bar, CA), with efforts initially focused on areas of known infarction or scar based on prior imaging. Using well-characterized bipolar voltage criteria of > 1.5 mV for identifying normal signal amplitude recorded from the LV endocardium,[19] we identify regions of bipolar voltage consistent with densely scarred myocardium or aneurysm (< 0.5 mV), border zone of scar (0.5–≤1.5mV), and healthy myocardium (> 1.5 mV). Similar criteria are utilized for bipolar RV mapping. The epicardial bipolar voltage cutoff for defining abnormal is kept at 1.0 mV.[13] Importantly, we recently found that unipolar voltage can also be helpful in revealing areas of deeper, that is midmyocardial or epicardial, substrate abnormalities (< 8.3 mV in the LV and < 5.5 mV in the RV).[20,21] After the bipolar voltage map is constructed, we then also examine the unipolar voltage, particularly when there is a disparately normal amount of endocardial bipolar voltage compared to the LVEF, or when the suspected VT exit occurs in an area of preserved bipolar voltage (**Figure 36.2**).

As the voltage map is being created, we also annotate regions of double potentials and/or LPs during sinus or

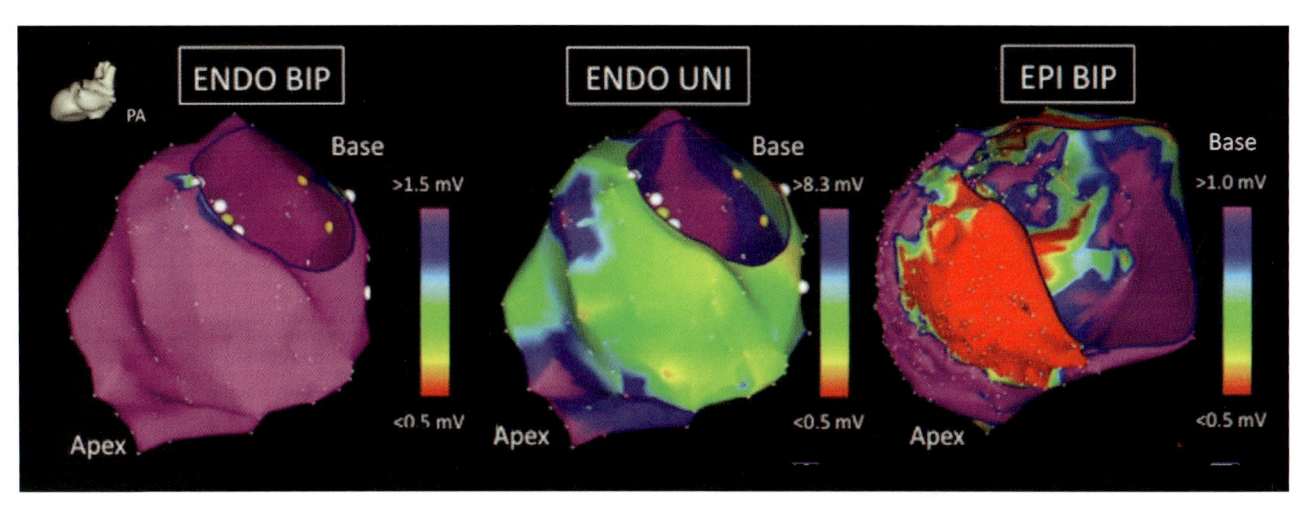

Figure 36.2 Shown are electroanatomic voltage maps of the left ventricle in posterior-anterior (PA) projection from a patient with nonischemic cardiomyopathy. The endocardial bipolar voltage (ENDO BIP) is normal. However, the endocardial unipolar voltage (ENDO UNI) map shows extensive periannular low voltage suggesting deeper (mid-myocardial and/or epicardial) scar and arrhythmia substrate. The subsequent epicardial bipolar voltage (EPI BIP) corroborates the abnormalities suggested by the ENDO UNI map. (Adapted from Hutchinson et al., Circ Arrhythm Electrophysiol. 2011;4:49–55, with permission.)

paced ventricular rhythm (**Figure 36.3**). LP are defined as distinct bipolar EGMs that are inscribed after the end of the surface QRS complex, and separated from the major initial component of the local ventricular EGM by an isoelectric interval. They are felt to represent delayed activation within diseased myocardium and have often been found at critical sites within reentrant VT circuits.[22,23] Often, pacing at these sites is performed to try to glean clues about potential exit or isthmus sites, based on (1) how well the pace map matches clinical VT 12-lead surface ECG or ICD EGM VT morphologies and (2) the time from pacing stimulus to QRS (stim-QRS).[24]

Pace mapping is also performed, regardless of presence of LP, from suspected site of origin or exit along border of the scar during sinus rhythm to identify site(s) at which the paced QRS morphology mimics that observed during VT (**Figure 36.4**). There are important limitations to recognize when using pace mapping to localize the VT exit site. The paced QRS morphology may not accurately reflect the VT site of origin and may not identify the appropriate sites for ablation. Bidirectional conduction from the pacing site during sinus rhythm may differ from the unidirectional wave front of activation during VT reentry. Furthermore, the output used to capture during pacing can influence the pattern of ventricular activation. Because of the increased size of the virtual electrode, higher outputs during pace mapping may produce a different-paced QRS morphology in sinus rhythm even when pacing within a critical site of the VT circuit. Nevertheless, pace mapping can approximate the exit site of the VT circuit as it leaves the border of the scar, and it is a generally accepted method for mapping when more detailed options are limited because of poor hemodynamic intolerance or noninducibility of VT.

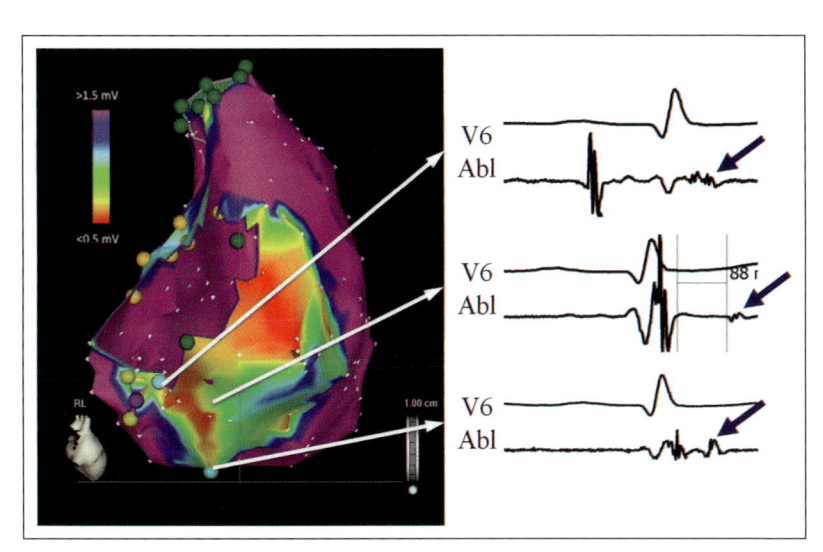

Figure 36.3 RL projection of a RV endocardial bipolar-voltage map is depicted from a patient with RV cardiomyopathy. Found within the area of low voltage around the lateral tricuspid annulus/RV free wall are examples of LPs.

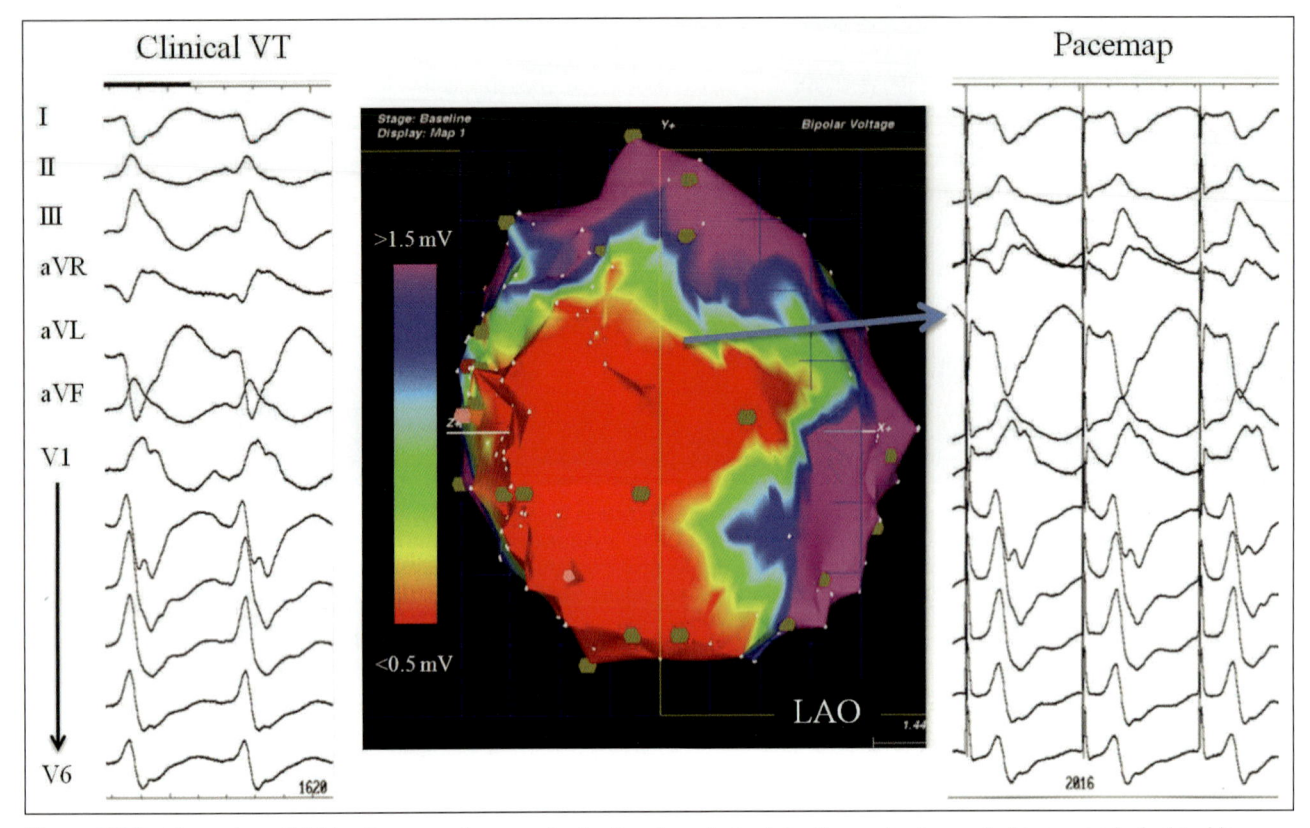

Figure 36.4 The endocardial LV voltage map from a patient with prior anterior infarction and antero-apical aneurysm is depicted in the middle panel (LAO projection). The patient's clinical VT is shown in the 12-lead ECG in the left panel. Coupling knowledge of the VT morphology and LV scar distribution, a VT exit along the anterior-lateral scar border zone (arrow) can be predicted. Indeed, pace map from the region of suspect exit resulted in a perfect match for the clinical VT.

Finally, in some cases, viable channels of conducting myocardium may be identified on the completed bipolar-voltage map by decreasing the color range, in order to highlight narrow channels of larger voltage surrounded by areas of extremely low voltage (**Figure 36.5**).[24,25] Such potential "conducting channels" can be more readily identified during RV pacing in the absence of ongoing VT.[26] Fractionated EGMs, with isolated delayed and/or multiple components, are often seen at isthmus sites; however, these low-amplitude signals may be obscured in sinus rhythm due to depolarization of the surrounding larger mass of more normal myocardium. Changing the direction of depolarization compared to sinus rhythm, for instance with pacing, has been observed to better elucidate these signals and potential channels of conduction, and we occasionally utilize this technique as an adjunct to the other mapping techniques described above.

Epicardial Mapping

In as many as 32% of cases, essential VT circuit components are localized to the subepicardium[27,28] and are not able to be eliminated with endocardial ablation, even using irrigated-tip energy. Features that compel us to proceed with epicardial mapping include (1) discovery of no or a small area of endocardial bipolar-voltage abnormalities, (2) discovery of a larger area of endocardial unipolar abnormalities compared to the bipolar-voltage abnormalities, (3) history of NICM, ARVC, or prior failed endocardial ablation, and/or (4) surface 12-lead ECG VT features[14,29,30] that suggest epicardial site of origin.

Methods for epicardial access are detailed in another chapter. We use the technique developed by Sosa and colleagues.[31] If LV endocardial ablation has been performed beforehand, or if patients are on chronic coumadin, anticoagulation is reversed completely. Once pericardial access has been confirmed, a long sheath (such as a short Agilis, St. Jude Medical) can be advanced with the dilator over the guide wire. Once the dilator and wire are removed, the ThermoCool catheter can then be inserted, and mapping and ablation can proceed.

Similar mapping techniques to those described for the endocardial approach are used, except that the bipolar-voltage cutoff for normal epicardial myocardium is > 1.0 mV.[13] The presence and typical distributions of epicardial fat should be considered in interpreting data. Low-voltage recordings in the absence of EGM fractionation or late potentials, particularly if in the predicted distribution of a major coronary artery or valve annulus, should lead one to suspect location within fat rather than abnormal epicardial tissue.[13]

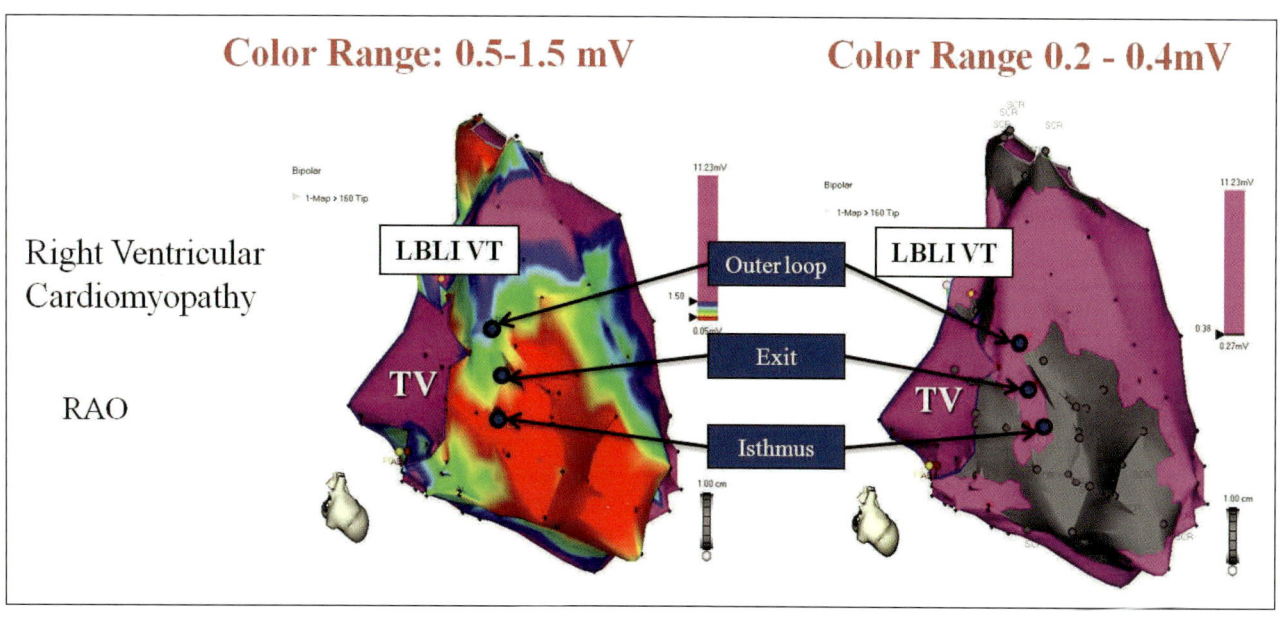

Figure 36.5 RAO projections of bipolar endocardial voltage maps are shown from a patient with right ventricular cardiomyopathy and a VT of left bundle, left axis, and inferiorly directed morphology (LBLI VT). Entrainment maneuvers identifying VT outer loop, exit, and isthmus sites are shown on the voltage map in the left panel, with standard bipolar color range cutoffs intended to display scar border zone (0.5–1.5 mV). After adjusting the voltage color range to better contrast relatively preserved voltage areas against more densely scarred areas (right panel), a channel of conduction corresponding to the sites of critical VT circuit elements is identified (Adapted from Hsia et al., *Heart Rhythm.* 2006;3:503–512, with permission from Elsevier.)

Ablation

The goal of ablation in unmappable VT is to modify the arrhythmogenic substrate. Specifically, we aim to create lines of block with ablation in order to interrupt zones of slow conduction within abnormal myocardium that may have given rise to the clinical VT(s) observed. We concentrate efforts in areas believed to be clinically important, including regions of LP, good pace maps within abnormal myocardium, and/or uncovered channels of slow conduction. Our approach is to create ablation lines through these regions, connecting the lines either to the border between abnormal tissue and healthy myocardium or to an anatomical barrier, such as dense, unexcitable scar or a valve annulus. Special care is made to avoid ablating in normal tissue. In addition to creating lines, we typically extend clusters of lesions around areas of interest and late potentials. When late potentials are targeted for ablation, we frequently will remap the same area afterward to document elimination of the progressively activated late potentials. For many patients, this approach results in an extensive lesion set that effectively dissects and homogenizes the abnormal myocardium to prevent VT recurrences.

For both endocardial and epicardial ablations, we titrate the energy delivered through an irrigated-tip catheter between 20 and 50 W, to a maximum temperature of 42°C to 45°C, and achieve a 12- to 18-ohm impedance drop over 1 to 2 minutes per lesion. We find that these settings are safe and effective within areas of scar. Although definitive proof of block with any line of ablation can be difficult, endpoints that we frequently employ include (1) inability to capture at maximal pacing output in areas that had lower threshold preablation; (2) change in paced morphology at a given site postablation compared to preablation; and (3) noninducibility with subsequent programmed stimulation. Total procedural times are usually in the 4- to 8-hour range, but can be longer, especially when a large anatomic substrate is present, multiple VTs are inducible, and/or both endocardial and epicardial ablation are performed.

When ablating on the epicardium, care is made to avoid damaging the coronary arteries or phrenic nerve. Our approach is to perform coronary angiography prior to any epicardial VT ablation, including ablation from the CS, as the LCx often closely follows the venous course. Typically, the ablation catheter is positioned at the site of interest on the epicardium during the angiogram so that direct visualization and distance estimations can be made. Generally, ablation within 12 mm of any proximal or large coronary artery is avoided. To avoid damaging the phrenic nerve, its position can be delineated with bipolar pacing at 20 mA/2 ms pulse-width, particularly when ablation is anticipated in its usual course along the lateral LV. Areas of diaphragmatic stimulation then are marked using the electroanatomic mapping system. Because the phrenic nerve is not adherent to the epicardial surface, it can be lifted away to avoid damage caused by ablation that would otherwise be too close in proximity. This can be accomplished either by using an inflated angioplasty balloon catheter or by insufflations of a combination of air and saline.[32,33] Finally, as intrapericardial fluid accumulation from the open-irrigated-tip ablation catheter can lead to tamponade (the increased pericardial effusion is usually obvious on ICE before hemodynamic compromise occurs), it is important to periodically aspirate excess fluid from the sheath side port, or to leave it connected to continuous suction throughout the case.

Particularly frustrating are cases in which mid-myocardial substrate is found or presumed to predominate, after extensive endocardial and epicardial mapping has been performed. Alternatively, sometimes other critical structures (eg, the coronary arteries) may preclude safe ablation in the exact region of interest. In these cases, we often ablate from 2 or more adjacent sides of the target area and stay on for longer durations (sometimes up to 3 minutes) in the hopes that multidirectional, irrigated-tip lesions may extend deeply enough to penetrate to the critical region of interest, or at least barricade it off.

Postprocedure Care

Recovery

After ablation is completed, catheters are removed, transseptal or long venous sheaths, if used, are pulled into the IVC, and heparin is discontinued. A final ICE survey is performed to monitor for pericardial effusion. If epicardial ablation has been performed, we infuse intrapericardial steroids (2 mg/kg triamcinolone or equivalent) to dwell for a period of 10 minutes, to help prevent pericarditis and secondary development of adhesions should a repeat epicardial attempt be required.[34] The epicardial sheath, with a pigtail drain inserted through it over a wire and then attached to bulb suction, is usually left in place overnight. Protamine is given to reverse anticoagulation if ACT is > 250 seconds, and sheaths are removed once the ACT is < 180 seconds. The ICD is reprogrammed to enable tachycardia therapies and bradycardia therapies as deemed appropriate.

During this period, if an IABP was inserted during the procedure, we also assess whether ongoing IABP support is needed. If stable hemodynamics are observed with intermittent or no counterpulsation, the IABP is maintained at 1:1 while anticoagulation is reversed to prevent clot formation, and it is removed at the same time as the other femoral sheaths.

Patients are confined to bed rest in supine position for 6 hours after sheaths have been removed and hemostasis with manual compression is achieved. If no significant bleeding has occurred, anticoagulation with heparin is resumed at that point to maintain a PTT of 50 to 70 seconds for a period of at least 24 hours (longer if other reasons for long-term therapeutic anticoagulation with Coumadin exist).

The epicardial sheath and the pigtail drain are removed the following day if (1) no significant pericardial bleeding has occurred; (2) echocardiography the following morning shows no significant pericardial effusion (occasionally the pigtail and sheath can become clogged and give the false impression that no fluid exists because none can be aspirated); and (3) repeat echocardiography 4 hours after heparin has been initiated continues to show no pericardial effusion.

Follow-up

In the acute postprocedural period, these patients are typically monitored on telemetry for several additional days for further medical optimization before discharge. If possible, we continue to withhold antiarrhythmic drugs or resume one preablation drug at a decreased dose. We then usually perform NIPS via the implanted device 2 to 3 days following ablation to (1) assess for inducibility of clinical VT; (2) assess the efficacy of anti-tachycardia pacing on any VTs induced; and (3) optimize programming of the ICD device as needed to treat future potential spontaneous events. This period appears to be critical for the adequate assessment of ablation efficacy in patients on amiodarone prior to the procedure, as it allows for further drug washout. We will also establish a template with ICD EGMs and 12-lead ECGs of all VTs that remain inducible to facilitate follow-up. In the uncommon patient with the clinical VT still inducible at the end of the ablation procedure, we will typically bring the patient back to the EP laboratory for a repeat ablation, unless clinical circumstances are unfavorable, given the high likelihood of arrhythmia recurrence.

After discharge, patients are usually followed closely. Clinic visits at 6 weeks, 3 months, 6 months, then every 6 months after ablation are typically scheduled, either in our clinic or with the referring electrophysiologist. Device interrogations and assessment of symptoms suggestive of recurrence are performed at each visit.

Repeat Ablations

Although the outcomes of VT ablations at our institution have improved with the introduction of irrigated-tip ablation,[9] challenges remain in achieving long-term efficacy and vary widely by institution.[10,35] At our center, repeat ablations are required in approximately 30% of patients. It is important to remember that many of these patients have had long-standing ventricular arrhythmias that have failed multiple trials of antiarrhythmic drugs, most including amiodarone, by the time they present for ablation. Recent data would suggest that earlier intervention with ablation may improve long-term outcomes.[11,36] Nevertheless, we find that the ventricular arrhythmia burden is significantly reduced after ablation, with resumption of low-dose amiodarone or other antiarrhythmic therapy reserved for the more challenging or refractory cases.

Based on consideration of each patient's clinical situation, repeat ablation procedures are pursued if (1) spontaneous VTs occur during the inpatient monitoring period, (2) the clinical VT is easily inducible on NIPS, or (3) VT recurs occur after discharge. In general, the approach to repeat procedures is the same as for the initial. Particularly in those with extensive scar burden, we often find that other reentrant circuits become active after the initial predominant VT(s) have been eliminated. Recurrent conduction of previously targeted tissue is also common, especially among patients with mid-myocardial substrate or areas of calcified scar. Repeat epicardial access may be more difficult due to areas of adherent pericardial tissue, even if intrapericardial steroid was administered during the first procedure, but these challenges usually can be overcome. For instance, a slightly different approach for access may be attempted, or careful blunt dissection of adhesions encountered after access is obtained using the ablation catheter, sometimes with the assistance of a short, steerable sheath.

Procedural Complications

With continuous and often invasive hemodynamic, ICE, and other monitoring as described above, many potential complications can be detected early and managed proactively. We observe a ~0.5% to 2% risk for each of the major complications that include pericardial effusion requiring drainage, embolic stroke, vascular complications (eg, pseudoaneurysm, AV fistula, or hematoma) necessitating transfusion and/or surgical intervention, and volume overload and/or progressive hemodynamic deterioration despite presence of sinus rhythm. Less common (< 0.5%) potential complications include phrenic nerve injury, myocardial infarction, and death.

Conclusions

We have developed a successful approach for catheter ablation of unstable VT. Most VT in this context arises because of presence of scar and is reentrant in mechanism. By combining careful preprocedural planning, including cardiac imaging, analysis of ECG and ICD intracardiac VT recordings, with detailed 3-dimensional electroanatomical mapping, the substrate for VT can usually be well delineated. Additional information acquired during mapping, including identification of late potentials, preferred channels of conduction, and pace mapping can further hone the approach for ablation. Our procedural endpoints include acute noninducibility and/or evidence for conduction block during or immediately after ablation, all of which usually can be achieved with diligence and perseverance.

Many improvements can be made in terms of current ablation endpoints and procedural outcomes. We and others remain invested in helping to invent and improve methods to advance this effort.

References

1. Zipes D, Camm A, Borggrefe M, et al. ACC/AHA/ESC 2006 guidelines for management of patients with ventricular arrhythmias and the prevention of sudden cardiac death: a report of the American College of Cardiology/American Heart Association task force and the European Society of Cardiology committee for practice guidelines. *J Am Coll Cardiol.* 2006;48:e247–e346.
2. Hsia HH, Callans DJ, Marchlinski FE. Characterization of endocardial electrophysiological substrate in patients with nonischemic cardiomyopathy and monomorphic ventricular tachycardia. *Circulation.* 2003;108:704–710.
3. Marchlinski FE, Zado E, Dixit S, et al. Electroanatomic substrate and outcome of catheter abative therapy for ventricular tachycardia in setting of right ventricular cardiomyopathy. *Circulation.* 2004;110:2293–2298.
4. Garcia F, Bazan V, Zado ES, Ren JF, Marchlinski FE. Epicardial substrate and outcome with epicardial ablation of ventricular tachycardia in arrhythmogenic right ventricular cardiomyopathy/dysplasia. *Circulation.* 2009;120:366–375.
5. Randomized antiarrhythmic drug therapy in survivors of cardiac arrest (The CASCADE study). The CASCADE investigators. *Am J Cardiol.* 1993;72:280–287.
6. Connolly SJ, Hallstrom AP, Cappato R, et al., on behalf of the investigators of the AVID C, and CIDS studies. Meta-analysis of the implantable cardioverter defibrillator secondary prevention trials. *Eur Heart J.* 2000;21:2071–2078.
7. Connolly SJ, Dorian P, Roberts RS, et al. Comparison of beta-blockers, amiodarone plus beta-blockers, or sotalol for prevention of shocks from implantable cardioverter defibrillators: the OPTIC study: a randomized trial. *JAMA.* 2006;295:165–171.
8. Mason JW. A comparison of seven antiarrhythmic drugs in patients with ventricular tachyarrhythmias. *N Engl J Med.* 1993;329:452–458.
9. Sauer WH, Zado E, Gerstenfeld EP, Marchlinski FE, Callans D. Incidence and predictors of mortality following ablation of ventricular tachycardia in patients with an implantable cardioverter-defibrillator. *Heart Rhythm.* 2010;7:9–14.
10. Stevenson WG, Wilber DJ, Natale A, et al. Irrigated radiofrequency catheter ablation guided by electroanatomic mapping for recurrent ventricular tachycardia after myocardial infarction: the multicenter thermocool ventricular tachycardia ablation trial. *Circulation.* 2008;181:2773–2782.
11. Reddy VY, Reynolds MR, Neuzil P, et al. Prophylactic catheter ablation for the prevention of defibrillator therapy. *N Engl J Med.* 2007;357:2657–2665.
12. Tzou WS, Zado ES, Lin D, et al. Sinus rhythm ECG criteria associated with basal lateral ventricular tachycardia substrate in patients with nonischemic cardiomyopathy. *J Cardiovasc Electrophysiol.* 2011;22(12):1351–1358.
13. Cano O, Hutchinson M, Lin D, et al. Electroanatomic substrate and ablation outcome for suspected epicardial ventricular tachycardia in left ventricular nonischemic cardiomyopathy. *J Am Coll Cardiol.* 2009;54:799–808.

14. Vallès E, Bazan V, Marchlinski FE. ECG criteria to identify epicardial ventricular tachycardia in nonischemic cardiomyopathy. *Circ Arrhythm Electrophysiol.* 2010;3:63–71.
15. Wagner A, Mahrholdt H, Holly TA, et al. Contrast-enhanced MRI and routine single photon emission computed tomography (SPECT) perfusion imaging for detection of subendocardial myocardial infarcts: an imaging study. *Lancet.* 2003;361:374–379.
16. Gaitonde RS, Subbarao R, Michael MA, Dandamudi G, Bhakta D, Mahenthiran J, Das MK. Segmental wall-motion abnormalities of the left ventricle predict arrhythmic events in patients with nonischemic cardiomyopathy. *Heart Rhythm.* 2010;7:1390–1395.
17. Nazarian S, Roguin A, Zviman MM, et al. Clinical utility and safety of a protocol for noncardiac and cardiac magnetic resonance imaging of patients with permanent pacemakers and implantable-cardioverter defibrillators at 1.5 tesla. *Circulation.* 2006;114:1277–1284.
18. Naehle CP, Strach K, Thomas D, et al. Magnetic resonance imaging at 1.5-t in patients with implantable cardioverter-defibrillators. *J Am Coll Cardiol.* 2009;54:549–555.
19. Marchlinski FE, Callans DJ, Gottlieb CD, Zado ES. Linear ablation lesions for control of unmappable ventricular tachycardia in patients with ischemia and nonischemic cardiomyopathy. *Circulation.* 2000;101:1288–1296.
20. Hutchinson MD, Gerstenfeld EP, Desjardins B, Bala R, Riley MP, Garcia FC, Dixit S, Lin D, Tzou WS, Cooper JM, Verdino RJ, Callans DJ, Marchlinski FE. Endocardial unipolar voltage mapping to detect epicardial VT substrate in patients with nonischemic cardiomyopathy. *Circ Arrhythm Electrophysiol.* 2010.
21. Polin GM, Haqqani H, Tzou W, Hutchinson MD, Garcia FC, Callans DJ, Zado ES, Marchlinski FE. Endocardial unipolar voltage mapping to identify epicardial substrate in arrhythmogenic right ventricular dysplasia/cardiomyopathy. *Heart Rhythm.* 2010;8(1):76–83.
22. Miller JM, Tyson GS, Hargrove WC, Vassallo JA, Rosenthal ME, Josephson ME. Effect of subendocardial resection on sinus rhythm endocardial electrogram abnormalities. *Circulation.* 1995;91:2385–2391.
23. Hsia HH, Lin D, Sauer WH, Callans DJ, Marchlinski FE. Relationship of late potentials to the ventricular tachycardia circuit defined by entrainment. *J Interv Card Electrophysiol.* 2009;26:21–29.
24. Brunckhorst CB, Delacretaz E, Soejima K, Maisel WH, Friedman PL, Stevenson WG. Identification of the ventricular tachycardia isthmus after infarction by pace mapping. *Circulation.* 2004;110:652–659.
25. Hsia HH, Lin D, Sauer WH, Callans DJ, Marchlinski FE. Anatomic characterization of endocardial substrate for hemodynamically stable reentrant ventricular tachycardia: identification of endocardial conducting channels. *Heart Rhythm.* 2006;3:503–512.
26. Arenal A, del Castillo S, Gonzalez-Torrecilla E, et al. Tachycardia-related channel in the scar tissue in patients with sustained monomorphic ventricular tachycardias: influence of the voltage scar definition. *Circulation.* 2004;110:2568–2574.
27. Kaltenbrunner W, Cardinal R, Dubuc M, et al. Epicardial and endocardial mapping of ventricular tachycardia in patients with myocardial infarction. Is the origin of the tachycardia always subendocardially localized? *Circulation.* 1991;84:1058–1071.
28. Sosa E, Scanavacca M. Epicardial mapping and ablation techniques to control ventricular tachycardia. *J Cardiovasc Electrophysiol.* 2005;16:449–452.
29. Bazan V, Bala R, Garcia F, et al. Twelve-lead ECG features to identify ventricular tachycardia arising from the epicardial right ventricle. *Heart Rhythm.* 2006;3:1132–1139.
30. Bazan V, Gerstenfeld EP, Garcia F, et al. Site-specific twelve-lead ECG features to identify an epicardial origin for left ventricular tachycardia in the absence of myocardial infarction. *Heart Rhythm.* 2007;4:1403–1410.
31. Sosa E, Scanavacca M, d'Avila A, Pilleggi F. A new technique to perform epicardial mapping in the electrophysiology laboratory. *J Cardiovasc Electrophysiol.* 1996;7:531–536.
32. Fan R, Cano O, Ho SY, et al. Characterization of the phrenic nerve course within the epicardial substrate of patients with nonischemic cardiomyopathy and ventricular tachycardia. *Heart Rhythm.* 2009;6:59–64.
33. Di Biase L, Burkhardt JD, Pelargonio G, et al. Prevention of phrenic nerve injury during epicardial ablation: comparison of methods for separating the phrenic nerve from the epicardial surface. *Heart Rhythm.* 2009;6:957–961.
34. D'Avila A, Neuzil P, Thiagalingam A, Gutierrez P, Aleong R, Ruskin JN, Reddy VY. Experimental efficacy of pericardial instillation of anti-inflammatory agents during percutaneous epicardial catheter ablation to prevent postprocedure pericarditis. *J Cardiovasc Electrophysiol.* 2007;18:1178–1183.
35. Calkins H, Epstein A, Packer D, et al. Catheter ablation of ventricular tachycardia in patients with structural heart disease using cooled radiofrequency energy. *J Am Coll Cardiol.* 2000;35:1905–1914.
36. Kuck KH, Schaumann A, Eckhardt L, et al. Catheter ablation of stable ventricular tachycardia before defibrillator implantation in patients with coronary heart disease (VTACH): A multicentre randomised controlled trial. *Lancet.* 2010;375:31–40.

CHAPTER 37

How to Map and Ablate Unstable Ventricular Tachycardia: The Brigham Approach

Usha B. Tedrow, MD, MSc; William G. Stevenson, MD

Introduction

Ventricular tachycardia is an important cause of morbidity and mortality in patients with structural heart disease. In patients with ICDs, shocks to terminate the arrhythmia decrease quality of life and cause significant emotional distress. In addition, shocks are associated with increased risk for exacerbation of heart failure and mortality, and have been suggested to have a causative role. Catheter ablation for VT is an increasingly important therapeutic modality for reducing shocks and reducing the need for antiarrhythmic drugs, which have their own toxicities. Ablation can be life-saving when VT is incessant.

Of patients with ICDs that are referred to us for ablation after failing antiarrhythmic drug therapy, fewer than one-third have VT that is sufficiently stable to allow mapping during VT. The majority have a combination of stable and unstable VTs, or only unstable VT. VT can be unstable for mapping due to hemodynamic intolerance, requiring immediate termination, inability to reliably induce VT, or inducibility of VT, which frequently and spontaneously shifts in morphology. Catheter ablation of VT requires mapping to locate the arrhythmogenic substrate. Catheter ablation techniques for stable VT rely on activation and entrainment mapping during sustained VT, which is only possible in a limited way in patients with unstable VT. There are many substrate mapping techniques that can address the substrate for these unstable VTs in these patients.

Preprocedural Planning

Underlying Substrate

All patients undergoing VT catheter ablation require evaluation of the underlying substrate prior to the procedure. Reentry related to ventricular scars from prior MI, cardiomyopathies, or surgical incisions is the most common cause of sustained monomorphic VT associated with structural heart disease. For this reason, when patients present with new episodes of VT, evaluation of possible new ischemic lesions with either stress testing or cardiac catheterization is essential to determine the safety of proceeding with catheter ablation, as well as the need for possible revascularization. It is important to note, however, that new ischemic lesions are rarely the sole cause of monomorphic VT.

For patients with underlying cardiomyopathic processes such as sarcoidosis, the extent of disease activity is important to consider. For those with active inflammation, immunosuppression may be a more prudent initial course than catheter ablation. Cardiac MRI (**Figure 37.1**) can also be helpful in patients without ICDs to identify arrhythmogenic processes such as giant cell arteritis, which may warrant other therapies and even consideration for LV assist device or transplantation rather than catheter ablation.

Approach to Ventricular Access

The ventricles can be approached from the endocardium or epicardium, and the LV endocardium can be approached via a retrograde aortic or transseptal route. Echocardiography is an essential component of the preprocedural evaluation of the patient. The first priority is to assess the presence of mobile thrombus in the left ventricle (▶ **Video 37.1**). If LV thrombus is present, an epicardial approach to the LV can still be considered, but endocardial LV mapping should be avoided, due to risk of embolic stroke. In addition, echocardiography can evaluate the possible presence of aortic stenosis that might make a retrograde aortic approach difficult. A mechanical aortic valve is a contraindication to a retrograde aortic approach. A transseptal approach is preferred for these situations as well as in instances of severe peripheral vascular disease or abdominal aortic aneurysm. Mitral stenosis or a mechanical valve prosthesis in the mitral position is a contraindication to a transseptal approach. Patients who have failed an endocardial attempt are reasonable candidates for an epicardial approach, independent of QRS morphology.

Procedure

Patient Preparation

Mapping and ablation may be performed with either conscious sedation or general anesthesia. An anesthesia consultation is obtained, and the majority of our patients with unstable VT undergo catheter ablation under general anesthesia. General anesthesia allows complete control of the patient during induction of arrhythmias that may require prompt cardioversion, in a patient who may require hemodynamic support with an IABP, pressors, or even urgent ventricular assist. It also ensures absence of movement during mapping, reducing the chance that patient movement invalidates an electroanatomic map. It is our impression, however, that hypotension occurs more promptly under general anesthesia as compared to conscious sedation. A urinary catheter is placed in all patients, since the volume of fluid given during the procedure with an external irrigated-tip catheter is often 2-4 liters.

Access in the RFV accommodates 2 venous sheaths, an 8-Fr to ultimately accommodate the ablation catheter if the RV is mapped endocardially, and a sheath for a custom hexapolar catheter with an intravascular electrode located 15 to 20 cm proximal to the tip. This can be positioned at

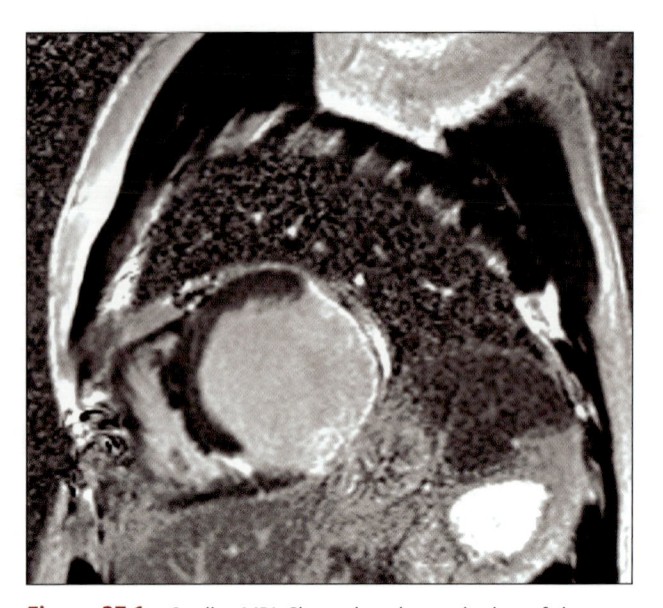

Figure 37.1 Cardiac MRI. Shown is a short-axis view of the heart by cardiac MRI. Normal areas of the heart appear dark and areas of ventricular scar by delayed hyperenhancement appear bright. Scar location can be a helpful adjunct to planning mapping and ablation.

the HB or in the right ventricle for pacing and recording. The LFV usually accommodates an 11-Fr sheath for the placement of a phased-array ICE catheter. An arterial line is often placed either radially or in the right femoral artery initially for hemodynamic monitoring. The 5-Fr femoral arterial sheath can be upsized to an 8-Fr sheath if a retrograde aortic approach to the LV endocardium is to be used. A long (35 cm) vascular sheath can help to negotiate tortuosities in the femoral arterial system and reduce risk of retrograde dissection.

Transseptal Puncture

All transseptal punctures are performed using ICE guidance. A large-curl steerable sheath (Agilis, St. Jude Medical, St. Paul, MN) is typically used because it allows the sheath to be buttressed against the posterior wall of the LA with good access to the mitral annulus with the ablation catheter due to the reach of the sheath. A view encompassing the IAS and *fossa ovalis* is selected on ICE. The sheath and needle are withdrawn from the SVC down the atrial septum until indentation of the fossa is seen. Blood is withdrawn from the LA and saline is flushed down the transseptal sheath, producing echocontrast that can be seen in the LA. A balanced heavyweight angioplasty wire is then advanced out the transseptal needle, though the LA and out the LSPV. The position of the wire is confirmed by fluoroscopy and ICE. The needle is then covered by the dilator, and the sheath is advanced over the dilator into the LA. Needle, sheath, and angioplasty wire are then carefully withdrawn as a unit. Heparin is administered peripherally and via continuous drip though the transseptal sheath to maintain ACTs of greater than 250 sec.

Hemodynamic Support

One option for approaching unstable VTs is with the use of percutaneous LV assist, or extracorporeal membrane oxygenation to support the circulation during mapping in VT. We have generally avoided these measures as a first approach. Deployment of these devices complicates vascular access and introduces the potential for complications related to the device. These may be considered when a substrate guided approach fails, or for severely compromised patients. More often, we consider placement of an IABP to provide some degree of support during mapping in sinus rhythm, and to facilitate hemodynamic recovery from VT that causes hypotension. Adjunctive inotropic medication is also often helpful.

Initial Mapping

Once vascular access has been obtained, the next step is usually to use programmed stimulation to induce VT. This serves several purposes. We confirm that the arrhythmia induced is indeed VT and not SVT with aberrancy or an antidromic tachycardia. We assess the possibility of bundle branch reentry, which may only require ablation of the right bundle branch. Most commonly this tachycardia has a LBBB-like configuration. Entrainment from the RVA usually reveals a postpacing interval that is within 50 ms of the TCL, and the VT is often easy to pace terminate. Analysis of H–H oscillations and confirming His-to-right bundle anterograde activation during a LBBB tachycardia further support the diagnosis. If the tachycardia is not due to bundle branch reentry, the QRS morphology influences the next step. LBBB-like tachycardias generally will warrant RV mapping to assess the possibility of RV scar. This may be done in a limited fashion, focusing on identifying whether scar is present in the region where the pace map approximates the VT QRS, if one can be identified. Even in patients with coronary artery disease and prior MI, RV tachycardias occasionally occur, possibly from RV infarction. If RV mapping does not suggest a scar-related RV tachycardia, or tachycardia has an RBBB-like configuration, we promptly focus on the LV. The next decision then relates to whether to obtain epicardial access prior to endocardial LV mapping and anticoagulation.

Epicardial Access

The possibility that percutaneous epicardial access may be needed is considered in all patients who have not had prior cardiac surgery. In particular, those who have failed an endocardial ablation attempt and patients with NICM are more likely to require this approach. We avoid percutaneous epicardial access in patients with prior cardiac surgery because residual adhesions frequently prohibit access. A surgical approach to the LV epicardium can be feasible, however. In patients with NICM, the QRS morphology can suggest an epicardial exit, but exceptions occur. In patients with prior MI, we have not been able to predict epicardial exits based on the QRS morphology of VT. If no prior ablation has been performed, limited transvenous mapping of brief, induced VT via the CS and accessible LV branches can suggest an epicardial VT circuit. Epicardial mapping can be considered as the first approach in patients with LV thrombus, if their anticoagulation can be safely interrupted for the procedure.[1]

We typically use a Touhey needle (Codman Inc.) with a soft-tipped wire with firm body such as a Benson wire (Cook Co.) for percutaneous epicardial access. Access is feasible in more than 90% of patients who have not had cardiac surgery. Skin entry is generally 2 to 3 cm below the xiphoid process. There are two approaches. Directing the needle superiorly at a relatively shallow angle, aiming for the RVA in the RAO projection, generally enters the pericardial space anteriorly over the RV. This approach may be more likely to avoid subdiaphragmatic vessels and facilitates access to the anterior aspect of the right and left ventricle. Directing the needle more posteriorly and toward the left shoulder, one enters the pericardium over the inferior aspect of the ventricles, such that the sheath typically tracks along the posterior aspect of the LV, as observed in the LAO projection. Biplane RAO and LAO fluoroscopy is used to facilitate the puncture. As the needle approaches the pericardium, injection of a small amount (< 1 cm^3) of contrast can help assess the relation of the needle to the parietal pericardium. Once tenting of the pericardium is seen, a slight advance achieves entry into the space and is palpable. Aspiration without blood indicates that the needle has not entered the RV. Injected contrast should layer in the pericardial space. The guide wire is then advanced generously into the pericardial space (▶ Video 37.2, A and B). It is essential to observe the wire in the LAO projection observing that it hugs the cardiac silhouette, crossing more than one chamber, circumferential to both the right and left heart. Observation in the RAO or anterior-posterior projection alone can be misleading, as a wire that enters the RV and passes into the RA or pulmonary artery can be misinterpreted as intrapericardial. The entire procedure is monitored by ICE, allowing for visualization of any accumulation of pericardial fluid that may occur, both during access and during the procedure (▶ Video 37.3). In addition, before ablation is performed, coronary angiography is often performed to ensure ablation is performed a distance from the coronary artery branches (**Figure 37.2**). We use a 5-mm cutoff for this safe distance.

Substrate Mapping

Once we have selected the chamber (RV, LV, or epicardial region) for initial evaluation, electroanatomic mapping is performed, influenced by the QRS morphology of the induced VT and that of any clinical VTs that are known. A LBBB-like configuration in lead V_1 indicates an exit in the RV or interventricular septum; dominant R waves in V$_1$ indicate a LV exit. The frontal plane axis points away from the exit. A superiorly directed axis indicates an inferior wall exit. An inferiorly directed axis indicates an anterior wall exit. The closer an exit is to a precordial lead, the more negative the S wave in that lead, providing an indication of exit location between the base and apex. Apical exits generate dominant S waves in leads V$_3$ and V$_4$. Basal exits generate dominant R waves in these leads. Epicardial reentry circuits produce VTs that typically have a relatively long QRS duration, slow QRS upstroke, producing pseudo–delta waves (**Figure 37.3**), possibly related to delayed activation of the endocardial Purkinje system as compared to endocardial VTs.

Areas of ventricular scar are characterized by low-amplitude bipolar EGMs (< 1.55 mV). Plots of peak-to-peak EGM amplitude displayed in electroanatomic mapping reconstructions are referred to as *voltage maps* (▶ **Video 37.4**, **Figure 37.4**). The low-voltage region is likely to contain the reentry circuit. In patients with prior infarction, these regions are often extensive, exceeding 20 cm in circumference in many patients. ICE (▶ **Video 37.5**) or preprocedure MRI (**Figure 37.5**) can be helpful to provide adjunctive information about scar location when integrated with electroanatomic voltage mapping. The scar border region typically extends along the scar margin defined by EGM amplitude between 0.5 and 1.5 mV. Exit regions are located along the scar border.

As low-voltage regions of potential scar are defined we make extensive use of pace mapping. Pacing in the exit

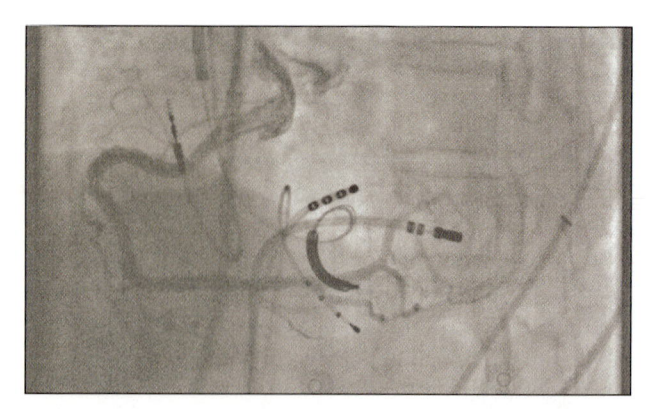

Figure 37.2 Coronary angiography during epicardial mapping. Shown is a still fluoroscopic image of a left anterior oblique projection during epicardial mapping of the posteroseptal region. Endocardial quadripolar catheters are seen in the His and RV location, and the ablation catheter tip is seen in the left posteroseptal region. The right coronary is being injected and one can see that the tip of the ablation catheter is located between distal branches of the posterior LV system.

region replicates the QRS morphology of VT (**Figure 37.6**). The interval between the stimulus and QRS onset is typically short, consistent with the exit location in the infarct border. Pacing in a channel produces a QRS that emerges after a delay (S–QRS > 40 ms) due to slow conduction through the channel.

EUS that are regions of fixed conduction block can be identified from a high pacing threshold (> 10 mA at 2 ms pulse width with unipolar pacing). In some low-voltage regions, marking EUS areas creates a visual map of

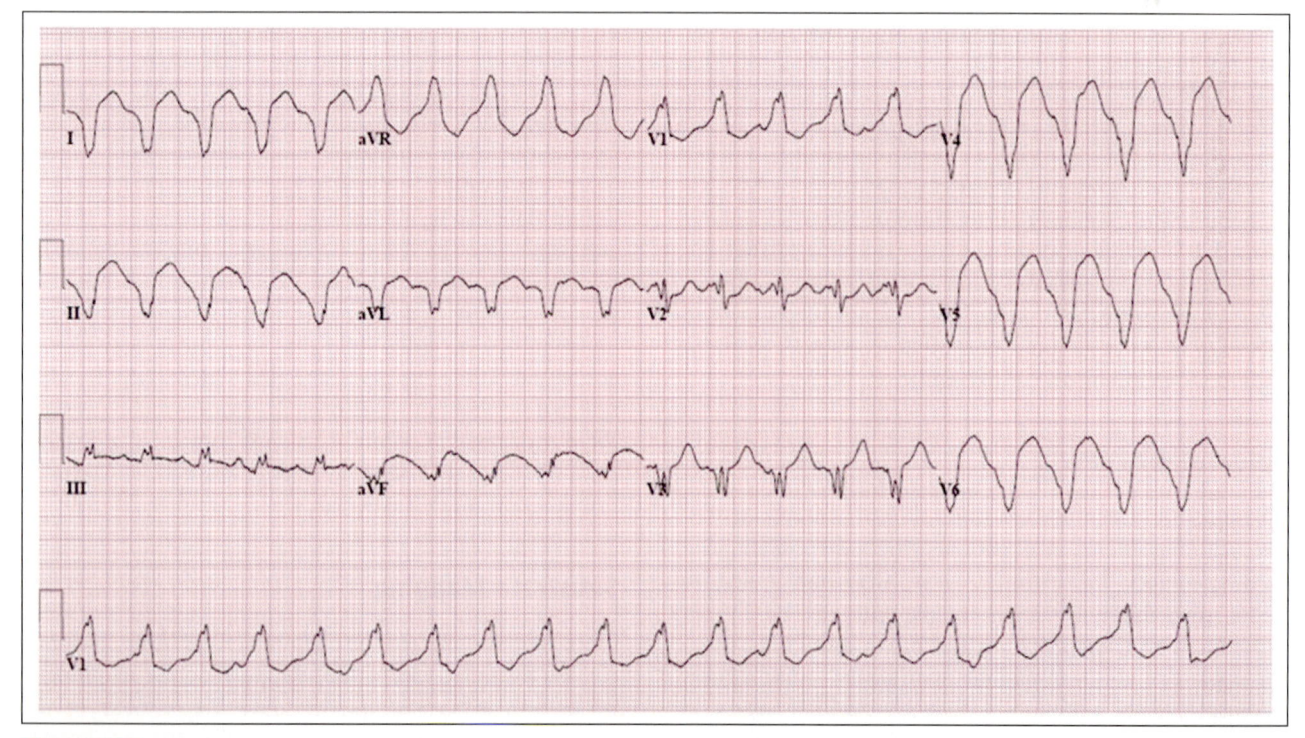

Figure 37.3 ECG of VT in epicardial location. Shown is a 12-lead ECG of an epicardial VT found in a patient with an inferoposterior LV scar. AV dissociation is seen during the rhythm strip, consistent with a diagnosis of VT.

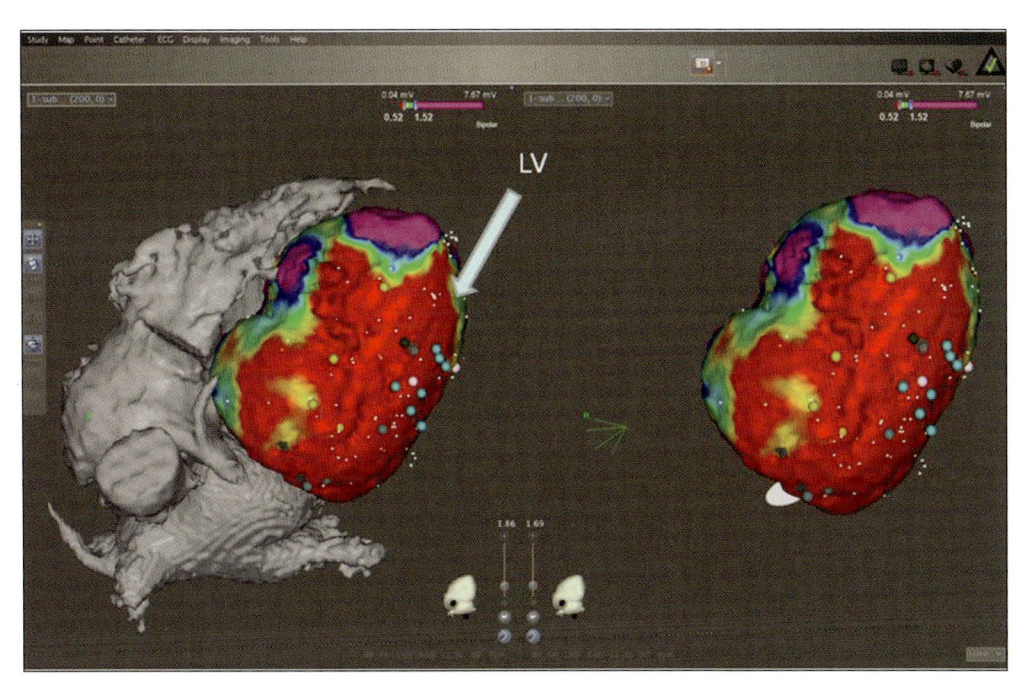

Figure 37.4 Voltage mapping. Shown here is electroanatomic voltage mapping performed on a shell of the LV (arrow) generated by cardiac MRI. The color coding depicts low voltages as red and increasing voltages through yellow, green, and blue, up to a normal voltage, which is purple (> 1.5 mV). Shown here is a large inferolateral scar region in red. The scar continues up to the mitral annulus, but the LVA is relatively spared.

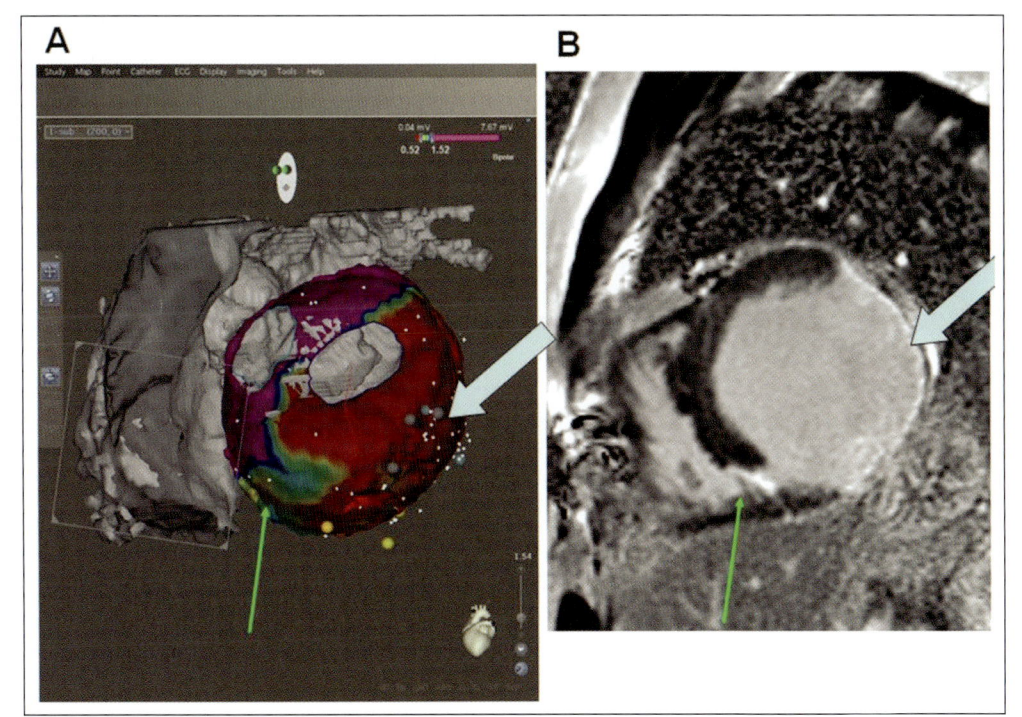

Figure 37.5 Scar thickness and voltage mapping. **A.** Anatomic MRI surface rendering incorporated into electroanatomic voltage mapping data from a catheter ablation procedure for ventricular tachycardia. Normal areas are purple, and abnormal areas are less than 1.5 mV coded in a color scale where red is the lowest voltage and voltages increase through yellow, green, and blue in the abnormal voltage range. **B.** Areas of bright delayed hyperenhancement (DHE). A partial thickness septal scar is indicated with the green arrow, and a large lateral dense thinned car is indicated with the heavy blue arrow.

potential channels. Narrow bands of fibrosis likely escape detection with this method. Inadequate electrode myocardial contact is also a potential source of error. EUS cannot be reliably detected based on EGM amplitude alone. Pacing captures at the majority of sites with very low EGM amplitude of < 0.25 mV. In contrast, some EUS sites have EGM amplitude > 0.5 mV, due to the presence of large far-field potentials. Thus, EGM characteristics and pacing techniques provide complementary information during substrate mapping.

Even in the case of unstable VT, limited activation mapping and potentially entrainment during VT can be helpful to confirm that an identified region is in a reentry circuit and to facilitate successful ablation with fewer ablation lesions.[2] Therefore, after substrate mapping has been performed and a candidate region is identified, the mapping catheter is positioned at a likely channel site. Programmed stimulation is used to induce VT. We are prepared to immediately assess EGMs, entrain the VT and ablate with RF energy in the hope of terminating VT,

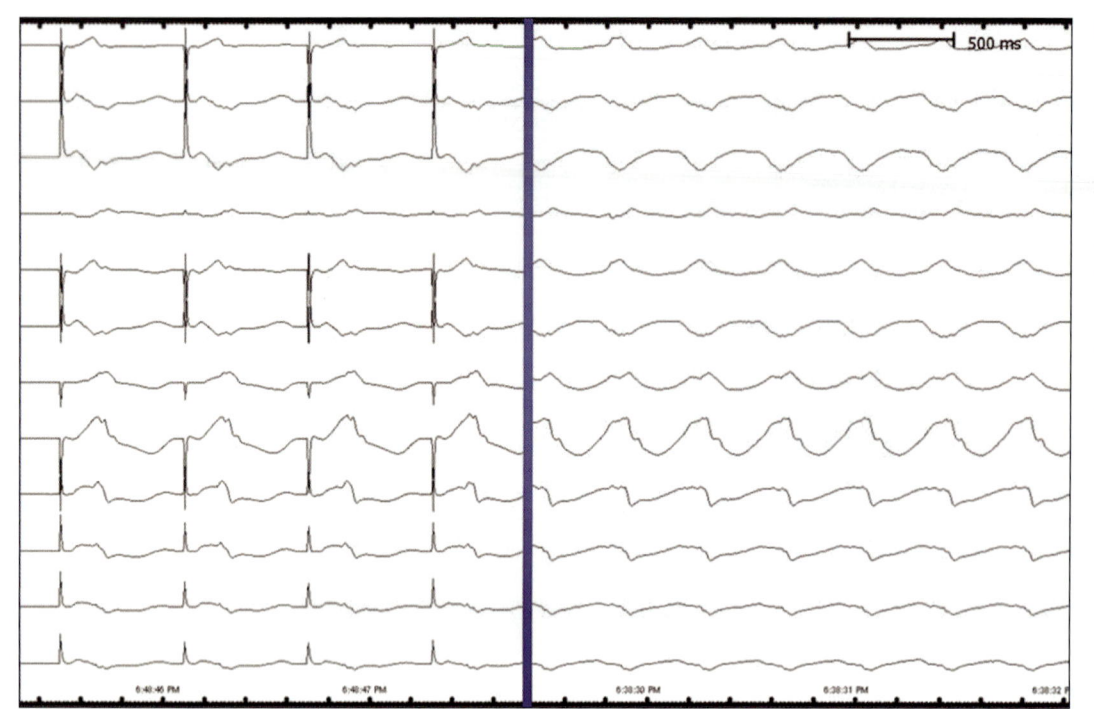

Figure 37.6 Pace mapping of clinical VT. Shown in the left panel is pacing from a candidate region, and shown on the right panel is the clinical VT. The pacing reproduces the morphology of the clinical VT with a small amount of delay, consistent with an area just proximal to the exit of the VT circuit.

or promptly perform burst pacing followed by external cardioversion, if needed, to terminate the VT. During VT, the circuit exit and isthmus have presystolic (prior to the QRS onset) and diastolic activation (**Figure 37.7**). Isolated diastolic potentials are often recorded at isthmus. Their timing is presystolic near the exit and progressively earlier relative to the QRS onset at sites further from the reentry circuit isthmus. Sites that are proximal in the circuit can be activated at the end of the QRS complex, without diastolic electrical activity, but can be identified by entrainment. In some patients, VT is not inducible after creation of the voltage map. Whether this reflects mechanical trauma to the circuit, or simply variability of programmed stimulation, is not clear. In some patients with poor ventricular function, even this limited induction of VT is deemed inadvisable due to concerns regarding patient stability. In these cases, RF lesions can be placed through presumptive exits and/or channels, followed by retesting for inducible VT.

Ablation

We typically perform ablation using an external irrigated 3.5-mm electrode-tip catheter, beginning with 30 W of energy and titrate to a maximum of 50 W, with a maximum temperature of 40°C and irrigation flow of 20 ml/min. In the situation where VT is induced and activation mapping/entrainment are favorable at the candidate site, ablation is often attempted in VT, with the goal of terminating the clinical VT. If this is not possible, we typically will perform RF ablation in areas of low EGM voltage with areas with long S-QRS delay that reproduce the QRS morphology of VT.[3] We perform pace mapping at 10 mA and 2 ms at the site prior to ablation and confirm loss of capture after ablation, to ensure adequate lesion formation. In some cases repeated RF applications over a small region are needed to render the area unexcitable. In other cases, inexcitability occurs with limited ablation. Areas are targeted in such a way as to connect areas of EUS and if possible to connect these areas with a valve annulus or other electrically nonconducting structure (**Figure 37.8**, ▶ **Video 37.6**).[4] After ablation, VT induction is performed again, and if inducible, further substrate modification is performed.

During epicardial ablation, we reduce the irrigated flow during mapping to 1 ml/min and increase it during ablation to 10–17 cm³/min. These lower flow rates, as compared to those used during endocardial mapping and ablation, are acceptable as thrombus formation does not pose a risk of embolization, and it is desirable to limit infusion of fluid into the pericardial space. It is important to periodically drain the pericardial space, after every few RF applications or every 15 to 20 minutes, to avoid accumulation of pericardial fluid from the irrigant. We accomplish this by using aspirating from the steerable sheath containing the ablation catheter, which has a larger diameter than the ablation catheter. ICE is very helpful to monitor for irrigant accumulation or unsuspected bleeding into the pericardial space as well (▶ **Video 37.3**).

Patients with unstable VT associated with heart disease often have poor ventricular function and other comorbidities. Close communication with the anesthesia team and monitoring of peripheral oxygen saturation and end tidal CO_2 are critical. Periodic arterial blood gas surveillance can be helpful in the tenuous patient. During the ablation

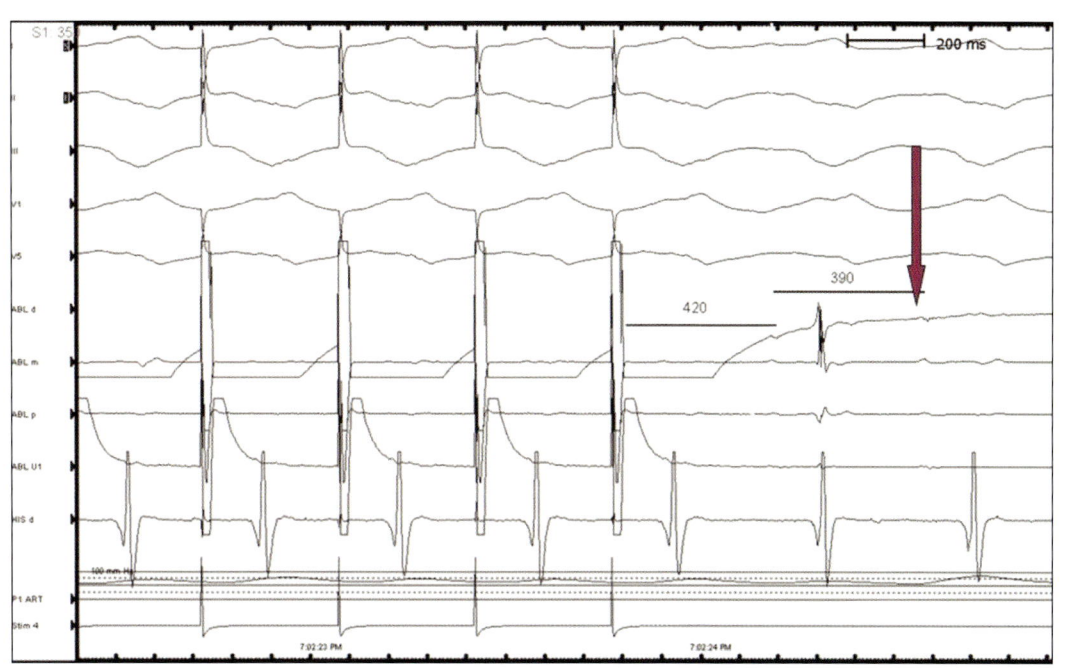

Figure 37.7 Entrainment of clinical VT. Shown is entrainment of the VT in Figure 37.6 from the candidate region. The tachycardia is accelerated to the paced cycle length with concealed fusion. The postpacing interval measured to the area of local activation (purple arrow) is +30 compared with the TCL. RF ablation in this region terminated VT.

procedure attention to fluid balance is critical, and diuresis is considered when a positive fluid balance exceeds 1 to 2 liters. Prompt recognition of any cardiorespiratory compromise and complications is of paramount importance.

Postprocedure Care

Recovery

Following ablation, protamine can be given to help reverse the heparin, and sheaths can be pulled once the activated clotting time is less than 200 seconds. We advocate closure of arterial access sites whenever possible, to reduce femoral bleeding complications. Many patients will have a large net-positive fluid balance when external irrigated-tip catheters are used, and diuretics can be administered accordingly. Patients will typically lie flat for 6 hours after sheaths are pulled due to the large sheaths used. For LV endocardial ablation, we typically start anticoagulation with unfractionated heparin 6 hours after sheath removal.

Further anticoagulation is guided by the extent of LV endocardial ablation and other indications for anticoagulation. For extensive LV endocardial ablation over an area of more than 3 cm, we typically recommend warfarin for 6 weeks. In patients treated with aspirin and thienopyridine antiplatelet agents, who are at risk of bleeding, warfarin is avoided. Patients for whom warfarin was discontinued prior to the procedure are given an IV heparin bridge until discharge. If warfarin is not needed, aspirin 325 mg daily for 6 weeks is administered, but prophylactic anticoagulation for deep venous thrombosis is employed until patients are ambulatory.

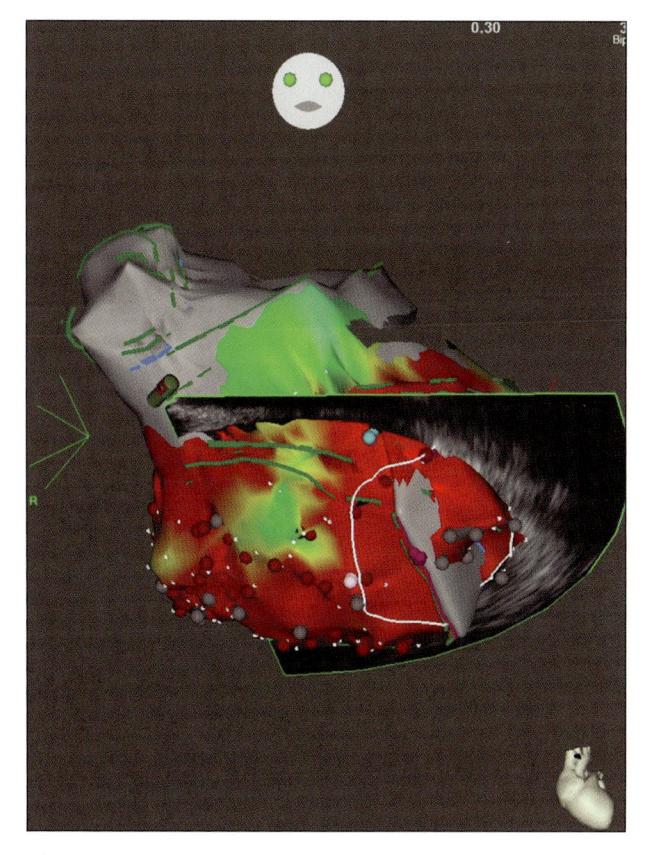

Figure 37.8 Electroanatomic mapping with ablation set in a patient with Dor LV reconstruction. Shown here is an LV endocardial voltage map performed on a shell of the LV assisted by ICE. The corresponding ICE image is shown in Video 37.6. Gray areas indicate EUS, and maroon dots indicate ablation sites. The white ring indicates the border of the Dor patch. Anchors for the ablation lesion set include the edge of the Dor patch and the mitral valve annulus in this case.

Patients are reassessed for the need for further diuresis and/or monitoring in the cardiac care unit postablation. Patients are usually monitored in hospital for a minimum of 2 days following ablation. Occasionally patients require inpatient rehabilitation after hospitalization. For those in whom inducibility or eradication of clinical VT is a concern, noninvasive programmed stimulation through their device is performed under conscious sedation prior to discharge to ensure VT remains noninducible.

Follow-up

Patients are followed closely following ablation. This often requires a joint approach between the patient's electrophysiologist and his or her cardiologist or heart failure specialist. Patients are generally seen within one week of discharge, and should undergo regular ICD follow-up to screen for recurrent arrhythmias.

Procedural Complications

Major complications are reported in 5% to 10% of patients including cardiac tamponade, shock, stroke (0%–2.7%), aortic valve injuries, vascular injuries, and AV block due to ablation of septal VTs. Procedure mortality, 2.7% in one multicenter trial, is often due to failure to control VT rather than complications of the procedure.[5]

In most series, previously ineffective antiarrhythmic drugs, frequently amiodarone, have been continued during follow-up. VT recurs in 19% to 50% of patients, although the frequency is reduced in the majority. Multiple morphologies of VT and unstable VTs are associated with a higher recurrence risk.[6]

During follow-up after ablation the annual mortality ranges from 5% to more than 20%, with death from progressive heart failure being the most common cause. This substantial mortality is consistent with the severity of heart disease, depressed ventricular function, and the observation that spontaneous VT is a marker for mortality and heart failure despite presence of an ICD. Older age and greater LV size and dysfunction are associated with worse mortality. The potential for ablation to adversely effect LV function is concerning, although assessment of LV ejection fraction after ablation has not shown deterioration. Confining ablation lesions to regions of low-amplitude scar, and attention to appropriate medical therapy for LV dysfunction, is prudent to avoid this theoretical concern.

During epicardial ablation, several precautions are important to avoid injury to adjacent structures. Over the lateral LV, pacing should be used to identify phrenic nerve capture, indicating where ablation might cause diaphragmatic paralysis. Phrenic nerve injury has been avoided in some cases by interposing a sheath, a balloon, or even air in the pericardium between the ablation site and the nerve. Overlying epicardial coronary arteries that can be identified by angiography may limit potential ablation sites, as direct application of RF ablation to a coronary artery can acutely occlude the vessel. A minimum of 5 mm is required between epicardial coronary vessels and the ablation catheter, and ensure that the catheter is not touching the vessel at any point of the cardiac cycle during angiography (**Figure 37.10**). There is the potential for injury to the esophagus, lungs, and great vessels. Symptomatic pericarditis is common, but usually mild, of limited duration, and often responds well to anti-inflammatory medications. Inflammatory pericarditis can render the epicardial space percutaneously inaccessible for repeat procedures due to the development of adhesions. Based on data from studies in animal models, we administer 0.5 to 1.0 mg/kg of methylprednisolone into the epicardial space at the end of the procedure to reduce the pericardial inflammatory reaction. All pericardial sheaths are removed at the end of the procedure unless there is concern for ongoing bleeding.

Advantages and Limitations

Catheter ablation for VT has the potential for controlling VT without potentially toxic antiarrhythmic drugs, or allowing control of VT to be achieved by a previously ineffective drug. A reduction in ICD therapies can be expected to translate into improvements in quality of life. Whether it also will reduce heart failure hospitalization and mortality is uncertain, but possible.

When ablation fails, there are often anatomic reasons. Intramural circuits are not accessible by endocardial and epicardial ablation techniques. These remain a major limitation to successful catheter ablation. Alcohol ablation can occasionally be effective when an appropriate coronary target can be found. New techniques dedicated to reaching and providing ablative therapies to VT involving intramural regions are needed.

Conclusions

Catheter ablation has an important role for reducing episodes of VT in patients with scar-related LV dysfunction and implantable defibrillators. Substrate mapping approaches have facilitated ablation despite the frequent presence of multiple and hemodynamically unstable VTs formerly considered "unmappable." Efficacy remains less than for ablation of many supraventricular arrhythmias. Failure of VT ablation often seems to be due to an anatomic difficulty, such as unreachable deep intramural reentry circuits in areas of thick myocardium. Further technologic developments are needed and will require careful assessment of risks and efficacy.

References

1. Tedrow U, Stevenson WG. Strategies for epicardial mapping and ablation of ventricular tachycardia. *J Cardiovasc Electrophysiol.* 2009;20(6):710-713.
2. Soejima K, Suzuki M, Maisel WH, et al. Catheter ablation in patients with multiple and unstable ventricular tachycardias after myocardial infarction: short ablation lines guided by reentry circuit isthmuses and sinus rhythm mapping. *Circulation.* 2001;104(6):664–669.
3. Brunckhorst CB, Delacretaz E, Soejima K, et al. Identification of the ventricular tachycardia isthmus after infarction by pace mapping. *Circulation.* 2004;110(6):652–659.
4. Soejima K, Stevenson WG, Maisel WH, et al. Electrically unexcitable scar mapping based on pacing threshold for identification of the reentry circuit isthmus: feasibility for guiding ventricular tachycardia ablation. *Circulation.* 2002;106(13):1678–1683.
5. Stevenson WG, Wilber DJ, Natale A, et al. Irrigated radiofrequency catheter ablation guided by electroanatomic mapping for recurrent ventricular tachycardia after myocardial infarction: the multicenter thermocool ventricular tachycardia ablation trial. *Circulation.* 2008;118(25): 2773–2782.
6. Aliot EM, Stevenson WG, Almendral-Garrote JM, et al. EHRA/HRS expert consensus on catheter ablation of ventricular arrhythmias: developed in a partnership with the European Heart Rhythm Association (EHRA), a registered branch of the European Society of Cardiology (ESC), and the Heart Rhythm Society (HRS); in collaboration with the American College of Cardiology (ACC) and the American Heart Association (AHA). *Heart Rhythm.* 2009;6(6): 886-933.

Video Descriptions

Video 37.1 LV apical thrombus. Shown is a TTE clip of an echocontrast-enhanced view of the LV apex in a patient with prior anteroapical infarction. The echocontrast reveals an egg-shaped mass in the apex of the LV. The mass had mobile components and was considered a contraindication to endocardial catheter ablation in this patient. Epicardial ablation, however, was successful. Echocontrast and ICE can be helpful to better define intracardiac thrombus when transthoracic views are inadequate.

Video 37.2 Epicardial access. Shown are right anterior oblique (**A**) and left anterior oblique (**B**) views of access to the epicardium. A residual blush of contrast material is seen in the pericardial space just inferior and lateral to the ICD lead. The guide wire is advanced generously into the pericardial space, crossing multiple cardiac chambers, confirming the wire is not inside a cardiac chamber.

Video 37.3 Monitoring the epicardial space for fluid accumulation. Shown is an electroanatomic map on the left and a corresponding ICE slice on the right. The view shown allows for monitoring of the amount of pericardial fluid during the case. The fluid can be the result of irrigation fluid, which is expected, or accumulation of unsuspected slow bleeding. The pericardial sheath should be periodically drained to prevent irrigant accumulation.

Video 37.4 Electroanatomic voltage mapping, an epicardial example. Shown here is electroanatomic voltage mapping performed on a shell of the heart generated by ICE and point-by-point mapping. The color coding depicts low voltages as red and increasing voltages through yellow, green, and blue, up to a normal voltage, which is purple (> 1.5 mV). Shown here is a discrete apical scar region in red. A multipolar catheter is also seen in gray, allowing assessment of activation in the scar from multiple regions simultaneously.

Video 37.5 LV shell construction using ICE. Shown here are slices generated by annotated ICE clips compiled to create a 3-dimensional shell of the endocardial surface of the LV. On the right, the ICE clip from a representative slice is shown.

Video 37.6 ICE clip in a patient with Dor LV reconstruction. Shown is a clip from the patient depicted in Figure 37.8. The Dor patch is the hyperreflective area seen from approximately 4 to 5 o'clock in the image. The ablation catheter is seen curving through the LV chamber with the tip at the septal aspect of the patch.

CHAPTER 38

How to Map and Ablate Ventricular Tachycardia Using Delayed Potential in Sinus Rhythm

Eduardo Castellanos, MD, PhD; Jesús Almendral, MD, PhD; Carlos De Diego, MD

Introduction

Catheter ablation of VT in patients with structural heart disease based on conventional mapping techniques (during VT) is limited to patients with stable, tolerated VT. For this reason, considerable research efforts have been devoted to the localization of the specific areas of the VT substrate in the absence of an ongoing VT. Such an approach represents significant progress since it permits catheter ablative therapies in patients with noninducible or poorly tolerated VT.

The theoretical base of this approach is as follows: VT in patients with structural heart disease has a reentrant mechanism that requires areas of slow conduction and arcs of block; areas of slow conduction and (maybe) arcs of block can be recognized by local EGM characteristics and pacing maneuvers in the absence of an ongoing VT; ablation of such areas may result in VT suppression.

The studies showing the feasibility of this methodology can be divided into 3 phases according to the tools that were used and the outcome data analyzed (**Table 38.1**) and started in the 1980s, when a surgical approach to VT therapy was developed.

In the first phase,[1-3] it was found that abnormal bipolar EGMs with low amplitude and long duration could be recorded in patients with VT and structural heart disease, but not patients with normal hearts. When the site of origin of VT, as detected during activation mapping, was studied during sinus rhythm, it typically displayed abnormal EGMs. However, abnormal EGMs were also found at many other sites unrelated to VT. Certain EGM characteristics (fractionated, delayed) were more closely associated to the VT site of origin but lacked sensitivity for its detection. The second phase, adding pacing techniques and response to RF ablation to improve VT localization,[4-6] described the so-called isolated potential during sinus rhythm (isoelectric line between 2 components) as a marker for the VT area of slow conduction, but again lacking sensitivity. With the hope that this lack of sensitivity could be overcome by a more detailed mapping with the aid of electroanatomic mapping tools, in recent years several groups have explored an ablation strategy based on targeting areas with abnormal EGMs suggestive of slow conduction[7,8] (generally referred to as LPs), or suggestive of boundaries between conductive and nonconductive tissue (arcs of block, channels, represented by unexcitable tissue or voltage gradients).[9-12] It should be mentioned that in all these studies pace mapping is added as a tool to select which EGMs are more likely to be related to VT. In general, results of these approaches have been encouraging although there is no controlled comparison with ablation based on conventional mapping during VT.

In addition, it has been shown that there are important differences in the substrate of patients with ischemic and NICM, associated with a different prevalence and location of LPs.[13-15]

Table 38.1 Chronological phases of studies on VT substrate in relation to tools used and outcome variables.

Chronological phase	1980s	Late 1990s, initial 2000	2000s
Mapping type	Activation during VT	Activation + entrainment	Activation + entrainment or NO VT mapping
VT type	Mappable	Mappable	Unmappable
Tools	Fluoroscopy	Fluoroscopy	Fluoroscopy + EA mapping
Ablation	No	Yes	Yes
Outcome variable	Compare SR with VT	Compare SR with VT	Clinical VT recurrence

Abbreviations: EA: electroanatomical; SR: sinus rhythm

Our present approach, as detailed in this chapter, is eclectic, involving an extensive study of EGM characteristics during sinus/paced rhythm, as well as an analysis of induced VT. A variety of scenarios can be encountered, as described below, and different strategies are proposed.

Preprocedural Planning

In all patients the preprocedure evaluation includes a detailed history and physical examination. It is always important to obtain and analyze 12-lead electrocardiograms during VT if they are available, since consideration of induced VT as clinical VT is based preferentially on the electrocardiogram. If this is not available or in addition to it, VTs documented in the stored EGMs of the ICD are also important references. In fact, with the increasing use of ICD for primary prevention, stored ICD EGMs tend to be the only documentation of clinical VT, and we pay attention not only to CL but also to EGM morphology.

All the patients are evaluated with a 2-dimensional echocardiogram to quantify the left ventricular ejection fraction and to rule out the presence of a left ventricular thrombus. Other studies include exercise testing or coronary angiography. In some patients, a cardiac magnetic resonance imaging is of interest before the EP study for quantification of left ventricular volumes, function, and scar tissue. This image can be integrated with the electroanatomical map during the EP study reducing the fluoroscopic and procedure time.

In patients with elective ablation the antiarrhythmic drugs are discontinued several days prior to the scheduled procedure.

Procedure

Electrophysiologic Study

After written, informed consent is obtained, the EP study is performed in the postabsorptive state, normally under conscious sedation or general anesthesia. A total of 2 or 3 5-Fr quadripolar catheters are introduced into the right femoral vein and positioned at the RA, HB area, and RVA. Having an atrial catheter is important to help distinguish between late ventricular potentials and atrial signals when the ablation catheter gets to annular positions, particularly during pacing. EGMs are filtered at 30 to 500 Hz and displayed simultaneously with 4 to 6 ECG leads and recorded and stored digitally (LabSystem™ PRO EP Recording System).

Our standard access to the left ventricle is via retrograde across the aortic valve, but in patients with significant atherosclerosis of the aorta or peripheral arteries, or in older people, we tend to increasingly choose the antegrade transseptal approach (▶ **Videos 38.1** and **38.2**). We use deflectable sheaths for LV access through a transseptal approach since they help in catheter control.

When the left heart is instrumented, anticoagulation with intravenous heparin is maintained throughout the procedure, maintaining the activated clotting time over 250 to 300 seconds. We tend to perform a full endocardial procedure as first-line study, and consider an epicardial approach only if the endocardial procedure fails, except in cases of previous failure at another institution, and also considering the underlying structural heart disease.

Epicardial access is achieved introducing the ablation catheter through an 8-Fr sheath into the pericardial space, using a subxiphoid approach, before the initiation of anticoagulation. Special attention is made to delimitate the course of the coronary arteries by coronary angiography or merged CT images.

Mapping Protocol

Electroanatomical mapping has become the standard for any type of substrate mapping. A detailed 3-dimensional voltage map of the ventricle is created using CARTO (Biosense Webster, Diamond Bar, CA) or NavX system (Ensite, St. Jude Medical, St. Paul, MN).

We prefer to use catheters with small electrodes to obtain a more local signal (3.5- or 4-mm-tip electrodes rather than 8-mm-tip electrodes). With CARTO, the bipolar EGMs are obtained normally using a 3.5-mm-tip open-irrigated ablation catheter (Navistar ThermoCool,

2-5-2 mm interelectrode spacing), with a fill threshold of 20 mm to ensure the representation of the entire endocardial surface of the ventricle. With the Ensite NavX 3-dimensional mapping system (St. Jude Medical, St. Paul, MN), any catheter can be used. Irrigated-tip ablation catheters tend to produce noisy signals in some laboratories, and in such cases, the use of a different catheter for mapping than for ablation can be considered.

Mapping is made using bipolar mode (filter 10–400 Hz) trying to identify areas of isolated delayed potentials, but voltage mapping is simultaneously performed. The peak-to-peak signal amplitude of the bipolar EGM is measured automatically to the largest component, and if an activation map is performed, we reannotate the local activation time to the EGM onset. The color display on the voltage map is set to a color range of 0.5 to 1.5 mV to distinguish the limits of the scar. Signals with an amplitude higher than 1.5 mV represent normal tissue, whereas the abnormal endocardium is defined as "dense scar" when the EGMs have amplitudes between 0.1 and 0.5 mV, and "complete scar" when the EGM voltage amplitude is lower than 0.1 mV. For the epicardial maps, the normal tissue voltage limit is changed to 1 mV, maintaining the limit of dense scar at < 0.5 mV.

Endocardial EGMs are recorded with the intention of fully defining the border zones and the scar region(s), trying to obtain a distance of < 1 cm between the mapped sites. A detailed mapping of the whole ventricular shape is required even if one scar area is detected because there may be more than one.

Our emphasis is in the identification of sites with abnormal signals, especially LPs that reveal local delayed activity in small isolated myocardial bundles within the scar. Isolated delayed potentials are defined as EGMs with some delayed low-voltage components separated from the early and usually larger components by an isoelectric segment of 20 to 50 ms (**Figures 38.1** and **38.2**). In general the delayed components are recorded after the QRS offset, but in our opinion this is not critical. Once a site with LPs is identified it is important to map adjacent sites in as detailed a manner as possible. We believe LPs are most significant when they are recorded over an area, not just a single point, although the area may be small. Some authors have differentiated between "moderate late potentials" and "very late potentials" if the onset of the EGMs after the QRS is shorter than 100 ms or longer, respectively,[10] and they consider more significant the latter.

We have observed that in some patients more LPs are detected during right ventricular pacing in comparison to sinus rhythm (**Figure 38.3**).[7] However, in some patients the opposite may be true. For that reason we usually perform the map during sinus rhythm, but also stimulate at

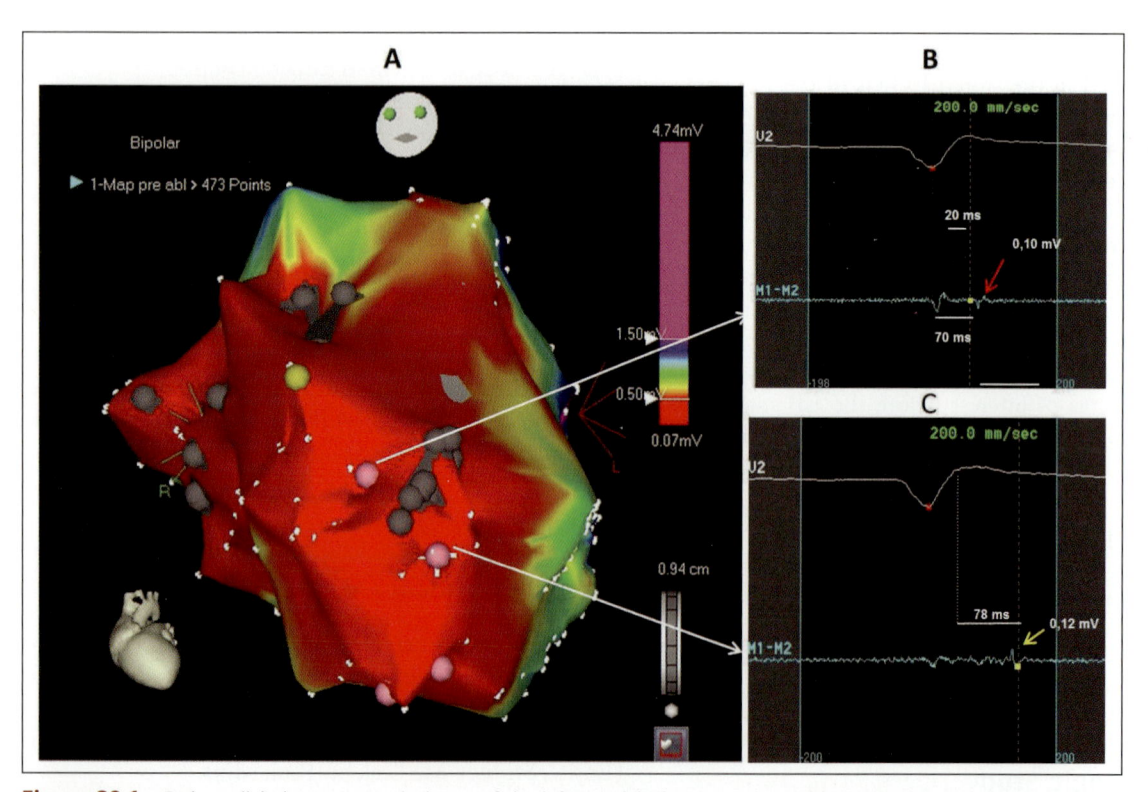

Figure 38.1 Endocardial electroanatomical map of the left ventricle from a patient with previous anterior myocardial infarction. **A.** The anteroposterior view shows the apical dense scar; the pink tags correspond with LPs recorded within the scar mapping during sinus rhythm, and the gray tags represent areas with voltage lower than 0.1 mV. **B.** An LP with an isoelectric segment of 70 ms between the ventricular EGM and the LP (red arrow) is shown. The amplitude of the LP is 0.10 mV, and the interval between the end of QRS and the LP is 20 ms. **C.** Another LP was recorded in the same area 78 ms after the end of the QRS (yellow arrow), with an amplitude of 0.12 mV. Two different ventricular tachycardias (VTs) were induced. After the ablation (see lesions in ▶ Video 38.6) VTs were not inducible. M1-M2 distal electrode pair of the ablation catheter.

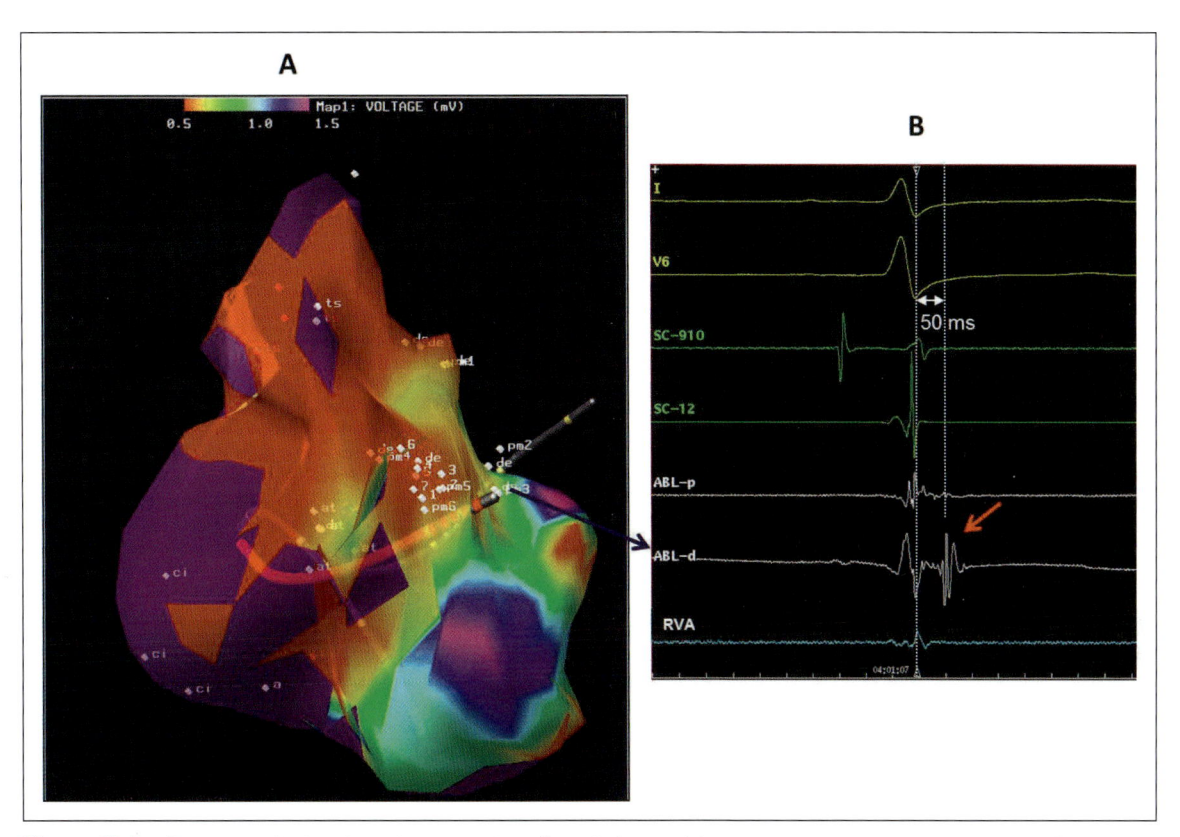

Chapter 38: Mapping/Ablating VT Using Delayed Potential in Sinus Rhythm • 353

Figure 38.2 **A.** Endocardial bipolar voltage map (RPM®; Real-Time Position Management System; Boston Scientific, S.A., Natick, MA) of the right ventricle in the left anterior oblique view showing an area of dense scar with an EGM amplitude lower than 0.5 mV (red color) in a patient with arrhythmogenic right ventricular dysplasia. **B.** A LP with an isoelectric segment of 50 ms between the ventricular EGM and the LP (red arrow) is shown.

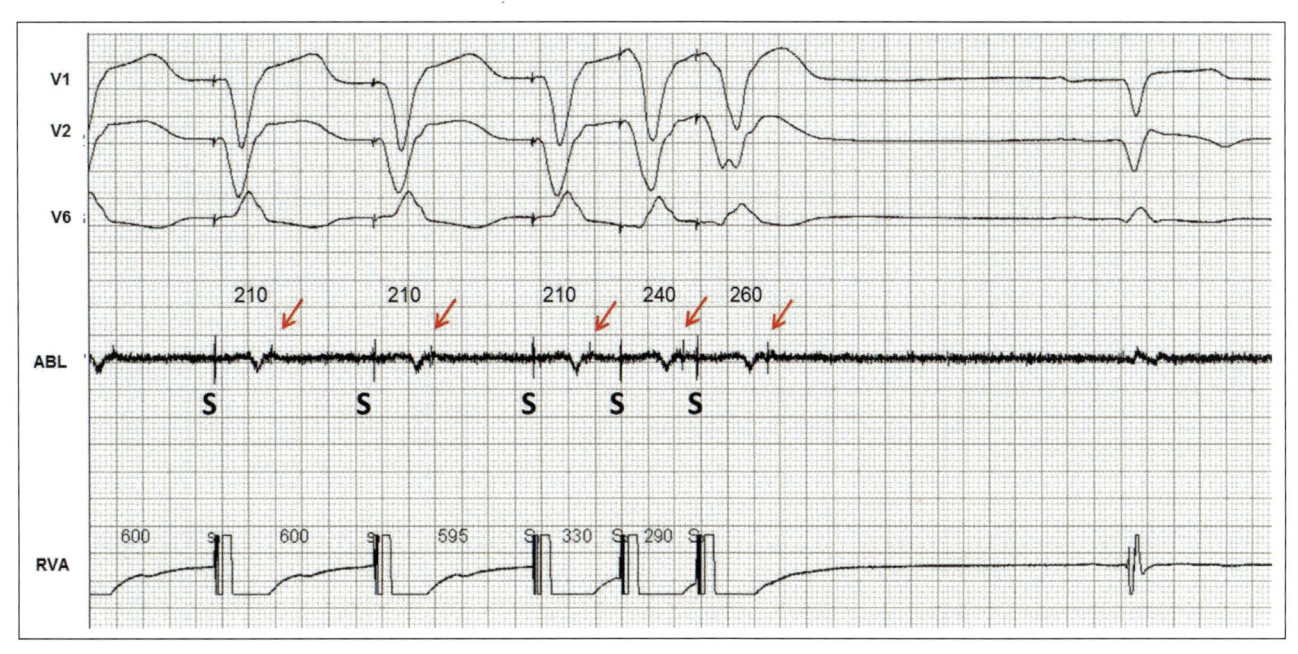

Figure 38.3 Recordings from surface leads V_1, V_2, and V_6 and intracardiac recordings from the mapping catheter (ABL) and right ventricular apex (RVA). A programmed ventricular stimulation protocol is performed with 2 extrastimuli pacing from RVA. The mapping catheter is located in an area of LPs where the pace mapping matched the clinical VT. The LPs in this area were more evident during pacing from RVA than in sinus rhythm (last beat), and showed delayed conduction with decremental properties.

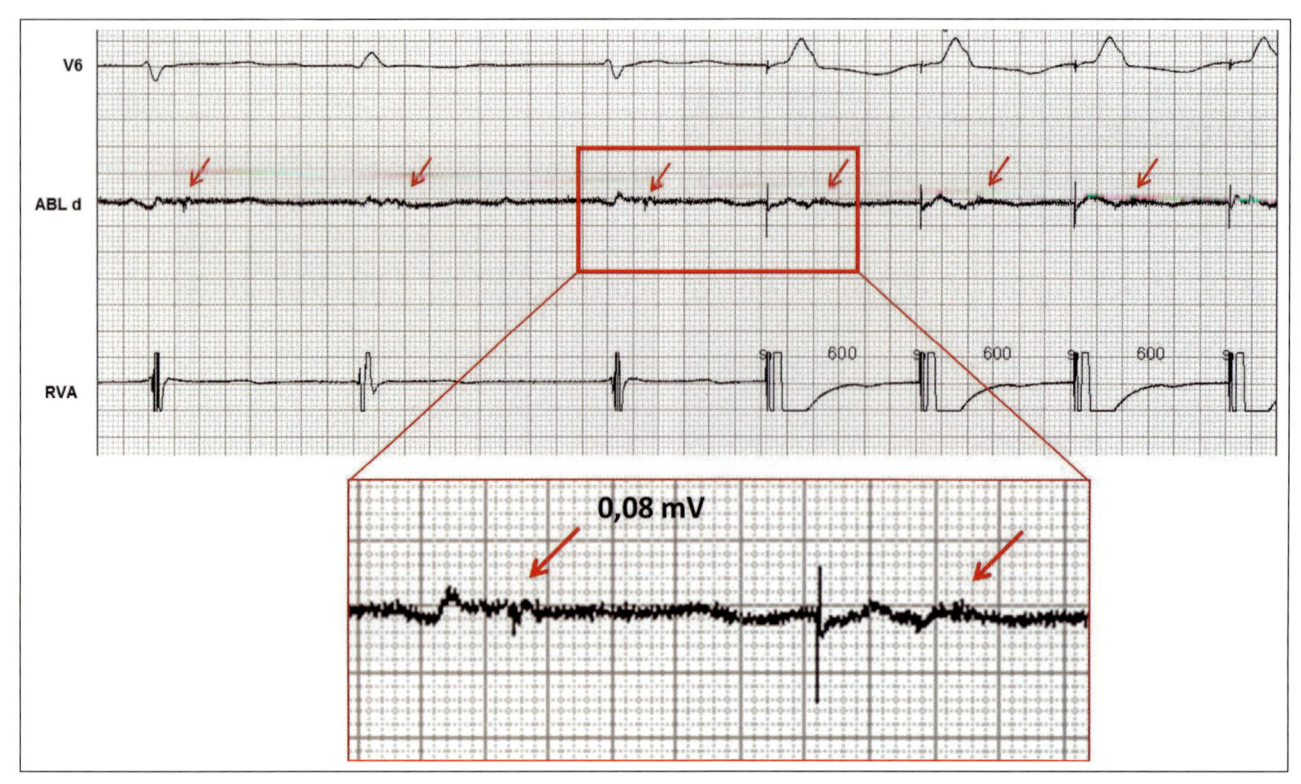

Figure 38.4. Recordings from surface lead V_6 and intracardiac recordings from the distal pair of the mapping catheter (ABL d) and right ventricular apex (RVA). The amplitude of the local EGM recorded by the mapping catheter is 0.14 mV. The local EGM recorded by the mapping catheter displays a LP (0.08 mV) evident during sinus rhythm and RVA pacing (oblique arrow).

each site (**Figure 38.4**) and tag if a site has an LP in any rhythms (▶ **Video 38.3**). An activation map is displayed too (▶ **Videos 38.4** and **38.5**).

Sometimes it is helpful to adjust the voltage cutoff values in different ways looking for voltage gradients that may represent channels of viable myocardium. The principle here is that if a small corridor of viable myocardium is surrounded by unexcitable tissue it is a potential protected isthmus of slow conduction during VT. An ablation strategy based on these assumptions have shown encouraging results.[11,12] However, according to a study that measured direct excitability by inability to direct pace capture, it is unclear what signal voltage represents unexcitable tissue.[10] We presently use this as an adjunctive finding, and voltage gradients are only considered important if the low-voltage areas have really low voltage (≤ 0.2 mV).

Pace Mapping

As a general strategy, when the voltage and activation map is completed, pace mapping is performed, pacing during sinus rhythm from the ablation catheter at the sites that displayed delayed potentials, starting at points with the latest isolated delayed potential recorded. A 12-lead ECG is obtained during pacing and compared to the surface QRS morphology of the clinical VT (**Figure 38.5**). We pay increasing attention to the morphology of the far-field ICD EGM and its timing to the bipolar ICD EGM as a template to which we compare pacing morphology of the ICD EGM during the ablation procedure, since we and others have shown its high sensitivity to discriminate between 2 different pacing sites or VT morphologies.[16-18] In the frequent situation, in patients with implanted ICD, that no 12-lead ECG VT has been recorded, the morphology and timing of ICD EGMs can be used as a template to which we compare the resultant ICD EGM from a paced site. The points at which the pace map matches the ECG morphology or ICD EGM morphology of the clinical VT, particularly if there is a delay between the stimulus and the onset of the QRS complex of ≥ 50 ms, are tagged in the navigation system as possible target points (protected isthmus of the circuit). However, if the pacing morphology matches the VT morphology without delay between the stimulus and the QRS onset, the site is likely to be close to the exit of the VT circuit. These sites are not our first option to target, but eventually could be targeted if VT remains inducible after other sites have been targeted.

Induction of VT and Catheter Ablation

When the ablation catheter is located at a potentially good target site, according to the previously discussed criteria, programmed ventricular stimulation protocol is performed with up to 3 extrastimuli, pacing from two right and eventually one left ventricular sites. VT is considered clinical if

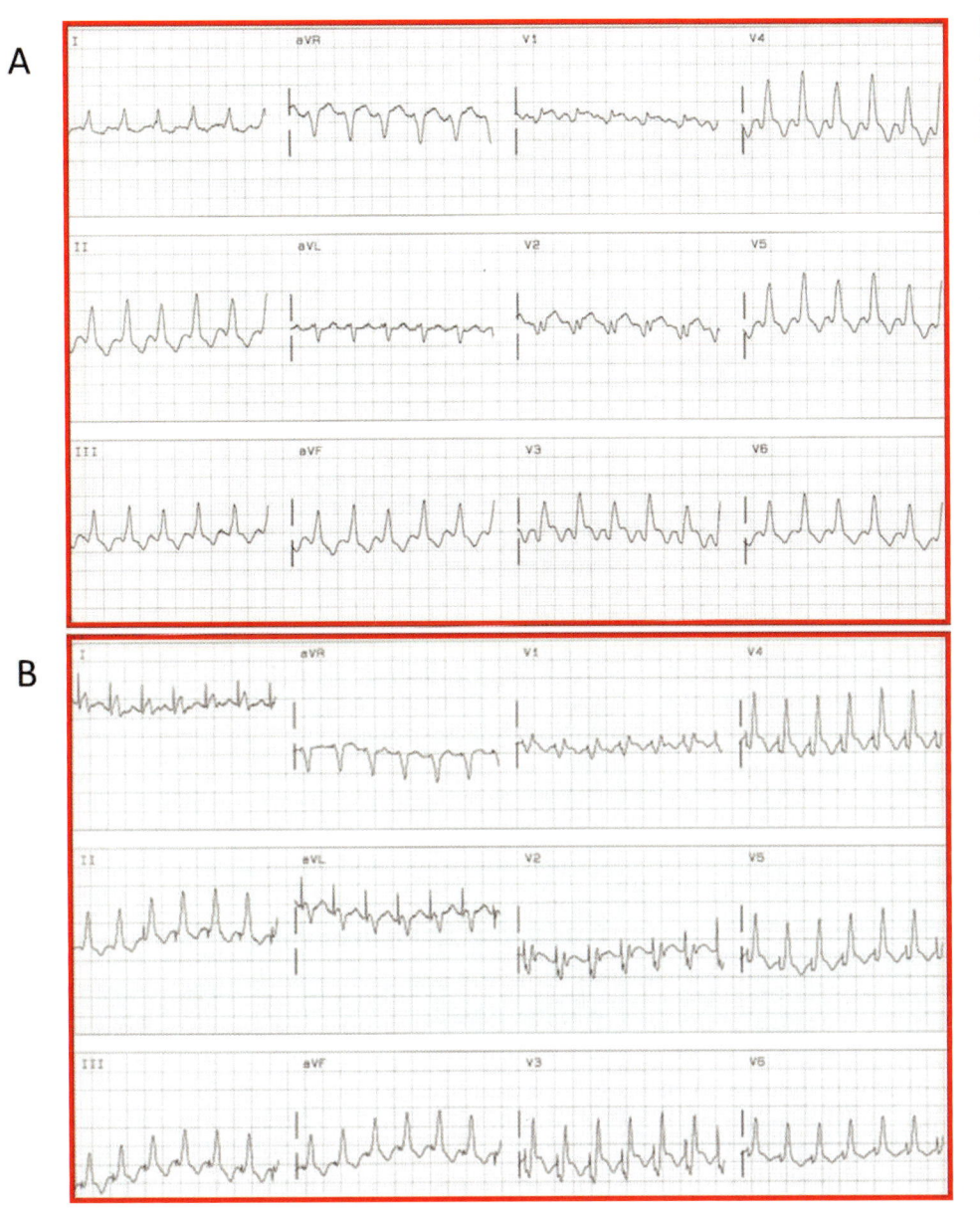

Figure 38.5 A. 12-lead ECG of a spontaneous ventricular tachycardia in a patient with previous inferior and anterior myocardial infarction. **B.** The 12 leads pacing during sinus rhythm at the TCL. Note that the morphology of the paced complex matched that of the spontaneous VT in all leads except V_2, in which minor differences are found.

the 12-lead morphology matches the previously documented VT. At this point, at least 3 scenarios are possible:

1. VT is hemodynamically tolerated and permits activation and entrainment mapping, delivering energy at points with diastolic potentials and adequate response to pacing maneuvers according to conventional criteria. Trains of 15 pacing stimuli are delivered at a CL 20 ms shorter than the VT CL. Pacing from outside and inside the circuit permit discrimination between a diastolic potential related with the critical isthmus of the VT or a bystander (**Figures 38.6** and **38.7**).

2. VT is associated with hemodynamic deterioration, defined as a decrease in systolic blood pressure to < 80 mm Hg for > 10 seconds. At this point it is important to check for the presence of mid-diastolic potentials during VT in the sites where the pace mapping was optimum, and try to entrain the tachycardia, at least once, pacing from the ablation catheter, measuring the PPI (difference between the PPI and the TCL). If all the parameters confirm that we are in the critical isthmus of the circuit, RF energy is delivered. If the tachycardia does not terminate within 30 seconds of RF delivery or the patient deteriorates hemodynamically, the tachycardia is terminated with overdrive pacing or electrical cardioversion.

3. VT is not inducible: substrate ablation is performed, concentrated in the area of isolated and delayed potentials.

For substrate ablation, the area over which the energy will be delivered is delineated targeting the areas with LPs

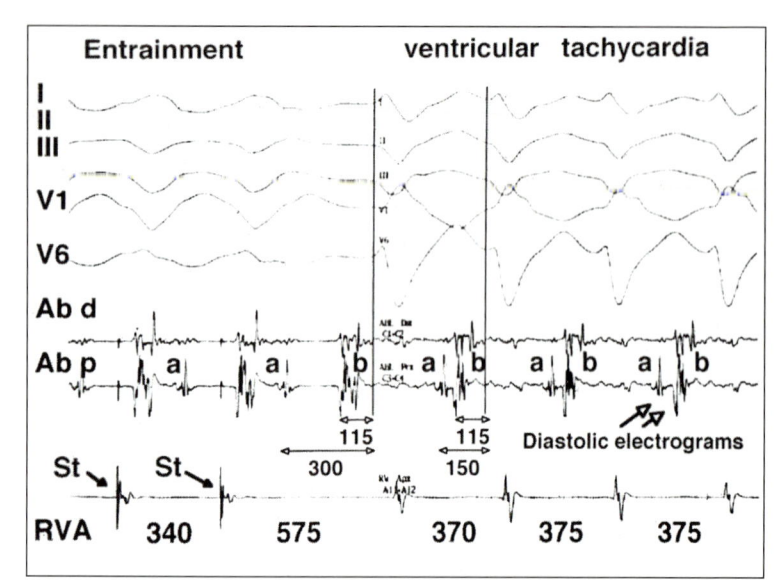

Figure 38.6 Identification of a diastolic potential unrelated to the tachycardia circuit pacing outside of the reentrant circuit. Surface ECG leads I, II, III, V_1, and V_6 and intracardiac recordings from a mapping LV catheter (Ab d: distal, Ab p: proximal) and the right ventricular apex (RVA) are shown during the last 2 paced beats of a pacing train (CL 340 ms) during VT resulting in transient entrainment. VT continues unaltered (last 4 QRS complexes). Two components ("a" and "b") are recorded at the mapping catheter: both are diastolic during VT. However, a different behavior is observed after the last paced beat. Component "a" precedes the onset of the VT QRS by 300 ms, totally different than the 150 ms interval with which it precedes QRS onset during the remaining VT beats. This suggests that this component is unrelated to the VT. In contrast component "b" precedes the onset of the VT QRS after the last paced beat by 115 ms, an interval identical to that with which it precedes QRS onset during the remaining VT beats. This is consistent with component "b" as being part of the VT circuit.

and good pace maps, and extending them to adjacent dense scar areas, so no potentially viable corridors are left. In the rather unusual case that all clinical VTs have been initiated and targeted successfully during VT, but LP areas remain, it is a matter of discussion whether they should be targeted as well.

In general, we prefer irrigated-tip technology for VT ablation in patients with structural heart disease, since it produces deeper and larger lesions resulting in more effective substrate modification and a higher success rate. RF energy is delivered as a continuous, unmodulated sine wave of 500 kHz between the distal electrode of the ablation catheter and a cutaneous patch electrode on the posterior chest. We deliver the applications with a temperature limit of 43°C at a cooling rate of 17 to 32 ml/min using a synchronized pump (EP shuttle, Cordis-Stockert Ltd., Freiburg, Germany) and starting power delivery at 35 W but adjusting power delivered during application in accordance with impedance fall, targeted to a decrease of 10 to 14 ohms in relation to the impedance measured at the initiation of the application.

After ablation, programmed ventricular stimulation is repeated at 2 right ventricular sites, whenever the clinical situation allows it. Successful catheter ablation is defined as termination of VT by application of RF energy and/or the subsequent inducibility suppression of the targeted VT. In cases with unmappable VT, we evaluate the disappearance of all recorded LPs in the area related to the clinical VT circuit.

Postprocedure Care

Patients are monitored for at least 12 hours in the intensive care unit. They receive an anticoagulant dose of low-molecular-weight heparin 4 hours after the procedure, and oral anticoagulation for 3 months (international normalized ratio > 2). During follow-up, patients are treated with the same antiarrhythmic drugs that they had been taking before the ablation procedure.

Previous to discharge from the hospital an echocardiogram is performed to rule out complications and quantify the ejection fraction of the left ventricle.

Procedural Complications

One of the most important complications is periprocedural pericardial tamponade related to myocardial perforation, or secondary to the transseptal approach when this is performed. Lesions of the coronary arteries during catheter manipulation in the aortic root, or associated with RF applications, can originate a myocardial infarction (in cases with epicardial approach). Other complications are linked to the vascular access resulting in bleeding, hematoma, and vascular injury associated with catheter manipulation inside the aorta, especially in patients with associated vascular disease. The risk of embolic complications, like stroke or systemic embolism, is not negligible, but this risk can be minimized with a precise anticoagulation protocol.

When the area of interest is close to the HPS, it is important to avoid the inherent risk of AV block secondary to RF applications.

During the ablation procedure the patients can develop acute left heart failure, related to the low ejection fraction and the extra volume received through the irrigation catheter; the use of diuretics, low-dose catecholamines, and mechanical ventilation may be needed to restore the hemodynamic equilibrium.

In some cases, the programmed stimulation protocol would induce rapid VT or ventricular fibrillation requiring external shocks. This is frequent and is not a complication. However, occasional patients develop incessant VT or

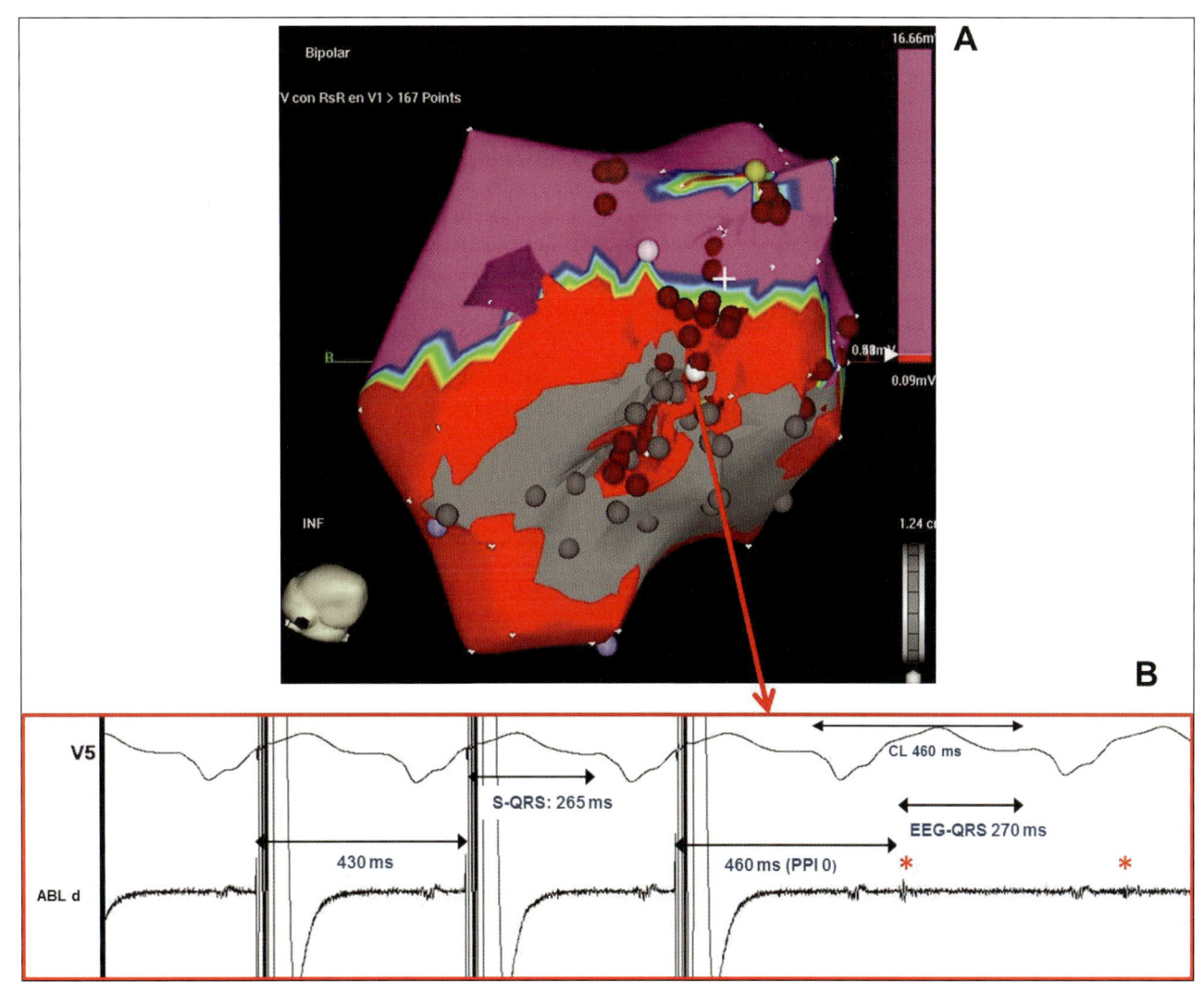

Figure 38.7 Entrainment from mapping catheter inside the reentrant circuit. **A.** Bipolar voltage map of the posterior aspect of the left ventricle showing a postero-inferior scar (complete scar in gray with EGM voltage amplitude ≤ 0.1 mV and dense scar in red with EGM's amplitude between ≥ 0.1 and ≤ 0.5 mV). The area of isolated, delayed potentials was close to the dense scar (white points). The VT was induced, and early diastolic potentials (red asterisks) during VT were recorded at this point. RF energy was delivered at points marked in red, and VT was interrupted. **B.** This figure shows the recordings from surface lead V_5 and intracardiac recording from the mapping catheter (Ab d). An LP related to the VT circuit is recorded by the mapping catheter. After entrainment of the VT the PPI is identical to VT CL. The interval from the stimulus to the onset of the following QRS complex during entrainment (S-QRS) is similar to the interval from EGM of the LP to the onset of the QRS complex (EEG-QRS) during VT.

deteriorate after cardioversion requiring support. In exceptional cases electromechanical dissociation and death have been described.

Advantages and Limitations

Substrate ablation based on the presence of isolated, delayed potential in sinus rhythm or during right ventricular pacing permits the ablation of unmappable or noninducible VTs, with a reasonably high efficacy with 60% to 70% of cases remaining free of VT recurrences over a 1-year period, and the majority of them showing a dramatic decrease in the frequency of ICD therapies. The identification of these characteristic potentials permits to increase the specificity in the identification of slow conduction zones, since these areas are relatively small in comparison with the total area of the scar, reducing the number of RF applications. In addition, substrate ablation could eliminate the substrate for different VTs otherwise not ablated by conventional strategies based on mapping during VT.

There are several limitations of this technique:

1. Limitations in specificity: the recording of delayed potentials during sinus rhythm or right ventricular pacing may relate with bystander tracts that are not critical for reentry.

2. Limitations in sensitivity: this is a more important limitation. One can never be sure that the whole ventricular endocardial surface has been mapped with adequate precision, so critical areas may have been missed due to difficulties in catheter manipulation; moreover, epicardial and/or intramural substrates could be missed despite adequate ablation of the endocardial substrate.

3. The endpoint is not well defined: one cannot rely on VT inducibility since VT may not be inducible (in the baseline) or uncertainty as to the significance of induced VT may be an issue; elimination of all recorded LPs is usually required, but this depends on how extensive the mapping procedure is performed after ablation.

Conclusions

Mapping in the absence of VT, based on the detection of areas of isolation and LPs during sinus rhythm or right ventricular pacing, identifies areas of slow conduction, corresponding with surviving tracts inside scar areas, in most patients with VT and structural heart disease. The combination of this information with pace mapping and entrainment techniques (whenever possible) allows ablation therapy that can be offered to most patients with unmappable VT with a reasonable outcome in terms of both efficacy and safety. It is important to consider that most of the experience has been gained with postmyocardial infarction VT and there are significant differences in the substrate of patients with ischemic and nonischemic heart disease. Whether a different approach should be routinely undertaken in the latter group of patients remains to be established.

References

1. Cassidy DM, Vassallo JA, Buxton AE, Doherty JU, Marchlinski FE, Josephson ME. The value of catheter mapping during sinus rhythm to localize site of origin of ventricular tachycardia. *Circulation*. 1984;69:1103–1110.
2. Cassidy DM, Vassallo JA, Buxton AE, Doherty JU, Marchlinski FE, Josephson ME. Catheter mapping during sinus rhythm: relation of local electrogram duration to ventricular tachycardia cycle length. *Am J Cardiol*. 1985;1;55:713–716.
3. Cassidy DM, Vassallo JA, Miller JM, et al. Endocardial catheter mapping during sinus rhythm: relation of underlying heart disease and ventricular arrhythmia. *Circulation*. 1986;73:645–652.
4. Harada T, Stevenson WG, Kocovic DZ, Friedman PL. Catheter ablation of ventricular tachycardia after myocardial infarction: relation of endocardial sinus rhythm late potentials to the reentry circuit. *J Am Coll Cardiol*. 1997;30:1015–1023.
5. Bogun F, Bender B, Li YG, Groenefeld G, et al. Analysis during sinus rhythm of critical sites in reentry circuits of postinfarction ventricular tachycardia. *J Interv Card Electrophysiol*. 2002;7:95–103.
6. Bogun F, Marine JE, Hohnloser SH, Oral H, Pelosi F, Morady F. Relative timing of isolated potentials during postinfarction ventricular tachycardia and sinus rhythm. *J Interv Card Electrophysiol*. 2004;10:65–72.
7. Arenal A, Glez-Torrecilla E, Ortiz M, et al. Ablation of electrograms with an isolated, delayed component as treatment of unmappable monomorphic ventricular tachycardias in patients with structural heart disease. *J Am Coll Cardiol*. 2003;41:81–92.
8. Bogun F, Good E, Reich S, et al. Isolated potentials during sinus rhythm and pace mapping within scars as guides for ablation of postinfarction ventricular tachycardia. *J Am Coll Cardiol*. 2006;47:2013–2019.
9. Marchlinski FE, Callans DJ, Gottlieb CD, et al. Linear ablation lesions for control of unmappable ventricular tachycardia in patients with ischemic and nonischemic cardiomyopathy. *Circulation*. 2000;101:1288–1296.
10. Soejima K, Stevenson WG, Maisel WH, Sapp JL, Epstein LM. Electrically unexcitable scar mapping based on pacing threshold for identification of the reentry circuit isthmus: feasibility for guiding ventricular tachycardia ablation. *Circulation*. 2002;106:1678–1683.
11. Arenal A, del Castillo S, Gonzalez-Torrecilla E, et al. Tachycardia-related channel in the scar tissue in patients with sustained monomorphic ventricular tachycardias: influence of the voltage scar definition. *Circulation*. 2004;110:2568–2574.
12. Hsia HH, Lin D, Sauer WH, Callans DJ, Marchlinski FE. Anatomic characterization of endocardial substrate for hemodynamically stable reentrant ventricular tachycardia: identification of endocardial conducting channels. *Heart Rhythm*. 2006;3:503–512.
13. Hsia HH, Callans DJ, Marchlinski FE. Characterization of endocardial electrophysiological substrate in patients with nonischemic cardiomyopathy and monomorphic ventricular tachycardia. *Circulation*. 2003;108:704–710.
14. Garcia FC, Bazan V, Zado ES, Ren JF, Marchlinski FE. Epicardial substrate and outcome with epicardial ablation of ventricular tachycardia in arrhythmogenic right ventricular cardiomyopathy/dysplasia. *Circulation*. 2009;120:366–375.
15. Nakahara S, Tung R, Ramirez RJ, et al. Characterization of the arrhythmogenic substrate in ischemic and nonischemic cardiomyopathy implications for catheter ablation of hemodynamically unstable ventricular tachycardia. *J Am Coll Cardiol*. 2010;55:2355–2365.
16. Almendral J, Atienza F, Rojo JL, et al. Spatial resolution of ICD electrograms to identify different sites of left ventricular stimulation. *Eur Heart J*. 2008;29:645 (abstract).
17. Yoshida K, Liu TY, Scott C, et al. The value of defibrillator electrograms for recognition of clinical ventricular tachycardias and for pace mapping of postinfarction ventricular tachycardia. *J Am Coll Cardiol*. 2010;56:969–979.
18. Almendral J, Marchlinski F. Is it the same or a different ventricular tachycardia? an additional use for defibrillator electrograms. *J Am Coll Cardiol*. 2010;56:980–982

Video Descriptions

Video 38.1 Right anterior oblique (RAO) view during the ablation procedure of a patient with recurrent ventricular tachycardia and multiple discharges by the ICD. Two diagnostic catheters were positioned at the RVA and the CS. The ablation catheter was progressed via transseptal approach to the left ventricle, using a long deflectable sheath. The tip of the ablation catheter is in the region of a big anteroapical calcified aneurysm.

Video 38.2 The left anterior oblique (LAO) view of the same patient shown in Video 38.1.

Video 38.3 Bipolar voltage map of the left ventricle. The color display is set to a color range of 0.5 to 1.5 mV to distinguish the limits of the scar; normal voltages (1.5 mV) are color coded in purple, and abnormal low-amplitude potentials are color coded in blue to red (the latter representing the lowest amplitudes). Complete scar is considered when the EGM's voltage amplitude is ≤ 0.1 mV (gray) and dense scar with an EGM amplitude between ≥ 0.1 and ≤ 0.5 mV (red). Pathological bipolar potentials and scar are found in the anteroapical region, consistent with a previous anterior myocardial infarction. The area of isolated LPs recorded within the scar mapping during sinus rhythm is labeled with pink dots.

Video 38.4 Activation map during sinus rhythm in the same patient displayed in Video 38.2. Note that the area where the LPs are recorded is activated lately, in comparison with the rest of the left ventricle.

Video 38.5 Propagation map during sinus rhythm in the same patient displayed in Videos 38.2 and 38.3.

Video 38.6 Bipolar voltage map of the left ventricle after ablation in the same patient shown in previous videos. Note that the area treated by RF applications is relatively small in comparison with the totality of the scar.

CHAPTER 39

How to Utilize Electroanatomical Mapping to Identify Critical Channels for Ventricular Tachycardia Ablation

Henry H. Hsia, MD; Kojiro Tanimoto, MD

Introduction

Catheter ablation in patients with recurrent VT requires identification of components of the reentrant circuit and is mostly limited to hemodynamically tolerated monomorphic VTs. However, most of the induced VTs are unstable, with multiple morphologies, and do not permit extensive pacing maneuvers during arrhythmia.

High-density electroanatomical mapping provides an accurate 3-dimensional characterization of the diseased myocardium and allows a paradigm shift in VT ablation. A substrate-based ablation strategy focuses on the identification of abnormal myocardium that participates as critical components of the reentry circuit. Pathological studies have suggested that zones of slow conduction/isthmus of the reentrant circuits are often located within myocardial scar, and EGM recordings from these sites may exhibit a higher signal voltage compared to the surrounding scar.[1,2] By careful analysis of the electroanatomical substrate and local voltage profiles, zones of slow conduction/isthmus can be detected.[3,4] By adjusting the color threshold on a voltage map, VT-related conducting channels can be identified that correspond to the zone of slow conduction within the reentry circuit. Such channels are defined as paths demonstrating contiguous EGMs with voltage higher than that of the surrounding areas, and participate in orthodromic activation during VT (**Figure 39.1**). Identification of such channels facilitates localization of potential reentrant circuit isthmuses that require additional mapping. Ultimately, it may allow ablation of multiple stable and unstable VTs in patients with scar-based reentry with limited arrhythmia induction.

Preprocedural Planning

Thorough preoperative assessment can facilitate procedural planning for efficient mapping and improves ablation outcomes. Defining patients' underlying arrhythmogenic substrate requires careful review of patients' history and data. In patients with coronary artery disease and prior myocardial infarction, the reentrant VTs often originate from subendocardial sites of infarcted myocardium, adjacent to the dense scar.[5,6] However, nonendocardial substrates in scar-related as well as in idiopathic VTs have recently been increasingly recognized.[7-9] In patients with dilated nonischemic cardiomyopathy, confluent areas of abnormal low-voltage scars (epicardial ≥ endocardial) are often located over the basal lateral left ventricle near the valve annulus. A prior history of open-chest coronary bypass grafting or valvular surgery is important if a percutaneous epicardial approach is being considered,[10] whereas a history of significant peripheral vascular disease, prior mechanical aortic prostheses, or mitral valvular prostheses may preclude a retrograde aortic or transseptal approach for endocardial intervention.

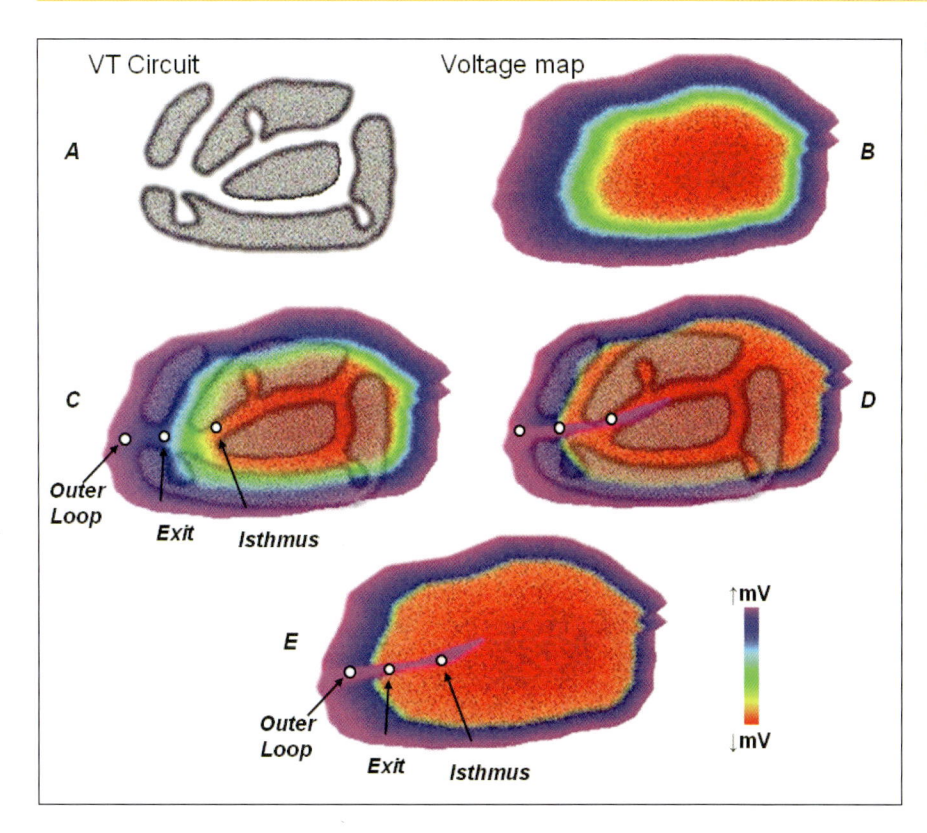

Figure 39.1 Channel identification with voltage color gradient adjustment. A reentrant VT circuit (**A**) is depicted by the illustrative cartoon of scar and multiple pathways. The circuit resides in the low-voltage scarred tissue. The baseline color gradient showed dense scar (red), normal tissue (purple), and the intermediate-colored border zone (**B**). The VT-related conducting channel represents the orthordromic activation during reentry (isthmus→exit→outer loop) and often corresponds to zone of slow conduction (**C**). Such channel may be visible by adjusting the color threshold on a voltage map (**D**). A VT-related conducting channel is defined as a path demonstrating contiguous EGMs with voltage higher than that of the surrounding areas (**E**).

Careful review of the ECG data is a critical step of the preprocedural planning. The presence of Q waves during sinus rhythm reveals the locations of myocardial scar and the potential arrhythmia substrate, particularly in patients with ICM. Analysis of the ECG patterns during VT or PVCs helps to regionalize the exit of the VT circuit. In addition, different electrocardiographic criteria for recognizing epicardial versus endocardial origins of arrhythmia have been described.[11-13]

In patients with ICDs, the stored intracardiac EGMs during the spontaneous arrhythmia episodes also provides valuable information. By comparing the real-time ICD EGM morphologies during the multiple induced VTs and the stored EGMs from the patient's spontaneous presenting arrhythmia, a diagnosis of the clinical VT may be confirmed, which helps the operator to focus the mapping effort during the procedure. Alternatively, a diagnosis of bundle branch reentry or fascicular reentry is suspected if similar ICD EGMs were recorded during the clinical VT episodes as that recorded during the baseline sinus rhythm, suggesting the participation of native HPS during arrhythmia.

Although ischemia does not cause recurrent monomorphic VTs, an adequate assessment of the ischemic burden is essential, particularly in elderly patients with history of ischemic heart disease and prior surgical/percutaneous interventions. From a procedural safety point of view, we have a low threshold to perform coronary angiograms to exclude potentially significant coronary arterial stenosis in this population with extensive structural heart disease.

A preoperative echocardiogram is also a part of the routine preprocedural planning. The presence of wall motion abnormalities or thinning suggests the locations of the scar substrate. The presence of a fresh, mobile, nonlaminated intracavitary thrombus is an absolute contraindication for endocardial catheter ablation. If significant aortic stenosis is present, a transseptal or an epicardial approach for left ventricular access needs to be planned.

Procedure

Patient Preparation

The majority of our patients who undergo VT ablation have multiple inducible ventricular tachyarrhythmias. Unique to VT mapping, ECG pattern recognition is crucial in localizing the VT exit and for pace mapping. Accurate placement of surface ECG electrodes is imperative. Erroneous ECG interpretations will lead to confusion, procedural delay, and failed outcome.

Our protocol recommends the use of the electroanatomic system for substrate mapping (CARTO, Biosense Webster, Diamond Bar, CA, USA). Care must be taken for placement of the reference patch to compensate for the dilated, leftward rotated left ventricles in most of our patients. The reference patch should be placed lower in the middle of the ventricular silhouette in the anterior-posterior projection to ensure proper registration of the electroanatomical navigational data. Although the St. Jude

Ensite NavX system (St. Jude Medical, St. Paul, MN) may also be used to construct the voltage maps, identification of VT-related conducting channels using this system has not been studied.

For the real-time ICD EGM recordings, a device-specific junction box (for example, Medtronic) may be obtained from the vendor that connects the programmer to the EP recording system (GE Prucka) in the analog channels for display.

In the majority of our patients with left ventricular VT ablation, the arterial access is through the right femoral artery with an 8- to 8.5-Fr sheath for retrograde aortic approach. In patients with significant peripheral vascular disease, a long sheath may be used for better support. A separate, redundant arterial line for hemodynamic monitoring may be necessary in patients with advanced heart disease and life-threatening arrhythmias. Many of our patients also undergo ICE imaging during either endocardial or epicardial VT ablation procedures. The right femoral vein is accessed to accommodate an 11-Fr sheath for the placement of a 10-Fr phased-array ICE catheter. Two right ventricular catheters are routinely placed at the RVA and near the HB. The RVA catheter marks the ventricular apex, and the His catheter marks the ventricular base, opposite to the aortic valve.

For procedures performed using an epicardial approach, or in patients who may have VTs that originate near the mitral annulus, an additional CS catheter, inserted either from the right internal jugular vein or from the femoral vein is used to outline the basal LV silhouette and to facilitate mapping.

Anesthesia

Although it is not necessary, the majority of our patients with scar-based VT who undergo ablation are under general anesthesia. Multiple episodes of poorly tolerated arrhythmias are often induced and require shock terminations. Among the many advantages, general anesthesia helps to control patients' discomfort, minimizes movement, and improves mapping accuracy. The disadvantage of general anesthesia is the abolition of the sympathetic tone for the compensatory vasoconstrictive response during rapid VTs. Nonetheless, close collaboration between the anesthesiologist and the electrophysiologist allows optimal hemodynamic management and respiratory support during the procedure.

Anticoagulation

Intravascular insertion and manipulation of catheters, creation of ablation lesions, activation of coagulation factors, and potential disruption of atherosclerotic plaques contribute to a risk of thromboembolism during and after catheter ablation. Patients with structural heart disease undergoing left heart catheterization have a risk of stroke or thromboembolism of ~1%. We recommend meticulous monitoring of the ACT every 20 minutes. The target ACT is maintained at ~300 seconds.

Mapping

Most patients who undergo VT ablation have significant structural heart disease and multiple inducible ventricular tachyarrhythmias (mean 4 ± 3 VT morphologies). A hybrid approach is needed, combining both the conventional mapping techniques and the substrate mapping approaches (**Table 39.1**).[14] A conventional mapping strategy consists of activation mapping and entrainment mapping, and both require sustained reentry and cannot be performed during poorly tolerated VT.

To optimize the result of substrate mapping during sinus/paced rhythm, areas of interest within the abnormal myocardium should be tagged, which helps to define the geometry of the circuit and its relationship to the underlying scar. Identification of conducting channels, along with other collaborative mapping strategies, helps to characterize the VT circuit (these include defining EUS, detecting LPs, and pace mapping [**Figure 39.2**]). Conventional mapping methods such as activation and/or entrainment/resetting response also complement the substrate mapping to confirm the functional significance of these conducting channels.

In any given patient, the mapping strategy has to be individualized. Detailed, high-density EGM recording is essential. The average number of sampled points per chamber should be at a minimum of 150 to 200 for adequate definition of anatomy and EP characterization of the VT substrate.

Our protocol recommends the use of the open irrigated radiofrequency ablation catheter (NaviStar ThermoCool, Biosense Webster, Diamond Bar, CA, USA). By cooling the electrode-tissue interface, irrigated electrodes allow for delivery of greater power without significant rise of impedance or catheter tip temperature. This consistently produces deeper and larger lesions compared to standard solid

Table 39.1 VT Mapping Techniques

Conventional Mapping Techniques	Substrate Mapping Techniques
Sinus rhythm mapping	Local electrogram voltage/amplitude
ECG analysis, pace mapping	Conducting channels (CC)
Activation mapping	Electrical unexcitable scar (EUS)
Entrainment mapping	Electrograms with isolated delayed components (E-IDC) or late potentials (LPs)
Personnel	Pace mapping

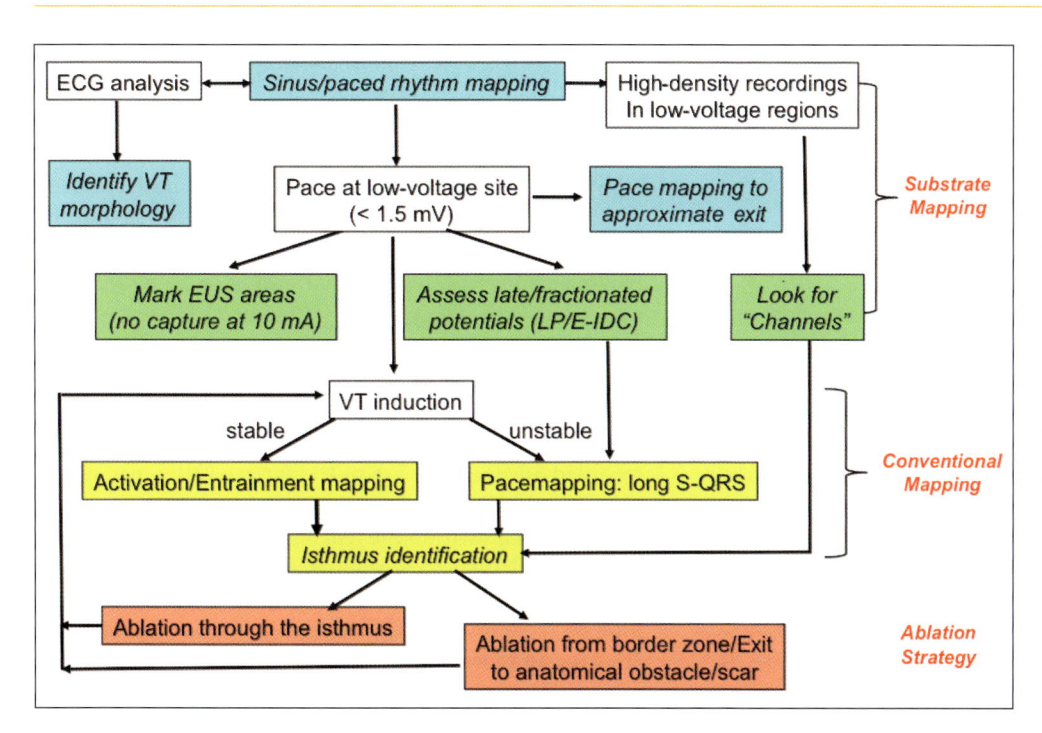

Figure 39.2 General approach to catheter mapping and ablation of VT. Identification of VT-related conducting channels is part of the overall strategy of VT ablation, particularly for substrate mapping. Careful sampling of local bipolar EGMs during sinus or paced non-VT rhythm is critical for construction of voltage maps and characterization of the electroanatomical substrate. Identification of EUS, LP/E-IDC, and pace mapping facilitates the detection of conducting channels.

electrodes, and is particularly important for relatively large circuits, and reentry pathways may be located deep in scarred myocardium.[15,16] In addition, the smaller distal mapping electrode pair (3.5 mm with 2-mm spacing) allows better spatial resolution compared to the standard 4- or 8-mm tip.

In order to identify the potential VT-related channels, we first must perform a detailed electroanatomical voltage map to characterize the local voltage profile of the substrate. Bipolar endocardial ventricular signals are recorded and filtered at 10 to 400 Hz on the CARTO system, and the peak-to-peak signal amplitude of the bipolar EGM is measured automatically. A 3-dimensional anatomical shell of the cardiac chamber is constructed, and the EGM signals are coupled and displayed as color gradients on a voltage map. Such voltage maps may be registered onto a previously constructed anatomical shell from the ICE images using the CARTOSound software. Valvular locations are tagged and excluded from the voltage analysis. Valvular sites are identified by fluoroscopic catheter tip positions that demonstrate simultaneous recordings of equal atrial and ventricular signal amplitudes. The voltage maps are then edited, and intracavitary points are eliminated.

The reference value for distinguishing normal and abnormal bipolar EGM amplitude has been previously established at 1.5 mV for the right ventricle and 1.8 mV for the left ventricle. The normal signal amplitude is defined as the value above which 95% of all bipolar signal voltages from the endocardium of normal ventricles are included. "Dense scar" is arbitrarily defined as areas with signal amplitude less than 0.5 mV. The "border zone" is defined as a transition zone between dense scar and normal tissue (0.5 to 1.5/1.8 mV).[17] For epicardial mapping, the "normal" epicardial signal amplitude is set at above 1.0 mV.

Isthmus sites have been shown to reside predominantly (> 80%) in the dense scar (< 0.5 mV) whereas most exit sites are located in the border zone (**Table 39.2**).[4] Pace mapping along the border zone (0.5–1.5 mV) is performed to approximate the exit of the VT circuit, which is defined by sites with a similar paced QRS morphology compared to that during spontaneous ventricular arrhythmia with a short stimulus-QRS interval, arbitrarily defined as < 40 ms.

Table 39.2 Local Electrogram Amplitude for Sites within the Reentrant Circuit

	Entrance	Central Isthmus	Exit	Outer Loop
Dense Scar (< 0.5 mV)	17	30	18	6
Border Zone (0.5–1.5 mV)	2	7	26	18
Normal (> 1.5 mV)	---	---	4	8
Total (136 sites)	19	37	48	32

(Modified with permission from Hsia et al., *Heart Rhythm.* 2006, 3: 503–512.)

Once the exit is identified, pace mapping and further mapping efforts should be directed progressively away from the abnormal border zone toward the center of the low-voltage dense scar (< 0.5 mV) for localizing the isthmus of the reentry circuit.

Identification of Conducting Channels (CCs)

The CARTO system displays the voltage maps and automatically selects the largest local component of the bipolar EGMs. The nominal setting for the color display of voltage maps has an upper threshold of 1.5 to 1.8 mV (purple) and a lower threshold of 0.5 mV (red). The border zone is the transition area between dense scar and normal tissue with intermediate colors.

Focusing on the low-voltage areas (< 1.5 mV), VT-related conducting channels can be identified by voltage color adjustment of the bipolar voltage maps during baseline rhythms without tachycardia induction. A "conducting channel" is defined by the presence of a "corridor" of consecutive EGMs differentiated by the higher signal voltage amplitudes than the surrounding area. The locations of such channels have been correlated to the reentrant circuit by entrainment mapping,[4] and may be observed on both endocardial and epicardial surfaces.

With the current versions of the software (CARTO XP or CARTO-3), color threshold enhancement can be performed by manually adjusting the color bar. First, the upper threshold of the color display is reduced toward 0.5 mV to minimize the intermediate colors and to maximize the color contrast between adjacent myocardium with different EGM voltages. Thereafter, both the upper and the low-color thresholds are decremented in small steps (0.1–0.2 mV) until a conducting channel could be identified or a minimal value of 0.05 mV was reached for the lower limit of the color range. A "scar" may also be designated and displayed as a solid gray area based on the specified voltage value by using the "scar setting" software feature (**Figure 39.3**).

It is important to note that the scar tissue is not homogeneous and there is a wide range of scar definition/voltage thresholds for best identifying the conducting channels. A single cutoff voltage threshold may not be feasible in all cases as VT-related complete (VTR-CCC) and incomplete (VTR-ICC) conducting channels are visualized at multiple voltage thresholds.[3] However, the majority of channels are identified when the scar voltage threshold is set around 0.2 to 0.3 mV, with a length ranging from 23 to 32 mm (**Figure 39.4**).

After the apparent conducting channels are identified, the relationship between the "channels" and the reentrant circuit must be confirmed by activation and/or entrainment mapping (**Figure 39.5**). In the majority of patients who do not have hemodynamically tolerated VTs, other surrogate markers for protected areas of slow conduction should also be investigated. These include (1) local capture during pacing with a long stimulus-QRS interval, and (2) fractionated LPs recorded deep within the channel that often are in proximity to (3) electrical unexcitable dense scar.

Scar mapping based on pacing threshold has been used to identify nonconducting tissue that borders viable myocardium during sinus rhythm.[18] Such EUS can be identified by noncapture with high-output pacing (> 10 mA), and is associated with a very low local bipolar EGM amplitude (< 0.25 mV). EUS is commonly located in proximity to the VT isthmus and the potential conducting channels (**Figure 39.6**).

Delayed local activation within the channels (LPs), recorded after completion of the surface QRS, may reflect slow impulse propagation within the scar-based reentrant VT circuit. LPs within the "channels" may be better identified during RVA pacing compared to sinus rhythm, with a change in the direction of the activation wave front that unmasks some areas of block and slows conduction (**Figure 39.7**).[19] Introduction of ventricular extrastimuli can also reveal decremental conduction delay of impulse propagation into a channel (**Figure 39.8**). The presence of such LPs has been associated with the VT isthmus, especially at sites with significantly prolonged local conduction delay (QRS-LP interval > 200 ms).[20]

Since the isthmus/zone of slow conduction can be defined by fixed or functional block, the conducting channels may also be correlated to the VT isthmus sites by pace mapping. During sinus or paced rhythm, selected pace mapping with local capture within the conducting channel should produce a QRS similar to that of VT, often with a longer stimulus-to-QRS interval (S-QRS) due to slow conduction within the channel.[21] Evidence of decremental delay of impulse propagation into the channels should be examined, which suggests the presence of a protected corridor of slow conduction (**Figures 39.7–39.10**).

Ablation

After visually identifying the potential VT-related channels, the functional significance of the channels should be confirmed by activation mapping and/or entrainment/resetting response (**Figure 39.10**). Locations of interest within the abnormal myocardium are tagged to define the geometry of the circuit and its relationship to the underlying scar. This is important in facilitating the design of the ablation lesion set(s). Linear ablation lesion sets to transact the channel/isthmus are performed to achieve a successful outcome.

Epicardial Approach

In general, epicardial mapping is similar to that of the endocardial surface, with some noticeable caveats. First, the normal epicardial bipolar voltage is identified as > 1.0 mV.[8,9] Second, care must be taken to distinguish true scar from

Chapter 39: EAM Channels for VT Ablation • 365

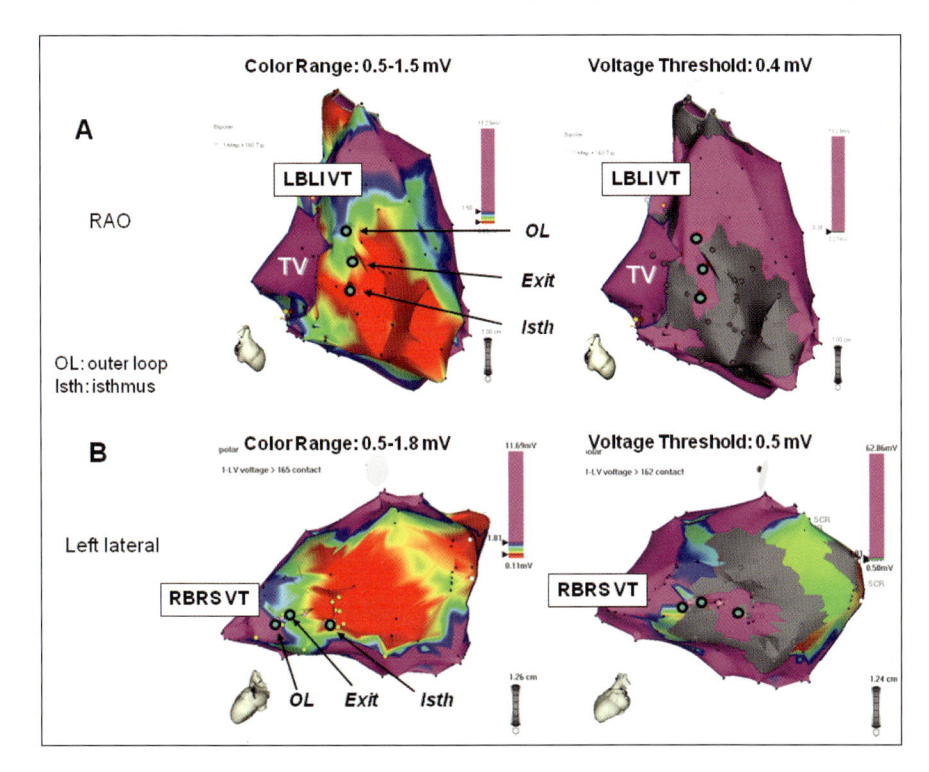

Figure 39.3 Identification of the conducting channels of reentrant VT circuits. Bipolar voltage maps in 2 patients with monomorphic VT are shown. Endocardial sites within the circuits were identified by entrainment mapping. The standard color range for the voltage maps was depicted on the left, and the maps after voltage threshold adjustment were depicted on the right. **A.** Right ventricular maps in a patient with a right ventricular cardiomyopathy and sustained LBLI axis VT. At a voltage threshold of 0.4 mV (dense scar is depicted by gray color at 0.38 mV), a conduit characterized by a higher voltage can be seen that follows the path defined by orthodromically activated VT sites. **B.** Left ventricular maps in a patient with an ischemic cardiomyopathy and prior infarction who presented with a RBRS axis VT. At a voltage threshold of 0.5 mV (dense scar is depicted by gray color at 0.4 mV), evidence of a conduit with a higher voltage that follows orthodromic activating sites during reentrant VT was identified. (Modified with permission from Hsia et al., Heart Rhythm. 2006;3:503–512.)

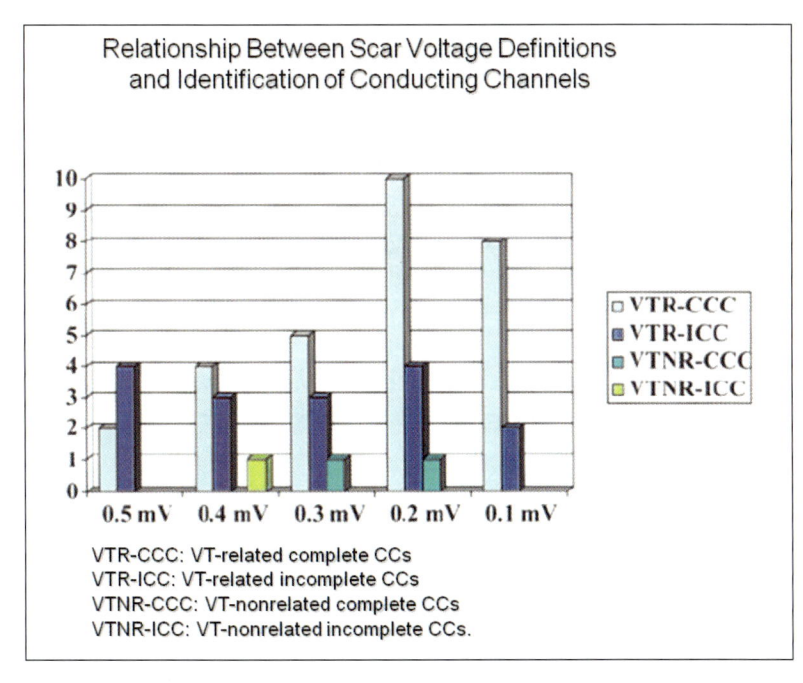

Figure 39.4 Relationship between scar voltage definitions and identification of conducting channels. Bar diagram presenting number of conducting channels recorded at each scar voltage definition. Some channels were defined at more than 1 voltage level. The VT-related complete (VTR-CCC) and incomplete (VTR-ICC) conducting channels are visualized at multiple voltage thresholds, and a single cutoff voltage threshold may not be feasible in all cases. The majority of channels were identified when the scar voltage was set around 0.2 mV. (Modified with permission from Arenal et al., Circulation. 2004;110:2568–2574.)

epicardial fat or poor contact/coronary arteries. Measurements of abnormal EGMs should demonstrate not only low amplitude but also discrete multicomponent, broad/split signals and/or LPs (**Figure 39.7**). Third, pace mapping or entrainment mapping with local capture may be difficult because of the elevated pacing threshold in the epicardium.

In the epicardial space, an open-irrigated catheter is essential for radiofrequency energy delivery. The use of ICE during percutaneous epicardial procedures is recommended. This provides real-time monitoring of the pericardial fluid accumulation and enhances procedural safety. Prior to ablation, high-output pacing to delineate the course of the phrenic nerve is important to avoid phrenic nerve injury and diaphragmatic paralysis. Acute or delayed coronary arterial injury/stenosis is a well-known complication of epicardial ablation, especially when the ablation energy is delivered within 5 mm of a vessel.

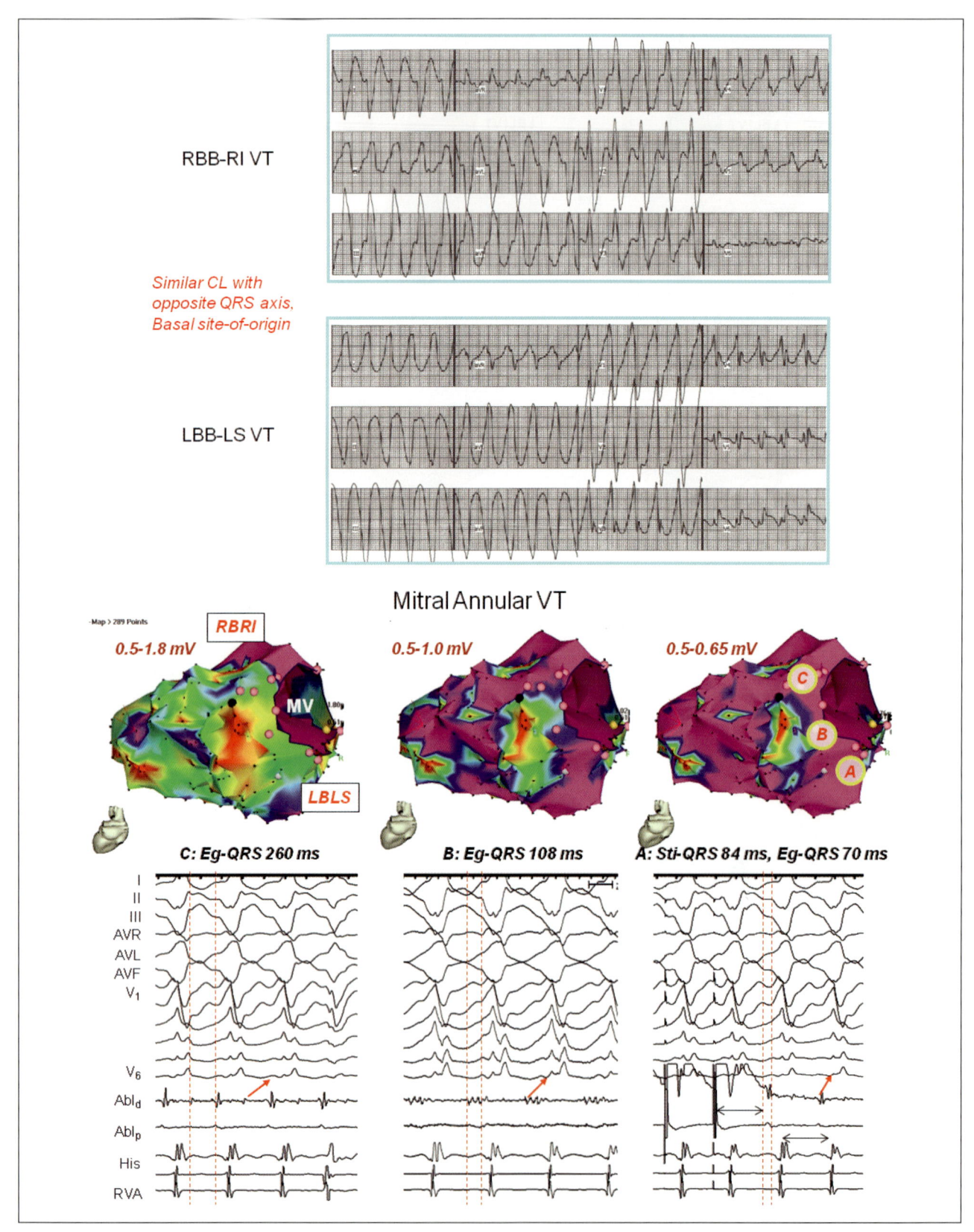

Figure 39.5 Identification of VT-related conducting channel in a patient with prior myocardial infarctions who presented with sustained VT. Two VTs were documented with RBRI and LBLS QRS morphologies. By carefully adjusting the upper and lower color voltage thresholds on the electroanatomic voltage map (0.5–1.8 mV, 0.5–1.0 mV, and 0.5–0.65 mV), a corridor demonstrating higher-voltage amplitude than that of the surrounding areas could be visualized. Entrainment with concealed fusion within the channel was noted at multiple sites (**A**, **B**, **C**) with progressively longer stimulus-QRS (Sti-QRS) intervals that equaled EGM-QRS intervals. This is an example of mitral annular VT with counterclockwise (LBLS) and clockwise reentry (RBRI) VTs around the mitral valve. (Modified with permission from Al-Ahmad AA, Callans DJ, Hsia HH, Natale A, Eds., *Electroanatomical Mapping: An Atlas for Clinicians*. Malden, MA: Wiley-Blackwell; 2008.)

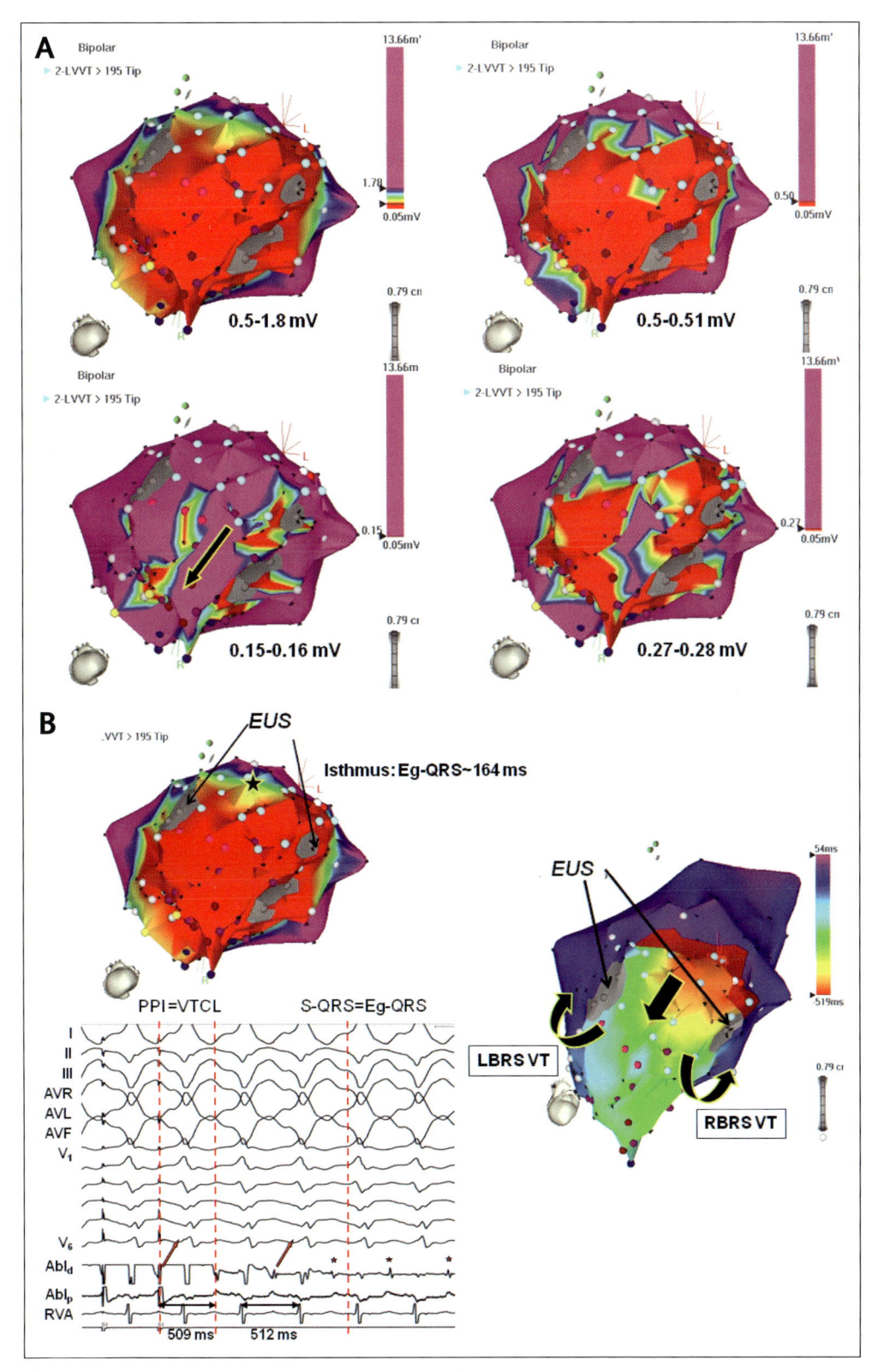

Figure 39.6 Conducting channels and electrically unexcitable scar. Electroanatomical mapping in a patient with a large anterior-lateral myocardial infarction and sustained monomorphic VT. **A.** Voltage map showed a large anterior lateral scar. The color gradients correspond to 0.5–1.8 mV, 0.5–0.51 mV, 0.27–0.28 mV, and 0.15–0.16 mV. EUS was identified by non-capture with high-output pacing and is depicted by the gray scar. VT-related conducting channel (arrow) is commonly located in dense scar tissues (< 0.5 mV) in proximity to the EUS. **B.** Activation mapping during VT showed a "figure-of-eight" reentry. Temporal isochronal color changes demonstrated an "early-meets-late" activation pattern with the red color representing early activation and the late area depicting the purple color. Two different VTs were induced, LBLS and RBRS QRS morphologies. Entrainment mapping with concealed fusion that identified the isthmus site that is between the EUS and within the channel (star). The EGM-QRS (164 ms) is equal to the stimulus-QRS intervals of 172 ms. (Modified with permission from Al-Ahmad AA, Callans DJ, Hsia HH, Natale A, Eds., *Electroanatomical Mapping: An Atlas for Clinicians*. Malden, MA: Wiley-Blackwell; 2008.)

368 • Ablation of VT

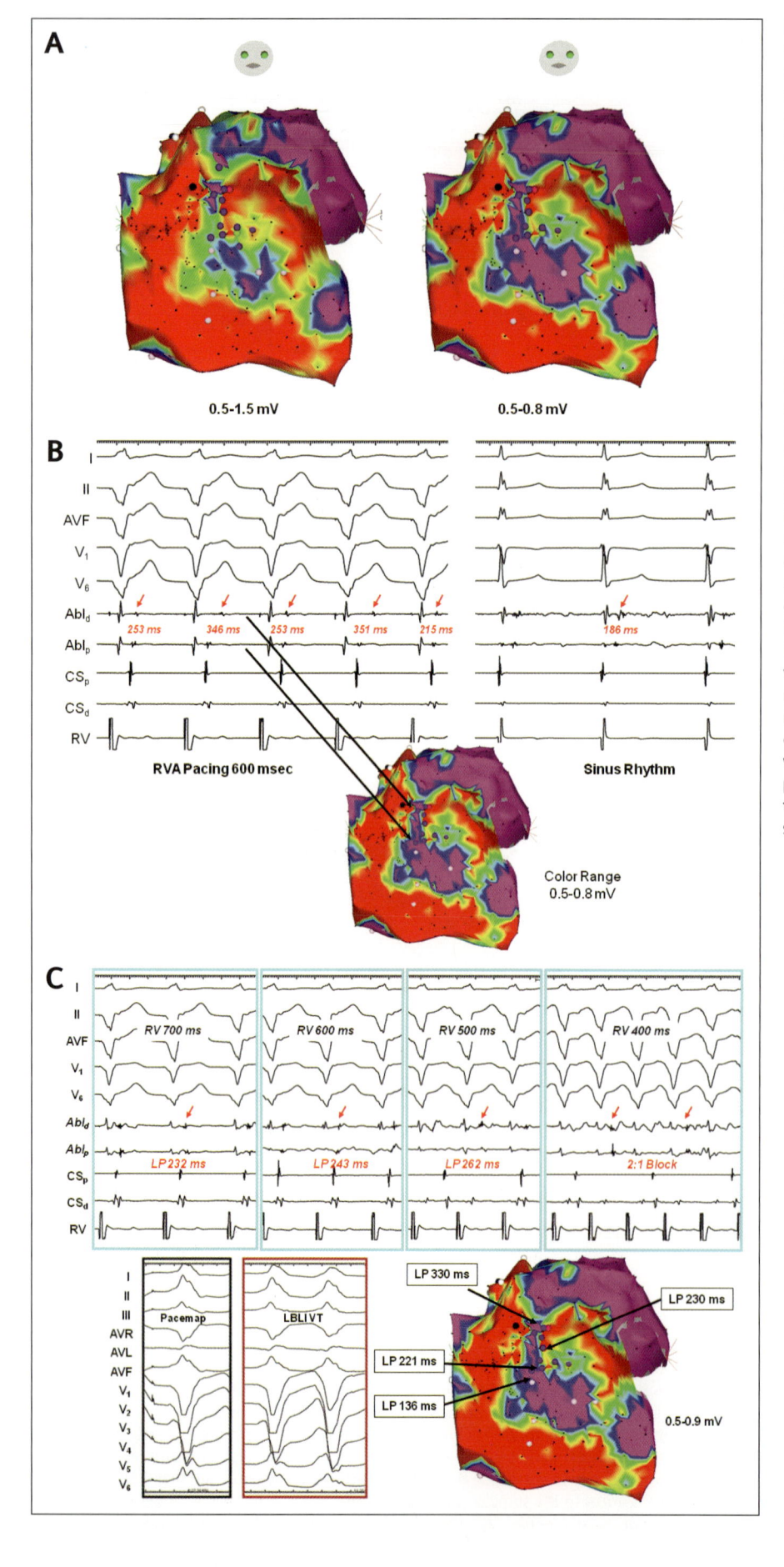

Figure 39.7 Epicardial voltage maps with VT-related conducting channels in a patient with an arrhythmogenic right ventricular cardiomyopathy (ARVC) and recurrent monomorphic VTs. His arrhythmia was refractory to multiple antiarrhythmic medications and a prior endocardial catheter VT ablation procedure. **A.** Epicardial voltage maps over the right ventricle in the LAO view. A channel is visible after color threshold adjustment from 0.5–1.5 mV to 0.5–0.8 mV. **B.** LPs are recorded within the putative VT-related channel during sinus rhythm, which becomes more obvious during RVA pacing at 600 ms. In addition, spontaneous oscillation of the QRS-LP intervals (arrows) are noted at the distal recording electrode pair but remain stable at the proximal electrodes. This suggests decremental conduction delay between the proximal and the distal recording electrodes during propagation of activation wave front from the RV apex. **C.** Demonstration of decremental conduction delay within the channel. Progressively prolonged QRS-LP intervals and 2-to-1 conduction block with faster pacing rate. The voltage map showed progressively delayed LP recordings deeper into the channel during RVA pacing. Pace mapping within the channel demonstrated a perfect pace map with a long stimulus-to-QRS interval compared to that of spontaneous VT.

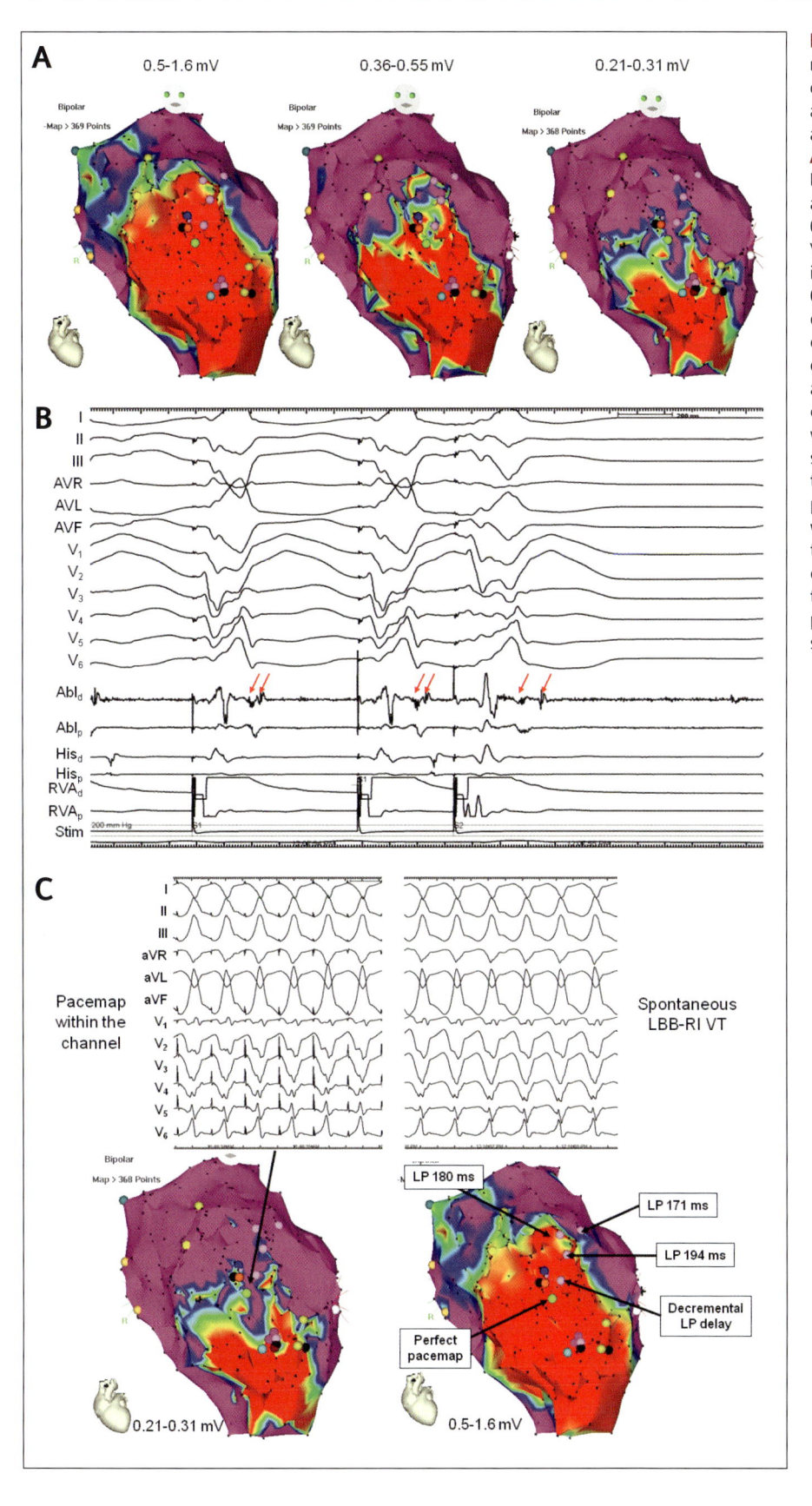

Figure 39.8 Endocardial voltage maps with VT-related conducting channels in a patient with a large anterior myocardial infarction and incessant monomorphic VTs. **A.** Endocardial voltage map showed a large anterior scar. The color gradient adjustments correspond to 0.5–1.6 mV, 0.35–0.55 mV, and 0.21–0.31 mV. A VT-related conducting channel can be identified at a color threshold at 0.21–0.31 mV. **B.** Decremental conduction delay within the channel with ventricular extrastimulation. E-IDC or LPs can be detected (arrows). There is delayed activation of the second potential of the multicomponent local EGMs with premature ventricular activation, suggesting delayed conduction into the channel. **C.** Voltage maps show progressively delayed LP recordings with decremental slow conduction from the border zone toward into the scar during RVA pacing. Pace mapping within the channel (arrow) demonstrated a perfect pace map compared to that of spontaneous LBB-RI VT.

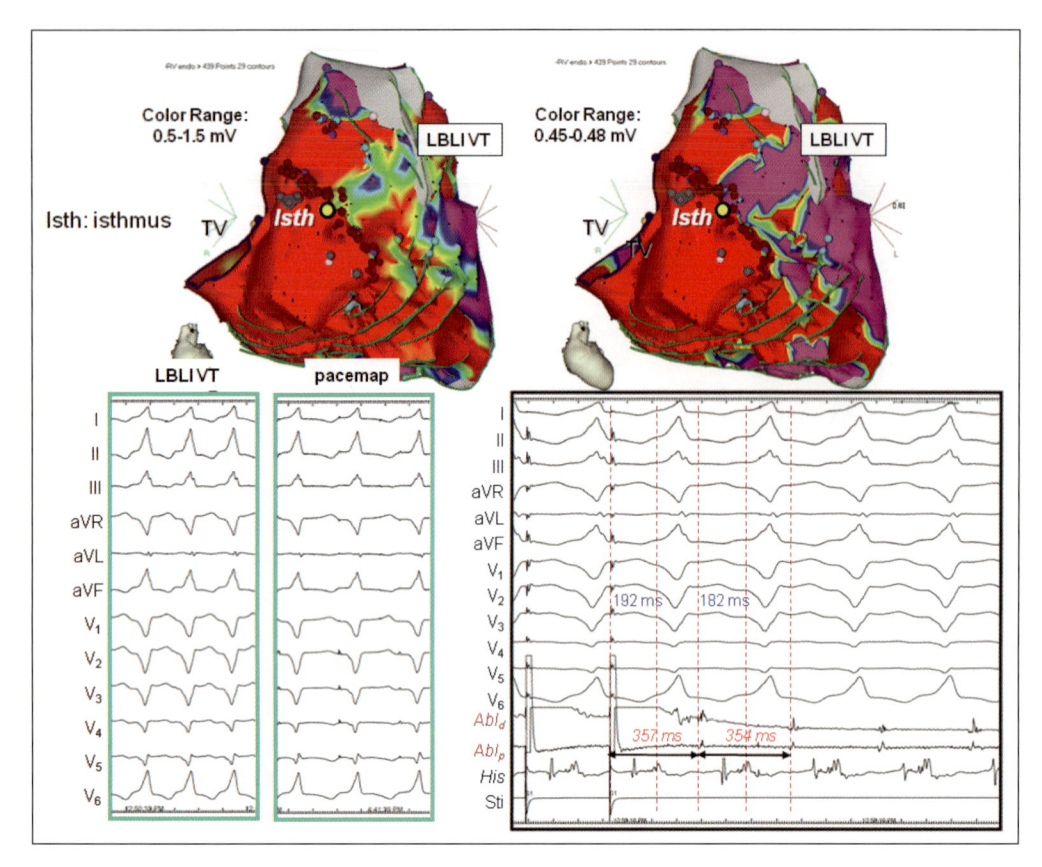

Figure 39.9 Identifying the VT-related channel in a patient with ARVC. Endocardial voltage maps of the right ventricle showed extensive dense scar involving nearly the entire lateral wall, extending from the annulus to the apex. A channel is visible after color threshold adjustment from 0.5–1.5 mV to 0.45–0.48 mV. Entrainment response within the channel is consistent with an isthmus location (yellow dot). Pacing within the channel demonstrated an excellent pace map.

Selective coronary angiography must be preformed prior to epicardial RF ablation to establish the distance between the ablation electrode and any adjacent major coronary vessels.

Postprocedure Care

Standard postoperative care protocol is recommended. Protamine may be given to help reverse the heparin, and access sheaths can be pulled once the activated clotting time is less than 180 seconds. A large net-positive fluid balance is expected when using irrigated-tip catheters for endocardial VT ablations. Additional diuretics are often required in patients with advanced ventricular dysfunction.

In patients who underwent left ventricular endocardial ablation procedures, postoperative anticoagulation is recommended for the duration of ~1 month. Oral warfarin or dabigatran can be started the day of the procedure for stroke prevention and minimizing thromboembolic complications. Lovenox, or low-molecular-weight heparin, is generally not required to bridge these patients. In all other patients (RV ablation, epicardial ablation, patients who are poor candidates for anticoagulation) aspirin 325 mg daily is recommended.

For epicardial VT ablation procedures, we generally leave a 5-Fr pigtail catheter for overnight drainage in the epicardial space. Follow-up transthoracic echocardiograms are performed after the procedure and at next day. We routinely administer steroid (Triamcinolone 2 mg/kg, diluted in 10–20 cm^3) into the epicardial space, with the pigtail catheter clamped for the first 4 hours before open to suction drainage.

Procedural Complications

Catheter ablation of VT is a complex intervention usually performed in patients with advanced heart disease. The incidence of major procedure-related complications reaches 8%, with up to 3% procedure-related mortality, often due to incessant VT.[22,14]

In order to reduce procedural complications, we try to minimize arrhythmia induction and procedural time. A hybrid approach is used with emphasis on substrate characterization during sinus/paced rhythm. Detailed and meticulous mapping techniques are essential to identify surrogate markers of slow conduction (channels, LPs, pace mapping) with limited VT induction.

Limitations

Despite comprehensive voltage maps with high-density sampling (> 150–200 points), VT-related conducting channels in the scarred substrate can only be identified in ~70% of patients with monomorphic VTs.[4] This may be

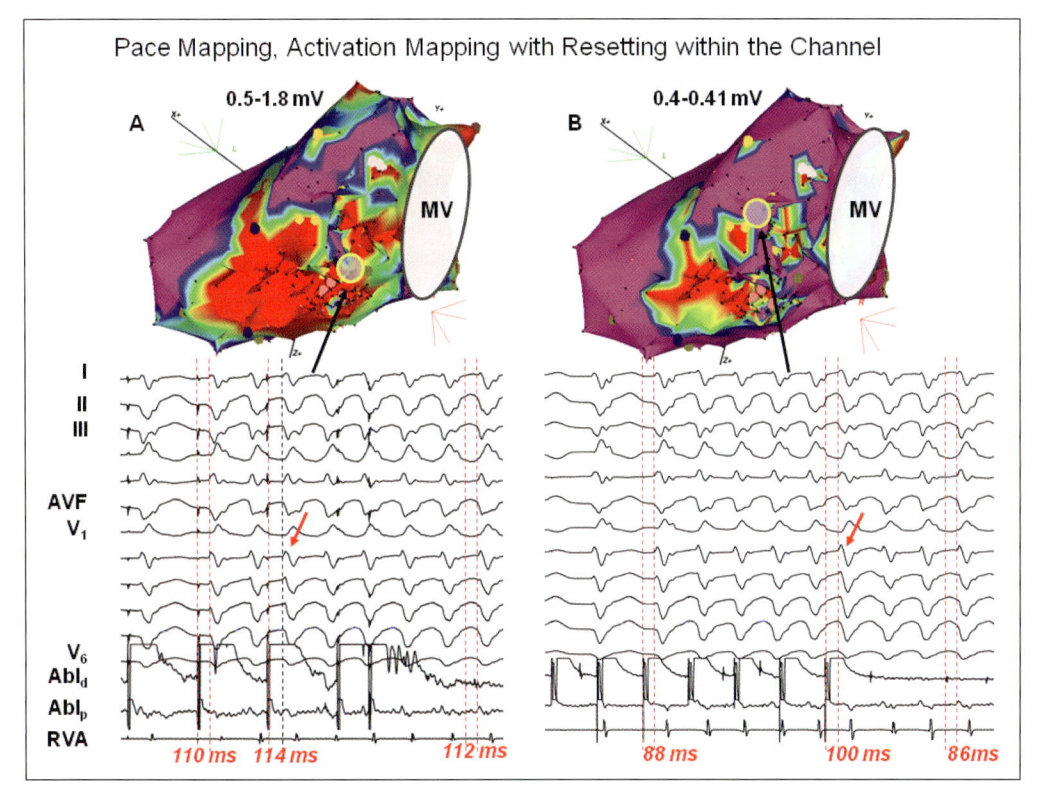

Figure 39.10 Endocardial voltage maps in a patient with a large inferior lateral myocardial infarction and recurrent VTs. **A.** Endocardial voltage map demonstrates a large inferolateral scar, extending from the base to the apex. The color thresholds are set at the nominal values of 0.5–1.8 mV. VT with RBBB-right-superior (RBRS) morphology is induced during the drivetrain of ventricular stimulation. The mapping catheter (yellow circle) is located deep in the scar, within a possible channel. The second VT beat is inadvertently reset (red arrow) by the pacing stimulus with a stimulus-QRS interval (114 ms) equals to the EGM-QRS interval (112 ms). Of note, the pace map also has a similar paced QRS as that during VT with a similar stimulus-QRS interval (110 ms). **B.** The color thresholds and scar definition have been adjusted to 0.4-0.41 mV that revealed a VT-related conducting channel within the large scar. The mapping catheter (yellow circle) has now moved along the channel toward the border of the scar. Again, a RBRS VT is induced during the drivetrain of ventricular stimulation. A VT beat is again reset (red arrow) with similar stimulus-QRS (100 ms) and EGM-QRS (86 ms) intervals. The paced map also shows a similar QRS morphology as that during VT with a stimulus-QRS interval of 110 ms. At this location, these intervals are shorter than those recorded deep inside the channel, suggesting activation propagating from inferior basal scar toward the lateral border of the scar. This figure demonstrates pace mapping, activation mapping with resetting all within the VT-related channel. Linear ablation transacting the channel is successful in eliminating the VT.

due to the fact that portions of the reentrant circuit are intramyocardial or epicardial. A slow VT with reentrant circuit resides in dense scar and significant conduction delay may favor the delineation and identification of critical channels, whereas nonuniform poorly tolerated rapid VTs may involve only small low-voltage areas without dense scar. Identification of VT-related channels thus may not be readily feasible in patients with small diffuse scar and rapid arrhythmias.

In our experience, identification of VT-related channels during substrate mapping is most applicable in patients with large low-voltage areas, particularly in those with dense (< 0.5 mV) scar (either endocardial or epicardial) (**Figures 39.7–39.10**). Commonly, only a single channel is observed that corresponds to the potential reentrant isthmus for a single morphology of VT. Occasionally, one conducting channel may be responsible for multiple VT morphologies (**Figure 39.5**).

Since the CARTO system automatically selects the largest local component of the bipolar EGMs, care must be given to measure the appropriate local signals and to exclude far-field recordings and pacing artifacts. In addition, sufficient sampling is essential for adequate delineation of the channel and electroanatomical characterization of the circuit.

Summary

The anatomic extent and location of components of reentrant VT circuits can be defined by detailed electroanatomic mapping. The anatomic size of the isthmus of slow conduction for VT is at least several centimeters long, with isthmus sites typically identified within densely scarred myocardium (0.2–0.3 mV). Conducting channels that correspond to zones of slow conduction within the circuit can be identified by adjusting the color thresholds of the display bipolar voltage maps made during sinus or paced rhythms in most patients. Identification of conducting channels should be considered as a major strategy for substrate mapping and ablation of VT, particularly in those patients with large, dense myocardial scar (either endocardial or epicardial).

To optimize the substrate mapping result during sinus/paced rhythm, multiple techniques are utilized to define areas of slow conduction as surrogate markers for the potential reentry circuit isthmus. Limited VT induction with activation or entrainment mapping may be performed for EP confirmation of the isthmus location. Placement of linear ablation lines, designed to transect preferred channels of conduction in more densely scarred regions of abnormal myocardium, may facilitate ablation of multiple stable and unstable VTs, even in the absence of VT induction.

References

1. Gardner P, Ursell P, Fenoglio J, Wit A. Electrophysiologic and anatomical basis for fractionated EGMs recorded from healed myocardial infarcts. *Circulation*. 1985;72(3):596–611.
2. de Bakker J, van Capelle F, Janse M, Tasseron S, Vermeulen J, de Jonge N, Lahpor J. Slow conduction in the infarcted human heart: "Zigzag" course of activation. *Circulation*. 1993;88(3):915–926.
3. Arenal A, del Castillo S, Gonzalez-Torrecilla E, et al. Tachycardia-related channel in the scar tissue in patients with sustained monomorphic ventricular tachycardias: influence of the voltage scar definition. *Circulation*. 2004;110: 2568–2574.
4. Hsia H, Lin D, Sauer W, Callans D, Marchlinski F. Anatomic characterization of endocardial substrate for hemodynamically stable reentrant ventricular tachycardia: identification of endocardial conducting channels. *Heart Rhythm*. 2006;3:503–512.
5. Horowitz L, Josephson M, Harken A. Epicardial and endocardial activation during sustained ventricular tachycardia in man. *Circulation*. 1980;61(6):1227–1238.
6. Harris L, Downar E, Mickeborough L, Shaikh N, Parson I. Activation sequence of ventricular tachycardia: endocardial and epicardial mapping studies in the human ventricle. *J Am Coll Cardiol*. 1987;10:1040–1047.
7. Schweikert R, Saliba W, Tomassoni G, et al. Percutaneous pericardial instrumentation for endo-epicardial mapping of previously failed ablations. *Circulation*. 2003;108: 1329–1335.
8. Cano O, Hutchinson M, Lin D, et al. Electroanatomic substrate and ablation outcome for suspected epicardial ventricular tachycardia in left ventricular nonischemic cardiomyopathy. *J Am Coll Cardiol*. 2009;54(9):799–808.
9. Garcia F, Bazan V, Zado E, Ren J, Marchlinski F. Epicardial substrate and outcome with epicardial ablation of ventricular tachycardia in arrhythmogenic right ventricular cardiomyopathy/dysplasia. *Circulation*. 2009;120:366–375.
10. Sacher F, Roberts-Thomson K, Maury P, et al. Epicardial ventricular tachycardia ablation: a multicenter safety study. *J Am Coll Cardiol*. 2010;55(21):2366–2372.
11. Miller J, Marchlinski F, Buxton A, Josephson M. Relationship between the 12-lead electrocardiogram during ventricular tachycardia and endocardial site of origin in patients with coronary artery disease. *Circulation*. 1988;77(4):759–766.
12. Berruezo A, Mont L, Nava S, Chueca E, Bartholomay E, Brugada J. Electrocardiographic recognition of the epicardial origin of ventricular tachycardias. *Circulation*. 2004;109: 1842–1847.
13. Daniels D, Lu Y, Morton J, Santucci P, Akar J, Green A, Wilber D. Idiopathic epicardial left ventricular tachycardia originating remote from the sinus of valsalva: electrophysiological characteristics, catheter ablation, and identification from the 12-lead electrocardiogram. *Circulation*. 2006;113: 1659–1666.
14. Aliot E, Stevenson W, Almendral-Garrote J, et al. EHRA/HRS Expert consensus on catheter ablation of ventricular arrhythmias. *Heart Rhythm*. 2009;6(6):886–933.
15. Nakagawa H, Yamanashi W, Pitha J, et al. Comparison of in vivo tissue temperature profile and lesion geometry for radiofrequency ablation with a saline-irrigated electrode versus temperature control in a canine thigh muscle preparation. *Circulation*. 1995;91(8):2264–2273.
16. Soejima K, Delacretaz E, Suzuki M, Brunckhorst C, Maisel W, Friedman P, Stevenson W. Saline-cooled versus standard radiofrequency catheter ablation for infarct-related ventricular tachycardias. *Circulation*. 2001;103(14):1858–1862.
17. Marchlinski F, Callans D, Gottlieb C, Zado E. Linear ablation lesions for control of unmappable ventricular tachycardia in patients with ischemic and nonischemic cardiomyopathy. *Circulation*. 2000;101:1288–1296.
18. Soejima K, Stevenson W, Maisel W, Sapp J, Epstein L. Electrically unexcitable scar mapping based on pacing threshold for identification of the reentry circuit isthmus: feasability for guiding ventricular tachycardia ablation. *Circulation*. 2002;106:1678–1683.
19. Arenal A, Glez-Torrecilla E, Ortiz M, et al. Ablation of electrograms with an isolated, delayed component as treatment of unmappable monomorphic ventricular tachycardias in patients with structural heart disease. *J Am Coll Cardiol*. 2003;41:81–92.
20. Hsia H, Lin D, Sauer W, Callans D, Marchlinski F. Relationship of late potentials to the ventricular tachycardia circuit defined by entrainment. *J Interv Card Electrophysiol*. 2009;26:21–29.
21. Brunckhorst C, Delacretaz E, Soejima K, Maisel W, Friedman P, Stevenson W. Identification of the ventricular tachycardia isthmus after infarction by pace mapping. *Circulation*. 2004;110:652–659.
22. Stevenson W, Wilber D, Natale A, et al. Irrigated radiofrequency catheter ablation guided by electroanatomic mapping for recurrent ventricular tachycardia after myocardial infarction: the multicenter thermocool ventricular tachycardia ablation trial. *Circulation*. 2008;118: 2773–2782.

CHAPTER 40

How to Use Noncontact Mapping for Catheter Ablation of Ventricular Tachycardia

Jason T. Jacobson, MD

Introduction

Noncontact mapping with the Array (St. Jude Medical, Minnetonka, MN) is an alternative to traditional contact mapping for the ablation of VT or frequent PVC in both the left and right ventricles. This unique and powerful tool can accurately locate exit sites for both idiopathic and scar-based VT and, at times, portions of the reentrant circuit within scar. This can greatly aid in mapping and ablation of VTs/PVCs that are nonsustained, infrequent, or not hemodynamically tolerated long enough to allow point-by-point catheter mapping. Proper utilization of this complex system requires a working knowledge of the scientific principles behind EGM reconstruction, and an intimate understanding of the advantages and limitations of the information it provides. This chapter will largely focus on the principles of mapping with the Array and using the information to guide ablation.

The Array consists of a gridwork of 64 0.003-inch wires mounted on a 7.5 cm^3 balloon. A 0.025-inch laser-etched insulation break is created on each wire to allow for signal reception from within the blood pool. The data from the Array is processed by the display system to "reconstruct" the unipolar EGM as they would appear at the endocardium. The system is also able to display the 12-lead ECG as well as signals from standard electrode catheters. The accuracy of EGM reconstruction decreases with distance from the equator of the Array, with 50 mm generally being the outer reaches of the Array. While fidelity starts to diminish at 34 mm, EGM reconstruction remains most accurate up to 40 mm.[1]

Preprocedural Planning

Ischemic Evaluation

Prior to pursuing a potentially prolonged ablation procedure, it is prudent to perform an ischemic evaluation. While ischemia is rarely an instigator of monomorphic VT, a patient's ability to tolerate the planned procedure may be impeded by active ischemia. Unless otherwise contraindicated, coronary angiography is the modality of choice in patients with cardiomyopathy, especially in the setting of VT storm. Patients with idiopathic VT or frequent PVC may undergo stress testing.

Ventricular Imaging

Preprocedural imaging is vital, not only to deduce ventricular morphology and function, but also to exclude endocardial thrombus and to aid in planning the ablation procedure. Preprocedural knowledge of substrate location may guide the approach taken for Array placement in the left ventricle. Lateral and anterior scarring may be better mapped with a transseptal placement, as a retrograde approach generally acheives a septal and more inferior Array location. Patients with acute ventricular clot would be at high risk for embolic events, especially with the introduction of the Array catheter. The use of the Array should be reconsidered in patients with severely enlarged ventricles, as the fidelity of the virtual unipolar EGM (VEGM) is limited beyond 50 mm from the equator of the Array.

Echocardiography

Chamber dimensions, wall motion abnormalities, and presence of thrombus can be well visualized with TTE, especially when a sonographic contrast agent is used. Areas of thinning and akinesis would harbor the substrate for VT. Patients in AF who have not been adequately anticoagulated should undergo TEE to exclude LAA thrombus. This information would be vital in the event that electrical cardioversion of VT was necessary during the procedure.

ICE is increasingly being used as an adjunct imaging modality in addition to fluoroscopy and electroanatomic mapping systems for VT ablations. The use of ICE is helpful for anatomical orientation, catheter placement, and tissue contact, as well as early identification of complications such as tamponade.

Magnetic Resonance Imaging (MRI)

In addition to elucidating chamber function and dimensions, cardiac MRI can be quite useful in defining VT substrate in patients with ICM and NICM. Late gadolinium enhancement can identify areas of scar and determine the extent of transmurality and mural location (endocardial, mid-myocardial, or epicardial). MRI can also identify ventricular thrombus.

Computed Tomography (CT)

As with echocardiography and cardiac MRI, cardiac CT can define chamber morphology, function, and areas of thinning and akinesis. While protocols to define ventricular scar are being investigated, no reliable method has been described.

Vascular Assessment/Access Planning

The Array is mounted on a 9-Fr catheter and can be placed through a 9-Fr sheath. Additionally, an 8- or 9-Fr sheath will be required for the ablation catheter and a 6- or 7-Fr sheath for a standard quadrapolar catheter for programmed stimulation. Consideration of vascular ultrasound should be given for patients with signs or symptoms of peripheral vascular disease in order to plan the access approach for LV procedures. Significant arterial stenoses or prosthetic aortic valves may preclude retrograde aortic access and necessitate a transseptal approach for both the Array and the ablation catheter.

Anesthesia and Hemodynamic Support

Depending on the clinical status of the patient, ablation can be performed with conscious sedation, monitored anesthesia care, or general anesthesia. Patients with significant heart failure should be optimized prior to ablation if possible, and general anesthesia support should be strongly considered. If a prolonged procedure is anticipated, or if VT is known to be hemodynamically intolerable and would require multiple cardioversions, general anesthesia support would be advisable.

Many new devices are available that can offer hemodynamic support during VT ablation for patients with significant refractory heart failure. All of these devices take up significant vascular access opportunities and may make the use of the Array problematic. IABP and PVAD require arterial access. These devices are most frequently utilized to provide hemodynamic support during VT to allow for traditional mapping, which is negated by use of the Array.

Antiarrhythmic Drugs

Short-acting antiarrhythmic drugs are generally stopped at least 5 half-lives prior to ablation if possible. Patients on chronic (approximately 2 weeks) oral amiodarone therapy are generally continued on this drug. Intravenous amiodarone is generally stopped prior to ablation.

Procedure

Patient Preparation

If ventricular ectopy is being targeted for ablation, 12-lead ECGs of the clinical PVC(s) are obtained with the EP recording system prior to the institution of any sedation, which may suppress triggered or automatic arrhythmias. A Foley urinary catheter is placed in most patients after sedation, especially those with cardiomyopathy and/or a history of congestive heart failure, since the volume of fluid given during the procedure with an irrigated-tip catheter can be significant.

Vascular Access/Approach for Array

Access for at least one RV quadrapolar catheter is obtained in either femoral vein, depending on which ventricle will be mapped and which approach to the left ventricle will be used. Access for the ablation catheter is usually via the right femoral artery or vein, as this affords the least tortuous route to the chamber of interest. The Array would be placed from the left femoral vessel (vein for RV mapping, artery for LV mapping). For anterior or lateral scar in a large LV, consideration to transseptal placement of the Array would be achieved from the right femoral vein. If a transseptal approach is required for both ablation catheter and Array, both will be placed via the right femoral vein. In this case, 2 short 8-Fr sheaths would be placed initially and changed out for the transseptal sheaths.

Array Preparation and Positioning

Array Preparation

First, an extension tubing (provided in the Array packaging) is attached to the Array lumen. This is then flushed with heparinized saline. The Array is placed into the "high-profile" (**Figure 40.1**, left panel) configuration (open), and the balloon is aspirated of any air with a 10 cm^3 syringe 2 times. Ten cm^3 heparinized saline is then instilled into the balloon and aspirated, taking care to remove any air bubbles from the balloon. Approximately 2 cm^3 saline remains in the lumen of the catheter. A mixture of 70% saline and 30% contrast is then instilled into the balloon. This too is aspirated as described above. The balloon stopcock is left open, and the Array is placed in "low-profile" (closed) to allow for introduction into the sheath (**Figure 40.1**, right panel).

Left Ventricle, Retrograde Approach

If a retrograde aortic approach is used for access to the LV, the Array can be placed through a 9-Fr arterial sheath. Care must be taken not to handle the Array itself as it is introduced into the sheath. Once in the sheath, the wire is advanced out the tip of the catheter so that the pigtail straightens. This wire should cross the aortic valve first and is manipulated to the apex if possible. The Array can then be advanced to the end of the wire (which is fixed in place). Most often, it is not possible to adequately position the wire while it is in the Array catheter. In these cases, the wire is first positioned in the LV apex with the aid of a standard pigtail catheter. Once the wire is in position, the pigtail is removed while taking care not to dislodge the wire. The Array is then back-loaded over the wire, across the aortic valve and placed with the pigtail end at the apex. The wire is then pulled back into the catheter shaft to allow the pigtail to assume its natural shape. The wire is not removed. A flush line is attached to the Array lumen port to prevent thrombus formation. The balloon Array is then deployed (see below).

Left Ventricle, Transseptal Approach

For a transseptal deployment of the balloon Array, a heparin bolus of 3000 U is typically given prior to crossing the septum, and the remainder of a 100 U/kg dose is given after transseptal access is obtained. The goal for ACT is 300 to 350 seconds, and is maintained with intermittent heparin boluses. The ACT is checked every 30 minutes during the procedure. Puncture for the Array is performed first to allow time for the ACT to reach therapeutic levels by the time the Array is deployed.

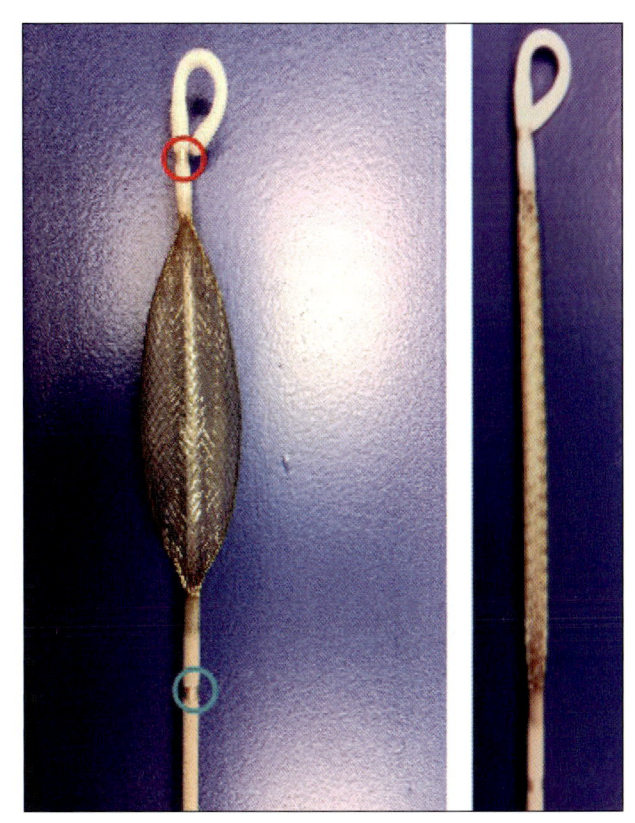

Figure 40.1 The balloon Array. The **left panel** shows the Array in "high-profile" while the **right panel** displays "low-profile." The proximal locator ring is circled in green, while the distal is circled in red.

A large curve deflectable sheath is often used to allow guidance of a stiff exchange-length 0.035-inch wire to the LV apex. This sheath is removed from the body, leaving the wire in place. Care *must* be taken to prevent dislodgement of this wire. After the transseptal sheath is removed, a 9-Fr short sheath is advanced over this wire to sit securely at the groin. This sheath is sutured in place to maintain Array position. Alternatively, a 9-Fr steerable sheath may be used for the Array puncture and left in place for placement of the Array. If transseptal access is performed for both the Array and the ablation catheter, puncture for the Array is performed first to allow time for the ACT to reach therapeutic levels by the time the Array is deployed (see below).

Right Ventricle

For right ventricular mapping, a wire can be positioned into the RVA or RVOT with the aid of a multipurpose coronary (or similar) catheter. For RVOT placement, the wire should be advanced across the pulmonic valve into the proximal left pulmonary artery. Once the wire is positioned, the multipurpose catheter can be removed, again taking care not to dislodge the wire. The Array is then back-loaded over the wire, across the tricuspid valve, and placed with the pigtail end at the RVA or RVOT. For apical positioning, the wire is then pulled back into the catheter shaft to allow the pigtail to assume its natural shape. For RVOT positioning, the wire is left in the pulmonary artery to ensure stability.

Array Deployment

Once the Array is in position, it is placed back into "high-profile" and the balloon is filled with 7 to 8 cm^3 saline/contrast (70% : 30%) mixture, depending on chamber size. It is important to note that the Array will be pulled back about 1 cm when placing in "high-profile" and will need to be advanced to its prior position. The shaft of the Array is then taped to the patient at its insertion into the groin sheath to ensure stability.

For the sake of efficiency, it is helpful to perform Array preparation just prior to insertion into the body. This allows the target ACT to be achieved without waiting idly by. The sequence of events would be:

1. Obtain groin access
2. Give initial heparin bolus, or obtain transseptal access if required, and give heparin as above
3. Position wire separately if required
4. Prepare the balloon Array
5. Check ACT; give additional bolus of heparin if needed
6. Position and deploy the Array

Mapping

Basic Principles

The mapping system is able to reconstruct 3360 VEGM over the endocardium by applying the inverse solution of Laplace's law to the potentials measured by the Array. As the Array is not in contact with the endocardium, these signals are essentially cavity potentials recorded from within the blood pool. Endocardial locations in 3-dimensional space are based on the geometry that is created by moving the ablation catheter throughout the chamber of interest, creating an endocardial "shell." The Array tracks the location of this catheter by sending out a 5.68-kHz locator signal from the ring electrodes located at the distal and proximal ends of the Array (Figure 40.1). It is important to realize that the Array is the "center of the universe" and that, if it were to move, the fidelity of VEGM reconstruction would be compromised, thus requiring a new geometry creation.

The system displays color-coded isopotential maps based on the reconstructed unipolar VEGM. The operator sets the color thresholds to display the negative voltage portion of the VEGM. By convention, all voltages > 0 mV (positive) are coded purple and are essentially negated. As the VEGM progresses into the negative and reaches its PNV, the display will progress through red, blue, green, yellow, white, and back through the reverse sequence to purple as resting potential returns (**Figure 40.2**). The system display relies on the assumption that the PNV indicates local activation of the unipolar VEGM. In actuality, it is the peak negative slope of the unipolar recording that marks local activation, but PNV is a reasonable surrogate. If desired, the system can display the VEGM with the most negative voltage at every step of the activation sequence as it is played back. This is termed the "tracking virtual" and is shown in an inset at the lower right corner of the display screen. On the map, a red asterisk localizes the location of this tracking virtual (▶ **Video 40.1**).

The system also has operator-defined high-pass (HP) and low-pass (LP) filters for the VEGM. The best use of the high-pass filter is to smooth out baseline wander of the signals. This usually can be achieved by setting the HP to 2 Hz. Care should be taken, however, as the unipolar VEGM takes on a different morphology at high HP settings. As such, the idea of the PNV as a surrogate for local activation is no longer valid. That said, higher HP filter settings might allow one to see low-voltage potentials within scar, such as mid-diastolic potentials during VT. The LP filter is generally set at 150 Hz and is not manipulated thereafter.

Scar Localization

The ability of the Array to locate low voltage areas in a single beat is a desirable goal that has not yet been fully realized. The system currenty employs a process termed "dynamic substrate mapping" (DSM) to mark areas of relatively low voltage as determined by the PNV alone, not the

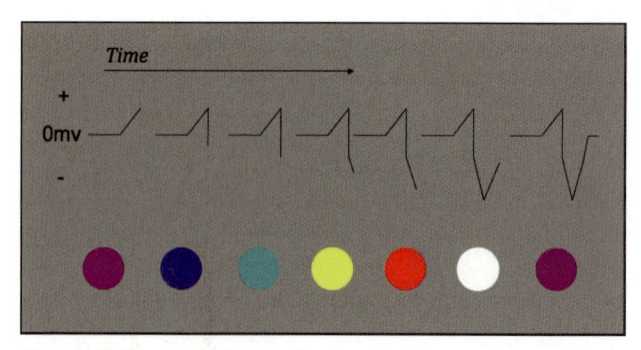

Figure 40.2 Color display of voltage for the array: A single VEGM in multiple time-steps displays the color progression as the PNV is reached. At voltages ≥ 0 mV, the VEGM site will be displayed in purple. As the voltage at this site becomes more negative, the color will change to blue, green, yellow, red, and finally, white. As the voltage becomes less negative and returns to 0 mV, the colors will cycle back in reverse until purple. It is important to note that the color scale is fully determined by the operator. By convention, purple is set to ≥ 0 mV, while white is often set to approximately half of the PNV seen in the chamber during the mapping interval. Therefore, not all sites will reach voltages displayed as white. mV = millivolts, VEGM = virtual electrogram, PNV = peak negative voltage.

peak-to-peak VEGM voltage. The operator defines the time period of interest (usually the QRS onset to offset) and defines a ratiometric threshold value for the definition of low voltage. This is based on the most negative PNV generated in the chamber during the time period chosen—the global peak negative (GPN) voltage (**Figure 40.3**). While this tool has been investigated in animal models of infarction with good results,[2,3] it has yet to be validated in human infarction. Additionally, it is unclear if DSM is valid in nonischemic cardiomyopathies as animal studies have not been performed. At this time, I cannot recommend DSM as the sole method for scar determination when using the Array. Fortunately, later versions of the system software (5.0 and later) allow for the overlay of a contact bipolar voltage map onto the geometry, allowing for accurate scar localization (**Figure 40.4**).

VT Mapping

One of the great strengths of the Array is for mapping idiopathic focal VT/PVC.[4] The system is able to display the entire activation wave front in a single beat of the tachycardia (▶ **Video 40.1**). As mentioned previously, it is important to record a 12-lead ECG of the clinical QRS morphology prior to introduction of any catheters. The Array can cause ectopy due to its size; therefore it is important to target the true arrhythmia and not catheter-induced ectopy. One way to distinguish between the 2 (if similar in morphology) is to look at the signals from the site of earliest activation. If the VEGM tracing is inscribed in purple, this indicates signal saturation due to contact of the Array with the endocardium (**Figure 40.5**). One must be aware that the pigtail of the Array can also cause ectopy (**Figure 40.6**). As electrode contact with the endocardium is not the cause, the signal would not be saturated.

The site of origin of VT/PVC should be at least 10–20 ms preQRS and display a QS unipolar VEGM morphology. This indicates the impulse originates at that point and moves away from it. An R wave on the VEGM indicates that the wave front approaches the site, which could not be the origin (**Figure 40.7**). The system has a review mode, which allows for playback at slower speeds to allow for acurate interpretation. Playback should be started prior to the QRS, and the first evidence of negative voltage generation (color other than purple) indicates possible activation. It is vital to look at the VEGM at this site to confirm it is a true activation and not due to repolarization or baseline noise (**Figure 40.8**). If the earliest site recorded with the Array is not preQRS and displays an R wave on the VEGM, the actual site of origin may be in the other ventricle, intramural, or epicardial. Prior to ablation, it is always advisable to confirm the Array findings with the contact catheter, as any Array displacement from the original geometry creation could render the data unusable. Of note, the Array cannot acurately map the aortic sinuses of valsalva, the coronary veins, or the epicardium in most cases, due to distance from the Array and intervening myocardial layers. That said, it can help locate the earliest endocardial activation, thereby guiding epicardial (including cusp and vein) mapping.

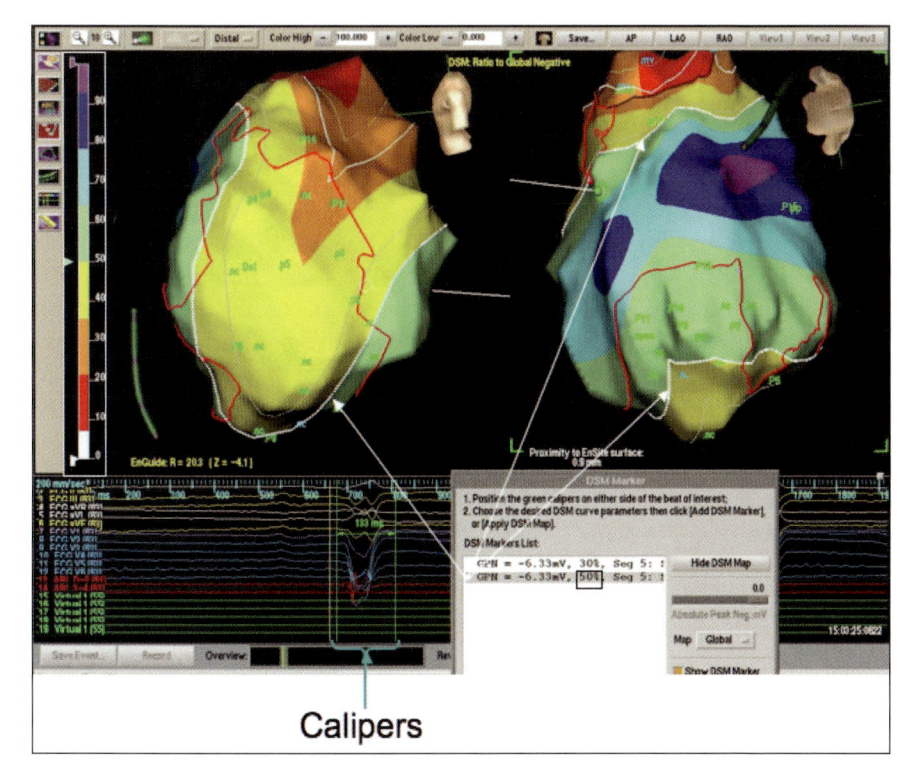

Figure 40.3 Dynamic substrate mapping (DSM) in a patient with an anterior infarction. An example of the DSM tool applied to sinus rhythm. The green calipers are placed around the QRS during sinus rhythm to identify the period of interest in which to apply DSM. The vertical color bar on the left side of the panel (white rectangle) displays the color coding for voltage normalized to the GPN voltage recorded during the time between the calipers. Fifty percent of the GPN is displayed as the border between yellow and green on the voltage maps. This low-voltage zone is circumscribed by a stippled white line in this figure (white arrows). Also seen is a DSM marker around the zone indicating voltages at 30% of GPN or less (solid white line in the brown area). The area circumscribed by the red line is the low-voltage area defined by bipolar contact mapping with a voltage of < 1.5 mV. Notice good, but not perfect, correlation between the DSM marker (50%) and the contact map. A significant source of error for the DSM map is the blending of the scar area with the mitral/aortic annular area, which is identified by the 30% DSM marker.

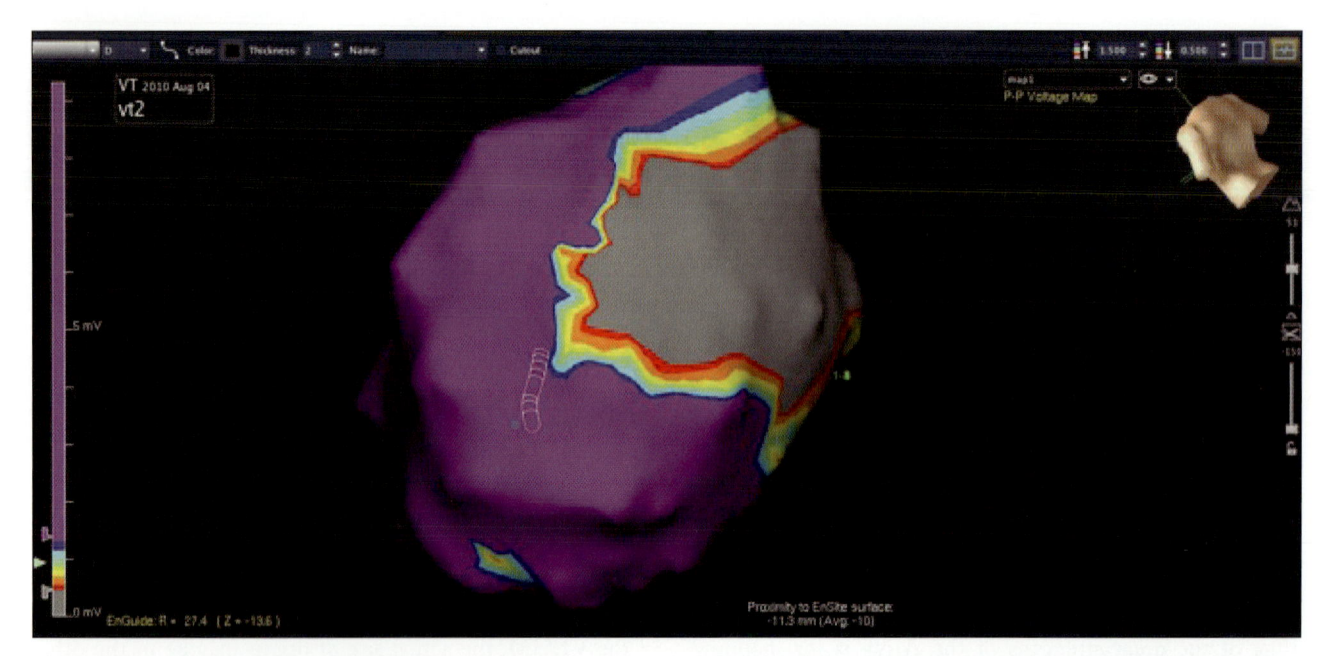

Figure 40.4 Bipolar contact voltage map. A posterobasal scar is displayed in a modified left-posterior oblique view. Normal voltage (1.5 mV and greater) is displayed in purple. Scar (0.5 mV and less) is displayed as gray. The torso in the upper right corner shows the orientation of the map. A color bar on the left of the screen displays the color scale. The ablation catheter is seen at mid-ventricular level.

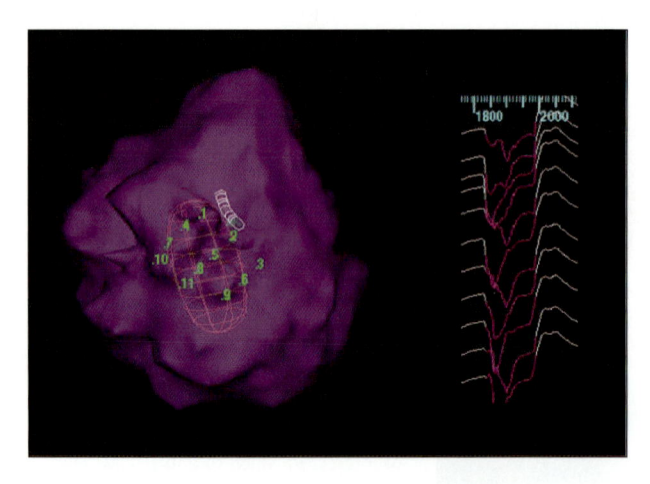

Figure 40.5 Saturated signal: A left ventricular geometry is shown with the outline of the array shown in the center as a yellow ellipse. A number of VEGM can be selected for display by swiping the cursor over the area of interest. In this example, a block of VEGM (green numbers 1–11) was selected on the septum, where the Array was in close physical apposition to the endocardium. To the right, these VEGM are displayed (top tracing is VEGM 1, bottom is VEGM 11). The purple portion of these VEGM indicates a saturated signal caused by the array bumping into the septum during ventricular contraction.

Exit sites for scar-based VT (in ischemic and non-ischemic substrates) can be accurately located with the Array in a similar process as described above for idiopathic VT/PVC. The VEGM morphology at the exit site will often display a QS with a more gradual slope, or a small R wave **[AQ2]** due to activation approaching from the distal isthmus (**Figure 40.9**, ▶ **Video 40.2**). The exit is defined by the onset of the surface QRS. If the first endocardial activation detected by the Array is after QRS onset, it is likely that the actual exit site of the VT is in the other ventricle, epicardial, or deeper in the myocardium. It is also important to note that most VT in patients with cardiomyopathy originates from scar, with the exception of bundle branch/fascicular reentry and cardiomyopathy due to frequent idiopathic VT/PVC. Therefore, care should be taken to identify areas of low voltage with a bipolar contact map and determine if the VT exits from a scarred area. If the exit site is remote from scar, one must consider the true exit may be in the other ventricle or epicardial in location.

In many instances (approximately 70% of VT), a portion of the VT isthmus (usually connected to the exit site) can be detected with the Array by recording the diastolic activity (**Figure 40.10**, ▶ **Video 40.3**).[5,6] To better detect these low-voltage signals, adjusting the HP to 8 Hz or above can filter out baseline noise, repolarization, and far-field signals that may obscure VEGM within scar (**Figure 40.11**).

Ablation

For idiopathic PVC/VT, ablation is performed at the site of earliest activation. For infrequent arrhythmia, pace

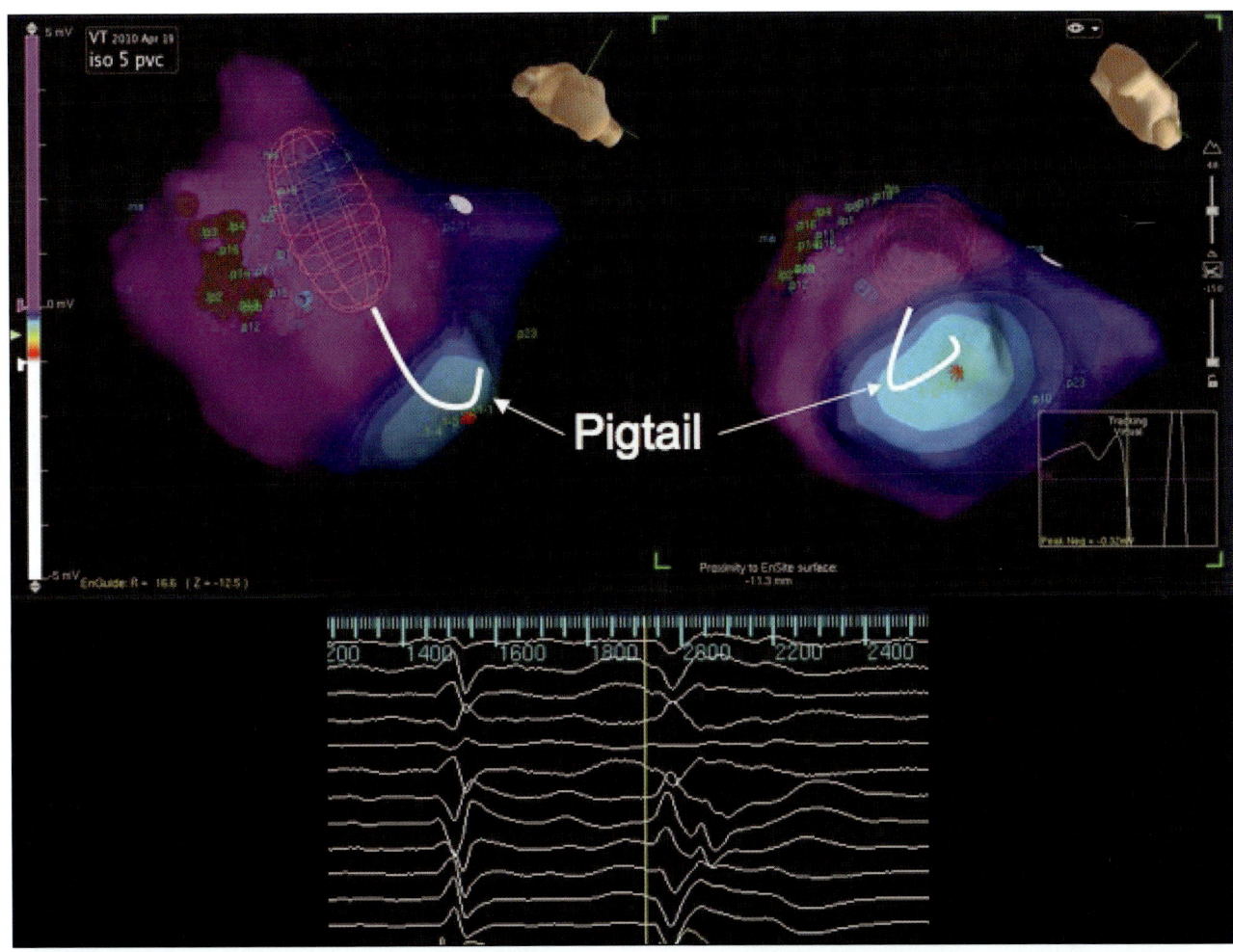

Figure 40.6 Mechanically induced PVC: A PVC caused by the pigtail portion of the Array (not displayed by the system, but is represented in this figure). Two views on the left ventricle are seen displaying the orientation of the Array (yellow ellipse) as placed via a retrograde approach. The blue area surrounding the red asterisk displays the site of origin of the PVC, which is where the pigtail would be expected to contact the endocardium. The bottom of the figure displays the ECG tracing. A sinus beat is followed by a PVC. The system displays the time step coinciding with the map by the yellow vertical line that is seen at the onset of the PVC. The VEGM that has reached the greatest negative voltage in that time step is displayed by the tracking virtual (the red asterisk on the isopotential map and the inset box at the lower right of the display). The brown disks indicate ablation lesions. PVC = premature ventricular contraction.

mapping can confirm ablation sites as well. A 4-mm ablation catheter is often adequate for these PVC/VT, although 8-mm and irrigated catheters can be used *with caution* in refractory cases.

When ablating scar-based VT, ablation lesions should be applied in the low-voltage areas. Irrigated-tip catheters offer the best efficacy for ablation within scar. If the distal isthmus is displayed by the Array within scar, a lesion set should be placed to transect this area. If only the VT exit is located, ablation should be performed in the scar border zone (bipolar voltage < 1.5 mV) adjacent to this exit site. Pace mapping in these locations not only can aid in confirming adequate ablation targets, but also provide a potential endpoint for ablation. If the paced wave front after ablation exits the scar from an anatomically distinct site from that prior to ablation, it is likely that the targeted VT exit will no longer conduct. Alternatively, this maneuver may also display a conduction gap in the ablation line (**Figure 40.12, ▶ Video 40.4**).

At this time, the resolution of the Array is not entirely clear. How the dimensions of the exit site as displayed by the system correlate to the length of the ablation line needed to achieve successful ablation is not known. Unipolar EGM are subject to far- and near-field voltage generated by myocardium that is not considered local to the recording site. The tracking virtual can be very helpful in locating a central position along the exit site as a starting point for ablation.

During mapping and ablation in patients with scar-based VT and cardiomyopathy, it is important to watch fluid status very carefully, especially when utilizing open-irrigated ablation catheters. In patients with very poor ventricular function, consideration for decreasing irrigant rate during ablation, or using closed-irrigation ablation catheters should be given.

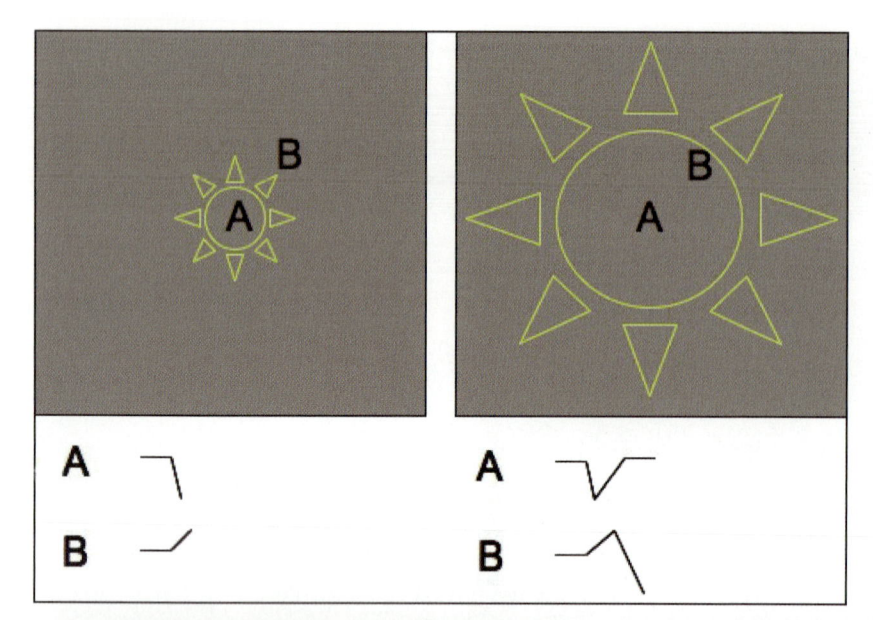

Figure 40.7 Directionality of the unipolar electrogram: The left panel displays the morphology of the unipolar EGM (bottom of figure) at 2 sites along a progressing wave front (yellow star). Site A is the site of origin. At this site, a steep negative deflection is inscribed as the wave front moves away from this site in all directions. Site B is distant from the origin. As the wave front approaches this site, a positive deflection is inscribed. The right panel shows the same 2 sites as the wave front moves out of the field of view of Site A. A QS EGM morphology is seen at Site A, indicating the wave front has never approached this site. Site B shows a positive deflection, followed by a negative deflection that is inscribed as the wave front passes through Site B. The point of maximal negative slope indicates the time of local activation. EGM = electrogram.

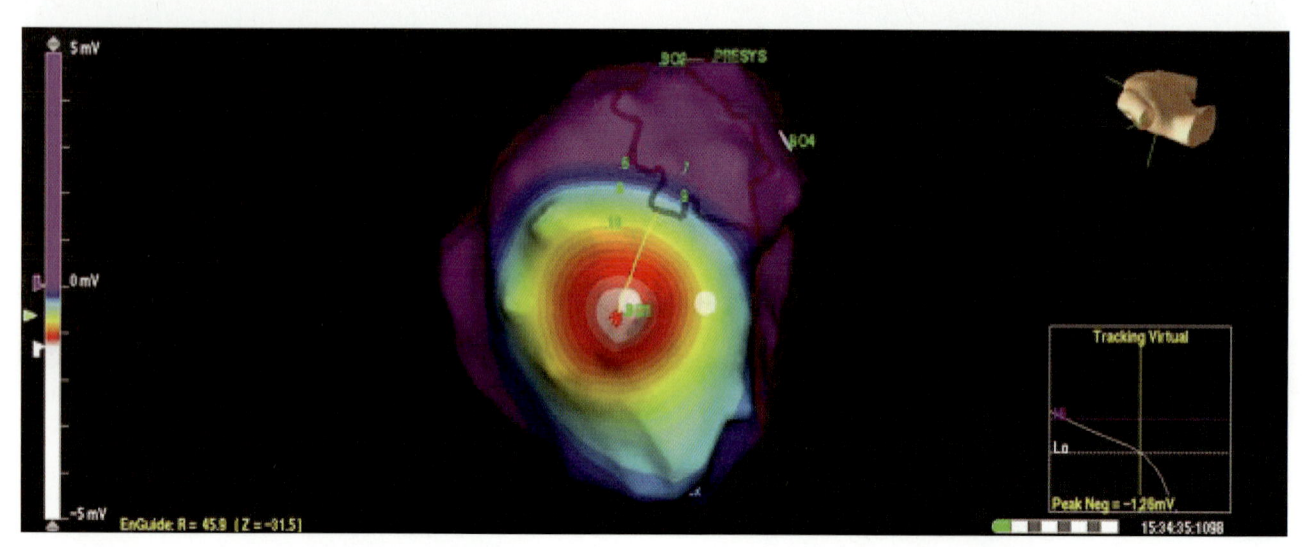

Figure 40.8 Focal origin of ventricular tachycardia: This VT originates in a site distant from scar (brown border) in this patient with non-ischemic cardiomyopathy. The asterisk denotes the tracking virtual. Note the QS complex being inscribed on the VEGM as the wave front progresses. The white dots represent the mapping points only.

Postprocedure Care

Immediate Postprocedure

Following ablation, contrast is fully aspirated from the balloon, and the Array is placed in low-profile. Keeping the balloon port open, the Array is removed, and heparin is stopped. Protamine can be considered to reverse anticoagulation, and sheaths are pulled when the ACT falls below 180 seconds. When arterial access is required, patients will need to lie flat for 6 hours after the groin sheaths are pulled. If extensive LV ablation is performed, or if patients have a history of LV thrombus, apical aneurysm, or AF that was cardioverted during the procedure, intravenous heparin can be started 6 hours after the sheaths are pulled. These patients are usually also placed on warfarin for 1 month after the ablation. This is usually started the night of the procedure.

Patients on short-acting antiarrhythmic drugs prior to ablation will often be taken off these medications prior to ablation (up to 5 half-lives, if time permits). Patients on chronic oral amiodarone are usually continued on this drug for about 1 month after the procedure, depending on the acute success of the ablation.

Long-Term

All patients are seen in clinic 2–4 weeks after the procedure. Patients with ICDs are followed every 3 months for device interrogation of arrhythmia events. Those with

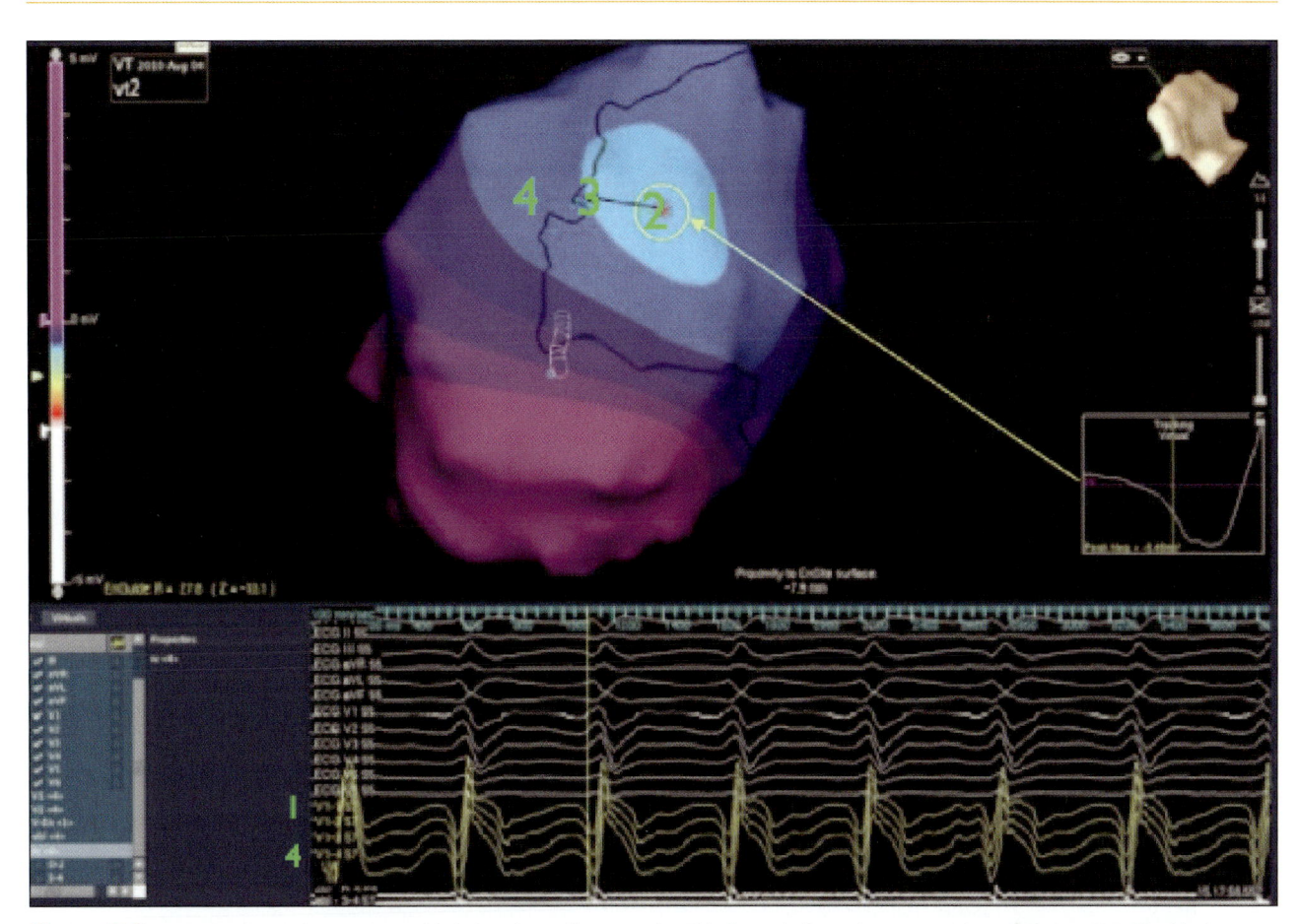

Figure 40.9 Exit site for VT in a patient with ischemic cardiomyopathy. This figure is from the same patient as Figure 40.3. The black border is the outline of the scar displayed in Figure 40.3. The system cannot display both contact bipolar maps and unipolar isopotential maps on the same display. The tracking virtual (red asterisk in yellow circle, also displayed as VEGM in the inset) shows activation within the scar adjacent to the exit site (indicated by black arrow). The bottom of the figure shows the 12-lead ECG (white tracings) and 4 VEGM (yellow tracings 1–4). The VEGM correspond to the green numbers 1–4 on the isopotential map. VEGM 3 is at the exit of the scar border. Note the steeper QS on this EGM as compared to the more gradual downslope on VEGM 1. See ▶ **Video 40.2** for the activation sequence of this VT.

idiopathic VT/PVC undergo Holter monitoring after 1 month to determine arrhythmia burden postablation. Warfarin can be discontinued at 1 month if there are no other indications for anticoagulation. Consideration can be given to discontinuing amiodarone if recurrent arrhythmia is not seen.

Procedural Complications

Given the girth of the balloon Array, care must be taken to avoid tamponade. Generally, the Array is not the source of perforation, but can instigate this complication due to difficulty maneuvering the ablation catheter around its perimeter. Use of ICE can aid in prevention and detection of this complication by visualizing the Array and identifying local tissue contact.

Thromboembolic complications can occur during any ablation procedure, but the Array provides an additional nidus for clot formation. As such, it is important to achieve and maintain a therapeutic ACT prior to and during deployment. As with all ablation procedures, vascular complications are the most common complication with the Array. For this reason, low-molecular-weight heparin is usually not used for postprocedure anticoagulation, especially when arterial access has been obtained.

As previously discussed, congestive heart failure in patients with cardiomyopathy must be aggressively prevented or treated due to the volume of irrigant often required during ablation.

Advantages and Limitations

No randomized investigation has been done comparing balloon Array-guided ablation with traditional approaches, although reported success rates are comparable.[4,6] Despite this, a major advantage to the Array is the ability to map an arrhythmia in a single beat. This can be significant when mapping hemodynamically intolerable VT or otherwise "unmappable" VT (infrequent, nonsustained, or difficult to induce).

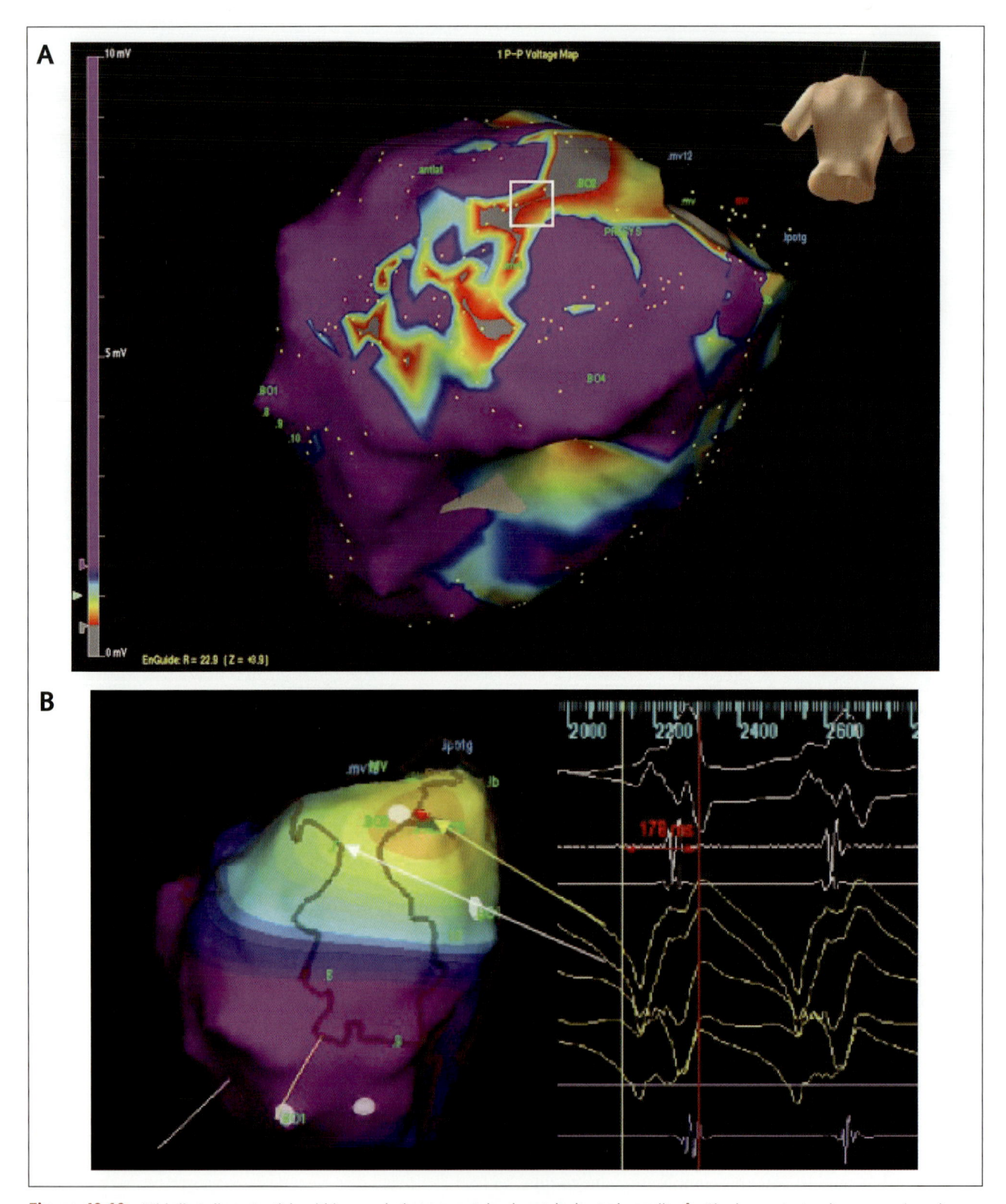

Figure 40.10 Mid-diastolic potentials within scar during nonsustained ventricular tachycardia: **A.** Bipolar contact voltage map (purple ≥ 1.5 mV, gray ≤ 0.5 mV) in a patient with non-ischemic cardiomyopathy. A small, somewhat patchy, posterobasal LV scar is seen. Note a relatively higher-voltage zone between 2 dense scar areas (white box). **B.** Isopotential map of VT. The right of the panel displays 2 ECG tracings (in white at the top), ablation catheter signals (next 2 white tracings), 4 VEGM (yellow tracings), and a right ventricular catheter (blue tracings at the bottom). This VT traverses the zone indicated by the white box in the top panel. VEGM 6-10 can be seen in green at different sites around the scar (brown border). Site 6 (yellow arrow) is at the tracking virtual as indicated by the red asterisk displaying notching in the downstroke of the VEGM (top yellow tracing at the right) that is approximately in the middle of diastole. The vertical yellow line indicates the time step that is displayed on the isopotential map to the left. Site 7 (white arrow) is the exit site of this VT and also displays presystolic notching on the VEGM (second yellow tracing from the top). See ▶ **Video 40.3** for the activation sequence of this VT. The white dots represent the mapping points only.

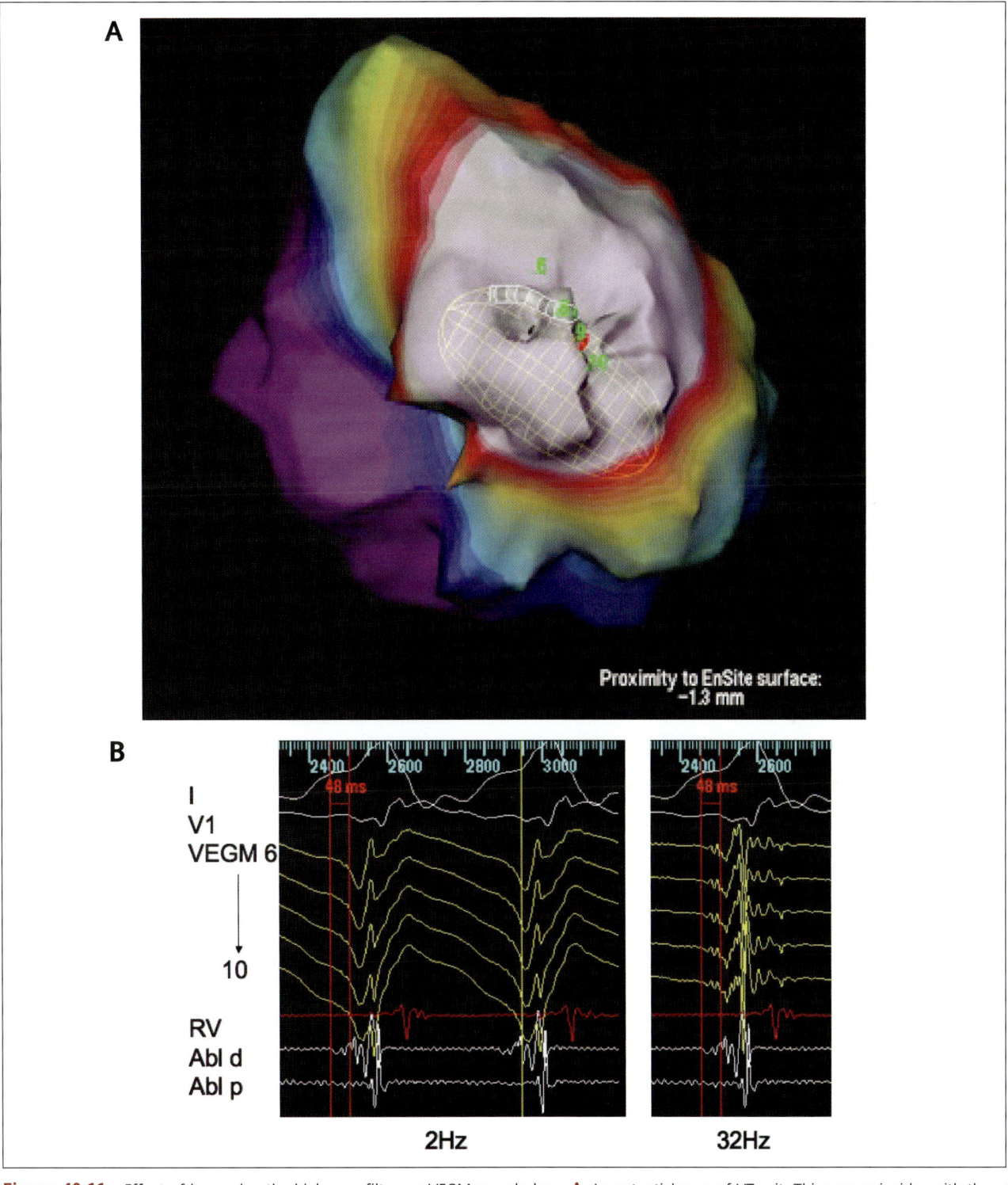

Figure 40.11 Effect of increasing the high-pass filter on VEGM morphology. **A.** Isopotential map of VT exit. This map coincides with the vertical yellow line in the left panel of Figure 40.11B. An ablation catheter is shown in outline with a green tip. **B.** VEGM with high-pass filter at 2 Hz (left) and 32 Hz (right). ECG leads I and V_1 are at the top. VEGMs 6–10 (corresponds to the green numbers on the isopotential map) as well as an RV catheter and distal and proximal electrode recordings from the ablation catheter (Abl d and Abl p) are displayed. Abl d is located at the same site as VEGM 8. At an HP filter of 2 Hz, the VEGMs show a gradual downslope with some notching. This is somewhat obscured by the repolarization waveform from the previous beat. The Abl d shows a multicomponent signal that begins 48 ms preQRS. At an HP filter of 32 Hz, the repolarization signal is effectively minimized, and the VEGM display the same late-diastolic multicomponent signal as the bipolar recordings of Abl d.

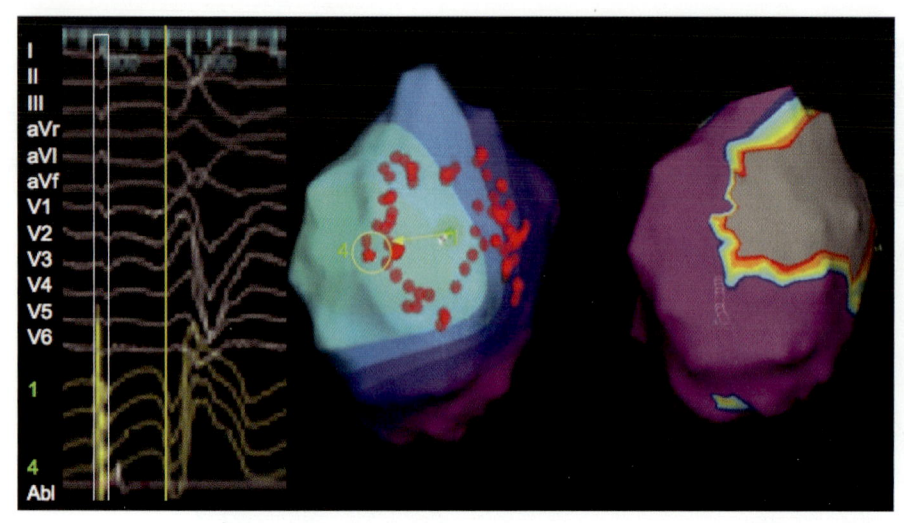

Figure 40.12 The leftward isopotential map displays the ablation lesion set for the same patient as Figures 40.3 and 40.9. Given the small size of the scar (displayed in a similar orientation in the rightward map) and multiple VT induced, ablation lesions were placed along the perimeter of the scar. Pacing within the scar at a site near the VT isthmus from Figure 40.9, the wave front exits the scar in a gap in the ablation line (yellow circle). The very left of the figure displays the 12-lead ECG (white tracings) and VEGM along the wave front (yellow signals, 1–4). The vertical yellow line indicates the time point that correlates to the isopotential map. Note the long stimulus (white rectangle) to QRS interval. Also note the similarity between the paced QRS morphology and that of the VT in Figure 40.9. See ▶ **Video 40.4** for the activation sequence of this paced wave front.

The main disadvantages to Array use can be divided into two types: physical and processing. Physical disadvantages include the time required to prepare and deploy the Array, the ectopy that can be induced by the Array, patient/Array size mismatch (Array occupies too much space), and difficulty maneuvering catheters around the Array. Processing disadvantages include the dependence of the reconstructed VEGM on the geometry fidelity and chamber size, the potential for the Array to move and render the geometry imprecise, the uncertain resolution of the Array, and the difficulty of detecting low-voltage potentials within scar.

Conclusions

Use of noncontact mapping for ablation of VT offers advantages to traditional mapping, especially for "unmappable" VT. Given the complexity of the Array, it is vital that the electrophysiologist be well versed in this technology and does not simply rely on the technologist or clinical engineer operating the system. Current limitations of the Array will hopefully be addressed in future iterations.

References

1. Schilling RJ, Peters NS, Davies DW. Simultaneous endocardial mapping in the human left ventricle using a noncontact catheter: comparison of contact and reconstructed electrograms during sinus rhythm. *Circulation.* 1998;98(9):887–898.
2. Jacobson JT, Afonso VX, Eisenman G, Schultz JR, Lazar S, Michele JJ, Josephson ME, Callans DJ. Characterization of the infarct substrate and ventricular tachycardia circuits with noncontact unipolar mapping in a porcine model of myocardial infarction. *Heart Rhythm.* 2006;3(2):189–197.
3. Reek S, Geller JC, Mittag A, Grothues F, Hess A, Kaulisch T, Klein HU. Noncontact mapping of ventricular tachycardia in a closed-chest animal model of chronic myocardial infarction. *Pacing Clin Electrophysiol.* 2003;26(12):2253–2263.
4. Ribbing M, Wasmer K, Monnig G, Kirchhof P, Loh P, Breithardt G, Haverkamp W, Eckardt L. Endocardial mapping of right ventricular outflow tract tachycardia using non-contact activation mapping. *J Cardiovasc Electrophysiol.* 2003;14(6):602–608.
5. Klemm HU, Ventura R, Steven D, Johnsen C, Rostock T, Lutomsky B, Risius T, Meinertz T, Willems S. Catheter ablation of multiple ventricular tachycardias after myocardial infarction guided by combined contact and non-contact mapping. *Circulation.* 200729;115(21):2697–2704.
6. Schilling RJ, Peters NS, Davies DW. Feasibility of a non-contact catheter for endocardial mapping of human ventricular tachycardia. *Circulation.* 1999;99(19):2543–2552.

Video Descriptions

Video 40.1 Activation map of RVOT PVC. Right anterior oblique (left) and posteroanterior (right) views of the RVOT display the anterior free wall as the site of origin of this PVC. The red asterisk denotes the tracking virtual, which is displayed in VEGM form in the inset at the bottom right of the display. His = His bundle location.

Video 40.2 Activation sequence of the VT described in the Figure 40.9 legend.

Video 40.3 Activation sequence of the VT described in the Figure 40.10 legend. Note the diastolic activation of the scar area prior to the onset of the surface QRS.

Video 40.4 Activation sequence of the paced wave front as it travels through a gap in the ablation line, as described in the Figure 40.12 legend.

CHAPTER 41

How to Use ICE to Aid in Catheter Ablation of Ventricular Tachycardia

Marc W. Deyell, MD, MSc; Mathew D. Hutchinson, MD; David J. Callans, MD

Introduction

The right and left ventricles are complex, 3-dimensional structures; integral to the ablation of ventricular arrhythmias is the ability to define this anatomy at the time of the procedure. The cornerstones of navigation in ventricular ablation are fluoroscopy and electroanatomic mapping systems; however, ICE is increasingly being used as an adjunct imaging modality. It provides invaluable complementary information that can improve both the efficacy and the safety of complex ventricular ablation.

At present, there are 2 types of commercially available ICE systems, radial and phased-array. Radial ICE (Ultra ICE™, Boston Scientific Co., San Jose, CA) has a transducer in the shaft of the catheter with a small ultrasound element at the tip, which is rotated by an external motor at 600 rpm. The ultrasound beam is emitted perpendicular to the longitudinal axis of the catheter, resulting in a circular image with the catheter at the center, similar to intravascular ultrasound imaging used in coronary interventions. The axial resolution with this catheter is excellent, but the tissue penetration is only 6 to 8 cm, and the catheter is nondeflectable, limiting its use in VT ablation.

Phased-array ICE catheters provide sector imaging, similar to transthoracic or transesophageal probes. In our laboratory we exclusively use the AcuNav™ probe (Acuson Corporation, Siemens Medical Solutions USA Inc., Malvern, PA) that is compatible with Siemens ultrasound platforms. This 8-Fr catheter has a forward-facing (perpendicular to tip), 64-element, phased-array transducer, which allows for scanning up to a 90° sector along the longitudinal axis of the catheter. It also has M-mode and pulsed or continuous-wave Doppler capabilities. The tissue penetration of the catheter is up to 16 cm, and the tip is deflectable in the anterior-posterior as well as the left-right plane, providing a flexible platform for ventricular imaging. St. Jude Medical (St. Paul, MN) produces a phased-array catheter (ViewFlex™ Plus ICE catheter) with a stand-alone, Phillips-based ultrasound platform (ViewMate II™), but we have not used this catheter to date. The ViewFlex transducer has full Doppler capabilities; however, deflection is limited to the anterior-posterior plane only.

Given its advantages for guiding ventricular ablation, the remainder of this chapter will focus solely on phased-array imaging (and, specifically, the AcuNav catheter). The transseptal approach for VT ablation is commonly used in our laboratory, and ICE is invaluable for guiding punctures; however, the use of ICE in transseptal puncture is discussed in detail in another chapter.

Preprocedural Planning

Setup

Insertion of the ICE catheter requires a dedicated femoral venous sheath that is 9 Fr. A 9-Fr sheath ensures easy passage of the ICE catheter and allows for intravenous infusions through the side port during the procedure. Where possible, the ICE catheter is placed through a left femoral venous sheath with the ablation catheter on the right side to allow for ease of manipulation of each catheter independently.

Controls and Settings

The AcuNav phased-array ICE catheter is capable of transmitting ultrasound at variable frequencies of 5.5, 7.5, 8.5, and 10 MHz. We typically start with 7.5 MHz, as this is adequate for most general ICE applications. Higher frequencies (8.5 and 10 MHz) are useful for better axial resolution when the structures of interest are near to the transducer, as is the case in outflow tract tachycardias. The lower frequency (5.5 MHz) may be required to visualize distant structures such as the inferior and lateral wall of the LV in a dilated heart. As lateral resolution declines with the width of the ultrasound beam, we use the minimum sector width required when focusing on a particular area of interest, such as a papillary muscle or the aortic cusps.

For optimal images, the operator must also have a good working understanding of the variable depth-compensation control that allows the relative gain to be adjusted throughout the image depth. Decreasing the near-field gain can be useful to overcome suppression from structures near to the probe, such as a thick IAS or a pacemaker lead, thereby allowing for better visualization of far-field structures.

By convention, ICE images are usually displayed with the marker on the left side of the image sector meaning the shaft of the catheter is to the left of the image and the top of the catheter is on the right. However, in our lab, we flip the image so the marker is on the right (**Figure 41.1**). We find this orientation is more intuitive for the operator in the EP laboratory as the "top" of the ICE image is in the same direction (left) as the patient's head when standing at the right side of the table. Most of the images in this chapter are shown in the conventional manner with the marker on the left and we have highlighted instances where the images are reversed.

Catheter Introduction and Manipulation

The ICE catheter can be advanced to the heart without fluoroscopy. As the ICE image is essentially perpendicular to the catheter plane, a small portion of the venous lumen and wall should be visible at all times while advancing the catheter. If resistance is encountered, or if visualization of the vessel is lost, the catheter is withdrawn slightly and rotated to visualize the lumen. Once the main vessel lumen is identified, the catheter can be deflected in the direction of the lumen and re-advanced to the heart.

Manipulation of the ICE catheter during the procedure can easily be performed by the same person performing the ablation, although a second pair of hands may be optimal when ablation catheter or ICE catheter stability is an issue. It is optimal to have a dedicated monitor for viewing the ultrasound images adjacent to the monitors displaying intracardiac EGMs, fluoroscopy and electroanatomic mapping information. An additional operator is required to manipulate the controls of the ultrasound platform and to record images. In our laboratory, this is frequently a fellow technologist or nurse. Adequate ultrasound training for this operator is therefore essential.

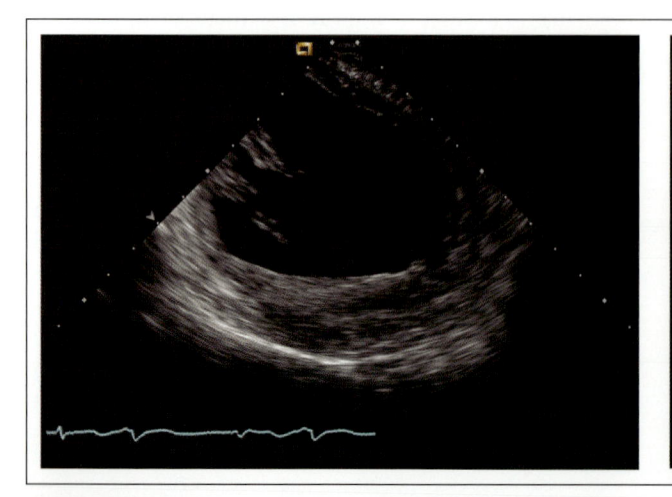

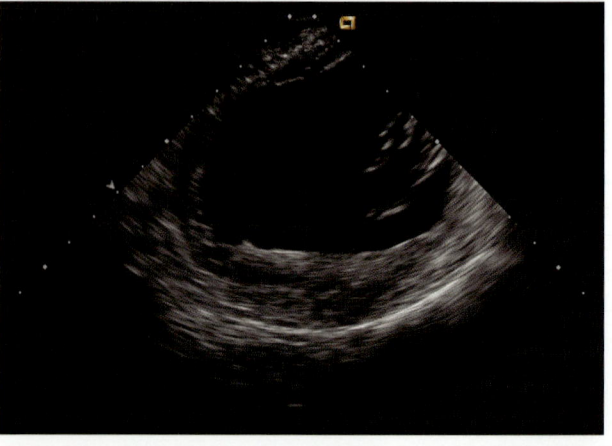

Figure 41.1 Long-axis view of the left ventricle from the right ventricle. The standard view is shown (left panel) with the marker on the left, denoting the shaft of the ICE catheter. In our laboratory we flip the images so the marker in on the right (right panel).

Procedure

Imaging of Ventricular Structures from the Right Atrium

In the next 2 sections, we review the components of a typical baseline ICE study for ventricular ablation, with emphasis on standard views for imaging of ventricular structures. However, given the maneuverability of ICE within the heart, these standard views can be modified as needed for the operator by deflecting the catheter to obtain optimal views of the structures of interest.

We always start our ICE studies from the "home" view with the ICE catheter in the neutral position in the mid-RA and oriented anteriorly to bring the tricuspid valve into view (▶ **Video 41.1A**). Here the proximal RVOT is also seen. Color Doppler imaging of the tricuspid valve is performed to quantify baseline tricuspid regurgitation (▶ **Video 41.1B**) and continuous wave (CW) Doppler of the jet is used to estimate baseline pulmonary artery systolic pressure. It is especially important to establish baseline pulmonary pressures in VT ablation of patients with impaired LV function. Advancement and (often) slight clockwise rotation of the catheter brings the RVOT and the pulmonic valve into view (**Figure 41.2**, ▶ **Video 41.2**). Further clockwise rotation reveals the aortic valve in long axis and LVOT (**Figure 41.3A**, ▶ **Video 41.3A**). The full LVOT is often slightly out of plane in the neutral position, but adjusting the left-right tilt can improve the image. Color Doppler is placed across the aortic valve to assess for baseline stenosis or regurgitation (**Figure 41.3B**, ▶ **Video 41.3B**). The mitral valve can be viewed in long axis with further slight clockwise rotation (**Figure 41.4A**, ▶ **Video 41.4A**). Again, some left-right tilt is usually required to bring the transducer parallel to the LV inflow. Baseline mitral regurgitation is assessed with color Doppler across the valve (**Figure 41.4B**, ▶ **Video 41.4B**).

Imaging of Ventricular Structures from the Tricuspid Valve And Right Ventricle

The ICE catheter can be advanced to the tricuspid annulus and right ventricles by deflecting it anteriorly, advancing it forward across the tricuspid valve then releasing the deflection back to the neutral position (▶ **Video 41.5**). Once the ICE catheter is in the body of the RV, it initially faces the inferior portion of the free wall and the adjacent pericardium (**Figure 41.5**, ▶ **Video 41.6**). Rotating the catheter clockwise brings into view the LV in long axis with visualization of the postero-medial papillary muscle and the mitral valve (**Figure 41.6A**, ▶ **Video 41.7A**). The anterolateral papillary is visualized with slight further clockwise rotation (**Figure 41.6B**, ▶ **Video 41.7B**). When imaging the left ventricle, clockwise rotation brings into view progressively more anterior structures. The ICE catheter can be advanced further into the RV to enhance visualization of the apex or withdrawn towards the

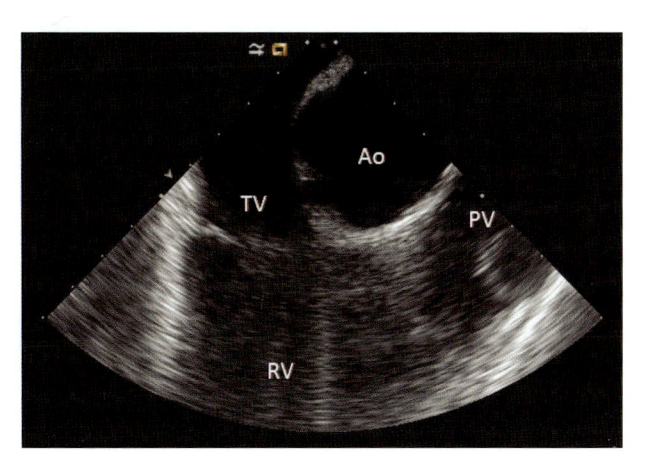

Figure 41.2 Advancing the ICE catheter from the home view position allows visualization of the right ventricular outflow tract (RVOT) and the pulmonary valve.

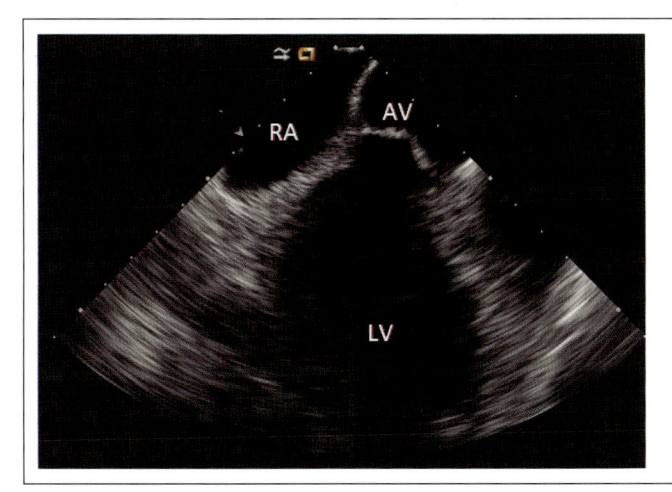

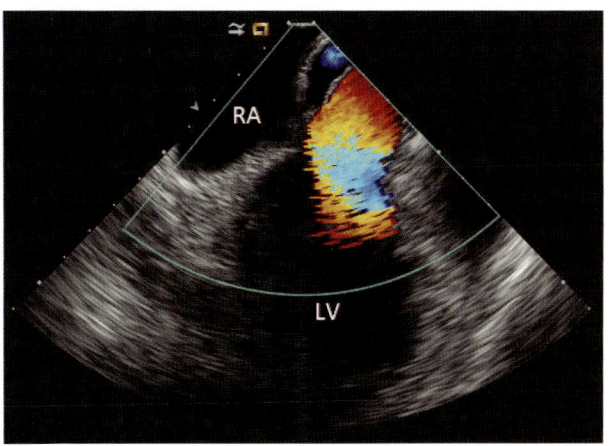

Figure 41.3 The aortic valve and left ventricular (LV) outflow tract viewed from the right atrium (RA) (left panel). Color Doppler across the aortic valve (right panel) shows largely laminar flow across the outflow tract.

388 • Ablation of VT

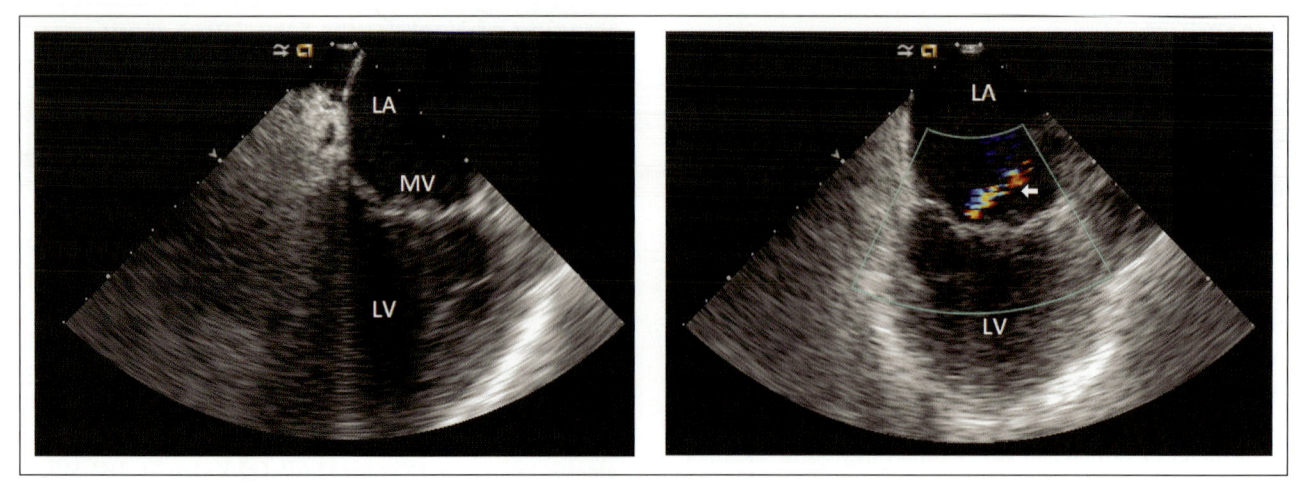

Figure 41.4 The left ventricle (LV) inflow and mitral valve (MV) viewed from the right atrium (RA) (left panel). Color Doppler across the MV (right panel) reveals mild regurgitation (arrow).

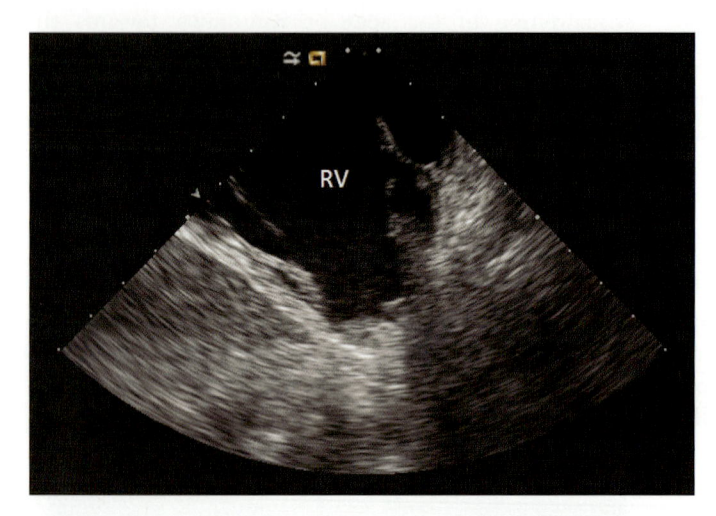

Figure 41.5 The initial image after insertion of the ICE catheter into the right ventricle (RV) shows the inferior RV free wall (bottom left) and apex. RV trabaculation can be identified (arrows).

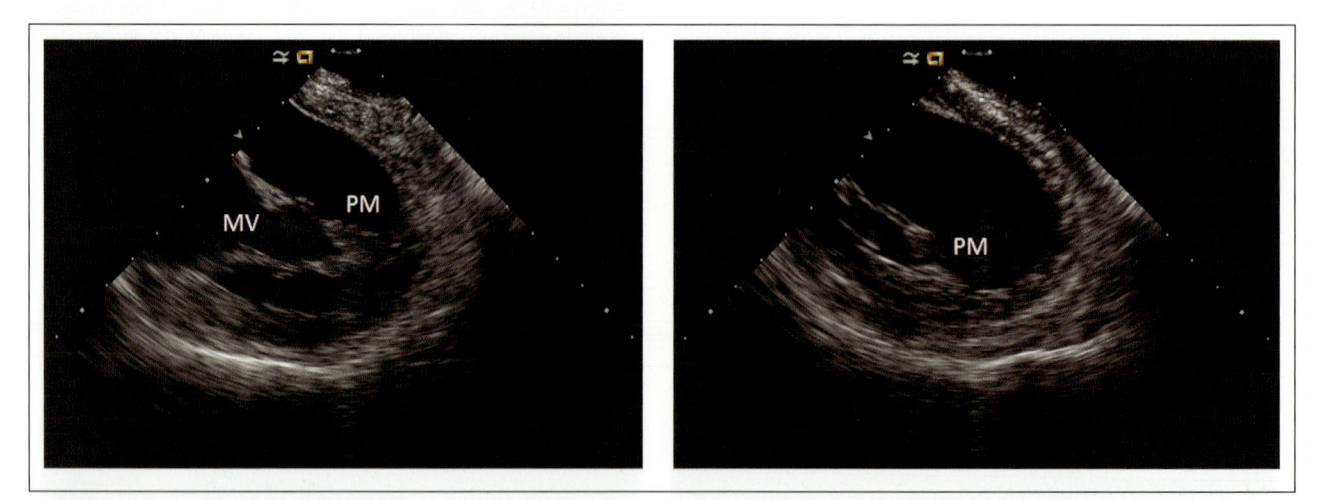

Figure 41.6 Long-axis view of the left ventricle (LV) with the postero-medial papillary muscle (PM) and MV (left panel). Smooth LV endocardium is noted without trabaculation. Further clockwise rotation of the ICE catheter brings the antero-lateral PM into view (right panel). Note each PM has 2 distinct heads. RV can be seen in the right upper corner.

tricuspid valve annulus to enhance more basal structures. Further clockwise rotation brings into view the aortic valve in short axis (**Figure 41.7A,** ▶ **Video 41.8A**), and color Doppler here is useful for assessment of regurgitation (**Figure 41.7B,** ▶ **Video 41.8B**). This view is essential for catheter mapping and ablation of aortic cusp arrhythmias. Slight advancement of the catheter into the RV in the same plane allows visualization of the pulmonic valve in long axis and the RVOT (**Figure 41.8, A and B,** ▶ **Video 41.9, A and B**). Continuous-wave Doppler of the pulmonic regurgitant jet can be used to assess pulmonary artery diastolic pressures. Additional clockwise rotation of the catheter then reveals the aortic valve in long axis and the ascending aorta (**Figure 41.9,** ▶ **Video 41.10**). This view of ascending aorta may identify atheroma that would preclude a retrograde approach to mapping of the LV (**Figure 41.10,** ▶ **Video 41.11, A and B**).

ICE to Guide Catheter Positioning and Lesion Formation

Stability of the ablation catheter tip and excellent tissue contact are the cornerstones of effective energy delivery during ablation. This is particularly important for tissue penetration in the thicker myocardium of the left ventricle. Achieving stability and contact in the ventricles can be challenging, especially in the presence of gross structural abnormalities such as scar or aneurysm.

Traditional markers of stability, including fluoroscopic appearance and EGM characteristics, are imperfect.

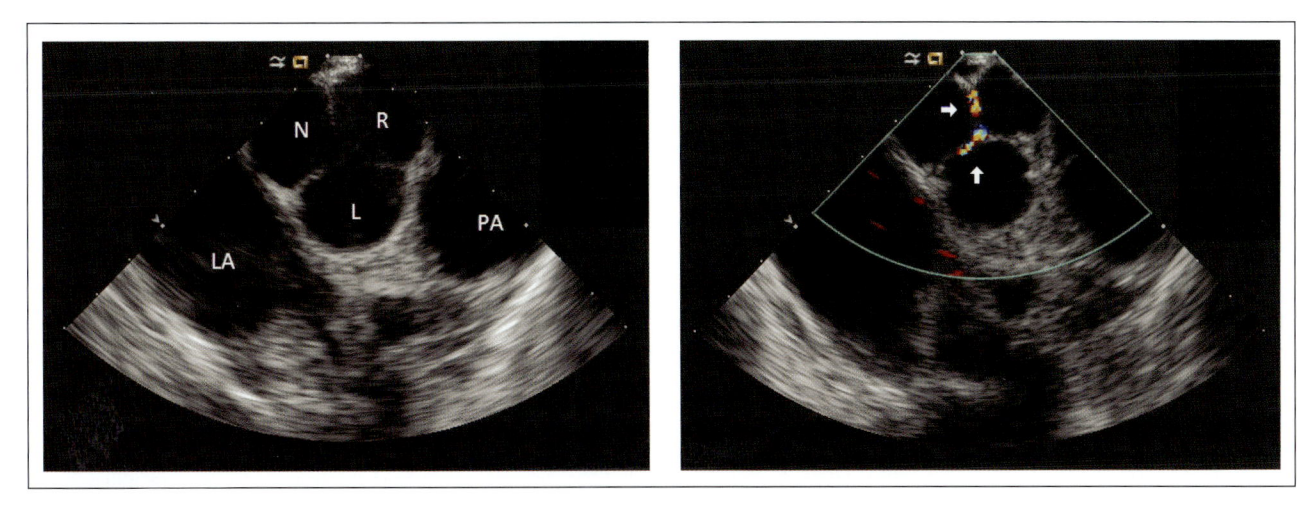

Figure 41.7 The aortic valve viewed in short axis from the right ventricle (RV). All 3 cusps (L = left, R = right, N = noncoronary) are seen (left panel). Color Doppler across the aortic valve reveals trace regurgitation (arrows, right panel). The pulmonary artery (PA) is seen on the right of the images.

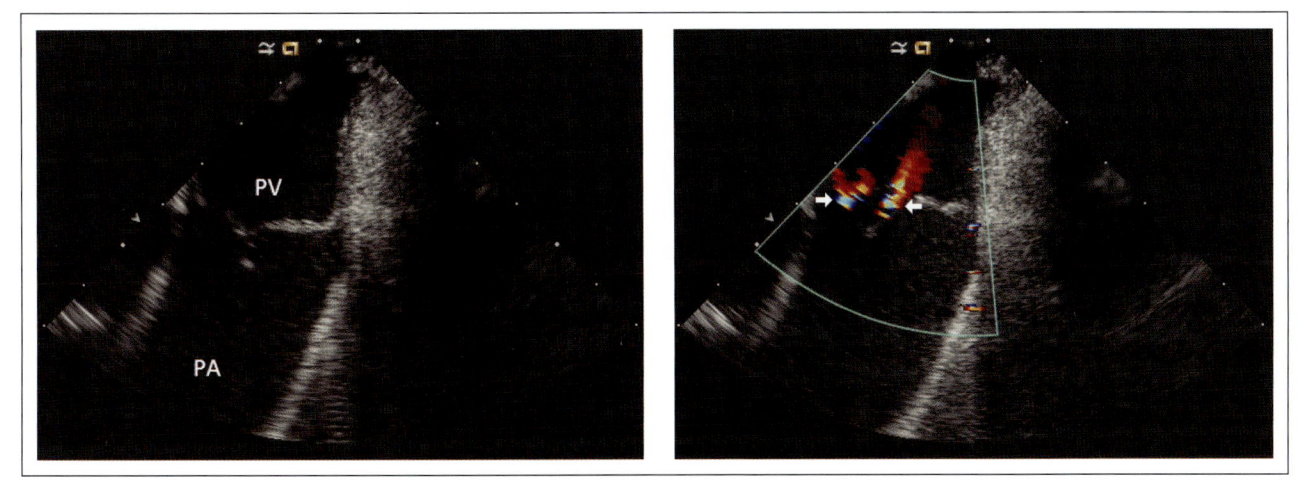

Figure 41.8 The pulmonary valve and artery (PA) viewed in long axis from the right ventricle (left panel). Color Doppler across the pulmonic valve reveals 2 jets of mild regurgitation (arrows, right panel).

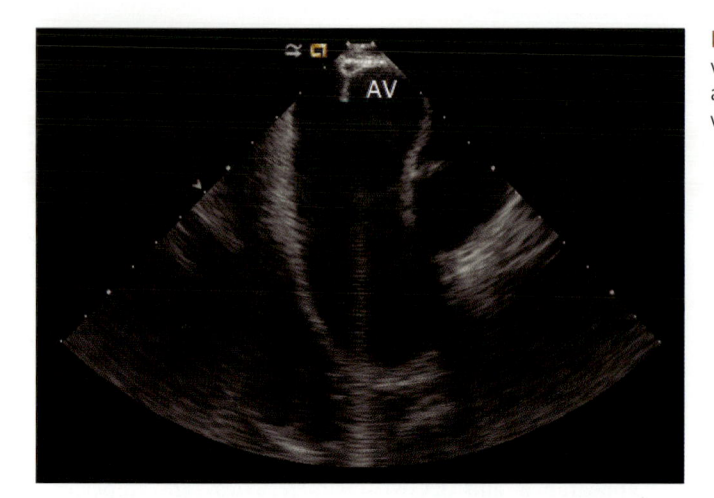

Figure 41.9 The aortic valve and ascending aorta as viewed from the right ventricle.

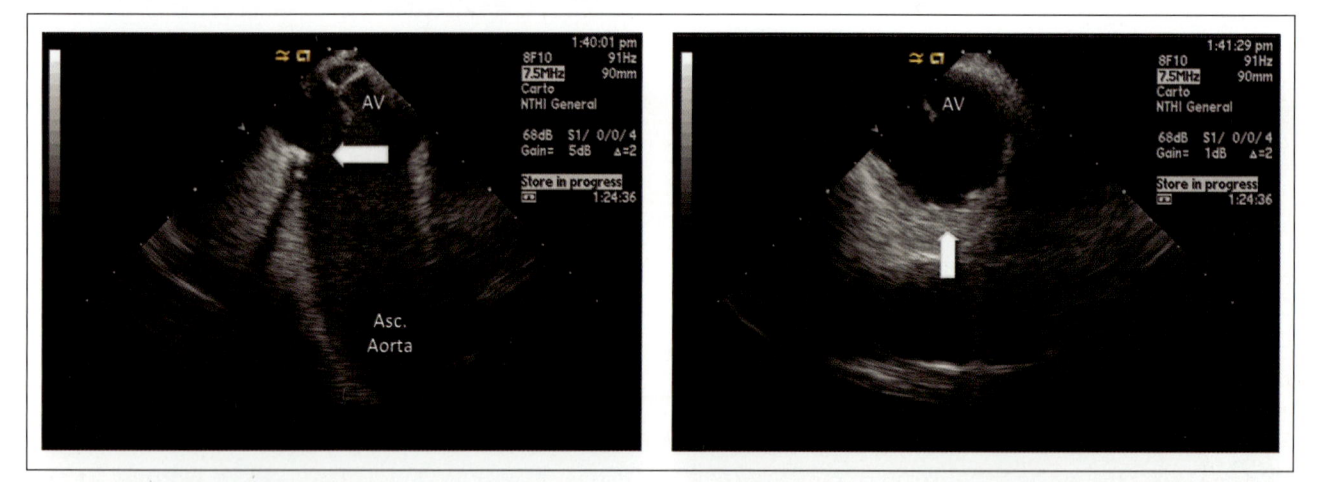

Figure 41.10 The ascending aorta is viewed in long axis (left panel) and obliquely (right panel) from the right ventricle. Focal atheroma at the sino-tubular junction is seen in the left panel (arrow) and more diffuse ascending aortic atheroma is seen in the right panel (arrow).

Electroanatomic mapping systems have been instrumental in better demonstrating the position of the ablation catheter tip in real time and even in assessing contact. However, these systems are also not without limitations as they are dependent on the geometry created during the procedure or obtained through prior imaging studies. They may be inaccurate if either the chamber geometry changes (as with differential volume loading) or there is a shift with respect to the mapping system reference. ICE offers the advantage of direct visualization of both the ablation catheter and the ventricular myocardium in real time (**Figure 41.11**, ▶ Video 41.12) and thus provides valuable adjunctive information to the electroanatomic mapping systems. Visualization of the myocardium allows for continuous assessment of catheter contact. This is particularly useful in areas with altered anatomy and/or diminished EGMs, such as dense scar.

The assessment of lesion formation during ablation can be challenging, particularly in areas of scar where EGM changes may be difficult to assess and impedance changes during ablation may not adequately reflect the true extent of myocardial damage. Increased echodensity of the myocardium, as visualized by ICE, has been previously correlated with lesion formation.[1,2] Further quantification of lesion formation by ICE remains a research tool at present, but the qualitative development of increased echodensity during ablation gives the operator reassurance that adequate lesions are being produced (**Figures 41.11** and **41.12**, ▶ Videos 41.12 and 41.13).

ICE in the Assessment of VT Substrate in Structural Heart Disease

The ability to directly visualize myocardium with ICE also allows for delineation of ventricular tachycardia substrate. Scar, particularly in ischemic heart disease, can be easily visualized as areas of hypocontractility or akinesis with accompanying thinning or effacement (**Figures 41.11** and **41.13**, ▶ Videos 41.12 and 41.14). Such areas, as seen with ICE, correlate well with the extent of endocardial bipolar voltage abnormalities.[3] Tissue Doppler imaging has now been incorporated into ICE catheters and may allow for even better quantification of the distribution of scar.

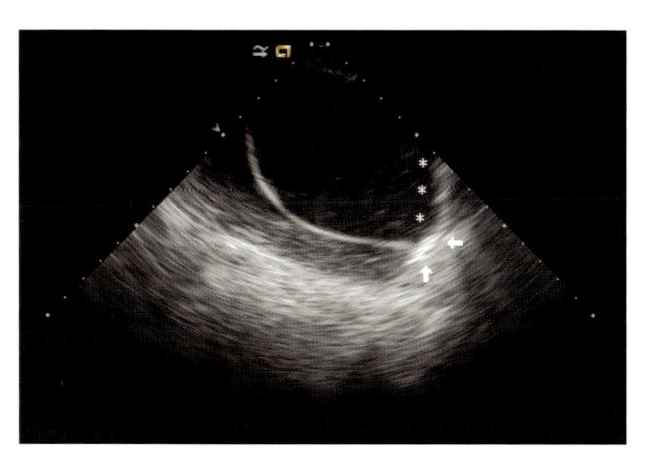

Figure 41.11 The ablation catheter in good contact with the endocardium at the border of an anteroapical infarct (asterisks). Note the ablation lesion is demonstrated by ICE as an area of increased echodensity (arrows).

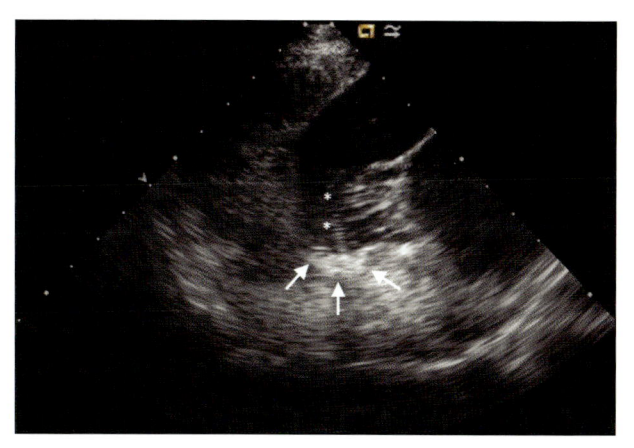

Figure 41.12 Ablation catheter (asterisks) with the tip on the basal lateral left ventricular endocardium. The ablation lesion is visualized as an area with increased echodensity (arrows). Note the image shown is reversed.

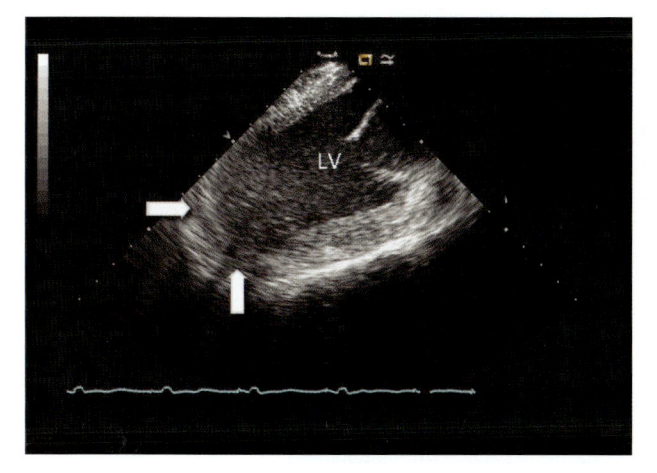

Figure 41.13 Long-axis view of the left ventricle (LV) with an apical aneurysm (arrows). There is spontaneous echo contrast in the aneurysm ("smoke"). Note the image shown is reversed.

Gross disturbances of ventricular anatomy, such as aneurysms, are challenging to delineate with only fluoroscopy and electroanatomic systems. ICE can easily visualize the location and extent of aneurysms and guide catheter mapping (**Figure 41.14**, Video 41.15). Safety is also greatly enhanced when the operator can directly visualize contact in these vulnerable areas, thereby avoiding inadvertent perforation.

In certain patients with NICM, ICE can also detect the presence of mid-myocardial and epicardial scar.[4] The scar may appear as an echodense lesion in the mid-myocardium or epicardium and is clearly separate from the parietal pericardium during systole (**Figure 41.15**, Video 41.16). These areas correlate well with the presence of epicardial bipolar abnormalities using voltage mapping. Visualization of such a lesion can help to focus mapping efforts during ablation of VT in NICM.

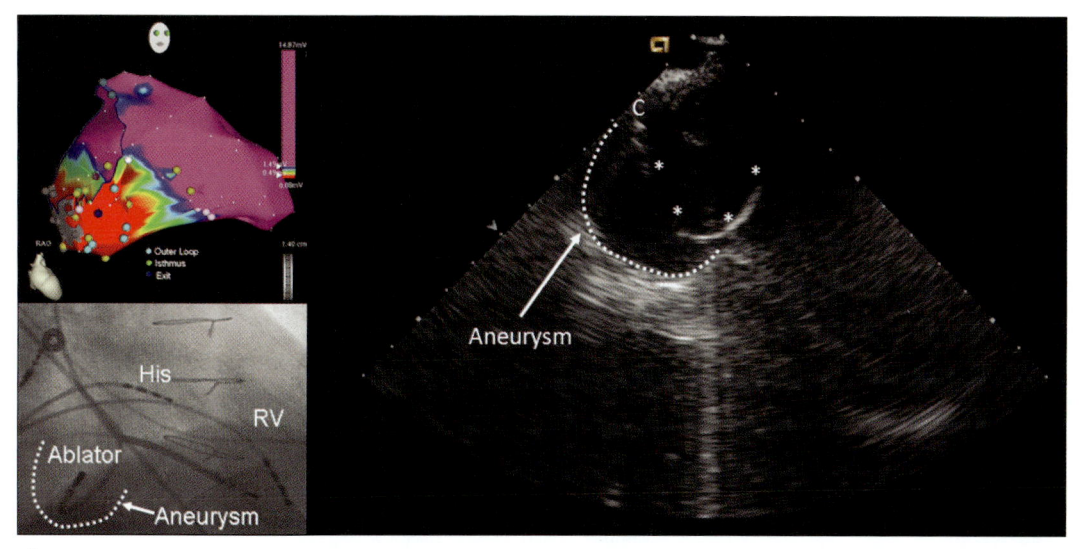

Figure 41.14 ICE imaging showing the extent of an infero-basal left ventricular aneurysm (right) with the ablation catheter positioned near the annulus (C = catheter tip, asterisks = shaft). The corresponding fluoroscopic right anterior oblique (RAO) image is shown on the bottom left with the outline of the aneurysm. The endocardial bipolar electroanatomic map is shown on the top left.

Integration of ICE with Electroanatomic Mapping Systems

Incorporation of the anatomical information provided by ICE into electroanatomic mapping systems can greatly enhance the accuracy of the maps or geometries created. Currently, direct integration of ICE data is only available using the CARTO™ mapping system with CARTOSound™ software (Biosense-Webster, Diamond Bar, CA). The ClearICE catheter is currently in development and integrates with the EnSite NavX mapping system (both by St. Jude Medical, St. Paul, MN) but is not yet commercially available.

The CARTOSound system employs a modified version of the AcuNav ICE catheter, the 10-Fr SoundStar™ catheter, that contains a location sensor allowing it to be visualized in the CARTO mapping system. Two-dimensional sector images obtained from the ICE catheter are displayed on the active map. Multiple images at various imaging planes are taken of the structure or chamber of interest. The endocardial border from each image is traced either manually or using edge-detection software (**Figure 41.16,** Video 41.17). These ICE images provide 2-dimensional contours that are integrated by the CARTOSound software to build into a 3-dimensional geometry.

The integration of ICE information into the mapping system can be used to create a quick geometry of the chamber of interest, without fluoroscopy and even before the ablation catheter is introduced. Many laboratories use

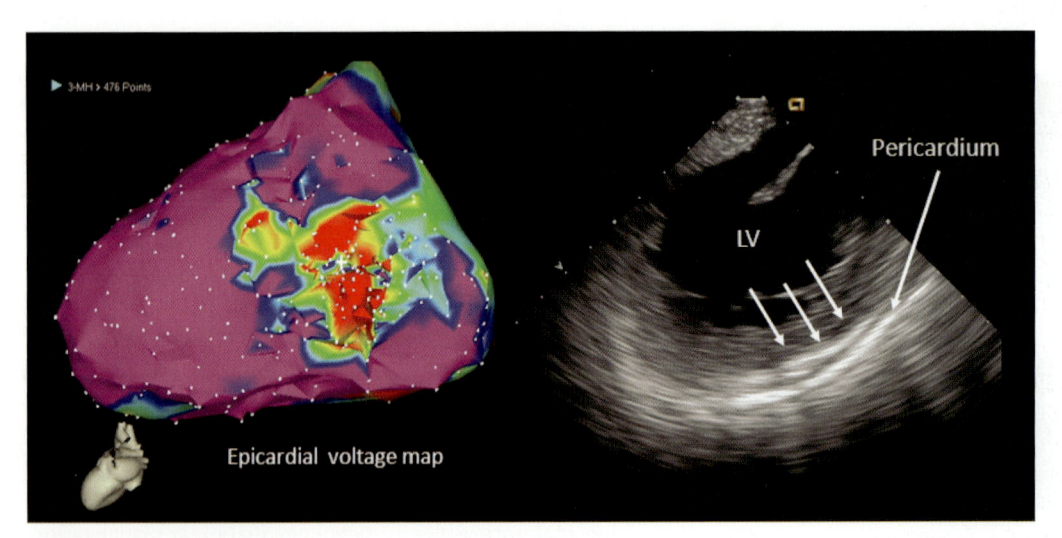

Figure 41.15 A linear area of increased echodensity near the epicardial surface on the lateral left ventricular (LV) wall (arrows) in a patient with NICM. The corresponding epicardial scar by electroanatomic mapping is shown on the left. Note the ICE image shown is reversed.

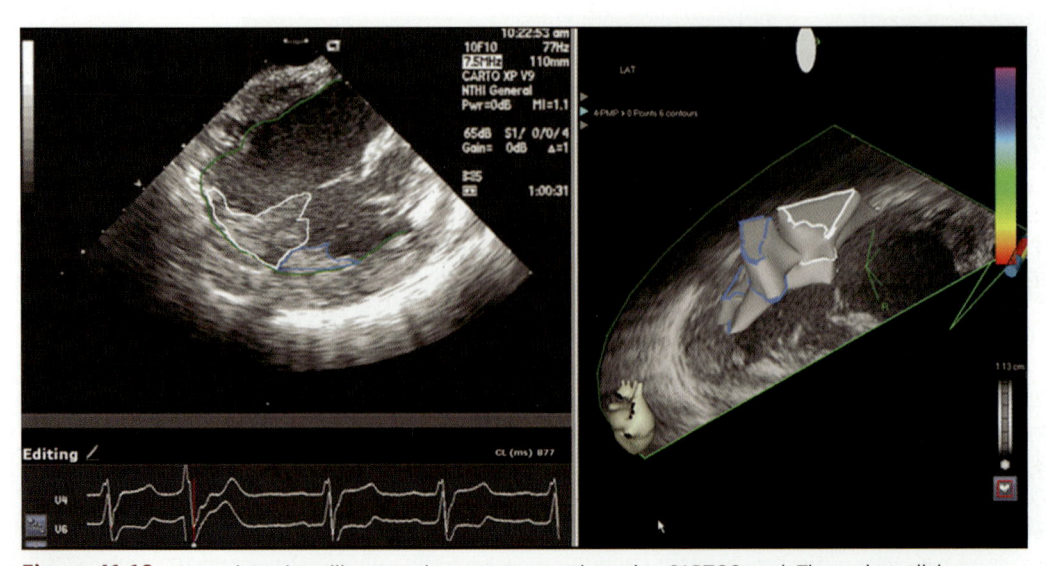

Figure 41.16 Anterolateral papillary muscle geometry creation using CARTOSound. The endocardial borders of each papillary muscle head on the ICE image (left) are manually traced. These contours are then incorporated into the 3-dimensional map (right) by the software. Note the ICE image shown is reversed.

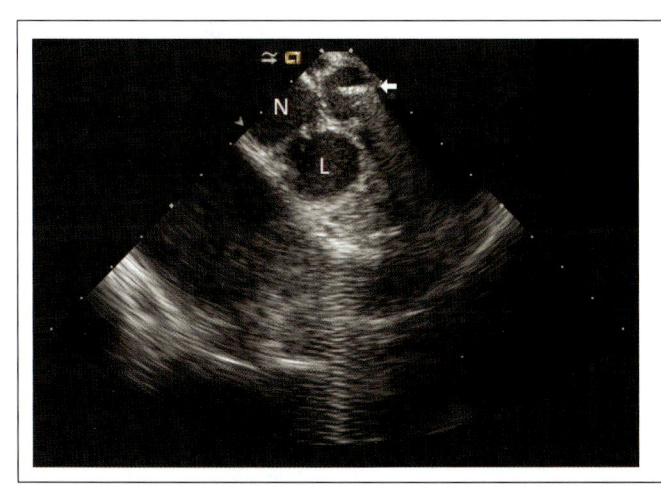

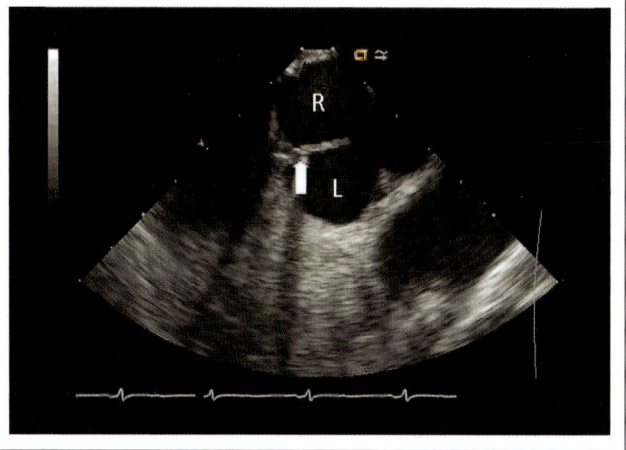

Figure 41.17 Short-axis view of the aortic valve (L = left coronary cusp, N = noncoronary cusp) from the right ventricle showing the ablation catheter in the right coronary cusp (arrow, left panel). A reversed image with the catheter (arrow) at the junction of the right (R) and left coronary cusps is shown in the right panel.

CARTOSound to create LV geometry prior to catheter mapping of left-sided VT or pulmonic valves. Integration of ICE is particularly useful in imaging complex structures, such as the aortic cusps or papillary muscles, where traditional electroanatomic mapping has difficulty delineating the anatomy. The use of CARTOSound in these situations is discussed further below.

Ablation of Arrhythmias Arising from the Coronary Cusps

It is increasingly recognized that many idiopathic VTs and pulmonic valves originate from the LVOT and can be successfully ablated from the coronary cusps. The anatomy of the aortic cusps and the sinuses of Valsalva is complex, and navigation by fluoroscopy can be difficult. ICE is invaluable for mapping and ablation in this region and is routinely used in our center.

The aortic cusps can be viewed in long axis and short axis with the ICE catheter in either the RA or RV. We typically place the ICE catheter in the RV as manipulation between the short-axis and long-axis views requires only minimal rotation and stability of the ICE catheter position is generally good. The short-axis view easily identifies which cusp the ablation catheter is positioned and facilitates manipulation to the junction of the right and left coronary cusps, a frequent site of origin of VTs and pulmonic valves (**Figure 41.17**, ▶ **Video 41.18, A and B**).[5] The long-axis view demonstrates the position of the catheter relative to the nadir of the cusp (**Figure 41.18**, ▶ **Video 41.19**). In ablation of VT or pulmonic valves arising from tissue adjacent to the cusps, the optimal and safest site for ablation is typically at the nadir or most inferior position or in the junction between the right and left cusps.

ICE and fluoroscopy alone can be used for mapping and ablation in this region, but we typically also employ electroanatomic mapping systems to provide added information, such as the site of earliest activation. The simplest approach for integration is to position the ablation catheter at each of the junctions using ICE, and then at the nadir of each cusp. Points tagged at these locations within the mapping system can then be used to create separate maps/geometries of each of the cusps. Alternatively, the ICE images can be integrated directly with the electroanatomic mapping system using CARTOSound. For the aortic cusps, multiple images at different planes are taken of the LVOT and cusps with the ICE catheter. Each cusp and the LVOT are created as separate "chambers" (**Figure 41.19**, ▶ **Video 41.20**). When mapping tolerated VT or frequent pulmonic valves, all ICE images are taken during VT or pulmonic valves to ensure accurate geometry

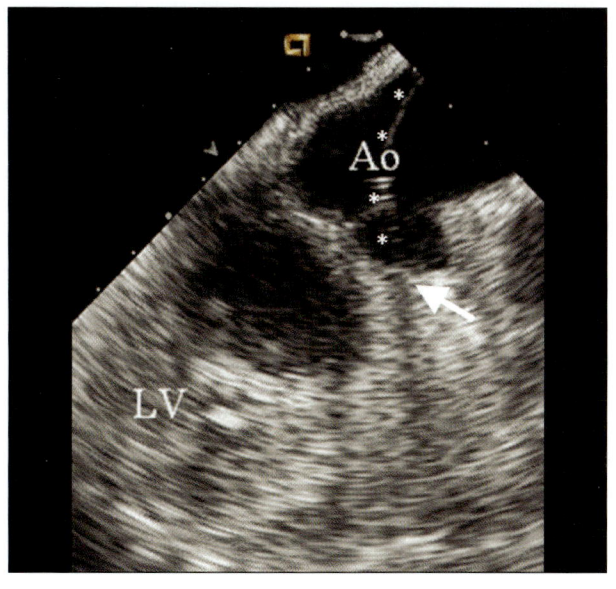

Figure 41.18 Long-axis view of the aortic valve from the right atrium (Ao, aorta; LV, left ventricle). The ablation catheter can be seen (asterisks) with the tip in the nadir of the left coronary cusp (arrow).

394 • Ablation of VT

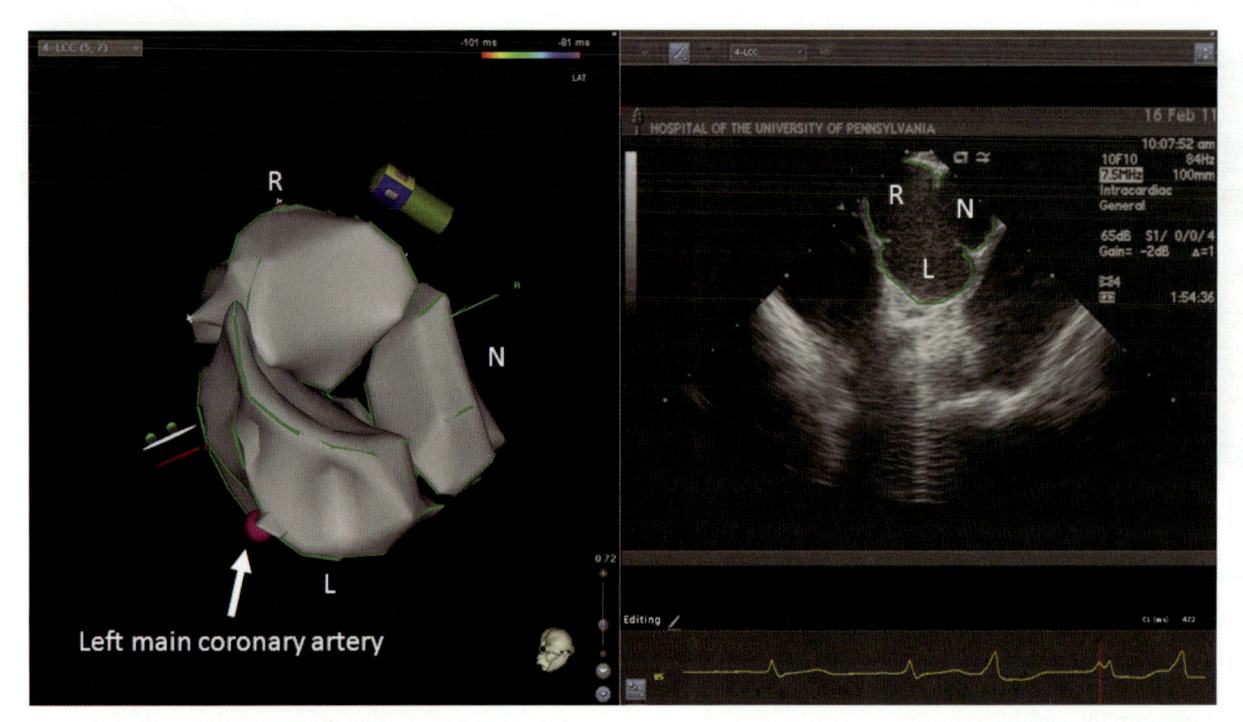

Figure 41.19 Maps of the aortic cusps using CARTOSound. The contours of each cusp (L = left coronary cusp, N = noncoronary cusp, R = right coronary cusp) are traced from the ICE image (right). Each traced contour is projected on the map view (left) and integrated into a 3-dimensional geometry. The left main coronary artery ostium was visualized on ICE and tagged on the map. Note the ICE image shown is reversed.

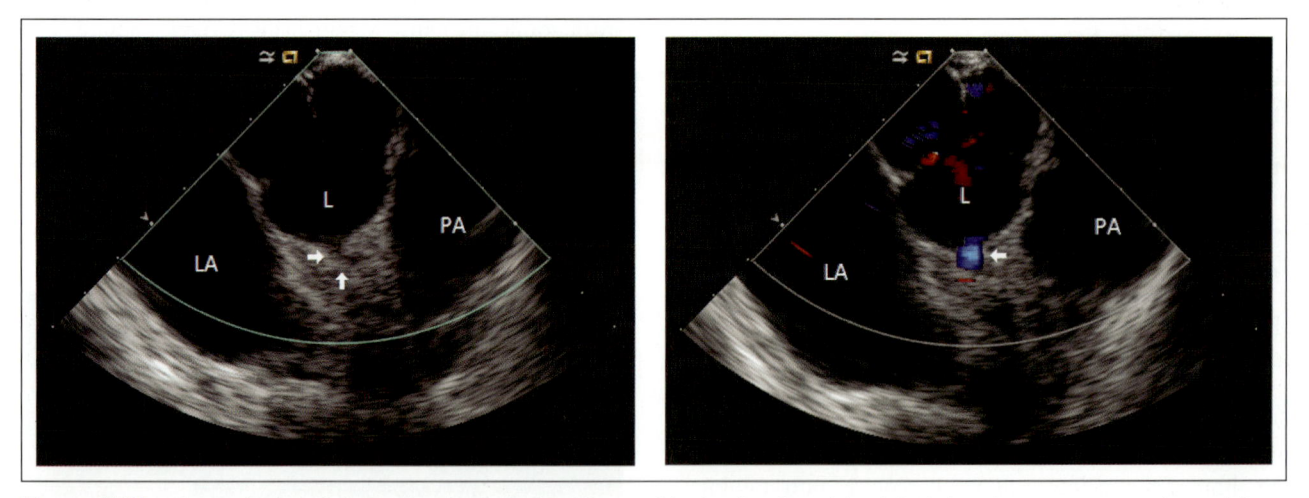

Figure 41.20 Short axis view of the aortic valve from the right ventricle showing the origin of the left main coronary artery (arrows) from the left coronary cusp (left panel = LA, left atrium; PA, pulmonary artery). Color Doppler can help visualize the origin of the coronary artery (arrow, right panel).

for activation mapping (as there is often a shift in the geometry between VT and sinus rhythm). In our experience, the anatomy is best created using short-axis images of the cusps only. Incorporating long-axis images for geometry creation frequently leads to distortion of the map as these images are mostly oblique views and slightly out of plane from the true longitudinal axis of the aorta. The rightward aspect of the noncoronary cusp is the most difficult to fully visualize from the RVOT with ICE, but this cusp is only rarely a site of earliest activation of VT or pulmonic valves.

A major concern of ablation in the coronary cusps is the proximity to a coronary artery ostium. In most centers, coronary angiography is undertaken to ascertain the distance between the ablation catheter tip and the coronary ostium. However, ICE alone often can accurately demonstrate that the catheter tip is at a safe distance (> 1 cm) from the coronary artery ostium. The left and right coronary ostia can frequently be visualized on ICE with careful manipulation (**Figure 41.20**, ▶ **Video 41.21**). If CARTOSound is used, ostia can then be tagged or created as separate geometries in CARTOSound. If the ablation catheter is in the nadir of a

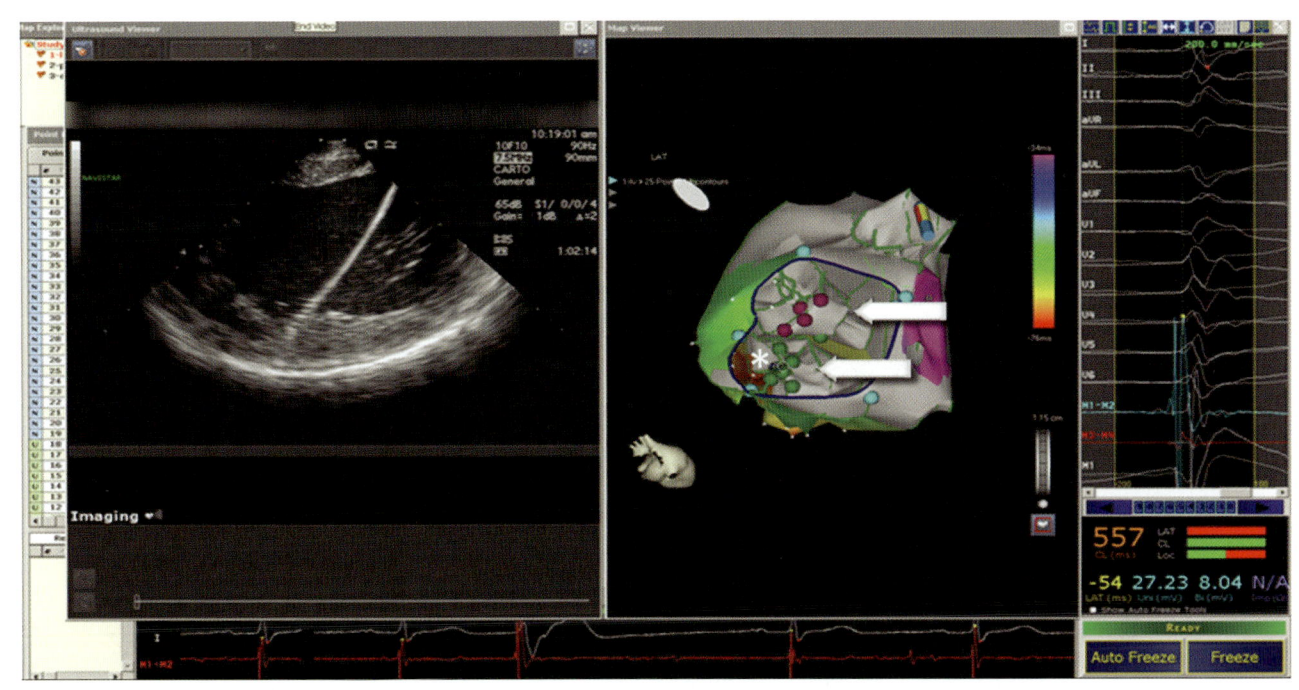

Figure 41.21 Maps of both heads of the anterolateral papillary muscle (arrows) created using CARTOSound. The map view (right) is through the mitral valve, into the left ventricular cavity. The ablation catheter can also be seen on the map (asterisk) and in real time on the ICE image (left). Note the ICE image shown is reversed.

cusp on the long-axis view, the ablation catheter is almost certainly > 1 cm from the ostium. Similarly, when ICE demonstrates the ablation catheter is near the junction of the left and right coronary cusps, the operator can be reassured that ablation can be performed safely, unless there is anomalous origin of the right coronary artery.

Ablation of Arrhythmias Arising from the Papillary Muscles

The papillary muscles present a unique anatomic challenge for mapping and ablation of VT or pulmonic valves, as they are highly complex. Ablation of arrhythmias arising from these structures is challenging as a consequence. Electroanatomic mapping systems rely on point-by-point sampling of the papillary muscles using an ablation catheter. Mapping in this fashion is difficult as ablation catheter stability on these mobile and intricate structures is tenuous. The papillary muscles are intracavitary, and representation of such structures can be difficult in the currently available mapping systems. As shown previously, the papillary muscles can be readily visualized with ICE (**Figure 41.6** and ▶ **Video 41.7**). Therefore, we typically use CARTOSound to create papillary muscle geometries when attempting ablation of pulmonic valves or VT localized to these areas on the basis of the ECG morphology. Multiple images of the papillary muscle of interest are taken at different planes with the ICE catheter in the RV. Each head of the papillary muscle is traced separately to create a geometry (**Figure 41.16,** ▶ **Video 41.17**). When mapping tolerated VT or frequent pulmonic valves, the map should be created during ectopic ventricular beats to ensure accuracy during activation mapping. Once the geometries are created, they can be displayed inside the LV map and the ablation catheter can be localized with better precision on the muscles (**Figure 41.21,** ▶ **Video 41.22**).

Postprocedure Care

Once the ablation procedure has finished, we routinely obtain postprocedure imaging with all mapping and ablation catheters removed from the heart. The primary focus of this examination is to identify procedural complications, which are discussed further below. We typically leave the ICE catheter positioned in the IVC until the patient has been extubated or recovered from sedation and is hemodynamically stable. This allows for rapid assessment of any delayed complications while still in the EP laboratory.

Procedural Complications

Identification of Procedural Complications with ICE

One of the primary advantages of ICE for guiding ventricular ablation is its ability to easily detect complications arising during the procedure. The continuous monitoring provided by ICE allows for the early identification of complications, which facilitates their management and limits adverse consequences.

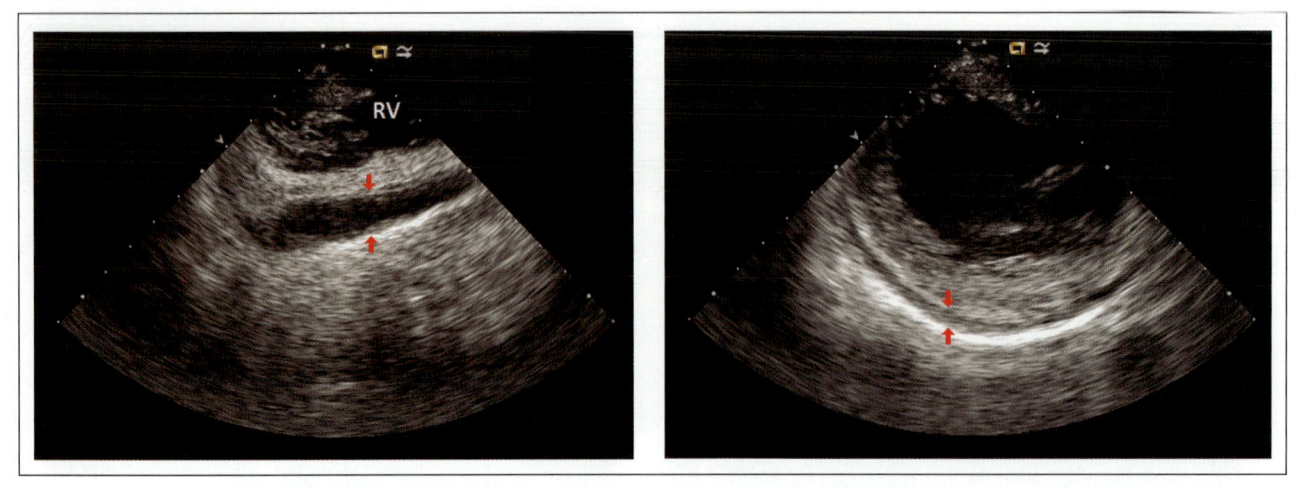

Figure 41.22 View of the right ventricular (RV) inferior free wall and pericardial effusion visible (arrows, left panel). The same effusion (arrows) viewed adjacent to the inferior left ventricular wall (right panel). Note the images shown are reversed.

Key to the identification of procedural complications is obtaining thorough baseline imaging before catheters are introduced into the heart. We have already outlined the key components to such an examination. Any interval change observed during the procedure can readily be compared to the baseline images. We obtain repeat images at regular intervals throughout the procedure and particularly if there are unexplained changes in the patient's clinical status.

Pericardial Effusion

Pericardial effusion can complicate VT ablation either from direct perforation of the ventricular myocardium from a mapping or ablation catheter or in the process of transseptal puncture, when this approach is used. ICE is very sensitive at detecting even minor amounts of pericardial fluid. This allows the electrophysiologists to intervene with reversal of anticoagulation and pericardiocentesis before the development of hemodynamic instability. Imaging of the pericardium is performed with the ICE catheter in the RV. The pericardium adjacent to the RV free wall and the LV inferior wall is examined for any evidence of pericardial effusion (**Figure 41.22**, ▶ Video 41.23, A and B). It is in these dependent areas where small pericardial effusions first become visible. Continuous monitoring of pericardial fluid is particularly useful in epicardial ablation using irrigated catheters to guide periodic drainage.

Cardiogenic Shock

VT ablation is often performed in patients with impaired ventricular function, and their hemodynamic status may be tenuous. Repeated inductions of VT, cardioversions, or defibrillations and volume loading from irrigated catheters may all contribute to worsening ventricular function and increased filling pressures during the procedure. ICE easily provides for rapid reassessment of RV and LV contractility. Repeat assessment of pulmonary pressures from the tricuspid and pulmonary regurgitant jets can also confirm elevation in filling pressures if a PA catheter is not in place. Thus ICE can help guide the appropriate management of cardiogenic shock in determining whether inotropes, diuretics, and/or mechanical support should be initiated.

Valvular Function

At the end of the procedure, each of the valves is examined again with 2-dimensional imaging and color Doppler to assess for any interval change in structure or regurgitation. For LV procedures, either retrograde or transseptal, particular attention is focused on the aortic and mitral valves, to ensure they were not damaged during mapping or ablation.

Other Complications

Thrombus formation on sheaths and catheters as well as at the site of ablation can be easily detected by ICE. Early detection of thrombus allows for intervention ideally before embolism has taken place. Once thrombus is detected, the operator can titrate the anticoagulation, attempt to aspirate the thrombus, and/or withdraw the offending equipment.

Coronary artery embolism is a rare complication of VT ablation and may occur as a result of air or thrombus. ICE can provide the diagnosis when a new wall motion abnormality is demonstrated in the setting of ST segment changes on the ECG.

Complications Directly Attributable to ICE

The rate of complications directly attributable to the ICE catheter is very low and is likely similar to the risk of complications from a diagnostic EP study, though no large ICE series has quantified this risk to date. Nonetheless, like any intravascular catheter, ICE is capable of causing damage to vascular or intracardiac structures, predominantly in the form of perforation. The risk of ICE can be mitigated by careful manipulation of the probe. The ICE catheter should only be advanced when the lumen of the vessel or chamber is readily visualized with the probe and no resistance is felt. Particular care must be taken when the ICE catheter is left in the RV during a procedure. Like any catheter, the probe can migrate during the case and perforation may result, and the catheter position should be assessed at regular intervals. The 10-Fr SoundStar catheter for use with the CARTOSound system is larger and stiffer than the 8-F catheter and therefore poses a slightly higher risk of perforation.

Advantages and Limitations

The chief advantage of ICE to guide ventricular ablation is the ability to visualize anatomy directly and in real time. ICE thus overcomes the major limitations of fluoroscopy and electroanatomic mapping systems where anatomy is viewed indirectly or inferred. The continuous anatomic information provided by ICE is integral to identification of substrate for ablation, assessment of catheter position and contact, mapping of complex structures, and identification of complications.

ICE also provides unique advantages over TEE. Most importantly, intubation or heavy sedation is not required to use ICE. This is critically important in the mapping of idiopathic VT and pulmonic valves that may be exquisitely sensitive to the patient's sympathetic tone. TEE is not practical in such situations. Unlike a TEE probe that must remain in the esophagus, the ICE catheter can be freely manipulated to all areas in the right heart, allowing almost unlimited viewing angles of structures of interest. The ICE probe is also manipulated by the electrophysiologist, eliminating the need for a second operator of the TEE probe.

The greatest limitation of ICE that impedes its widespread use is the cost of the catheters. Each catheter can cost in excess of $2000.00 US, though actual cost depends on the location and the volume of purchase. Limiting this cost is the fact that ICE catheters have no lumen and can be gas-resterilized up to 3 times. The reprocessing cost for an ICE cathter is less than half that of a new catheter. We routinely resterilize our ICE catheters, though this is accompanied by some noticeable degradation in image quality. Hopefully as more vendors of ICE probes emerge, competition will further reduce catheter cost. The AcuNav catheter has the additional advantage that it integrates into existing Siemens platforms used for TTE and TEE. This may obviate the need for purchasing a separate ultrasound workstation.

Conclusions

ICE can easily be integrated into the EP laboratory and provides invaluable additional information for ventricular ablation. We routinely use ICE for all of our left-sided VT and pulmonic valve cases. The real-time anatomical information and catheter visualization may improve the success of ablation, particularly in difficult areas such as the aortic cusps and papillary muscles. ICE has also reduced our reliance on fluoroscopy, thereby limiting the radiation exposure to the patient and operator. Most important of all, ICE allows for the early recognition and treatment of procedure-related complications and enhances the safety of ablation in these often-vulnerable patients.

As competition among ICE vendors increases, hopefully catheter costs will continue to decrease, allowing for more widespread use of ICE in EP procedures. There will also undoubtedly be many advances in ICE technology in the near future. Already, forward-looking phased-array catheters are in development as are combination ICE/EP catheters capable of simultaneous imaging and mapping.[6,7] Undoubtedly, 4-dimensional ICE catheters, allowing 3-dimensional imaging in real time, will also be soon commercially available. These catheters may provide even greater anatomic visualization of complex ventricular structures.

References

1. Callans DJ, Ren JF, Narula N, Michele J, Marchlinski FE, Dillon SM. Effects of linear, irrigated-tip radiofrequency ablation in porcine healed anterior infarction. *J Cardiovasc Electrophysiol.* 2001;12(9):1037–1042.
2. Ren JF, Callans DJ, Schwartzman D, Michele JJ, Marchlinski FE. Changes in local wall thickness correlate with pathologic lesion size following radiofrequency catheter ablation: an intracardiac echocardiographic imaging study. *Echocardiography.* 2001;18(6):503–507.
3. Khaykin Y, Skanes A, Whaley B, Hill C, Beardsall M, Seabrook C, et al. Real-time integration of 2D intracardiac echocardiography and 3D electroanatomical mapping to guide ventricular tachycardia ablation. *Heart Rhythm.* 2008;5(10):1396–1402.
4. Cano O, Hutchinson M, Lin D, Garcia F, Zado E, Bala R, et al. Electroanatomic substrate and ablation outcome for suspected epicardial ventricular tachycardia in left ventricular nonischemic cardiomyopathy. *J Am Coll Cardiol.* 2009; 54:799–808.
5. Bala R, Garcia FC, Hutchinson MD, Gerstenfeld EP, Dhruvakumar S, Dixit S, et al. Electrocardiographic and electrophysiologic features of ventricular arrhythmias originating from the right/left coronary cusp commissure. *Heart Rhythm.* 2010;7(3):312–322.
6. Hijazi ZM, Shivkumar K, Sahn DJ. Intracardiac echocardiography during interventional and electrophysiological cardiac catheterization. *Circulation.* 2009;119(4):587–596.
7. Stephens DN, O'Donnell M, Thomenius K, Dentinger A, Wildes D, Chen P, et al. Experimental studies with a 9F forward-looking intracardiac imaging and ablation catheter. *J Ultrasound Med.* 2009;28(2):207–215.

Video Descriptions

Video 41.1 The "home view" of the RV inflow and tricuspid valve viewed from the RA (Video A). The proximal RVOT is also seen. The aortic valve is visible but slightly out of plane. Note the presence of an RV defibrillator lead. Color Doppler of the tricuspid valve (Video B) reveals mild regurgitation with 2 jets visible.

Video 41.2 Advancing the ICE catheter from the home view position allows visualization of the RVOT and the pulmonary valve.

Video 41.3 The aortic valve and LVOT are viewed from the RA (Video A). Color Doppler across the aortic valve (Video B) shows largely laminar flow across the outflow tract with only physiologic regurgitation.

Video 41.4 The LV inflow and mitral valve viewed from the RA (Video A). Color Doppler across the mitral valve (Video B) reveals mild regurgitation (arrow).

Video 41.5 Starting from the home view visualizing the tricuspid valve, the catheter is anteflexed keeping the tricuspid valve in view. The catheter is then advanced across the tricuspid valve into the RV. Once in the RV, the anteflexion of the catheter is released.

Video 41.6 The initial image after insertion of the ICE catheter into the right ventricle (RV) shows the inferior RV free wall (bottom left) and apex.

Video 41.7 Long-axis view of the LV with the posteromedial papillary muscle and mitral valve (Video A). Further clockwise rotation of the ICE catheter brings the anterolateral papillary muscle into view (Video B). Note each papillary muscle has 2 distinct heads.

Video 41.8 The aortic valve viewed in short-axis from the RV. All 3 cusps (L = left, R = right, N = noncoronary) are seen (Video A). The left main coronary artery ostium can be visualized as well. Color Doppler across the aortic valve reveals trace regurgitation (arrows, Video B).

Video 41.9 The pulmonary valve and artery in long axis as seen from the right ventricle (Video A). Color Doppler across the pulmonic valve reveals two jets of mild regurgitation (arrows, Video B).

Video 41.10 The aortic valve and ascending aorta as viewed from the right ventricle.

Video 41.11 The ascending aorta is viewed in long-axis (Video A) and obliquely (Video B) from the right ventricle. Focal atheroma at the sinotubular junction is seen in Video A (arrow), and more diffuse ascending aortic atheroma is seen in Video B (arrow).

Video 41.12 The ablation catheter in good contact with the endocardium at the border of an akinetic anteroapical infarct (superior to catheter tip). Note the ablation lesion is demonstrated by ICE as an area of increased echodensity (arrows). Bubbles from the irrigated ablation catheter can also be seen.

Video 41.13 Ablation catheter with the tip on the basal lateral LV endocardium. The ablation lesion is visualized as an area with increased echodensity (arrow). Note the image shown is reversed.

Video 41.14 Long-axis view of the LV with an apical aneurysm (arrows). There is spontaneous echo contrast in the aneurysm ("smoke"). Note the image shown is reversed.

Video 41.15 ICE imaging showing the extent of an inferobasal LV aneurysm with the ablation catheter positioned near the mitral annulus (arrow).

Video 41.16 A linear area of increased echodensity near the epicardial surface on the lateral LV wall (arrows) in a patient with NICM. Note the image shown is reversed.

Video 41.17 Anterolateral papillary muscle geometry creation using CARTOSound. The endocardial borders of each papillary muscle head on the ICE image (left) are traced. The software then incorporates the surfaces into the CARTO map (right). Note the ICE image shown is reversed.

Video 41.18 Short-axis view of the aortic valve (L = left coronary cusp, N = noncoronary cusp) from the RV showing the ablation catheter in the right coronary cusp (arrow, Video A). A reversed image with the catheter (arrow) at the junction of the right (R) and left coronary cusps is shown in Video B.

Video 41.19 Long-axis view of the aortic valve from the RA (Ao, aorta; LV, left ventricle). The ablation catheter can be seen with the tip in the nadir of the left coronary cusp (arrow).

Video 41.20 Maps of the aortic cusps using CARTOSound. The contours of each cusp (L = left coronary cusp, N = noncoronary cusp, R = right coronary cusp) are traced from the ICE image (right). Each traced contour is projected on the map view (left) and integrated into a 3-dimensional geometry. The left main coronary artery ostium was visualized on ICE and tagged on the map (arrow). Note the ICE image shown is reversed.

Video 41.21 Short-axis view of the aortic valve from the right ventricle showing the origin of the left main coronary artery (arrows) from the left coronary cusp. Note the blue color on Doppler, indicating blood flow away from the transducer into the artery.

Video 41.22 Maps of both heads of the anterolateral papillary muscle (arrows) created using CARTOSound. The map view (right) is through the mitral valve, into the LV cavity. The ablation catheter can also be seen on the map and in real time on the ICE image (left). Note the ICE image shown is reversed.

Video 41.23 View of the RV inferior free wall and pericardial effusion visible (Video A). An RV defibrillator lead is seen at the RVA (arrow). The same effusion viewed adjacent to the inferior LV wall (Video B). Note the images shown are reversed.

CHAPTER 42

How to Perform an Epicardial Access

Mauricio I. Scanavacca, MD, PhD; Sissy Lara Melo, MD, PhD;
Carina A. Hardy, MD; Cristiano Pisani, MD; Eduardo Sosa, MD, PhD

Introduction

Subepicardial myocardial fibers may be the source of origin of cardiac arrhythmias in patients with[1,2] or without[3] structural heart diseases, and one of the reasons for unsuccessful RF catheter ablation in patients, in which endocardial ablation was unable to reach such fibers.

Electrophysiologists have been searching subepicardial fibers by two techniques: exploring the coronary sinus, as well as the great cardiac vein and its branches,[4] and using the direct access to the pericardial space through the subxiphoid approach.[5,6] The transvenous access is very useful when the target fibers are related to the mitral annulus or located close to the coronary vascular system. The subxiphoid access has been useful to access beyond those places, exploring extensive areas of the epicardial surface of the heart. **Figure 42.1** shows a combination of endocardial and epicardial electroanatomic map and a scar-related VT that is predominantly subepicardial. In these cases, RF epicardial ablation is very effective to interrupt the macroreentrant circuit and render VT no more inducible.

In this chapter, we will focus on how to perform and to avoid complications when performing the percutaneous subxiphoid access to the pericardial space, and also how to solve the most common related problems.

Before Scheduling the Pericardial Space Access

Before scheduling a patient for an epicardial procedure, there are three important points to consider:

1. Whether epicardial access should be performed in the first procedure, or should be scheduled after an unsuccessful endocardial approach;

2. Whether adequate technical conditions are present to perform the epicardial access procedure safely; and

3. Whether a review of clinical data and image evaluation exams could anticipate problems during the procedure.

In patients with ventricular arrhythmias referred to catheter ablation, clinical characteristics, image exams evaluation, ECG patterns,[7] and results of previous procedures[3] give us the probability of the subepicardial myocardial fibers as the source of origin in a given patient. Patients with structural heart disease and recurrent sustained VT related to nonischemic diseases, such as Chagas disease and dilated cardiomyopathy (excluding bundle

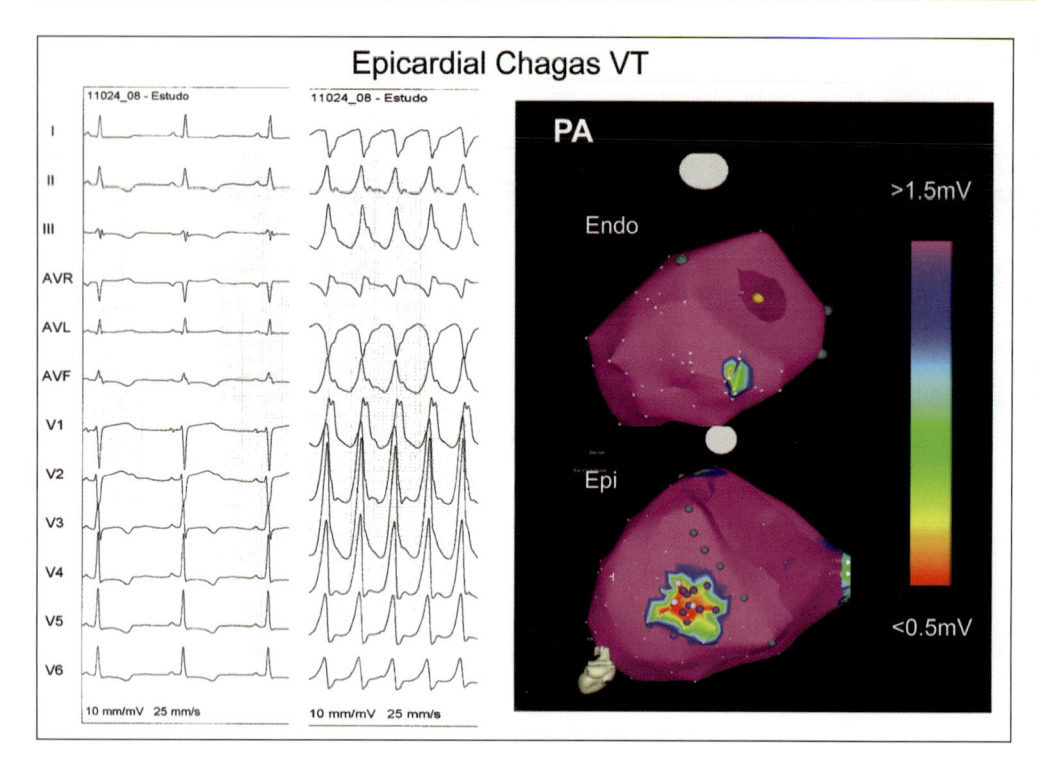

Figure 42.1 A case of a patient with Chagas disease and recurrent sustained VT and preserved LV function. Left panel: 12-lead ECG in sinus rhythm. Middle panel: 12-lead ECG in sustained VT. Right panel: Substrate mapping—endocardial (upper) and epicardial (inferior) electroanatomic maps in sinus rhythm. Note that the scar-related VT is predominantly subepicardial.

branch reentry), usually have multiple morphologies and high probability of any associated epicardial VT.[8] Substrate image evaluations, either by MRI with gadolinium and late enhancement or CT scan in patients with ICDs, are also useful for identifying epicardial substrate related to those arrhythmias. In patients with a high probability of epicardial source of origin, we usually schedule an epicardial mapping in the first procedure. Patients presenting with VT late after myocardial infarction with inferior scar,[9] very wide QRS, pseudo–delta wave pattern, and prolonged deflection time index are also scheduled to the epicardial mapping in the first procedure. Patients with idiopathic VTs also can undergo epicardial mapping when the regular exploration at RVOT, aortic cusps, and CS and its branches[3] were unsuccessful. The VT morphology on the ECG also helps to make this decision. Other patients are usually referred to epicardial mapping after an unsuccessful endocardial approach, mainly when adequate endocardial EP signals were not found in the first procedure.

Despite the subxiphoid epicardial access being a usually safe procedure and the rarity of severe complications, ventricular perforation and pericardial bleeding can happen, and the EP lab must be prepared for this complication. Then, just in case, it is important to have a cell-saver system to infuse the pericardial bleeding safely and a surgical team available.

Pericardial adhesions can make the pericardial access difficult or impossible. Then an echocardiogram or preferentially an MRI is useful to evaluate the status of pericardial membranes when evaluating the arrhythmia's substrate. The knowledge of coronary anatomy is also required before the procedure (angiography, MRI, or CT scans). Based on VTs 12-lead ECG, we can anticipate the plausible area that we will have to approach and estimate the risks for damaging coronary circulation during catheter ablation. During the procedure a new angiography will be performed again to confirm the safety for RF delivery. Liver and colon can be in risk of perforation during subxiphoid epicardial access. Clinical data and abdominal examination are important in order to identify patients with possible liver enlargement (heart failure) or colon dilatation (Chagas disease, idiopathic dilatation), and complementary evaluation with abdominal ultrasound, X-ray, or CT scan also may be useful for better investigation.

Preventing Complications

There are 2 main concerns when one decides to access the pericardial space through the subxiphoid approach. The first is how to make the puncture while avoiding injury to intraabdominal organs; the second is how to introduce the needle in such small pericardial space without promoting cardiac damage and pericardial bleeding.

When deciding to perform the subxiphoid puncture, it is important to remember that before reaching the pericardial space, the needle introduced through the subxiphoid approach will cross the upper peritoneal cavity, trespassing an area with potential risk of intraabdominal organ injury. **Figure 42.2** shows a thoracic and abdominal sagittal CT scan view demonstrating the relationships between heart, liver, and transverse colon, the main intraperitoneal organs in risk of perforation when subxiphoid puncture is

Figure 42.2 Thoracic and abdominal CT scan showing the 3 main organs in risk of perforation when we perform the subxiphoid access: liver, stomach, and colon.

performed. The left lobe of the liver has a close relation to diaphragmatic aspect of the ventricles, and it is always in risk during such procedure, mainly when patient has heart failure and liver enlargement. The stomach and transverse colon are usually in a deeper position and are not in risk in normal conditions. When needle is positioned at 45° and puncture is performed laterally to the xiphoid appendix, close to the ribs, it usually will reach safely the cardiac border (**Figure 42.3**). However, there is a considerable risk of liver or even colon perforation if this angle is maintained and puncture is performed below this area. Thus, diminishing the angle of puncture to 30° or 15° is safer to avoid intraperitoneal structures (**Figure 42.4**). The problem is that the needle tip may hit the ribs if it is too close to the ribs' border. To avoid this situation, it is important to compress the epigastric area with the left hand in order to create a space before performing needle penetration (**Figure 42.5**). In general, performing the puncture 1 to 2 cm from the rib border, with a small angle, makes possible a comfortable needle introduction, with low risk of intraabdominal injury. However, patients with significant colon dilatation present a considerable risk of perforation independently of the needle position. This is a common situation in South America, where Chagas disease is frequent and megacolon may be present in 10% of the patients referred for VT ablation. **Figure 42.6A** shows an example in which we were not able to perform a safe subxiphoid puncture because of a megacolon. For safety, we asked for a surgeon to introduce 2 sheaths in the pericardial space through a small subxiphoid window before we initiated the procedure.

Stomach air insufflations are frequently observed in patients undergoing VT ablation under anesthesia (**Figure 42.6B**). In general, some air reaches the esophagus and the stomach during anesthesia induction, and a substantial stomach insufflation is observed, increasing the risk of stomach perforation. Aspirating air through an oral

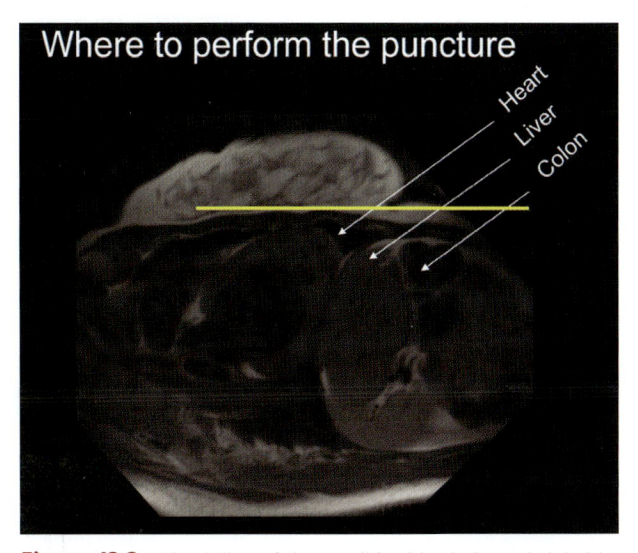

Figure 42.3 Simulation of the possible risks during subxiphoid needle introduction. When needle is positioned at 45° and puncture is performed close to the ribs, it usually will reach the cardiac border. However, there is a considerable risk for liver or even colon perforation if this angle is maintained and puncture is performed lower.

gastric tube easily solves this situation. Although there are potential risks of intraperitoneal organ perforation during subxiphoid approach, we have not observed any of those complications in our series. However, unreported cases of stomach and colon perforation during these procedures have been observed, in general, during initial learning curve.

How to Access the Pericardial Space Safely

What worries most electrophysiologists attempting to access the pericardial space is that this space is almost virtual, and there is a considerable risk of ventricular perforation. This is why we have been using the Tuhoy

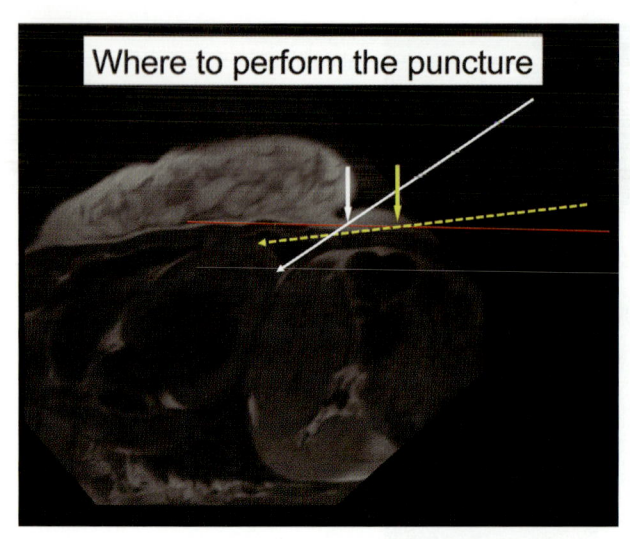

Figure 42.4 Different angles for the needle to reach the pericardial space through the subxiphoid approach. Puncture close to the ribs' border will reach the inferior wall. To reach the anterior wall the puncture is performed a little bellow, but with shallow angle.

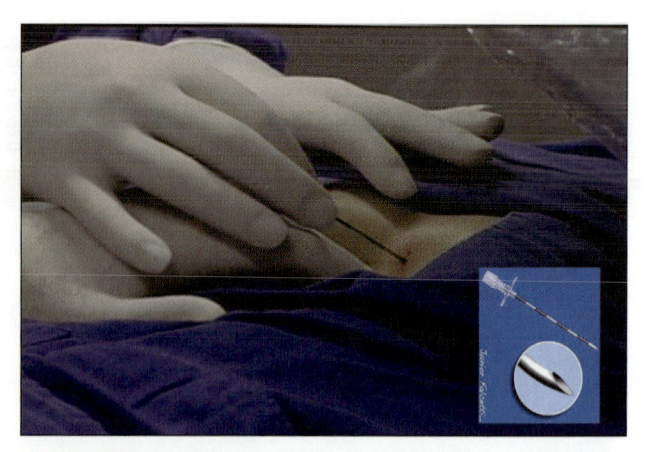

Figure 42.5 Pressing gently the epigastric area allows that a good space under the rib border be found to perform the subxiphoid puncture.

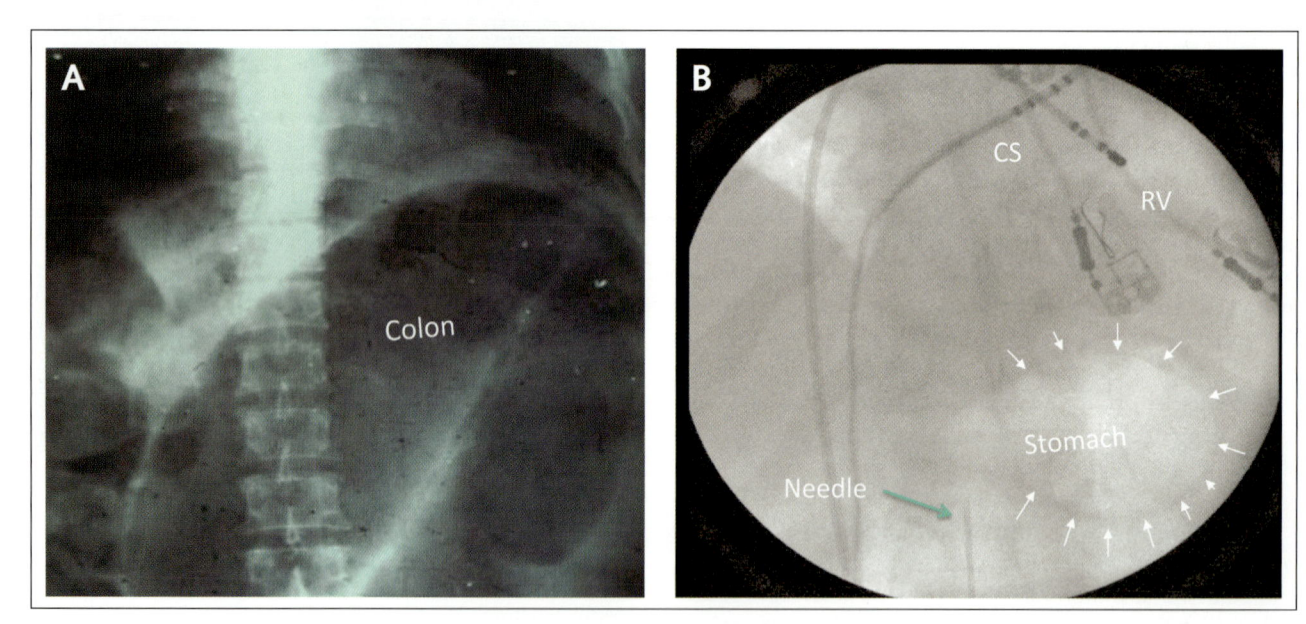

Figure 42.6 **A.** Abdominal X-ray shows a Chagas megacolon. **B.** Fluoroscopic view revealed a stomach dilatation by air swallowed during the anesthesia. In such cases there is a considerable risk of colon or stomach perforation during subxiphoid puncture. In the first case (A), it is recommended to perform a surgical pericardial window. In the second (B), a gastric tube easily empties the stomach.

needle that was developed by the anesthesiologists to access the epidural space, also a virtual space. When we access the pericardial space through the subxiphoid approach, the needle tip will be directed toward the RV in most cases. RV has a thin wall compared to the left ventricle and is relatively easy to perforate. An easy way to understand the technique is simulating it with a hand wearing 2 gloves, in which the hand is the heart and the 2 gloves are the visceral and parietal pericardial membranes (**Figure 42.7**). If we want to introduce a needle between the 2 gloves (**Figure 42.7A**), what should we do to avoid hurting ourselves? If we introduce the needle straight and fast, probably the needle tip will reach the hand (**Figure 42.7B**). But if the needle is introduced slowly, and tangentially to the border of the hand, it can be introduced without any damage (**Figure 42.7C and D**).

Depending on the needle's entry position in the pericardial space, the mapping catheter will be directed to 2 different ventricular walls: the anterior or posterior (**Figure 42.8**). The anterior access allows the catheter to be moved easily over the RV anterior wall, toward the LAA. The posterior access allows the catheter to reach easily the

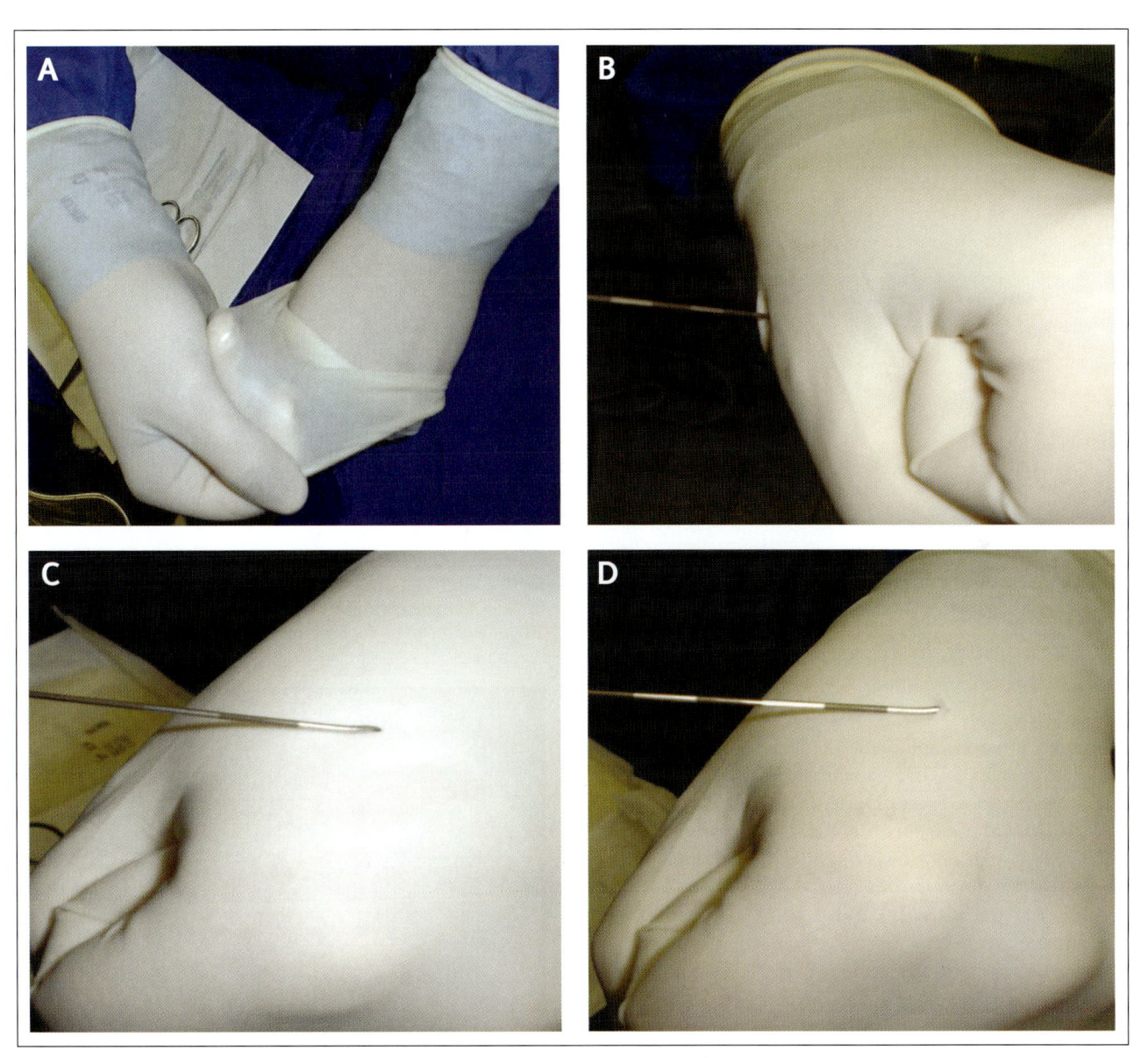

Figure 42.7 Simulation model for accessing a virtual space between 2 membranes. **A.** The hand simulates the heart, and 2 gloves simulate the pericardial membranes. **B.** Introducing the needle tip perpendicular to the cardiac border increases the risk for perforation. **C.** and **D.** Advancing the needle tangentially to the cardiac border decreases the perforation risk.

posterior LA to explore the oblique sinus. The anterior access is obtained when the needle tip is directed tangentially to the right ventricle wall with the opening side in upward position. To obtain the posterior access, we must introduce the needle tip towards the inferior and apical aspect of the ventricles with the opening side twisted inferiorly. It helps to direct the guide wire, the sheath, and the catheter to the ventricle's inferior wall.

Despite such maneuvers, an unexpected RV perforation may occur in approximately 10% of the cases. Once this accident is recognized, the needle must be moved back slowly and the guide wire repositioned in the pericardial space. It often results in a small pericardial bleed that, in general, does not require interruption of the procedure. The problem occurs when the perforation is not recognized and the electrophysiologist goes on introducing the sheath in the right ventricle, as shown in **Figure 42.9**. The contrast in the RA confirms the wrong position of the sheath. The most important maneuver to avoid this complication is to check the guide wire position before introducing the sheath. To be sure that the guide wire is in the pericardial space, it is essential to see its position on the left border of the cardiac silhouette, better visualized in LAO fluoroscopic view (**Figure 42.10**).

Performing the Subxiphoid Epicardial Access Step by Step

▶ **Videos 42.1** and **42.12** present the main steps we have used to perform an epicardial access. These videos also

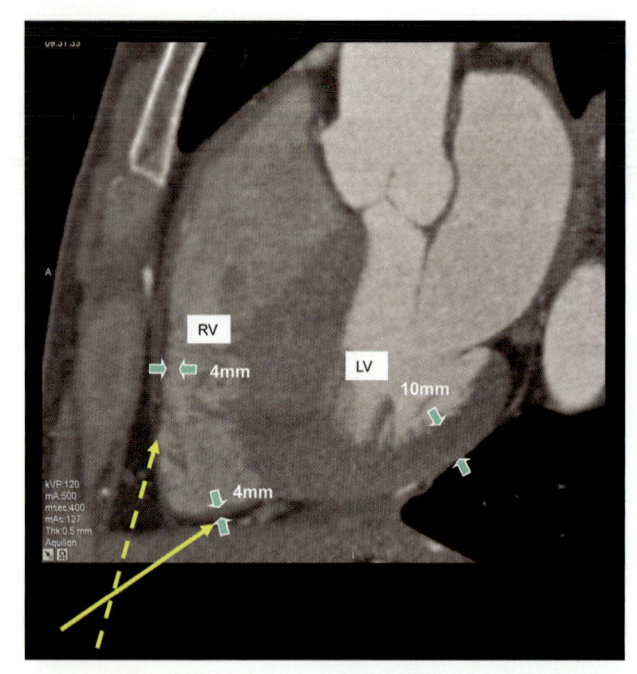

Figure 42.8 Thorax CT scan showing 2 different ways to access the pericardial space. Depending on the needle direction, anterior or posterior, the needle will puncture the anterior or posterior pericardial face of the ventricles.

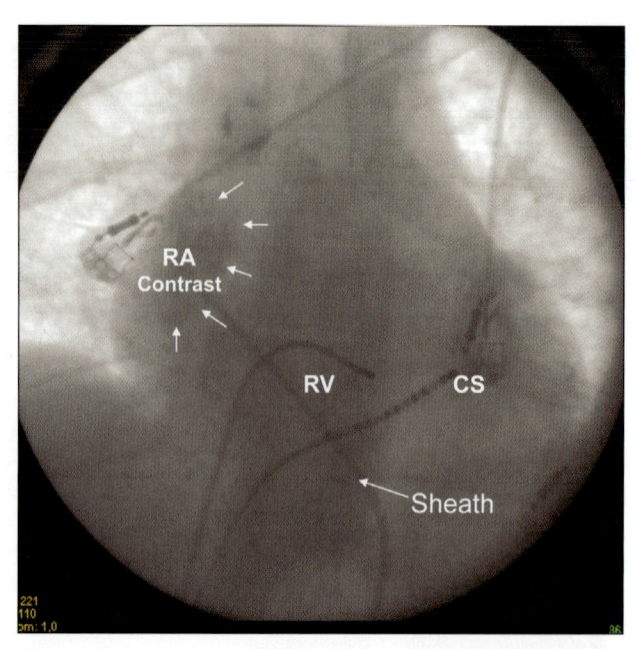

Figure 42.9 Puncture accident during subxiphoid approach. The catheter introducer (sheath) transfixed the RV. Its tip is in the right atrium confirmed by contrast injection on fluoroscopy.

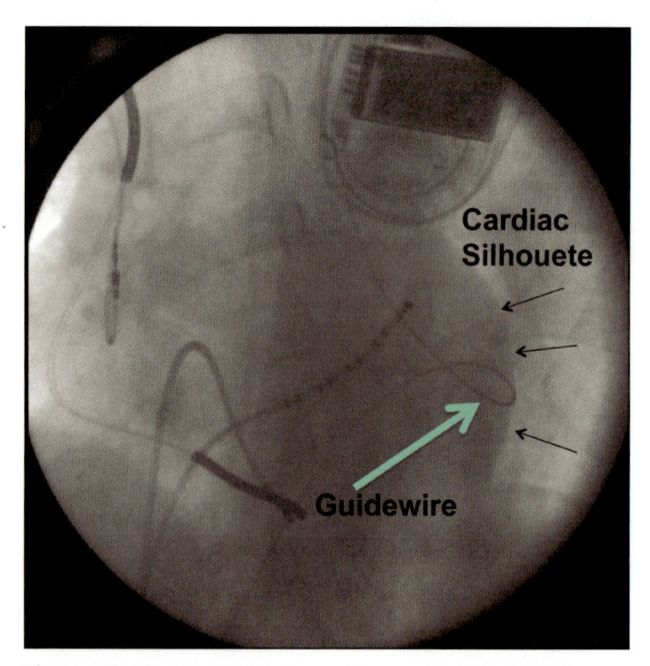

Figure 42.10 The guide wire position on the lateral border of the cardiac silhouette confirms the right position into the pericardial space (LAO view).

represent a noncomplicated, combined epicardial and endocardial mapping in a patient with recurrent sustained VT secondary to Chagas disease.

In our institution, this procedure is performed under anesthesia. We usually use 2 multipolar catheters as landmarks for the puncture, 1 in the CS (▶ Video 42.1) and the other at the RVA (▶ Video 42.2). We prepare the pericardial space access, exploring manually the epigastric area, looking for a space to introduce the Tuhoy needle and additionally to exclude liver enlargement (▶ Video 42.3) and colon and gastric dilatations, confirmed by fluoroscopy. Local anesthesia with lidocaine is performed (▶ Video 42.4) with a small needle to confirm if there is a convenient space to introduce the long needle under and between the xiphoid process and left ribs' border. We also perform a small incision on the skin (▶ Video 42.5), in order to reduce the resistance when introducing the Tuhoy needle. It seems that we can better feel when the needle tip is crossing the pericardial membranes without the skin resistance. The Tuhoy needle is positioned toward the anterior or posterior border of the ventricles, depending on the operator's usual practice; the needle is progressively and slowly advanced until the cardiac beats can be felt at the needle. Positioning the opening side of the needle anteriorly, it will direct the guide wire to the anterior wall; otherwise, twisting it posteriorly, the guide wire will be directed to inferior wall when the needle tip reaches the pericardial space. A funny sensation is felt when the needle tip crosses the pericardial space (▶ Video 42.6). To confirm its position in the pericardial space, we used to inject some contrast media. However, in some conditions too much contrast is injected, so that it becomes difficult to visualize the needle tip and guide wire. Thus, we have used just the guide wire to confirm intrapericardial position of the needle. The more important maneuver to confirm it is positioning the fluoro in LAO view and confirming the guide wire position at the left border of the cardiac silhouette (▶ Video 42.7). After introducing a 7-Fr or 8-Fr regular sheath, and before removing the guide wire, we check for pericardial bleeding aspirating the sheath

(▶ Video 42.8) and also confirm how far the sheath has been introduced in the pericardial space by infusing some contrast (▶ Video 42.9). Longer and deflectable sheaths are also used to stabilize the catheter during RF delivery. The guide wire is then removed, and the mapping and ablating catheter introduced in the pericardial space (▶ Video 42.10), enabling the free movement of the catheter through several positions on the epicardial space (▶ Video 42.11). After epicardial mapping and ablation, the pericardial space is aspirated again to check for pericardial bleeding, and if none is found, catheter and sheaths are removed (▶ Video 42.12). If there was some small bleeding, we change the catheter for a pigtail catheter and control the draining for next 6 to 24 hours, when the system is finally removed.

How to Manage Pericardial Access Complications

The first question is, what should be done when we do not realize that the guide wire was not in the pericardial space but in the RV? In general, it is not a great problem: the guide wire can be removed and repositioned into the pericardial space with transitory small pericardial bleeding. More problematic is what to do when it was supposed that the guide wire was well positioned, but in fact it was inside the ventricle so that the sheath was also advanced inside the RV? When this has occurred, we have removed the sheath successfully, resulting in a small bleeding, without any clinical consequence. However, before removing the sheath, it is important to have another sheath positioned in the pericardial space to drain the bleeding, thus avoiding cardiac tamponade, and to have a surgical team standing by. **Figure 42.11** shows a case in which the operator was not able to access the pericardial space after many attempts and the patient underwent cardiac surgery. During the surgery, important pericardial adhesions were observed that explained the difficulties to access the pericardial space. This patient had no history of previous cardiac surgery and the echocardiogram performed before ablation did not demonstrate the adhesions.

How to Manage Pericardial Bleeding

Detecting a pericardial bleeding after accessing the pericardial space is always problematic. It is in general a small amount (less than 100 ml) and stops spontaneously in 10 to 30 minutes, allowing the procedure to continue. However, sometimes bleeding persists. In this situation, we have infused the aspirated blood through the femoral vein while waiting for spontaneous bleeding to stop without significant problems. When the bleeding does not stop after 30 minutes and a significant amount of blood has already been

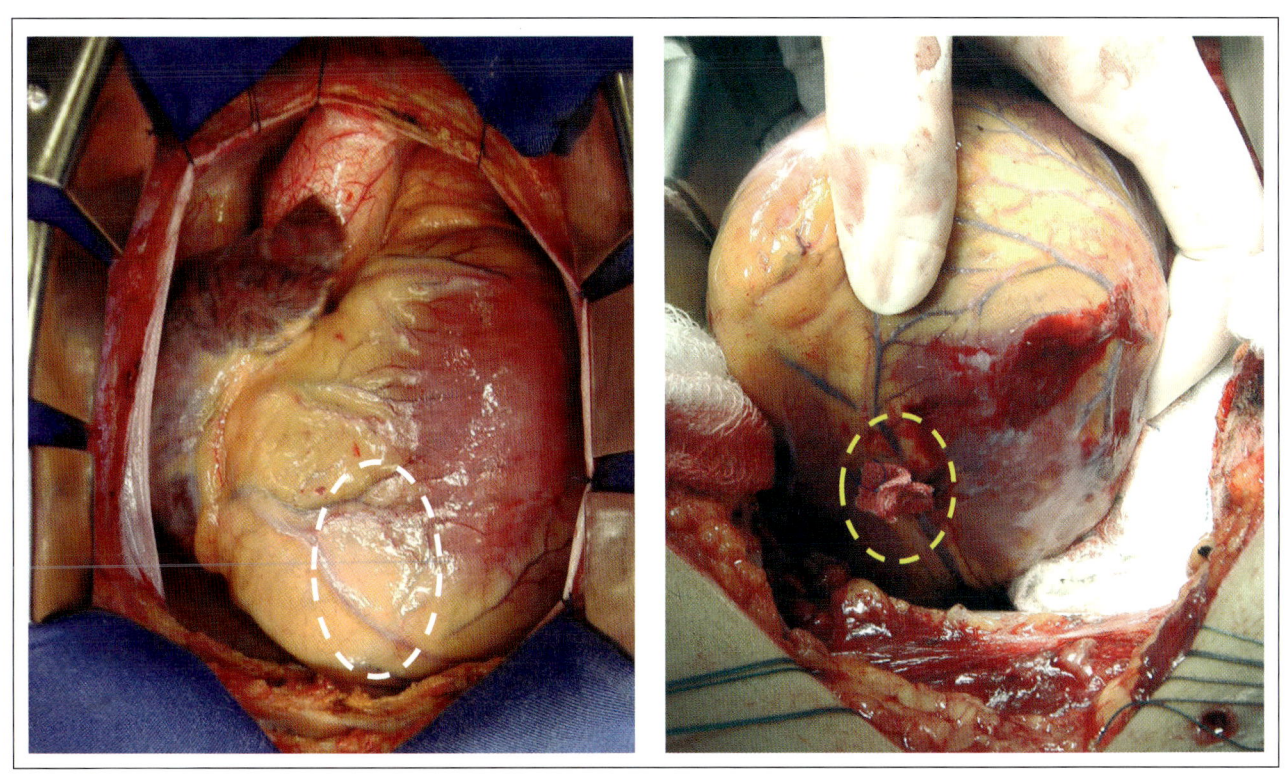

Figure 42.11 Left panel: open-chest surgery aspect, showing coronary arteries and veins crossing the area that is usually accessed by the needle during pericardial puncture. The right panel shows the surgical aspect of a patient who underwent open-chest surgery after continuous pericardial bleeding in consequence of an interventricular vein rupture.

drained (> 300 ml), we use the cell-saver system to reinfuse the drained blood in a safer way. In some cases, a surgical repair is necessary. Surgery is considered when significant bleeding persists after 1 hour of continuous drainage. In a series involving 373 patients, 10% of the cases presented 100 ml or more bleeding volume. Three (0.8%) patients underwent surgical repair. In 1 of these patients, there were 2 perforations in the RV, suggesting that the needle had transfixed the right free wall. In the other 2 patients, surgical exploration recognized that pericardial bleeding resulted from a coronary vein rupture. In the left panel of Figure 42.11, you can see an open-chest surgical aspect, showing the coronary arteries and veins crossing the area that is usually accessed by the needle during pericardial puncture. Figure 42.11 shows the surgical aspect of a patient who underwent open-chest surgery after continuous pericardial bleeding in consequence of an interventricular vein rupture. Thus, although open-chest surgery is rarely necessary during an epicardial ablation, it is essential to have a team prepared as a safety support.

Conclusion

In conclusion, the percutaneous epicardial approach can be performed safely and might improve the results of endocardial ablation in selected patients. Despite being the simplest technique to explore widely the epicardial surface of the heart, the subxiphoid puncture carries some risks of injury to intraperitoneal organs, as well as to ventricular perforation, coronary vessel damage, and consequent pericardial bleeding. Following a standard method, potential complications can be identified and avoided. However, a support system for blood reinfusion and an open-chest surgical team support is always recommended.

References

1. Brugada J, Berruezo A, Cuesta A, Osca J, Chueca E, Fosch X, et al. Nonsurgical transthoracic epicardial radiofrequency ablation: an alternative in incessant ventricular tachycardia. *J Am Coll Cardiol*. 2003;41(11):2036–2043.
2. Soejima K, Stevenson WG, Sapp JL, Selwyn AP, Couper G, Epstein LM. Endocardial and epicardial radiofrequency ablation of ventricular tachycardia associated with dilated cardiomyopathy: the importance of low-voltage scars. *J Am Coll Cardiol*. 2004 May 19;43(10):1834–1842.
3. Schweikert RA, Saliba WI, Tomassoni G, Marrouche NF, Cole CR, Dresing TJ, et al. Percutaneous pericardial instrumentation for endo-epicardial mapping of previously failed ablations. *Circulation*. 2003 Sep 16;108(11):1329–1335.
4. Daniels DV, Lu YY, Morton JB, Santucci PA, Akar JG, Green A, et al. Idiopathic epicardial left ventricular tachycardia originating remote from the sinus of Valsalva: electrophysiological characteristics, catheter ablation, and identification from the 12-lead electrocardiogram. *Circulation*. 2006;113(13):1659–1666.
5. Sosa E, Scanavacca M. Epicardial mapping and ablation techniques to control ventricular tachycardia. *J Cardiovasc Electrophysiol*. 2005;16(4):449–452.
6. Sosa E, Scanavacca M. Images in cardiovascular medicine: percutaneous pericardial access for mapping and ablation of epicardial ventricular tachycardias. *Circulation*. 2007;115(21): e542–e544.
7. Berruezo A, Mont L, Nava S, Chueca E, Bartholomay E, Brugada J. Electrocardiographic recognition of the epicardial origin of ventricular tachycardias. *Circulation*. 2004; 109(15):1842–1847.
8. Sosa E, Scanavacca M, D'Avila A, Bellotti G, Pilleggi F. Radiofrequency catheter ablation of ventricular tachycardia guided by nonsurgical epicardial mapping in chronic Chagasic heart disease. *Pacing Clin Electrophysiol*. 1999;22 (1 Pt 1):128–130.
9. Sosa E, Scanavacca M, d'Avila A, Oliveira F, Ramires JA. Nonsurgical transthoracic epicardial catheter ablation to treat recurrent ventricular tachycardia occurring late after myocardial infarction. *J Am Coll Cardiol*. 2000;35(6):1442–1449.

Video Descriptions

Video 42.1 Landmarks to guide subxiphoid puncture: coronary sinus catheter.

Video 42.2 Landmarks to guide subxiphoid puncture: right ventricle apex catheter.

Video 42.3 Manually exploring the epigastric area.

Video 42.4 Local anesthesia with lidocaine is performed with a small needle, in order to look for a space to introduce the Tuhoy needle and additionally to exclude liver enlargement.

Video 42.5 Small incision on the skin, in order to reduce the resistance when introducing the Tuhoy needle.

Video 42.6 Tuhoy needle on subxiphoid approach is advanced until the needle passes pericardium.

Video 42.7 Guide wire is used to confirm intrapericardial position of the needle by demonstrating (LAO) it at the left border of the cardiac silhouette.

Video 42.8 Sheath introduced over the guide wire followed by aspiration of the content to evaluate if there was any accident on the puncture.

Video 42.9 Small amount of contrast through the sheath to confirm how long is the sheath introduced in the pericardial space.

Video 42.10 Mapping and ablating catheter introduced in the pericardial space.

Video 42.11 Movements of the catheter through several positions on the epicardial space.

Video 42.12 At the end of the procedure, pericardial space is aspirated again using a pigtail catheter to check for pericardial bleeding, and if none is found, the catheter and sheaths are removed.

CHAPTER 43

Transcoronary Ethanol Ablation for Ventricular Tachycardia

Karin K. M. Chia, MBBS; Paul C. Zei, MD, PhD

Introduction

Incessant ventricular tachycardia (VT) has presented a therapeutic challenge over the years. After animal studies demonstrating successful termination of VT by intracoronary injection of phenol or ethanol by Inoue and colleagues,[1] interruption of coronary flow to arrhythmogenic substrates by balloon occlusion and the infusion of antiarrhythmic drugs or obliterative agents like ethanol[2-4] were developed as treatment options for VT uncontrolled by antiarrhythmic or device therapy.

Interest in transcoronary ethanol ablation (TCEA) decreased as endocardial RF catheter ablation matured into a successful treatment option for drug-resistant VT. However, many VT circuits are intramural or epicardial. Intramural circuits are potentially difficult to damage endocardially even with the use of irrigated catheters for increased depth of energy delivery. While epicardial access can be attained by percutaneous pericardial puncture with relative ease by a subxiphoid approach, this approach may be precluded by adhesions from previous cardiac surgery or pericardial fat, preventing adequate energy delivery to the myocardium. In addition, an epicardial approach does not allow access to circuits deep in the septum. For these patients, one option is ablation through chemically induced necrosis of the involved myocardium by the instillation of corrosive agents through the associated vasculature. Hence there has been renewed interest in and use of TCEA.

An understanding of how instillation of ethanol into coronary arteries results in permanent damage to tachycardia substrates through myocardial necrosis and scarring comes largely from animal studies, with limited confirmatory evidence in human pathological specimens.[5] Ethanol results in a coagulative necrosis of the myocardium that can be seen as early as 5 minutes after instillation in canine coronary arteries.[6] Necrotic tissue is eventually replaced by scar late after ablation.[5] Ethanol also has a direct cytotoxic sclerosant effect on arteries and a denaturing effect on blood components, resulting in fixation of blood and development of acute vascular occlusion by intraluminal necrotic debris, even in the absence of intimal injury.[1] This intraluminal occlusion causes an ischemic infarction distally, which contributes further to coagulative necrosis of the subtended myocardium. While one would expect the extent of infarcted tissue to be predicted by the perfusion bed of the targeted artery, this correlation is not perfect. Pathological examination has demonstrated areas of resultant necrosis to be variably focal, confluent, and nonconfluent. Studies in pigs have demonstrated ablated tissues to be smaller than the areas perfused. This may be a result of collateral blood supply at the watershed of the perfusion bed of the selected artery.[7] Reflux of ethanol into nontargeted vascular beds also contributes to the potential imprecision of the created infarct. The concentration of ethanol used can also influence the size of the ablative lesion.[8] The purpose of this review is to detail the practical aspects of performing the procedure of TCEA for VT.

Preprocedural Preparation

As with all invasive procedures, due diligence must be taken in appropriate selection of patients and general preparation for the procedure of TCEA. Here we review the requirements and preprocedural processes that should be undertaken.

Patient Selection

Suitable patients are those with a monomorphic VT or premature ventricular complexes, with likely scar-based substrates. The majority of patients with scar-based VT will have an underlying pathology of CAD. The VT circuit(s) in these patients are most often located subendocardially, given the typical location of coronary arterial watershed areas, and therefore, these substrates are typically amenable to endocardial ablation. Nonischemic pathologies underlying scar-based VT, on the other hand, have no particular predilection for the endocardial portion of the ventricular myocardium, and therefore are often considered for TCEA. One exception is CAD-associated scar involving the septal myocardium, particularly in the basal portion of the septum, which is relatively thick. Nonischemic pathologies considered for TCEA have included idiopathic dilated cardiomyopathy, ARVC, and infiltrative cardiomyopathies.[9]

The most common treatment algorithm that leads to TCEA is as follows:

1. Patients undergo endocardial mapping and attempted ablation.

2. After endocardial ablation fails, a determination is made that the likely substrate location is intramural or epicardial, most commonly based on mapping information obtained during the initial ablation attempt.

3. An epicardial approach to mapping and ablation is attempted if the substrate is thought to be potentially accessible through such an approach.

4. If an epicardial attempt is unsuccessful because the substrate is thought to be intramural rather than epicardial, or if the substrate is thought to be septal and intramural after the initial ablation attempt, TCEA is then considered as a therapeutic strategy.

Additional patient groups in whom TCEA is considered earlier are those in whom epicardial access is difficult, most commonly due to a prior sternotomy and resultant adhesions, and/or patients in whom endocardial access is precluded due to the presence of mechanical aortic and/or mitral valves.

Review of ECG Morphology

ECGs of suitable VTs typically appear to have a septal origin, or if nonseptal, intramural or epicardial. ECG characteristics of a septal origin VT include a left or right bundle branch morphology and possibly a narrow QRS from early engagement of the HPS. The frontal plane axis, as well as the precordial transition, may vary, depending on the site of exit along the septum. The ECG morphology of VT substrates outside of the septum considered for TCEA will often demonstrate a relatively slow intrinsic deflection.[10]

Discontinuation of Antiarrhythmic Drugs

As with all arrhythmias, inducibility and sustainability are necessary for optimal mapping of VTs. This is particularly important in TCEA, as mapping for the involved coronary artery typically relies on termination of sustained VT with test infusions. Hence, as much as can be tolerated, antiarrhythmic drugs should be discontinued for at least 5 half-lives prior to the procedure. If necessary, the patient can be admitted to hospital for this drug washout.

Preprocedural Imaging

Cardiac imaging should be undertaken and/or reviewed if previously performed for several reasons. First, VT circuits are often located within or adjacent to scarred myocardium that manifests as areas of decreased contractility, decreased enhancement, and decreased perfusion on echocardiography, MRI, and nuclear imaging. Hence, all preprocedural imaging should be reviewed carefully to predict the likely target of ablation. Secondly, the risk of complications can be minimized by assessing left ventricular function, identifying the presence of thrombus, and localizing areas of excessively thinned myocardium.

Review of Previous Endocardial and/or Epicardial VT Mapping

Data from all prior endocardial and epicardial ablation attempts should be reviewed carefully. Electroanatomical data should be reviewed to identify low-voltage areas and electrically unexcitable scar. Pace mapping and entrainment mapping from previous studies should be reviewed to identify the likely exit and possible isthmi of the VT circuits.

Intraoperative Requirements

General Anesthesia

While not absolutely necessary, performing the procedure under general anesthesia is advisable in view of the need for recurrent VT inductions and associated potential cardioversions. In addition, the associated infarction and accompanying chest pain induced with ethanol infusion does present analgesic requirements that may be optimally managed with general anesthesia. These considerations must be balanced against the cardiosuppressive effects of general anesthesia and the fact that many VTs may be more difficult to induce in an anesthetized state.

Intraprocedural Fluoroscopy and Mapping Requirements

The EP laboratory should be equipped for electroanatomical mapping. Standard techniques for delineating the VT anatomic substrate include "substrate" mapping to define low-voltage areas and abnormal diastolic potentials corresponding to putative scar, entrainment mapping to delineate the reentrant circuit, and activation mapping to localize an automatic focus. In addition, the fluoroscopy resolution requirements are higher than for a standard EP study as the terminal branches of coronary arteries, and occasionally the coronary venous system, are commonly targeted with 0.014" guide wires and over-the-wire infusion balloon catheters. Hence fluoroscopy and acquisition needs to be performed at a higher frame rate than is used in typical EP procedures. A suggested frame rate would be 15 frames per second (fps) for fluoroscopy and 30 fps for acquisition.

Operators

An electrophysiologist experienced in the mapping and ablation of scar-based VT is required. In addition, an experienced interventional cardiologist facile in the technique of TCEA, most commonly applied to hypertrophic cardiomyopathy septal ablation, needs to be involved.[11]

Vascular Access

Femoral venous access is typically obtained for placement of diagnostic catheters. Catheters required are typically a quadripolar catheter that can be manipulated to the RVA and RVOT for programmed stimulation for induction of VT, and a His catheter for marking the location of the HB and septum, in part to allow for closer monitoring of AV conduction. Femoral arterial access is necessary both for arterial blood pressure monitoring and for placement of the coronary angiography catheters (6- to 7-Fr) through which TCEA is performed.

Procedure

The initial mapping depends on whether the VT is stable and tolerated. Nonetheless, voltage mapping in sinus rhythm is typically undertaken first to delineate the likely scar substrate for the VT, if not previously performed. This will usually have been undertaken during a prior endocardial and epicardial attempt and can be used to guide higher-resolution mapping in the area of interest during the TCEA procedure. If the VT is hemodynamically stable and sustained, termination mapping and more classical mapping methods can be employed for localization of the target vessel. VT originating from an automatic focus may be activation-mapped as well.

VT Induction

VT induction should be attempted with programmed electrical stimulation from multiple ventricular sites, at different pacing cycle lengths, with multiple extrastimuli. The ease of inducibility is also important for determining the endpoint of the procedure on postablation testing.

IV Heparin

Similar to the requirement for percutaneous coronary intervention, intravenous heparin at a dose of 60 to 100 IU/kg should be administered once the coronary arteries are cannulated. The ACT should be maintained at > 250 seconds.[12]

Selective Coronary Angiography

Using in part the VT morphology to predict the location of scar and VT substrate, the relevant coronary artery should be selected using an 0.014" angioplasty guide wire. An over-the-wire balloon catheter that has been sized to be larger than the angiographic diameter of the target vessel to allow occlusion of its ostium when deployed is passed over the wire using standard percutaneous techniques.[13]

Contrast Sonography

To confirm that the target myocardium is supplied by the suspected vessel, echocardiography may be performed and sonographic contrast agent injected through the over-the-wire infusion catheter to confirm the territory supplied by the target vessel.

Mapping

After a candidate target vessel is selected, the VT still needs to be mapped to the corresponding coronary vessel before any ethanol is instilled to perform the ablation. More commonly, mapping by termination of the tachycardia is undertaken; however, there are ways to undertake more classical EP mapping through the target vessel.

Mapping by Termination

After having intubated the suspect vessel, the VT is reinduced. The balloon of the infusion catheter is fully inflated to occlude the ostium of the artery and prevent retrograde flow of infusate. Two to 3 ml of ice-cold sterile saline is then injected through the central lumen. If the VT terminates (**Figure 43.1**) with the injection and without evidence of potential associated complications such as PR prolongation or AV block, that artery is suitable for ethanol injection. Termination may also be assessed with injection of contrast media[14] or lidocaine in place of saline.[15] These methods result in transient termination of blood flow to the potential target tissue, which should result in transient conduction block and termination of arrhythmia as a result. The arrhythmia may or may not spontaneously reinitiate. If the clinical VT is not inducible during EP study, or if it is unstable, precise localization of the ideal target coronary vessel will be difficult. In fact, strong consideration should be made whether or not to proceed further with ablation, as targeting the incorrect vessel will not only fail to terminate the clinical VT, but given the relatively large area of myocardial damage induced, a significant unwanted myocardial infarct may result.

Classical Mapping

Mapping by termination to select the appropriate arterial branch for ethanol injection is limited by the inability to record EGMs from the target artery, hence precluding classical mapping techniques to confirm that the arterial branch subtends the critical portion of the VT circuit. In order to circumvent this issue, one can record and pace from a multielectrode catheter or electrically active guide wire placed within the vessel, or by placing a conventional endocardial mapping catheter as closely adjacent to the target vessel either endocardially or epicardially.

Utilizing a Multielectrode Catheter

A small-caliber multielectrode mapping catheter such as a Pathfinder (Cardima, CA), which unfortunately is not in production at the time of publication, can be passed down the lumen of a coronary artery toward its terminal branches (**Figure 43.2**). Utilizing the array of recording electrodes on such a catheter, one can map for late potentials during sinus rhythm, and pace mapping can be performed to identify the branches that may subtend the exit of the VT circuit. During VT, diastolic potentials can be mapped, and entrainment mapping can also be performed. Compared to utilizing a 0.014" guide wire as detailed below, a multielectrode mapping catheter is limited to passage within the main coronary arteries or their initial branches. Nonetheless, this may allow gross localization to part of the coronary vasculature such as the proximal versus distal septal perforators when the catheter is placed within the left anterior descending artery. Placement of a mapping catheter within a coronary vessel may increase the risk of complications, including coronary arterial dissection, spasm, or thrombus.

Intracoronary Guide Wire Mapping

An 0.014" angioplasty guide wire may be advanced into branches of a coronary artery and then connected to a channel of a conventional electrophysiology amplifier and monitoring system to record unipolar signals against an

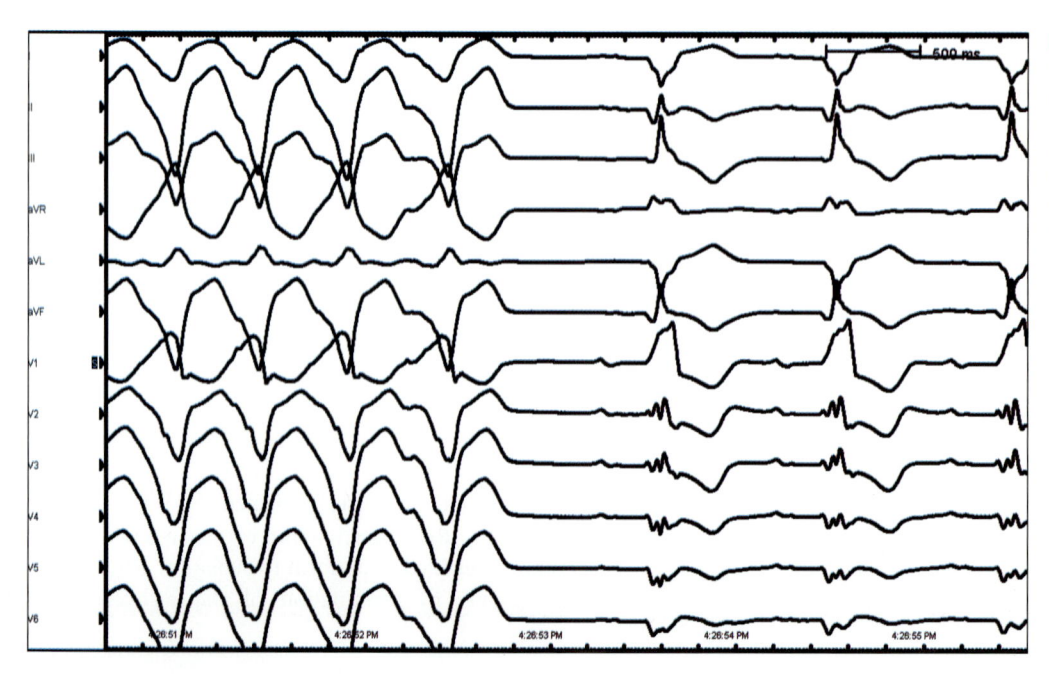

Figure 43.1 Mapping by termination of VT with instillation of ice-cold saline through an infusion catheter in the distal LAD after inflation of the balloon to occlude the vessel proximally.

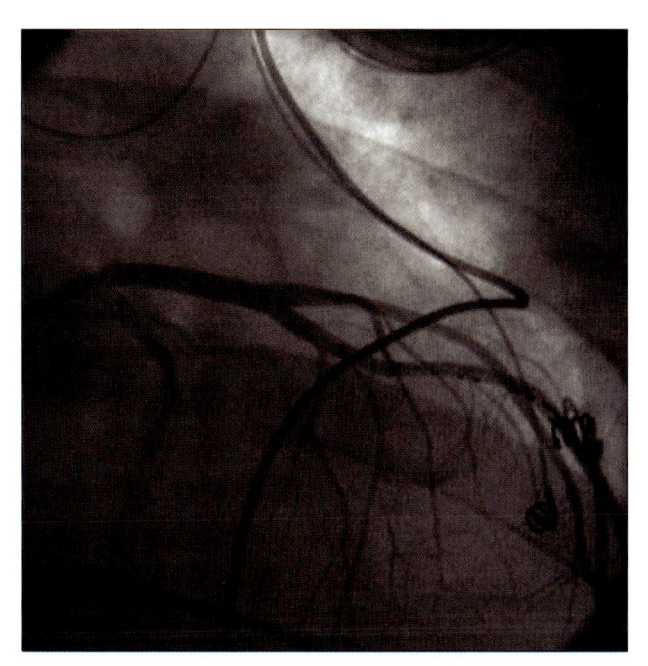

Figure 43.2 Multipolar Cardima catheter within the LAD allowing for activation and pace mapping to localize VT circuit in relation to different septal arterial branches.[16] (Reproduced with permission from HMP Communications, LLC.)

indifferent electrode within the IVC. In order to insulate the proximal portion of the wire, an uninflated angioplasty balloon can be advanced over the wire to expose only the distal tip. The insulated wire can then be advanced to different branches and be used functionally like a mapping catheter. During tachycardia, it can be used to locate mid-diastolic or presystolic potentials for activation mapping. Pacing can be performed for entrainment mapping during tachycardia and pace mapping during sinus rhythm. In this way, conventional EP mapping methods can be used to confirm the target coronary artery for ablation.[16] This method of mapping in the circumflex artery has also been used to guide RF ablation in the adjacent coronary venous system.

Conventional Mapping / Catheter-Based Mapping

Using fluoroscopic imaging, a standard steerable EP mapping catheter may be placed as close as possible to the target vessel either endocardially or epicardially. This approximates the electrical signal that would be observed in the arrhythmic substrate of interest. The significant distance separating the mapping catheter and the deep intramural substrate may introduce error that must be taken into consideration.

Ablation

After the appropriate target vessel has been identified, the over-the-wire infusion catheter is deployed as distally as possible within the selected coronary arterial branch (**Figure 43.3**). The balloon is then fully inflated. A small volume of contrast is infused to ensure that there is no backwash into more proximal coronary vessels. Once the contrast has diffused, which may require deflation and reinflation of the balloon, the corrosive agent is injected. Phenol has previously been used. Currently, as with ablation for hypertrophic cardiomyopathy, absolute ethanol (96%) is infused as a volume of 1 ml.[9] The balloon is left inflated for 5 to 10 minutes, after which contrast is injected to assess the patency of the target vessel. As a precaution, 10 ml of saline can be infused through the infusion catheter to washout the ethanol before deflating the balloon to prevent backflow of the ethanol. In addition, the saline infusion promotes tissue penetration of the ethanol.[16] If contrast injection demonstrates persistent perfusion in the target vessel, additional ethanol is infused after balloon inflation for another 10 minutes, repeating up to 5 ml of ethanol per artery.[9]

As is the case for endocardial ablations, the endpoint of a successful ablation is termination of the VT during chemical ablation and failure of reinducibility of the VT. Theoretically, because the final region of scar formation may not completely match the initial area of tissue injury and necrosis, the targeted VT substrate may or may not be adequately damaged after the procedure has been completed.

Complications and Safety

In addition to the vascular and infectious complications that may accompany all EP procedures, there are additional complications that are particular to TCEA that should be considered.

Coronary Artery Dissection, Perforation, and Thrombus Formation

The use of angioplasty guide wires in percutaneous coronary interventions comes with a risk of coronary perforation. This risk has been reported at 0.4% in the context of angioplasty in complex CAD.[17] This risk in TCEA is likely to be similar or lower than this. This procedure should be performed by an experienced coronary interventionalist to minimize these risks. The use of mapping catheters within the coronary vasculature may increase the risk of intracoronary complications. Due to the thrombogenic nature of guide wires, plus the possibility of endothelial disruption by guide wire passage or balloon inflation, occlusive or nonocclusive intracoronary thrombus may form. This risk is managed with intraprocedural therapeutic anticoagulation.

AV Block

A recognized complication of the procedure is the development of permanent AV block, even after prior iced

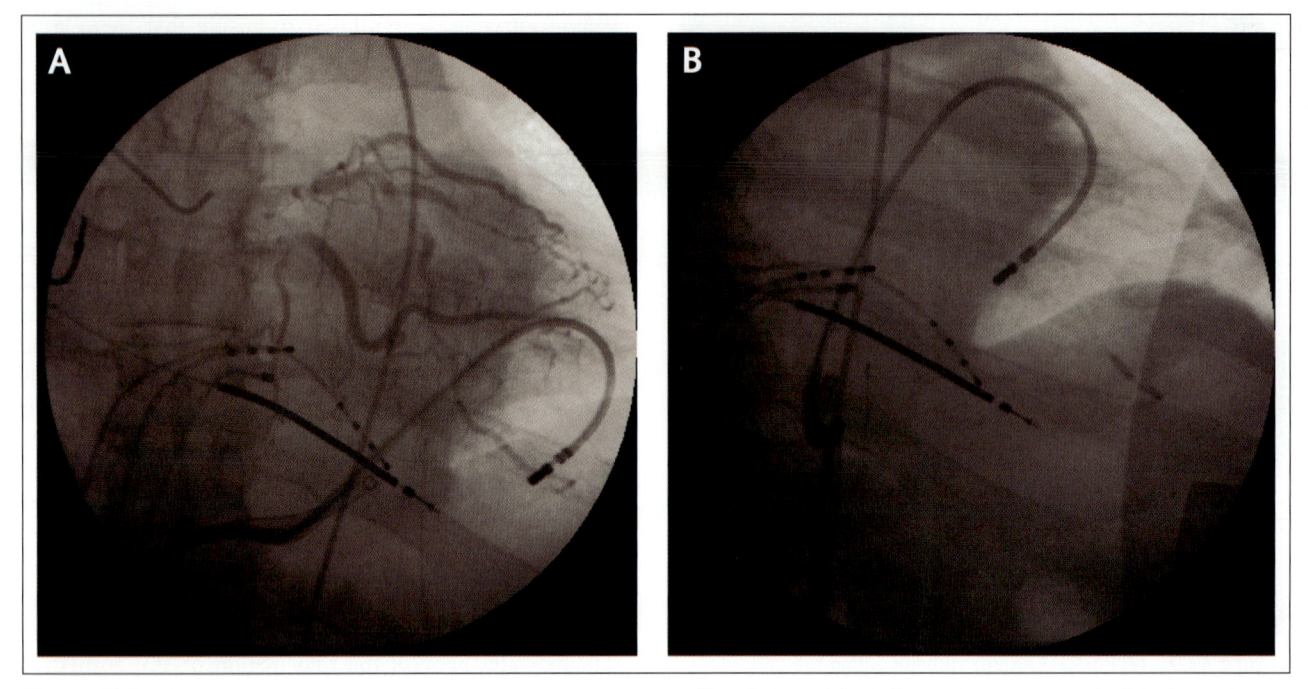

Figure 43.3 A. Coronary angiogram of the LCA in a near-AP projection. **B.** Inflation of the balloon of an over-the-wire infusion catheter with injection of contrast demonstrating no retrograde efflux of contrast into proximal non-VT–related coronary vessels prior to injection of ethanol.

saline test injections. Depending on the arterial supply to the AV node, AV block has been reported with injection to branches of the RCA and the left circumflex artery and has also been demonstrated transiently or permanently with injection into septal perforators of the left anterior descending artery.[9,14] Ensuring that ethanol does not efflux into nontarget vessels during the ablation can help minimize this risk.

Significant Myocardial Infarction and Decompensated Heart Failure

The infarction created by ethanol injection has the potential for causing sufficient myocardial damage leading to impairment of ventricular function and worsening of heart failure symptoms. In addition, ablation of areas containing Purkinje fibers can result in conduction system disturbance and mechanical dyssynchrony. Hence, TCEA has the risk of causing decompensated heart failure. To minimize the risk, the smallest arterial branch where repeated cold saline injection results in VT termination should be selected. Care should be given to ensure adequate placement and inflation of the balloon to ensure proximal occlusion of the branch prior to ethanol injection. In order to track the extent of myocardial injury, serial determination of cardiac markers of injury or echocardiography may be considered postprocedurally.

Myocardial Dissection and Rupture

The injection of ethnanol into the target vessel is aimed at producing coagulative necrosis in the arrhythmogenic focus, essentially creating a small myocardial infarction. Ethanol injection may, however, produce an uncontrolled infarction, which may result in myocardial dissection, leading to tamponade with free wall rupture or VSD with septal rupture. This complication may be delayed[18] necessitating close postprocedural hemodynamic monitoring and a low index of suspicion for this catastrophic complication.

The reported mortality during follow-up of patients has been reported as high as 33% in some small case series.[9] However, this patient population tends to be critically ill, with preceding refractory VT likely either to directly contribute to hemodynamic deterioration or to serve as a marker of the underlying degree of illness.

Efficacy

Due to the rare indication for the procedure, the efficacy for TCEA can only be drawn from the limited number of small case series that have been published. The initial series published by Brugada and colleagues in 1989 detailed the variable long-term follow-up of 3 patients. After repeat procedures, one patient was free of VT after 9 months, another had no recurrences after 6 months, and a third was free of VT after 2 months.[4] A later case series of 10 patients who underwent TCEA by Kay and colleagues demonstrated acute success defined as noninducibility at follow-up electrophysiology study at 5 to 7 days in 9 out of 10 patients.[14] Longer-term follow-up of a mean of 372 ± 210 days demonstrated 5 out of the 10 patients to be free of VT without antiarrhythmic drugs. The most recent series published by Sacher et al. followed 9 patients for a mean of 29 ± 23 months. Four patients remained free of all VT, while 1 had a dramatic decrease in episodes. One cause of recurrences that may warrant repeat selective angiography is the development of collateral blood supply after occlusion of the target coronary vessel.[4]

Conclusions

Transcoronary ethanol ablation is a therapeutic option that, though rarely used, has a moderate degree of efficacy. It is a complex procedure, requiring the appropriate personnel and preparation, with potential significant complications. While not to be considered as a first-line option, it may be a life-saving consideration for patients with drug-refractory VT with septal and/or deep intramural circuits that are resistant to endocardial and/or epicardial ablation.

References

1. Inoue H, Waller B, Zipes DP. Intracoronary ethyl alcohol or phenol injection ablates aconitine-induced ventricular tachycardia in dogs. *J Am Coll Cardiol.* 1987;10:1342–1349.
2. Brugada P, de Swart H, Smeets JL, Bär FW, Wellens HJ. Termination of tachycardias by interrupting blood flow to the arrhythmogenic area. *Am J Cardiol.* 1988;62:387–392.
3. Friedman PL, Selwyn AP, Edelman E, Wang PJ. Effect of selective intracoronary antiarrhythmic drug administration in sustained ventricular tachycardia. *Am J Cardiol.* 1989;64:475–480.
4. Brugada P, de Swart H, Smeets J, Wellens H. Transcoronary chemical ablation of ventricular tachycardia. *Circulation.* 1989;79:475–482.
5. Baggish AL, Smith RN, Palacios I, Vlahakes GJ, Yoerger DM, Picard MH, Lowry PA, Jang IK, Fifer MA. Pathological effects of alcohol septal ablation for hypertrophic obstructive cardiomyopathy. *Heart.* 2006;92:1773–1778.
6. Slezak J, Tribulova N, Gabauer I, Styk J, Slezak, J Jr, Danelisen I, Singal PK. Ethanol ablation of myocardial tissue: early histochemical and ultrastructural changes. *Kuwait Med J.* 2004;36(4):256–263.
7. Haines DE, Verow AF, Sinusas AJ, Whayne JG, DiMarco JP. Intracoronary ethanol ablation in swine: characterization of myocardial injury in target and remote vascular beds. *J Cardiovasc Electrophysiol.* 1994;5:41–49.
8. Haines DE, Whayne J, DiMarco JP. Intracoronary ethanol ablation in swine: effects of ethanol concentration on lesion formation and response to programmed ventricular stimulation. *J Cardiovasc Electrophysiol.* 1994;5:422–431.
9. Sacher F, Sobieszczyk P, Tedrow U, et al. Transcoronary ethanol ventricular tachycardia ablation in the modern electrophysiology era. *Heart Rhythm.* 2008;5:62–68.
10. Daniels DV, Lu Y-Y, Morton JB, et al. Idiopathic epicardial left ventricular tachycardia originating remote from the sinus of Valsalva: electrophysiological characteristics, catheter ablation, and identification from the 12-lead electrocardiogram. *Circulation.* 2006;113:1659–1666.
11. Aliot EM, Stevenson WG, Almendral-Garrote JM, et al. EHRA/HRS expert consensus on catheter ablation of ventricular arrhythmias: developed in a partnership with the European Heart Rhythm Association (EHRA), a Registered Branch of the European Society of Cardiology (ESC), and the Heart Rhythm Society (HRS); in collaboration with the American College of Cardiology (ACC) and the American Heart Association (AHA). *Heart Rhythm.* 2009;6:886–933.
12. Narins CR, Hillegass WB, Jr, Nelson CL, et al. Relation between activated clotting time during angioplasty and abrupt closure. *Circulation.* 1996;93:667–671.
13. Baim D, ed. *Grossman's Cardiac Catheterization, Intervention and Angiography* (7th ed.). Baltimore, MD: Lippincott Williams & Wilkins, 2005.
14. Kay GN, Epstein AE, Bubien RS, Anderson PG, Dailey SM, Plumb VJ. Intracoronary ethanol ablation for the treatment of recurrent sustained ventricular tachycardia. *J Am Coll Cardiol.* 1992;19:159–168.
15. Hartung WM, Lesh M, Hidden-Lucet F, et al. Transcatheter subendocardial infusion of ethanol (abstract). *Circulation.* 1994;90:I–487.
16. Segal O, Wong T, Chow A, et al. Intra-coronary guide wire mapping–A novel technique to guide ablation of human ventricular tachycardia. *J Interv Card Electrophysiol.* 2007;18:143–154.
17. Gunning MG Williams IL, Jewitt DE, Shah AM, Wainwright RJ, Thomas MR. Coronary artery perforation during percutaneous intervention: incidence and outcome. *Heart.* 2002;88:495–498.
18. Verna E, Repetto S, Saveri C, Forgione N, Merchant S, Binaghi G. Myocardial dissection following successful chemical ablation of ventricular tachycardia. *Eur Heart J.* 1992;13:844–846.

CHAPTER 44

How to Perform Epicardial Ablation in Postcardiac Surgery Patients

Sheldon M. Singh, MD; James O. Coffey, MD; Andre d'Avila, MD, PhD

Introduction

Pericardial access with subsequent epicardial mapping and ablation of VT is an important tool in the armamentarium of invasive electrophysiologists. Sosa and colleagues first reported the percutaneous method of accessing the pericardial space to perform epicardial ventricular mapping and ablation in 1996.[1] This approach, described in detail in a previous chapter, relies on the insertion of a needle into a "virtual space"—that is, the space between the parietal and visceral pericardium. Unfortunately, adhesions related to prior cardiac surgery or pericarditis may obliterate this space, thereby complicating pericardial access and mapping after open-heart surgery. The magnitude of this problem, that is, the need for epicardial access in patients with prior cardiac surgery, is significant. Approximately 30% of patients with VT related to coronary artery disease have had prior coronary artery bypass surgery,[2] and some patients with NICM have undergone prior valve replacement. Thus, electrophysiologists at high-volume centers should be expected to encounter this problem frequently. In this chapter, we will describe our approach to obtaining epicardial access and mapping/ablation in patients who have undergone cardiac surgery. In this situation, 3 options exist for epicardial mapping and ablation: (1) limited epicardial mapping via the coronary venous system, (2) percutaneous access, and (3) surgical epicardial access.

Limited Epicardial Mapping from the Coronary Venous System

In select patients who have undergone prior cardiac surgery, mapping the coronary venous system may be beneficial given the epicardial nature of this structure. For example, Obel[3] reported on the utility of this approach for the ablation of idiopathic outflow tract VTs, whereas Doppalapudi reported on the utility of this approach for the ablation of idiopathic VTs originating from the crux of the heart.[4] While potentially valuable, this approach has significant limitations including partial access to the left ventricle based on individual variation in the CS anatomy. Moreover, even when a target is located, potential complications of ablation such as venous stenosis, rupture, thrombosis, or collateral injury to an adjacent coronary artery may limit the use of this approach. Reduction of RF power applications (to 20–25 W) during ablation may improve the safety of ablation with this approach. While this approach does allow one to undertake limited epicardial mapping when all else fails, in many patients, the region of interest is not accessible with coronary venous system mapping, particularly in scar-related VT. In these circumstances, access to the pericardial space is necessary.

Percutaneous Access with Limited Epicardial Mapping

Pericardial adhesions frequently develop after cardiac surgery and limit entrance to and mapping within the pericardial space. In general, the anterior aspect of the pericardium is opened during cardiac surgery. As such, dense adhesions tend to form particularly in this anterior region. Thus, the key to obtaining pericardial access in these patients is to select an inferior approach angle with the needle in order to enter adjacent to the inferior wall of the heart[5]—a region that typically has fewer adhesions. Furthermore, it is our experience that fewer adhesions tend to form along the AV groove as compared to the more apical portion of the pericardial space. Thus, one should make sure the inferior puncture is guided toward the base of the heart, parallel and close to the CS catheter, which constitutes an excellent landmark to guide the puncture. Practically speaking, the use of a left anterior oblique, anteroposterior, or lateral view can aid the operator in positioning the needle inferiorly prior to entering the pericardial space (**Figure 44.1A**). If necessary, a RAO view should be used to confirm a basal rather than apical epicardial entrance point.

As with the traditional approach described in a previous chapter, once the pericardial space is entered, contrast is injected to confirm the location and a guide wire advanced (**Figure 44.1B**). In this situation, the contrast injection forms a pool of contrast along the inferior wall of the heart (**Figure 44.1C**) instead of quickly spreading around the heart silhouette, which typically happens when one approaches the pericardial space free of adhesions. It is also important to note that it may be impossible to advance the guide wire to encircle the entire cardiac shadow—a fluoroscopic sign that is frequently used to confirm that the pericardium is entered. As such, one must be confident that the pericardium is entered prior to advancing the sheath in order to avoid inadvertent sheath placement in the right ventricle. Thus, it is reasonable to advance a 5-Fr introducer over the wire, which will allow for further injection of small amounts of contrast in order to confirm pericardial access and/or allow for further manipulation of the guide wire.

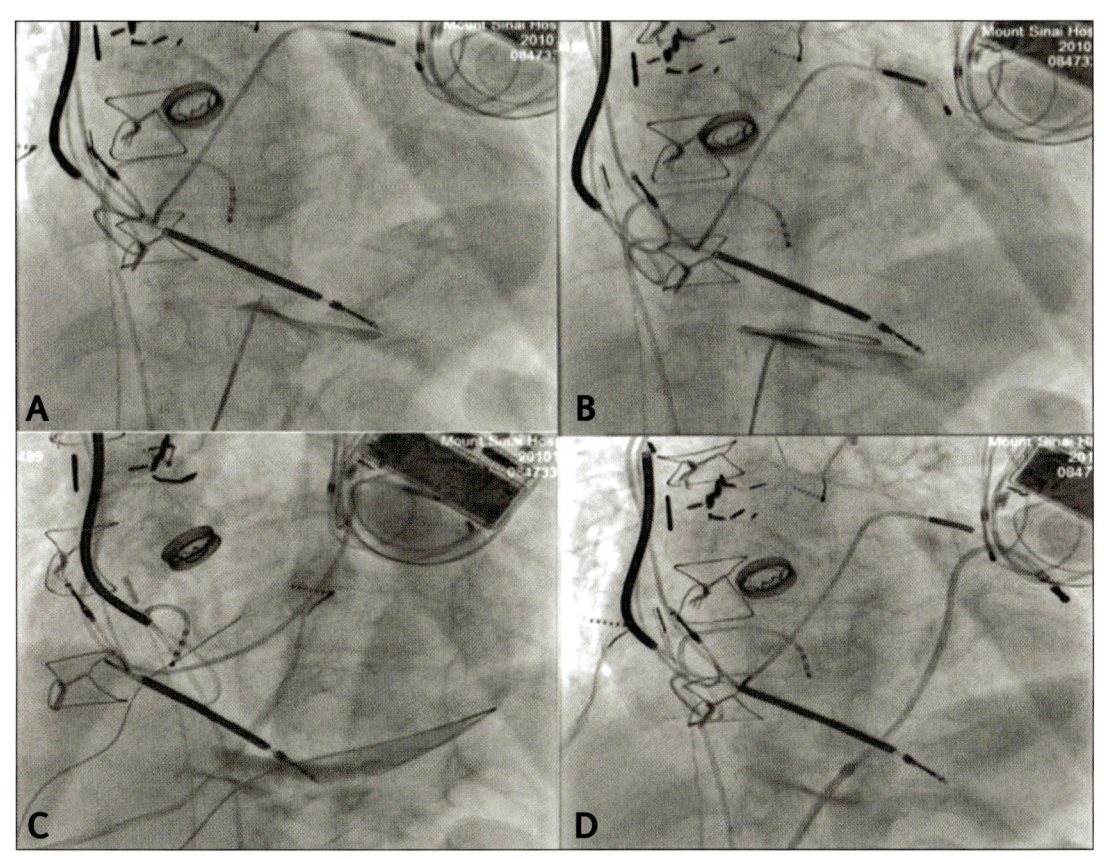

Figure 44.1 The inferior puncture is guided toward the base of the heart, parallel to the CS CRT lead, which constitutes an excellent landmark to guide the puncture in RAO (**A** and **B**). Once inside the pericardial space, contrast is injected (**B**), forming a pool of contrast along the inferior wall of the heart (**C**) instead of quickly spreading around the heart silhouette. In order to confirm the location the position of the wire is checked in the LAO projection (**C** and **D**). Deflection and extension of the ablation catheter can typically break these inferiorly located adhesions (**D**).

Adhesions may be present along the inferior surface of the heart. In general, these adhesions tend to be "looser" than the dense anterior adhesions. The operator may increase the region available to map by breaking these adhesions with the ablation catheter. Deflection and extension of the ablation catheter can typically break these inferiorly located adhesions (**Figure 44.1D**). While one may attempt this maneuver anterolaterally, it is frequently less successful given the density of the adhesions in this location; however, it is not unreasonable to attempt this as it may increase the mappable region.

A percutaneous route is our first option for postsurgical patients requiring epicardial mapping. Despite the limited region available to map, this approach is still quite valuable as epicardial VT circuits in the setting of coronary artery disease are more prevalent in patients with prior inferior infarction,[6] a region that may be accessed with this approach. Additionally, this approach is less "invasive" than the surgical approach described below.

Surgical Access with Limited Epicardial Mapping

Occasionally postsurgical adhesions may be so dense resulting in total obliteration of the "virtual space" between the visceral and parietal pericardium. In this situation a surgical approach to expose the pericardial space may be the only available option as percutaneous access will be impossible in the absence of this "virtual space." Two approaches have been described: a subxyphoid approach and limited anterior thoracotomy.[7,8]

The experience of Soejima and colleagues with the surgical subxyphoid approach is similar to ours (**Figure 44.2**).[7] This approach can be carried out in the EP laboratory employing general anesthesia and a sterile technique. We always enlist the help of our cardiac surgical colleagues when this access is required. Briefly, an incision (approximately 3 inches) is made in the midline epigastrium and carried down to the linea alba. This incision is usually made to the left of the xyphoid process, although in some cases it may be necessary to remove the xyphoid process in order to obtain improved access. Once the pericardium is identified, a pericardiotomy is performed and extended to ensure adequate visualization of the ventricle. Blunt dissection, sometimes with the surgeon's finger, is performed under direct visualization to lyse adhesions, thereby exposing as much of the inferior and posterior epicardial surface of the ventricle. At this point, an 8-Fr sheath is then placed in the pericardial space to allow placement of the ablation catheter within this region for mapping and ablation. This approach usually adds an additional 30 to 40 minutes of time to the procedure.

The subxyphoid surgical approach is frequently sufficient as the majority of epicardial circuits in patients with coronary artery disease occur in the setting of inferior scar. However, access to the anterior epicardial surface may sometimes be necessary. In this situation a limited anterior thoracotomy approach may be required to expose the anterolateral epicardial surface. Although we seldom employ this approach, others have reported their experience with this.[8,9] Again, general anesthesia is required. Double lumen endotracheal intubation is performed to allow for deflation of the left lung, which is necessary to access the heart. An incision is made over a selected rib space, which is in close proximity to the region where one would like to perform epicardial mapping. The incision is then carried down through the intercostal space. The pericardium is then identified and dissected off to expose the region one is interested in mapping. One may be able to map by directly placing the ablation catheter in the area of interest, depending on the extent of the exposure obtained.

At the end of either surgical approach, the site is closed. We typically leave a pericardial drain in for at least 12 hours. This drain is removed when clinically indicated.

Preprocedural Planning

Thoughtful preprocedural assessment is vital prior to performing epicardial procedures in the postsurgical patients. As many individuals referred for epicardial ablation do not have a critical epicardial isthmus, it is important that the operator review available 12-lead ECGs of the VT or imaging studies such as MRI to determine the pretest probability that epicardial mapping is indicated or whether further detailed endocardial mapping is necessary.

We frequently perform CT or coronary angiography in patients with prior coronary artery bypass surgery in order to identify the location of bypass grafts to minimize injuring them. While surgical pericardial dissection is performed under direct visualization, the release of adhesions with catheter deflection using a percutaneous approach is performed in a relatively blind fashion, which potentially places these grafts at risk of injury. Although dense adhesions, which typically form around coronary grafts, offer some degree of protection against disruption, knowledge of their location will help minimize their injury, which may result in significant bleeding necessitating conversion to a sternotomy. CT angiography has the additional benefit of allowing image integration of the 3-dimensional reconstructed image of the left ventricle and bypass grafts with the electroanatomic map created, which may be of help when navigating in the pericardial space and prior to performing ablation by ensuring that the region ablation is > 5 mm away from a coronary artery.

Anesthesia consultation is obtained on all patients undergoing VT ablation procedures at our institution as the majority of our ventricular tachycardia ablation procedures are performed using general anesthesia. General anesthesia allows one to control respiration during the percutaneous and surgical approaches. Additionally, the use of general anesthesia allows for additional control

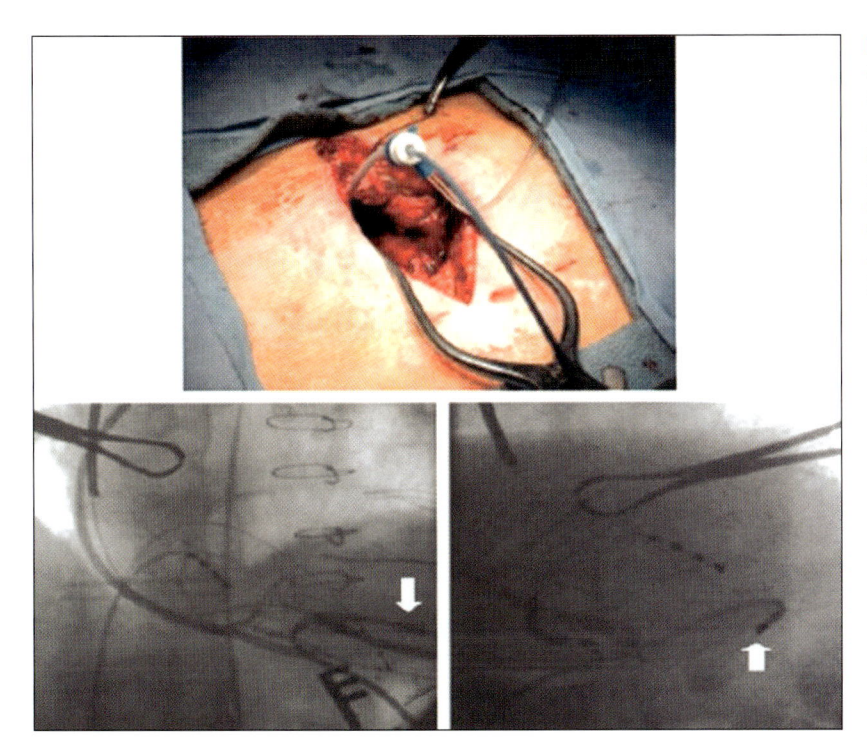

Figure 44.2 The surgical subxyphoid window is shown. A 3-inch incision is made and the pericardial space entered with direct visualization. An 8-Fr sheath is then placed in the pericardial space (shown) to allow placement of the ablation catheter. Fluoroscopic images demonstrating mapping of the inferior wall with this approach. (Reprinted with permission from Soejima et al. *Circulation*. 2004;110:1197–1201.)

should a complication arise requiring urgent sternotomy and/or the use of cardiopulmonary bypass.

Intraprocedure Considerations

We always administer prophylactic antibiotics (for example cephazolin, vancomycin, or clindamycin) to provide coverage against skin flora prior to obtaining epicardial access. Patients continue to receive prophylactic antibiotics at the appropriate frequency postprocedure as long as a pericardial drain remains in situ.

Access to the epicardium is typically obtained at the start of the procedure prior to administering anticoagulation. This approach minimizes significant bleeding, which would be magnified should a complication occur with therapeutic anticoagulation. Should epicardial access be desired subsequent to the administration of heparin, protamine is administered to reverse the ACT to less than 200 seconds.

We typically place an 8-Fr Brite-tip sheath in the pericardial space to stabilize the ablation catheter. However, the use of deflectable sheaths (Agilis, St. Jude Medical, Minnesota, MN) may allow for improved stability during mapping and also assist with loosening adhesions.

We currently perform epicardial ablation using an irrigated tipped catheter (Navistar Thermocool, Biosense Webster, Diamond Bar, CA). When performing epicardial ablation, the ablation mode on the Stockert Generator (Biosense Webster, Diamond Bar, CA) is set to "Manual Unipolar" rather than "Thermocool" mode, which is typically employed during irrigated endocardial ablation. With this setting, the flow rate through the irrigated catheter can be manually adjusted. We typically set the flow rate in this mode to 5 cm^3/min. Power is initially set at 15 W and uptitrated, aiming for a 10- to 15-ohm impedance drop. Prior to ablation, the location of the catheter in relation to the coronary vessels (or grafts) is assessed with either real-time coronary angiography or overlay of the 3-dimensional reconstructed CT image. Additionally, we do assess for phrenic nerve capture, although it is rare that access to the lateral aspect left ventricle (where the phrenic nerve courses) is achieved.

Complications

It is not unusual for patients to experience symptoms of pericarditis after epicardial mapping and ablation. At the end of the procedure we typically instill steroids (Solumedrol 150 mg/m^2 of body surface area) into the pericardial space to minimize symptomatic pericarditis. Additional use of oral anti-inflammatory agents may be necessary to aid with symptom relief.

Injury to subdiaphragmatic vessels may occur when access is obtained percutaneously regardless of whether patients have undergone cardiac surgery. One needs to be vigilant for intra-abdominal bleeding in the setting of a drop in hematocrit or blood pressure with the absence of pericardial fluid.

Complications specific to obtaining pericardial access in patients with prior cardiac surgery include the formation of loculated pericardial effusions. In patients where a percutaneous approach is taken, we often remove the pericardial drain at the end of the procedure, whereas we typically leave a drain in place overnight for patients who undergo a surgical approach. We recommend obtaining an echocardiogram within 24 hours postprocedure to ensure the absence of any procedure-related effusion.

Additionally, injury to the phrenic nerve may occur during anterolateral ventricular dissection with the limited anterior thoracotomy approach. Patients need to be made aware of this potential complication with this approach.

Conclusion

In summary, pericardial access is feasible in patients who have undergone prior cardiac surgery. Proper preprocedural planning and collaboration with surgical colleagues may increase the ease of obtaining this important access.

References

1. Sosa E, Scanavacca M, D'Avila A, Pilleggi F. A new technique to perform epicardial mapping in the electrophysiology laboratory. *J Cardiovasc Electrophysiol.* 1996;7:531–536.
2. Connolly SJ, Gent M, Roberts RS, Dorian P, Sheldon RS, Mitchell LB, Green ms, Klein GJ, O'Brien B. Canadian implantable defibrillator study (CIDS): A randomized trial of the implantable cardioverted defibrillator against amiodarone. *Circulation.* 2000;101:1287–1302.
3. Obel OA, d'Avila A, Neuzil P, Saad EB, Ruskin JN, Reddy VY. Ablation of left ventricular epicardial outflow tract tachycardia from the distal great cardiac vein. *J Am Coll Cardiol.* 2006;48:1813–1817.
4. Doppalapudi H, Yamanda T, Ramaswamy K, Ahn J, Kay GN. Idiopathic focal epicardial ventricular tachycardia originating from the crux of the heart. *Heart Rhythm.* 2009;6:44–50.
5. Sosa E, Scanavacca M, D'Avila A, Antonio J, Ramires F. Nonsurgical trans-thoracic epicardial approach in patients with ventricular tachycardia and previous cardiac surgery. *J Interv Card Electrophysiol.* 2004;10:281–288.
6. Sosa E, Scanavacca M, d'Avila A, Oliveira F, Ramires JAF. Nonsurgical transthoracic epicardial catheter ablation to treat recurrent ventricular tachycardia occurring late after myocardial infarction. *J Am Coll Cardiol.* 2000;35: 1442–1449.
7. Soejima K, Couper G, Cooper JM, Sapp JL, Epstein LM, Stevenson WG. Subxiphoid surgical approach for epicardial catheter-based mapping and ablation in patients with prior cardiac surgery or difficult pericardial access. *Circulation.* 2004;110:1197–1201.
8. Michowitz Y, Mathuria N, Tung R, et al. Hybrid procedures for epicardial catheter ablation of ventricular tachycardia: value of surgical access. *Heart Rhythm.* 2010;7(11): 1635–1643.
9. Sacher F, Roberts-Thompson K, Maury P, et al. Epicardial ventricular tachycardia ablation: a multicenter safety study. *J Am Coll Cardiol.* 2010;55:2366–2372.

CHAPTER 45

How to Perform Endocardial/Epicardial Ventricular Tachycardia Ablation

J. David Burkhardt, MD; Luigi Di Biase, MD, PhD; Matthew Dare, CEPS; Pasquale Santangeli, MD; Andrea Natale, MD[1]

Introduction

Ablation therapy for VT has advanced significantly in the last decade. Mapping techniques such as substrate mapping, pace mapping, and entrainment mapping, as well as improvements in ablation technology such as irrigated RF ablation, have improved the success rates in VT ablation, making this therapy a viable option in drug-refractory patients.[1-3] Recent innovations include the technique of epicardial ablation via a minimally invasive subxiphoid approach.[4] This technique allows ablation on the outer surface of the heart, which may be the focus of some ventricular arrhythmias. This area may not be accessible by even the deepest endocardial ablation lesions.

Preprocedure Planning

History and Evaluation

Prior to the ablation procedure, it is important to obtain a detailed history, including any history of prior cardiac surgeries, pericarditis, and device implantation. If the patient has had pericarditis, previous coronary artery bypass grafting, or other cardiac surgery, subxiphoid access to the pericardial space may be very difficult to impossible. In such cases, the pericardial sac may fibrose to the epicardial surface, which does not allow free access to the space. Occasionally, catheters can be introduced, but manual techniques are required to break through fibrotic areas. This process can be difficult and bloody. In most cases of patients who have had coronary artery bypass surgery and who need epicardial ablation, an open-chest procedure with a cardiac surgeon is likely the best approach.

During the physical examination, one should focus on the shape of the chest, xiphoid process, and abdominal contents near this area. During insertion of the needle, abdominal contents can be injured. In patients with splenomegaly or hepatomegaly, these structures may cross the midline and lie in the preferred area for needle insertion.

If the patient has an ICD implanted, this is very valuable information, which can be used for procedural planning. The ICD should be interrogated. The CLs of the clinical VTs should be noted. Also, the morphology of the tachycardia on the RV lead and other available EGMs should be saved. If the rhythms are pace terminable, then the scheme should also be saved for the procedure. This information can be used to determine if the induced arrhythmias at the time of EP study are clinically relevant.

---

1. Disclosure/Conflict of Interest: Dr. Di Biase is a consultant for Hansen Medical and Biosense Webster. Dr. Natale is a consultant for Biosense Webster and has also received a research grant from St. Jude Medical and received speaker honoraria from St. Jude Medical, Medtronic, Boston Scientific, Biotronik, and Biosense Webster.

It is also important to ensure that the patient is not better served by a simultaneous surgical procedure. An echocardiogram and stress test should be updated. If the patient requires coronary artery bypass grafting or valvular repair, then ablation can be performed at the time of the surgical procedure. The echocardiogram may also show segments of scar or hypokinesis that may yield clues as to the location of the tachycardias. The presence of LV clot may necessitate the delay of any procedure. Of course, an ECG during tachycardia is invaluable. This yields localization and CL information. If not in tachycardia, the location of previous myocardial infarctions may suggest potential locations. Although not necessary, cardiac CT or MRI may be used to define areas of scar and can be imported into the electroanatomic mapping system.

If patients are on warfarin anticoagulation, this is usually stopped 5 days prior to the procedure. Any antiarrhythmics are held for 5 half-lives if possible. If the patients are concerned or having frequent episodes, they may be admitted to the hospital for observation while the medications are being washed out. Of course, some patients are already hospitalized for VT storms or frequent ICD shocks.

Procedure

Patient Preparation

Most patients undergoing endocardial and epicardial VT ablation are sedated with moderate to deep sedation, usually using propofol. During the time in which sheaths are being placed, the patient may be deeply sedated; however, some patients need to be more responsive to fully awake to induce the target arrhythmia. Also, the blood pressure tends to be higher when patients are not under general anesthesia. It is important to have an anesthesiologist who is familiar with ablation and cardiovascular drugs for such procedures. Some anesthetics have antiarrhythmic properties, and occasionally, vasopressor medications are required to support the blood pressure when performing activation mapping during tachycardia. Of course, the anesthesiologist must also be comfortable and understand that VT mapping may require long periods of sustained tachycardia. They are also important in recognizing complications early.

Most patients have a Foley catheter placed after anesthesia is started. If the patient has an ICD, it is interrogated and reprogrammed to turn detections off. If possible, ventricular pacing is minimized to allow for any substrate map to be acquired during sinus rhythm. The EGMs, morphologies, and CLs of the clinical tachycardias are noted. Paper printouts of the EGM morphologies are obtained for review during tachycardia induction. In general, a person is assigned to manage the implanted device during the procedure for pacing, internal cardioversion, or defibrillation.

The patient is prepped from the carotid notch to the groin bilaterally. Using ultrasound guidance, arterial and venous access is obtained. If the patient has a very enlarged heart and there are no significant arterial pathologies such as aortic aneurysm or aortic valve replacement, then the retrograde aortic approach is used. For all other cases, a transseptal approach is used. In the case of the retrograde aortic approach, an 8-Fr short sheath is used in the right femoral artery for passing the ablation catheter and pressure monitoring. If the ileofemoral system is tortuous, a long stainless steel 24-cm sheath is used. If the transseptal approach is used, a 4-Fr short sheath is placed in the femoral artery for arterial pressure monitoring, and 8- and 11-Fr sheaths are placed in the right femoral vein. All sheaths are flushed with heparinized saline, and the arterial sheath is connected to pressure monitoring. A venous sheath is connected to an IV pump for delivery of medications. Through the 11-Fr sheath, an intracardiac ultrasound catheter is placed into the RA. It is set to a depth of 160 mm and retroflexed across the tricuspid valve to view a long-axis shot of the LV. This view shows pericardial effusion and the septal and posterior walls of the left ventricle as well as the mitral apparatus (**Figure 45.1**).

Epicardial Access

At this point, epicardial access is the next procedure. A towel is placed over the femoral sheaths. The equipment needed for this includes a 7-cm epidural needle, contrast dye, a 180-cm 0.032-inch diameter wire, a short 8-Fr introducer, and a 24-cm stainless steel sheath. The fluoroscope is placed into the LAO 18° position. In this view the needle should not violate the left or right side of the spine. The operator palpates the xiphoid process and plans to puncture slightly to the patient's left and about 2 cm inferior. This area is infiltrated with lidocaine. It is preferable that the patient is anesthetized so only shallow slow breathing is seen, or else deep breathing can pull the heart

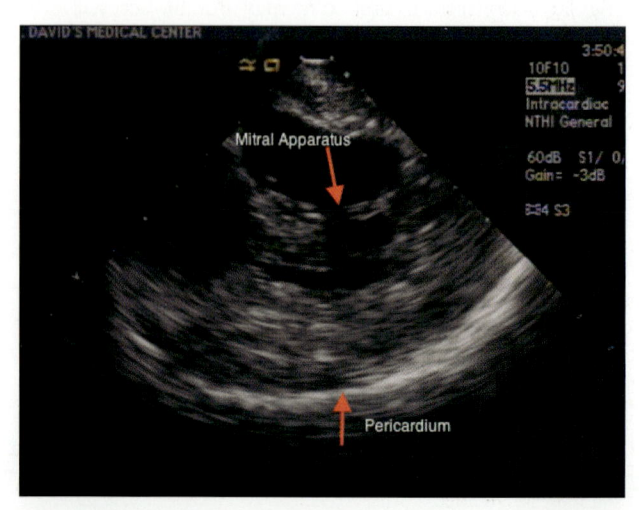

Figure 45.1 ICE image showing the long-axis LV and mitral valve, without pericardial effusion.

downward. The needle is placed on top of the chest under fluoroscopy to the level of the cardiac border to approximate the distance needed once inside the patient. The needle is advanced from the selected site toward the left side of the spine at a 40° angle to the skin. The needle should advance smoothly. Once any resistance or cardiac pulsation is felt, or the needle tip is at the cardiac border, the stylet is removed from the needle, and contrast is attached. A small amount (< 0.5 cm^3) of contrast is infused. If one is near the pericardium, tenting is seen. The needle should be advanced until it pops through this tented area. A palpable "pop" may be felt. After popping through, more contrast is infused that should layer around the heart (**Figure 45.2** and **Video 45.1**). If one is not in the correct area, contrast will simply diffuse into the tissue. If the needle has punctured the heart, the contrast will swiftly move away. Usually PVCs are seen during advancement in this situation. The needle should be withdrawn into the pericardial space if felt to be intracardiac. Occasionally, a tenting is seen when the diaphragm is punctured. The pericardial surface is just past this location. Once the needle is confirmed to be in the pericardial space, the guidewire is advanced through the needle. During this process, the needle can be pushed out due to breathing. Slight advancement will re-engage the space. The wire should advance easily. A very long segment of wire should be advanced into the space so that large loops are seen around the heart. These loops should cross multiple chambers, confirming epicardial location (**Figure 45.3** and **Video 45.2**). A sheath should not be inserted over the wire unless it is seen crossing multiple chambers. At this point, the needle is removed, and the sheath is placed over the wire into the space. If difficulty is met at the cardiac border due to a sharp angle, a short dilator may be inserted first. Once the sheath is inserted well into the space, the dilator and wire are removed. The side arm of the sheath is aspirated, and any fluid removed is examined for blood content (**Figure 45.4** and **Video 45.3**). Some blood may be expected, but it is usually dilute. All fluid removed from the space is tabulated, as well as any fluid infused from the ablation catheter. The ICE catheter is used to monitor for pericardial effusion. The side arm is aspirated every 20 minutes or more frequently during ablation.

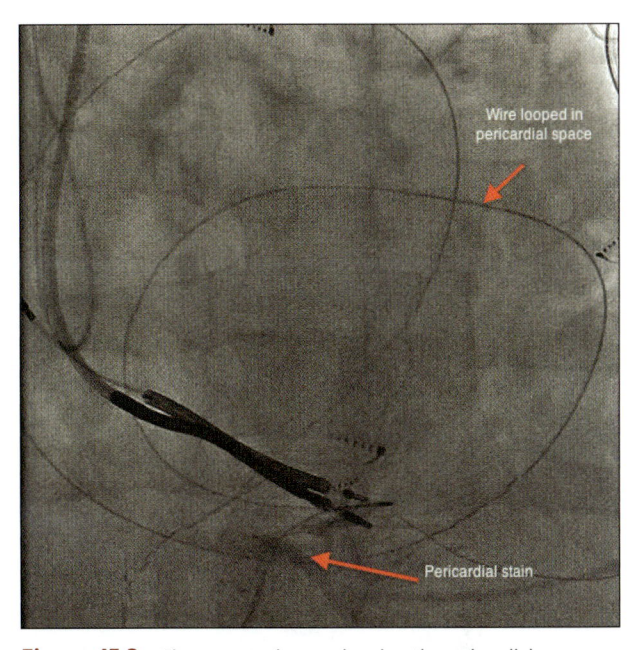

Figure 45.3 Flouroscopy image showing the epicardial guidewire covering multiple chambers confirming the epicardial location.

Figure 45.2 Fluoroscopy image showing the epicardial tenting with contrast.

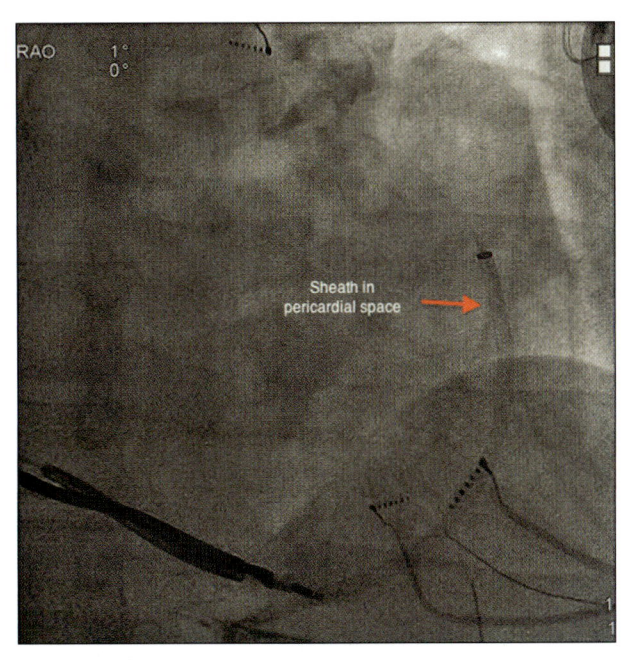

Figure 45.4 Flouroscopy image showing the sheath in the endocardial space.

Approach

After all sheaths are placed, anticoagulation is started. A weight-based heparin bolus is given to achieve a goal ACT of 300 seconds. If a transseptal approach is to be used, the short sheath is exchanged for a Mullins transseptal sheath. This sheath is advanced over the guidewire into the SVC. A transseptal needle is placed inside, and the system is withdrawn to the septum. The puncture is performed under ICE guidance. The puncture is performed in the fossa ovalis, which is slightly anterior to the puncture for AF ablation. The LAA is in view on the ICE monitor. Once the puncture is performed and dilator and needle removed, the catheter is advanced to the mid-mitral valve location. This allows for optimal support during mapping. A 3.5-mm ablation catheter is advanced through the sheath into the LV for mapping (**Figure 45.5**).

In the case of the retrograde aortic approach, the ablation catheter is advanced to the subclavian artery. A loop is made in the catheter, and it is advanced to the aortic valve. It is prolapsed through the valve into the LV.

Mapping

The first goal is to construct a detailed endocardial substrate map. The catheter is directed throughout the ventricle to reconstruct its geometry and collect electrical data. All points should be collected in sinus rhythm. Maneuvers such as advance and retract, clockwise and counter-clockwise torque, and looping may be required to navigate the entire ventricle (▶ **Video 45.4**). The voltage meter should be set to 0.5 mV on the lower end (which is usually just above the baseline noise level) and the upper level to 1.5 mV. Areas of fractionated potentials, late potentials, and His or bundle branch potentials should be annotated with special notations. Areas of scar should receive the most detailed mapping, particularly the scar border (▶ **Video 45.5**). Areas of completely healthy tissue need just enough detail to complete the map without holes. The fill threshold (fill threshold setting at 15 mm) should not be changed to complete the map. A complete map, generally, requires at least 250 points and as many as 500 to 700 points before ablation. After completion, the map should be checked. All internal and incorrect points should be deleted and any holes should be filled (**Figure 45.6**).

At this point, endocardial activation mapping may begin. We use the ablation catheter for induction, since other catheters may introduce unwanted extra beats. Pacing is enabled through the ablation catheter or through the ICD. Single extrastimuli are initially used until the ventricular effective refractory period is determined or the arrhythmia induced. Further extrastimuli are added to facilitate induction. Once an arrhythmia is induced, the patient is evaluated for hemodynamic stability. A minute may be required for the patient to adjust to the arrhythmia and for anesthesia to support the blood pressure if needed.

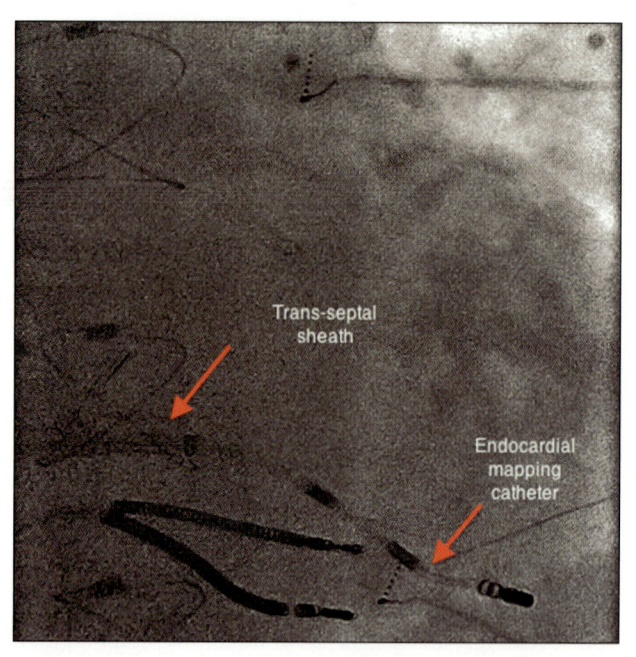

Figure 45.5 Fluoroscopy image of the mapping/ablation catheter in the epicardial space.

If unstable, the patient is cardioverted or pace terminated. The induced arrhythmia is analyzed to see if it correlates with the clinical arrhythmia based on the previously obtained clinical and ICD information (ICD EGM morphologies and rate). If it appears to be a clinical tachycardia, then a probable location is inferred from the 12-lead ECG. This should correlate with the area of scar that was identified. Short periods of activation mapping can be performed if tolerated, to confirm that the location is correct.

If the tachycardia is tolerated, then a detailed activation map is created (**Figure 45.7**). The map should, once again, recreate the ventricular geometry without holes or gaps. Areas of late activation can be less detailed, while areas of early activation require more detailed mapping. One must ensure that all points are taken during the same tachycardia. Areas of mid-diastolic potentials, as well as continuous or fractionated EGM signals recorded during tachycardia, require special annotation. Once the map is completed, incorrect and internal points are deleted. Further mapping may be required to complete the map. The same maneuvers performed during substrate mapping are used for activation mapping. Entrainment mapping may be performed from areas of earliest activation. This map should be made to overlay the substrate map to confirm the area that will need to be ablated. Usually, the areas of early activation will be in or on the border of the scar seen in the substrate map. Any other induced clinical tachycardia should be handled the same way.

Now the epicardial surface is ready to be mapped. A new ablation catheter is placed through the stainless steel sheath. In the same way, a substrate map of the epicardial surface is performed. Movement in this space is much easier since there are no structures that hinder the catheter

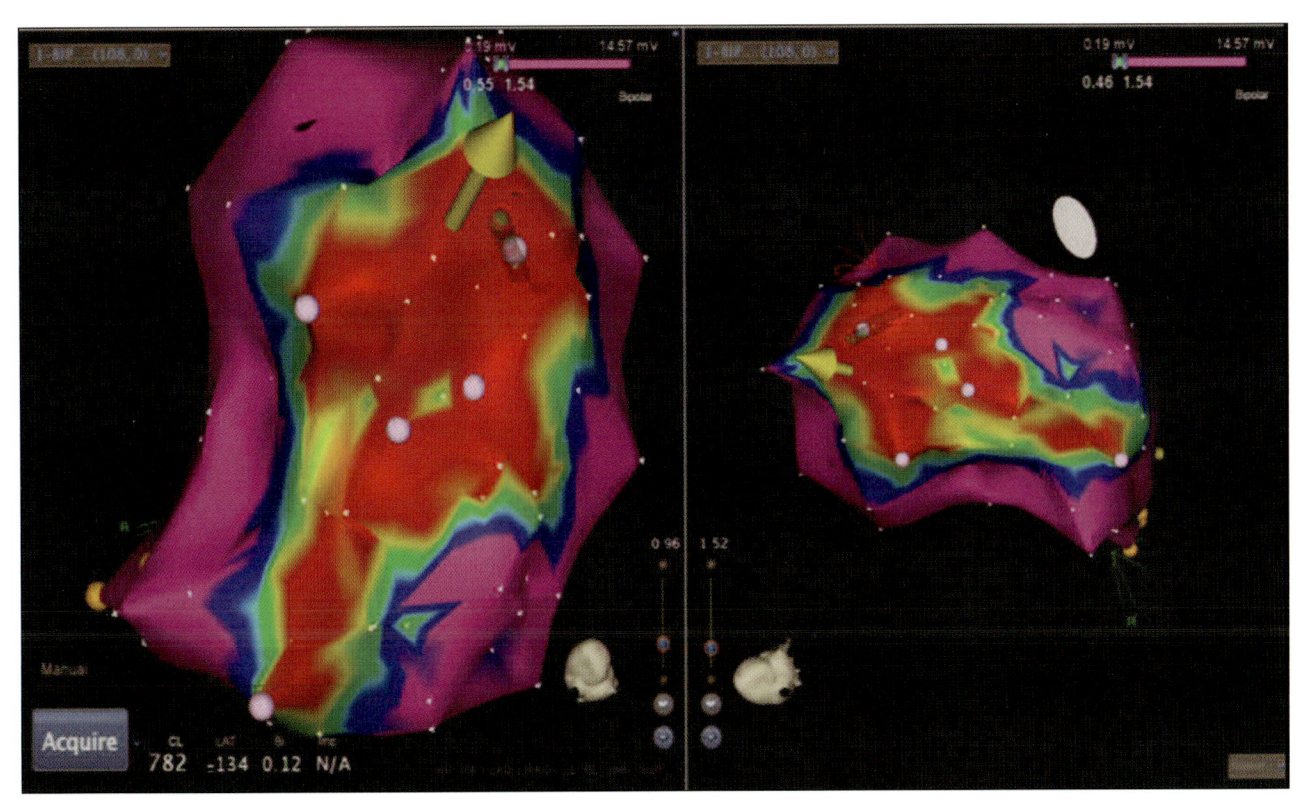

Figure 45.6 Electroanatomic map of the endocardial substrate.

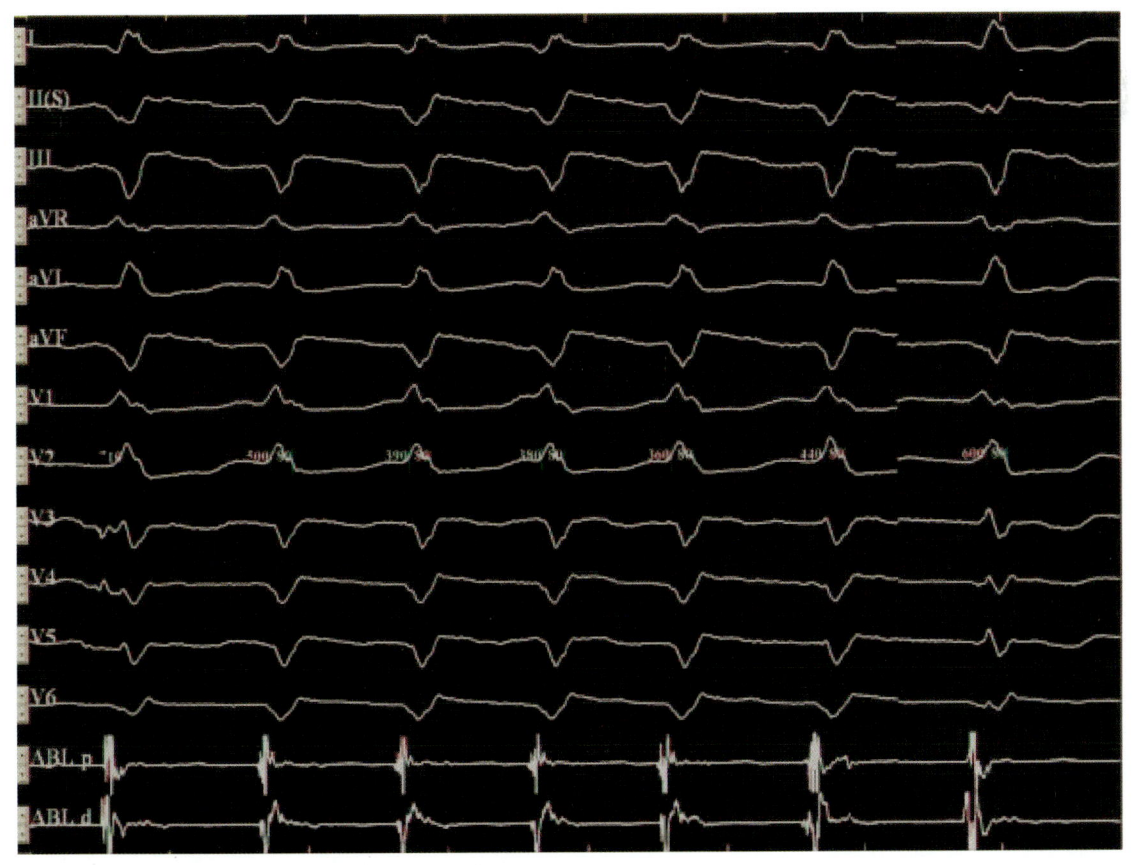

Figure 45.7 Twelve-lead ECG and mapping catheter signals on the recording system during a stable VT.

424 • Ablation of VT

(**Figure 45.8** and ▶ **Videos 45.6** and **45.7**). However, techniques of rotation and torque do not work as well. In general advancing and retracting the catheter is the main movement. Loops can be made and may be required to reach certain areas. One must use the pericardial reflections to direct the catheter to a certain point. The substrate map is performed in the same manner, with the same settings. One may notice areas of low voltage that do not correlate and do not exhibit fractionated potentials. This is usually due to epicardial fat. The areas of scar should correlate with the endocardial map. One additional requirement with epicardial mapping is to locate the left phrenic nerve. High output pacing is performed along the left lateral border. Areas of diaphragmatic capture are annotated on the map.

After this, epicardial activation mapping of the clinical tachycardia is performed in the same fashion as the endocardial activation map (**Figure 45.9**). The larger areas of the epicardial surface usually require more points on the map. Once completed, this map is compared to the epicardial voltage map, as well as the endocardial maps (**Figures 45.7** and **45.10**).

Ablation

Once all of the maps are completed, an ablation strategy is formulated. This strategy should have the goal of homogenizing the entire scar, that is ablating all signals above the noise level within areas of scar, and including the scar border and areas of early activation.[5] This is performed on both the endocardial and epicardial surfaces. If desired, ablation can be performed during tachycardia in the early activation areas, to observe for CL prolongation and termination (▶ **Videos 45.7** and **45.8**, respectively); however, termination does not end the procedure. Completion of the scar ablation and lack of inducibility is the goal

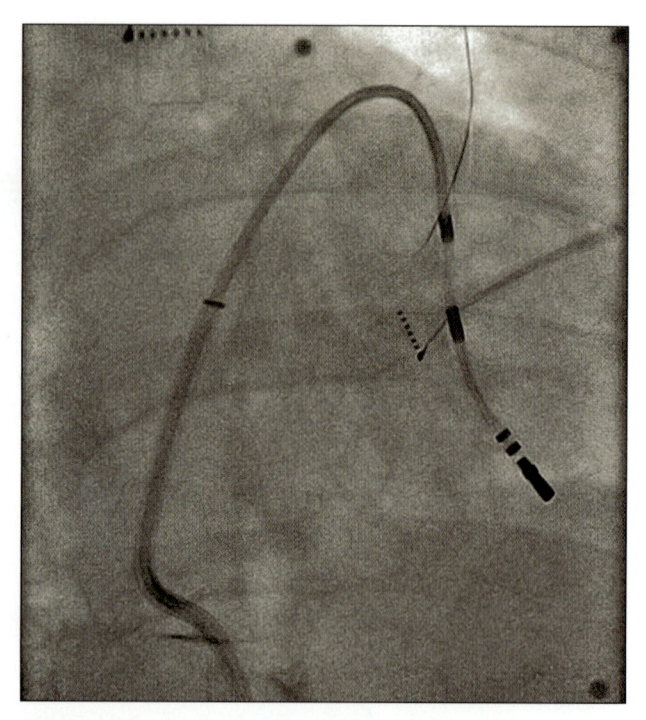

Figure 45.8 Fluoroscopic image of the mapping/ablation catheter in the epicardial space.

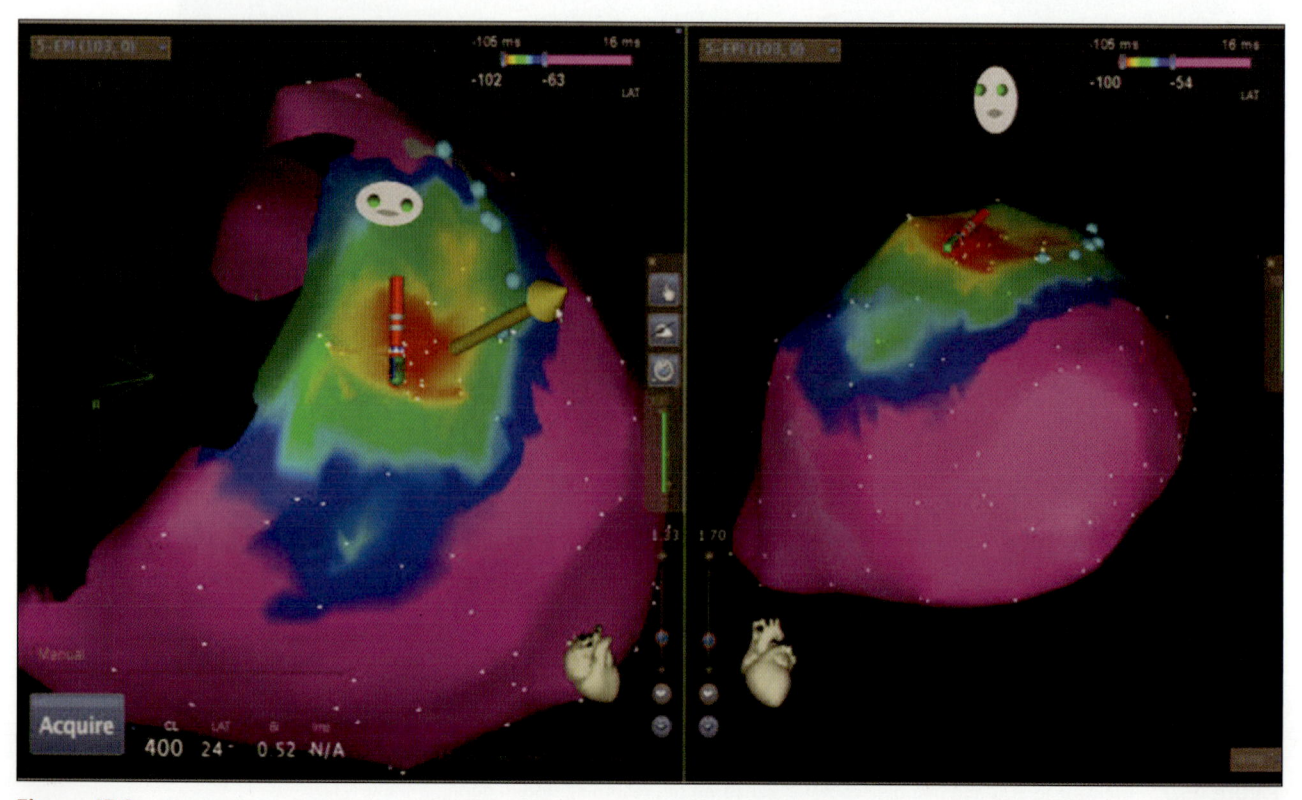

Figure 45.9 Electroanatomic epicardial activation map.

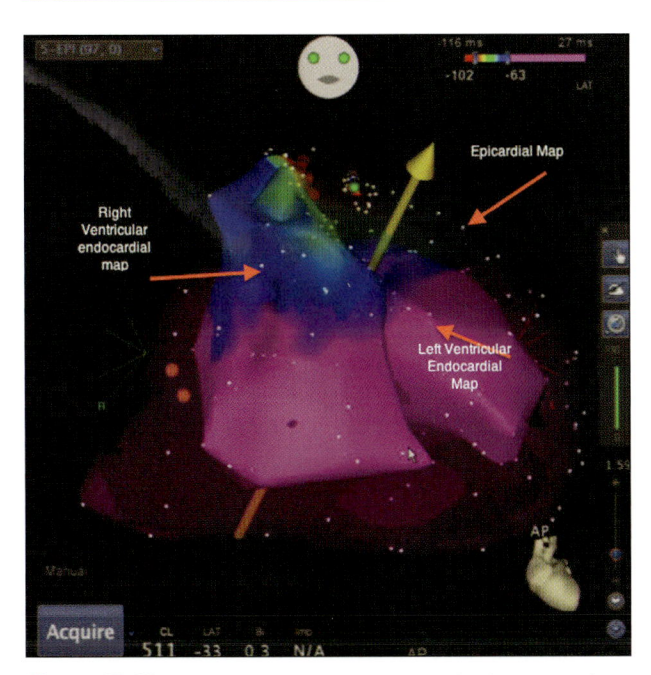

Figure 45.10 Combined electroanatomic activation maps of endocardial RV, LV, and epicardial LV with ablation points.

(**Figure 45.11**). Ablation should be performed in and around the scar on both surfaces. Ablation is performed at 40 W with lesions at a single point for about 20 seconds. If the tip temperature rises above 40°C, then the catheter should be moved. If the temperature rises above 42°C, then ablation should be terminated because this may predict a steam pop. The catheter is moved while ablation is performed continuously. Ablation annotations should meet each other without gaps. During epicardial ablation the side arm of the sheath should be frequently aspirated to remove fluid, which allows better contact. This fluid should be visually inspected for bloody content. After ablation is completed, repeat stimulation should be performed to confirm lack of inducibility of the clinical tachycardia. If tachycardia is still inducible, further mapping and ablation should be performed. Cryoablation may be considered if epicardial RF ablation appears unsuccessful.

After the procedure is completed, catheters should be removed from the arterial system, and protamine given to fully reverse the anticoagulation. Once the ACT is less than 180 seconds, sheaths can be removed. If the pericardial sheath is still draining fluid or blood despite reversing anticoagulation and draining the pericardial space, the drain should be left in overnight and monitored for drainage. An echocardiogram should be performed the next day prior to removal to confirm the absence of fluid.

If the drain is not draining fluid at the end of the procedure, it may be removed. A last look on fluoroscopy and ICE should be performed prior to removal (▶ **Video 45.9**). Sometimes air may be present in the pericardial sac. It should be removed along with any residual fluid. A pigtail catheter can be placed through the sheath for this purpose. The pigtail can be wrapped around the heart to remove any air or fluid, while suction is being applied with an attached 20-cm^3 syringe.

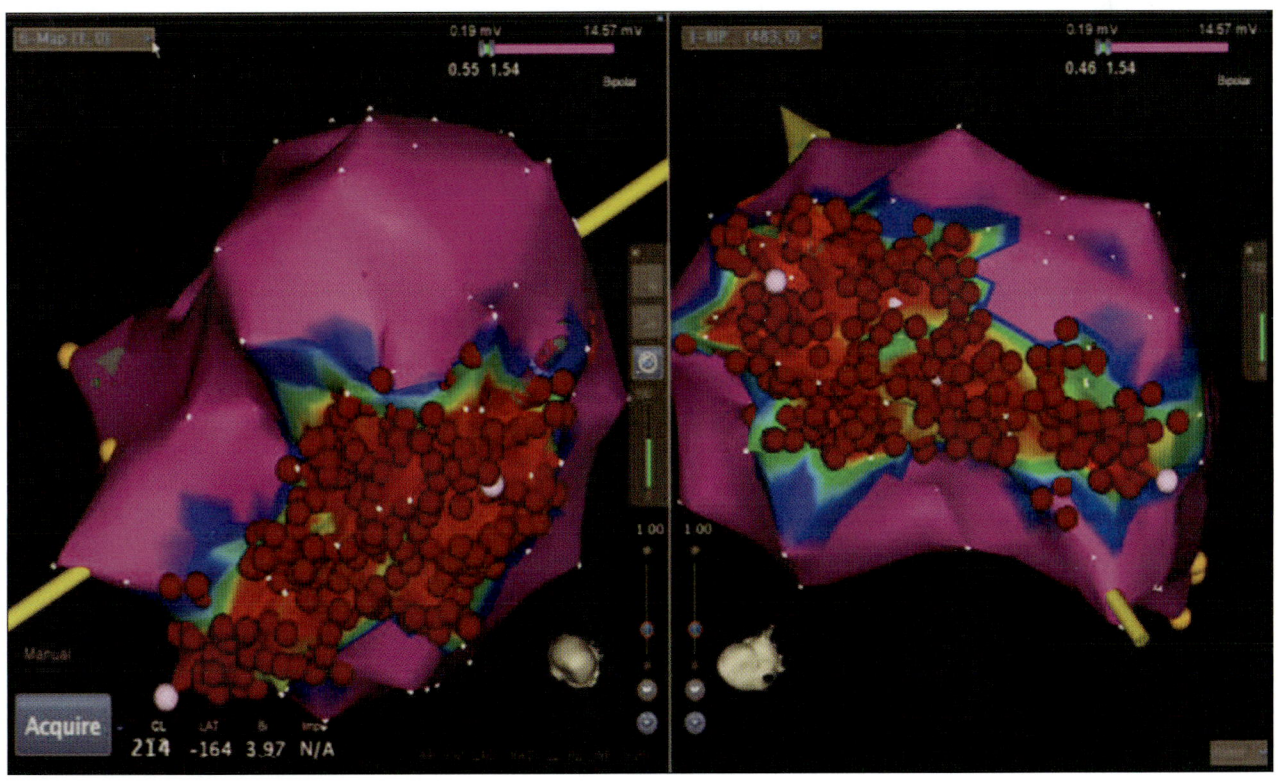

Figure 45.11 Electroanatomic ablation map showing homogenization of the endocardial scar.

Prior to leaving the laboratory, the ICD should be checked and reprogrammed to detections on. Reprogramming of VT zones may be necessary based on the results of EP testing for monitoring of arrhythmias.

While the patient remains in the hospital, he or she may experience pericarditis-type pain. Ibuprofen should be given to all patients who can tolerate it. Ketorolac can be given for severe pain. The patient should be given ibuprofen regularly for 2 weeks if possible. We do not routinely use steroids in our patients.

Generally, patients who have had the epicardial sheaths removed may be discharged the next day. If the patient has continued drainage and has a sheath in place, it is usually removed the day after the procedure, and the patient stays another night in the hospital.

Follow-up

Patients are followed at 3-month intervals if they are experiencing no arrhythmias or difficulties. If the patient has an ICD, this is interrogated at each visit. If the patient does not have an ICD, he or she is given an event monitor for 30 days after the procedure.

Repeat Ablations

Patients with recurrent arrhythmias are offered repeat ablation procedures. Repeat epicardial access can usually be performed as in the first case unless the patient has significant pericarditis. Repeat ablation has the same goals as the initial ablation procedure. Rarely, if the focus is felt to be very deep in the tissue, a surgical ablation may be required.

Complications

Most complications associated with the ablation can be discovered or prevented during the procedure. Phrenic nerve paralysis can be avoided in many cases by high-output pacing in areas near the phrenic nerve, although this is not always reliable. Pericardial bleeding occurs on occasion, but this is usually limited. The use of peripheral angioplasty balloon, air, and saline are also being described to avoid phrenic nerve injury.[6] Interestingly, ST elevation myocardial infarction appears to be rare. The coronary arteries appear to be protected by epicardial fat. Pericarditis is common but usually limited and treatable with ibuprofen. Severe cases may require steroid therapy.[7,8]

Other structures border the heart in the chest, such as the lung, esophagus, and great vessels. Based on animal studies these are certainly receiving RF energy, but reports of significant clinical effects are rare. The most common complication is groin vessel bleeding or damage. Using ultrasound, guided punctures may reduce rate of this complication.

Advantages and Limitations

Endocardial and epicardial ablation for ischemic VT has several advantages. It appears to be significantly more effective than medical therapy and appears to have few long-term complications. Reducing ICD therapies may also relieve patients of anxiety associated with potential shocks. The addition of epicardial ablation seems to augment the success associated with endocardial ablation.[9] Most patients are candidates for endocardial ablation. Currently, ablation is being evaluated as a preventative strategy in patients being evaluated for ICD therapy.[10]

Unfortunately, limitations do exist for this approach. Patients who have had previous bypass surgery, significant pericarditis, or other cardiac surgery may not be candidates for the minimally invasive subxiphoid approach.[11] These patients who still require epicardial ablation need an open-chest procedure. Also, the epicardial approach is not a routine procedure and requires significant expertise. Also, the tools that are currently available for ablation are not optimal. Even the lesions created with irrigated RF ablation are not typically transmural, and there are no tools specifically made for the epicardial approach. New technology may improve the success and acceptance of this procedure.

Conclusion

Endocardial and epicardial mapping and ablation of ischemic VT can be a meticulous and challenging procedure. Significant mapping and ablation are required to achieve optimal results. Homogenization of the myocardial scar improves the success rate of the procedure, and the addition of epicardial ablation may further improve the outcomes. The effort required for such a procedure may benefit patients who suffer from these difficult to treat arrhythmias.

References

1. Azegami K, Wilber DJ, Arruda M, Lin AC, Denman RA. Spatial resolution of pacemapping and activation mapping in patients with idiopathic right ventricular outflow tract tachycardia. *J Cardiovasc Electrophysiol.* 2005;16:823–829.
2. Coggins DL, Lee RJ, Sweeney J, et al. Radiofrequency catheter ablation as a cure for idiopathic tachycardia of both left and right ventricular origin. *J Am Coll Cardiol.* 1994;23: 1333–1341.
3. Tanner H, Hindricks G, Volkmer M, et al. Catheter ablation of recurrent scar-related ventricular tachycardia using electroanatomical mapping and irrigated ablation technology: results of the prospective multicenter euro-vt-study. *J Cardiovasc Electrophysiol.* 2010;21:47–53.

4. Di Biase L, Santangeli P, Astudillo V, et al. Endo-epicardial ablation of ventricular arrhythmias in the left ventricle with the remote magnetic navigation system and the 3.5-mm open irrigated magnetic catheter: results from a large single-center case-control series. *Heart Rhythm.* 2010;7: 1029–1035.
5. Di Biase L, Santangeli P, Burkhardt DJ, et al. Endo-epicardial homogenization of the scar versus limited substrate ablation for the treatment of electrical storms in patients with ischemic cardiomyopathy. *J Am Coll Cardiol.* 2012;60:132–141.
6. Di Biase L, Burkhardt JD, Pelargonio G, et al. Prevention of phrenic nerve injury during epicardial ablation: comparison of methods for separating the phrenic nerve from the epicardial surface. *Heart Rhythm.* 2009;6:957–961.
7. Sacher F, Roberts-Thomson K, Maury P, et al. Epicardial ventricular tachycardia ablation a multicenter safety study. *J Am Coll Cardiol.* 2010;55:2366–2372.
8. Bai R, Patel D, Di Biase L, et al. Phrenic nerve injury after catheter ablation: Should we worry about this complication? *J Cardiovasc Electrophysiol.* 2006;17:944–948.
9. Pokushalov E, Romanov A, Turov A, Artyomenko S, Shirokova N, Karaskov A. Percutaneous epicardial ablation of ventricular tachycardia after failure of endocardial approach in the pediatric population with arrhythmogenic right ventricular dysplasia. *Heart Rhythm.* 2010;7:1406–1410.
10. Tung R, Josephson ME, Reddy V, Reynolds MR. Influence of clinical and procedural predictors on ventricular tachycardia ablation outcomes: an analysis from the Substrate Mapping and Ablation in Sinus Rhythm to Halt Ventricular Tachycardia Trial (SMASH-VT). *J Cardiovasc Electrophysiol.* 2010;21:799–803.
11. Roberts-Thomson KC, Seiler J, Steven D, et al. Percutaneous access of the epicardial space for mapping ventricular and supraventricular arrhythmias in patients with and without prior cardiac surgery. *J Cardiovasc Electrophysiol.* 2010;21: 406–411.

Video Descriptions

Video 45.1 Fluoroscopy of the epidural needle tenting the pericardium and puncture.

Video 45.2 Fluoroscopy of wire advancing into pericardial space.

Video 45.3 Fluoroscopy of sheath introduction into epicardial space.

Video 45.4 Fluorosopy of navigation of the ablation catheter within the left ventricle with the Stereotaxis system.

Video 45.5 Electroanatomic map generation using a Navistar® RMT with the Stereotaxis system.

Video 45.6 Catheter navigation within the pericardial space (fluoroscopy).

Video 45.7 Video of combined right ventricular, left ventricular, and epicardial maps with ablation points.

Video 45.8 Video of recording system signals and VT termination during ablation.

Video 45.9 ICE video showing no significant residual effusion.

CHAPTER 46

How to Ablate Ventricular Fibrillation Arising from the Structurally Normal Heart

Shinsuke Miyazaki, MD; Ashok J. Shah, MD;
Michel Haïssaguerre, MD; Mélèze Hocini, MD

Introduction

Ventricular fibrillation (VF) is a challenging arrhythmia with only a limited number of treatment options. Based on the results of large randomized trials, most patients with VF are treated with ICDs. Defibrillators deal with the ongoing arrhythmia rather than abolishing the arrhythmia trigger, therefore leading to multiple ICD shocks.

Due to its strikingly lethal characteristics and transient presence, VF has been mapped and studied, by and large, in animal hearts or models. Moreover, VF is mechanistically varied in comparison to the sustained monomorphic reentrant ventricular arrhythmias. Reentry involving the Purkinje-myocardium junction and the migratory propagation of vortices are the likely mechanisms occurring during the maintenance of arrhythmia. The trigger for VF in the majority of cases is acute ventricular ectopy similar to AF, which led to the concept of ablation of the trigger to treat VF. This chapter focuses on strategies, techniques, and results of ablation of primary VF (excluding VF occurring due to degeneration of VT) at our center.

Preprocedural Planning of VF Ablation

Exclusion of Underlying Structural Heart Disease

Recognition of the underlying heart disease is essential before deciding the treatment strategy in patients with VF. Briefly, on the basis of the published guidelines, structural heart disease is ruled out by echocardiography, exercise testing, coronary angiography, and other imaging techniques including MRI. Primary electrical disorders associated with VF include the long- or short-QT syndrome (corrected QT interval [QTc] more than 440 ms or less than 300 to 320 ms at baseline, respectively), the Brugada syndrome (right bundle branch block and ≥ 0.2 mV ST-segment elevation in ≥ 2 precordial leads from V_1 to V_3, with or without provocative drugs), the catecholaminergic arrhythmias (ventricular arrhythmias during catecholamine infusion or exercise testing), and the early repolarization syndrome (at least 0.1 mV J-point elevation in 2 contiguous leads other than V_1 to V_3 with terminal QRS slur/notch).

Indication of VF Ablation

Although implantation of an ICD remains the primary treatment for secondary and primary prevention of VF, the underlying heart disease should be considered for deciding the treatment strategy. For those patients who have multiple, recurrent episodes of VF resistant to antiarrhythmic drugs, with frequent, triggering PVCs, RF ablation can be a good option.

Documentation of PVCs Triggering VF

Prior to ablation, it is essential that there is an accurate 12-lead ECG documentation of the triggering PVCs. All morphologies of PVCs should be recorded and analyzed beforehand. We perform continuous 12-lead ECG monitoring of the patient during the preprocedural period to identify Purkinje PVCs (duration of QRS, polymorphic or monomorphic, right or left; **Figure 46.1**).

Scheduling the Procedure

Due to unpredictable nature of the triggering beats, the optimal time for ablation is often the time within 3 days following an electrical storm, when the PVCs tend to be frequent. The procedure is known to be less successful when the ablation is undertaken in the absence of clinical ectopy. We attempt to perform the procedure during the period of electrical storm. If this is not possible, patients are studied soon thereafter or at the time of frequent PVCs. Emergent need for the procedure should always be borne in one's mind. It is also important to determine if the episode of VF is situational and if any provocation of PVCs/VF is possible.

Organizing the Procedure

Stable intraprocedural hemodynamic state is necessary for a successful procedure. It is important to have a therapeutic or prophylactic circulatory support for the patients experiencing electrical storms and multiple shocks from a defibrillator before the procedure can be undertaken safely. At our center, we obtain the help of cardiac surgeons whenever necessary to ensure stable hemodynamics through the procedure. Usual support devices include extracorporeal membrane oxygenator and left ventricular assist device. The VF ablation procedure is therefore performed by a very closely interacting team of cardiac electrophysiologist, cardiac anaesthesiologist, cardiac surgeon, and intensivist.

Procedure

Due to the rapidly lethal nature of the arrhythmia, trigger mapping remains largely restricted to the area of interest. For the same reason, invasive mapping of the initiation of

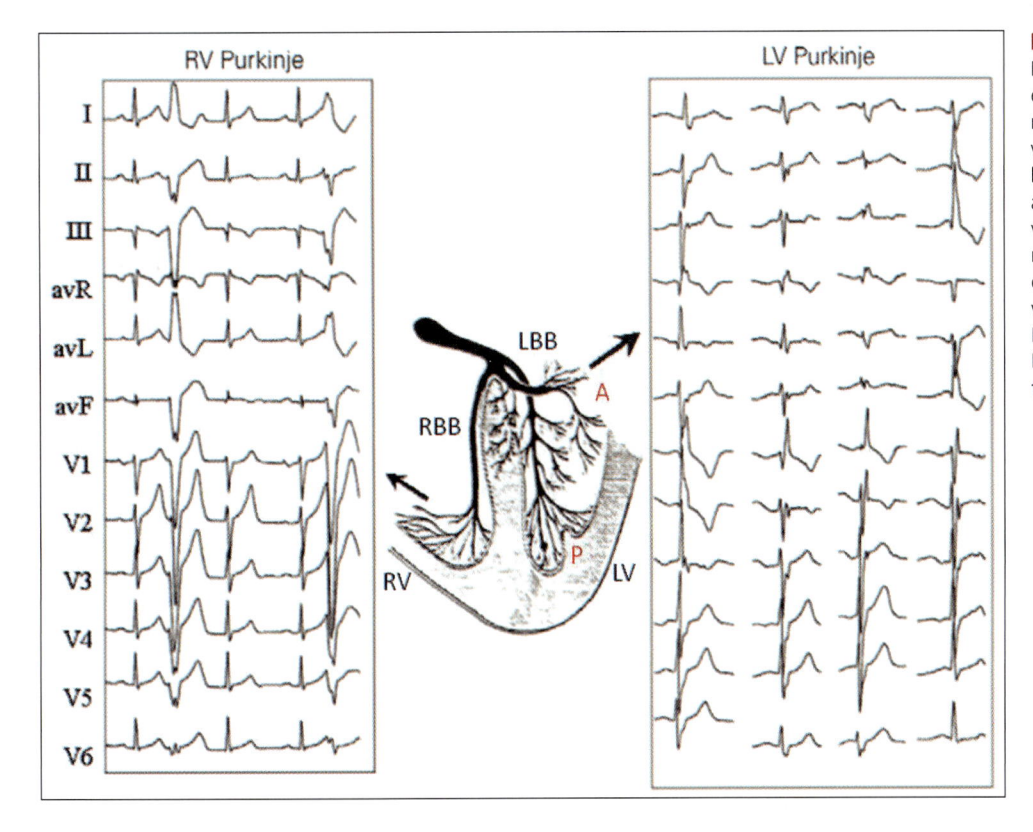

Figure 46.1 Typical 12-lead ECG pattern of ectopic beats originating from the left and right Purkinje network. Right ventricular Purkinje beats have an LBBB pattern in V_1 and are usually wide. Left ventricular Purkinje beats are narrow, and have a left, right, or intermediate axis. RV: right ventricle, LV: left ventricle, RBB: right bundle branch, LBB: left bundle branch, A: anterior fascicle, P: posterior fascicle.

these arrhythmias is difficult during ongoing arrhythmia. However, during periods of silence in between the episodes of arrhythmia, isolated or repetitive premature beats with the morphology identical to those triggering fibrillation allow mapping of their origin. Based on the currently available evidence, majority of such initiating ventricular complexes could be mapped to various locations in the His-Purkinje tree as indicated by sharp potentials preceding local muscle EGM during sinus rhythm as well as during ectopy (**Figures 46.2** and **46.3**). If the site of origin of the ectopic beat is not preceded by a sharp potential during sinus rhythm, the trigger source is considered to be the local myocardium, although the ectopic beat may be preceded by the sharp potential.

On-Table Preparation

Defibrillation patches should be applied to the patient for immediate external defibrillation. Biphasic electrical shock is recommended. Although the ventricular arrhythmia sensing and management function of the implanted defibrillator is switched off, it can be used for emergency bailout defibrillation.

Recording System and Mapping/Ablation Catheters

Surface ECG and bipolar endocardial EGMs (filtered from 30 to 500 Hz) are continuously monitored and stored on a computer-based digital amplifier/recorder system (Labsystem Pro, Bard EP, Lowell, MA). High-gain mapping (1 mm = 0.1 mV) is useful to clearly identify Purkinje potentials.

Deflectable decapolar or/and quadripolar catheter (2–5–2 mm electrode spacing, Xtrem, ELA Medical, France) can be used for various purposes. It is useful for mapping the His-Purkinje tree when the catheter is placed inside the ventricle (**Figure 46.4**), and also useful as a stable reference when the catheter is placed inside the CS.

A multispline catheter (PentaRay, Biosense Webster, Diamond Bar, CA) is also useful for the mapping process over a wide area of ventricular endocardium (**Figures 46.4** and **46.5**). This deflectable-tip 7-Fr catheter provides high-density contact mapping (20-pole unit). The internal orientation of splines is guided by radiopaque markers (**Figure 46.5**). Care needs to be taken not to "bump" the right or left bundle with the catheters as this conceals ipsilateral Purkinje activation during sinus rhythm. It is also possible for catheter bump to abolish the clinical PVCs. Therefore, it is important that mapping is done especially gently and carefully (**Figure 46.6**).

Ablation is performed using externally irrigated 3.5-mm tip-catheter (Thermocool, Biosense Webster) under direct fluoroscopy guidance.

Mapping and Ablation Technique

Mapping is undertaken after overnight fasting and under conscious sedation using midazolam and nalbuphine in an elective procedure. Left ventricular access is preferably obtained both transseptally and retrograde. An intravenous bolus dose of 50 U/kg of heparin is administered,

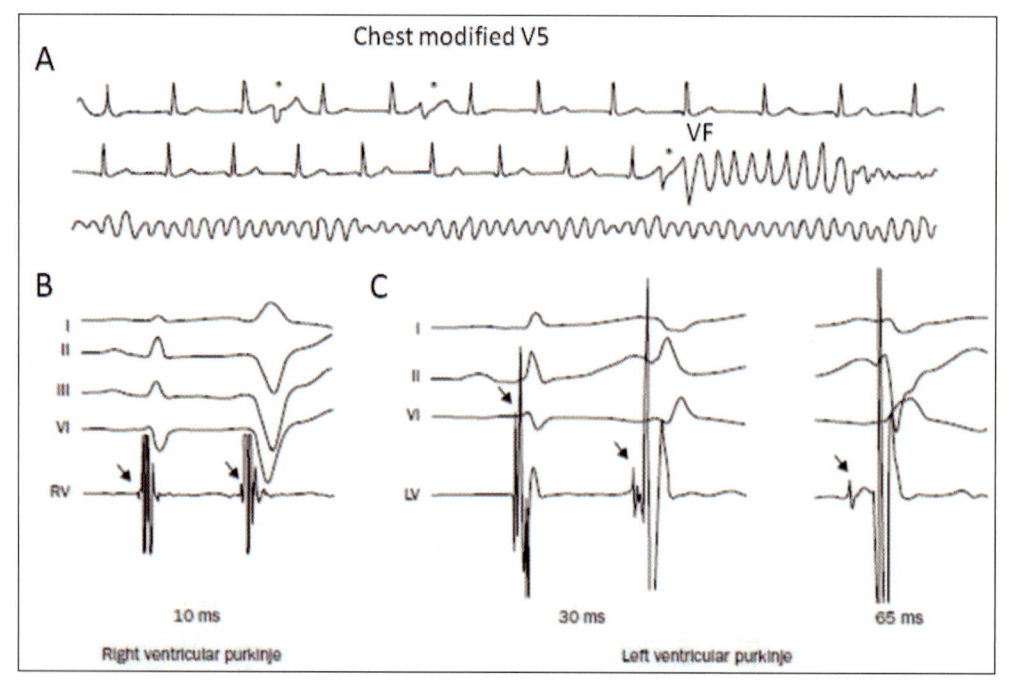

Figure 46.2 A. The initiating beat is identical to preceding isolated premature beat (*; upper). **B.** A premature beat originating from the right ventricular Purkinje system is indicated by a sharp potential (arrow), which also precedes activation during sinus rhythm. **C.** Two morphologically distinct premature beats originate from the left ventricular Purkinje system (arrow) with different conduction times to local muscle.

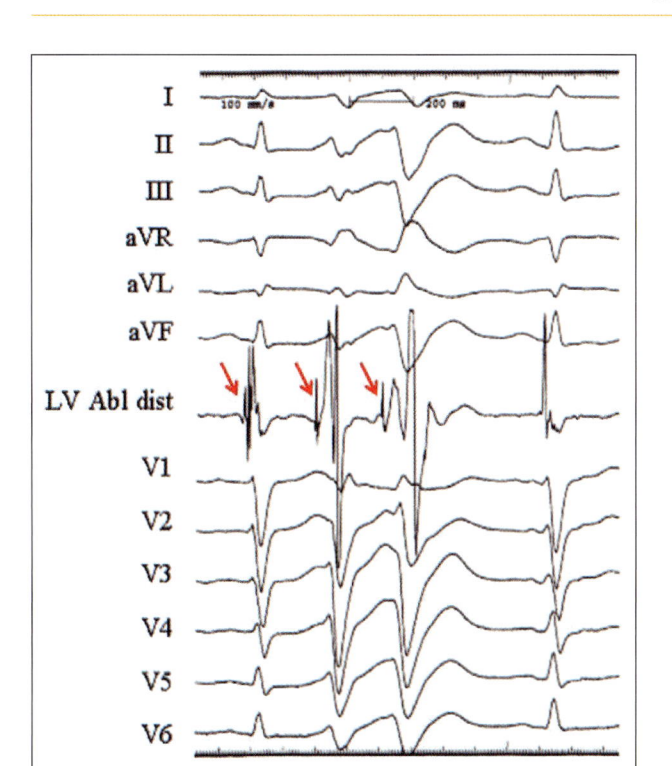

Figure 46.3 Left ventricular Purkinje-triggered couplet in a patient with idiopathic VF. Purkinje potentials are seen before each QRS, and varying conduction times between the Purkinje potential and local muscle are associated with varying QRS morphology.

Activation mapping is performed to localize the earliest EGM relative to the onset of the ectopic QRS complex in the chamber of interest, which is the target of catheter ablation. During sinus rhythm, the location of the mapping catheter on the distal Purkinje network is indicated by initial sharp potentials (< 10 ms in duration) preceding the onset of QRS complex by ≤ 15 ms, whereas longer intervals indicate proximal Purkinje fascicle activation. Fascicular block frequently occur by the application at this site (Figure 46.6). During ectopic activity, such EGMs are distinctly earlier (≥ 15 ms) from the onset of ectopic QRS suggestive of initiation of ectopy from the distal Purkinje arborisation (Figures 46.2 and 46.3). The absence of a Purkinje potential at the site of earliest ectopic/sinus beat indicates the ventricular myocardium as the origin of the ectopy. Whenever required, ectopies are induced by the use of pacing maneuvers post pauses (at twice the diastolic threshold and 2 ms of pulse width). If these measures are ineffective, pace mapping is used to identify the site of origin of clinical ectopy (appropriate targets are selected by matching at least 11 or 12 leads on the surface ECG). Note that mechanical manipulation and RF application at critical site provoke clinical ectopy frequently.

Ablation is performed using RF energy with a target temperature of 45°C and a maximum power of 30 W with an externally irrigated 3.5-mm tip-catheter. Manual titration of the saline perfusate ranging from 10 to 60 ml/min is undertaken to achieve the required power. Ablation is extended approximately 1 cm² around the target site.

thereafter. Usually, the femoral vein is punctured twice and accessed using 1 short and 1 long sheath (Preface multipurpose, Biosense-Webster or SL0, St. Jude, MN, USA). The long sheath is continuously perfused with heparinized saline. A decapolar catheter is positioned in the CS. Multipolar ablation catheters like Pentaray™ I and II are used for detailed mapping of the triggers arising from the distal Purkinje system.

Procedural Endpoint

The procedural endpoint is abolition of all clinical ventricular ectopies and unstable ventricular arrhythmias and

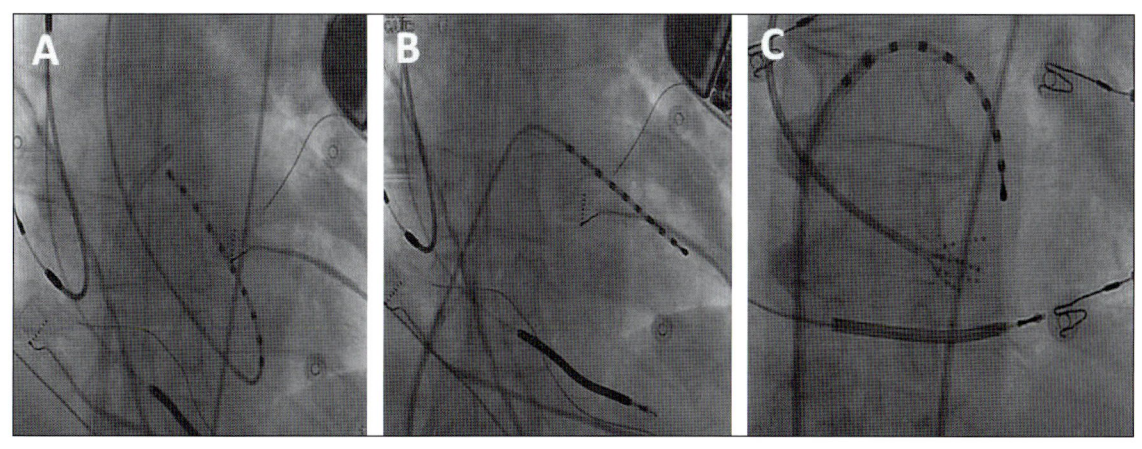

Figure 46.4 Various catheter positions for left ventricular mapping. **A.** Decapolar catheter is positioned in LV retrogradely. **B.** Decapolar catheter is positioned in LV through transseptal hole. **C.** Twenty-pole multielectrode catheter is positioned in LV retrogradely, and decapolar catheter is positioned through transseptal hole.

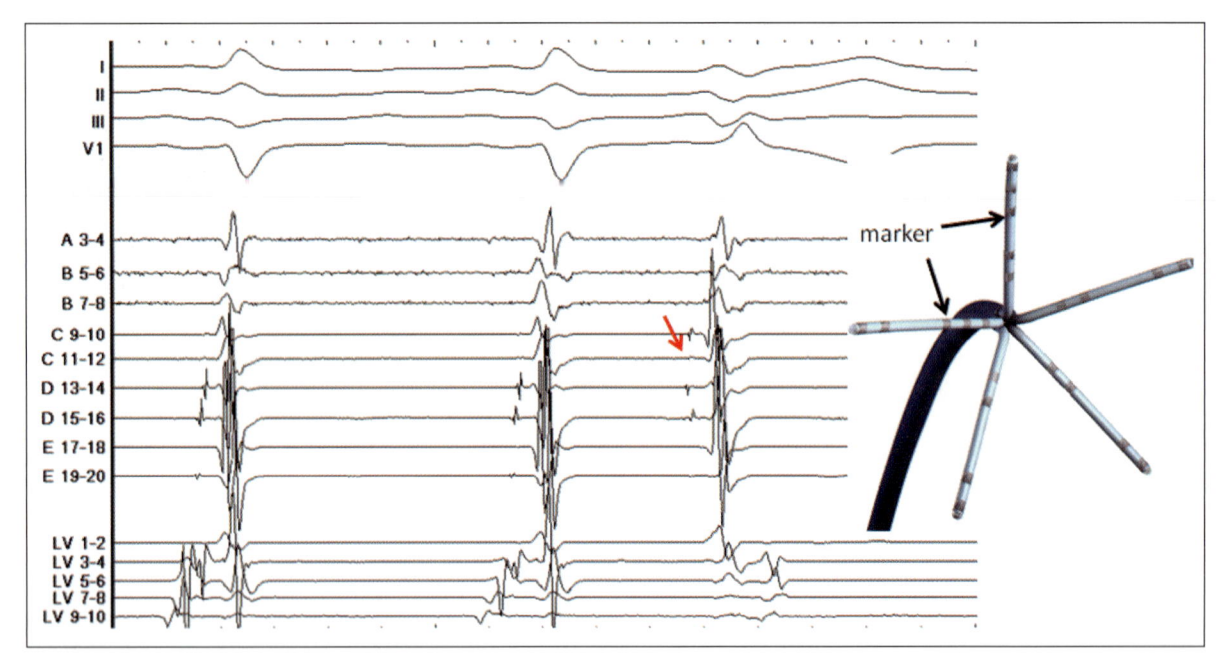

Figure 46.5 A premature beat (third beat) originating from the left ventricular Purkinje system is indicated by a sharp potential on 20-pole multielectrode catheter, which also precedes local activation during sinus rhythm (first and second beats). **Inset:** A 20-pole multispline catheter with splines A and B being recognized by radio-opaque markers (encircled). The marker on spline A is in proximity of the external 2 electrodes, and on spline B, it is in proximity of the internal 2 electrodes. (Copyright Biosense Webster, Inc. 2011. Used with permission.)

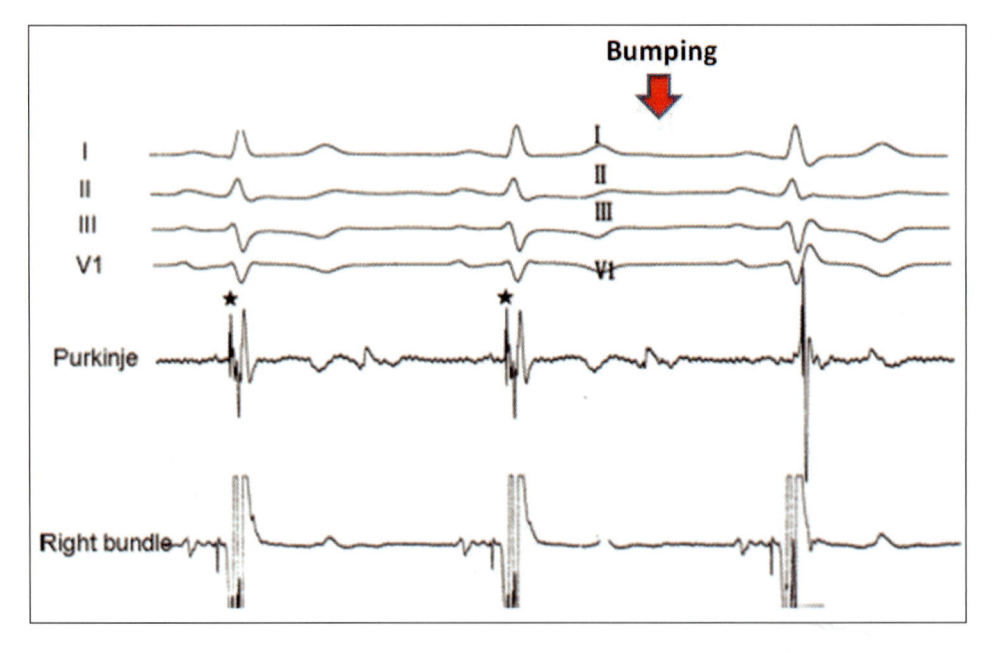

Figure 46.6 A mechanical "bumping" of the right bundle branch results in a typical right bundle branch pattern on the 12-lead ECG and the disappearance of the Purkinje potential (asterisks). Local Purkinje fiber gets activated retrogradely, and therefore the potential is obscured by the ventricular EGM.

elimination of local Purkinje potentials (**Figure 46.7**). We wait at least 30 minutes after the last energy application to ensure the attainment of procedural endpoint.

Follow-up After VF Ablation

After the procedure, patients are intensively monitored for at least 4 days in the hospital. Antiarrhythmic drugs are discontinued before ablation. At interval follow-up, clinical history, ECG, and Holter monitoring are undertaken on a regular basis to look for clinical PVCs and/or VF besides device interrogation. The ICD serves as a reliable long-term monitor besides providing a therapeutic backup after successful ablation.

Procedural and Clinical Outcome

We describe the procedural and clinical results of ablation of VF in patients with idiopathic, long QT, Brugada, and early repolarization syndromes at our center.

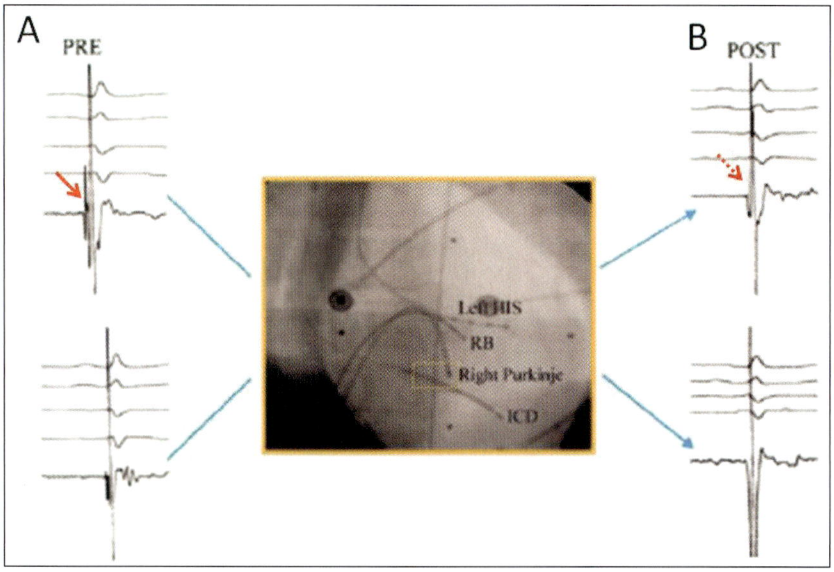

Figure 46.7 Anterior-posterior radiographic image showing the ablation area in the right ventricle as well as the location of the right bundle and left-sided His (to reduce the risk of mechanical injury to the right bundle) recordings. Right and left panels show 2 recording sites before **(A)** and after **(B)** local RF delivery in the right Purkinje network. Besides abolition of the local Purkinje potential, note the slight delay in the local ventricular EGM with regard to the QRS onset.

Idiopathic VF

Ablation of monomorphic ectopy was performed in 38 patients with idiopathic VF (Purkinje network in 33 patients and myocardium in 5).[1-3] The median duration of RF energy delivery, fluoroscopy, and total procedural time was 14 minutes, 28 minutes, and 135 minutes, respectively. Thirty patients (81%) had clinical ectopy at the time of the procedure, whereas 8 patients (19%) did not. Of 5 patients with myocardial-origin ectopies, 4 patients were successfully ablated in the RVOT. A mean of 1.7 ± 2.0 ectopic morphologies was targeted per patient. Ectopies were abolished successfully in all patients. Ablation at successful sites resulted in polymorphic VT and/or VF. After ablation, 1 patient developed transient LBBB. Six patients developed intraventricular conduction defects not meeting the established criteria for BBB. None of the patients developed any other complications.

All patients were followed for a median duration of a little over 5 years. Thirty-one patients did not have recurrence off antiarrhythmic drugs. Repeat ablation procedures were required after a median of 2 years in 5 of 7 patients with frequent VF recurrence refractory to antiarrhythmic medication. Four patients had new morphology ectopy, whereas 1 patient had the same clinical morphology of the ectopy triggering VF as previously ablated. These patients had no subsequent recurrence of VF or documented ectopies over a follow-up period of median 28 months. One of the 2 patients with VF recurrence who were not reablated responded to previously ineffective quinidine therapy. Arrhythmia resolved spontaneously in the other.

Electrical storm (3 or more separate episodes of sustained VT/VF within 24 hours, each requiring termination by an intervention) recurred in 3 of 12 patients who presented with storm before undergoing ablation. Ectopic beats recurred in 3 patients, one of whom underwent successful reablation for symptoms. In the other 2 patients, ectopies continued to persist without initiating arrhythmia on verapamil and quinidine therapy respectively.

Long QT and Brugada Syndrome

Ablation has been reported in 7 patients experiencing polymorphic VT/VF associated with long QT and Brugada syndromes.[2] The procedural and fluoroscopy durations were 169 ± 57 minutes and 42 ± 21 minutes, respectively.

Long-QT Syndrome

Ventricular ectopy initiating the arrhythmia originated in the Purkinje arborisation in 3 out of 4 patients (distal arborisation: 2, and posterior fascicle: 1). In the remaining patient, the ventricular ectopy originated from the RVOT myocardium and was successfully ablated by 6 minutes of RF application. Ablation of Purkinje ectopies was preceded by a flurry of ectopies and polymorphic VT before complete elimination of ectopic activity. Different morphologies were progressively eliminated by ablation at multiple sites using 12 to 24 minutes of RF application. Postablation, Purkinje potential was not observed preceding the local EGM. There was no evidence of block within the HPS or ventricular conduction delay on surface ECG. We have a mean follow-up of more than 4 years (unpublished data), at present. One patient died unexpectedly during sleep after 5 years of freedom from VF, syncope, or sudden death. All others have remained free from recurrent VF, syncope, or sudden cardiac death. One patient also continues to take beta blockers.

Brugada Syndrome

In 3 patients, RVOT myocardial triggers responsible for originating the arrhythmia were successfully ablated by 7 to 10 minutes of RF application. VF that was induced previously from the RVA could not be induced with up to 2 extrastimuli. No conduction disturbances were observed. After a mean period of more than 4 years of follow-up duration, all patients are free from recurrent VF, syncope, or sudden cardiac death. In one of the patients, the ECG became normal, and the Brugada pattern disappeared immediately after ablation. The ECG continues to remain normal after almost 7 years of ablation, suggestive of a potential role for ablation in both trigger and substrate abolition in Brugada syndrome.

Early Repolarization Syndrome

Ablation has been reported in 8 patients experiencing recurrent, drug-refractory VF associated with early repolarization syndrome[5] without any structural cardiac abnormality. A total of 26 ectopic patterns were mapped either to the ventricular myocardium (16 patterns) or to the Purkinje tissue (10 patterns). In 6 subjects with early repolarization recorded only in the inferior leads, all ectopic beats originated from the inferior ventricular wall. In 2 subjects with widespread early repolarization, as recorded in both inferior and lateral leads, ectopic beats originated from multiple regions.

Catheter ablation eliminated all ectopic beats in 5 subjects but failed to control them in 3 subjects. Multiple morphologies of ectopic beats and widespread presence of triggering foci in a small number of patients with early repolarization syndrome treated with catheter ablation may make catheter ablation therapy less appealing. We don't have long-term follow-up data in the patients with early repolarization syndrome who underwent VF ablation.

Conclusion

Implantation of an ICD remains the primary treatment for VF. For those patients who have multiple recurrent episodes of VF, with a limited number of triggering premature ventricular ectopic beats, RF ablation appears to be a promising therapy. Advances in technology, including new catheter designs and mapping systems, would help further improve the clinical success rate of VF ablation.

References

1. Haïssaguerre M, Shah DC, Jaïs P, et al. Role of Purkinje conducting system in triggering of idiopathic ventricular fibrillation. *Lancet.* 2002;359:677–678.
2. Haïssaguerre M, Shoda M, Jaïs P, et al. Mapping and ablation of idiopathic ventricular fibrillation. *Circulation.* 2002;106:962–967.
3. Knecht S, Sacher F, Wright M, et al. Long-term follow-up of idiopathic ventricular fibrillation ablation: a multicenter study. *J Am Coll Cardiol.* 2009;54:522–528.
4. Haïssaguerre M, Extramiana F, Hocini M, et al. Mapping and ablation of ventricular fibrillation associated with long-QT and Brugada syndromes. *Circulation.* 2003;108:925–928.
5. Haïssaguerre M, Derval N, Sacher F, et al. Sudden cardiac arrest associated with early repolarization. *N Engl J Med.* 2008;358:2016–2023.

CHAPTER 47

HOW TO ABLATE VENTRICULAR TACHYCARDIA IN PATIENTS WITH CONGENITAL HEART DISEASE

Katja Zeppenfeld, MD, PhD

Introduction

The number of patients with severe congenital heart disease (CHD) who are entering the adult population is increasing, likely due to surgical progress resulting in lower morbidity and mortality. The current estimated prevalence of adults with severe congenital heart disease is 0.38 per 1000 adults.[1] Patients at high risk for monomorphic VT are those who have undergone a ventriculotomy and patching of a ventricular septal defect (VSD) and VT after repair of tetralogy of Fallot (TOF) can serve as a paradigm for these postoperative arrhythmias. Ventricular arrhythmias can also occur in the setting of a more generalized myopathic process without discrete ventricular scars. This is typical for aortic valve disease or a failing RV after the Mustard or Senning procedure for transposition of the great arteries. These patients are at high risk for sudden cardiac death. Polymorphic VT and VF are the most common documented arrhythmias, whereas monomorphic VT suitable for catheter ablation is less common.

The feasibility of catheter ablation of VT in patients after repair of CHD has been demonstrated, and accordingly, more than 80% of all treated patients were patients after repair of TOF, with an additional 10% having undergone closure of a VSD.

After repair of TOF, the incidence of VT is 11.9% by 35 years of follow-up. The majority of these late VTs are fast and often unstable due to hemodynamic intolerance, therefore requiring a substrate-based ablation approach.[2]

Case reports and small series of intraoperative and catheter mapping have demonstrated macroreentry as the underlying mechanism of VT after repair of TOF.[3,4] We previously demonstrated that the critical reentry circuit isthmus of a significant number of these macroreentrant VTs is located within anatomically defined isthmuses bordered by unexcitable tissue.[5] Approaches that identify and target these anatomical isthmuses, containing the critical isthmus of the VT without the need for mapping during VT, have been associated with favorable results.[5,6]

Preprocedural Planning

Step 1: Knowledge of the Malformation and Review of Operation Records

The potential anatomic isthmuses containing critical parts of the reentry circuit are determined by the malformation and the type of surgical repair. Knowledge of the anatomy and the type of repair is therefore mandatory. We usually make a big effort to obtain all operation records, which are then carefully reviewed. It might be helpful to discuss unclear cases with a surgeon experienced in repair of congenital heart disease or a colleague specialized in grown-up congenital heart disease (GUCH) patients.

The most common underlying disease, TOF, is characterized by a subpulmonary stenosis, a VSD, a dextroposed and overriding aortic orifice, often associated with a clockwise rotation (viewed from the apex) of the aorta resulting in a leftwards displacement of the RCC, and RV hypertrophy. However, it is important to keep in mind that the malformation represents a morphologic spectrum. Reparative surgery involves closing of the VSD, which is subaortic and perimembranous in the majority of TOF patients. The posterior-inferior border of the VSD in these cases is made up of the mitral-tricuspid fibrous continuity, thus unexcitable tissue (**Figure 47.1A**). In a minority, the defect has a muscular postero-inferior rim (**Figure 47.1B**). The RVOT obstruction is typically due to an infundibular or subpulmonary stenosis caused by (1) anterior displacement of the outlet septum and (2) hypertrophy of septoparietal trabeculations (anterior) and/or of the trabecula septomarginalis, which requires sometimes extensive resection of the hypertrophied myocardium (**Figure 47.1A**). A stenosis of the pulmonary orifice, often accompanied by valvular abnormalities, can be relieved by a transannular patch, which disrupts the integrity of the pulmonary valve annulus (**Figure 47.2A**). Rarely, the stenosis is exclusively infundibular with a pulmonary orifice of normal size. In these cases a RVOT patch might be necessary to augment the restrictive RVOT, sparing the pulmonary valve annulus (**Figure 47.2B**).

Until 1993, repair was often performed through a right longitudinal (majority) or transverse ventriculotomy. Since then, a combined approach through the RA and the pulmonary artery is used, thereby avoiding a RVOT incision, which can serve as a potential boundary of an anatomical isthmus. A limited RV incision is added, if patch augmentation for the RVOT or pulmonary annulus is needed.

Based on the detailed information on the malformation and the performed reparative surgery, the anatomical boundaries consisting of unexcitable tissue can be predicted; these include the tricuspid annulus, the pulmonary valve, patch material, and surgical incisions. The 4 potential anatomical isthmuses include the isthmus between (1) tricuspid annulus and scar/patch in the anterior RV outflow; (2) pulmonary annulus and the RV free wall scar/patch; (3) pulmonary annulus and septal scar/patch; and (4) septal scar/patch and tricuspid annulus (**Figure 47.3**).

Step 2: Evaluation of the Status of the Patient and Assessment of Residual Lesions

As in other patients with structural heart disease who present with VT, a complete workup of the patient is important. This should be performed in specialized GUCH centers. In particular, significant pulmonary

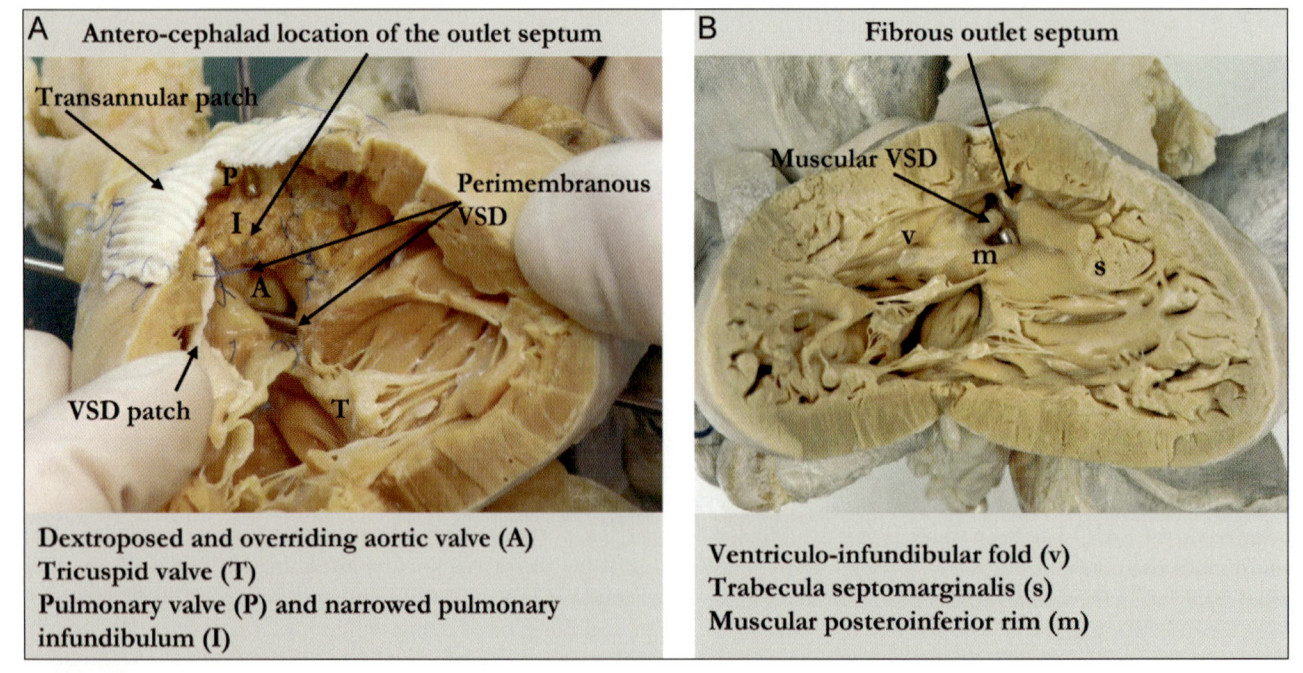

Figure 47.1 Postmortem specimens with tetralogy of Fallot (TOF), view from the RVA. **A.** Specimen with previous repair of TOF consisting of a transannular patch and patch closure (folded back) of a perimembranous ventricular septal defect (VSD). **B.** Specimen with TOF consisting of a muscular VSD (the ventriculo-infundibular fold is in muscular continuity with the trabecular septomarginalis) and an extreme displacement of a fibrous outlet septum almost obliterating the pulmonary infundibulum (modified from Zeppenfeld et al. VT/VF Summit SCA: The Present and the Future, Heart Rhythm Society, 2008).

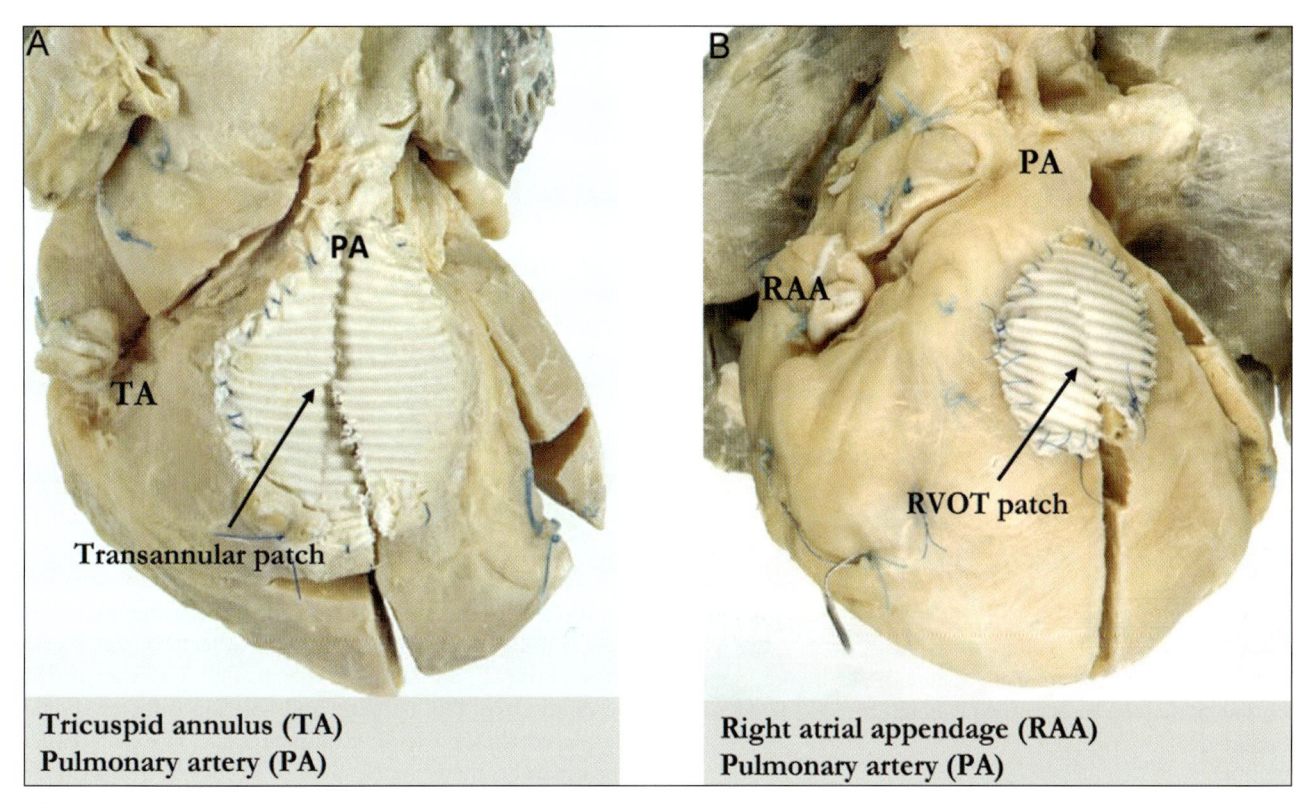

Chapter 47: Ablation of VT in Congenital Heart Disease Patients • 437

Figure 47.2 Anterior view of 2 specimens after repair of TOF. **A.** Large transannular patch that disrupts the integrity of the pulmonary valve annulus. **B.** RVOT patch to augment the restrictive RVOT sparing the pulmonary valve annulus (modified from Zeppenfeld et al. VT/VF Summit SCA: The Present and the Future, Heart Rhythm Society, 2008).

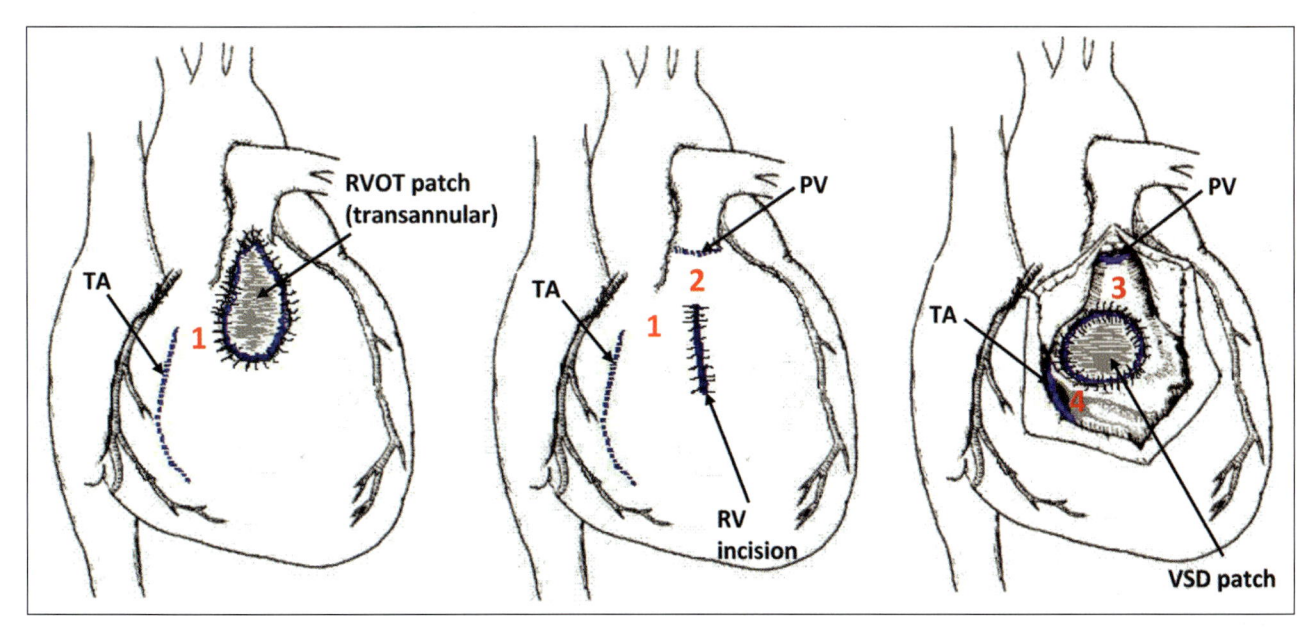

Figure 47.3 Schematic of the localization of anatomical boundaries (blue lines) and the resulting anatomical isthmuses (number 1 to 4). TA = tricuspid annulus; RVOT = right ventricular outflow tract; PV = pulmonary valve; VSD = ventricular septal defect (modified from Zeppenfeld et al.[5]).

regurgitation, which nearly always occurs after transannular patching with subsequent RV enlargement, is a common finding (**Figure 47.4**, ▶ **Video 47.1**). It is also important to look for residual RVOT obstruction and a residual VSD, which may lead to RV pressure overload and LV volume overload, respectively (**Figure 47.5**, ▶ **Video 47.2**). These patients may require surgery. Although pulmonary regurgitation is associated with occurrence of VT, simply replacing the pulmonary valve does not appear to eliminate the underlying VT substrate. Therefore, intraoperative ablation should be considered in close cooperation between congenital cardiologist, congenital surgeon, and electrophysiologist.

All patients should undergo cardiac imaging prior to ablation. Although echocardiography is usually helpful, MRI is currently the reference standard to evaluate associated pathology such as branch pulmonary artery stenosis or hypoplasia. Assessment of RV and LV function before ablation helps to identify patients in whom prolonged mapping during VT should be avoided, even if the VT seems to be hemodynamically tolerated. Finally, additional cardiac pathology such as CAD should be considered and excluded.

Step 3: Review of the 12-Lead ECG of the Clinical VT

As in other scar-related VT, the morphology of the 12-lead VT QRS is determined by the VT exit site. However, it is important to keep in mind that each anatomical isthmus can be activated clockwise or counterclockwise, resulting in a different QRS morphology. In some patients, 2 VTs are documented that are morphologically different but share the same anatomical isthmus (**Figure 47.6**). In these cases, the VT cycle length is often similar or even identical. The precordial transition is usually earlier (eg, V_2), and a QR in V_1 is typically present in counterclockwise reentry VTs that use isthmus 3 bordering high on the septum. However, VTs with clockwise wave front propagation through the same isthmus might have a LBBB-like morphology with a late transition (eg, V_5).

In addition, in the increasing number of patients who have received an ICD for primary or secondary prevention, information on the clinical VT is often restricted to EGM data available from ICD interrogation.

Procedure

Patient Preparation

We usually perform the procedure in conscious sedation achieved with fentanyl and midazolam. The right femoral vein is punctured at least twice and accommodates 1 or 2 sheaths of 6 Fr and an 8-Fr sheath. The 8-Fr sheath that accommodates the mapping and ablation catheter should be placed through its own puncture site to enable easier sheath and catheter manipulation. The 8-Fr sheath can be later replaced with a long sheath. We prefer a long sheath (Swartz™ Braided Transseptal Guiding Introducer [SR-0], St. Jude Medical, St. Paul, MN) for catheter stability in the majority of patients; in patients with severe RV enlargement and/or RVOT aneurysms, we use steerable sheaths (Agilis™ NxT Steerable Introducer, St. Jude Medical, St. Paul, MN) (**Figure 47.7**).

We use a 5-Fr sheath placed in the right femoral artery for hemodynamic monitoring. This sheath can be easily replaced by an 8-Fr sheath if a retrograde aortic approach becomes necessary. After vascular access a heparin bolus of

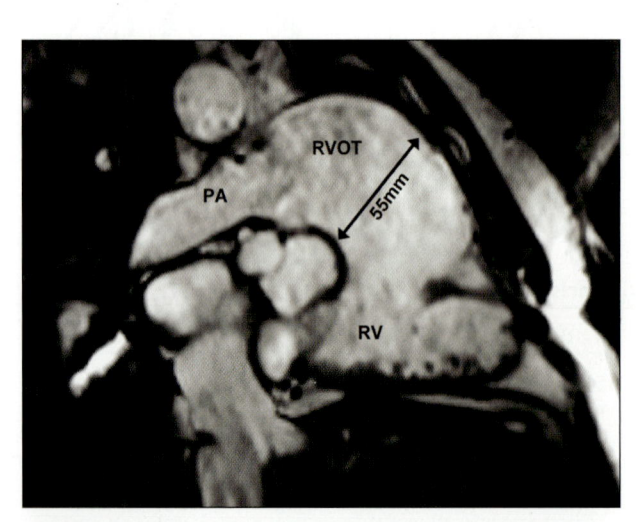

Figure 47.4 MRI, oblique view. Aneurysmatic dilatation (arrow indicates the maximal diameter) of the RVOT due to a prior transannular patch; PA = pulmonary artery, RV = right ventricle. (Courtesy H.M. Siebelink, LUMC, Leiden, the Netherlands.)

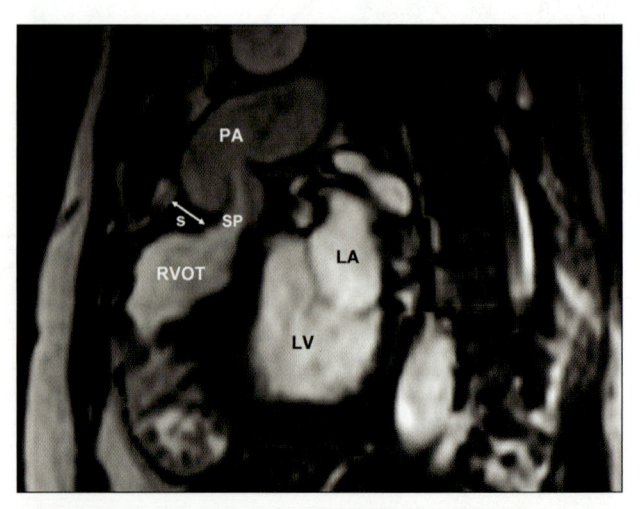

Figure 47.5 MRI, oblique view. Subpulmonary stenosis (SP) mainly due to the severe hypertrophy of septoparietal trabeculations (S); PA = pulmonary artery, LA = left atrium, LV = left ventricle, RVOT = right ventricular outflow tract. (Courtesy H.M. Siebelink, LUMC, Leiden, the Netherlands.)

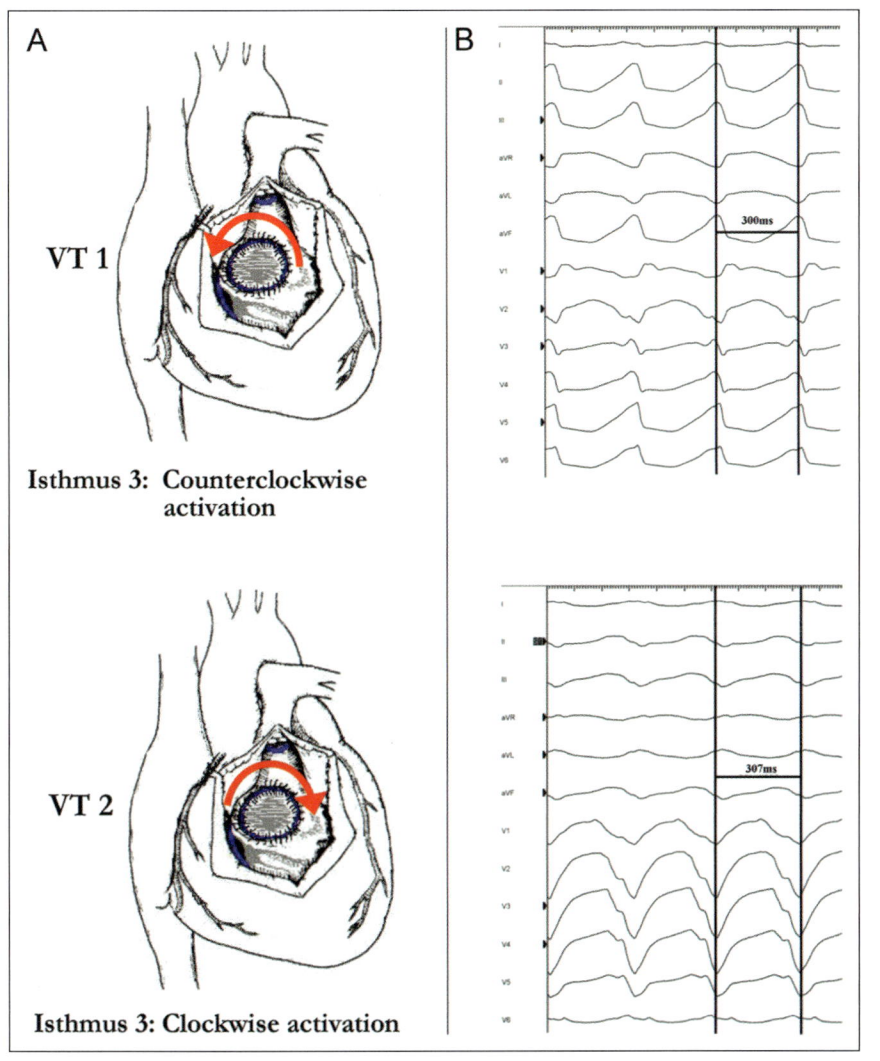

Chapter 47: Ablation of VT in Congenital Heart Disease Patients • 439

Figure 47.6 A. Schematic of counterclockwise and clockwise propagation through isthmus 3 (viewed from anterior) bordered by a VSD patch and the pulmonary valve during ventricular tachycardia. **B.** Twelve-lead surface ECGs of the documented and induced VTs. Counterclockwise propagation during macroreentrant VT results in VT morphology 1 (CLs 300 ms, QR in precordial lead V_1, transition in precordial lead V_3); clockwise propagation results in VT morphology 2 (similar cycle lengths, left-bundle-block-like morphology in V_1, transition in V_6).

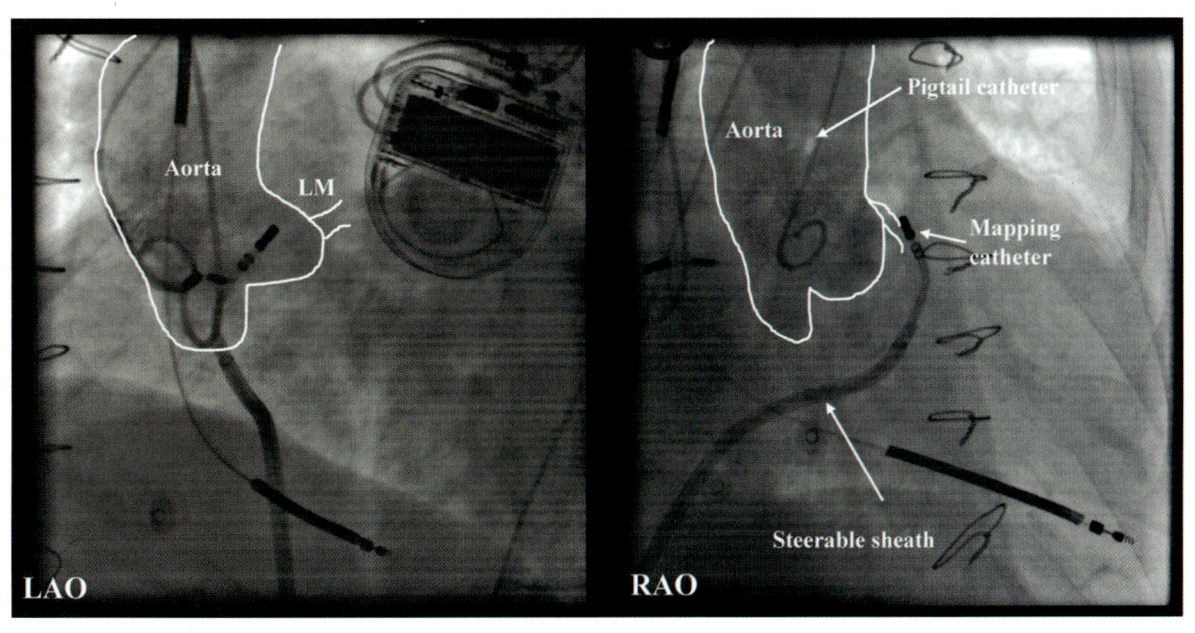

Figure 47.7 Typical biplane fluoroscopic views: LAO, 45° and RAO, 35°. A pigtail catheter is placed in the aortic root, and contrast is injected to visualize the position of the left main in close relationship to the mapping catheter in the posteroseptal aspect of the RVOT, inserted through a steerable introducer. Note the dextroposition of the aortic root.

100 U/kg is given. An additional bolus of 50 U/kg is given to achieve an ACT of 250 to 300 seconds, which is checked every 30 minutes. Standard 4-polar catheters are positioned in the HRA and in the RV for VT induction. For mapping and ablation, we usually use a 3.5-mm irrigated-tip quadripolar mapping catheter with an F-curve (2-5-2 mm interelectrode spacing, Navistar ThermoCool, Biosense Webster Inc, Diamond Bar, CA).

First Step: VT Induction

The first step in each case is VT induction to obtain the 12-lead VT QRS morphology. We use a standard programmed stimulation protocol with 3 drive-cycle lengths (600, 500, and 400 ms) at no fewer than 2 RV sites, including one high septal site and up to 3 extrastimuli. We also use incremental burst pacing and repeat the stimulation protocol following isoprotenerol (2–8 mcg/min) infusion if necessary. Even if hemodynamically tolerated we immediately terminate the VT and proceed with substrate mapping.

Twelve-lead surface ECGs and intracardiac EGMs are recorded simultaneously with a 48-channel acquisition system (Cardio-Lab 4.1; Prucka Engineering, Houston, TX). The 12-lead QRS template of the induced VT is displayed in the second review window of the electrophysiological recording system to allow for immediate comparison of the VT QRS morphology with the paced QRS morphology during substrate mapping.

Second Step: Substrate Mapping

We always perform electroanatomical bipolar voltage and activation mapping using a 3-dimensional nonfluoroscopic mapping system (CARTO XPTM, Biosense Webster, Inc.) during sinus rhythm or RV pacing to obtain a 3-dimensional reconstruction of all potential VT isthmuses by identifying the anatomic boundaries. During mapping, the RV catheter is withdrawn from the RV, and the maximum positive or negative peak deflection of a surface QRS complex is used as a reference. The onset of the window of interest is usually set before or at the onset of the QRS complex, and its duration should extend beyond the QRS duration to allow for annotation of local EGMs occurring late after the QRS complex.

Peak-to-peak bipolar EGM amplitudes recorded from the distal electrode pair of the mapping catheter (filtered at 30–400 Hz) are displayed color-coded with EGMs greater than 1.5 mV defined as normal voltage and displayed in purple.[7] We do not define unexcitable tissue by voltage criteria, but use EGMs with amplitudes of less than 0.5 mV, which are displayed in red, as a rough road map for pacing. At these sites we perform bipolar pacing with 10 mA at 2-ms pulse widths. Although bipolar pacing has the potential drawback of anodal capture, the safety settings of the CARTO™ system do not allow easily unipolar pacing from the ablation catheter. If pacing does not capture, the site is tagged as scar or unexcitable tissue likely consistent with an anatomic boundary, and these sites are displayed as gray tags on the map.[8] If pacing captures, we can at the same time compare the paced QRS morphology with the VT QRS morphology.

We define tricuspid annulus sites by atrial and ventricular EGMs of approximately equal amplitudes (**Figure 47.8**). The pulmonary valve is identified by advancing the catheter in the pulmonary artery and withdrawing the catheter until we obtain the first RV EGM. It is also helpful to annotate the position of the His bundle to assess the spatial relationship with the anatomical isthmuses, in particular if isthmus 4 bordered by the tricuspid annulus and the VSD patch is targeted.

All maps are carefully reviewed to avoid annotation sites without wall contact (internal points) and after or during a spontaneous or catheter-induced PVC. **Figure 47.9** and ▶ **Video 47.3** give examples of the 3-dimensional reconstruction of the anatomical isthmuses. During the review process local activation time is set at the first sharp positive or negative peak deflection of the bipolar EGM. Double potentials, defined as EGMs separated by an isoelectric period, may be indicative for an area of conduction block and are tagged on the map. In case of local conduction block, for example, due to a surgical incision, adjacent normal voltage EGMs with slightly earlier local activation time are usually present. Late potentials, defined as EGMs recorded after the QRS and fragmented EGMs consistent with slow conduction, are also indicated on the map, and at these sites pace mapping is performed. Of importance, characteristics of the isthmuses, such as isthmus widths and evidence of slow conduction during sinus rhythm, vary between anatomic isthmuses and patients. Narrow isthmuses with slow conduction during sinus rhythm may be more likely to contain critical reentry circuit isthmus sites and require shorter ablation lines.

Third Step: Identification and Ablation of Reentry Circuit Isthmus Sites

After the reconstruction of the anatomic substrate we try to identify the location of the critical reentry circuit isthmus of the induced VT(s). We usually start detailed pace mapping at narrow isthmuses with slow conduction during sinus rhythm. For unstable VTs, reentry circuit isthmuses within an already identified anatomic isthmus are defined by pace mapping as a site where the QRS morphology matches that of the VT with an S-QRS of more than 40 ms.[9] If we move the catheter in the direction of the assumed VT exit site, we expect a decrease in stimulus-to-QRS interval, but the same paced QRS morphology (**Figure 47.10**). However, it is important to recognize that a pace map that does not resemble VT does not necessarily indicate that the site is remote from the reentry circuit. In some patients isthmuses are short, and therefore small movements of the catheter may result in completely different paced morphologies due to the change in exit sites, and the S-QRS interval might be sometimes shorter than 40 ms. During pacing, wave fronts also might emerge from the scar at different locations producing a different QRS morphology than during VT (**Figure 47.11**).

If VT is briefly tolerated, we terminate the VT and perform pace mapping as in untolerated VT. We then move the catheter to the presumed isthmus site, and we reinduce the VT to confirm the position within the circuit either by entrainment mapping or by termination during RF delivery (**Figure 47.12**).

In stable or briefly tolerated VTs, reentry circuit isthmus sites are defined by entrainment mapping with a difference between the VTCL and the PPI of less than 30 ms and a stimulus-to-QRS interval of less than 70% of VTCL or as site with diastolic activity during VT and termination and prevention of reinduction by RF energy application.

RF energy application with the open irrigated-tip catheter is usually set to deliver from 20 to 45 W, with a flow rate of 20 ml/min up to 30 ml/min, targeting a maximum temperature of 43°C and an impedance fall of 10 to 15 ohms. Power depends on the ablation target area and should be set with caution when ablation is performed at free wall sites in aneursymatic dilated RVOT. In contrast, the infundibular septum can be very thick requiring deeper lesions and high-power settings.

If VT terminates or slows during RF application within an anatomical isthmus, we connect the anatomic boundaries during sinus rhythm by a linear lesion until we have reached the endpoint of ablation.

Fourth Step: Endpoint of Ablation

No Capture Along the Line

The first endpoint for a linear lesion connecting 2 anatomical boundaries is no capture along the ablation line. We start at 1 anatomical boundary, and we slightly draw the catheter back and perform pacing with high output

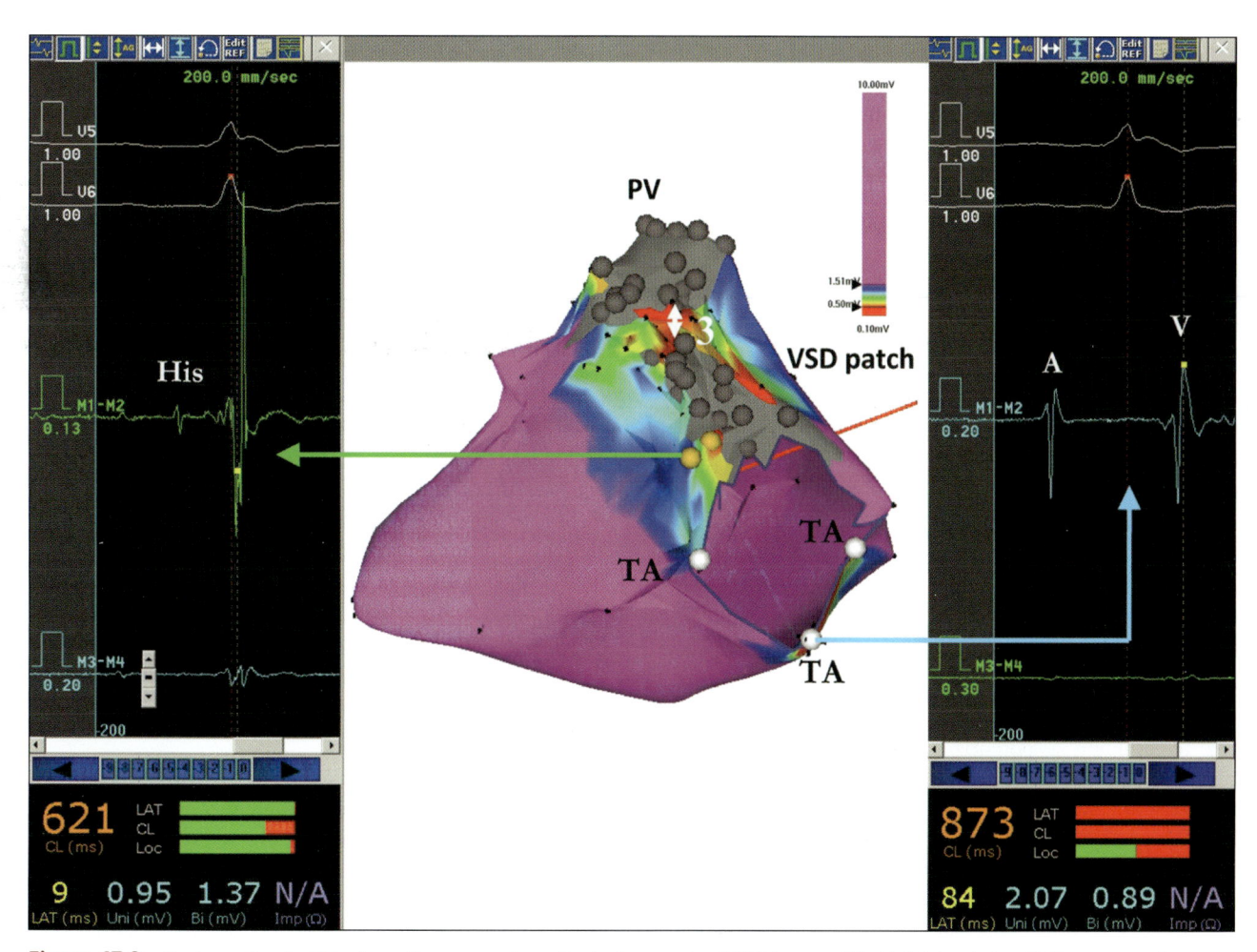

Figure 47.8 Electroanatomical bipolar voltage map of a patient after repair of TOF in a modified left lateral view. Voltages are color coded according to the color bar. Gray areas indicate unexcitable tissue. Yellow tags indicate sites with recording of a His bundle EGM (left panel); white tags indicate sites with recording of an atrial and ventricular EGM of approximately equal amplitude, typical for tricuspid annulus sites (right panel). The anatomical isthmus 3 is bordered by the pulmonary valve and the VSD patch.

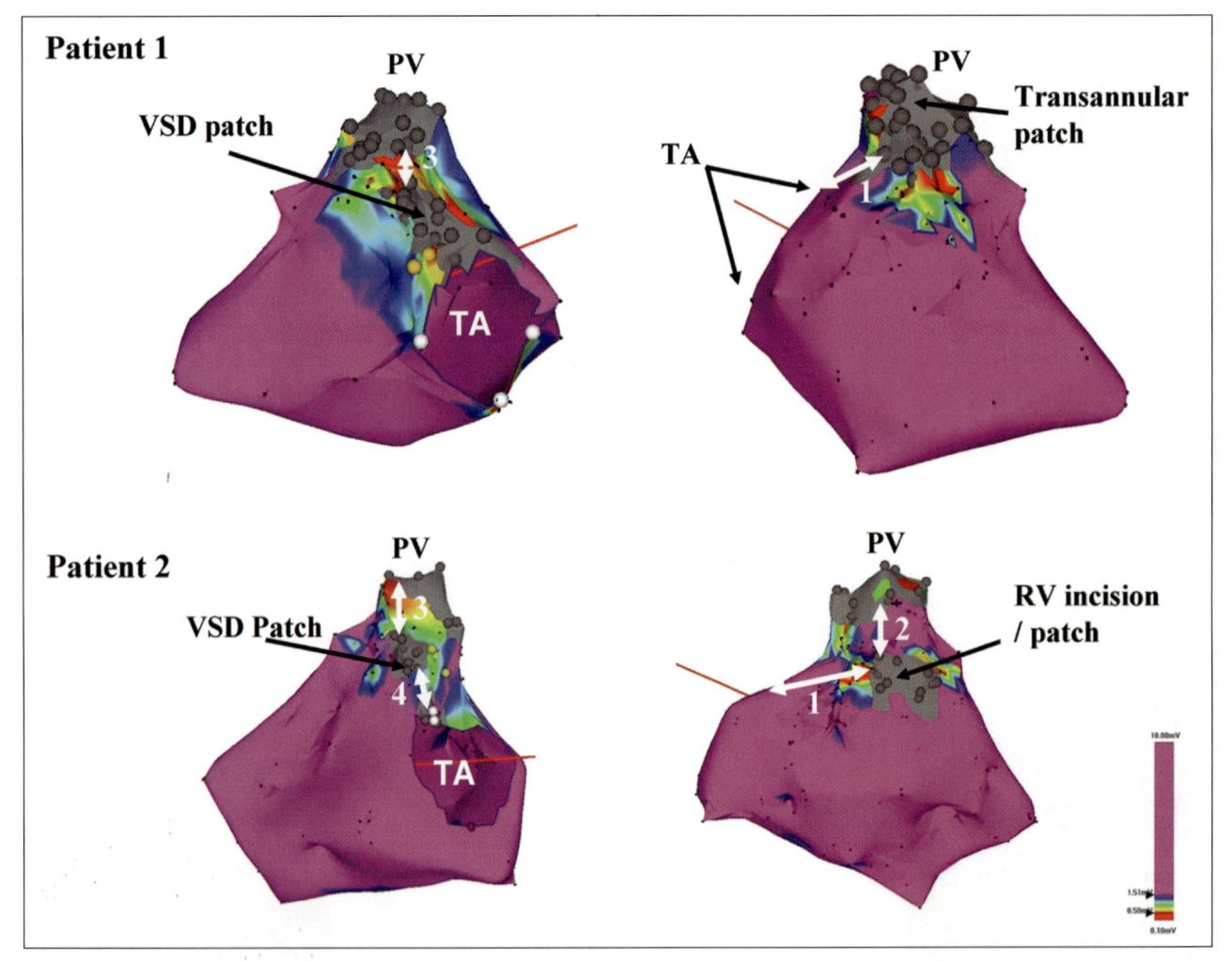

Figure 47.9 Bipolar electroanatomical voltage maps in a modified left lateral view (left) and an anterior view (right) of 2 patients after repair of TOF. Voltages are color coded according to the color bar. Gray areas indicate sites where high-output pacing did not capture. Identified anatomical isthmuses include: Isthmus 1 is between the anterior RV incision or the transannular patch and the tricuspid annulus; isthmus 2 is between the pulmonary valve and the RV incision or patch; isthmus 3 is between the pulmonary valve and the VSD patch; isthmus 4 is between the VSD patch and the tricuspid annulus. Patient 1 had only isthmus 1 and 3; while patient 2 had isthmus 1, 2, 3, and 4.

(10 mA, 2 ms) at each site until we have reached the second anatomical boundary.

Change in Local Activation Sequence

We then perform limited reactivation mapping on both sides of the ablation line during sinus rhythm or RVA pacing to evaluate a potential change in the activation sequence on both sides of the line. With complete block along the line, wave front propagation during sinus rhythm or RVA pacing should be directed toward the transected isthmus on both sides of the line. This is particularly helpful, if we have demonstrated continuous activation through the isthmus prior to ablation (**Figure 47.13**). However, propagation toward the isthmus may be observed before ablation if 2 activation wave fronts originating close to the septum during sinus rhythm or the RVA during pacing propagate in the same direction reaching the line at the same or similar time (**Video 47.4**). Furthermore, even if a change in the activation sequence after ablation is observed, this unfortunately does not prove conduction block but may also occur if ablation has resulted in further conduction delay through the isthmus.

Differential Pacing

In selected patients, we try to perform differential pacing to test for conduction block along the RF line. This is similar to the testing performed after ablation for cavotricuspid isthmus or mitral isthmus dependent flutter. For this purpose we use a 6-Fr 4-polar steerable catheter for pacing. The mapping catheter is first positioned on 1 side and adjacent to the ablation line. This site is tagged on the map, and we then place the 6-Fr catheter in that same position guided by fluoroscopy (pacing site 1 on **Figure 47.14**). From the 6-Fr catheter, pacing is then

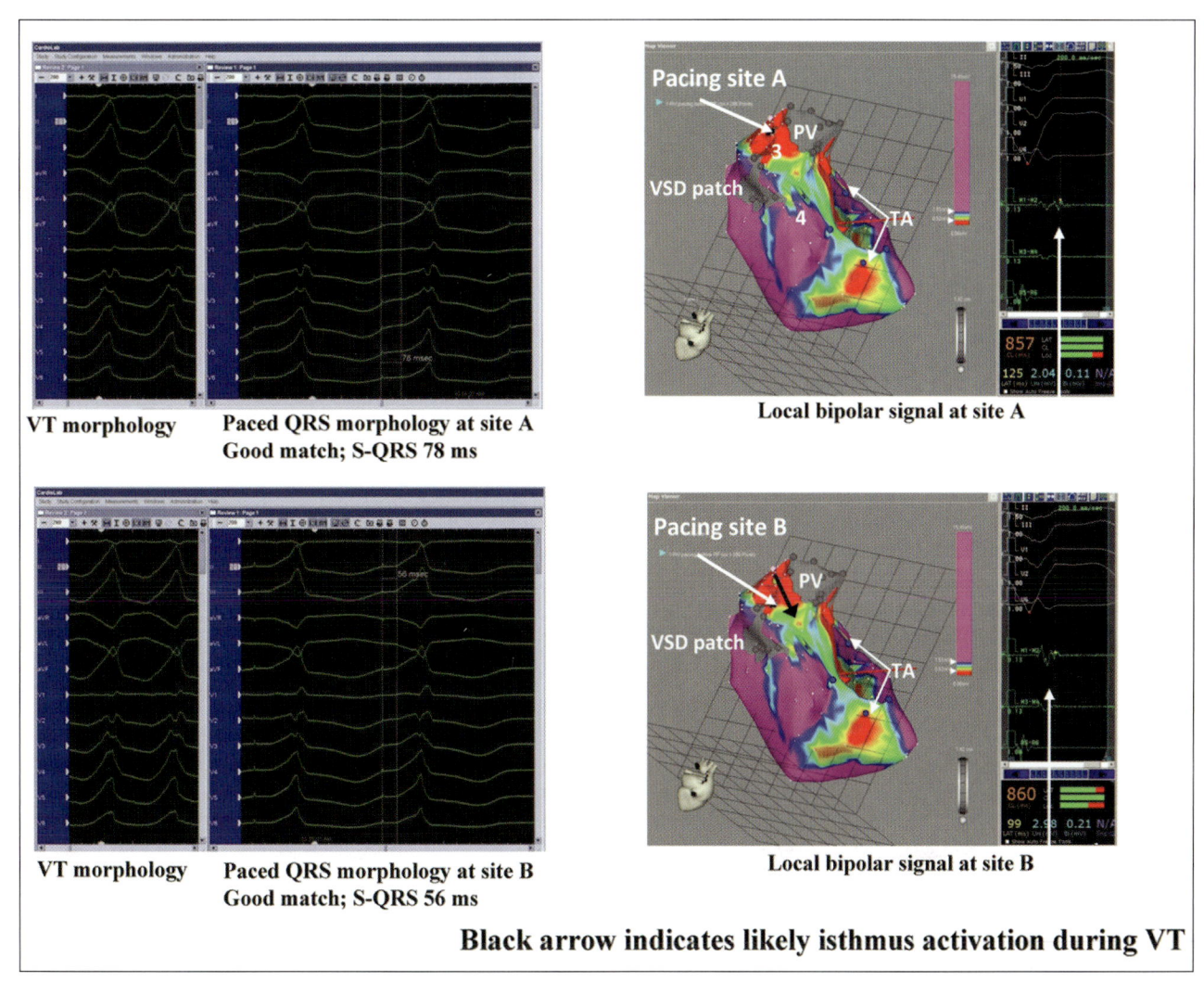

Figure 47.10 The template of the 12-lead VT morphology allows for comparison with the paced QRS morphology. Electroanatomical voltage map in a modified left lateral view of a patient after repair of TOF showed anatomical isthmus 3 (bordered by the pulmonary valve and the VSD patch) and isthmus 4 (bordered by the VSD patch and the tricuspid annulus [indicated by blue tags]). Pace mapping was started at pacing site A with a 12-lead pace-match of the VT and a stimulus-to-QRS (S-QRS) of 78 ms. Pacing at site B resulted in an identical pace map with a decrease of the S-QRS interval to 57 ms suggesting that during VT isthmus 3 is activated counterclockwise (viewed from anterior). (Figure is modified from Zeppenfeld et al. VT/VF Summit SCA: The Present and the Future, Heart Rhythm Society, 2008.)

performed with a CL of 600 ms. The resulting stimulus-to-EGM interval is measured on both sides of the ablation line as recorded with the mapping catheter. The mapping catheter is then placed at a second site (pacing site 2) with a distance of 1 to 2 cm from the first site, which can be confirmed by tagging the position on the map, and the 6-Fr steerable pacing catheter is brought to that position. Pacing from this position is performed, and the stimulus-to-EGM interval is again measured on both sides of the ablation line (**Figure 47.15**). In case of unidirectional conduction block, the stimulus-to-EGM interval should be longer at the pacing site adjacent to the line (pacing site 1), and shorter when pacing is performed further away to the line (pacing site 2). The same maneuver is then performed from the other side of the ablation line.

However, it is important to realize that conduction delay across the isthmus might be significantly longer than activation from the other direction, thereby mimicking conduction block.

Noninducibility of Any Monomorphic VT

In our experience, the reproducibility of VT induction in patients after repair of CHD who present with VT is very high. This is in line with prior data showing that only 16% of patients who had documented sustained VT were not inducible by programmed stimulation.[10] Of importance, patients who are rendered noninducible for any VT after ablation have a low risk for VT recurrence during follow-up.[5,6] In addition, induction of sustained VT was a powerful predictor of VT recurrence in a large multicenter

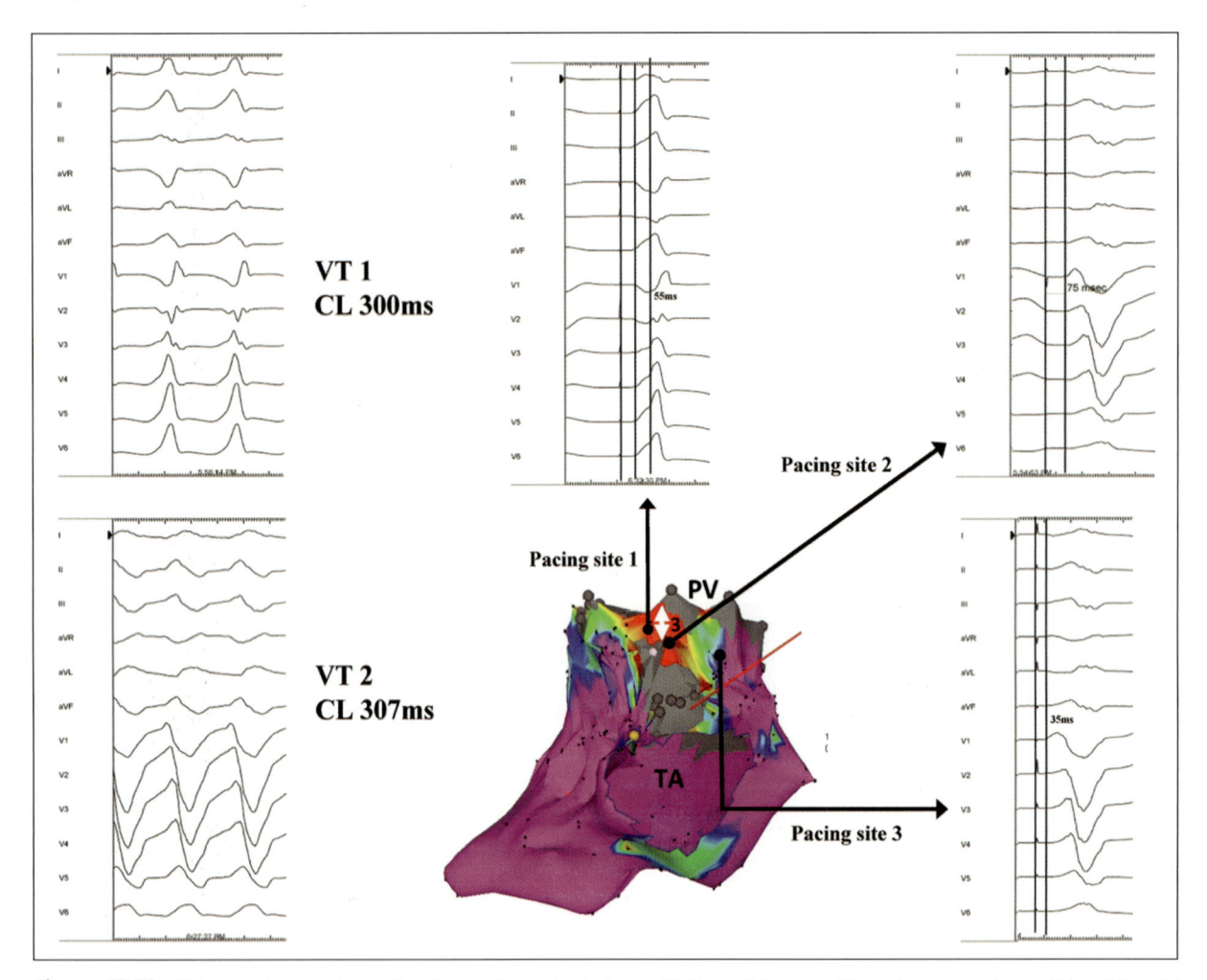

Figure 47.11 Two ventricular tachycardias sharing the same anatomical isthmus 3 between the pulmonary valve and the VSD patch (see Figure 47.4). Pacing sites during sinus rhythm are indicated on the electroanatomical voltage map shown in a modified left lateral view. Pacing at site 1 results in a poor pace map for VT 1 with a stimulus-to-QRS (S-QRS) interval of 55 ms, although entrainment mapping confirmed that during VT 1, site 1 was a central isthmus site. This finding suggests that during pacing the wave front emerges from different sites than during VT. Moving the catheter slightly toward the free wall (pacing site 2) results in a good pace map for VT 2 with an S-QRS of 75 ms. Further catheter movement to site 3 results in a similar paced morphology with a decrease in S-QRS. TA = tricuspid annulus.

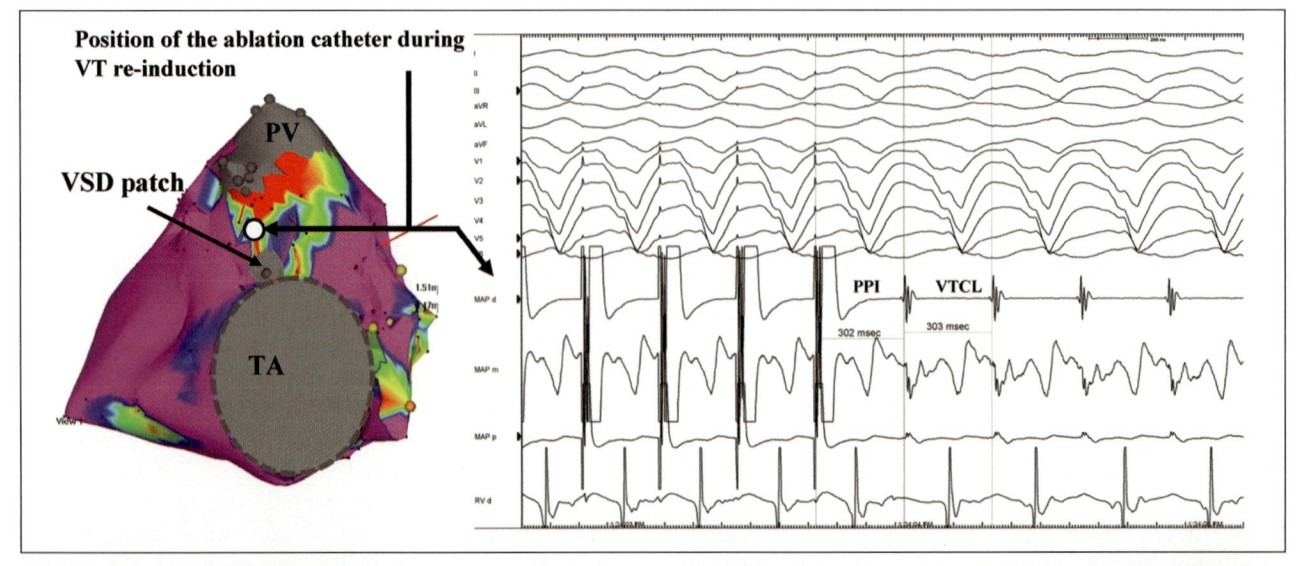

Figure 47.12 The ablation catheter is moved to a pace-match site (indicated by the white tag) within anatomical isthmus 3 bordered by a small VSD patch and the pulmonary valve. With the catheter in place, VT was reinduced and entrainment mapping performed. Pacing entrained the VT with concealed fusion and the PPI = VTCL.

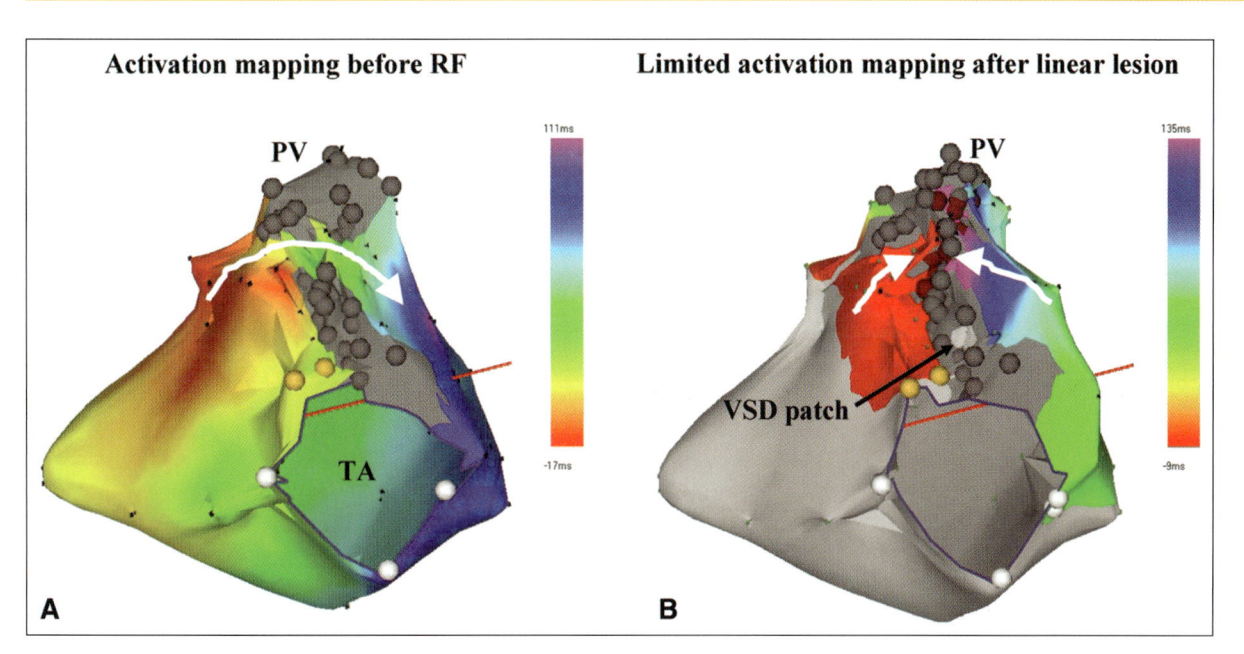

Figure 47.13 Electroanatomical activation maps during sinus rhythm before (**A**) and after (**B**) a linear ablation lesion connecting the pulmonary valve (PV) with the ventricular septal defect (VSD) patch. Red tags indicate radiofrequency (RF) ablation sites. Gray tags indicate sites that did not capture at high-output pacing. Note that after ablation no capture along the line was observed. Before ablation counterclockwise (from an anterior view) propagation through the isthmus was observed from the septal to the free wall site during sinus rhythm. After the linear RF lesion, wave front propagation was directed toward the transected isthmus at the septal and the free wall site.

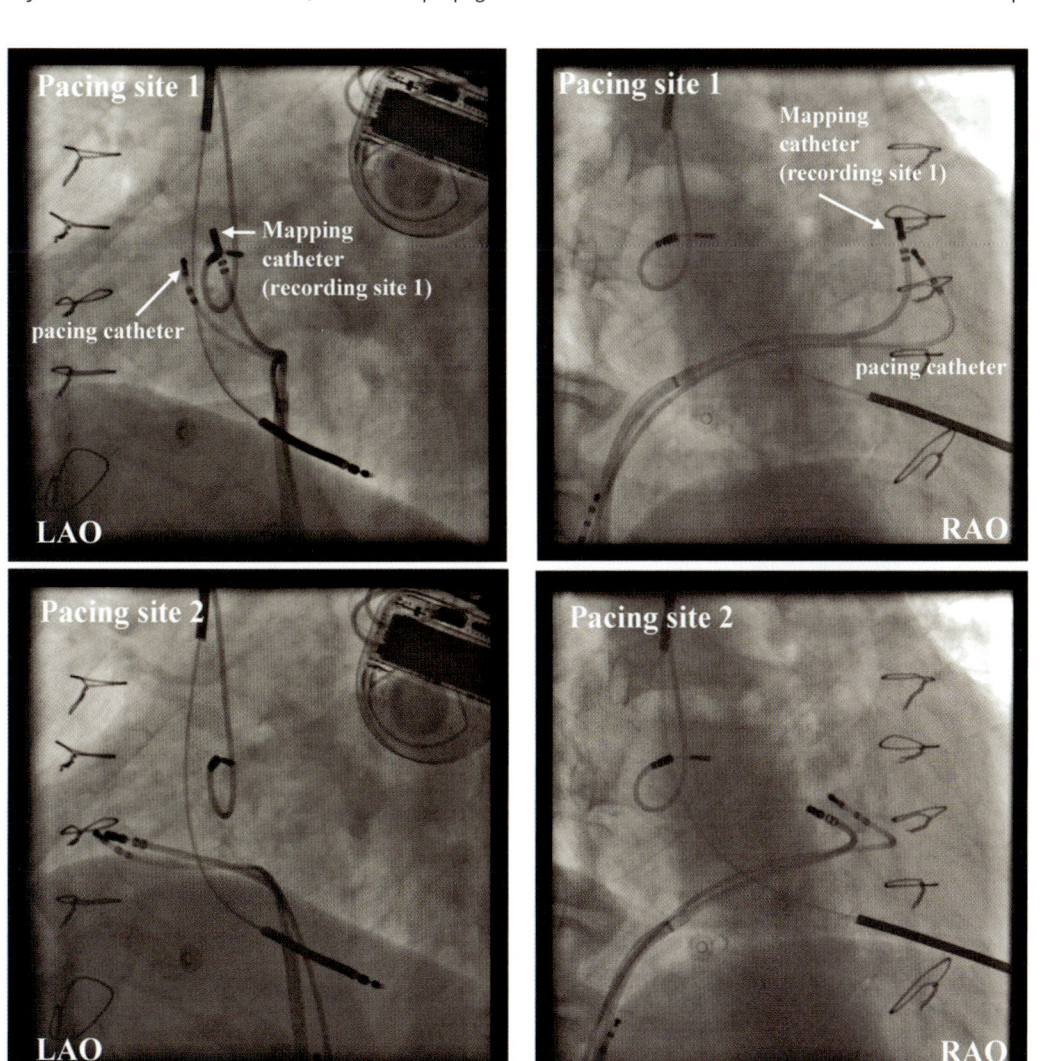

Figure 47.14 Fluoroscopic LAO and RAO views during differential pacing at the free wall site of isthmus 3 (see also Figure 47.13). First, the mapping catheter is placed close to the ablation line, and the position is tagged on the map. The pacing catheter is then brought in the same position (pacing site 1), and the stimulus-to-EGM interval recorded from the mapping catheter is measured at both sites of the ablation line. Second, the mapping catheter is moved away from the ablation line to position 2, the site is tagged on the map, and the pacing catheter is positioned at site 2. During pacing from site 2 the stimulus-to-EGM interval is measured at both sites of the line (not shown).

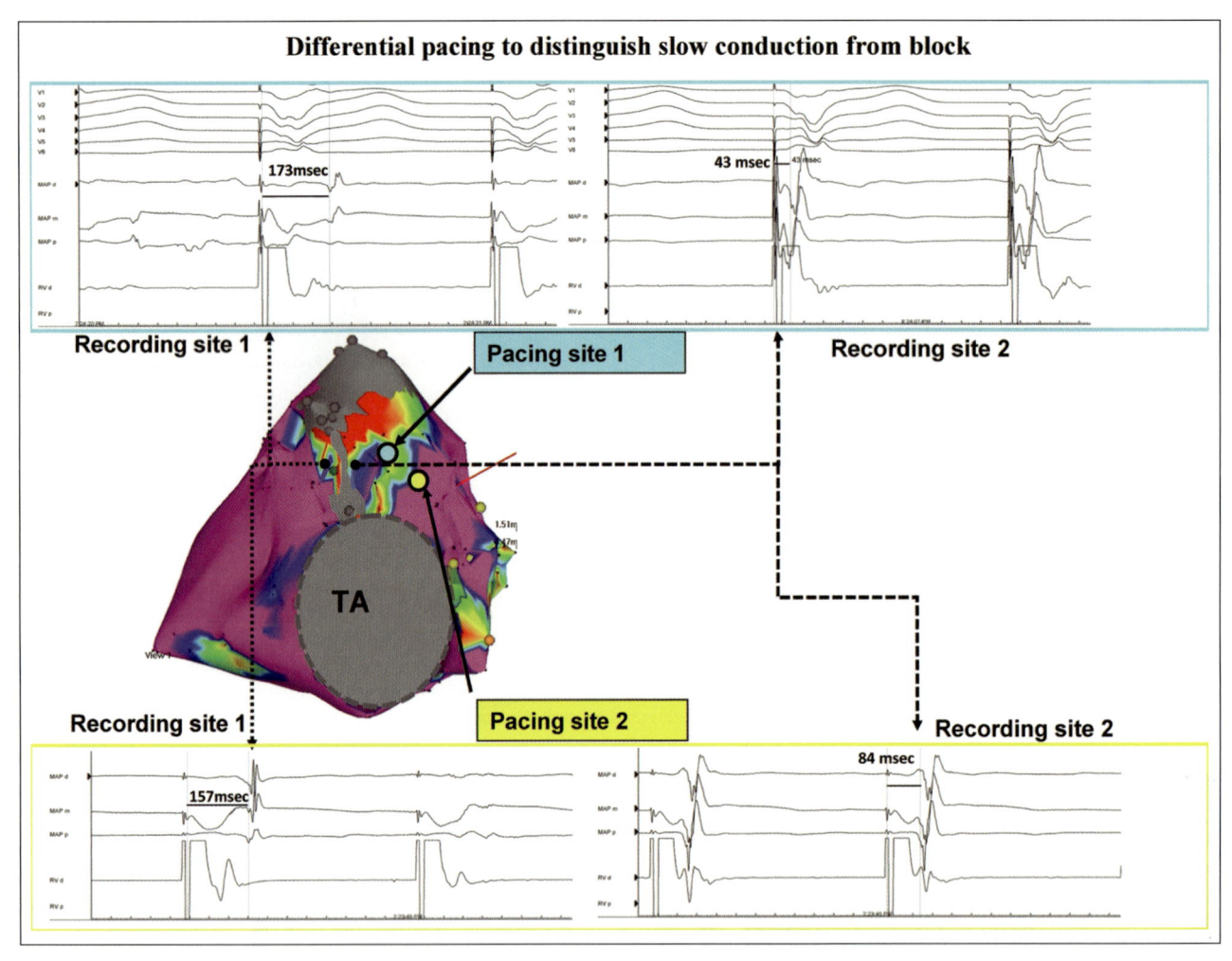

Figure 47.15 During pacing at site 1 the stimulus-to-EGM interval was 173 ms at recording site 1 and 43 ms at recording site 2. Pacing at site 2 resulted in a stimulus-to-EGM interval of 157 ms at recording site 1 and of 84 ms at recording site 2 suggesting complete unidirectional block.

study.[10] Therefore noninducibility of any VT is considered as 1 important endpoint of ablation in our laboratory. After linear ablation lesions, we therefore repeat the entire induction protocol in at least 2 RV pacing sites. If we induce a different VT, we try to identify the location of the specific reentry-circuit isthmus site, which is facilitated by the 3-dimensional reconstruction already obtained, and proceed as described.

Additional Linear Lesions

Although not supported by clinical data yet, we empirically transect short isthmuses with significant conduction delay during sinus rhythm or RV pacing as a potential substrate for macroreentrant tachycardias, even if we have not induced a VT that might use this isthmus, provided that the ablation can be performed safely. It is important to avoid RF lesions in the proximity to the AV conduction system. AV block is more likely if ablation is performed to transect isthmus 4 between a muscular VSD patch and the tricuspid annulus, and we usually keep away from this area.

Postprocedure Care

Recovery

Following ablation, the long sheaths are pulled back in the caval vein, and all sheaths are removed once the ACT is less than 200 seconds. Anticoagulation with low-molecular-weight heparin is instituted 6 hours after hemostasis is achieved and continued for 12 hours. Patients usually lie flat for 6 hours after the sheaths are removed, and the puncture site is carefully evaluated for hematomas and new murmurs. In case of a new murmur, we perform an ultrasound study. All patients undergo routine TTE 12 to 18 hours after the procedure to rule out pericardial effusion and are discharged the next day. Following the procedure we administer aspirin, 100 mg daily for 12 weeks.

ICD Implantation

Patients considered being at risk for sudden cardiac death receive an ICD, usually the day after the procedure. Regardless of the outcome of the ablation procedure, survivors of cardiac arrest, patients with significant RV dilatation and impaired RV function, patients with impaired LV function, and patients in whom the ablation procedure has failed undergo ICD implantation. However, patients who present with a hemodynamically tolerated VT in the absence of residual lesions and with a preserved RV and LV function, and whose VT is rendered uninducible after ablation, are discharged without ICDs.

Follow-up

All patients are followed at our institute. We typically see patients 3 months after discharge. Evaluation includes careful history of symptoms suspicious for arrhythmias, exercise testing, 24-hour Holter registration, and TTE. Further periodic follow-up is done in cooperation with the cardiologist specialized on GUCH, usually annually. ICD recipients are followed according to our institute protocol twice a year.

Procedural Complications

In our experience serious complications are uncommon. Vascular complications such as femoral hematomas, AV fistula, and pseudoaneursyms may occur. A potential risk is cardiac tamponade, which may become evident acutely during the procedure due to mechanical perforation or tissue disruption during RF delivery, resulting in hypotension and bradycardia. Occasionally tamponade may happen several hours after the procedure; therefore, every episode of hypotension should lead to immediate echocardiographic evaluation.

Advantages and Limitations

In most of the series reporting on VT ablation after repair of CHD, the targeted VTs were slow and approachable by conventional mapping techniques such as activation and entrainment mapping during ongoing VT, with an acute success rate of 68% and a recurrence rate of 33%. However, in our experience the majority of patients present with fast VTs that are only briefly tolerated. The strong link between anatomically defined isthmuses and reentry circuit isthmuses allows for mapping and ablation during sinus rhythm resulting in an acute success rate of 91% and a recurrence rate of 18%.[5,6] However, despite these promising results, it is important to consider that some isthmuses are more difficult to transect than others. In particular, the anatomical isthmus between the RVOT patch and the tricuspid annulus often requires steerable sheaths to achieve catheter stability and contact. At this location, catheter and sheath manipulation must be performed with caution, as some parts of the RV free wall might be aneurysmatic and thinned.

Severe hypertrophy of the RVOT myocardium, which might be detected by MRI, sometimes prevents isthmus transection and is an important reason for procedure failure. In these cases careful review of the 3-dimensional map can be helpful to identify a second isthmus that might be used during tachycardia. The mapping catheter can then be positioned within this potential anatomic isthmus during sinus rhythm. We then reinduce the VT and perform limited entrainment mapping to prove or rule out that this region is part of the macroreentrant tachycardia.

In selected cases transection of the isthmuses 3 or 4 requires RF lesions applied from the aortic root or the LV (**Figure 47.16**). However, in these cases it is important to recognize the location of the His bundle and the left fascicle to avoid total AV block.

An important limitation to transect isthmus 3 is recognized in patients who have undergone pulmonary valve replacement and is the main reason for ablation failure in our patient population. In these patients parts of the homograft with the valve placed at the position of the original valve cover the distal RVOT. The lower border of the graft often reaches the VSD patch thereby preventing RF lesions between the former pulmonary valve and the patch. Therefore it is important to evaluate patients who undergo pulmonary valve replacement prior to surgery to identify patients who might require intraoperative ablation.

Conclusions

The prevalence of severe CHD in adults increases, and VT becomes a central issue in the management of patients, in particular after repair of TOF. The majority of VT after repair of TOF is monomorphic, fast, and poorly tolerated and requires ICD shocks for termination in those who have received ICDs for primary or secondary prevention.[2] Patients are usually young and active, in particular if prior surgery has resulted in a good functional status. Therefore therapies that prevent VT recurrence regardless of ICD implantation are necessary. The suggested approach to ablation of all and in particular untolerated VT relies on identification of the underlying substrate by electroanatomical voltage and activation mapping during sinus rhythm or RV pacing in those patients who are pacemaker dependent.

Although this substrate-based approach was only performed in small groups of patients, acute results and low recurrence rates are encouraging. In addition, advances in our understanding and identification of the underlying substrate may also be helpful to guide surgical ablation

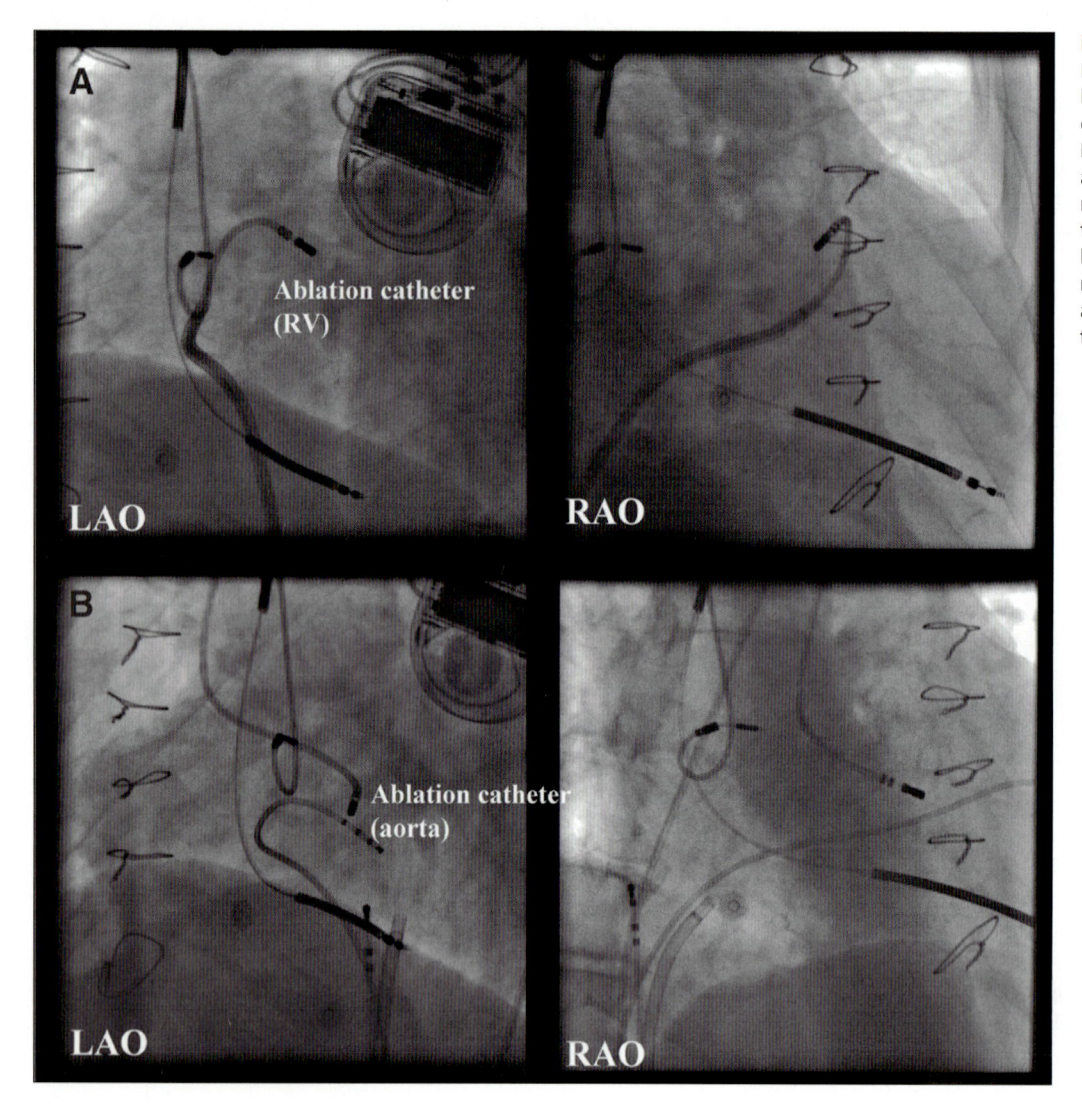

Figure 47.16
Fluoroscopic views in left and right anterior oblique views (LAO, RAO). **A.** Isthmus 3 is approached from the right ventricle (RV) first. **B.** Completing the line and preventing VT reinduction required additional lesions from the aortic root.

during reoperation. Close cooperation between the cardiologist who follows GUCH, the surgeon experienced in initial repair and consecutive operations, and the electrophysiologist performing the ablation procedure is mandatory.

References

1. Marelli AJ, Mackie AS, Ionescu-Ittu R, Rahme E, Pilote L. Congenital heart disease in the general population: changing prevalence and age distribution. *Circulation*. 2007;115:163–172.
2. Khairy P, Harris L, Landzberg MJ, et al. Implantable cardioverter-defibrillators in tetralogy of Fallot. *Circulation*. 2008;117:363–370.
3. Horton RP, Canby RC, Kessler DJ, et al. Ablation of ventricular tachycardia associated with tetralogy of Fallot: demonstration of bidirectional block. *J Cardiovasc Electrophysiol*. 1997;8:432–435.
4. Chinushi M, Aizawa Y, Kitazawa H, Kusano Y, Washizuka T, Shibata A. Successful radiofrequency catheter ablation for macroreentrant ventricular tachycardias in a patient with tetralogy of Fallot after corrective surgery. *Pacing Clin Electrophysiol*. 1995;18:1713–1716.
5. Zeppenfeld K, Schalij MJ, Bartelings MM, et al. Catheter ablation of ventricular tachycardia after repair of congenital heart disease: electroanatomic identification of the critical right ventricular isthmus. *Circulation*. 2007;116:2241–2252.
6. Kriebel T, Saul JP, Schneider H, Sigler M, Paul T. Noncontact mapping and radiofrequency catheter ablation of fast and hemodynamically unstable ventricular tachycardia after surgical repair of tetralogy of Fallot. *J Am Coll Cardiol*. 2007;50:2162–2168.
7. Marchlinski FE, Callans DJ, Gottlieb CD, Zado E. Linear ablation lesions for control of unmappable ventricular tachycardia in patients with ischemic and nonischemic cardiomyopathy. *Circulation*. 2000;101:1288–1296.
8. Soejima K, Stevenson WG, Maisel WH, Sapp JL, Epstein LM. Electrically unexcitable scar mapping based on pacing threshold for identification of the reentry circuit isthmus:

feasibility for guiding ventricular tachycardia ablation. *Circulation.* 2002;106:1678–1683.
9. Brunckhorst CB, Stevenson WG, Soejima K, et al. Relationship of slow conduction detected by pace mapping to ventricular tachycardia reentry circuit sites after infarction. *J Am Coll Cardiol.* 2003;41:802–809.
10. Khairy P, Landzberg MJ, Gatzoulis MA, et al. Value of programmed ventricular stimulation after tetralogy of fallot repair: a multicenter study. *Circulation.* 2004;109:1994–2000.

Video Descriptions

Video 47.1 Dynamic MRI showing severe pulmonary valve regurgitation and RVOT enlargement in a patient late after repair of tetralogy of Fallot including a transannular patch. (Courtesy H.M. Siebelink, LUMC, Leiden, the Netherlands.)

Video 47.2 Dynamic MRI showing severe subpulmonary obstruction due to hypertrophy of the septoparietal trabeculations that encircle the subpulmonary infundibulum. (Courtesy H.M. Siebelink, LUMC, Leiden, the Netherlands.)

Video 47.3 Three-dimensional electroanatomical voltage map of a patient who presented with VT late after repair consistent of a transannular patch, resection of infundibular muscle, and patch closure of a muscular ventricular septal defect. Three anatomical isthmuses could be identified.

Video 47.4 Electroanatomical propagation map obtained during RVA pacing. Activation wave fronts are reaching the 3 isthmuses from different directions at a similar time.

CHAPTER 48

Catheter Ablation of Ventricular Tachycardia in Sarcoidosis / Hypertrophic Cardiomyopathy

Kyoko Soejima, MD; Akiko Ueda, MD; Masaomi Chinushi, MD, PhD

Introduction

Sarcoidosis is a multisystem disorder of unknown etiology characterized by the accumulation of T lymphocytes, mononuclear phagocytes, and noncaseating granulomas in involved tissue. Most frequently, lungs are affected (90%), and up to 30% have extrapulmonary disease, such as skin involvement (20%), ocular involvement (20%), peripheral lymphadenopathy (40%), hepatomegaly (20%), and cardiac involvement (5%). However, autopsy studies indicate that substantial subclinical cardiac involvement is present in 20% to 30% of cases.[1] In Japanese patients, it has been reported that up to 70% of patients had cardiac involvement by autopsy.[2] Roberts et al. reported that sudden death was the most common manifestation of cardiac sarcoidosis, involving more than 60% of patients.[3]

Substrate

The common mechanism of VT in cardiac sarcoidosis is reentry due to the increased fibrosis, which gives rise to the slow zigzag conduction as in ICM. However, initial presentation of active sarcoidosis can be VT. The mechanism of VT during the acute phase of cardiac sarcoidosis was carefully evaluated by Furushima et al.[4] In their series of 8 patients, 22 VTs were induced, and 15 of these VTs (68%) were reentrant. Interestingly, EP study was repeated in active and inactive phases of sarcoidosis; most reentrant VTs were induced during the active phase, which may suggest that the slow conduction zone might be present during the acute inflammation stage, and not only the chronic inactive stage. If the cardiac involvement is confirmed without spontaneous sustained ventricular arrhythmia, EP study should be considered. Aizer et al. reported that inducible ventricular arrhythmias with programmed stimulation predicted subsequent life-threatening arrhythmias.[5] In patients with spontaneous or inducible sustained VT, appropriate ICD therapy was observed in 50% in less than 1 year of follow-up. In their series, programmed stimulation was performed only in patients with symptoms (palpitations, presyncope, syncope, or sudden death) and EP abnormalities (PVC, nonsustained VT, or sustained VT, or VF), but only 20% of the patients had reduced LVEF of less than 30%. Therefore, in a general patient population with the apparent cardiac sarcoidosis, whether to use EP study for risk stratification remains to be evaluated in the future.

If the patients have frequent VT episodes, it would be necessary to perform the catheter ablation or use antiarrhythmic agents prior to the ICD implant to prevent electrical storm. Optimal timing to start corticosteroid is also an important issue. In most cases, patients are required to have lifetime corticosteroid therapy, which may increase the risk for the acute device infection. Therefore, if the device is required, it should be implanted prior to the steroid treatment, and once the wound is healed, the steroid therapy can be started.

Catheter Ablation

If patients present with frequent VT episodes, catheter ablation or antiarrhythmics should be considered in addition to the device implantation. Recently, prophylactic catheter ablation has been demonstrated to have a benefit in patients who had ICD implantation for sustained VT associated with ICM.[6] It may also benefit cardiac sarcoidosis patients with spontaneous VT to have catheter ablation in addition to device implantation.

Using the electroanatomical mapping system, Koplan et al. identified multiple low-voltage areas, which may represent fibrosis or granulomatous tissue, and all VTs were demonstrated to originate from these areas.[7] In their series, 50% of patients who underwent ablation for VT were free of recurrent VT at long-term follow-up (range; 6 months to 7 years), but complete elimination of VT was difficult to achieve. Their study suggested that VTs in sarcoidosis tended to be more difficult to control due to diffuse and heterogeneous ventricular involvement and potential deep intramural circuits.

The largest series of catheter ablation of VT in patients with sarcoidosis was reported by Jefic et al.[8] In their study, 42 patients were diagnosed with cardiac sarcoidosis, and when VT occurred, a stepwise approach was used: ICD implant, followed by immunosuppressive agents, antiarrhythmic agents, then catheter ablation if refractory. In 9 of 42 patients, VT was not controlled by medical therapy, and RF ablation was performed. A total of 44 VTs (348 ± 78 ms) were induced. Endocardial ablation was performed in 8 patients (5 in RV, 3 in LV), and epicardial ablation was performed in 1 patient. Seventy percent of VTs were abolished by the RF ablation. The most frequent reentrant circuit location was peri-tricuspid circuit. This type of VT was eliminated in all patients. VT events decreased from 271 ± 363 events prior to the ablation to 4.0 ± 9.7 postablation.

Using an imaging study, such as cardiac MRI, identification of the distribution of the scar can guide us to the location of the reentry circuit. With the use of open-irrigated catheters and electroanatomical mapping systems, optimal results can be pursued to control the VT.

Finally, it is sometimes difficult to diagnose cardiac sarcoidosis correctly, especially in its diffuse, chronic phase. One important differential diagnosis is ARVD/C. Vasaiwala et al. report a series of patients referred for evaluation of LBBB VT and suspected ARVD/C.[9] The patients were evaluated prospectively with standardized protocol including right ventricle cineangiography-guided myocardial biopsy. Sixteen patients had ARVD/C, and 4 had probable ARVD/C. Three patients were found to have noncaseating granulomas on biopsy consistent with sarcoid. Age, systemic symptoms, findings on chest X-ray or MRI, type of ventricular arrhythmia, RV function, ECG abnormalities, and the presence or duration of LPs did not discriminate between sarcoid and ARVD/C. Left ventricular dysfunction (ejection fraction < 50%) was present in 3 of 3 patients with cardiac sarcoid, but only 2 of 17 remaining patients with definite or probable ARVD/C ($P = 0.01$). Hence, it is important to suspect sarcoidosis in these patients, as some may respond to steroid therapy.

An external irrigation catheter is recommended for the catheter ablation of VT associated with sarcoidosis. Usually 1- to 2-minute RF application was made with maximum power of 50 W, provided that the temperature recorded from the electrode remained < 50°C. We use 30 W to start and usually titrate it up to 50 W. RF application is terminated immediately if temperature exceeds 50°C or an impedance increase > 10 ohm. Impedance should be monitored carefully to avoid the pop or charring of the tissue. We usually use the retrograde approach to map the LV. However, if the stability of the catheter is the issue, transseptal access to the LV using the deflectable sheath (Agilis NxT, St. Jude Medical, Minneapolis, MN) should be considered. In some labs, both the retrograde and antegrade access are obtained. However, in sarcoidosis, it is not unusual to have the reentry circuit in RV as well. If clinical situation allows, cardiac MRI will help to guide where the substrate of VT is located and plan for the mapping and ablation.

Case Study

In a case report published by Chinushi and colleagues,[10] a 64-year-old male with a history of complete AV block at the age of 48 was referred for catheter ablation for frequent ICD shocks. Patient had spontaneous VT episodes at the age of 56, and was found to have developed a LV aneurysm. He has a probable diagnosis of cardiac sarcoidosis, but neither biopsy nor gallium scintigraphy was positive. Pacemaker was upgraded to ICD, and he now presented with frequent ICD shocks.

His baseline paced rhythm (atrial sensed, ventricular paced) is shown in **Figure 48.1A**. Two different VTs with identical CL were induced during the EP study (**Figure 48.1, B** and **C**). VT1 was RBBB morphology and +105° of frontal axis. VT2 was LBBB morphology and −55° of frontal axis. A large aneurysm was detected by CT at the base of both ventricles, extending from the superior base to the septum, and the abnormal low-voltage area (local EGM amplitude < 1.5 mV) was identified by mapping (**Figure 48.2A**). Delayed potentials (arrows) were recorded at multiple sites inside the low-voltage zone during RV paced rhythm. With programmed stimulation, 2 types of stable VTs were induced and both VTs were mapped. **Figure 48.3, A** and **B** show the activation map during each VT. Same circuit was observed for both VTs with opposite activation. Presystolic potential was recorded at the same site for both VTs. Entrainment mapping at this site demonstrated concealed fusion, S-QRS/VTCL of 20%, and postpacing interval close to VTCL, suggesting the site being the exit sites for both VTs (**Figure 48.4, A** and **B**). RF application at this site during VT1 terminated VT immediately (**Figure 48.4C**) and VT2 was no longer inducible as well.

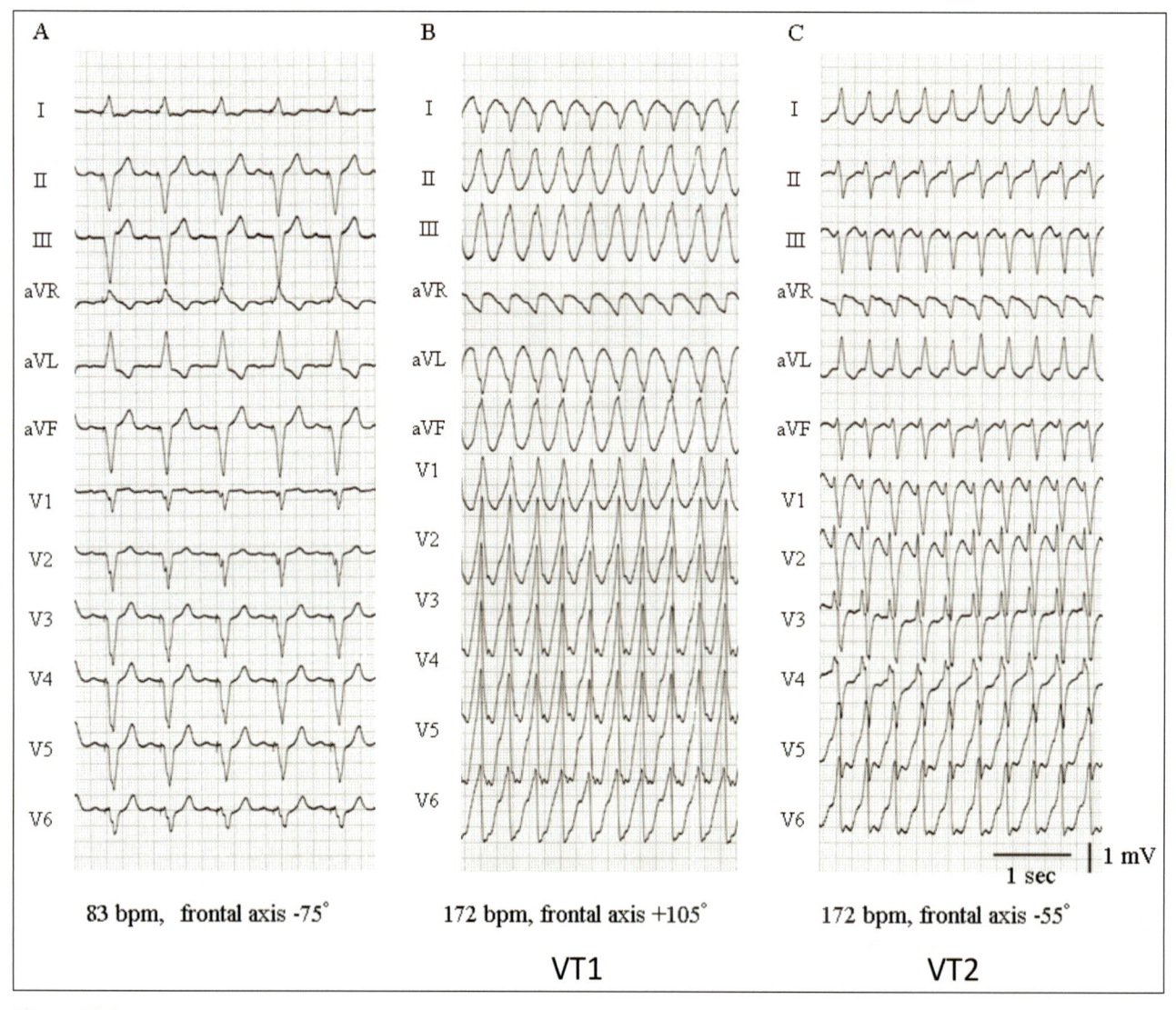

Figure 48.1 Baseline ECG and induced 2 VTs. **A.** Baseline ECG is shown. The baseline rhythm is atrial sensed and ventricular paced with his DDD pacemaker. **B.** Twelve-lead ECG of VT1 is shown. The morphology is RBBB with inferior axis, suggesting the exit of the VT is basolateral of LV. **C.** Twelve-lead ECG of VT2 is shown. The morphology is LBBB with superior axis, suggesting the exit of the VT is septum. (Chinushi M, Izumi D, Furushima H, Aizawa Y. Catheter ablation of ventricular tachycardias due to forward and reverse propagation across a reentrant circuit inside a nonischemic biventricular aneurysm. *J Cardiovasc Electrophys.* 2011;22(4):467–471. With permission.)

Hypertrophic Cardiomyopathy

Hypertrophic cardiomyopathy (HCM) is an autosomal-dominant genetic disorder, characterized by a LV hypertrophy. Mutations in genes encoding sarcomere protein cause extensive myocyte hypertrophy, myocardial fibrosis, and disarray. Asymmetrical hypertrophy in basal septum and subaortic region is the most common type and causes LVOT obstruction. Other forms include apical hypertrophy and mid-ventricular obstruction with or without apical aneurysms. Some patients progress to a dilated-phase, the so-called "burned-out type" of HCM, which resembles dilated cardiomyopathy.

Although most of the patients are asymptomatic and their clinical courses are benign, HCM is one of the major causes of sudden cardiac death in young people. The mechanisms of sudden cardiac death and syncope in HCM are severe heart failure, thromboembolic events, LVOT obstruction, myocardial ischemia, and ventricular arrhythmias. It had been believed that VF and polymorphic VT were more common,[11] and sustained monomorphic VT was less frequent. However, ICD recording showed that monomorphic VT is more frequent than previously estimated.[12,13] It might have been underestimated, as VT degenerates into VF in early phase.[14] Furushima et al. reported that 28% of hospitalized HCM patients had monomorphic VTs, and most of the patients had mid-ventricular obstruction.[15]

Imaging Study

The mechanism of sustained monomorphic VTs is thought to be reentry. Myocyte disarray and interstitial fibrosis associated with HCM can create the dispersion of

Chapter 48: Ablation of VT in Sarcoidosis/Hypertrophic Cardiomyopathy • 453

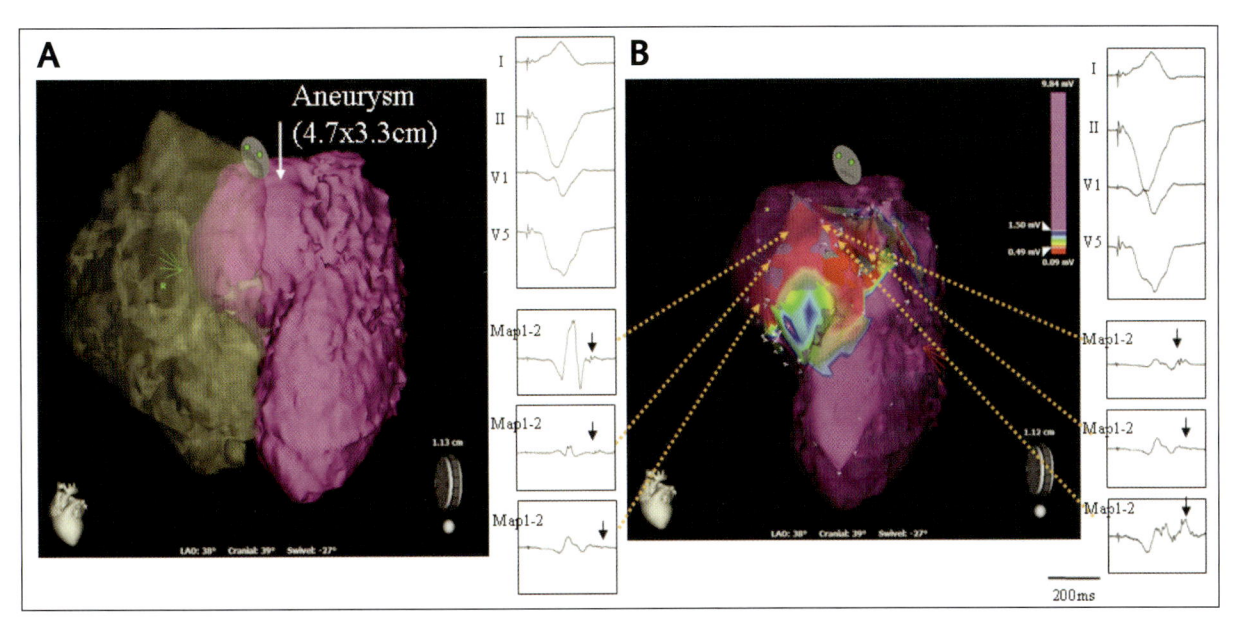

Figure 48.2 Three-dimensional CT image **A.** Three-dimensional CT image of the left (purple) and the right (gray) ventricles is shown. A large interventricular septal aneurysm is shown. **B.** Substrate mapping during paced rhythm shows the abnormal low-voltage area, compatible with the aneurysm. Along the border of the aneurysm, sites with delayed components of recorded potentials are observed. Voltage is set for 1.5 mV as maximal voltage and 0.5 mV as minimal voltage. (Chinushi M, Izumi D, Furushima H, Aizawa Y. Catheter ablation of ventricular tachycardias due to forward and reverse propagation across a reentrant circuit inside a nonischemic biventricular aneurysm. *J Cardiovasc Electrophys.* 2011;22(4):467–471. With permission.)

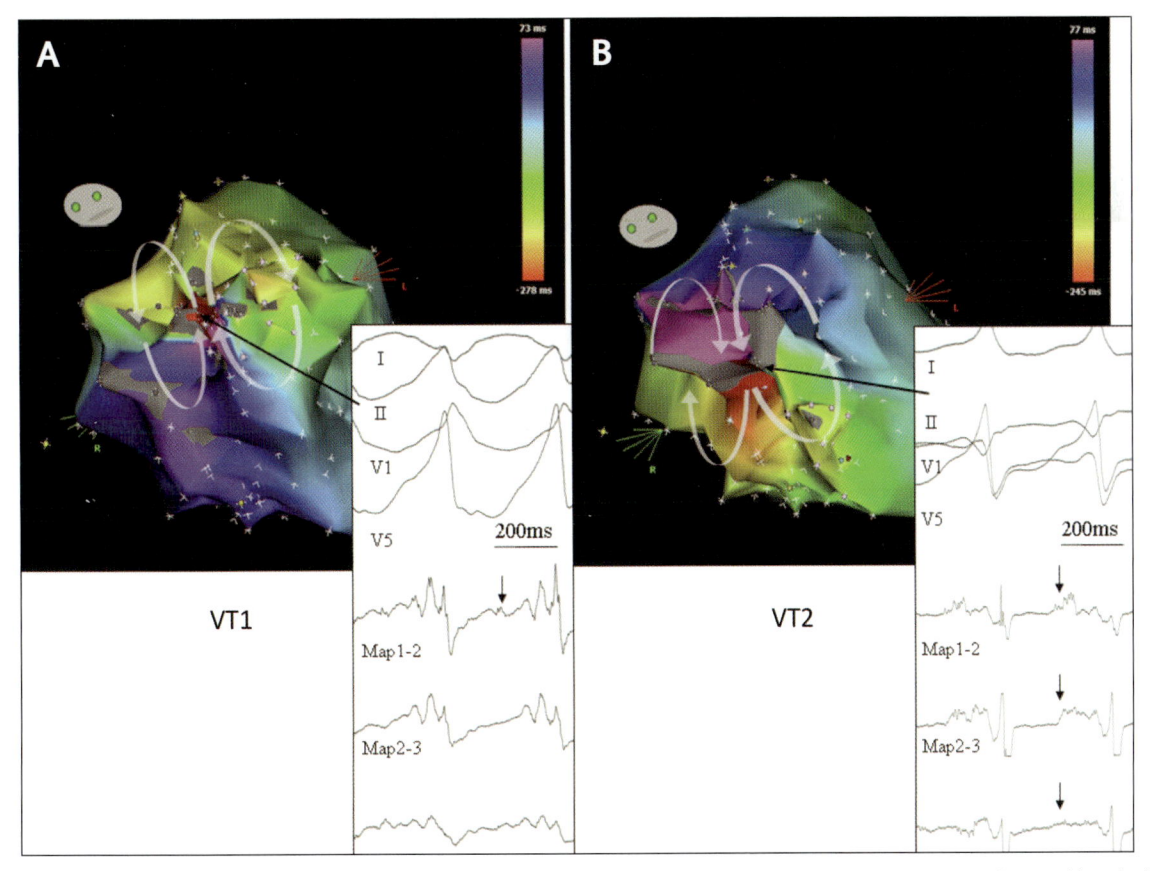

Figure 48.3 Activation map using the electroanatomical mapping system for each VT. Earliest activation is shown with red, then yellow, green, blue, and purple. The color range covers most of the VTCL (333 ms out of 352 ms). **A.** Activation map of the VT1 is shown. Activation front goes up from the aneurysm, and figure-eight reentrant circuit is observed. In between the dense scars, small channel is identified, which shows the mid-diastolic potential. **B.** Activation map of the VT2 is shown. Activation front goes down from the aneurysm, and figure-eight reentrant circuit with opposite direction is observed. In the channel, presystolic potential is recorded. (Chinushi M, Izumi D, Furushima H, Aizawa Y. Catheter ablation of ventricular tachycardias due to forward and reverse propagation across a reentrant circuit inside a nonischemic biventricular aneurysm. *J Cardiovasc Electrophys.* 2011;22(4):467–471. With permission.)

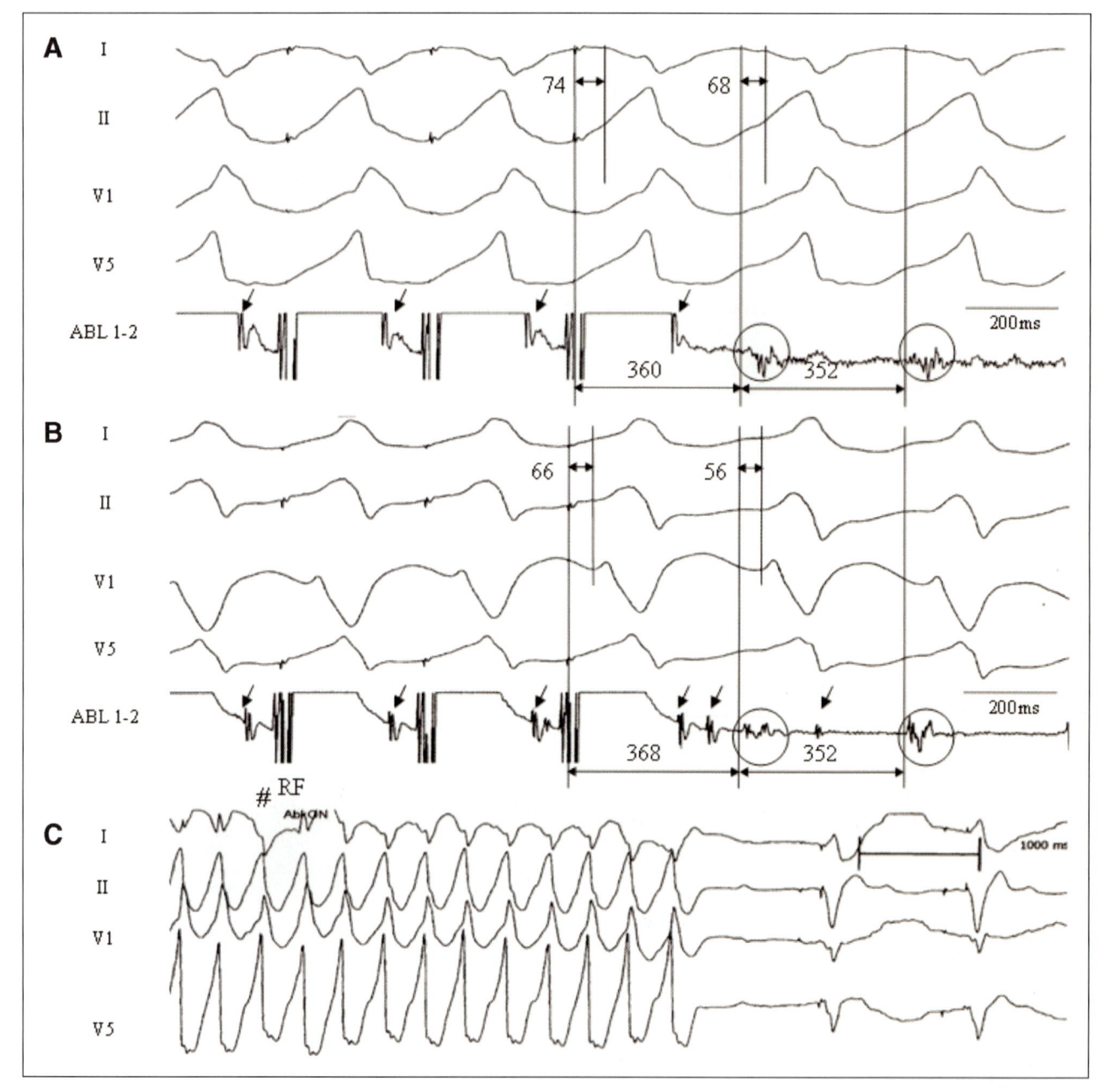

Figure 48.4 Entrainment mapping and RF application. **A.** Entrainment mapping during VT1 is shown. Concealed fusion, postpacing interval (360 ms) similar to the VTCL (352 ms), and S-QRS less than 30% of VTCL suggest the site being at the exit of the reentrant circuit. **B.** Entrainment mapping during VT2 is shown. Again, concealed fusion, postpacing interval similar to the VTCL, and S-QRS less than 30% of the VTCL suggest the site being the exit of the reentrant circuit. The arrows point to the local artifacts. **C.** RF application terminated VT1 following the prolongation of the VTCL. (Chinushi M, Izumi D, Furushima H, Aizawa Y. Catheter ablation of ventricular tachycardias due to forward and reverse propagation across a reentrant circuit inside a nonischemic biventricular aneurysm. *J Cardiovasc Electrophys.* 2011;22(4):467–471. With permission.)

depolarization and repolarization, promoting the reentrant tachycardia. Distribution and extent of myocyte disarray and fibrosis depend on types of gene mutations in HCM patients. There has been a report that sudden deaths in patients with severe myocyte disarray could be caused by ischemia due to the abnormal blood pressure response rather than the arrhythmia.[16] However, others report that the myocyte disarray and disorganization of intercellular junctions can serve as arrhythmogenic substrate.[17]

Cardiac MRI can provide very important structural information,[18] such as the presence of aneurysm, global or regional systolic and diastolic function, degree of outflow obstruction, and mitral regurgitation. Delayed contrast-enhancement MRI can evaluate the location and distribution of the scar, and is useful for planning the ablation method. The extent of late gadolinium enhancement has good pathological correlation with distribution of collagen tissue.[19] These areas can be arrhythmogenic,[20-22] and the usefulness of MRI as a predictor of malignant cardiac event and VT inducibility has been reported.[22,23]

Mapping and Ablation Strategy

The electroanatomical mapping system is of great use for the mapping of VT associated with structural heart disease. It can identify the abnormal low-voltage area, which contributes to the reentrant tachycardia. Carefully merged CT or MRI can guide the mapping and ablation. During the sinus rhythm, substrate mapping can be reconstructed, and sites with delayed potential or fractionated potential can be tagged as sites of interest. If the VT is hemodynamically stable and can therefore be mapped, a activation map can be reconstructed, and entrainment mapping during VT can identify the isthmus of the VT. In the case of unstable VTs, pace mapping can be used to approximate the exit of the VT circuit.

Patients with mid-ventricular-obstruction-type HCM usually have low-voltage area with unexcitable scar in the apical aneurysm, and require detailed mapping in the aneurysm for the ablation of VT.[24-26] Characteristic ECG morphology of VT arising from the apical aneurysm is usually RBBB with superior axis. Advancing the mapping catheter via the narrow neck of the aneurysm can be challenging and needs special attention. LV thrombus should be ruled out prior to the procedure. Preprocedural LV angiography, CT, or MRI is useful for the mapping. Recently, effectiveness of epicardial ablation in these types of VT has been reported.[27,28]

Patients with apical HCM also have arrhythmogenic substrates in LVA. Inada et al. reported 3 apical HCM patients had sustained monomorphic reentrant VT originating from the apical wall.[29] Two of these patients required endocardial and epicardial ablations, and the other required transcoronary ethanol ablation for the deep intramural reentrant circuit.

In a large series of HCM patients with relatively low ejection fraction, Santangeli et al. reported the most common location of reentry circuits were RV-LV junctions at the level of basal (42%) or apical (18%) segments.[27] They emphasized the efficacy of epicardial ablation with an open irrigated catheter because most scars were located at deep intramural myocardium or epicardium. Their procedures eliminated VTs successfully in more than two-thirds of the patients. However, VTs were not curable in some cases with extremely thick wall or with scars originating from the interventricular septum. In such cases, transcoronary chemical ablation might be considered.

Usually an irrigation catheter is used to make the larger and deeper lesion. A D-curve catheter is used frequently for VT ablation, but if the ventricle is dilated, it is an F-curve catheter that provides the longer reach to the wall.

Alcohol Ablation

Although the open-irrigated catheter makes deeper lesions, VTs can originate from the deep intramural area in thick LV wall. In this situation, another alternative ablation method, such as chemical ablation or surgical ablation, might be required. EHRA/HRS consensus on catheter ablation of ventricular arrhythmias states that ethanol ablation should be considered only in unstable cases refractory to endocardial and epicardial ablation.[30] The mechanism of chemical ablation is cytotoxic myocardial damage and ischemic injury by ethanol. The target coronary vessel supplying blood to the arrhythmogenic area has to be identified, and it has traditionally been based on the empirical use of cold saline or contrast injection that results in termination of VT. However, a significant limitation of this method was the inability to record electrograms from the target coronary artery, which precludes the use of entrainment and pace mapping to confirm that site is a critical portion of the VT circuit. Recently, a novel method of recording the EGM and pacing from the guide wire was reported.[31] Intracoronary guide wire is advanced into the vessel, and its proximal portion is covered by the intracoronary balloon except the distal several millimeters, and the distal tip of the guide wire can be used to perform pace mapping or entrainment mapping (unipolar pacing). It is important to use the noncoated wire to record the EGM. Cold saline can then be injected into the target coronary artery to demonstrate VT termination. After confirmation of the target vessel, highly concentrated ethanol (1–2 ml) is injected during VT or sinus rhythm. It is crucial to occlude proximal portion of the target artery to prevent the reflux of ethanol. The potential risks of alcohol ablation are complete AV block (common in septal lesion), pericarditis, infarction of unintended myocardium due to ethanol reflux, and worsening of heart failure.

Cases

Case 1

A 49-year-old male with mid-ventricular-obstruction-type HCM presented with frequent VT episodes. Obstruction and the apical aneurysm can be demonstrated clearly with cardiac MRI and LV angiogram (**Figure 48.5**). Substrate for the VT with extensive scar tissue can also be identified with delayed enhancement at the apex (**Figure 48.5C**). Typical 12-lead ECG for the apical origin VT can be recorded, and an ablation catheter was carefully advanced into the aneurysm (**Figure 48.6, A and B**). In the aneurysm, the site with presystolic potential (**Figure 48.6C**) was identified during VT, and entrainment with concealed fusion was demonstrated (**Figure 48.6D**). RF application at this site terminated VT immediately (**Figure 48.6E**).

Case 2

A 57-year-old male with dilated phase of HCM presented with frequent ICD shocks (**Figure 48.7**). Endocardial substrate mapping demonstrated almost normal voltage in the whole chamber, and the activation sequence during the VT showed a focal VT pattern, although the mechanism of VT was clearly reentry. Epicardial mapping was then

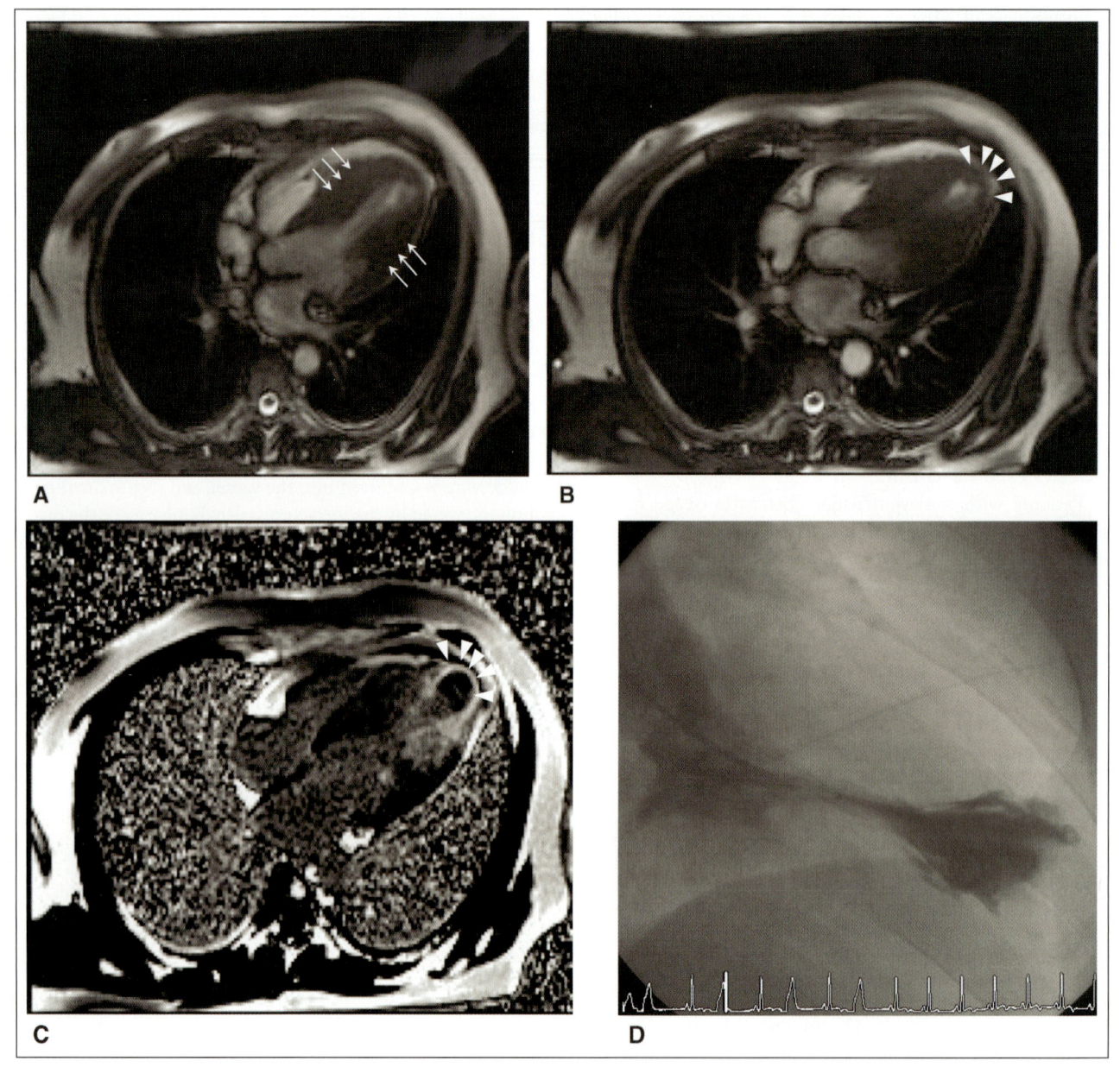

Figure 48.5 Mid-ventricular obstruction HCM. Cardiac MRI (cineT2, long-axis) of a 49-year-old male with apical aneurysm in mid-ventricular obstruction type HCM is shown. (**A**) The extremely hypertrophied LV mid-portion (white arrows) during diastole and complete LV obstruction of the apical aneurysm (arrow heads) during systole. (**B**) Delayed contrast-enhancement cardiac MRI (**C**) showed the delayed enhancement of the aneurysm (arrow heads). LV angiography (**D**) also indicated a large apical aneurysm. MRI = magnetic resonance image; HCM = hypertrophic cardiomyopathy; LV = left ventricle

performed, and relatively large scar was identified. Activation map of the VT demonstrated small epicardial reentrant circuit, and RF application abolished VT.

Case 3

A 69-year-old male with dilated phase of HCM presented with frequent ICD shocks. Endocardial and epicardial mapping was performed simultaneously and demonstrated the septal origin of VT. RF application from the right and left side of the septum was performed in addition to the epicardial application without effect (**Figure 48.8**, A–C). The decision to perform ethanol septal ablation was then made on the following day due to the inability to control the VT episodes. Using the guide wire, activation mapping and entrainment mapping were performed, and the responsible branch was identified. Cold saline was injected during VT, which demonstrated the termination of the VT. Then 2 cm³ of ethanol was injected during sinus rhythm, and VT became noninducible.

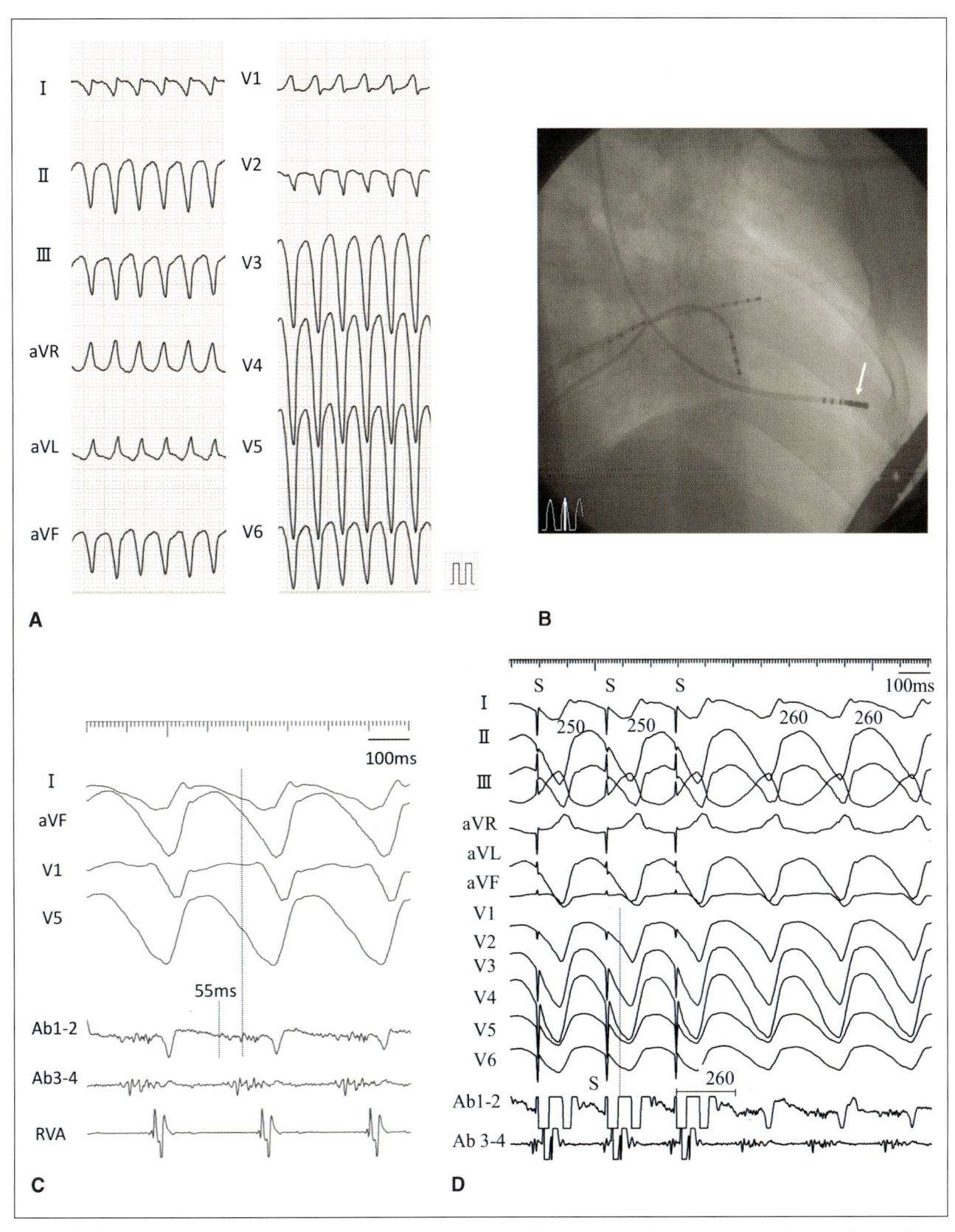

Figure 48.6 Mapping and ablation of VT. ECG of the clinical VT is shown (**A**) in the same patient as Figure 48.5. Fluoroscopic view (**B**) shows the ablation catheter (arrow) inserted into the aneurysm. Small and fractionated potentials preceding the QRS onset by 55 ms is recorded (**C**), and entrainment mapping at this site demonstrated concealed fusion (**D**). Postpacing interval was same as VTCL.

(Continued on next page)

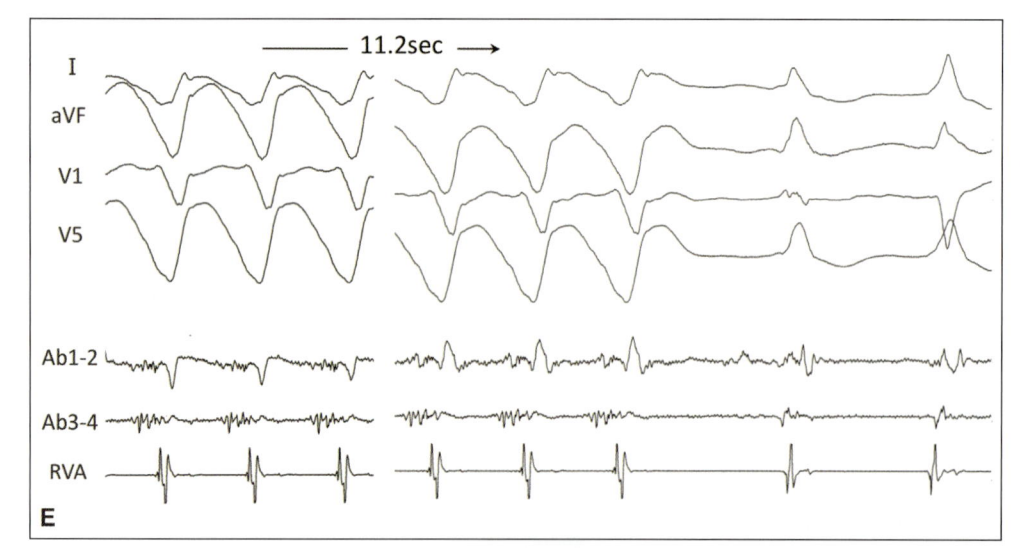

Figure 48.6 (continued) RF energy application successfully terminated the VT in 11 seconds (**E**). ECG = electrocardiogram; PPI = postpacing interval; VTCL = VT cycle length; RF = radiofrequency.

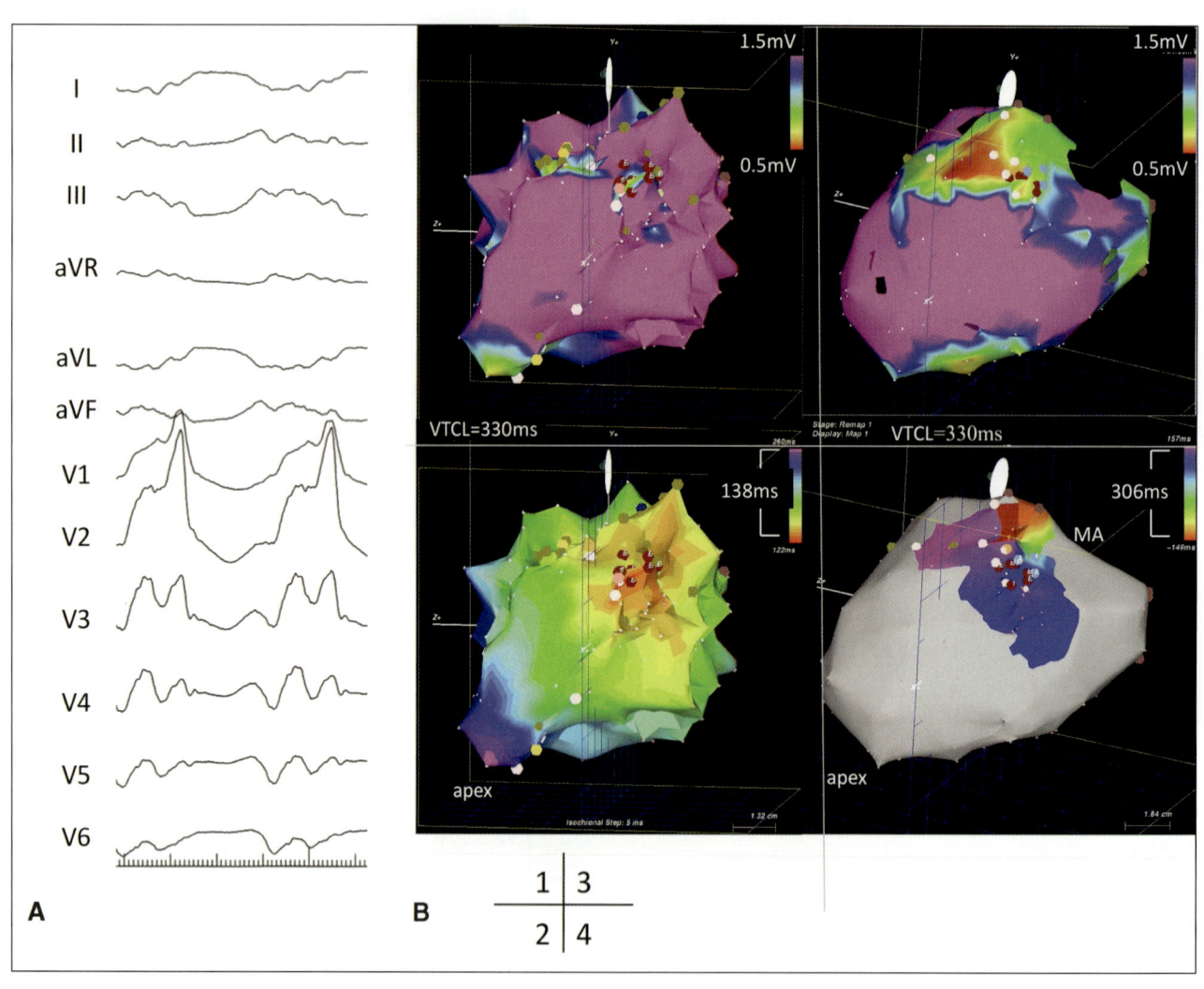

Figure 48.7 Dilated-phase HCM. ECG of spontaneous sustained monomorphic VT (**A**) in a 57-year-old man with dilated-phase HCM is shown. Endocardial voltage map (**B-1**) demonstrates almost normal voltage, and the activation map during the VT (**B-2**) shows focal activation pattern, covering only the small portion of the VTCL (138ms/330ms). RF application at the earliest endocardial site did not terminate the VT. Epicardial mapping was then performed. Epicardial voltage map shows abnormal low-voltage area at the basal-lateral LV (**B-3**). More than 90% of VTCL was covered (306 ms/330 ms) in the activation map (**B-4**). Ablation at the low-voltage area successfully terminated the VT. MA = mitral annulus. (Ueda A, Fukamizu S, Soejima K, et al. Clinical and electrophysiological characteristics in patients with sustained monomorphic reentrant ventricular tachycardia associated with dilated-phase hypertrophic cardiomyopathy. *Europace*. 2012;14(5):73. Used with permission from Oxford University Press.)

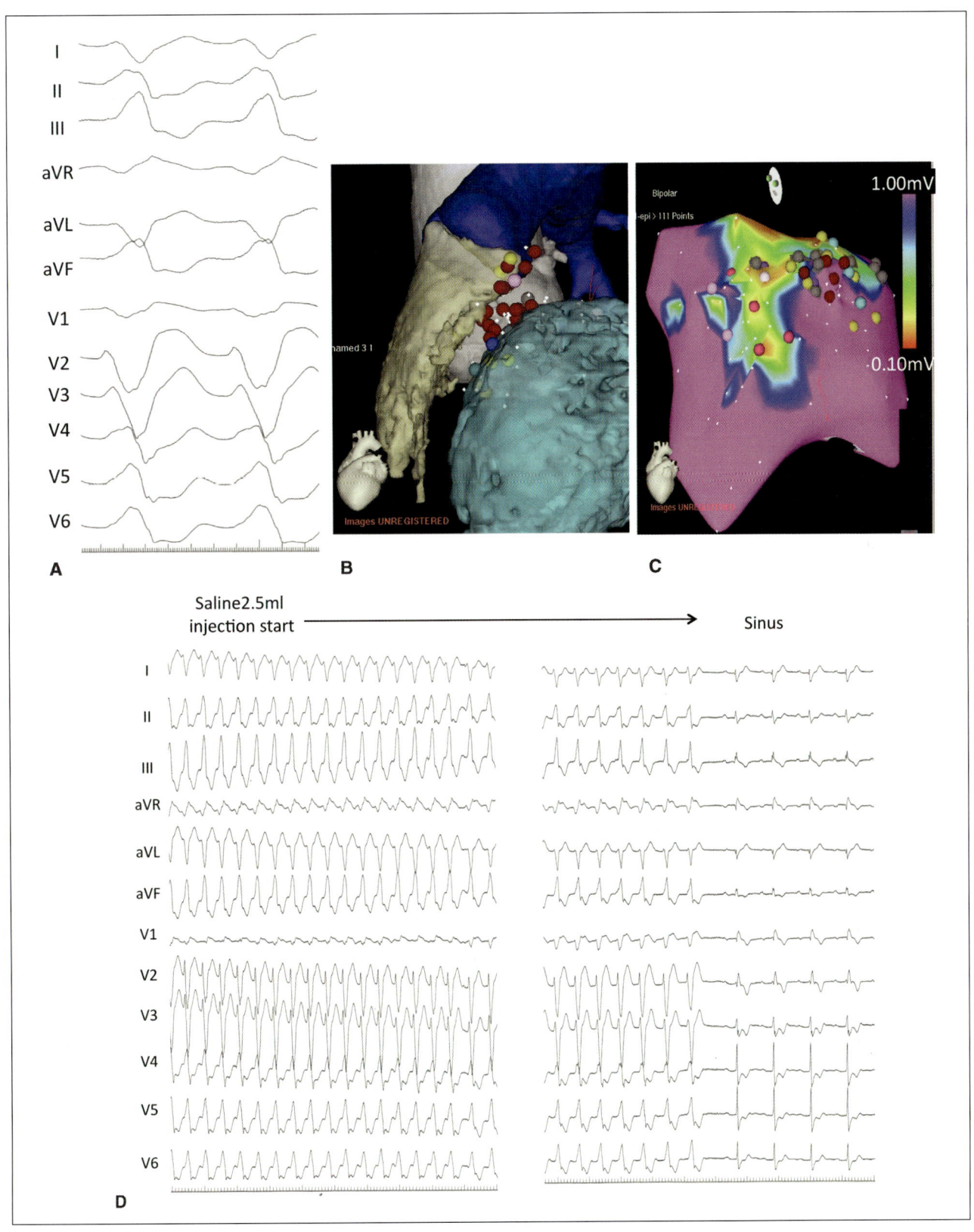

Chapter 48: Ablation of VT in Sarcoidosis/Hypertrophic Cardiomyopathy • 459

Figure 48.8 Dilated-phase HCM. ECG of the clinical monomorphic VT in a 69-year-old man with dilated-phase HCM is shown (**A**). Earliest activation site is located at the ventricular septum, and RF applications from the LV, RV, and epicardium were not effective. Red tags in CARTO map (**B**, LV septum and RV outflow, and **C**, epicardium) represent ablation sites. Epicardial voltage map (**C**) shows the abnormal low-voltage area in the outflow area. Intracoronary (first septal branch) cold saline injection successfully terminated the VT reproducibly (**D**), and it was confirmed to be the responsible branch for the VT. A total of 2 ml of ethanol was injected into the branch during sinus rhythm. After the injection, VT was no longer inducible.

(Continued on next page)

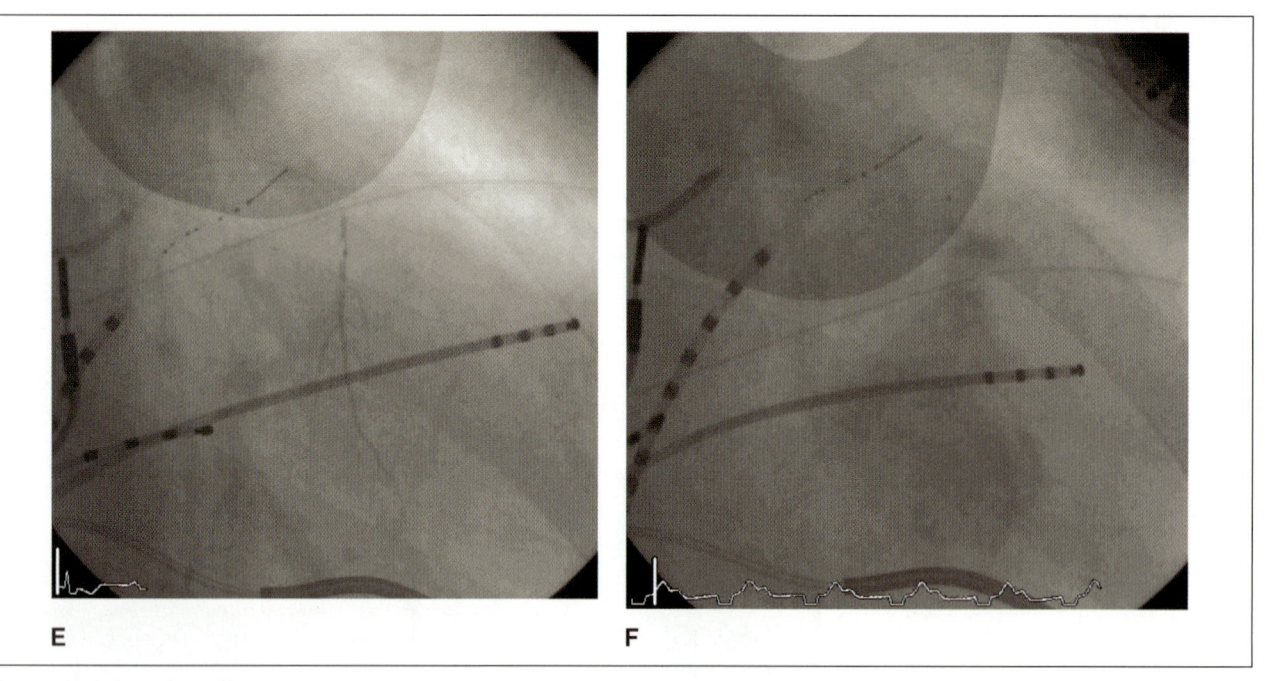

Figure 48.8 (continued) **E** and **F** show the pre- and postangiography. Contrast stain with no coronary flow is observed after ethanol injection (**F**). (Ueda A, Fukamizu S, Soejima K, et al. Clinical and electrophysiological characteristics in patients with sustained monomorphic reentrant ventricular tachycardia associated with dilated-phase hypertrophic cardiomyopathy. *Europace*. 2012;14(5):73. Used with permission from Oxford University Press.)

Summary

The common mechanism of VT in cardiac sarcoidosis is reentry due to the increased fibrosis, which gives rise to the slow zigzag conduction as in ICM. Ventricular tachycardia in sarcoidosis tends to be more difficult to control due to the diffuse and heterogeneous ventricular involvement and potential deep intramural circuits. Most frequently, the reentry circuit is located in the peritricuspid area. If clinical situation allows, cardiac MRI will help to guide where the substrate of VT is located and plan for the mapping and ablation.

For HCM, the mechanism of sustained monomorphic VTs is thought to be reentry. Myocyte disarray and interstitial fibrosis associated with HCM can create the dispersion of depolarization and repolarization, promoting the reentrant tachycardia. Locations of the reentry circuits varied depending on the types of HCM, such as apical aneurismal type, dilated phase, or apical HCM. Cardiac MRI can provide very important structural information, such as the presence of aneurysm, global or regional systolic and diastolic function, degree of outflow obstruction, and mitral regurgitation. Delayed contrast-enhancement MRI can evaluate the location and distribution of the scar, and is useful for planning the ablation method. Most common locations of reentry circuits were RV-LV junctions at the base or apex.

In both clinical entities, an irrigation catheter should be used for the larger and deeper lesion, and some cases require epicardial ablation. VTs are not curable in some cases with extremely thick wall or with scars originated from interventricular septum. In such cases, transcoronary chemical ablation or cardiac surgery may be required to abolish VTs.

References

1. Iwai K, Sekiguti M, Hosoda Y, DeRemee RA, Tazelaar HD, Sharma OP, Maheshwari A, Noguchi TI. Racial difference in cardiac sarcoidosis incidence observed at autopsy. *Sarcoidosis*. 1994;11(1):26–31.
2. Iwai K, Takemura T, Kitaichi M, Kawabata Y, Matsui Y. Pathological studies on sarcoidosis autopsy. II. Early change, mode of progression and death pattern. *Acta Pathol Jpn*. 1993;43(7-8):377–385.
3. Roberts WC, McAllister HA, Jr., Ferrans VJ. Sarcoidosis of the heart. A clinicopathologic study of 35 necropsy patients (group (1) and review of 78 previously described necropsy patients (group 11). *Am J Med*. 1977;63(1):86–108.
4. Furushima H, Chinushi M, Sugiura H, Kasai H, Washizuka T, Aizawa Y. Ventricular tachyarrhythmia associated with cardiac sarcoidosis: its mechanisms and outcome. *Clin Cardiol*. 2004;27(4):217–222.
5. Aizer A, Stern EH, Gomes JA, Teirstein AS, Eckart RE, Mehta D. Usefulness of programmed ventricular stimulation in predicting future arrhythmic events in patients with cardiac sarcoidosis. *Am J Cardiol*. 2005;96(2):276–282.
6. Reddy VY, Reynolds MR, Neuzil P, et al. Prophylactic catheter ablation for the prevention of defibrillator therapy. *N Engl J Med*. 2007;357(26):2657–2665.

7. Koplan BA, Soejima K, Baughman K, Epstein LM, Stevenson WG. Refractory ventricular tachycardia secondary to cardiac sarcoid: electrophysiologic characteristics, mapping, and ablation. *Heart Rhythm.* 2006;3(8):924–929.
8. Jefic D, Joel B, Good E, Morady F, Rosman H, Knight B, Bogun F. Role of radiofrequency catheter ablation of ventricular tachycardia in cardiac sarcoidosis: report from a multicenter registry. *Heart Rhythm.* 2009;6(2):189–195.
9. Vasaiwala SC, Finn C, Delpriore J, et al. Prospective study of cardiac sarcoid mimicking arrhythmogenic right ventricular dysplasia. *J Cardiovasc Electrophysiol.* 2009;20(5):473–476.
10. Chinushi M, Izumi D, Furushima H, Aizawa Y. Catheter ablation of ventricular tachycardias due to forward and reverse propagation across a reentrant circuit inside a nonischemic biventricular aneurysm. *J Cardiovasc Electrophysiol.* 2011;22(4):467–471.
11. Fananapazir L, Chang AC, Epstein SE, McAreavey D. Prognostic determinants in hypertrophic cardiomyopathy. Prospective evaluation of a therapeutic strategy based on clinical, Holter, hemodynamic, and electrophysiological findings. *Circulation.* 1992;86(3):730–740.
12. Cha YM, Gersh BJ, Maron BJ, et al. Electrophysiologic manifestations of ventricular tachyarrhythmias provoking appropriate defibrillator interventions in high-risk patients with hypertrophic cardiomyopathy. *J Cardiovasc Electrophysiol.* 2007;18(5):483–487.
13. Maron BJ, Spirito P. Implantable defibrillators and prevention of sudden death in hypertrophic cardiomyopathy. *J Cardiovasc Electrophysiol.* 2008;19(10):1118–1126.
14. Gilligan DM, Missouris CG, Boyd MJ, Oakley CM. Sudden death due to ventricular tachycardia during amiodarone therapy in familial hypertrophic cardiomyopathy. *Am J Cardiol.* 1991;68(9):971–973.
15. Furushima H, Chinushi M, Iijima K, Sanada A, Izumi D, Hosaka Y, Aizawa Y. Ventricular tachyarrhythmia associated with hypertrophic cardiomyopathy: incidence, prognosis, and relation to type of hypertrophy. *J Cardiovasc Electrophysiol.* 2010;21(9):991–999.
16. Varnava AM, Elliott PM, Baboonian C, Davison F, Davies MJ, McKenna WJ. Hypertrophic cardiomyopathy: histopathological features of sudden death in cardiac troponin T disease. *Circulation.* 2001;104(12):1380–1384.
17. Sepp R, Severs NJ, Gourdie RG. Altered patterns of cardiac intercellular junction distribution in hypertrophic cardiomyopathy. *Heart.* 1996;76(5):412–417.
18. Duarte S, Bogaert J. The role of cardiac magnetic resonance in hypertrophic cardiomyopathy. *Rev Port Cardiol.* 2010;29(1):79–93.
19. Moon JC, Reed E, Sheppard MN, Elkington AG, Ho SY, Burke M, Petrou M, Pennell DJ. The histologic basis of late gadolinium enhancement cardiovascular magnetic resonance in hypertrophic cardiomyopathy. *J Am Coll Cardiol.* 2004;43(12):2260-2264.
20. Rickers C, Wilke NM, Jerosch-Herold M, Casey SA, Panse P, Panse N, Weil J, Zenovich AG, Maron BJ. Utility of cardiac magnetic resonance imaging in the diagnosis of hypertrophic cardiomyopathy. *Circulation.* 2005;112(6): 855–861.
21. Mahrholdt H, Wagner A, Judd RM, Sechtem U, Kim RJ. Delayed enhancement cardiovascular magnetic resonance assessment of nonischaemic cardiomyopathies. *Eur Heart J.* 2005;26(15):1461–1474.
22. Leonardi S, Raineri C, De Ferrari GM, Ghio S, Scelsi L, Pasotti M, Tagliani M, Valentini A, Dore R, Raisaro A, Arbustini E. Usefulness of cardiac magnetic resonance in assessing the risk of ventricular arrhythmias and sudden death in patients with hypertrophic cardiomyopathy. *Eur Heart J.* 2009;30(16):2003–2010.
23. Bruder O, Wagner A, Jensen CJ, et al. Myocardial scar visualized by cardiovascular magnetic resonance imaging predicts major adverse events in patients with hypertrophic cardiomyopathy. *J Am Coll Cardiol.* 2010;56(11):875–887.
24. Rodriguez LM, Smeets JL, Timmermans C, Blommaert D, van Dantzig JM, de Muinck EB, Wellens HJ. Radiofrequency catheter ablation of sustained monomorphic ventricular tachycardia in hypertrophic cardiomyopathy. *J Cardiovasc Electrophysiol.* 1997;8(7):803–806.
25. Lim KK, Maron BJ, Knight BP. Successful catheter ablation of hemodynamically unstable monomorphic ventricular tachycardia in a patient with hypertrophic cardiomyopathy and apical aneurysm. *J Cardiovasc Electrophysiol.* 2009;20(4): 445–447.
26. Mantica M, Della Bella P, Arena V. Hypertrophic cardiomyopathy with apical aneurysm: a case of catheter and surgical therapy of sustained monomorphic ventricular tachycardia. *Heart.* 1997;77(5):481–483.
27. Santangeli P, Di Biase L, Lakkireddy D, et al. Radiofrequency catheter ablation of ventricular arrhythmias in patients with hypertrophic cardiomyopathy: safety and feasibility. *Heart Rhythm.* 7(8):1036–1042.
28. Dukkipati SR, d'Avila A, Soejima K, Bala R, Inada K, Singh S, Stevenson WG, Marchlinski FE, Reddy VY. Long-term outcomes of combined epicardial and endocardial ablation of monomorphic ventricular tachycardia related to hypertrophic cardiomyopathy. *Circ Arrhythm Electrophysiol.* 4(2):185–194.
29. Inada K, Seiler J, Roberts-Thomson KC, Steven D, Rosman J, John RM, Sobieszczyk P, Stevenson WG, Tedrow UB. Substrate characterization and catheter ablation for monomorphic ventricular tachycardia in patients with apical hypertrophic cardiomyopathy. *J Cardiovasc Electrophysiol.* 2011;22(1):41–8.
30. Aliot EM, Stevenson WG, Almendral-Garrote JM, et al. EHRA/HRS Expert Consensus on Catheter Ablation of Ventricular Arrhythmias: developed in a partnership with the European Heart Rhythm Association (EHRA), a Registered Branch of the European Society of Cardiology (ESC), and the Heart Rhythm Society (HRS); in collaboration with the American College of Cardiology (ACC) and the American Heart Association (AHA). *Europace.* 2009;11(6):771–817.
31. Segal OR, Wong T, Chow AW, Jarman JW, Schilling RJ, Markides V, Peters NS, Wyn Davies D. Intra-coronary guide wire mapping-a novel technique to guide ablation of human ventricular tachycardia. *J Interv Card Electrophysiol.* 2007;18(2):143–154.

CHAPTER 49

How to Ablate Ventricular Tachycardia in Patients with Arrhythmogenic Right Ventricular Cardiomyopathy/Dysplasia

Fermin C. Garcia, MD; Victor Bazan, MD, PhD

Introduction

Arrhythmogenic right ventricular cardiomyopathy/dysplasia (ARVC/D) is a heart muscle disorder characterized by fibrofatty replacement of the RV myocardium. The term arrhythmogenic was formally introduced in a reported series of 24 adult cases with RV dysplasia associated with RV tachycardia as a principal manifestation of this disease.[1] The pathological process leading to a partial replacement of the right ventricular musculature by fatty and fibrous tissue was initially referred as "dysplasia." However, this developmental defect of the RV free-wall myocardium may only represent a low proportion of ARVC/D patients. Lately, the term "cardiomyopathy" is being more widely used as it reflects the (progressive) loss of myocardial cells within the RV free wall, with a variable incidence of familiar cases, followed by a peculiar fatty or fibro-fatty replacement. Overall, it is considered that ARVC/D includes a wide spectrum of pathologic disorders affecting the RV free wall myocardium, some of which are genetically determined.

The RV myocardial abnormalities favoring the occurrence of VT are concentrated to the RV free-wall, usually sparing the RV septum. The affected regions are usually the anterior infundibular portion of the RV, the basal inferior RV (in the proximity of the acute angle of the heart) and the RVA, completing the so-called triangle of dysplasia.[1,2] Interestingly, although histologically affected, the RVA is not a frequent site of origin of VTs in the setting of ARVC/D, unlike the two former regions.[3]

Patients with ARVC/D represent a unique subset of scar-related VT. A left bundle branch (LBBB) VT QRS morphology with a late R-wave progression throughout the precordial ECG leads is the characteristic ECG pattern of the ventricular arrhythmias registered in this population. In concordance to the most frequent sites of origin of VT in the setting of ARVC/D (the anterior and inferior aspect of the tricuspid valve, periannular, free-wall regions), the VT QRS complex will show a prominent R wave in lead I, a notched R or S wave in the inferior leads, and absence of a negative concordance in the precordial leads, with R/Rs/rS complexes beyond leads V_2 to V_6.[4,5]

Although endocardial VT mapping and ablation frequently results in adequate arrhythmia control, notorious discrepancies have aroused with regard to the long-term outcome of these patients. In this sense, VT recurrences after endocardial catheter ablative therapy are very variable among the different series, ranging from 11% to 95%.[3,6-8] These conflicting results may be related to different variables, among which include patient selection, the percentage of targeted VTs out of the total number of induced VTs, the use of irrigated-tip catheters and/or electroanatomical mapping techniques. Nevertheless, beyond these discrepancies, it is accepted that an epicardial approach is a reasonable alternative to enhance adequate arrhythmia control in those ARVC/D patients presenting with VT not amenable to successful endocardial ablation.[3]

Indeed, the potential need for an epicardial approach to eliminate VT in this setting appears to be justified from both histological and electrophysiological standpoints. The importance of the epicardial and subepicardial right ventricular layers for the initiation and maintenance of RV-VT in the setting of ARVD/C was first suggested by Fontaine and colleagues.[1,2] The pathological process of myocardial replacement by fatty and fibro-fatty tissue advances from the epicardium toward the endocardial surface of the RV. During this process the strands of myocytes responsive for slow conduction and arrhythmogenicity may be concentrated toward the epicardial surface.[1,2] This phenomenon, together with a resulting local increase in the wall thickness and the presence of subendocardial fibrosis may preclude for endocardial RF lesions to reach VT circuits located deeper in the RV myocardium toward the epicardial surface.[1,2,9]

Therefore, a somewhat low threshold to perform epicardial access and mapping of VT in the setting of ARVC/D appears necessary. In this sense, we have demonstrated that the epicardial substrate favoring the occurrence of VT may be more prominent as opposed to its endocardial counterpart, frequently containing critical portions of the tachycardia circuit that cannot be mapped and ablated from the endocardial approach.[9] In this particular setting, epicardial ablation will result in a more favorable long-term arrhythmia control.[9] It is suggested that epicardial ablation should be strongly considered in the event of a limited (or even absent) endocardial low voltage area (a surrogate of endocardial RV scar) as detected during electroanatomical mapping, late VT termination during endocardial ablation, or early VT recurrences after endocardial ablation. An epicardial origin of the right ventricular arrhythmia will also be suspected upon the identification of some ECG clues associated to epicardial right ventricular tachycardia.[10] These ECG clues are based on the assessment of the initial vector of ventricular depolarization traveling from the epicardium toward the endocardium during epicardial VTs, and are region-specific in their ability to identify this subset of ventricular arrhythmias. Of note, previously reported interval criteria based on the measurement of the initial pseudo-delta wave that is registered during epicardial LV tachycardia do not apply to RV-VTs.[10]

During this chapter, we shall discuss how to ablate ventricular tachycardia occurring in the setting of ARVC/D, including patient and preprocedural preparation, endocardial and epicardial ablation techniques and indications and management of complications related to this procedure.

Preprocedural Planning

Recognition of ARVC/D as the underlying pathological condition in a patient presenting with RV tachycardia is crucial in order to enhance adequate long-term arrhythmia control by means of catheter ablative therapy. This especially applies to those right VTs originated remote from the RVOT region, in which an accurate characterization of the myocardial RV scar area will help defining an appropriate radiofrequency lesion set strategy. It is acknowledged that the diagnosis of ARVC/D is based upon reported task force criteria, including RV dilatation and dysfunction (**Figure 49.1**) and identification of multiple RV tachycardia morphologies and baseline ECG abnormalities.[11] These baseline ECG signs include incomplete or complete RBBB, T-wave inversion in the anterior precordial leads (V_1 to V_4), postexcitation Epsilon waves and selective prolongation (> 25 ms) of the QRS duration in leads V_1 to V_3 as compared to lead V_6.

When catheter ablative therapy is considered in an ARVC/D patient presenting with RV-VT, the first step consists of an individualized preparation of the mapping and ablation strategy on the basis of a careful initial clinical evaluation. Special attention must be paid to the particular hemodynamic characteristics, including the degree of RV and/or LV function and optimization of fluid status in order to minimize the incidence of intra-procedural complications related to pump failure. In this sense, it also appears mandatory to assess for the hemodynamic tolerance of the clinical VT in order to anticipate the possibility of intra-procedural collapse.

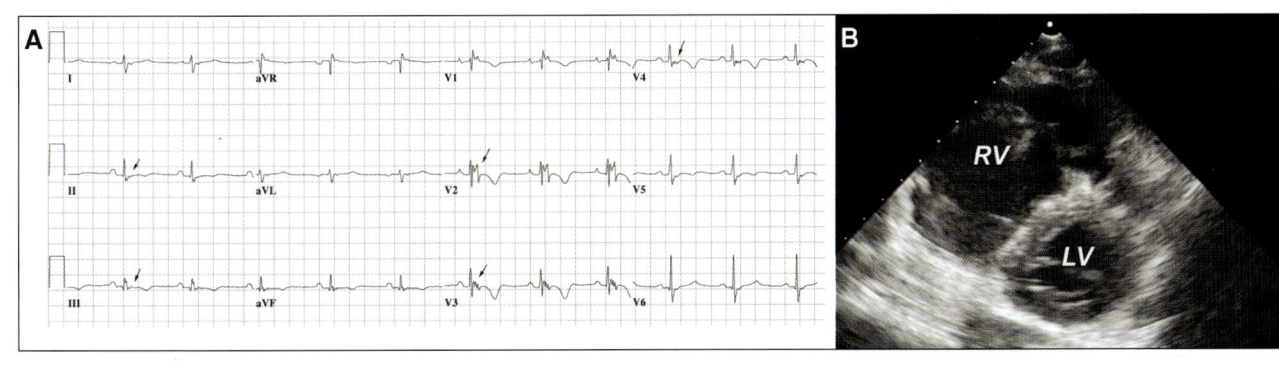

Figure 49.1 **A.** Characteristic baseline 12-lead ECG in a patient with ARVC/D. Note the abnormalities in depolarization (Epsilon waves, arrow) and T-wave inversion across the precordium. **B.** Two-dimensional echocardiogram shows enlarged RV and normal LV in the same patient.

Twelve-lead ECG documentation of all VT morphologies, whenever feasible, is of high interest. In this sense, extensive electroanatomical mapping, especially in the setting of large RV myocardial scars, will be accompanied by the identification of critical parts of tachycardia circuits (circuit isthmuses and exit sites) in which a particular VT QRS morphology is reproduced during pace mapping, mimicking that obtained during spontaneous clinical VT. These specific areas become a potential target for RF energy delivery. Additionally, surface electrocardiographic recording (12-lead ECG or limited telemetry tracings) as well as intracardiac defibrillator (ICD) EGMs, if available, are used to compare spontaneous and induced VT during the procedure. The 12-lead ECG characteristics are important predictors of the location of the arrhythmia and aid in preparing upfront for an early epicardial approach, for which specific patient's preparation, including the need for general anesthesia, is of special concern.[4,5,10]

Ablation Procedure

Endocardial Electroanatomical Voltage Mapping

In those cases in which incessant hemodynamically tolerated VT is not the baseline rhythm, the first step of the ablation procedure should consist of a detailed characterization of the endocardial electroanatomical voltage map (**Figure 49.2**; ▶ **Video 49.1**). We usually insert a long introducer (LAMP 90, St. Jude Medical, St. Paul, MN) from the right femoral vein and position it in the inflow aspect of the RV. We consider this essential, as a long catheter sheath will dramatically enhance catheter stability and support, which is usually a matter of special concern when dealing with patients with ARVC/D, who usually present with dilated right atria and significant tricuspid regurgitation. We further deploy an ICE catheter in the right heart that permits for real-time monitoring, in order to anatomically guide the mapping and ablation procedures.

Careful identification of valvular structures during RV-VT ablation is critical. The tricuspid valve is identified at the base of the RV by means of the fluoroscopic typical valvular motion, by the registering of bipolar recordings demonstrating both atrial and ventricular signals of approximately equal amplitude in the mapping catheter, and upon echocardiographic confirmation by ICE imaging. The pulmonic valve is identified by advancing the mapping catheter into the pulmonary artery and slowly withdrawing it back into the RV, until a bipolar ventricular EGM is identified, along with consistent pacing capture. We then confirm the mapping catheter position under direct visualization by ICE. These valvular sites are given a location only tag in the electroanatomical map, in order to avoid their influence in the bipolar voltage color map for identifying areas of RV scar tissue. Intracavitary points should also be usually excluded from the final map, with the exception of those points representing true anatomic structures (ie, papillary muscle or moderator band), as confirmed by direct visualization by ICE.

Detailed electroanatomic mapping of the endocardial RV surface is performed in a point-by-point fashion. Peak to peak signals aligned with the QRS are measured automatically and manually confirmed for each point. The reference values for normal endocardial voltage are represented in a color scale and set at > 1.5 mV.[12] Abnormal signals representing diseased myocardial tissue and border zone are considered between 0.5 to 1.5 mV. Myocardial RV dense scar is represented below 0.5 mV and is usually associated with noncapture at 10 mA and 2-second pulse

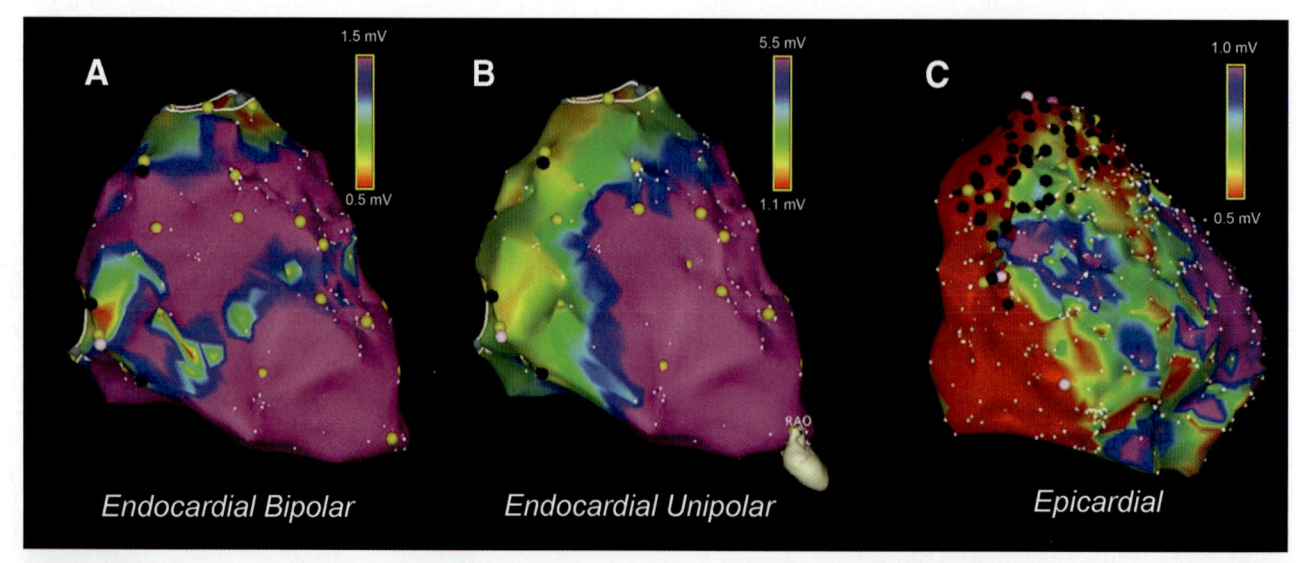

Figure 49.2 **A.** Endocardial bipolar voltage map in a patient with ARVC/D shows limited areas of abnormal EGMs in the lateral wall at the level of tricuspid valve. **B.** The endocardial unipolar voltage map suggests a much larger abnormal substrate in the epicardium. **C.** The epicardial bipolar voltage map confirms a very extensive abnormal substrate in the epicardium, as opposed to the endocardial counterpart.

width.[12,13] Fractionated and late potentials extending beyond the QRS are tagged in the map and are of particular utility when pace mapping is used to correlate the arrhythmia with the diseased myocardium that incorporates a critical portion of the reentrant VT circuit. Common areas of abnormal voltage usually involve perivalvular structures within the free wall of the RV, and it is emphasized that high density mapping around these areas should be performed (**Figures 49.3** and **49.4**).

It should be noted that endocardial bipolar voltage abnormalities might underestimate the degree of abnormal myocardium. The myocardial substrate favoring the occurrence of VT in ARVD/C patients may spare the endocardium and be more concentrated to the epicardial surface in some cases.[1,2,9] In this sense, endocardial unipolar mapping may serve to identify areas of RV scar tissue located deep in the intra-myocardial layers, toward the epicardial surface.[14] We have noted the unipolar voltage representation of the endocardial surface to be predictive of the epicardial voltage characteristics and to accurately correlate with the RV epicardial bipolar voltage map. Once the endocardial voltage map is finished the voltage is adjusted to a unipolar mode with the cutoff set at > 5.5 mV for normal tissue (**Figures 49.2** and **49.4**; ▶ **Video 49.2**). Noteworthy, early suspicion of epicardial abnormalities combining electrocardiographic criteria and unipolar voltage mapping allows for early planning for epicardial access.[10,14]

Electrophysiology Study and Arrhythmia Induction

In those patients not presenting with incessant VT, a comprehensive electrophysiological study (EPS) should be performed once the electro-anatomical substrate map has been elaborated. The EPS should initially include both baseline atrial and ventricular stimulation. Once the ventricular effective refractory period is defined, programmed ventricular stimulation (PES), including ventricular drive trains at 600 and 400 ms with up to triple extrastimuli at least at 2 different sites should be performed. All surface ECG and the real-time intracardiac EGMs from the ICD registering of the induced VT are recorded and compared to the clinical arrhythmias. The induced ventricular arrhythmias may not be hemodynamically tolerated, thus precluding for performance of entrainment and/or activation mapping techniques. This is especially true when general anesthesia is used, frequently when a probable need to an epicardial approach is established in advance. It is therefore recommended that, regardless of the suspicion

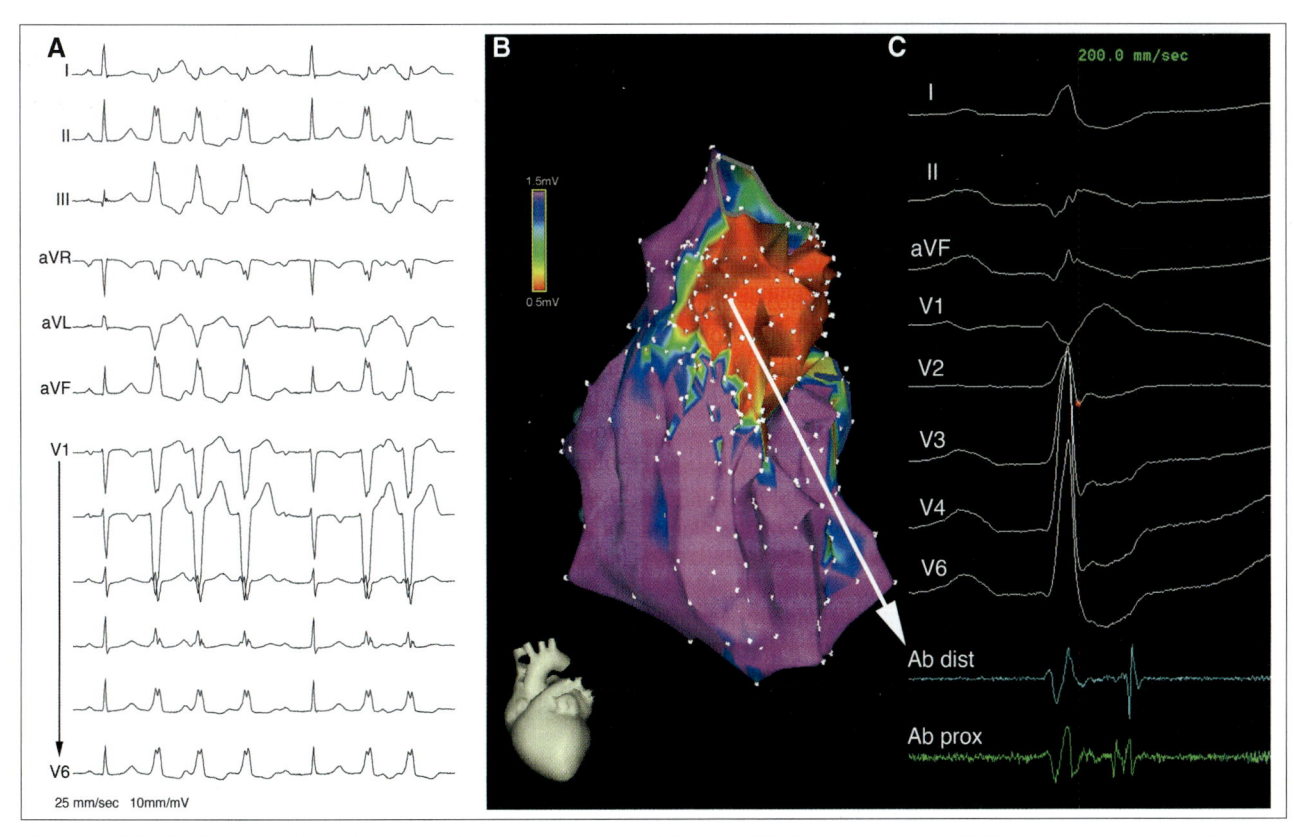

Figure 49.3 **A.** The 12-lead ECG during spontaneous nonsustained VT in an ARVC/D patient shows a LBBB morphology transitioning in V$_4$, with inferior and leftward axis. **B.** The endocardial voltage map abnormalities are consistent with abnormal myocardium in the RVOT region, where VT originates. **C.** Noteworthy, the low-voltage region is associated with fractionated and late EGMs as the myocardial substrate favoring the occurrence of VT in this setting.

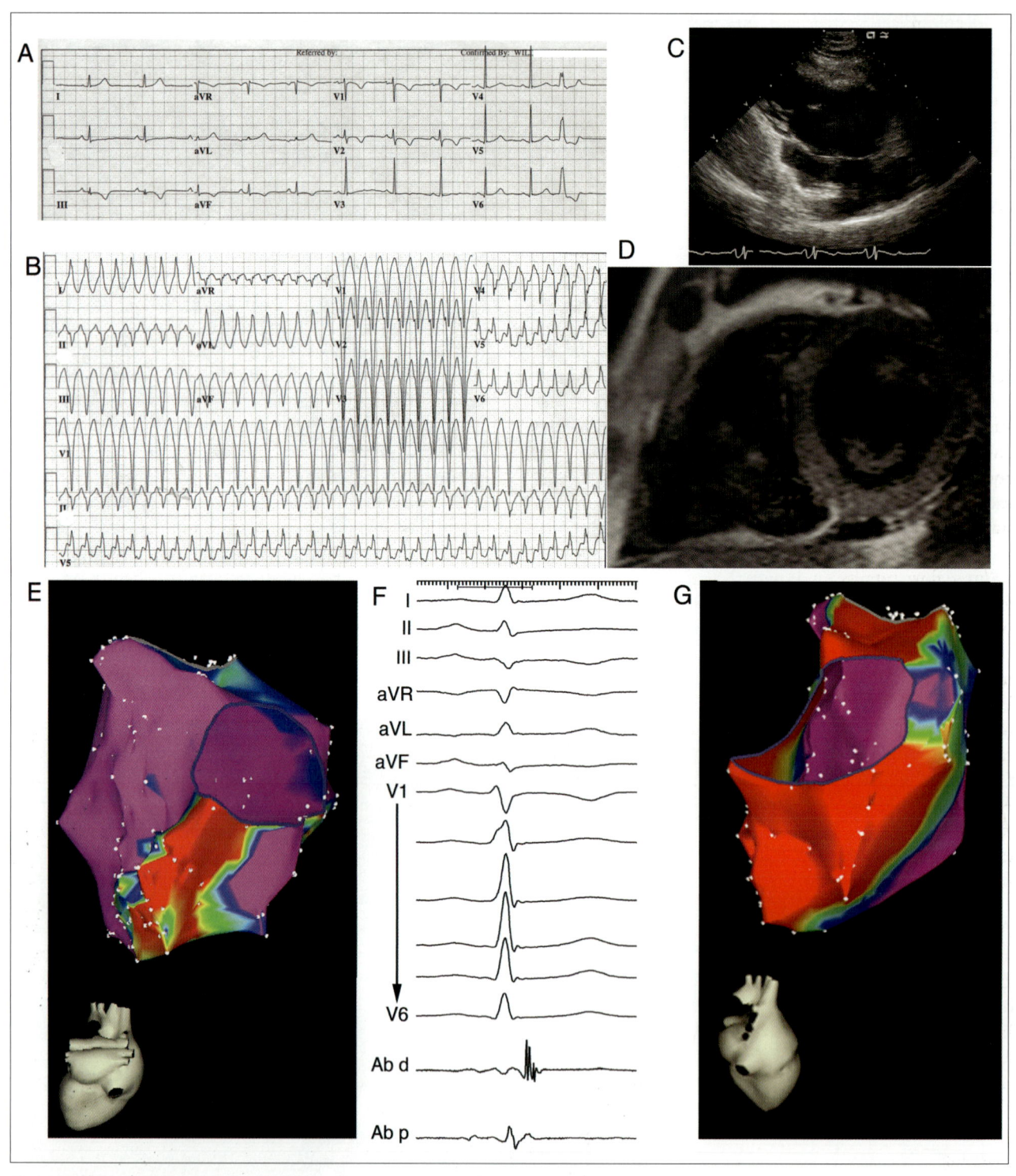

Figure 49.4 **A.** Sinus rhythm 12-lead ECG in a patient with ARVC/D showing T-wave inversion in the precordial and inferior leads. **B.** The 12-lead ECG during VT is consistent with origin around the inferior tricuspid valve annulus. **C.** The 2-dimensional echocardiogram image identified an area of akinesis and myocardial thining at the RV base next to the tricuspid valve (arrow). **D.** This abnormality is also apparent in the short-axis view of the cardiac MRI (small arrows). **E.** Bipolar endocardial voltage map shows an area of abnormal voltage and scar (0.5 to 1.5 mV) corresponding to the same are captured by the imaging methods. **F.** Low voltage EGMs and late potentials are recorded from this area. **G.** Interestingly, unipolar endocardial representation suggests a much larger epicardial substrate.

of an epicardial origin of the ventricular arrhythmia, the first part of the procedure during which PES and VT induction are performed should be attempted under conscious sedation, thus favoring the use of entrainment and activation mapping as preferred techniques to guide the ablation procedure.

Endocardial Mapping and Ablation

In the setting of ARVC/D, we typically utilize an open-irrigated 3.5-mm catheter allowing for electroanatomical mapping and ablation. It is preferred to perform activation and entrainment mapping during VT as the most reliable techniques to precisely identify the exact VT site of origin and critical portions of the circuit. However, in the event of VT hemodynamic intolerance or self-termination, substrate mapping and pace mapping techniques will serve as guidance in order to approximate the target for successful ablation.[3,9] This usually includes the identification of fragmented/abnormal signals registered in the 1 to 2 cm area surrounding the best pace map site.[12]

We usually commence RF applications at 30 W with 30 ml/min flow rate and a temperature limit of 45°C. We gradually titrate the power to a 12 to 16 ohm impedance drop depending on the starting impedance, and aim for 120-second applications. Catheter contact and lesion formation are monitored with the use of ICE, and effective lesion creation is indexed by bipolar signal attenuation, increase in local pace-capture threshold, and, very importantly, by the disappearance of isolated potentials or high frequency late EGM components after ablation.[3,12] These endpoints for individual lesion delivery are often very difficult to achieve in the presence of thick RV scar, which exerts an insulating effect against RF current flow, even with irrigated-tip ablation.

Mappable VTs are targeted until noninducible. Aggressive ablation of all induced VTs on the endocardial and epicardial surfaces of the RV has become the goal of the ablation procedure in our center. Certainly, all regions of low bipolar voltage scar associated to spontaneous or induced VT morphologies are targeted. Isolated and very late potentials are also comprehensively identified and targeted, particularly those clustered together in apparent networks, and those displaying long stimulus to QRS times and good morphology matches during pace mapping.

For unmappable VTs, the endocardial lesion set is designed to incorporate as many target sites (as identified by pace mapping and EGM morphology) within the low-voltage zone as possible (substrate ablation), with the aim to eliminate the critical components of all potential VT circuits.[12] Linear lesions that cross through the entire endocardial low voltage area, beginning at VT exit sites based on pacing at the border of the low voltage area and terminating at the valve plane, are frequently employed.

More commonly, clusters of lesions are delivered targeting areas demonstrating LPs, particularly those in which pacing produces a long stimulus to QRS interval and a pace map that matches of the VT QRS complex.

Again, for unmappable VTs the main procedural endpoint is also VT noninducibility with aggressive programmed stimulation protocol. Noninvasive programmed stimulation via the ICD is performed 1 to 2 days later to ensure absence of remnant inducibility of all VT morphologies.

Epicardial Mapping and Ablation

An epicardial origin for RV tachycardia in the setting of ARVC/D should be suspected upon recognition of 12-lead ECG characteristics during VT suggesting an epicardial origin, along with a late termination of VT during endocardial ablation or inability to eliminate VT from the endocardium. Additionally, when analysis of unipolar endocardial signals suggest a more prominent epicardial substrate, access to the epicardium for catheter mapping and ablation should be considered.[3,9,10,14]

Percutaneous epicardial access (⏵ Video 49.3) is obtained by using the techniques described by Sosa and colleagues.[15] In summary, the technique consists of advancing an epidural needle under fluoroscopic guidance to the pericardial space, as confirmed by contrast injection. A guide wire is then introduced through the needle, and an 8-French introducer is subsequently inserted into the pericardial space through the guide wire. A steerable introducer can be used as an alternative to enhance detailed epicardial mapping and catheter contact. A diagnostic quadrapolar catheter is usually inserted endocardially to the RVA in order to fluoroscopically guide the pericardial puncture. Alternatively, the ICD lead tip, usually positioned to the RVA, may serve as the anatomical guidance. The procedure is usually performed under general anesthesia, due to the high-risk nature of the patients and also because RF energy applications in the epicardial surface are painful.[16] The fluoroscopic view of choice for the pericardial puncture is usually the LAO. The posterior approach to pericardial puncture is preferred, as a dilated RV may increase the risks associated with an anterior needle pass. Careful attention has to be placed to the orientation of the needle, given the potential risk of liver damage as the needle is directed deeper in the subxiphoid area. Detailed epicardial substrate mapping (**Figure 49.2**) is then performed using a similar technique to the endocardium but with the voltage cut-off for normal myocardium set at 1.0 mV.[17] In the low voltage area, notable attention is paid to identification of isolated late potentials and fractionated EGMs, since these characteristics are paramount of scar tissue and differentiate abnormal areas from interposed fat tissue or epicardial vessels when voltage value is used as the sole criterion. Pace mapping to identify channels and potential exit sites are tagged. Close attention is also paid to sites of apparently greater separation of the endocardial and epicardial shells on the electroanatomic map and ICE as suggested regions of increased wall thickness, where the VT substrate may be more likely to reside.[9] Programmed ventricular stimulation is then repeated and any stable VTs are then mapped as described before using an irrigated-tip catheter.

On the epicardium, we employ similar biophysical parameters for lesion delivery, although usually at a lower irrigation flow rate (10–17 ml/min). Intermittent or continuous aspiration of fluid from the side-arm of the pericardial introducer is performed. As on the endocardium, epicardial fat and thick fibro-fatty replacement tissue can again hamper efforts to create transmural lesions (**Figure 49.5**).

Before RF energy is delivered at the target RV epicardial sites, performance of coronary angiography is mandatory. Following coronary artery definition, RF energy can be delivered at candidate sites identified by entrainment mapping to terminate tolerated VT, always keeping a > 10 mm safety distance from the coronary epicardial vasculature.

In the event of epicardial unmappable VTs, it is noteworthy that the tricuspid valve plane marks a region in proximity to the right coronary artery. Therefore, extensive linear lesions are usually discouraged. As compared to endocardial lesions, epicardial linear lesions in this setting will connect areas of pacing inexcitability and cross through the best pace map sites.

Procedural Complications

Complications of ventricular tachycardia ablation can be prevented by careful preprocedural preparation and patient individualization.[18] Fluid status, ventricular function and hemodynamic condition are evaluated noninvasively and invasively prior to the mapping and ablation procedure.

Whether the pathological process is confined to the RV or not, there is no conclusive data that the risk of RV perforation and cardiac tamponade during VT ablation is higher in patients with ARVC/D in comparison to other conditions. Careful attention to the hemodynamics and constant monitoring under ICE to assess catheter position, and early recognition of a pericardial effusion are essential. By these means, early drainage of pericardial fluid and anticoagulation reversal will prevent cardiac tamponade.

Pulmonary embolism from clots formed in sheaths and catheters may have significant hemodynamic consequences in a patient with limited RV reserve. For this reason, we give low-level anticoagulation (a 5000 U bolus of unfractionated heparin, usually not increasing ACT above 250 seconds) while mapping the endocardium, which will need to be reversed with protamine once the pericardial access is attempted.

During pericardial access, the posterior route is preferred in order to avoid laceration of the anterior wall of a dilated RV. All patients are type and crossed, and blood transfusion is available if necessary. Close attention to a subxiphoid area of pericardial access away from the abdomen is critical to limit the potential damage to the liver, which could be especially enlarged in the setting of ARVC/D due to chronic right heart failure. Once in the pericardium, RV perforation has to be ruled out before advancing the sheath. In this sense, a guide wire has to be advanced through the needle and confirmed into the pericardial space, giving a characteristic fluoroscopic image of the wire wrapping around the cardiac silhouette in the left anterior oblique view. In case of a laceration to the RV with uncontrollable intrapericardial bleeding, early detection and surgical intervention are essential.

Once in the pericardial space, both a steerable sheath and presence of a small amount of fluid may facilitate catheter movement. Careful attention to ECG recording is important since local contact with coronary arteries may result in vasospasm. Coronary angiography and high output pacing should be performed before any RF lesion is deployed on the epicardial RV surface. Of particular interest in these cases is the location of the RV marginal artery (or arteries) which usually runs diagonally down the midfree wall of the RV, therefore usually allowing for the possibility of ablating the epicardium overlying the acute inferior angle of the RV, where VT exit sites and substrate are often located. Assessment for phrenic nerve capture, although less frequently observed as compared to epicardial LV mapping and ablation, is also recommended but usually not a limitation for energy delivery.

Postprocedure Care

Acute pericarditis, with its common signs and symptoms, is frequent after pericardial mapping and ablation. Treatments of pericarditis after ablation focus on pain relief and inflammation control. The cornerstone for the treatment is nonsteroidal anti-inflammatory drugs (NSAID), with ibuprofen being the preferred medication (high dose, 1200 to 1300 mg, administered in 3 or 4 divided doses for a few days, and at lower doses for a week). Other oral NSAIDS less commonly used are indomethacin, aspirin, and colchicines. If the patient has not started oral intake, intravenous ketorolac is used. Pain control is also managed with intravenous infusion of opioids. Intrapericardial administration of corticosteroids, usually triamcinolone (2 mg/kg or up to 300 mg/m^2) immediately upon completion of the case while pericardial access is still available has been reported to effectively decrease inflammation and is routinely used in our laboratory for pericardial mapping procedure.[19,20]

A pericardial sheath (small pigtail catheter) is left in place for 12 hours for drainage of any pericardial effusion,

Chapter 49: Ablation of VT in ARVC/D • 469

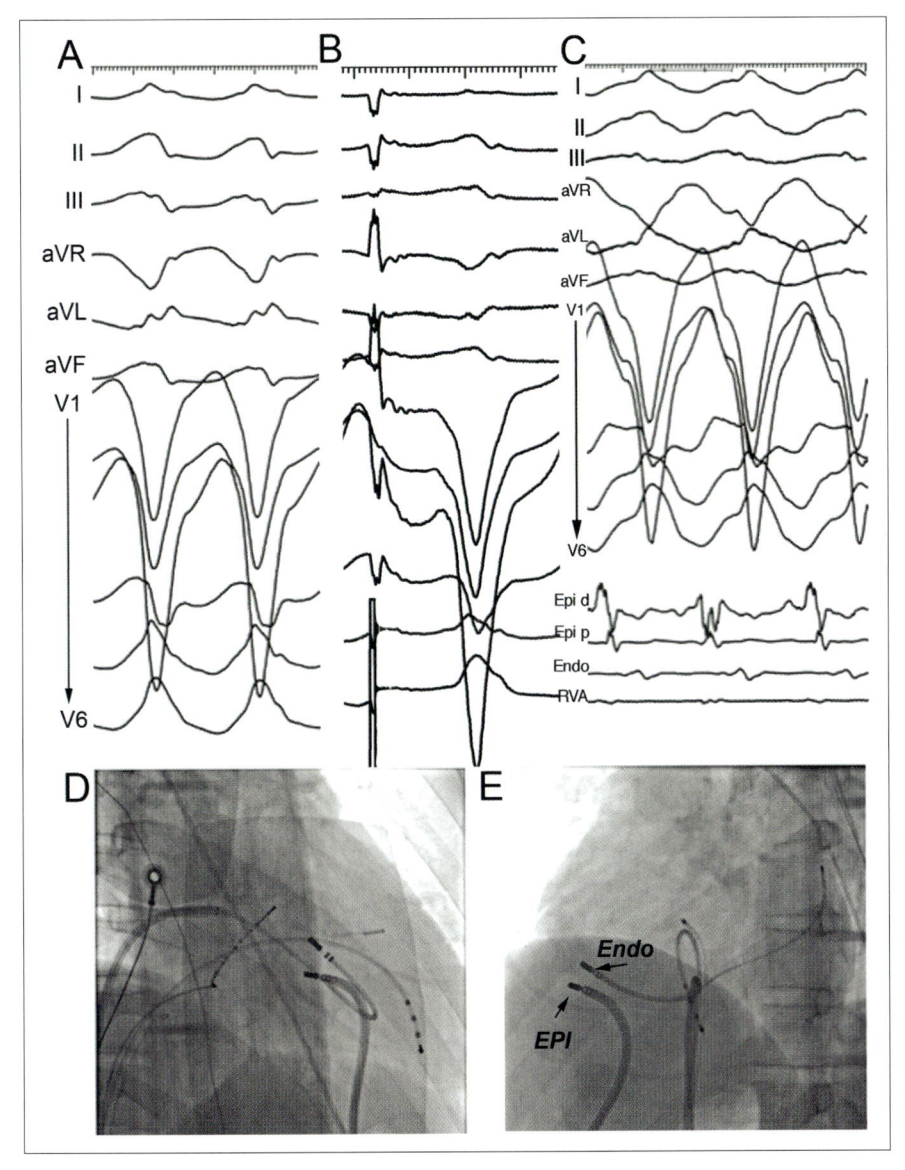

Figure 49.5 Ventricular tachycardia arising from the epicardial aspect of the anterior RV free-wall. **A.** A QS pattern in leads V1 to V3 is suggestive of an epicardial site of origin for VTs originated from this particular RV region. **B.** Pace mapping from the best endocardial site resulted in a poor QRS match and a long stimulus-to-QRS is demonstrated, together with an initial small R wave in leads V1 through V3. **C.** During VT, the epicardial mapping catheter (epi distal and proximal) shows earlier epicardial activation as opposed to the best endocardial site (endo distal), which is consistent with an epicardial exit site of the ventricular arrhythmia. **D, E.** The epicardial exit site was proved to be located just opposite to the endocardial best site, and ablation from this particular location resulted in VT elimination.

and removed after echocardiographic confirmation of absence of any significant pericardial fluid accumulation. The patient is observed in critical care unit for 12 to 24 hours.

Before hospital discharge, all patients undergo either non-invasive programmed electrical stimulation via their implanted defibrillators, or a single catheter electrophysiological study and programmed ventricular stimulation. Early ambulation and diuresis are the focus of postoperative care, paying close attention to continuous telemetry for the next 24 to 48 hours after ablation.

Conclusions

Endocardial and epicardial electroanatomical mapping and ablation is a safe and effective therapy in the treatment of RV arrhythmias occurring in the setting of ARVC/D.

Activation and entrainment mapping are the preferred techniques to identify critical parts of VT circuits and targeted for ablation. In the event of unmappable VTs, substrate mapping and pace mapping will help identifying the potential surrogate markers and landmarks that will serve as references for linear ablation. Aggressive endocardial irrigated-tip catheter ablation may be enough to achieve VT elimination and adequate long-term arrhythmia control. However, if late-termination of VT during ablation, VT reinducibility or early arrhythmia recurrences are documented, epicardial ablation is strongly encouraged, especially upon accomplishment of VT QRS characteristics suggestive of an epicardial VT site of origin. In addition, epicardial intervention should be considered when the endocardial voltage mapping suggests a prominent epicardial VT substrate. Strict hemodynamic monitoring during the ablation procedure will help minimizing the complications associated to endocardial and epicardial VT ablation.

References

1. Marcus FI, Fontaine GH, Guiraudon G, et al. Right ventricular dysplasia: A report of 24 adult cases. *Circulation.* 1982;65:384–398.
2. Fontaine G, Fontaliran F, Hébert JL. Arrhythmogenic right ventricular dysplasia. *Annu Rev Med.* 1999;50:17–35.
3. Marchlinski FM, Zado E, Dixit S, et al. Electroanatomic substrate and outcome of catheter ablative therapy for ventricular tachycardia in setting of right ventricular cardiomyopathy. *Circulation.* 2004;110:2293–2298.
4. Josephson ME, Callans DJ. Using the twelve-lead ECG to localize the site of origin of ventricular tachycardia. *Heart Rhythm.* 2005;2:443–446.
5. Tada H, Tadokoro K, Ito S, et al. Idiopathic ventricular arrhythmias originating from the tricuspid annulus: Prevalence, electrocardiographic characteristics, and results of radiofrequency catheter ablation. *Heart Rhythm.* 2007;4:7–16.
6. Dalal D, Jain R, Tandri H, et al. Long-term efficacy of catheter ablation of ventricular tachycardia in patients with arrhythmogenic right ventricular dysplasia/cardiomyopathy. *J Am Coll Cardiol.* 2007;50:432–440.
7. Reithmann C, Hahnefeld A, Remp T, et al. Electroanatomical mapping of endocardial right ventricular activation as a guide for catheter ablation in patients with arrhythmogenic right ventricular dysplasia. *Pacing Clin Electrophysiol.* 2003;26:1308–1316.
8. Verma A, Kilicaslan F, Schweikert RA, et al. Short- and long-term success of substrate-based mapping and ablation of ventricular tachycardia in arrhythmogenic right ventricular dysplasia. *Circulation.* 2005;111:3209–3216.
9. Garcia FC, Bazan V, Zado ES, et al. Epicardial substrate and outcome with epicardial ablation of ventricular tachycardia in arrhythmogenic right ventricular cardiomyopathy/dysplasia. *Circulation.* 2009;120:366–375.
10. Bazan V, Bala R, Garcia FC, Sussman JS, Gerstenfeld EP, Dixit S, Callans DJ, Zado ES, Marchlinski FE. Twelve-lead ECG features to identify ventricular tachycardia arising from the epicardial right ventricle. *Heart Rhythm.* 2006;3:1132-9.
11. Marcus FI, McKenna W, Sherill D, et al. Diagnosis of arrhythmogenic right ventricular cardiomyopathy/dysplasia: proposed modification of the Task Force criteria. *Circulation.* 2010;121;1533–1541.
12. Marchlinski FM, Callans DJ, Gottlieb CD, et al. Linear ablation lesion for control of unmappable ventricular tachycardia in patients with ischemic and nonischemic cardiomyopathy. *Circulation.* 2000;101;1288–1296.
13. Callans DJ, Ren JF, Michele J, et al. Electroanatomic left ventricular mapping in the porcine model of healed anterior myocardial infarction: correlation with intracardiac echocardiography and pathological analysis. *Circulation.* 1999;100:1744–1750.
14. Polin GM, Haggani H, Tzou W, et al. Endocardial unipolar voltage mapping to identify epicardial substrate in arrhythmogenic right ventricular dysplasia/cardiomyopathy. *Heart Rhythm.* 2011;8(1):76–83.
15. Sosa E, Scanavacca M, d'Avila A. A new technique to perform epicardial mapping in the electrophysiology laboratory. *J Cardiovasc Electrophysiol.* 1996;7:531–536.
16. Sosa E, Scanavacca M. Epicardial mapping and ablation techniques to control ventricular tachycardia. *J Cardiovasc Electrophysiol.* 2005;16:449–452.
17. Cano O, Hutchinson M, Lin D, et al. Electroanatomic substrate and ablation outcome for suspected epicardial ventricular tachycardia in left ventricular nonischemic cardiomyopathy. *J Am Coll Cardiol.* 2009;54;799–808.
18. Garcia FC, Valles E, Dhruvakumar S, et al. Ablation of ventricular tachycardia. *Herzschrittmacherther Elektrophysiol.* 2007;18:225–233.
19. D'Avila A, Neuzil P, Thiagalingam A, et al. Experimental efficacy of pericardial installation of anti-inflammatory agents during percutaneous epicardial catheter ablation to prevent postprocedure pericarditis. *J Cardiovasc Electrophysiol.* 2007;18:1178–1183.
20. Maisch B, Seferovic PM, Ristic AD et al. Guidelines on the diagnosis and management of pericardial diseases. Executive summary: the Task Force on the Diagnosis and Management of Pericardial Diseases of the European Society of Cardiology. *Eur Heart J.* 2004;25:587–610.

Video Descriptions

Video 49.1 Endocardial bipolar voltage map in ARVCM/D that showed limited low voltage abnormalities at the basal inferior tricuspid annular area.

Video 49.2 Endocardial unipolar voltage map in ARVCM/D. The unipolar endocardial recordings showed a large low voltage abnormality a the inferiobasal tricuspid annulus, suggesting ther presence of a larger epicardial scar substrate.

Video 49.3 Epicardial puncture (courtesy of David Lin, MD. Hospital of the University of Pennsylvania).

CHAPTER 50

How to Perform Hybrid VT Ablation in the Operating Room

Paolo Della Bella, MD; Giuseppe Maccabelli, MD; Francesco Alamanni, MD

Introduction

The onward growth of the curative function of catheter ablation in patients with ICDs underlines the need of a complementary role of catheter ablation in patients with structural cardiomyopathy and ICD.[1,2] This group includes patients with ICM in whom catheter ablation can achieve good results as well as patients with idiophatic dilated cardiomyopathy (IDCM), in whom the success rate is lower. Since failure of catheter ablation provides an independent positive predictive value of mortality, it is mandatory to resort to more effective procedures.

In the last few years, a great deal of effort has been made to understand the mechanism causing arrhythmias. This has emphasized how the intramural or epicardial layers are often critical areas for the reentry circuits, particularly in patients with NICM.

In the past, the first approach at the epicardium was performed by surgeons.[3,4] Patients with ischemic or primary cardiomyopathy with intractable ventricular arrhythmia were subjected to a surgical treatment performed with epicardial, transmural, and endocardial mapping techniques. The identification of the earliest local activation during the arrhythmia was followed by surgical excision that interrupts potential reentrant circuits included in the myocardial wall with the subsequent elimination of the rhythm disturbance.[5] Instead of the surgical excision, Gallagher et al.[6] proposed the use of the cryoablation, which offered some advantages, such as the possibility of testing the effect of reversible block over the arrhythmia before proceeding to irreversible ablation. Thus, surgical resection in addition to cryoablation has allowed the removal of sustained monomorphic VT in about 69 to 95% of patients.[7-14]

The surgical mapping experience provides a 3-dimensional view of the substratum of the VT and the evidence that the subepicardial or the intramural layers can be involved in a minor but still substantial number of cases.[15-18] Despite good results, surgery may have some complications, and the mortality rate commonly related to pump failure is not insignificant. On the other hand, catheter ablation with pacing maneuvers like pace mapping, entrainment, and the new computerized mapping system have permitted achievement of very good results in the settings of VT ablation. The only important limitation is related to the depth of the lesions created with RF energy, which may render it useless in case of epicardial circuits. The use of cooled-tip RF catheter ablation can increase the lesions' size and depth[19,20]; however, in cases of truly epicardial circuits, present in different proportion in ischemic, dilated, and Chagas disease, ablation performed from the endocardial surface is always ineffective.[21-23]

In 1996, Sosa et al.[24] proposed an innovative technique to access the pericardial space through a subxyphoidal puncture. An epidural needle is advanced in the pericardial space under fluoroscopic control. With an 8- to 9-Fr introducer, an ablation catheter may be inserted into the pericardial space to achieve epicardial mapping and ablation. This technique has gradually spread, although its complexity and potential risk have limited its diffusion in only a few centers in the world that have used this technique in a widespread mode with good results in different types of cardiomyopathy.

Despite the important improvement in the endocardial mapping and ablation technique and the capability to perform these procedures in the epicardial surface, there are some situations where these tools are unable to solve the arrhythmic problems. The option of using a fast and precise computerized mapping system in the operating theatre has permitted the surgical ablation in these selected although infrequent cases with reduced procedural time and good results.

Indications for Surgical Ablation

Although surgical ablation provides the possibility to treat patients with VT successfully, it must be emphasized that indications to this procedure are quite limited.

Lack of Percutaneous Approach

The first situation where surgical ablation may be considered is in circumstances in which it is impossible to perform an epicardial procedure in the EP laboratory using a conventional percutaneous approach. Patients presenting with aortic and mitral mechanical prosthesis, with previous cardiac surgery, or with pericardial adhesion due to old inflammatory processes may be considered for a surgical ablation. The approach would be different in relation to the characteristics of the patient and the supposed origin of the ventricular arrhythmia.

In patients with previous cardiac surgery or epicardial adhesion, the surgical approach should be considered only after a previous percutaneous endocardial mapping and ablation attempt. In this setting, careful evaluation of the anatomy of the pericardium must be performed before planning the surgical procedure, and a Marfan window could be considered as first attempt before sternotomy. Thus, the only limitation is provided by the complexity and extension of the adherences and by the presence and course of the coronary artery bypass.

Failure of Percutaneous Approach

Another situation where surgical ablation may be considered is the inefficacy of a previous endo- or epicardial ablation performed in the EP lab. The reasons for such failures may differ.

One of the current limitations of the RF energy is the ability to reach circuits located deep within the ventricular wall. In these situations, commonplace in a hypertrophic left ventricle, the possibility of applying cryoenergy directly on the epicardial surface through purposely designed large surgical probes enhances the likelihood of achieving deeper lesions.

Other situations that can determine failure of percutaneous procedure are:

1. Presence of epicardial fat
2. Coronary arteries located in the critical part of the arrhythmia circuit
3. Presence of the phrenic nerve

Fat is usually present in the epicardial surface of the heart, particularly along the coronary arteries' course and at the base of the heart. The latter may be a problem for patients with IDCM, in which scars and arrhythmic circuits are more frequently located in basolateral LV epicardial surface.[25,26] Moreover, fat is increased and is correlated positively with age and waist circumference,[27] and is significantly increased in ischemic patients.[28] Several experimental contributions have demonstrated in the past that RF energy, even though irrigated, has limited efficacy in the presence of fat. Cooled-tip RF ablation with 2.6 ± 1.2 mm thick layers of fat can determine lesions of 4.1 ± 2 mm in depth, but in the presence of a fat layer of more than 3.5 mm, it is unable to produce lesions. Currently pericardial fat can be evaluated with echocardiography, CT scan, and MRI, but no software is available to translate information obtained with these diagnostic tools to the EP mapping system. Moreover, bipolar voltages recorded over a fat surface can be of lower amplitude (< 0.5 mV) if myocardial tissue is normal, making the evaluation of the maps obtained quite difficult.

Another important problem related to closed-chest epicardial ablation is the presence of coronary arteries that sometimes lie quite near or over a critical part of the circuit suitable for RF ablation. Since RF energy delivery over a coronary artery could induce damage,[29] ranging from replacement of the media with extracellular matrix to severe intimal hyperplasia with intravascular thrombosis, careful evaluation of the position of the ablating catheter as regards to the coronary artery must be performed with angiography. Future development of imaging techniques could probably reduce these problems, allowing precise and detailed navigation of the catheter tip along the coronary arteries, but at the present time, in relation to the complexity of the arrhythmic circuit or the deviousness of the artery, safer delivering of RF energy may be difficult or impossible.

Also, the presence of the phrenic nerve may be an obstacle to the RF energy delivery. Unlike the right phrenic nerve, the intrathoracic course of which doesn't represent an obstacle for the epicardial ablation, the left nerve can run in a changeable way from the sternocostal to the lateral epicardial surface.[30] The presence of the phrenic nerve can be easily detected with high-intensity pacing, and its course annotated over an electroanatomical map. In this setting, RF energy delivery in a site where pacing causes diaphragmatic contraction can produce damage to the phrenic nerve and permanent diaphragmatic paralysis. In the past few years, some tricks have been published to avoid damage to the phrenic nerve. Some of these,[31] such as the use of a balloon or the creation of hydropneumopericardium to create a space between the pericardial surface and the nerve, seem effective to permit safe RF energy delivery. These techniques are not simple to use, however, and require further evaluation before inserting them in the current practice.

Concomitant Need for Heart Surgery

In patients with ventricular arrhythmias and contemporary indication to heart surgery, if an endocavitary study excludes an endocardial origin of the ventricular arrhythmias, an EP evaluation must be planned during surgery. If available, the ability to perform an electroanatomical epicardial evaluation of the arrhythmic substrate without the usual risk factors that usually come with the percutaneous approach must always be taken into account. The condition where this approach is more frequently necessary is the LV aneurysm repair, where the usual presence of endocardial calcification can impede a percutaneous endocardial ablation.

Surgical EP Room Setting

In view of the inconsistent inducibility of the target ventricular arrhythmia in the open-heart surgical setting, high-density sinus rhythm epi- and/or endocardial mapping should be undertaken to localize areas with abnormal EGMs, with special reference to low-amplitude fragmented or even isolated LPs. For this reason, the availability of an electroanatomical mapping system is essential.

A CARTO system with Version 9 software is used in our surgical theater. Prior to the system installation, it is necessary to perform the technical evaluation of the room to guarantee that the system will work correctly; this evaluation must be performed with a special metal-free bed. The system is usually connected with the patient with an ECG cable with all peripheral leads and selected precordial leads (usually V_1, V_5, V_6 in case of median sternotomy, or V_1-V_2-V_3 in lateral approach procedures).

X-ray availability must be taken into account because it is necessary at the beginning of the surgical procedure for the proper positioning of the skin reference patch. This is usually placed on the back of the patient in correspondence with the central area of the LV as evaluated with x-ray. Unlike the usual placement performed in EP room, it is important to remember that in an open-heart surgical setting, the left ventricle is vertically positioned. For this reason, the patch must be located more toward the AV groove than usual. This operation is extremely important because a perfect location of the patch is necessary to have the entire epicardial surface included in the active magnetic field; potential incorrect positioning cannot be recovered once the chest is open.

Other tools required for the surgical procedure are an EP recording system with the availability to perform programmed ventricular stimulation. Cryoenergy is delivered by a Frigitronics® Cryosurgical CCS-200 unit (**Figure 50.1**).

Mapping and Ablation Procedure

The mapping and the ablation procedure is not different from that used in EP room. A dedicated mapping EP catheter (Navistar, Biosense-Webster, Diamond Bar, CA) is used for the procedure. During the mapping, it is important to use gentle movements, maintaining the tip of the catheter in firm contact with the myocardial surface, avoiding excessive pressure that could modify the position of the heart. Due to the different position of the heart in the surgical setting, at the beginning, it is important to tag the coronary arteries for 3-dimensional spatial orientation. We usually tag with a different color the left anterior descending coronary artery, the left circumflex and marginal arteries, and the right posterior descending artery. A supplementary reference is acquired on the apex of the heart. The mapping procedure is then performed using conventional cutoff value suggested for the epicardial surface: > 1.5 mV for healthy tissue, 1.5 to 0.5 mV for the border zone, and < 0.5 mV for the true scar area. In fact, Cano[32] recently suggested that in the setting of NICM, the use of a more restrictive cutoff of 1 mV to distinguish normal from scarred myocardium. With this technique, it is possible to obtain high-density maps to define scar areas and LPs that are the usual target for the ablation. When the map is complete, we usually try to induce the clinical VT. Normally the induction of a VT in this particular setting is quite difficult because the anesthesia, the abnormal position of the heart and the mild hypothermia. For these reasons, multiple attempts are usually made with endocardial pacing, epicardial pacing in basal state, during and after isoproterenol infusion. Hemodynamic support is usually provided to enhance tolerance of the induced VT, after that activation mapping is performed to identify the diastolic pathway. Cryoenergy is applied (–60°C, 3 minutes) to achieve termination of the ongoing arrhythmia. Additional applications are usually delivered during sinus rhythm to achieve complete disappearance of any delayed or fragmented potentials on the preoperative sinus rhythm map. A similar strategy of LPs abolition during sinus rhythm is undertaken in those instances in which no VT can be induced, or if the induced arrhythmia is not tolerated or if it degenerates in VF. A final remap during sinus rhythm is required to prove the complete disappearance of the LPs after the complete set of cryoablation lesions has

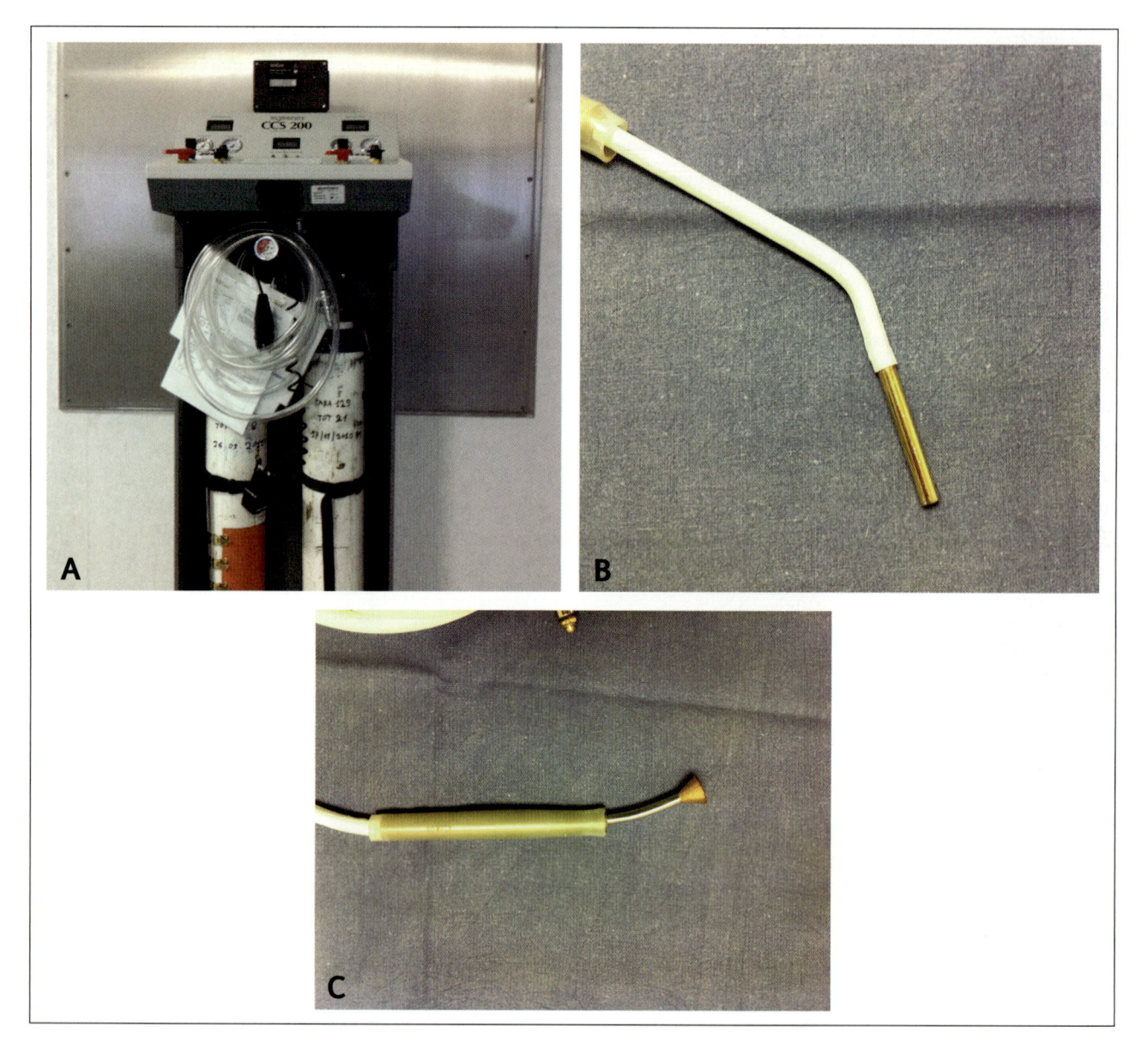

Figure 50.1 The Frigitronics unit (**A**) performs cryolesion through interchangeable probes: linear 35 × 5 mm (**B**) and conical with 15-mm diameter flat face (**C**). Freezing is assured by N_2O delivery and may reach a stable 60°C temperature. It is provided with temperature and gas pressure monitoring. To obtain deep, clean-edged and complete necrosis, cryoenergy is applied for at least 3 minutes.

been delivered. The prevention of VT induction is also required for the termination of the procedure. In all cases, at the end a remap is undertaken to confirm the abolition of all LPs, and a further attempt to induce VT is then performed. Different shapes and angles of the cryoprobes may be required to reach all the segments involved easily. Any application is maintained for about 3 minutes after reaching an efficacy temperature of at least −60°C. It is important to apply a moderate pressure over the epicardium, particularly in the presence of fat, to reach the deeper subepicardial layers. A back pressure on the other side of the heart may limit the heart movements. As the heart is likely to move away from its initial position, it is important to put a reference (staple) in the critical areas that are to be ablated in such a way as to be able to proceed should this occur.

Different Approaches

Marfan Window

The epicardial approach performed with a subxyphoidal puncture is not always feasible in patients with previous inflammatory processes due to the presence of adherence (**Figure 50.2**). In this situation, before an open chest procedure, we try to perform the procedure with a Marfan window.

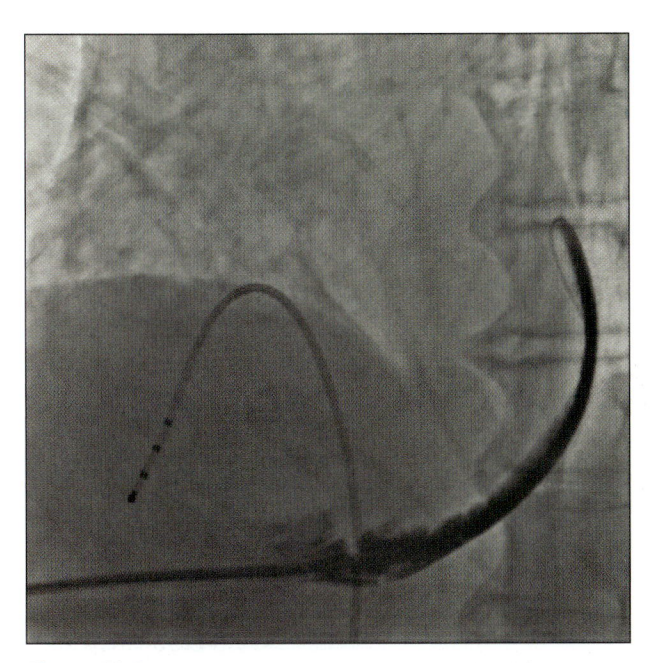

Figure 50.2 Percutaneous approach via subxyphoidal puncture is shown. Due to the presence of adherence, the guide wire does not proceed inside the pericardial space, and the contrast media does not diffuse, but remains localized in a small portion of the pericardial space.

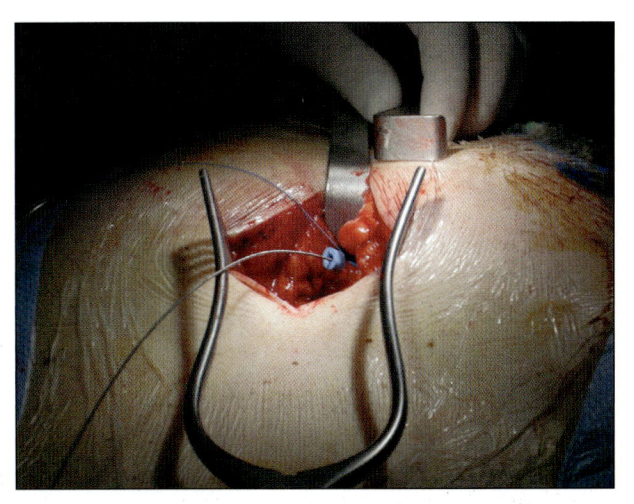

Figure 50.3 Marfan window with a sheath (9-Fr, 12 cm.) introduced in the pericardial space. Because the pericardial space is finally closed, a drainage system is connected to the side port to allow drainage of fluids as in a normal percutaneous pericardial approach.

Surgical subxiphoid approach is performed with 4- to 5-cm cutaneous incision just below the xiphoid process (**Figure 50.3**). The linea alba is longitudinally divided, and we access to the pericardial space below the caudal sternum, taking care not to damage the RV. Adherences are carefully divided, and an arterial 5- to 6-Fr introducer can be advanced in the pericardial space. The linea alba is then closed and the EP procedure may follow as usual. Femoral vessels are cannulated with introducers for a quick percutaneous cannulation if cardiopulmonary support is needed.

Case 1

This patient with IDCM and moderate LV function was referred to our centre for life-saving epicardial ablation of an incessant VT causing hemodynamic decompensation. With a conventional subxyphoidal puncture, the pericardial space was reached, but mapping was not possible because of strong and widespread pericardial adherences. Through surgery, a bipolar voltage map of the epicardial surface could be obtained. The map with conventional cut-off values showed a big area of scar (**Figure 50.4A**), but with more restrictive criteria, a channel was discovered inside (**Figure 50.4B**). Concealed entrainment (**Figure 50.4C**) performed on site 1 was indicative of a proximal part of a reentry circuit, and RF delivery on this site (**Figure 50.4D**) resulted in prompt termination of the clinical VT during RF delivery performed on the same site. After that, additional RF applications were performed along the channel to destroy it and to remove all LPs discovered (**Figure 50.5**).

At the end of the procedure, programmed ventricular stimulation was unable to induce VT both in basal state and during isoproterenol infusion.

Median Sternotomy

With a median sternotomy, it is possible to access the entire epicardial surface (both right and left) to obtain a complete electroanatomical epicardial map. If an endocardial map is necessary, this setting permits the team to perform it either with a conventional percutaneous approach or with a surgical approach. In the presence of previous heart surgery, sternotomy must be evaluated carefully; the surgical trauma is significant and can involve very serious risks, particularly considering the extremely compromised clinical and functional status frequently present in these patients. Moreover, postsurgical adherence can make the correct exposure of the heart difficult or impossible.

In the organization of a surgical ablation it is important to plan a circulatory support with the cardiopulmonary bypass that is necessary for three main reasons. First, it can support the patient during the presence of VTs, which for the peculiar clinical setting are frequently untolerated. These arrhythmias can be present spontaneously or can be induced during the EP study, and the ability to sustain the arrhythmia allows activation mapping.

Second, it is necessary to utilize cardiac tilting during the procedure. The technique is comparable to that used for the bypass beating-heart surgery and is impossible to apply in patients with severe dilated cardiomyopathy without serious hemodynamic effects.

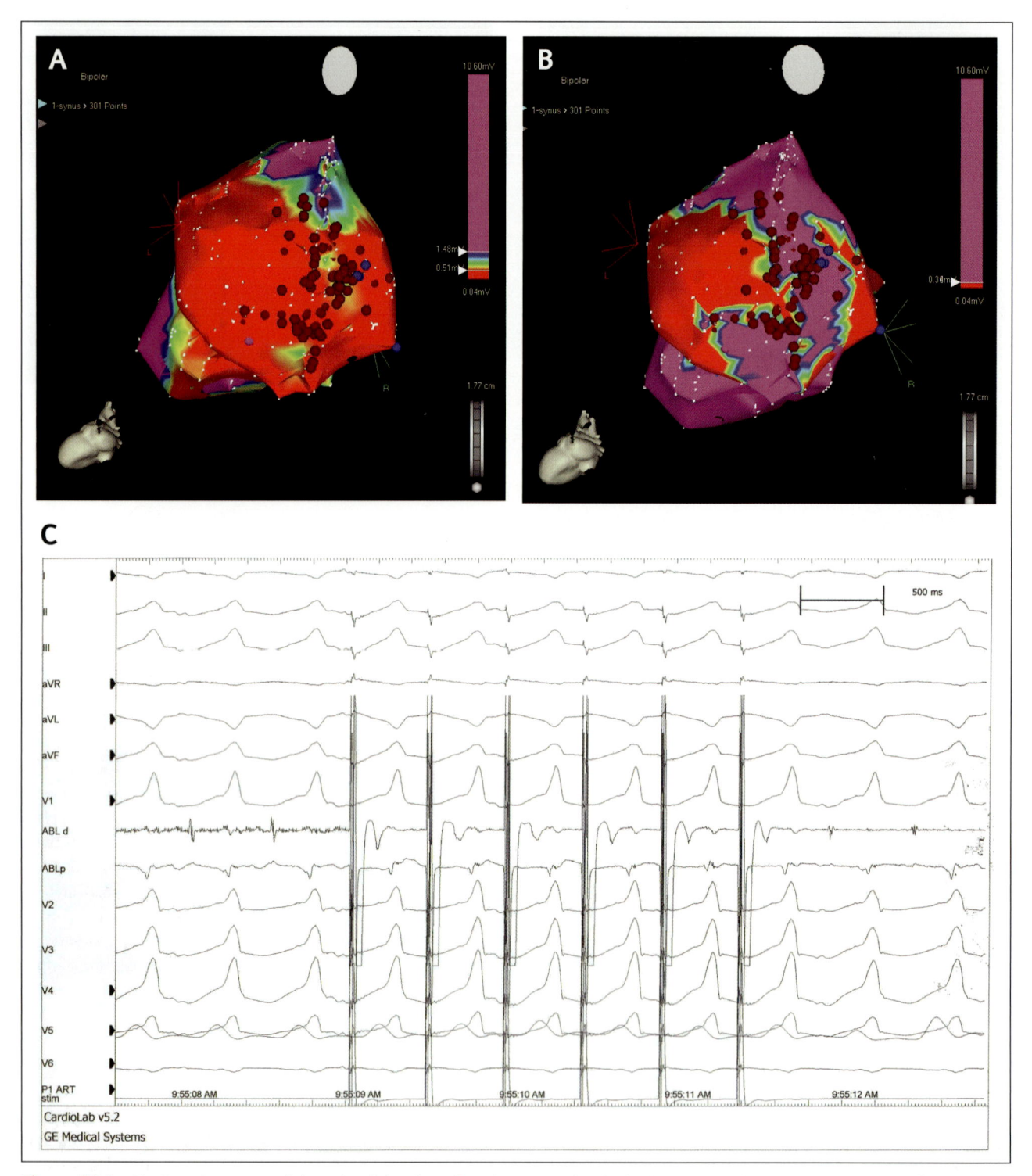

Figure 50.4 Bipolar voltage map of the epicardial surface. **A.** Using conventional criteria, the map showed a large scar area. **B.** Use of more restrictive criteria revealed a channel inside. **C.** Concealed entrainment performed on site 1 was indicative of a proximal part of a reentry circuit.

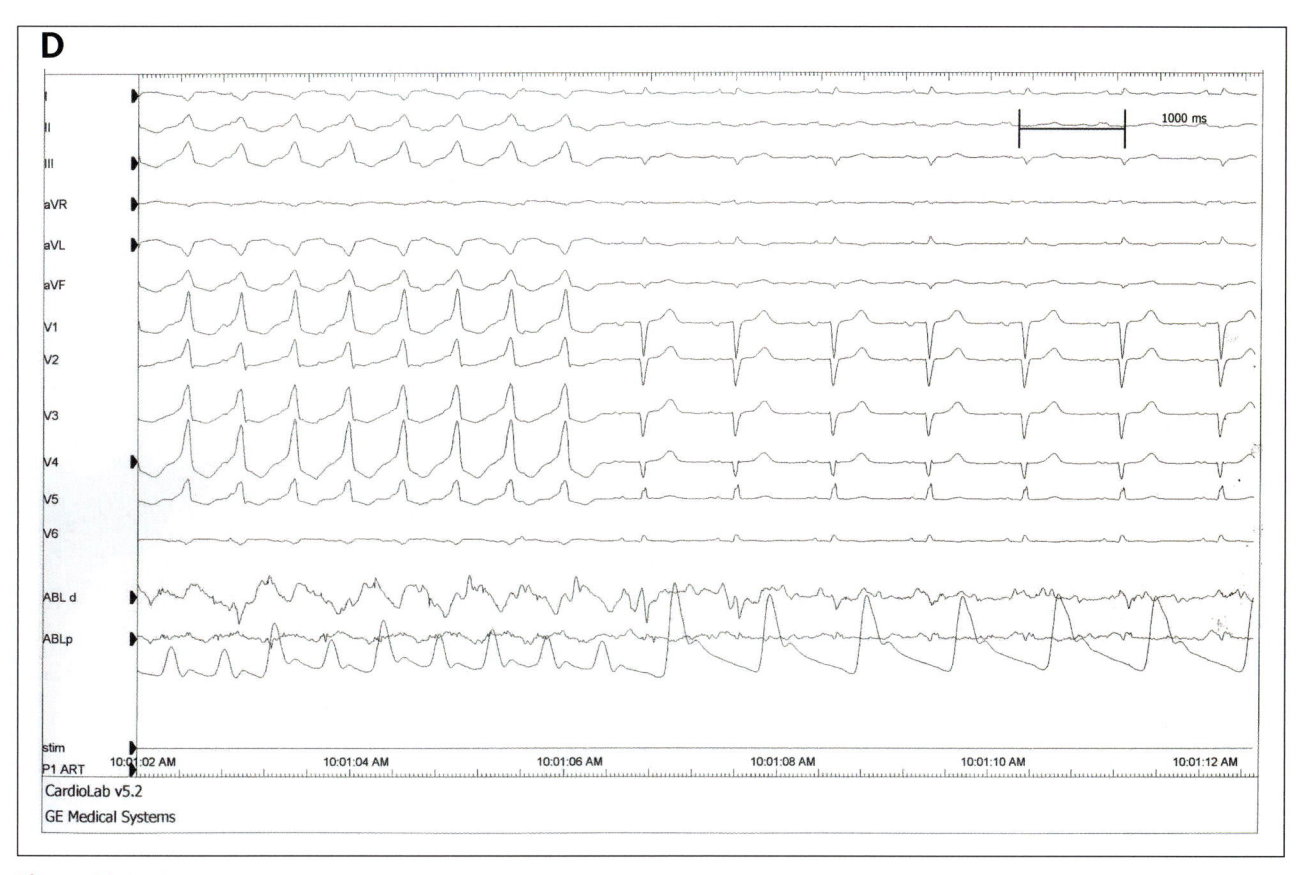

Figure 50.4 D. RF delivery on this site in panel C resulted in prompt termination of the clinical VT.

Third, endocardial surgical access is obviously impossible without a cardiopulmonary bypass. The skin incision is made from the jugular notch to just below the xyphoid process. The sternum is divided longitudinally in the midline and, after placement of a sternal spreader, the timic fat is divided up to the level of the left brachiocefalic vein. The pericardium is opened in an inverted T-shaped incision. The lateral extension is exaggerated in order to facilitate mobilization of the apex of the heart and to create increased space for the RV during positioning. Intrapericardial adherences, if present, are completely and carefully dissected out to obtain optimal exposure and to prevent bleeding. The cardiopulmonary bypass is carried out with a single cavoatrial cannula (two stages), typically introduced via RAA. The application of a vacuum-assisted venous drainage allows the use of smaller-diameter cannula in order to facilitate subsequent heart positioning. In these cases, the distal ascending aorta is the preferred cannulation site for the systemic arterial flow line. To obtain a good heart exposure for achieving a complete and stable electroanatomical map, deep pericardial traction sutures (Lima stitch) are used to subluxate the heart and to visualize the complete lateral and posterolateral LV surface. These deep pericardial traction sutures elevate and rotate the heart by placing tension on the posterior pericardial wall. In addition to Lima stitch, some cotton strips may be used in order to have a stable spatial positioning of the heart during the construction of a stable electroanatomical map. In selected cases in which the apical map is not useful for the EP procedure, an apical suction device can be used, allowing positioning and manipulation of the heart by creating a vacuum-type seal to the apical epicardial surface. During this phase, it is frequently necessary to start with a cardiopulmonary bypass to maintain a good hemodynamic control in patients often affected with dilated cardiomyopathy. At this point, the CARTO mapping may be started.

Case 2

Male, 62 years old, presented with obstructive hypertrophic cardiomyopathy with normal coronary arteries. The patient had multiple episodes of VT initially responsive to amiodarone and beta blockers. For these reasons, the patient underwent to ICD implantation. Subsequently he had an arrhythmic storm with 48 episodes of VT/VF uncontrolled by antiarrhythmic drugs, for which he was referred to our center for an ablation procedure. This patient had 5 different morphologies of VT and was initially treated with an endo-epicardial ablation performed in the EP room. Upon creation of the electroanatomical voltage map, the endocardial surface was normal. However,

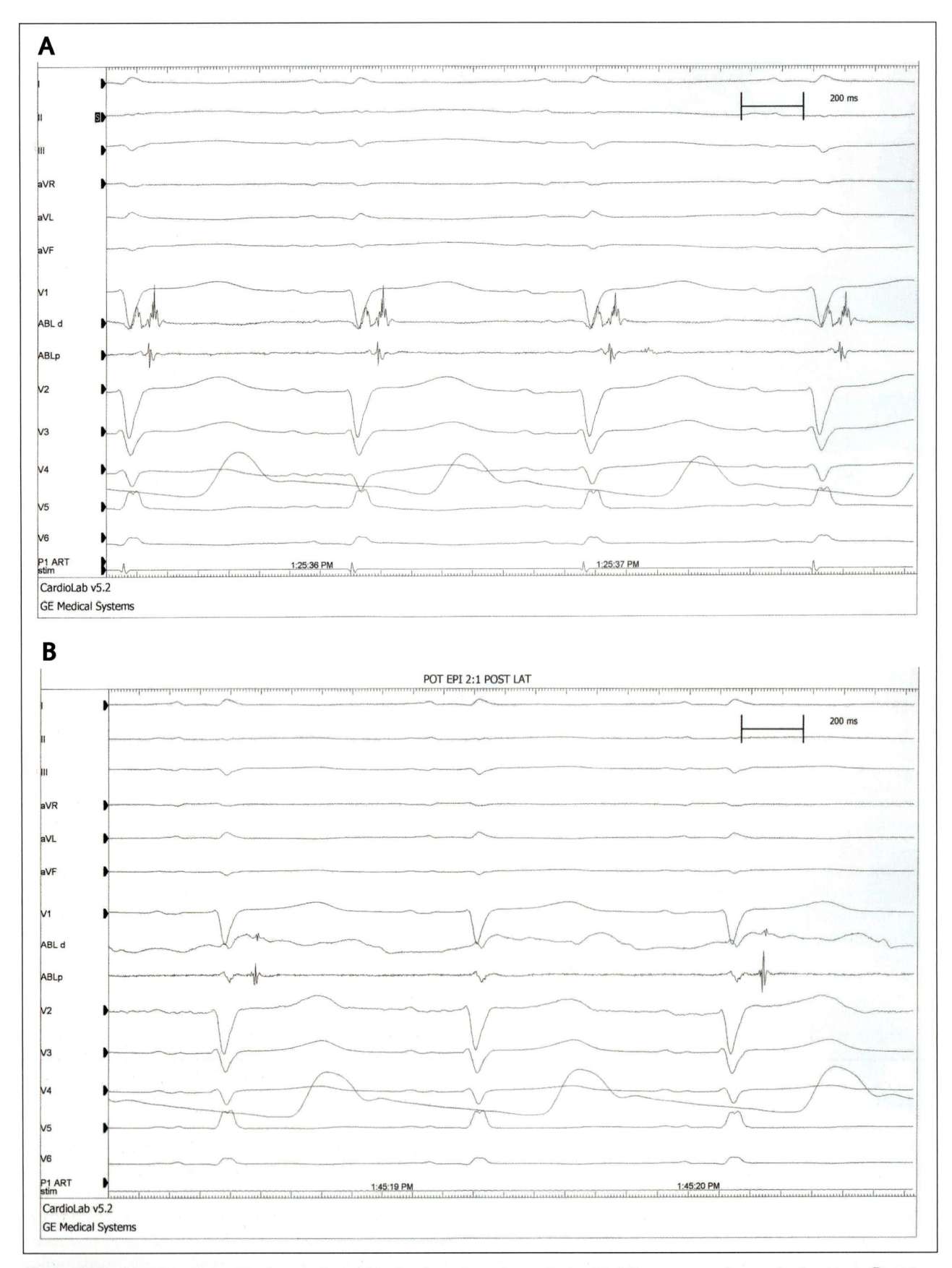

Figure 50.5 (**A**) LPs registered in sinus rhythm within the channel are shown. During RF delivery, progressive conduction block (**B**) with final disappearance of the LP (**C**).

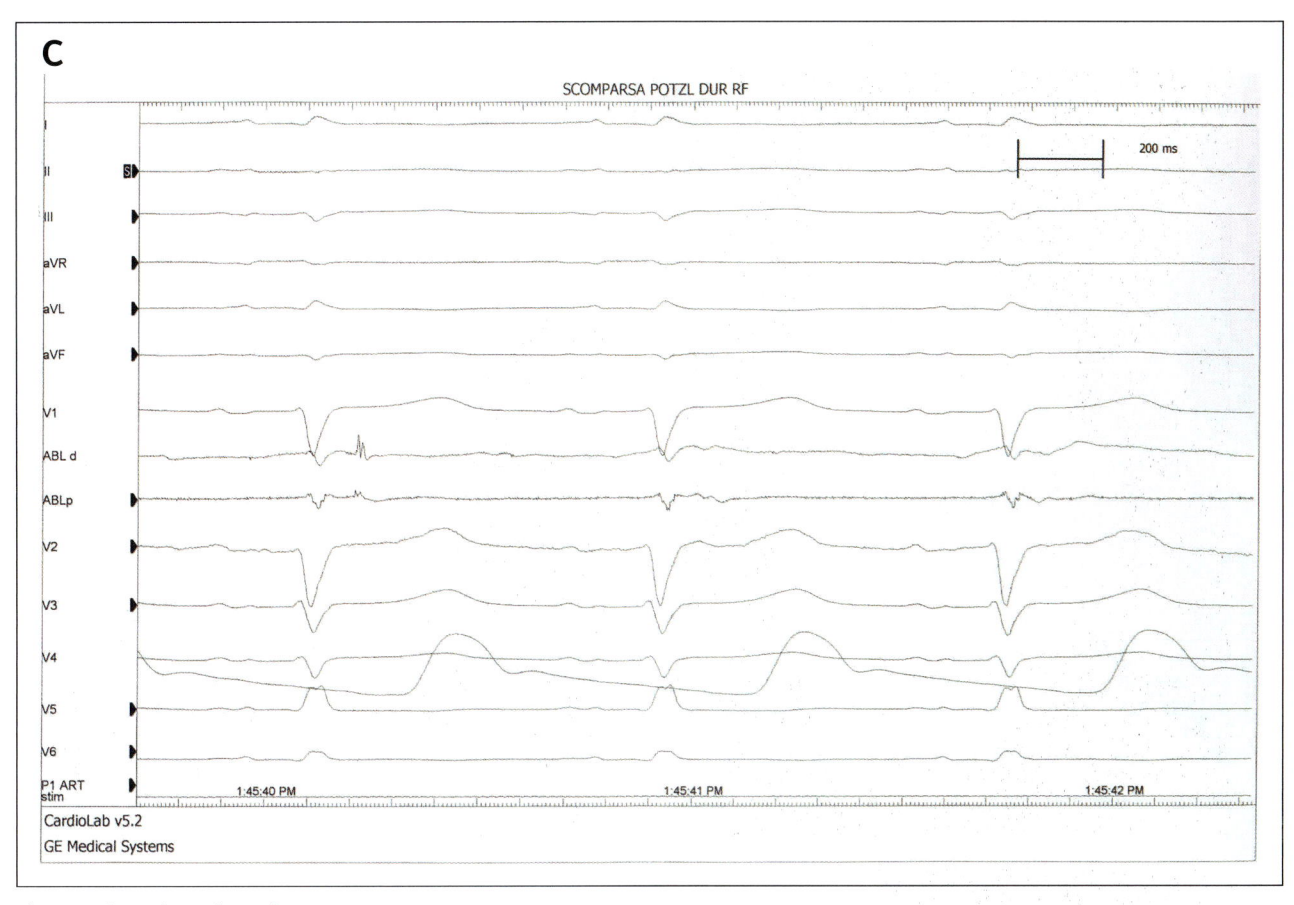

Figure 50.5 (continued)

a large area of scar was discovered on the anterior layer of the epicardial surface and RF ablation was then performed on this site with acute success. After 5 days, the patient had recurrence of arrhythmic storm, which required deep sedation and emergency surgical ablation. The surgical procedure highlighted a heart with fatty epicardium (**Figure 50.6**). An electroanatomical bipolar voltage map obtained during surgery showed the same area of scar identified with the previous procedure where the applications of RF energy were unable to obtain effective and stable results, probably due to the presence of a hypertrophic myocardial wall and the layer of thick fat (**Figures 50.7** and **50.8**).

Patient was then discharged with beta blocker therapy 10 days after the ablation. No significant differences with preoperative data were present at the echocardiography performed predischarge. No arrhythmia recurrences have been reported after 9 months of follow up.

Left Anterior Thoracotomy

In patients with previous heart surgery where the median sternotomy may be extremely difficult and dangerous, it is possible to consider a thoracotomic approach (**Figure 50.9**) that is also usable for the previously described endocardial

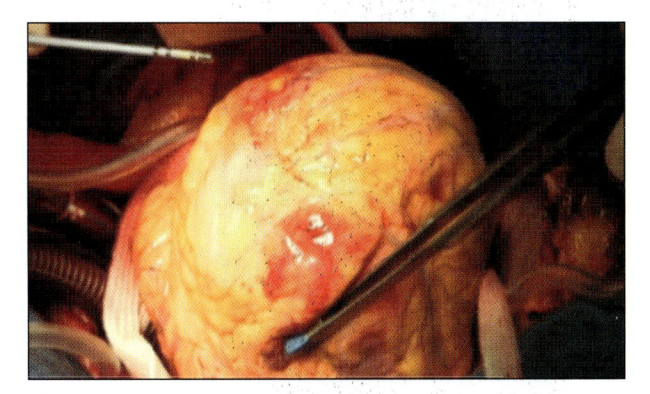

Figure 50.6 This picture shows the position of the heart before starting with the mapping procedure. A large amount of fat is present that probably caused the failure of a previous percutaneous approach. In the inferoapical surface, a hemorrhagic area caused by the previous percutaneous subxyphoidal pericardial approach is visible.

approach. In this situation, for the reduced exposition of the heart that is achievable with this technique, it is quite important to perform a careful analysis of the surface ECG and of the myocardial substrate to identify the hypothetical site of origin of the VT and the possibility of exposing it for the mapping process. The procedure is usually simpler in the presence of a LV aneurysm. The left anterior

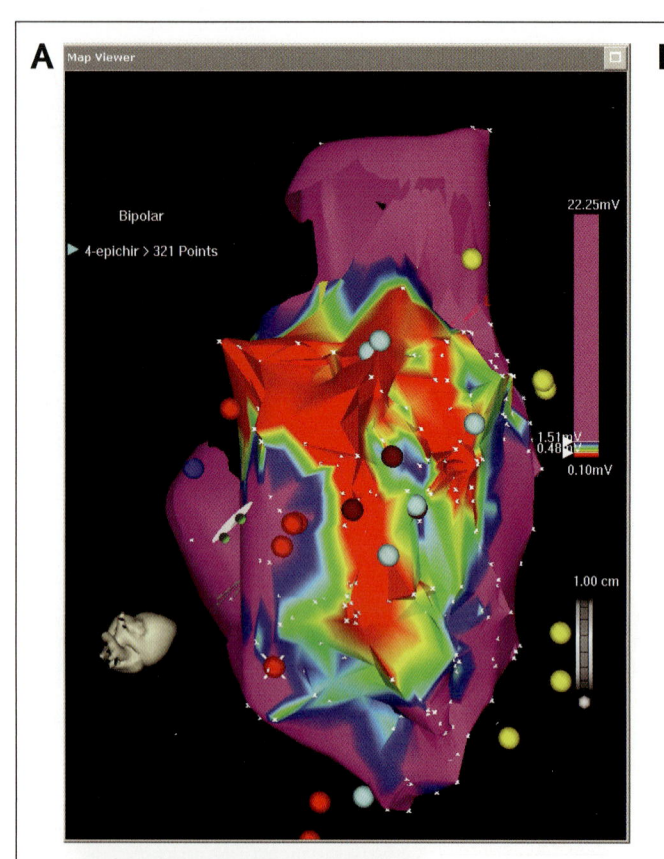

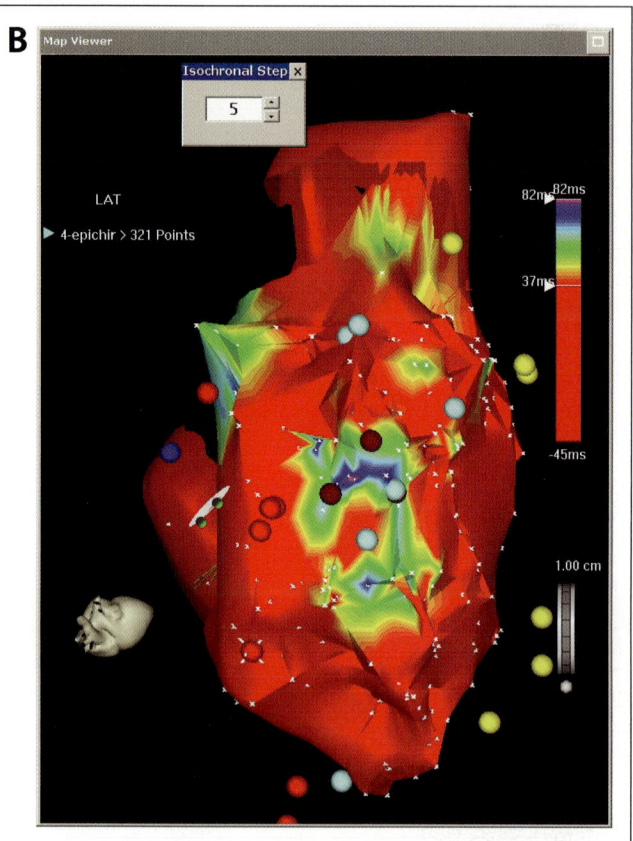

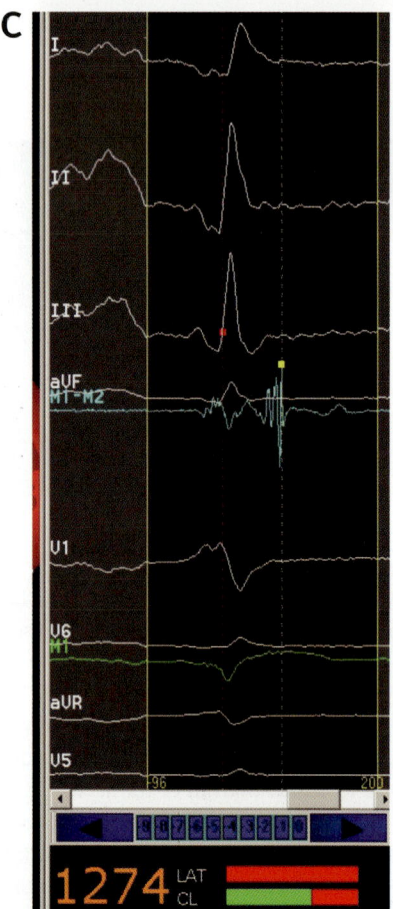

Figure 50.7 **A.** Bipolar voltage map of the epicardial surface obtained in surgical theatre. A big area of scar that is extended from the base to the apex is present on the anterior surface. **B.** Map of LPs. Inside the scar area there are a lot of LPs identified with colors ranging from yellow to purple. **C.** shows an example of LPs registered in the scar area.

Chapter 50: Hybrid Ablation of VT • 481

Figure 50.8 Comparison of the two maps obtained in the EP room (**A**) and in the surgical theatre (**B**) is shown. The two maps are quite similar and similar are the points where the ablation was performed (red dot for RF energy, blue dot for cryoablation).

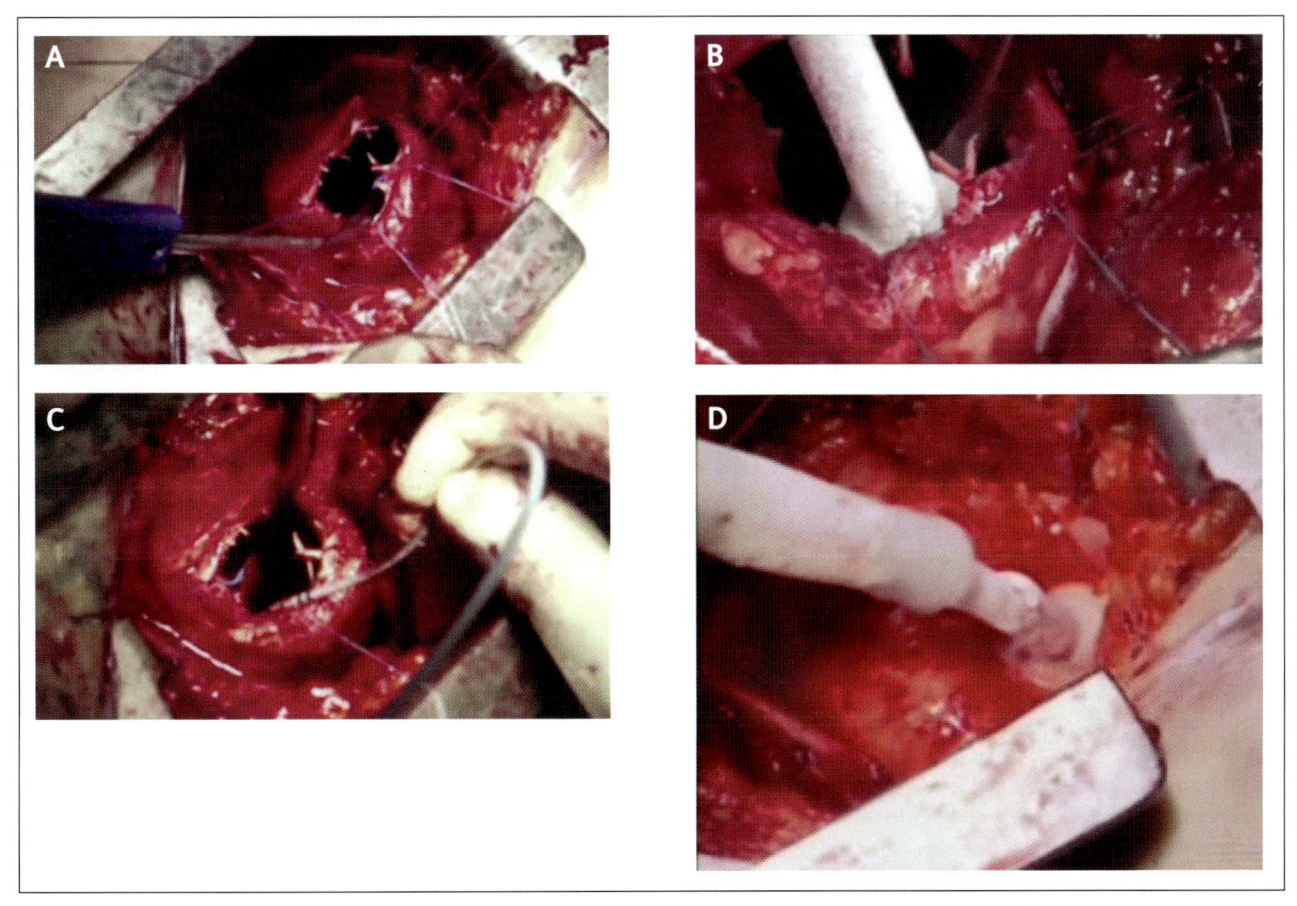

Figure 50.9 Surgical procedure via left anterior thoracotomy is shown. **A.** Surgical opening of an aneurysm. **B.** Endocardial cryoablation. **C.** Electroanatomical mapping of the neck of the aneurysm. **D.** Epicardial cryoablation.

thoracotomy permits the visualization of the necrotic apex and with appropriate traction point the boundary with the healthy myocardium. The mapping and ablation procedure is then performed with availability of percutaneous extracorporeal circulation in case of hemodynamic instability.

After the induction of general anesthesia and insertion of a double lumen endotracheal tube, the left thorax is slightly elevated. Femoral vessels are cannulated with Introducer for a quick cardiopulmonary bypass start. It is important to remember in this approach to predispose an external plaque for DC shock should it be necessary. For the frequent occurrence of cardiomegaly and subsequent heart displacement in the thorax, the level of the thoracotomy must be guided by the echocardiographic identification of the cardiac apex. The origin of clinical tachycardia must be taken in to account to understand which part of the periapical heart must be better exposed. An 8- to 10-cm skin incision is performed and the pleural space is opened. Possible adherences between lung and pericardium are divided. The pericardium is opened anteriorly to the phrenic nerve and the cardiac apex is exposed. In case of previous cardiac surgery, care must be taken to gently dissect epicardial adherences. Epicardial dissection must continue until the healthy, viable myocardium around the anterior scar and/or the suspected origin of tachycardia are completely exposed. During dissection we can induce VT that may be interrupted with external DC shock or with the activation of the ICD (if present). Activation map or control of any hemodynamical instability may be easily accomplished via the starting of the cardiopulmonary support. Pericardial-free borders are held up with traction stitches in order to have a stable positioning for CARTO electroanatomical mapping. With the exposure of the apex, we can perform epicardial and endocardial EP procedures as usual.

Endocardial Mapping

During surgical ablation, there are some isolated cases where an endocardial approach is necessary. A previous failed endocardial approach, particularly for deep septal scars or in the presence of endocardial calcification and a presence of a double mechanical valve, are the main reasons where this approach is mandatory. In these cases, there are two possible solutions.

Ventriculotomy is pinpointed in the area of full-thickness scar, the border of which can also be defined with the epicardial CARTO mapping. During beating-heart cardiopulmonary bypass, we obtain a ventricular emptying and the area of scarred, thinned ventricular wall suddenly subsides, finally identifying the target area for the ventriculotomy. A linear ventriculotomy is performed, paying attention to coronary artery course. Possible mural thrombi or endocardial calcification (**Figure 50.10**) are carefully

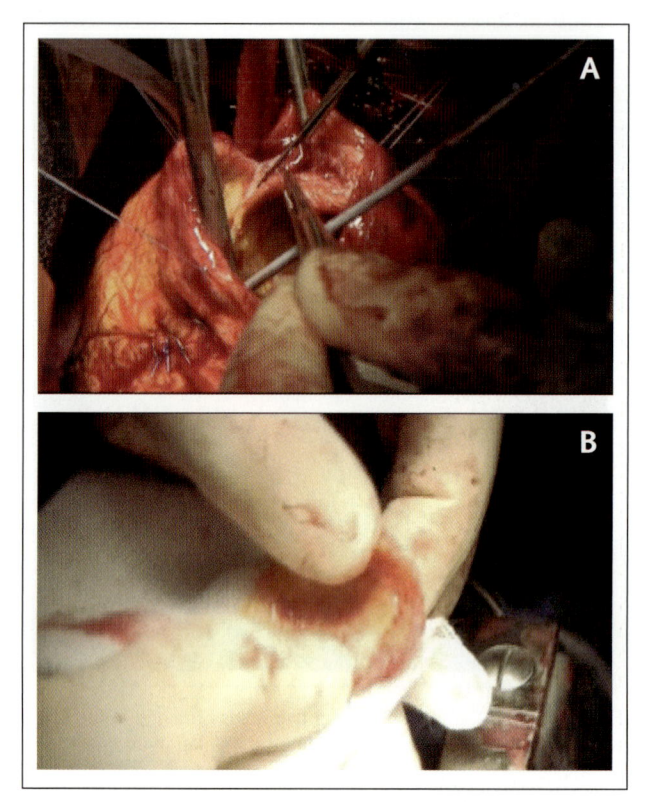

Figure 50.10 **A.** Ventriculotomy in a patient with apical aneurysm and endocardial calcification is shown. **B.** The endocardial calcification that made the previous endocardial ablation ineffective.

identified and removed. After obtaining a stable position, with some traction stitches into the cardinal points of the incision, we perform an endocardial electroanatomical mapping and subsequent cryoablation (**Figure 50.11**), either on target and/or all around the scar neck.

The endocardial mapping is performed with the same maneuvers used for the epicardial mapping. In this setting the space for the access to the endocardial surface may be little making the catheter movements quite difficult. For the highly possible displacement of the heart, we suggest limiting the mapping process to the area of interest building different maps for any segment. Since the inducibility of a VT in this setting is really difficult or impossible, a substrate mapping approach is mandatory. The cryoablation is then performed in the same way as the epicardial ablation and at the end it is always important to check the ablated area with a remap procedure. Subsequent repair of LV aneurysms may be accomplished with various techniques; we prefer to continue with a beating-heart procedure, as we can touch and see the border between the contractile muscle and the scar. Usually we perform a no-patch reconstruction with multiple purse-strings to approach the healthy contractile muscle wall, and finally we close over the fibrous rim. We have to keep in mind that after this surgery a further endocardial transcatheter

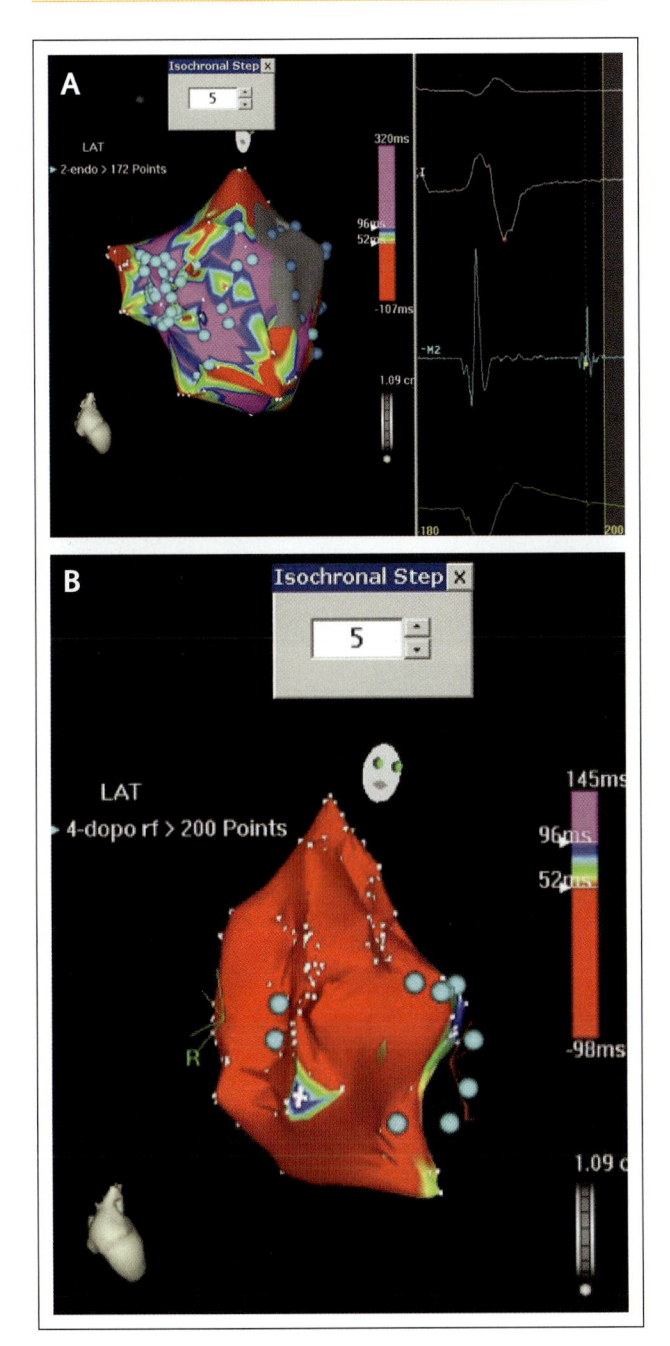

Figure 50.11 An endocardial mapping performed after a left ventriculotomy is shown. **A.** Map of LPs identified by the purple area and azure dots. Blue dots identify the ventriculotomy. An example of LP is shown. **B.** Remap performed after cryoablation. The geometrical map of the same area is different due to the displacement of the heart determined by the ablation procedure. The absence of purple color with a same cutoff value of the scale suggests the absence of LPs.

procedure is virtually impossible, so the ablation process must be as complete as possible. In the absence of a clearly visible ventricular scar, a conventional endocardial mapping can be achieved through a conventional catheter and a short sheath inserted directly in the LV (**Figure 50.12**).

In this case, the procedure is performed with the aid of the mapping system and of the X-ray, and the ablation is conventionally performed with RF energy.

Conclusions

Surgical ablation of VT is an effective procedure that can be considered in a few, highly selected cases but offers a very high rate of long-term cure.

Although the popularity of ventricular arrhythmia surgery has decreased over the years due to the advent of ICD and catheter ablation, the need for an effective curative strategy could lead to its resurgence in specialized centers, where a strong VT program is in place. Aside from the conventional indications in the setting of postinfarction VTs, an emerging indication is the open chest–closed heart cryoablation treatment.

Because it is a one-shot procedure, it must be planned with great attention to detail, and strict cooperation between the surgeon and the electrophysiologist is mandatory. Conventional preoperative routine exams for heart surgery must be performed. Sometimes a CT scan can be useful for the surgeon to understand the anatomical relationship of the cardiac structures and the course of the cardiac bypass, if present.

In our experience, there is no detrimental effect on the cardiac function after the procedure, and time spent in the recovery room is similar to that for the routine heart surgery. In high-volume centers, it is possible that recourse to this procedure may account for 5% to 6% of the all VT ablations. Future development of epicardial mapping and ablation techniques would probably reduce the need for this particular approach.

References

1. Reddy VY, Reynolds MR, Neuzil P. Prophylactic catheter ablation for the prevention of defibrillator therapy. *N Engl J Med*. 2007;357(26):2657–2665.
2. Carbucicchio C, Santamaria M, Trevisi N. Catheter ablation for the treatment of electrical storm in patients with implantable cardioverter-defibrillators: short- and long-term outcomes in a prospective single-center study. *Circulation*. 2008;117(4):462–469.
3. Fontaine G, Guiraudon G, Frank R. Epicardial cartography and surgical treatment by simple ventriculotomy of certain resistant re-entry ventricular tachycardias. *Arch Mal Coeur Vaiss*. 1975;68(2):113–124.
4. Spurrell RA, Yates AK, Thorburn CW. Surgical treatment of ventricular tachycardia after epicardial mapping studies. *Br Heart J*. 1975;37(2):115–126.
5. Wittig JH, Boineau JP. Surgical treatment of ventricular arrhythmias using epicardial, transmural, and endocardial mapping. *Ann Thorac Surg*. 1975;20(2):117–126.

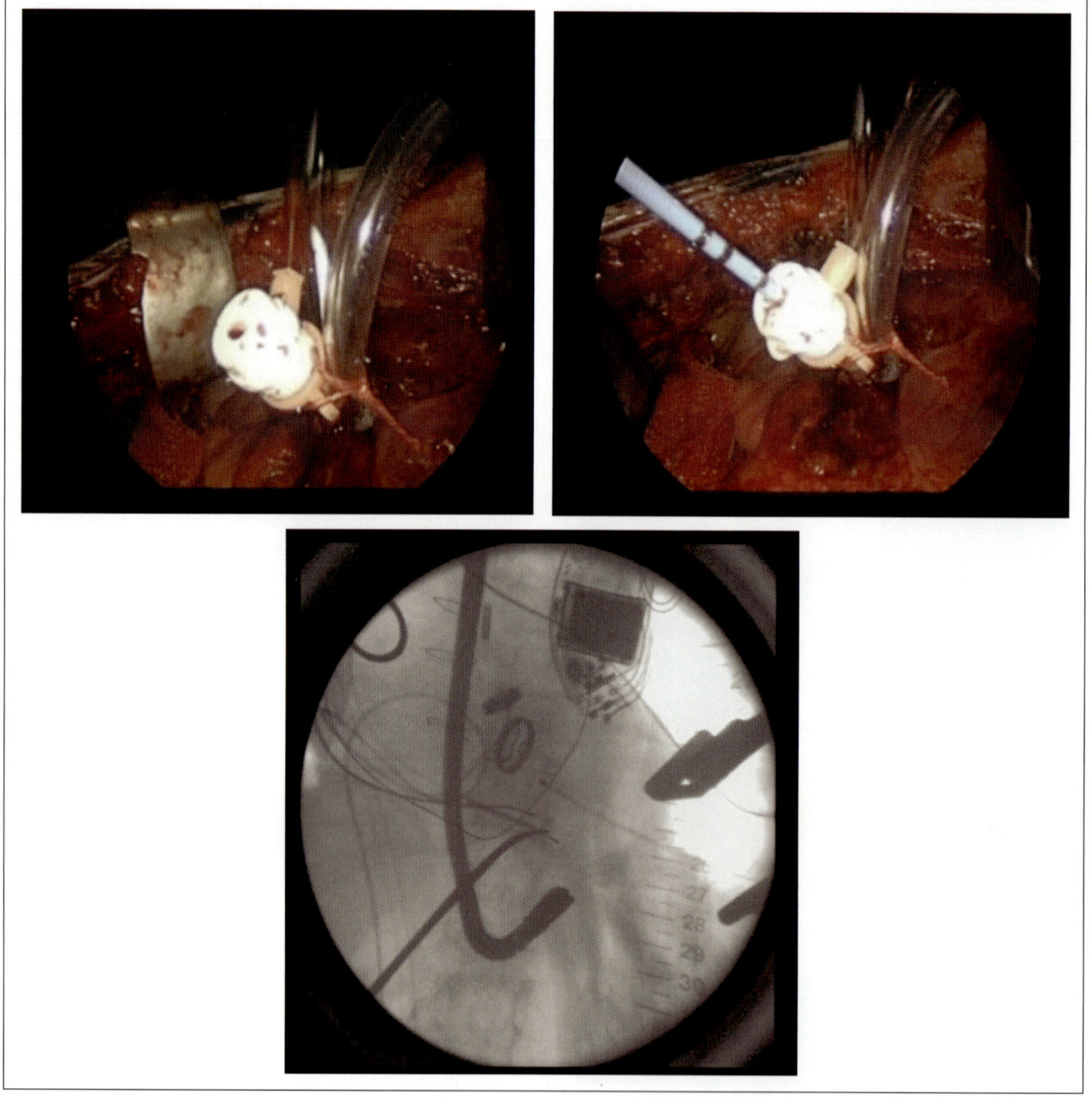

Figure 50.12 Endocardial mapping achieved with a conventional catheter inserted in the LV through an apical sheath in a patient with double mechanical valve.

6. Gallagher JJ, Anderson RW, Kasell J. Cryoablation of drug-resistant ventricular tachycardia in a patient with a variant of scleroderma. *Circulation*. 1978;57:190–197.
7. Cox JL. Patient selection criteria and results of surgery for refractory ischemic ventricular tachycardia. *Circulation*. 1989;79(Suppl I):I-163–I-177.
8. Niebauer MJ. Kirsh M, Kadish A, et al. Outcome of endocardial resection in 33 patients with coronary artery disease: correlation with ventricular tachycardia morphology. *Am Heart J*. 1992;124:1500–1506.
9. Manolis AS. Raslegar H. Payne D, et al. Surgical therapy for drug-refractory ventricular tachycardia; Results with mapping-guided subendocardial resection. *J Am Coll Cardiol*. 1989;14:199–208.
10. Mittleman RS. Candinas R. Dahlberg S, et al; Predictors of surgical mortality and long-term results of endocardial resection for drug-refractory ventricular tachycardia. *Am Heart J*. 1992;124;1226–1232.
11. Hargrove WC, Miller JM. Risk stratification and management of patients with recurrent ventricular tachycardia and other malignant ventricular arrhythmias. *Circulation*. 1989:79(Suppl I):I-178–I-181.
12. Saksena S, Gielchinsky I, Tullo NG. Argon laser ablation of malignant ventricular tachycardia associated with coronary artery disease. *Am J Cardiol*. 1989;64:1298–1304.
13. Trappe H-J, Klein H, Frank G, et al. Role of mapping-guided surgery in patients with recurrent ventricular tachycardia. *Am Heart J*. 1992;124:636–644.

14. Mickleborough L, Harris L, Downar E, et al. A new intraoperative approach for endocardial mapping of ventricular tachycardia. *J Thorac Cardiovasc.* 1988;95:271–280.
15. Kaltenbrunner W, Cardinal R, Dubuc M. Epicardial and endocardial mapping of ventricular tachycardia in patients with myocardial infarction. *Circulation.* 1991;84:1058–1071.
16. Littman L, Svenson RH. Gallagher JJ, et al. Functional role of the epicardium in post-infarction ventricular tachycardia. Observations derived from computerized epicardial activation mapping, entrainment, and epicardial laser photoablation. *Circulation.* 1991;83:1577–1591.
17. Svenson RH, Littmann L, Gallagher JJ, et al. Termination of ventricular tachycardia with epicardial laser photocoagulation: A clinical comparison with patients undergoing successful endocardial photocoagulation alone. *J Am Coll Cardiol.* 1990;15:163–170.
18. Harris L. Downar E, Michelborough L, et al. Activation sequence of ventricular tachycardia; Endocardial and epicardial mapping studies in the human ventricle. *J Am Coll Cardiol.* 1987;10:1040–1047.
19. Calkins H, Epstein A, Packer D, et al. Catheter ablation of ventricular tachycardia in patients with structural heart disease using cooled radiofrequency energy: results of a prospective multicenter study. Cooled RF Multi Center Investigators Group. *J Am Coll Cardiol.* 2000;35:1905–1914.
20. Callans DJ, Ren JF, Narula N, et al. Effects of linear, irrigated-tip radiofrequency ablation in porcine healed anterior infarction. *J Cardiovasc Electrophysiol.* 2001;12:1037–1042.
21. Blanchard SM. Walcott GP. Wharton JM, et al. Why is catheter ablation less successful than surgery for treating ventricular tachycardia that results from coronary artery disease? *Pacing Clin Electrophysiol.* 1994;17:2315–2335.
22. Gonska BD. Cao Keijiang, Schaumann A, et al. Catheter ablation of ventricular tachycardia in 136 patients with coronary artery disease: Results and long-term follow-up. *J Am Coll Cardiol.* 1994;24:1506–1514.
23. Morady F. Harvey M. Kalblleisch SJ, et al. Radiofrequency catheter ablation of ventricular tachycardia in patients with coronary artery disease. *Circulation.* 1993;87:363–372.
24. Sosa E, Scanavacca M, D'Avila A. A new technique to perform epicardial mapping in the electrophysiology laboratory. *J Cardiovasc Electrophysiol.* 1996;7:531–536.
25. Hsia HH, Callans DJ, Marchlinski FE. Characterization of endocardial electro- physiological substrate in patients with nonischemic cardiomyopathy and mono- morphic ventricular tachycardia. *Circulation.* 2003;108:704–710.
26. Cano O, Hutchinson M, Lin S. Electroanatomic substrate and ablation outcome for suspected epicardial ventricular tachycardia in left ventricular nonischemic cardiomyopathy. *J Am Coll Cardiol.* 2009;54(9):799–808.
27. Silaghi A, Piercecchi-Marti MD, Grino M. Epicardial adipose tissue extent: relationship with age, body fat distribution, and coronaropathy. *Obesity.* (Silver Spring) 2008;16(11): 2424–2430.
28. Ahn S-G, Lim H-S, Joe D-Y. Relationship of epicardial adipose tissue by echocardiography to coronary artery disease. *Heart.* 2008;94 (3):e7.
29. d'Avila A, Gutierrez P, Scanavacca M. Effects of radiofrequency pulses delivered in the vicinity of the coronary arteries: implications for nonsurgical transthoracic epicardial catheter ablation to treat ventricular tachycardia. *Pacing Clin Electrophysiol.* 2002;25:1488–1495.
30. Sánchez-Quintana D, Cabrera JA, Climent V. How close are the phrenic nerves to cardiac structures? Implications for cardiac interventionalists. *J Cardiovasc Electrophysiol.* 2005; 16(3):309–313.
31. Di Biase L, Burkhardt JD, Pelargonio G. Prevention of phrenic nerve injury during epicardial ablation: Comparison of methods for separating the phrenic nerve from the epicardial surface. *Heart Rhythm.* 2009;6:957–961.
32. Cano O, Hutchinson M, Lin D. Electroanatomic substrate and ablation outcome for suspected epicardial ventricular tachycardia in left ventricular nonischemic cardiomyopathy. *J Am Coll Cardiol.* 2009;54(9):799–808.

INDEX

A

A-A-V. *See* atrial-atrial-ventricular
accessory pathways
    ablation of
        localization before, 64
        mapping before, 64–67
        technique for, 67–70
    antegrade, 67
    anteroseptal, 74–75, 79
    atriofascicular, 82–83
    in Ebstein's anomaly. *See* Ebstein's anomaly
    epicardial posteroseptal, 68–70
    left-lateral. *See* left-lateral accessory pathway ablation
    midseptal, 75, 79
    oblique course of, 65
    posteroseptal, 66, 68–70, 72, 75–76, 79
    right-sided
        anteroseptal, 74–75
        classification of, 72
        description of, 72
        free-wall, 72–74, 79
        midseptal, 75
        posteroseptal, 75–76
ACT. *See* activated clotting time
activated clotting time, 121, 338
activation mapping, 236–237, 246, 251, 320
adenosine-sensitive ventricular tachycardia, 286, 288
AF. *See* atrial fibrillation
AFCL. *See* atrial fibrillation cycle length
AFL. *See* atrial flutter
alcohol ablation, of ventricular tachycardia in hypertrophic cardiomyopathy, 455
amiodarone, 13
antegrade conduction, 68
anteroseptal pathways, 74–75, 79
anticoagulation
    description of, 13
    pulmonary vein antrum isolation, 127
    before transseptal puncture, 99
aortic sinus cusps, 292–300, 393–394

aortic valve, 387, 389–390, 393
AP. *See* accessory pathway
Array (St. Jude Medical), 373–375, 384
arrhythmogenic right ventricular cardiomyopathy/dysplasia
    definition of, 462
    description of, 285, 313, 462–463
    ventricular tachycardia ablation in
        ablation procedure, 464–468
        complications of, 468
        electroanatomical voltage mapping, 464–465
        electrophysiology study, 465–467
        endocardial mapping and, 467
        epicardial mapping and, 467–468
        overview of, 462–463
        postprocedure care, 468–469
        preprocedural planning for, 463–464
"Artis zeego" system, 131
Artisan catheter, 261–262, 264
ARVC/D. *See* arrhythmogenic right ventricular cardiomyopathy/dysplasia
ASC. *See* aortic sinus cusps
ascending aorta, 390
ASD. *See* atrial septal defect
AT. *See* atrial tachycardia
atrial drive pacing, 52
atrial electrograms
    complex fractionated. *See* complex fractionated atrial electrograms, atrial fibrillation ablation by targeting of
    types of, 141
atrial entrainment, 8–9
atrial fibrillation
    ablation of. *See* atrial fibrillation ablation
    characteristics of, 248
    left atrial appendage triggering of, 165
    left atrial ganglionic plexi in
        catheter ablation of, 227–232
        endocardial high-frequency stimulation for localization of, 229–230
    length of, 186
    paroxysmal. *See* paroxysmal atrial fibrillation
    perpetuators of, 139

    persistent
        atrial tachycardia associated with, 211
        Bordeaux approach for. *See* Bordeaux approach
        hybrid endocardial-epicardial technique for. *See* hybrid endocardial-epicardial technique
atrial fibrillation ablation
    advances in, 129–131
    atrial tachycardia
        ablation of, 216–218
        activation mapping, 236–237, 246
        circuits, 211–212
        classification of, 211
        description of, 155, 210
        diagnosis of, 212–216
        drug therapy for, 211
        electroanatomic mapping of, 234–247
        electrophysiologic diagnosis of, 213–215
        focal, 244–245
        incidence of, 210–211
        mechanism of, 211
        mitral isthmus-dependent atrial flutter, 237–240
        postprocedure care, 245–246
        prevention of, 218
        surface electrocardiogram diagnosis of, 212–213
        3-dimensional entrainment mapping for, 220–226
        three-dimensional mapping of, 215–216
    balloon cryoablation for. *See* balloon cryoablation
    Bordeaux approach to. *See* Bordeaux approach
    circumferential pulmonary vein ablation. *See* circumferential pulmonary vein ablation
    complex fractionated atrial electrogram targeting for. *See* complex fractionated atrial electrogram
    description of, 129

dominant-frequency mapping used in
    limitations of, 256
    nonparoxysmal atrial fibrillation, 254–255
    paroxysmal atrial fibrillation, 253
    procedure, 251–255
    reliability and stability of, 249–250
    technological considerations, 248–249
frequency analysis used in, 248–257
hybrid epicardial-endocardial technique for
    ablation technique, 198
    alternatives to, 200
    atrial floor line, 192–193
    atrial flutter induction and tracking, 196–198
    atrial roof line, 192–193
    complex fractional atrial electrograms, 198
    complications of, 200
    electrophysiologic procedure, 194
    epicardial block, 190–194
    ganglia/ganglia ablation, 191, 193
    goals of, 189–190
    heparin, 194
    left atrial appendage lesion, 193–194
    left-sided entry and setup, 193
    mitral isthmus line, 193
    patient selection, 190
    phased-array intracardiac echocardiography, 195–196
    postprocedure care, 198, 200
    pulmonary vein isolation, 191–193
    recovery after, 198, 200
    right atrial lesions, 192–193
    summary of, 189–190
    surgical procedure, 190–194
    transseptal puncture, 194
intracardiac echocardiography use for optimal safety and efficacy during. *See* intracardiac echocardiography
new technologies for, 129–131
pulmonary vein isolation
    antrum. *See* pulmonary vein antrum isolation
    stepwise technique, 149–150
pulmonary venous narrowing after, 117
remote, 131–132
remote magnetic navigation for
    advantages of, 273
    complications of, 273
    follow-up, 273
    limitations of, 273
    postprocedure care, 272–273
    preprocedural planning, 267–268
    procedure, 268–272
stepwise
    Bordeaux approach to, 148–157
    complications of, 157
    electrogram-based ablation, 150–152
    electrophysiological study, 160–161
    follow-up after, 165–166
    left atrial imaging, 148
    linear ablation, 152–155
    Natale approach, 159–166
    outcomes of, 157
    patient preparation, 148
    patient selection for, 147–148
    postprocedural care, 155–157, 165–166
    preprocedural planning of, 147–148, 159
    pulmonary vein angiography used in, 149
    pulmonary vein antrum isolation, 161–163
    radiofrequency delivery, 149
    right atrial ablation, 155
    stroke prevention, 148
    targets of, 163–165
    transseptal puncture, 148–149
surgical/endocardial procedure
    advantages of, 187
    endocardial procedure, 185
    limitations to, 182
    overview of, 182
    thoracoscopic, 182–183
    transdiaphragmatic, 183–184
transesophageal echocardiography before, 108, 140, 159, 235
transseptal puncture for. *See* transseptal puncture
atrial fibrillation cycle length, 149
atrial fibrillation nest, 250–251
atrial flutter
    ablation of
        adjunctive, 13
        advantages of, 31
        amiodarone versus, 13
        anticoagulation before, 13
        bidirectional block after, 19, 21, 30–31
        catheters, 13–14, 17–18
        complications of, 21, 31
        electroanatomic mapping, 15
        endpoints for, 19, 29–31
        fluoroscopic orientation of catheters, 14–15
        indications for, 12–13
        lack of inducibility after, 30
        limitations, 21, 31
        postprocedure care, 21, 31
        postsurgical, 23–32
        preprocedure planning, 13
        procedure, 13–15
        repeat, 21
        technique, 18
        troubleshooting, 19–21
        vascular access, 13–14
    activation of, 16
    anatomy and physiology of, 11–12
    atypical, 127
    cavotricuspid isthmus-dependence in, 16–17
    description of, 11
    differential pacing of, 19
    electrocardiogram of, 12
    electrophysiologic study of, 16–17
    induction of, 196–197
    initiation of, 16
    mitral isthmus-dependent, 237–240
    perimitral, 217–218
    postsurgical
        ablation of, 23–32
        activation mapping of, 23
        mapping of, 26–31
    stroke risks associated with, 13
    terminology associated with, 11
    3-dimensional entrainment mapping for, 220–226
    tracking of, 197–198
atrial pacing, 9
atrial remodeling, 137
atrial septal defect, 104
atrial tachycardia
    ablation of, 216–218
    in atrial fibrillation ablation. *See* atrial fibrillation ablation, atrial tachycardia
    centrifugal, 215
    classification of, 33, 211
    in congenital heart disease patients. *See* congenital heart disease
    diagnosis of, 212–216
    drug therapy for, 211
    electroanatomic mapping of, 234–247
    electrophysiologic diagnosis of, 213–215
    entrainment of, 214
    focal. *See* focal atrial tachycardias
    imaging of, 40–41
    macroreentrant. *See* macroreentrant atrial tachycardias
    mechanism of, 3, 211
    postablation, 137–138
    prevention of, 218
    recurrence of, 48
    small-reentrant, 243–244
    surface electrocardiogram diagnosis of, 212–213
    3-dimensional entrainment mapping for, 220–226
    three-dimensional mapping of, 215–216
atrial-atrial-ventricular response, 7
atrial-ventricular response, 7
Atricure surgical component, 187
atriofascicular conduction fibers, 81–84
atriofascicular pathways, 76, 81–84
atrioventricular block
    atrioventricular nodal reentry tachycardia ablation as cause of, 56–57
    transcoronary ethanol ablation as cause of, 411–412
atrioventricular nodal reentry tachycardia
    ablation of
        anatomic approach, 55
        atrioventricular block secondary to, 56–57
        complications of, 56–57
        efficacy of, 56
        endpoints, 56
        energy application, 55–56
        lesion formation with, 51
        mapping before, 52–53
        preprocedural preparation, 51–52
        procedure, 52, 54–55, 93
        slow pathway, 55–56
    age at presentation, 3
    characteristics of, 3
    cryoablation of, 56
    description of, 51
    diagnosis of, 52–54
    dual atrioventricular nodal pathways, 52–53
    electrocardiography of, 51–52

electrophysiological testing of, 52
fast-fast, 51, 54
fast-slow, 54
focal atrial tachycardia versus, 33–34, 36
induction of, 53
left-sided, 54
prevalence of, 3
retrograde atrial activation sequence in, 6
septal accessory pathway versus, 7–8
slow-fast, 51, 53–54
slow-slow, 51, 53–54, 57
spontaneous termination of, 7
summary of, 57
termination of, 7
types of, 51
atrioventricular reciprocating tachycardia
    atriofascicular conduction fibers as cause of, 81–84
    characteristics of, 6
    focal atrial tachycardia versus, 36
    gender and, 3
    orthodromic, 75
AVNRT. *See* atrioventricular nodal reentry
AVRT. *See* atrioventricular reciprocating tachycardia

B

Bachmann's bundle, 243
balloon cryoablation
    advantages of, 172–173
    complications of, 172
    cryoablation balloon, 168–169
    disadvantages of, 173
    follow-up after, 171
    limitations of, 172–173
    overview of, 167
    postprocedure care, 170–172
    preprocedure planning, 167–168
    procedure, 168–170
    recovery from, 170–171
    repeat, 171–172
basal ventricular tachycardias, 286, 288
BBB. *See* bundle branch block
BBVRT. *See* bundle branch reentrant ventricular tachycardia
biantral ablation, 208
bidirectional block, 19, 21
Bordeaux approach
    complications of, 157
    electrogram-based ablation, 150–152
    left atrial imaging, 148
    linear ablation, 152–155
    outcomes of, 157
    patient preparation, 148
    patient selection for, 147–148
    postprocedural care, 155–157
    preprocedural planning of, 147–148
    pulmonary vein angiography used in, 149
    radiofrequency delivery, 149
    right atrial ablation, 155
    stroke prevention, 148
    transseptal puncture, 148–149
Brigham approach, to unstable ventricular tachycardia ablation, 341–348
Brockenbrough needle, 102–103
Brugada syndrome, 433–434
bundle branch block
    left, 6
    right, 87
bundle branch reentrant ventricular tachycardia, 283–284

C

CAD. *See* coronary artery disease
calcium transient triggered firing hypothesis, 228
cardiac tamponade, 157
cardiogenic shock, 396
CARTO system, 43, 78, 130, 132, 143, 277–278, 306, 363, 392, 440, 473
catheters
    atrial flutter ablation, 13–14, 17–18
    bidirectional, 17
    focal atrial tachycardia mapping, 35
    irrigated, 46
    left-lateral accessory pathway ablation, 61–63
    pulmonary vein isolation using. *See* laser catheter ablation
    supraventricular tachycardia, 4
    transseptal puncture, 97–98, 102
cavotricuspid isthmus
    ablation of
        adjunctive, 13
        amiodarone versus, 13
        anticoagulation before, 13
        catheter configuration for, 13–14
        description of, 170
        electroanatomic mapping, 15
        fluoroscopic orientation of catheters, 14–15
        imaging of, 115
        indications for, 12–13
        preprocedure planning, 13
        procedure, 13–15
        technique, 18
        troubleshooting, 19–21
        vascular access, 13–14
    anatomy of, 11–12
    bidirectional block, 19, 30–31
    description of, 11
    physiology of, 11–12
centrifugal atrial tachycardia, 215
CFAE. *See* complex fractionated atrial electrograms
Chagas disease, 400
circumferential pulmonary vein ablation
    atrial remodeling, 137
    coronary sinus disconnection, 133
    efficacy of, 136–137
    endpoints, 133–135, 138
    operating room for, 132
    overview of, 129, 132
    procedure, 132–138
    pulmonary vein electrical isolation, 133
    remapping after, 134–135
    rhythm outcome of, 136
    targets of, 135–136
    vagal denervation, 134
CL. *See* cycle length
complex fractionated atrial electrograms,
    atrial fibrillation ablation by targeting of
        ablation technique, 142–144
        adjunctive use of, 145, 255
        advantages of, 144
        complications of, 144
        description of, 33, 139, 150–152
        electrophysiologic mechanisms underlying, 141–142
        follow-up after, 144
        guiding sheaths for, 140
        intracardiac echocardiography application, 143
        limitations of, 144–145
        mapping, 140–144
        patient preparation, 140
        postprocedure care, 144
        preprocedural planning, 139–140
        procedure for, 140–142, 164
        after pulmonary vein antrum isolation, 164
        regional distribution of, 142
        right atrial, 163
        transseptal puncture for, 140
computed tomography, 275–276, 374
concealed entrainment, 16, 26
congenital heart disease
    atrial tachycardia ablation in
        advantages of, 49
        anatomic shell, 44
        anticoagulants, 41
        biventricular repairs, 47
        catheters used in, 43
        complications of, 48–49
        electroanatomical mapping, 41
        electrocardiogram before, 40
        electrograms, 45
        empiric strategies, 47–48
        imaging before, 40–41
        irrigated catheters for, 46
        lesion confirmation, 47
        limitations of, 49
        long vascular sheaths, 42
        mapping in, 43
        overview of, 39
        postprocedure care, 48
        preprocedural planning of, 39–41
        procedure, 41–48
        recurrence risks, 48
        repeat, 48
        targeted ablation, 43–47
        transseptal puncture, 42
        vascular access, 41–42
    ventricular tachycardia ablation in
        advantages of, 447
        complications of, 447
        differential pacing, 442–443
        electrocardiographic studies, 438
        endpoint, 441–446
        implantable cardioverter-defibrillator implantation after, 447
        limitations of, 447
        overview of, 435
        postprocedure care, 446–447
        preprocedural planning of, 435–438
        procedure for, 438–446
        recovery after, 446
        reentry circuit isthmus sites, 440–441
        residual lesion assessments, 436–438

contrast-induced nephropathy, 279
coronary angiography, 409
coronary artery disease, 284–285, 313–314
coronary artery dissection, 411
coronary artery embolism, 396
coronary artery mapping, 92
coronary artery ostium, 394
coronary cusps, arrhythmias from, 393–394
coronary sinus
    description of, 68, 165
    Marshall bundle connection with, 203
    mitral isthmus and, 240
coronary sinus angiography, 70
crista terminalis, 23–24
cryoablation
    atrioventricular nodal reentry tachycardia, 56
    balloon. *See* balloon cryoablation
CS. *See* coronary sinus
CT. *See* computed tomography
CTI. *See* cavotricuspid isthmus
cycle length, 7

D

decompensated heart failure, 412
"destructive" mapping, 24–25
diaphragmatic paresis, 49
differential pacing, 19, 442–443
differential right ventricular pacing, 6
direct thrombin inhibitors, 13
dominant frequency mapping
    limitations of, 256
    nonparoxysmal atrial fibrillation, 254–255
    paroxysmal atrial fibrillation, 253
    procedure, 251–255
    reliability and stability of, 249–250
    technological considerations, 248–249
double potentials, 26
dual atrioventricular nodal pathways, 52–53
duodecapolar catheter, 91
dynamic substrate mapping, 376

E

early repolarization syndrome, 434
Ebstein's anomaly
    accessory pathway ablations in
        advantages of, 94
        catheters, 89
        complications, 94
        coronary artery mapping, 92
        electrocardiography, 87
        electrophysiology study, 90–92
        incidence of, 86
        limitations of, 94
        mapping before, 90–92
        physical examination of, 88
        postprocedure care, 93
        preprocedural planning, 87–88
        procedure for, 89–94
        repeat ablations for, 93
        technique, 92
    anatomy of, 85–86
    electrophysiology study of, 86–87
    hemodynamic effect of, 85
    right bundle branch block associated with, 87
    valve displacement effects, 86
ECG. *See* electrocardiogram
ectopic beats, 434
EGM. *See* electrograms
E-IDC. *See* electrograms with isolated delayed components
electrical storm, 433
electrical unexcitable scar, 317–319, 344, 367
electroanatomic mapping
    arrhythmogenic right ventricular cardiomyopathy/dysplasia, ventricular tachycardia ablation in, 464–465
    atrial tachycardia after atrial fibrillation ablation, 234–247
    description of, 15, 26, 275
    endocardial substrate, 423
    fascicular ventricular tachycardias, 306–308
    image registration using, 275–280
    intracardiac echocardiography and, 109, 112, 392–393
    in ventricular tachycardia, for identifying critical channels
        ablation technique after, 364
        anesthesia for, 362
        anticoagulation, 362
        complications of, 370
        conducting channels, 364–370
        epicardial approach, 364–365, 370
        limitations of, 370–371
        mapping technique, 362–364
        overview of, 360
        patient preparation for, 361–362
        postprocedure care, 370
        preprocedural planning, 360–361
        procedure, 361–370
electrocardiogram
    accessory pathways in Ebstein's anomaly, 87
    atrial flutter, 12
    atrial tachycardia in congenital heart disease patients, 40
    atrioventricular nodal reentry tachycardia, 51–52
    focal atrial tachycardias, 34–35
    unstable ventricular tachycardia, 331–332
    ventricular tachycardias
        hemodynamically tolerated, 314
        left ventricular outflow tract, 292–293
        localization of, 283–290, 292–293
        right ventricular outflow tract, 292–293
electrograms
    complex fractionated atrial. *See* complex fractionated atrial electrograms
    dominant-frequency mapping as guidance for. *See* dominant-frequency mapping
    focal atrial tachycardias, 36–37
    implantable cardioverter-defibrillator, 332, 354
    Marshall bundle, 203
    spectral analysis used to characterize, 250
electrograms with isolated delayed components, 317
electrogram-to-QRS interval, 324–325
electrophysiology study
    arrhythmogenic right ventricular cardiomyopathy/dysplasia, ventricular tachycardia ablation in, 465–467
    atrial flutter, 16–17
    atrial tachycardia, 213–215
    atriofascicular pathways, 82–83
    Ebstein's anomaly, 86–87, 90–92
    focal atrial tachycardias, 35–38
    ligament of Marshall, 203–205
    Marshall bundle, 203–205
    supraventricular tachycardia. *See* supraventricular tachycardia
endocardial ablation
    for atrial fibrillation, 185, 187
    for ventricular tachycardia. *See* ventricular tachycardia, endocardial/epicardial ablation of
endocardial high-frequency stimulation, for left atrial ganglionic plexi localization, 229–230
endocardial lesions, 28–29
endocardial mapping, of ventricular tachycardia
    in arrhythmogenic right ventricular cardiomyopathy/dysplasia, 467
    surgical ablation, 482–483
    unstable ventricular tachycardia, 334–336
entrainment, 137
    atrial tachycardia, 214
    concealed, 16, 26
    definition of, 321
    "N+1" method of, 325
    response, assessment of, 26–27
    3-dimensional entrainment mapping, 220–226
entrainment mapping, for hemodynamically tolerated ventricular tachycardia ablation, 320–322
EP. *See* electrophysiology
epicardial ablation
    complications of, 417–418
    endocardial technique and. *See* hybrid endocardial–epicardial technique
    ventricular tachycardia
        complications of, 417–418
        description of, 364–365, 370–371
        in postcardiac surgery patients, 414–418
        preprocedural planning, 416–417
epicardial access
    complications of, 400–401, 405–406
    considerations before, 399–400
    subxiphoid, 403–405
epicardial atrioventricular groove, 89
epicardial mapping, of ventricular tachycardia
    arrhythmogenic right ventricular cardiomyopathy/dysplasia, 467–468
    description of, 414–416
    unstable, 336
epicardial posteroseptal accessory pathways, 68–70
epicardial ventricular tachycardias, 289
EUS. *See* electrical unexcitable scar

F

fascicular ventricular tachycardias
　ablation of
　　advantages of, 311
　　complications of, 311
　　electroanatomic mapping, 306–308
　　limitations of, 311
　　postprocedure care, 308, 311
　　preprocedural planning, 302–303
　　procedure, 303–310
　　repeat, 311
　definition of, 286, 302
　diagnosis of, 303–306
　electroanatomic mapping of, 306–308
　inducement of, 306–307
　left anterior, 302
　left posterior, 302, 305
　left upper septal, 302
　subtypes of, 302
fast-fast atrioventricular nodal reentry tachycardia, 51, 54
fast-slow atrioventricular nodal reentry tachycardia, 54
first-degree atrioventricular block, 87
focal atrial ectopy, 35
focal atrial tachycardias
　ablation of, 35, 37–38, 217
　anatomic locations of, 34
　after atrial fibrillation ablation, 244–245
　atrioventricular nodal reentry tachycardia versus, 33–34, 36
　diagnostic confirmation of, 33–34, 36
　differential diagnoses of, 33–34, 36
　electrocardiography of, 34–35
　electrograms of, 36–37
　electrophysiological study of, 35–38
　incidence of, 33
　inducement of, 36
　in left atrium, 34
　macroreentrant atrial tachycardia versus, 36
　mapping of, 35–37
　P-wave morphology of, 34–35
　in right atrium, 34
　surface electrocardiography of, 34–35
focal ventricular tachycardias, 377
free-wall pathways, 72–74, 79
frequency analysis, 248–257

G

ganglionic plexi
　description of, 142
　left atrial
　　catheter ablation of, 227–232
　　endocardial high-frequency stimulation for localization of, 229–230
gender, 3

H

HA. See His-atrial
Hansen robotic catheter navigation system
　ablation lesion sets, 264–2655
　Artisan catheter, 261–262, 264
　background of, 259–260
　catheter stability, 263–264
　components of, 260–261
　description of, 260–262
　titration of contact, 263–264
　transseptal access, 262–264
HB. See His bundle
HB-RB. See His bundle-right bundle branch
hemodynamically tolerated ventricular tachycardia ablation
　activation mapping, 320
　acute effect of, 327
　anesthesia for, 316
　anticoagulation before, 316
　cardiac function evaluations, 314
　complications of, 328
　conducting channels, 317
　description of, 313
　electrical unexcitable scar, 317–319
　electrocardiogram before, 314
　endpoint, 327–328
　follow-up, 328
　late potentials, 317
　mapping
　　activation, 320
　　description of, 318, 320
　　entrainment, 320–323, 326
　　postpacing interval, 322–324
　　QRS fusion, 324
　　stimulus-to-QRS interval, 324–326
　　substrate, 316–318
　patient preparation for, 314–316
　postprocedure care, 328
　preprocedure planning of, 313–314
　procedure, 314–316
　substrate mapping, 316–318
　target site for, 326
　wall motion abnormalities, 314
hemodynamics, 103
heparin, 89, 409
heparin "bridging," 41
His bundle-right bundle branch, 5
His-atrial, 5–6
His-Purkinje system, 356
His-refractory premature ventricular contractions, 8–9
His-refractory PVCs, 8–9
HPS. See His-Purkinje system
HRP. See His-refractory PVCs
hybrid endocardial-epicardial technique
　for atrial fibrillation ablation
　　ablation technique, 198
　　alternatives to, 200
　　atrial floor line, 192–193
　　atrial flutter induction and tracking, 196–198
　　atrial roof line, 192–193
　　complex fractional atrial electrograms, 198
　　complications of, 200
　　electrophysiologic procedure, 194
　　epicardial block, 190–194
　　ganglia/ganglia ablation, 191, 193
　　goals of, 189–190
　　heparin, 194
　　left atrial appendage lesion, 193–194
　　left-sided entry and setup, 193
　　mitral isthmus line, 193
　　patient selection, 190
　　phased-array intracardiac echocardiography, 195–196
　　postprocedure care, 198, 200
　　pulmonary vein isolation, 191–193
　　recovery after, 198, 200
　　right atrial lesions, 192–193
　　summary of, 189–190
　　surgical procedure, 190–194
　　transseptal puncture, 194
　for ventricular tachycardia ablation
　　ablation technique, 424–426
　　advantages of, 426
　　complications of, 426
　　epicardial access for, 420–421
　　follow-up for, 426
　　limitations of, 426
　　mapping, 422–424
　　patient preparation, 420
　　preprocedure planning, 419–420
　　procedure, 420–426
　　repeat, 426
hypertrophic cardiomyopathy
　definition of, 452
　ventricular tachycardia in, 452–460
hypotension, 116

I

IABP. See intra-aortic balloon pump
IART. See intra-atrial reentrant tachycardia
IAS. See interatrial septum
ICD. See implantable cardioverter-defibrillator
ICE. See intracardiac echocardiography
IDCM. See idiopathic dilated cardiomyopathy
idiopathic dilated cardiomyopathy, 471, 475
idiopathic ventricular fibrillation, 433
idiopathic ventricular tachycardias, 285–289
image registration, using electroanatomic mapping systems, 275–280
implantable cardioverter-defibrillators, 313, 332, 341, 419, 447
inferior vena cava, 268
informed consent, 168
interatrial septum, 102
intra-aortic balloon pump, 338
intra-atrial reentrant tachycardia
　definition of, 23
　mapping of
　　entrainment response, 26
　　lines of block, 25–26
　　preprocedure planning for, 24
　　procedure, 24–29
intracardiac echocardiography
　advantages of, 117–118, 397
　anatomical characterizations, 107–108
　baseline imaging using, 108–112
　catheter positioning and contact, 113–114
　complex fractionated atrial electrogram application, 143
　complications of, 114–117, 396–397
　costs of, 118, 397
　description of, 107

electroanatomic mapping and, 109, 112, 392–393
hypotension evaluations, 116
intracardiac thrombus secondary to, 116–117
learning curve in performing, 108
left atrial thrombus detection, 108
left atrium, 112
left pulmonary artery, 111
left pulmonary veins, 111
limitations of, 117–118, 397
pericardial effusion during atrial fibrillation ablation identified using, 114–115
phased-array catheters, 108, 110, 114, 195–196, 385
phased-array transducer, 107–108
postprocedure care, 116–117
preprocedure planning of, 107–108
procedural imaging, 108–116
pulmonary valve stenosis reductions using, 116
radial transducers, 107
real-time monitoring uses of, 115
repeat, 116
right atrium, 98, 100, 387
right ventricle, 387–389
transducers, 107
transesophageal echocardiogram/echocardiography versus, 397
transseptal puncture guidance using, 98–99, 102, 104, 108, 112–113, 117–118
vascular access, 108
ventricular tachycardia
advantages of, 385, 395, 397
catheter introduction and manipulation, 386, 389–390
complications of, 395–397
electroanatomic mapping and, 392–393
limitations of, 397
phased-array catheters, 385
postprocedure care, 395
preprocedural planning, 386
procedure for, 387–395
systems, 385
intracardiac thrombus, 116–117
intracardiac ultrasound, 278
irrigated catheters, 46, 245
isoproterenol, 16, 185
IVC. See inferior vena cava

L

LA. See left atrium
LAA. See left atrial appendage
LAO. See left anterior oblique
laser catheter ablation
advantages of, 181
background of, 175–176
endoscopic view used in, 178
equipment, 175–176
laser energy levels, 178
left atrium access, 176–178
left pulmonary vein ablation, 179
lesion visualization software, 178–179
right pulmonary vein ablation, 180
Lasso catheter, 122–123
LBBB. See left bundle branch block
left anterior fascicular ventricular tachycardia, 302
left anterior oblique, 285, 296, 333
left anterior thoracotomy, 479, 482
left atrial appendage
atrial fibrillation triggers from, 165
description of, 100, 110–111, 114, 152
imaging of, 199
isolation of, 165–166
left atrial roof, 152
left atrial thrombus, 104, 108, 148, 267
left atrium
ablation of, 162
cardiac segmentation surface of, 131
intracardiac echocardiography of, 112
laser catheter ablation access, 176–178
macroreentrant atrial tachycardias of, 237–245
Marshall bundle connections with, 203–205
transseptal catheterization of, 97
left bundle branch block
orthodromic reentrant tachycardia and, 6
ventricular tachycardia, 284, 292
left femoral vein, 342
left inferior pulmonary vein, 170, 179
left posterior fascicular ventricular tachycardia, 302, 305
left pulmonary artery, 111
left pulmonary veins
description of, 111, 114
laser catheter ablation of, 179
left superior pulmonary vein, 228
left upper septal fascicular ventricular tachycardia, 302
left ventricle
Array deployment in, 375
epicardial surface of, 298
imaging of, 98
left ventricular outflow tract
intracardiac echocardiography of, 387
ventricular tachycardia
ablation of, 292–300, 393
electrocardiography of, 288–289, 292–293
left-lateral accessory pathway ablation
catheter for, 61–63
complications of, 63
description of, 59
energy delivery for, 62
mapping before, 60–61
patient preparation for, 60
postprocedure care, 63
preprocedural planning, 59
procedure for, 60–63
recovery from, 63
success of, 63
transseptal puncture, 60
LFV. See left femoral vein
ligament of Marshall
ablation of, 193
anatomy of, 202–203
definition of, 202
description of, 184
electrophysiological characteristics of, 203–205
variations of, 203
linear block, 241–243
lipomatous hypertrophy, 97, 104
LIPV. See left inferior pulmonary vein
liver, 401
LOM. See ligament of Marshall
long-QT syndrome, 433
LPA. See left pulmonary artery
LPV. See left pulmonary vein
LSPV. See left superior pulmonary vein

M

MAC. See monitored anesthesia care
macroreentrant atrial tachycardias
after atrial fibrillation ablation
description of, 211, 217
multi-loop tachycardia, 243
small-reentrant atrial tachycardias, 243–244
description of, 33, 36
left atrial, 237–245
multi-loop, 243
roof-dependent, 240–241
macroreentrant ventricular tachycardias, 320
magnetic navigation, remote
advantages of, 273
complications of, 273
follow-up, 273
limitations of, 273
postprocedure care, 272–273
preprocedural planning, 267–268
procedure, 268–272
magnetic resonance imaging, 275–276, 374, 454–455
Mahaim tachycardias, 76–78
mapping
accessory pathways
in Ebstein's anomaly, 90–92
left-lateral, 60–61
technique for, 64–67
atrial tachycardia ablation
in congenital heart disease, 43
focal, 35–37
atriofascicular pathways, 83
"destructive," 24–25
dominant-frequency. See dominant-frequency mapping
electroanatomic. See electroanatomic mapping
focal atrial tachycardias, 35–37
intra-atrial reentrant tachycardia, 24–29
left-lateral accessory pathway, 60–61
Marshall bundle, 205–207
multisite, 24
pulmonary vein antrum isolation, 123
right ventricle, 294
ventricular fibrillation ablation, 430–431
ventricular tachycardia
in hypertrophic cardiomyopathy, 452–460
transcoronary ethanol ablation, 409–411

using delayed potential in sinus rhythm, 350–359
Marfan window, 474–475
Marshall bundle
　ablation of, 207–208
　connections, 203–205
　definition of, 202
　electrophysiological characteristics of, 203–205
　mapping of, 205–207
MB. *See* Marshall bundle
MDP. *See* mid-diastolic potential
median sternotomy, 475, 477–479
MI. *See* myocardial infarction
mid-diastolic potential, 320
midseptal pathways, 75, 79
mitral annulus, 101, 214
mitral isthmus, 152, 155, 237
mitral isthmus-dependent atrial flutter, 237–240
mitral valve, 388
monitored anesthesia care, 332
monomorphic ventricular tachycardia, 313, 443, 446
MRI. *See* magnetic resonance imaging
multi-loop tachycardia, 243
multisite mapping, 24
Mustard procedure, 47
myocardial dissection, 412
myocardial infarction
　transcoronary ethanol ablation and, 412
　ventricular tachycardia after, 284
myocardial rupture, 412

N

"N+1" entrainment, 325
Natale approach
　anesthesia protocol, 160
　electrophysiological study, 160–161
　follow-up, 165–166
　postprocedural care, 165–166
　preprocedural management, 159
　pulmonary vein antrum isolation, 161–163
　repeat procedures, 165
　superior vena cava isolation, 161–163
　targets, 163–165
　transseptal puncture, 160
NavX system, 43, 130, 278, 306, 373
negative predictive value, 4
nephrogenic systemic fibrosis, 279
NICM. *See* nonischemic cardiomyopathy
Niobe system, 79
noncontact mapping, for ventricular tachycardia ablation
　ablation technique, 378–380
　advantages of, 381
　anesthesia, 374
　antiarrhythmic drugs, 374
　complications of, 381
　description of, 373
　limitations of, 381, 384
　mapping technique, 376–378
　postprocedure care, 380–381
　preprocedural planning, 373–374
　procedure, 374–379
　vascular access, 374–375
nonischemic cardiomyopathy, 414
nonsteroidal anti-inflammatory drugs, 468
NPV. *See* negative predictive value

O

ORT. *See* orthodromic reentrant tachycardia
orthodromic atrioventricular reciprocating tachycardia, 75
orthodromic reentrant tachycardia
　description of, 3
　diagnosis of, 6
　left bundle branch block associated with, 6
　termination of, 7
outflow tract ventricular tachycardias
　ablation of, 292–300
　electrocardiography of, 286, 288–289, 292–293
overdrive pacing, 321–323

P

P wave, 26
pace mapping, 354–355
pacing
　atrial, 9
　differential, 19, 442–443
　entrainment, 46
　ventricular, 7–8
papillary muscles
　arrhythmias arising from, ablation of, 388
　imaging of, 388
parahisian pacing, 5–6, 67, 76
paroxysmal atrial fibrillation
　atrial fibrillation nest analysis in, 254
　description of, 125, 210
　dominant-frequency mapping in, 253
　pulmonary vein isolation for, 211. *See also* pulmonary vein isolation
paroxysmal supraventricular tachycardia
　definition of, 3
　mechanism of, 4
patent foramen ovale, 262
percutaneous access with limited epicardial mapping of ventricular tachycardia, 415
pericardial adhesions, 400, 416
pericardial effusions
　during atrial fibrillation ablation, intracardiac echocardiography of, 114–115
　description of, 63, 93
　ventricular tachycardia ablation affected by, 396
pericardial sheath, 468
pericardial space access
　bleeding management during, 405–406
　complications of, 400–401, 405–406, 417
　considerations before, 399–400
　technique for, 401–403
pericardial tamponade, 356
pericarditis, 21, 348
perimitral flutter, 217–218
permanent junctional reciprocating tachycardia, 78

PFO. *See* patent foramen ovale
phased-array transducer, 107–108
phrenic nerve paralysis, 157, 172, 418
PJRT. *See* permanent junctional reciprocating tachycardia
positive predictive value, 4
posteroseptal pathways, 66, 68–70, 72, 75–76, 79
postpacing interval, 26, 137, 237, 322–324, 355
postpacing interval minus the tachycardia cycle length, 7, 223, 305
PPI. *See* postpacing interval
PPI-TCL. *See* postpacing interval minus the tachycardia cycle length
PPV. *See* positive predictive value
protamine, 272
PSVT. *See* paroxysmal supraventricular tachycardia
pulmonary embolism, 468
pulmonary stenosis, 116
pulmonary valve, 389
pulmonary vein
　description of, 112
　electrical isolation of, 133
pulmonary vein angiography, 149
pulmonary vein antrum isolation
　adjunctive ablation sites, 125–126
　advantages of, 127
　anticoagulation after, 127
　complex fractionated atrial electrogram after, 164
　complications of, 127
　definition of, 120
　follow-up after, 126–127
　general anesthesia for, 121
　goals of, 123–125
　guiding sheaths for, 123–124
　left atrial imaging, 120
　lesions delivered with, 124
　limitations of, 127
　mapping for, 123
　Natale approach, 161–163
　patient preparation, 121
　postprocedure care, 126–127
　preprocedural planning, 120–121
　procedure for, 121–126, 161–163
　repeat ablation, 127
　stroke prevention, 120–121
　summary of, 127–128
　transseptal puncture, 123–124
pulmonary vein isolation
　atrial fibrillation ablation using, 149–150, 167
　complex fractionated atrial electrogram ablation as adjunct to, 145
　description of, 107, 113–114, 139
　frequency analysis before, 248–257
　laser catheter ablation for. *See* laser catheter ablation
pulmonary vein potentials, 126
pulmonary venous narrowing, 117
Purkinje-associated ventricular tachycardia, 286–287
PV. *See* pulmonary vein
PVAI. *See* pulmonary vein antrum isolation
PVI. *See* pulmonary vein isolation
P-wave morphology, 34–35, 235

Q

Q waves, 314
QRS fusion, 324
QRS-T subtractions, 249

R

RAA. *See* right atrial appendage
RAAS. *See* retrograde atrial activation sequence
radial transducers, 107
radiopaque contrast, 102
RAO. *See* right anterior oblique
RCA. *See* right coronary artery
remote ablation, of atrial fibrillation, 131–132
remote magnetic navigation
    advantages of, 273
    complications of, 273
    follow-up, 273
    limitations of, 273
    postprocedure care, 272–273
    preprocedural planning, 267–268
    procedure, 268–272
retrograde atrial activation sequence, 5–6
retrograde conduction, 68
RFV. *See* right femoral vein
right anterior oblique, 285, 296
right atrial ablation, 155
right atrial appendage, 155
right atrium, intracardiac echocardiography of, 100, 387
right bundle branch block
    in Ebstein's anomaly, 87
    ventricular tachycardia, 284, 292
right coronary artery, 73, 89, 92
right femoral vein, 342
right inferior pulmonary vein, 111, 177
right pulmonary vein
    description of, 113
    laser catheter ablation of, 180
right superior pulmonary vein, 111, 183
right ventricle
    Array deployment in, 375–376
    imaging of, 98
    intracardiac echocardiography of, 387–389
    mapping of, 294
right ventricular apex, 303
right ventricular outflow tract
    catheter ablation in, 298–299
    description of, 66, 99, 116
    ventricular ectopy from, 433
    ventricular tachycardia, 288–289, 292–300
RIPV. *See* right inferior pulmonary vein
robotic catheter navigation system. *See* Hansen robotic catheter navigation system
roof-dependent macroreentrant atrial tachycardias, 240–241
rotational angiography, 276
R-P tachycardia, 4
RPV. *See* right pulmonary vein
RSPV. *See* right superior pulmonary vein
RV. *See* right ventricle
RVA. *See* right ventricular apex
RVOT. *See* right ventricular outflow tract

S

sarcoidosis, ventricular tachycardia in, 450–452, 460
Senning procedure, 26, 42, 47
septal accessory pathway
    atrioventricular nodal reentry tachycardia versus, 7–8
    differential right ventricular pacing for, 6
slow-fast atrioventricular nodal reentry tachycardia, 51, 53–54
slow-slow atrioventricular nodal reentry tachycardia, 51, 53–54, 57
small-reentrant atrial tachycardias, 243–244
spectral analysis, 250
"spot burn" technique, 18
stepwise ablation, of atrial fibrillation
    Bordeaux approach to, 148–157
    complications of, 157
    electrogram-based ablation, 150–152
    electrophysiological study, 160–161
    follow-up after, 165–166
    left atrial imaging, 148
    linear ablation, 152–155
    Natale approach, 159–166
    outcomes of, 157
    patient preparation, 148
    patient selection for, 147–148
    postprocedural care, 155–157, 165–166
    preprocedural planning of, 147–148, 159
    pulmonary vein angiography used in, 149
    pulmonary vein antrum isolation, 161–163
    radiofrequency delivery, 149
    right atrial ablation, 155
    stroke prevention, 148
    targets of, 163–165
    transseptal puncture, 148–149
stimulus-to-QRS interval, 324–326
stomach air insufflations, 401
stroke
    atrial flutter as risk factor for, 13
    prevention of, 120–121, 148
structural heart disease
    exclusion of, before ventricular fibrillation ablation, 428–429
    ventricular tachycardia in, 390–391
subepicardial myocardial fibers, 399
substrate mapping
    description of, 255
    dynamic, 376
    hemodynamically tolerated ventricular tachycardias, 316–318
    unstable ventricular tachycardia ablation, 343–346
    ventricular tachycardia, 316–318, 343–346, 372, 422–423, 440
subxiphoid epicardial access, 403–405, 416
subxiphoid puncture, 400
superior vena cava, 73, 161–163
supraventricular tachycardia
    atrioventricular block during, 7
    causes of, 3, 86
    characteristics of, 6–7
    differential diagnosis of, 3
    electrocardiography of, 4
    electrophysiologic study of
        baseline observations, 4–6
        catheter placement, 4
        differential right ventricular pacing, 6
        parahisian pacing, 5–6
        preprocedure planning for, 3–4
        sedation for, 4
        vascular access for, 4
    gender and, 3
    pacing maneuvers during, 7–9
surgical/endocardial ablation
    for atrial fibrillation
        advantages of, 187
        endocardial procedure, 185
        limitations to, 182
        overview of, 182
        thoracoscopic, 182–183
        transdiaphragmatic, 183–184
    for ventricular tachycardia
        endocardial mapping, 482–483
        indications for, 472–473
        left anterior thoracotomy, 479, 482
        mapping procedure, 473–474
        Marfan window, 474–475
        median sternotomy, 475, 477–479
        overview of, 471–472
        percutaneous approach failure as reason for, 472–473
        procedure, 473–474
        room setting, 473–474
        ventriculotomy, 482
sustained ventricular tachycardias, 313
SVC. *See* superior vena cava
SVT. *See* supraventricular tachycardia

T

tachycardia
    atrial. *See* atrial tachycardia
    Mahaim, 76–78
    multi-loop, 243
    permanent junctional reciprocating, 78
    spontaneous termination of, 7, 29
    supraventricular. *See* supraventricular tachycardia
    ventricular. *See* ventricular tachycardia
tachycardia cycle length, 6, 26, 236, 322
TCEA. *See* transcoronary ethanol ablation
TCL. *See* tachycardia cycle length
TEE. *See* transesophageal echocardiogram/echocardiography
tetralogy of Fallot, 435–437
3-dimensional entrainment mapping, 220–226
thromboembolism, 381
thrombus, 396
TIA. *See* transient ischemic attack
Touhey needle, 343
transcoronary ethanol ablation
    ablation technique, 411
    atrioventricular block caused by, 411–412
    complications of, 411–412
    efficacy of, 412–413
    intraoperative requirements, 409
    mapping, 409–411
    overview of, 407–408
    preprocedural preparations, 408
    procedure, 409–411
    vascular access, 409

transdiaphragmatic surgical procedure, for atrial fibrillation ablation, 183–184
transesophageal echocardiogram/echocardiography
    before atrial fibrillation ablation, 108, 140, 159
    intracardiac echocardiography versus, 397
transient ischemic attacks, 172
transisthmus conduction, 16
transseptal puncture
    advantages of, 104
    alternative techniques, 102
    anticoagulation before, 99
    atrial septal defect persistence after, 104
    atrial septum tenting before, 124
    atrial tachycardia ablation in congenital heart disease, 42
    baseline imaging before, 98–99
    Bordeaux approach to persistent atrial fibrillation, 148–149
    catheter placement, 97–98, 102
    complex fractionated atrial electrograms, 140
    complications of, 103–104
    equipment for, 98
    intracardiac echocardiography guidance of, 98–99, 104, 108, 112–113, 117–118
    left-lateral accessory pathway ablation, 60
    limitations of, 104
    needle advancement, 102
    pitfalls to avoid, 102–103
    postprocedure care, 103
    preprocedure planning, 97
    procedure, 97–102
    pulmonary vein antrum isolation, 123–124
    second, 101–102
    sheath placement, 97–98, 103
    unstable ventricular tachycardia ablation, 334
transthoracic echocardiogram/echocardiography, 374
tricuspid valve, 387–389
    annulus of, 24, 89–90
    displacement of, 86
    Ebstein's anomaly of. See Ebstein's anomaly
TTE. See transthoracic echocardiogram/echocardiography

U

University of Pennsylvania approach, to unstable ventricular tachycardia ablation, 331–339
unstable ventricular tachycardia ablation
    advantages of, 348
    Brigham approach to, 341–348
    catheter placement for, 333
    complications of, 339, 348
    endocardial mapping, 334–336
    epicardial access, 343
    epicardial mapping, 336
    follow-up, 338, 348
    goal of, 337
    hemodynamic support, 343
    implantable cardioverter-defibrillator electrogram, 332
    induction of, 334
    left ventricular access, 334
    limitations of, 348
    mortality rates, 348
    noninvasive imaging of, 332
    patient preparation, 332–333, 342
    postprocedure care, 338, 347–348
    preprocedural planning for, 331–333, 341–342
    procedure for, 332–336, 342–347
    recovery from, 338, 347–348
    repeat, 338–339
    substrate identification before, 341–346
    surface electrocardiogram of, 331–332
    transseptal puncture, 334, 342
    University of Pennsylvania approach to, 331–339
    vascular access for, 333
    ventricular access, 342

V

VA. See ventriculo-atrial
vein of Marshall, 203
ventricular contractions, 8–9, 296, 377, 429
ventricular ectopy, 433
ventricular fibrillation ablation
    endpoint for, 431–432
    follow-up after, 432
    idiopathic, 433
    mapping, 430–431
    outcome of, 432–434
    overview of, 428
    preprocedural planning of, 428–429
    procedure for, 429–432
    structural heart disease exclusion before, 428–429
ventricular pacing, 7–8
ventricular tachycardia ablation
    adenosine-sensitive, 286, 288
    aortic sinus cusps, 292–300
    in arrhythmogenic right ventricular cardiomyopathy/dysplasia
        ablation procedure, 464–468
        complications of, 468
        electroanatomical voltage mapping, 464–465
        electrophysiology study, 465–467
        endocardial mapping and, 467
        epicardial mapping and, 467–468
        overview of, 462–463
        postprocedure care, 468–469
        preprocedural planning for, 463–464
    basal, 286, 288
    bundle branch reentrant, 283–284
    conducting channels in, 364–370
    in congenital heart disease
        advantages of, 447
        complications of, 447
        differential pacing, 442–443
        electrocardiographic studies, 438
        endpoint, 441–446
        implantable cardioverter-defibrillator implantation after, 447
        limitations of, 447
        overview of, 435
        postprocedure care, 446–447
        preprocedural planning of, 435–438
        procedure for, 438–446
        recovery after, 446
        reentry circuit isthmus sites, 440–441
        residual lesion assessments, 436–438
    in coronary artery disease, 284–285
    delayed potential in sinus rhythm used to map, 350–359
    electroanatomical mapping used to identify critical channels in
        ablation technique after, 364
        anesthesia for, 362
        anticoagulation, 362
        complications of, 370
        conducting channels, 364–370
        epicardial approach, 364–365, 370
        limitations of, 370–371
        mapping technique, 362–364
        overview of, 360
        patient preparation for, 361–362
        postprocedure care, 370
        preprocedural planning, 360–361
        procedure, 361–370
    electrocardiographic localization of, 283–290
    electrophysiologic study of, 351
    endocardial/epicardial
        ablation technique, 424–426
        advantages of, 426
        complications of, 426
        epicardial access for, 420–421
        follow-up for, 426
        limitations of, 426
        mapping, 422–424
        patient preparation, 420
        preprocedure planning, 419–420
        procedure, 420–426
        repeat, 426
    epicardial, 289
        complications of, 417–418
        description of, 364–365, 370–371
        in postcardiac surgery patients, 414–418
        preprocedural planning, 416–417
    epicardial mapping of, 414–416
    fascicular. See fascicular ventricular tachycardias
    focal, 377
    hemodynamically tolerated. See hemodynamically tolerated ventricular tachycardia ablation
    in hypertrophic cardiomyopathy, 452–460
    idiopathic, 285–289
    induction of, 354–356, 409, 440, 465
    intracardiac echocardiography
        advantages of, 385, 395, 397
        catheter introduction and manipulation, 386, 389–390
        complications of, 395–397
        electroanatomic mapping and, 392–393
        limitations of, 397
        phased-array catheters, 385
        postprocedure care, 395
        preprocedural planning, 386

procedure for, 387–395
systems, 385
left bundle branch block, 284
left ventricular outflow tract, 288–289
mapping
    delayed potential in sinus rhythm for, 350–359
    endocardial/epicardial ablation, 422–424
    epicardial, 414–416
    intracoronary guide wire, 410–411
    multielectrode catheter for, 410
    noncontact. See ventricular tachycardia, noncontact mapping
    pace, 354–355
    substrate, 422–423, 440
monomorphic, 313, 443, 446
noncontact mapping
    ablation technique, 378–380
    advantages of, 381
    anesthesia, 374
    antiarrhythmic drugs, 374
    complications of, 381
    description of, 373
    limitations of, 381, 384
    mapping technique, 376–378
    postprocedure care, 380–381
    preprocedural planning, 373–374
    procedure, 374–379
    vascular access, 374–375
outflow tract
    ablation of, 292–300, 393
    electrocardiography of, 286, 288–289, 292–293
postmyocardial infarction, 284
Purkinje-associated, 286–287
right bundle branch block, 284
right ventricular outflow tract, 288–289
in sarcoidosis, 450–452, 460
in structural heart disease, 390–391
substrate
    ablation, 350–358
    intracardiac echocardiography assessment of, 390–391
    mapping of, 422–423, 440
surgical
    endocardial mapping, 482–483
    indications for, 472–473
    left anterior thoracotomy, 479, 482
    mapping procedure, 473–474
    Marfan window, 474–475
    median sternotomy, 475, 477–479
    overview of, 471–472
    percutaneous approach failure as reason for, 472–473
    procedure, 473–474
    room setting, 473–474
    ventriculotomy, 482
sustained, 313
transcoronary ethanol ablation for
    ablation technique, 411
    atrioventricular block caused by, 411–412
    complications of, 411–412
    efficacy of, 412–413
    intraoperative requirements, 409
    mapping, 409–411
    overview of, 407–408
    preprocedural preparations, 408
    procedure, 409–411
    vascular access, 409
unstable. See unstable ventricular tachycardia
verapamil-sensitive, 286, 303–304
ventriculo-atrial interval, 66
ventriculotomy, 482
verapamil-sensitive ventricular tachycardia, 286, 303–304
video-assisted thoracoscopic surgery, 200
voltage mapping, 317
VOM. See vein of Marshall
VT. See ventricular tachycardia

W

warfarin, 126, 148
Wolff-Parkinson-White syndrome, 59
WPW. See Wolff-Parkinson-White syndrome

Z

zones of transition, 6